THE SANA DIET

Health Resilience and Dementia Prevention

AN ANTI-INFLAMMATORY LIFESTYLE FOR A HEALTHY GUT AND LIFELONG PHYSICAL, MENTAL, AND COGNITIVE WELL-BEING

CHARLES LEWIS, MD, MPH

First Edition
1.01

Psy Press
Est. 1978

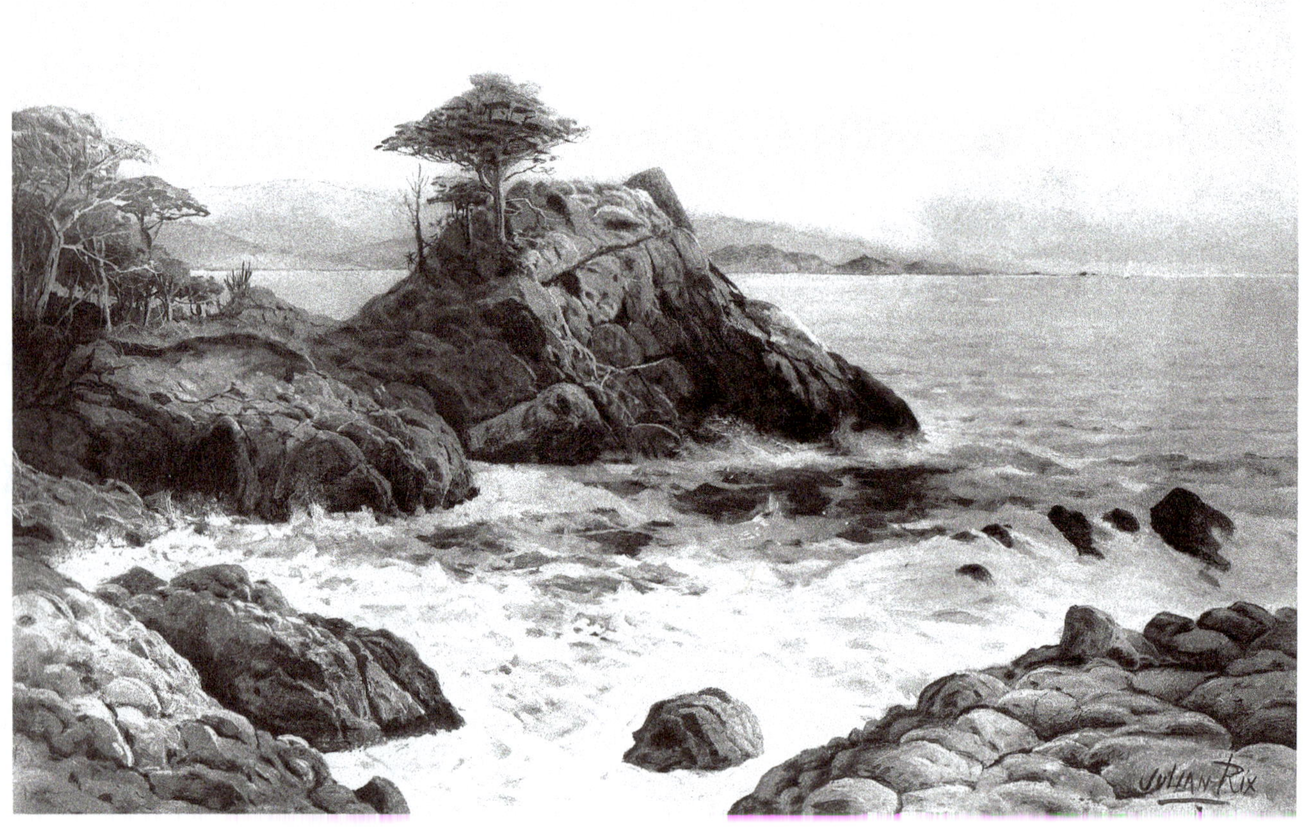

Psy Press
Carrabelle Florida
PsyPress[illegible]mail.com
Edition: 1.01 2025

ISBN 978-1-938318-09-2

TABLE OF CONTENTS

Author's preface to the first edition: This is personal. My father died of Alzheimer's disease, as did his only brother. At least one of my brothers has ApoE4/4, putting him at a very high risk of the disease, and indicating that my mother was also a risk carrier. I had mentioned my intent to write a book on Alzheimer's disease prevention to a sibling nearly a decade ago, and she reminded me repeatedly that it was time to get on with it. Despite my disrelish and aversion to spending a year or more of full-time effort on the project, the need was clear and present, despite my personal delusions of invulnerability.

After years of active study and research, and writing on the topic, I had felt that I had a pretty good idea of what a healthy, anti-inflammatory diet should be. Nevertheless, researching and writing a book like this is an exploration. I let my research lead me wherever it went. Many things were as I expected, some were unfamiliar, and a considerable amount was new and unforeseen. In this book, I challenge several aspects of nutritional orthodoxy, including polyunsaturated fats being healthy and the need to avoid cholesterol and salt.

Ma sha Allah, I have not underestimated the fallout of calling things as I see them. Galileo promoted the notion that the sun is at the center of the solar system, for which he was found "vehemently suspect of heresy," and was sentenced to house arrest for the remainder of his life. I suppose I could live with that (as long as I can walk and run on the beach). Prometheus had a much worse fate; for sharing enlightenment and knowledge with humanity, Zeus condemned him to eternal torment. He was chained to a rock and had an eagle eat his liver every day (his liver would regenerate overnight). But I am not too worried. If history is prologue, nearly no one will ever read this, and I shall remain free to pursue my happiness and the pursuit of understanding the true nature of nature.

1: Introduction

What is a Healthy Diet?

The traditional Mediterranean diet is well-known for being one of the healthiest on the planet. Its inspiration comes from the traditional dietary consumption habits of countries bordering the Mediterranean Sea, where residents are known for their longevity and relatively low risk of heart disease in comparison to the rest of Europe. The diet has common aspects shared by people from Greece, Italy, and Spain. There is plenty of fresh fruits and vegetables, whole grains, fish, and olive oil is commonly used. Poultry and dairy products such as yogurt and many forms of cheese are included. Meat is eaten, but less than in the typical Western diet. There is moderate consumption of alcohol, mostly as wine. The "Medi" diet has been the basis for several other diets.

Another set of healthy diets is the "Blue Zone" diets. The diets and the Blue Zone Food Guidelines derived from them try to emulate the diet in communities that have an unusually high number of centenarians. If people live healthy lives to age 100, they must be doing most things right and few things wrong, at least when it comes to health.

Thus, the conceptual underpinnings for understanding what constitutes a healthy diet are to emulate these diets; thus, providing a dietary paradigm for long, healthy lives.

The Dash (Dietary Approach to Stop Hypertension) diet is a diet designed to lower blood pressure. It was designed to be an improvement over the Mediterranean diet (Medi diet) by restricting red meat, sugar, and salt. It promotes a diet based on the consumption of plant-based foods and additionally limits the intake of saturated fatty acids, total fat, cholesterol, and sodium. It has been shown to reduce *risk factors* for cardiovascular disease.

Another method for discerning what foods are healthy is to compare different diets. This is what has been done in the "Adventist Studies". The Seventh-day Adventists are encouraged, but not required, to eat a vegan or vegetarian diet. Some do, some don't. For over thirty years, thousands of Adventists have participated in health studies, and thus we have learned that vegans have the lowest rates of cancer, followed by vegetarians and semi-vegetarians; meanwhile, meat eaters have the highest rates of most chronic diseases. Thus, there is strong evidence that a plant-based diet is healthy, and there is agreement among most health professionals who are concerned with diet that a plant-based diet is a great improvement over the Western diet.

The Western diet is not what they serve in saloons in the cowboy movies, but it is perhaps not too different. Sometimes referred to as the "Standard American Diet" (SAD), the Western diet is consumed in many parts of the industrialized world, including North America, most of Europe, and increasingly other areas with the rise of industrialization of the food market and a rise in the standard of living. Thus, it might be referred to as the Industrialized Diet. Of the many countries that have industrialized, Japan seems unique in not having adopted the Western diet or something similar to the SAD diet.

Numerous studies (thousands) have examined what (millions of) people eat, using detailed food questionnaires, and then follow up after several years to see which and how long subjects survived, who got sick, who died, and what diseases they succumbed to. These studies provide information on what foods and diets help prevent and promote disease. We know that processed meat is associated with higher rates of cancer, and that yellow vegetables decrease the risk of certain cancers. We have data on which types of food are associated with the risk of heart disease, diabetes, dementia, and death.

The Medi and Dash diets are associated with a lower risk of dementia than the typical Western diet consumed in the U.S. and northern Europe. The MIND diet (Mediterranean-DASH Intervention for Neurodegenerative Delay) was developed to take dementia prevention a step further. In preliminary studies, the MIND diet appeared to reduce the incidence and progression of AD and Parkinson's Disease, in comparison to the Western diet;[1] [2] however, in a more comprehensive and longer-term study, the MIND diet intervention failed to show significant benefit as compared to patients on a control diet with mild caloric restriction.[3]

We can be confident that the Western diet from the year 2000 increases the risk of dementia and other chronic diseases, and there is evidence that the average American diet has improved since then. When the MIND diet failed, this improvement in the diet was cited as a possible reason for the lack of difference in disease progression between participants on the MIND or control diet. The MIND diet, which was specifically envisioned to prevent the progression of dementia, was not significantly more helpful or harmful than the typical American diet. One of the findings from various studies and trials using the MIND diet was that the consumption of vegetables was helpful in slowing dementia progression, but that fruit consumption was not. In other MIND diet studies, the consumption of fruits was not helpful except for berries.

It's a simple question, for which one might expect a simple answer. Does the consumption of fruits lower the risk of Alzheimer's disease (AD)? The simple answer from population studies is that they do not. If this is correct, can we assume that the consumption of fruit does not lower the risk of heart disease, cancer, or other chronic diseases?

Let me suggest that this dietary dilemma is the outcome of asking the wrong questions. The better question is "Are there fruits that, when frequently consumed, are associated with a lower risk of Alzheimer's disease?". Here, the answer is yes.

If you ask whether eating vegetables lowers the risk of AD (or most other chronic diseases of aging, including diabetes, heart disease, cancer, and strokes), the answer is yes. But is that answer helpful? Potatoes are vegetables. They are, in fact, the most abundantly consumed vegetable in the American diet. Nearly half of all potatoes are eaten as fries or potato chips. When studying diet, what is a fruit? There is no question of whether or not apples are a fruit. Does apple juice count? What about apple pie and apple sauce?

What the MIND, DASH, and Medi diets miss is the details of diet: how the individual foods, their preparation, and additives impact health. These are critical details in an industrialized diet. Details matter.

The SANA Diet

The SANA Program takes a different approach to provide dietary and lifestyle recommendations. It assesses the impact of how individual foods and their preparation impact health.

The SANA (Symbiotic Anti-inflammatory Nutritional Agenda) diet was initially developed as a means for the prevention of dementia; however, it also lowers the risk of many other chronic diseases. A central focus of the SANA diet is to prevent dysbiosis and leaky gut, which are underlying causes of dementia and other chronic diseases. The diet is anti-inflammatory. The diet emphasizes the inclusion of nutritional compounds from foods that are important to brain and overall health. Additionally, the diet focuses on the strategic use of dietary components that promote adaptive mechanisms that prevent disease by making us more resilient to oxidative and other metabolic injury.

An underlying, but not exclusive, goal of the diet is to promote a healthy oral and intestinal microbiome while providing balanced nutrition and an anti-inflammatory impact on the body. Other goals include supplying protective molecules, such as antioxidants, including lycopene and certain phenolic compounds, particularly those that cross the blood-brain barrier (BBB).

The SANA warns against foods that are harmful, and ranks foods according to their relative benefits so that better choices can be made, while trying to maintain choice and options. The SANA diet pays close attention to the PPPs (proper procedures of preparation) that have a strong impact on digestion and the intestinal microbiome.

The traditional Medi-diet does not have much fried food, the DASH diet limits saturated fats, and the MIND diet avoids fried food, but other than this, cooking technique is not a focus. In contrast, food preparation is a critical aspect of the SANA diet. Fried food is not part of the SANA diet, but it does allow that some foods may be gently air-fried.

Like other healthy diets, the SANA diet is predominantly plant-based. It is designed to be a long-term diet, and thus, a dietary regimen that is as easy to comply with as possible.

- Eat fresh when possible
- Avoid manufactured foods
- A pleasurable menu is key to success
- Planning meals ahead aids in fruition

The SANA diet can be a vegan, lacto-ovarian-vegetarian diet, pesco-ovarian, and may even include some meat in the diet. Its design goal was to be inclusive by being granular. That is, to take a close look at each food and determine its effect on promoting or preventing dysbiosis and inflammation, and in doing so, prevent the underpinnings of many chronic diseases.

The gut microbiota's influence on systemic disorders like Alzheimer's disease (AD) is increasingly recognized, with findings suggesting that microbial compositions in AD patients differ from those in healthy individuals, potentially affecting neuroinflammatory processes and neurodegeneration. Recent research on the impact of the intestinal microbiome on AD highlights its role in disease pathology and progression and showing evidence of bacterial toxins from the gut present in the brains of patients dying with AD.[4] Studies emphasize the microbiota-gut-brain axis as a crucial link, where dysbiosis can promote neuroinflammation.[5] [6] Systemic inflammation and vascular disease, which are risk factors for AD, are widely recognized to be impacted by the intestinal microbiome.

Another recognized risk factor for AD is type 2 diabetes, also recognized as an inflammatory disease for which dysbiosis is an underlying risk factor. The DAD diet can help prevent and reverse type 2 diabetes (T2D). T2D used to be called adult-onset diabetes, but it has become common in children as a result of unhealthy lifestyles and obesity. Sadly, I have diagnosed "adult-onset diabetes" in obese 6-year-old children. By healing dysbiosis and reversing the inflammation leading to diabetes, the disease can be managed and potentially minimize diabetic sequela and thwart disease progression. If done early enough, the disease can be reversed.

The SANA diet (with some minor adaptations) can be recommended to control Inflammatory Bowel Disease (IBD), including ulcerative colitis (UC) and Crohn's disease. Some of the insights into the prevention of dysbiosis that were used to develop the SANA diet were adopted from inflammatory bowel disease research.[7 8 9]

There is considerable evidence that ADHD is a lifestyle disease. Although not yet formally tested, there is supporting evidence, and I am confident that the SANA diet, along with its recommended lifestyle, would improve this condition.

Here is a partial list of diseases associated with dysbiosis: [10 11 12 13 14 15 16]

- Alzheimer's Disease,
- Parkinson's Disease
- Amyotrophic Lateral Sclerosis
- Crohn's disease and Ulcerative colitis
- Irritable bowel syndrome (IBS)
- Heart disease (TMAO, phenylacetylglutamine)
- Kidney disease (TMAO)
- Anxiety and depression
- Obesity
- Behavioral disorders (including exacerbation of Autistic Spectrum Disorder (ASD) related behaviors
- Allergies, Atopic asthma
- Type 2 diabetes mellitus (T2D)
- Autoimmune disease, including Multiple Sclerosis
- Major depressive disorder, Schizophrenia, Chronic stress
- Chronic Migraines
- Polycystic ovary syndrome (PCOS – caused by insulin resistance)
- Thyroid disorders
- Sjögren's syndrome

The list goes on.

As will be explained in the coming chapters, the SANA diet is a nutritious, low-fat, low-added sugar diet, rich in fiber. But beyond that, it is an anti-inflammatory diet that protects against dysbiosis. The SANA program goes beyond just providing guidance as to which food classes to eat and avoid. It ranks foods so the best choices can be selected and the worst foods avoided. Further, the SANA diet provides essential information on the impacts of food preparation methods.

Prevention vs. Reversal

Many chronic health conditions can improve with lifestyle and diet. Coronary artery disease and plaque in the carotid arteries can be reversed with diet and lifestyle changes, as demonstrated by the Ornish Lifestyle Medicine Program. Metabolic syndrome can be reversed, along with type 2 diabetes and fatty liver disease, as long as the damage is not too far gone. Retinal receptors lost from glaucoma do not recover with treatment. After hepatic sclerosis, infarcted heart muscle, renal failure, and strokes, there can be functional recovery from adaptation of surviving tissues, but the dead tissues do not recover.

Clearly, AD, vascular dementia (VaD), Parkinson's disease (PD), and many other forms of dementia are preventable. The best time to do this is before there is injury and cognitive decline, which typically gets started in middle age, if not sooner. Protein markers of AD and PD have been detected in the brains of teenagers who lived in areas with high levels of air pollution. The ability to prevent dementia does not necessarily mean that once dementia has started, its progression can be stopped. Many forces are in play, including epigenetic programming, (inflammatory) activated microglia in the brain, the buildup of toxic compounds, and continued aging, that continue to drive cognitive decline. Nevertheless, there is epidemiologic data that show that certain interventions do slow cognitive decline. Unfortunately, I have found no long-term interventional studies that have stopped disease progression in those with mid to late-stage dementia.

It is a considerably more difficult and perhaps impossible task to reverse dementia. There are some small interventional studies that have shown improvement in cognitive functioning in AD. These should likely be seen to be similar to the impact of getting a smoker with emphysema to quit smoking. Their breathing and exercise tolerance will improve as the inflammation in their lungs subsides and their physical conditioning improves. They will function better. Will their bodies repair the lung tissue that smoking destroyed? Will new alveoli grow in the lung? Medical and lifestyle interventions meant to reanimate lost or dead tissue are a considerably more monumental task than preventing the disease. Unfortunately, many dementia studies try to do this, and when they fail, it is interpreted to mean that the intervention was futile, rather than understanding that it has just been applied too late.

Is it possible for AD and other forms of dementia to be reversed? I am an optimist, and the brain is designed to learn and make new connections. I think that interventions, such as the SANA program and other treatments, can improve cognitive function and improve the lives of those with dementia and of their caregivers. I think early on, Parkinson's Disease may potentially be reversible. Nevertheless, the focus should be on prevention. Waiting until the diagnosis of dementia or even mild cognitive impairment to address this disease is a fool's errand.

Outro

Disclaimer: I have done my best to research the topic of this book with an open mind and make recommendations according to my understanding of the science. Although the basic concepts of the diet coincide with the Mediterranean and other healthy diets, many restrictions and recommendations that resulted from this research were unanticipated. Thus, they were not a product of preconceived notions.

Many recommendations are made as to which foods to avoid and which are preferentially encouraged. Recommendations are made for cooking processes. References are given to provide interested readers with sources. The diet recommendations are made to avoid health risks and, as much as possible, provide the most benefit and be relatively easy to comply with. When reading this text, it is important to keep in mind that nutritional science is constantly evolving. This book covers many areas for which the science is uncertain, and tries to move things forward. It is not unlikely that I may have gotten some details wrong, such as the exact ratings of some foods. In an attempt to keep concepts practical, some overgeneralizations creep in. For example, as a rule, the untreated skin of root vegetables is disallowed on the diet. There may be some root vegetables whose skin does not promote dysbiosis.

I am confident that the recommendations will act as reliable guideposts for most people and that the recommendations will provide far more benefit than harm. This does not guarantee that all individuals will respond in the same way to any single food or any diet. This book should not be considered medical advice. For that, consult your doctor.

This Book provides the research and reasoning underlying the SANA Program, as well as an assessment of the impacts of various food ingredients on health or disease. Under separate cover is a user's guide, *Wellness with the SANA Diet*. *Wellness* is an abridged, condensed version of the diet, meant as a quick reference, which also contains sample recipes. While this book focuses on the scientific support for the SANA Program in preventing dementia and other chronic diseases, *Wellness* is presented as a healthy diet for everyone, for growing children, and health throughout adult life.

Table 1A: The Mediterranean, DASH, and MIND Diets (Adapted from van den Brink[17]), Compared to the SANA Program.

	Mediterranean Diet	DASH Diet	MIND Diet	SANA Diet
High amounts	Olive oil	—	Olive oil	
	Fish	—	Fish	
	Breads and other forms of cereals	Grains	Whole grains	Properly prepared, germinated grains, oats, and rice, Nixtamalized corn
	Fruits	Fruits	Berries	Certain Fruits
	Vegetables	Vegetables	Green leafy vegetables	Certain vegetables
	—	—	Other vegetables	
	Legumes	Legumes	—	Properly prepared Legumes
	Nuts	Nuts	Nuts	
	Beans	—	Beans	Properly prepared Beans
	Seeds	Seeds	—	
	—	Low-fat dairy products	—	Low-whey dairy
	—	—	Poultry	Properly Prepared Eggs
Moderate amounts	Dairy products	—	—	Oily fish
	Poultry	Poultry	—	Certain Nuts
	Alcohol	—	Alcohol/wine	
	—	Fish	—	Salt
Restricts amounts	Red meat	Red meat	Red meat and products	Poultry, white fish
	Processed meat	—	—	
	Sweets	Sweets	Pastries and sweets	Sweets, sugar, fruit juice
	—	Saturated fat	—	Fats and vegetable oils
	—	Total fat	—	Total Fat
	—	Cholesterol	—	Alcohol
	—	Sodium	—	
	—	—	Cheese	
	—	—	Butter/margarine	
	—	Salt	Fast-fried foods	Air-fried foods
Prohibits				Sweet beverages
				Red meat, all animal skin
				Skin of certain fruits and root vegetables
				Some vegetables
				Certain food additives
				Most wheat and corn products
				Margarine, vegetable oils

Table 1B: Comparing the Blue Zone Recommendations with the SANA Program Diet

Food	Blue Zone Guidelines	SANA Program
Meat	2 oz. or less, about 5 times a month	No mammalian meat. Chicken breast is not recommended, but occasionally allowed.
Dairy	Reduce	Avoid milk and whey; hard cheese and Greek yogurt are allowed
Sugar	Limit to 28 grams of added sugar per day.	Up to 0.7 grams per kg of ideal body weight of added sugar in solid foods for non-diabetics. No sugar-sweetened beverages.
Eggs	No more than 3 per week	Fine, but they must be properly prepared
Fish	Less than 3 oz. 3 times per week	Only certain fish, up to 10 oz per week
Nuts	1 – 2 handfuls a day	Only certain nuts, 16 grams per day
Beverages	Water 7 glasses per day, coffee and tea in moderation.	Water – yes. Coffee and tea, and herbal teas, when properly prepared, are encouraged.
Wine	In moderation	50 ml, every other day
Beans	½ to 1 cup per day	½ to 1 cup per day, properly prepared
Whole Foods	Single ingredient, raw, cooked, ground, fermented, not highly processed	Other than a few fruits and vegetables, most foods require preparation. Avoid foods with added non-nutritive compounds.
	95 – 100% plant-based	Mostly a plant-based diet, with a granular selection of foods recommended or proscribed.
Fruits and vegetables		At least 6 servings of recommended fruits and vegetables each day.

[1] MIND diet associated with reduced incidence of Alzheimer's disease. Morris MC, Tangney CC, Wang Y, Sacks FM, Bennett DA, Aggarwal NT. Alzheimers Dement. 2015 Sep;11(9):1007-14. doi: 10.1016/j.jalz.2014.11.009. Epub 2015 Feb 11. PMID: 25681666

[2] MIND and Mediterranean Diets Associated with Later Onset of Parkinson's Disease. Metcalfe-Roach A, Yu AC, Golz E, Cirstea M, Sundvick K, Kliger D, Foulger LH, Mackenzie M, Finlay BB, Appel-Cresswell S. Mov Disord. 2021 Apr;36(4):977-984. doi: 10.1002/mds.28464. Epub 2021 Jan 6. PMID: 33404118

[3] Trial of the MIND Diet for Prevention of Cognitive Decline in Older Persons. Barnes LL, Dhana K, Liu X, Carey VJ, Ventrelle J, Johnson K, Hollings CS, Bishop L, Laranjo N, Stubbs BJ, Reilly X, Agarwal P, Zhang S, Grodstein F, Tangney CC, Holland TM, Aggarwal NT, Arfanakis K, Morris MC, Sacks FM. N Engl J Med. 2023 Aug 17;389(7):602-611. doi: 10.1056/NEJMoa2302368. Epub 2023 Jul 18. PMID: 37466280

[4] Bridging the Gap between Gut Microbiota and Alzheimer's Disease: A Metaproteomic Approach for Biomarker Discovery in Transgenic Mice. Ayan E, DeMirci H, Serdar MA, Palermo F, Baykal AT. Int J Mol Sci. 2023 Aug 15;24(16):12819. doi: 10.3390/ijms241612819. PMID: 37629000

[5] Microbiome Alterations and Alzheimer's Disease: Modeling Strategies with Transgenic Mice. Biomedicines López-Villodres JA, Escamilla A, Mercado-Sáenz S, Alba-Tercedor C, Rodriguez-Perez LM, Arranz-Salas I, Sanchez-Varo R, Bermúdez D.. 2023 Jun 27;11(7):1846. doi: 10.3390/biomedicines11071846. PMID: 37509487; PMCID: PMC10377071.

[6] Gut Microbiota is an Impact Factor based on the Brain-Gut Axis to Alzheimer's Disease: A Systematic Review. Zou B, Li J, Ma RX, Cheng XY, Ma RY, Zhou TY, Wu ZQ, Yao Y, Li J. Aging Dis. 2023 Jun 1;14(3):964-1678. doi: 10.14336/AD.2022.1127. PMID: 37191418

[7] Diet, Food, and Nutritional Exposures and Inflammatory Bowel Disease or Progression of Disease: an Umbrella Review. Christensen C, Knudsen A, Arnesen EK, Hatlebakk JG, Sletten IS, Fadnes LT. Adv Nutr. 2024 May;15(5):100219. doi: 10.1016/j.advnut.2024.100219. PMID: 38599319

[8] Dietary risk factors for inflammatory bowel disease in Shanghai: A case-control study. Mi L, Zhang C, Yu XF, Zou J, Yu Y, Bao ZJ. Asia Pac J Clin Nutr. 2022;31(3):405-414. doi: 10.6133/apjcn.202209_31(3).0008. PMID: 36173212

[9] Dietary Guidance from the International Organization for the Study of Inflammatory Bowel Diseases. Levine A, Rhodes JM, Lindsay JO, Abreu MT, Kamm MA, Gibson PR, Gasche C, Silverberg MS, Mahadevan U, Boneh RS, Wine E, Damas OM, Syme G, Trakman GL, Yao CK, Stockhamer S, Hammami

MB, Garces LC, Rogler G, Koutroubakis IE, Ananthakrishnan AN, McKeever L, Lewis JD. Clin Gastroenterol Hepatol. 2020 May;18(6):1381-1392. doi: 10.1016/j.cgh.2020.01.046. Epub 2020 Feb 15. PMID: 32068150

[10] https://www.webmd.com/digestive-disorders/ss/slideshow-how-gut-health-affects-whole-body

[11] The gut microbiome: Relationships with disease and opportunities for therapy. Durack J, Lynch SV. J Exp Med. 2019 Jan 7;216(1):20-40. doi: 10.1084/jem.20180448. Epub 2018 Oct 15. PMID: 30322864

[12] Mind, Mood and Microbiota-Gut-Brain Axis in Psychiatric Disorders. Toader C, Dobrin N, Costea D, Glavan LA, Covache-Busuioc RA, Dumitrascu DI, Bratu BG, Costin HP, Ciurea AV. Int J Mol Sci. 2024 Mar 15;25(6):3340. doi: 10.3390/ijms25063340. PMID: 38542314

[13] Gut Symptoms, Gut Dysbiosis and Gut-Derived Toxins in ALS. Lee A, Henderson R, Aylward J, McCombe P. Int J Mol Sci. 2024 Feb 3;25(3):1871. doi: 10.3390/ijms25031871. PMID: 38339149

[14] Association of dietary and lifestyle inflammation score (DLIS) with chronic migraine in women: a cross-sectional study. Bakhshimoghaddam F, Shalilahmadi D, Mahdavi R, Nikniaz Z, Karandish M, Hajjarzadeh S. Sci Rep. 2024 Jul 16;14(1):16406. doi: 10.1038/s41598-024-66776-6. PMID: 39013951

[15] A Narrative Review of Intestinal Microbiota's Impact on Migraine with Psychopathologies. Francavilla M, Facchetti S, Demartini C, Zanaboni AM, Amoroso C, Bottiroli S, Tassorelli C, Greco R. Int J Mol Sci. 2024 Jun 17;25(12):6655. doi: 10.3390/ijms25126655. PMID: 38928361

[16] Severe intestinal dysbiosis is prevalent in primary Sjögren's syndrome and is associated with systemic disease activity. Mandl T, Marsal J, Olsson P, Ohlsson B, Andréasson K. Arthritis Res Ther. 2017 Oct 24;19(1):237. doi: 10.1186/s13075-017-1446-2. PMID: 29065905

[17] The Mediterranean, Dietary Approaches to Stop Hypertension (DASH), and Mediterranean-DASH Intervention for Neurodegenerative Delay (MIND) Diets Are Associated with Less Cognitive Decline and a Lower Risk of Alzheimer's Disease-A Review. van den Brink AC, Brouwer-Brolsma EM, Berendsen AAM, van de Rest O. Adv Nutr. 2019 Nov 1;10(6):1040-1065. doi: 10.1093/advances/nmz054. PMID: 31209456

2: New Prescripts

The SANA diet is not just a diet, but rather is a lifestyle prescription that includes proper sleep, sufficient exercise, sidestepping stress, and enjoying life. Without quality of life, extreme longevity does not provide much of a blessing. Some central concepts underlie the SANA program beyond promoting a nutritious and balanced diet.

While this book focuses on reducing the risk of dementia, the SANA program also helps promote overall health, aids in the recovery from type 2 diabetes (T2D), inflammatory bowel disease (IBD), and lowers the risk of most chronic diseases present in industrialized countries.

The Pillars of Health

Although a balanced, healthy, non-toxic diet and a healthy microbiome are the central focus of this book, several pillars of health keep the heavy marble ceiling of the temple from toppling down upon us. These are the pillars of health that should not be ignored.

I A balanced, healthy, diverse diet. Provides our bodies with the essential nutrients needed to function properly.
II A healthy, supportive microbiome. A healthy community of gut bacteria plays a vital role in digestion, immunity, and overall health. A healthy oral microbiome is also important.
III Stimulation of adaptive mechanisms to maintain vitality; includes dietary, immune, and physical and emotional adaptive mechanisms.
IV Sufficient, appropriate level, physical activity. Regular vigorous exercise helps maintain physical fitness, improves mood, and reduces the risk of chronic diseases.
V Sufficient, quality sleep. Getting enough restful sleep is essential for cognitive function, physical recovery, and overall well-being.
VI A healthy, supportive, social environment. Strong social connections provide emotional support and a sense of purpose and belonging.
VII Love and intimacy. Emotional connection fosters happiness, helps resolve distress, and contributes to overall well-being.
VIII Play, intellectual, and environmental stimulation. Engaging in stimulating activities keeps the mind sharp, reduces stress, and improves cognitive function.
IX Avoidance of toxic stress. Chronic stress harms both physical and mental health.
X A clean, healthy, quiet, non-toxic, physical environment. Minimizing exposure to environmental toxins and noise can help reduce the risk of chronic diseases.

Each of these areas is important to health and impacts the risk of neurodegenerative disease, and thus is integral to the SANA protocol. Most of the volume of this book concerns diet and nutrition; exercise and sleep are also discussed. Emotional health and stress will only be briefly covered; this is not to minimize their importance, but rather because they deserve a full, in-depth discussion.

Humans are social creatures; studies have shown that social isolation, loneliness, or living alone increases mortality by approximately 30% overall and by 43% in seniors.[1 2] Loneliness was found to be associated with as much as a 15-year decrease in lifespan; an impact comparable to smoking 15 cigarettes a day or being obese. Loneliness has been associated with an increased risk of cancer, cardiovascular disease, and impaired immunity.[3] Loneliness can be painful and is highly prevalent in the U.S., especially among older adults. Humans need social interaction for health.

Social interaction is a health habit; join a club, volunteer, or mentor. Meet and interact with new people. Social interaction is as important to health as exercise is. Get a twofer by exercising with a buddy.

Anger is deadly. A study examined 826 million tweet messages from 1,347 counties that encompassed more than 88% of the U.S. population. The study looked at county-level socioeconomic, demographic, and health variables. The tweets were categorized by their emotional content based on the words used, and then mapped to location data, resulting in 148 million mapped tweets. The emotional content was mapped and correlated to the prevalence of atherosclerotic heart disease (AHD) in these counties. Counties that were high in tweets with hostility, aggression, hate, interpersonal tension, and disengagement had higher levels of AHD. Counties that were high in tweets showing positive interpersonal relationships and emotions and social engagement had significantly lower rates of AHD. The emotional content of Twitter (now X) tweets was more predictive of the county's AHD rates than were income, smoking, diabetes, hypertension, obesity, education level, income, and racial demographic factors combined.[4] This was a single ecological study that should not be assumed to imply causation, but it is not unreasonable to consider anger and ire as addictive and poisonous.

Matthew 15:17-19 (New Living Translation): *"Anything you eat passes through the stomach and then goes into the sewer. But the words you speak come from the heart—that's what defiles you."*

Our words define us. Be careful what you say.

Adaptive Mechanisms

The SANA program also focuses on adaptive mechanisms that protect the body and brain from injury and promote repair. This includes foods that promote the expression of antioxidant enzymes, for example. A compound or other stimuli that "promotes expression" triggers the transcription of a specific area of the DNA so that the protein encoded by those genes can be made in a cell. Compounds in certain foods, such as green tea and blueberries, are well known to contain phenolic compounds that promote health through these mechanisms. These adaptation-promoting food components are discussed in Chapters 19 to 23. Exercise also promotes the expression of genes that promote brain and physical health; exercise is an essential component in the SANA program, discussed in Chapter 29. Sleep is discussed in Chapter 30.

Emotional adaptation is also essential. We can practice this through social engagement with empathy, internal honesty, and kindness.

Environmental Toxins

A clean, healthy, non-toxic, physical environment is essential for neurologic and general health, and minimizing exposure to environmental toxins can help reduce the risk of neurodegenerative and other chronic diseases. Pillar ten, however, is sufficiently complex that it merits discussion beyond the scope of this book. In contrast to diet, exercise, and sleep hygiene, which are under the agency of the individual and as such are the major focus of the SANA program, individuals generally have limited control over their exposure to environmental toxins outside of their homes.

There are a couple of environmental toxins that the individual does have some control over, as examples.

- Living in an area of high levels of fine particulate matter air pollution (at $PM_{2.5}$ 10μg/m3) increases the risk of Alzheimer's disease (AD) two to three times.[5]

If one lives in an area of elevated PM air pollution, the use of HEPA filters in your home, moving to a cleaner environment, and banging on the door of your congressman to push him or her to remedy this may help. Control of indoor air pollution is discussed in Chapter 32.

- Many pesticides are intentionally neurotoxic, as that is one method of killing insects. We share some neurotransmitters with insects, and thus we can be poisoned by insecticides that target these neurotransmitters. Other insecticides are neurotoxic, just like general toxins. In a meta-analysis, those with higher levels of pesticide exposure were found to be 34% more likely to develop AD.[6] Certain pesticides are used in research to create animal models of Parkinson's disease.
- In the 2013 – 2014 National Health and Nutrition Examination Study (NHANES), 84% of elderly Americans were found to have detectable levels of glyphosate (Roundup weed killer) in their urine. Those with higher exposure levels were more likely to score poorly on cognitive tests.[7]

Those who live in agricultural areas are generally at higher risk of exposure to pesticides, but household and landscape pesticide exposure is also a risk. Using minimally-toxic insecticides, such as boric acid, using baits and traps rather than sprays, and keeping the home clean, helps avoid household exposure to insecticides. The use of herbicides in the garden is not a requirement.

Environmental toxins and their impact on the brain are beyond the scope of this book, but are a subject of another book by this author, *Neurodevelopment and Intelligence*.

The DAD Scoring System

The SANA diet takes a detailed approach to diet, rating each food and its preparation. There is a myriad of different food combinations, so each brand of spaghetti sauce cannot be rated. Rather, the most commonly consumed food ingredients are scored and given a nine-point Dietary Antiinflammatory and Digestibility (DAD) rating from exceptional to disastrous, with numbers being positive and letter grades negative. For example, each of the thirty most commonly consumed vegetables in commerce is rated.

The DAD ratings go in descending order from 4 to zero and then from A to D, from most beneficial to highly detrimental.

- 4: Exceptionally beneficial to gut and general health. When possible, select foods with a score of 4. When there is a choice, choose one rated four.
- 3: Excellent. Highly rated food for general and GI health. If there is a choice, a 3 is better than a 2.

❋ 2: Very good: A great food choice. Most of the diet should come from foods scoring 2 or above.

❋ 1: OK. These foods provide moderate benefits for GI health. They are acceptable foods on the SANA diets and do not need to be avoided; however, some may need to be consumed in moderation. When a higher-rated choice is available, take it.

☺ 0: These foods have little positive or negative impact on the GI microbiome. They are neither helpful nor harmful for GI health. They are not top choices, but are not banished from the diet. Many of the items that are rated zero are flavorings or ingredients used in cooking other foods. Sugar, baking soda, and starch are, for example, rated zero. The SANA diet allows restricted amounts of sugar. Of course, the amounts are very restricted for diabetics.

💣 A: Is for Avoid. Foods rated A should only be consumed occasionally, for example, on special occasions. For individuals who have active symptoms of dysbiosis, it is best to avoid these altogether. After stabilizing on the SANA diet and the remission of dysbiosis, occasional consumption of A-rated items should not cause problems if the rest of the diet is well balanced, with most of the foods rated 2 or more. For example, chicken, which gets a DAD score of A, may occasionally be eaten if properly prepared. If a person needs to cheat, it should be done rarely, and the cheating limited to foods rated A.

💣 B: B is for bad. B-rated foods are worse than A-rated foods. These foods upset the intestinal microbiome and should be kept out of the diet as much as possible and consumed in only small amounts when they cannot be avoided.

💣 C: Is for condemned: These foods go contrary to any work that has been done to improve microbiome health. They are convicts that will contaminate the colon's copasetic comfort and corrupt its condition. Cancel the consumption of these foods.

☠ D: Is for disastrous, destructive, and don't down. Foods rated D are prohibited from the SANA diet. Some of the items rated D are not even foods, but are things put into foods to increase shelf life. Others are foods that many consider healthy, but still mess up the intestinal microbiome or are otherwise problematic.

Foods rated C or D are prohibited from the SANA diet.

A key component of the SANA program is to provide better choices. As an example, the diet promotes the frequent consumption of legumes. However, some legumes provide more benefit than others for the microbiome and general health, and the method of preparation has a large impact on the DAD score. The SANA diet rates fruits, vegetables, grains, legumes, and other foods, and teaches their proper preparation to provide the highest value for health, nutrition, and the enterobiome.

While the MIND diet for the prevention of dementia does not recommend the consumption of fruit (other than berries) for Alzheimer's disease prevention, as studies have failed to show any benefit, the SANA diet offers an explanation of why fruits failed to slow AD progression in the MIND study, and provides a means to overcome this failure. The reason is simple; the fruits most commonly consumed (bananas, apples, and strawberries) are unhelpful; nevertheless, many fruits are helpful. The SANA diet provides a rating of the health impact of fruits.

Thus, food selection is rated within categories to show which foods are the most helpful and which should be avoided. The goal is to help people select foods they enjoy that are helpful.

A Diet for Flourishing

A flourishing diet is one that makes people feel energetic and clearer-minded. The SANA diet is designed to do this. Whole food, plant-based diets are associated with lower chronic disease risk, including a low risk of obesity, diabetes, heart disease, cancer, and dementia. They also appear to be associated with improved mental health. People who eat more fruits and vegetables have been found to have a lower incidence of depression and anxiety.[8] Here, however, I refer to mental health as *health* rather than the absence of affective disease or thought disorders.

An analysis of data from 80,000 Brits assessed metrics of well-being, including happiness, life satisfaction, mental well-being, and perception of overall health, as well, assessed feelings of "low", nervous, or suffering from mental disorders. Those with the highest level of well-being were those consuming around seven portions of fruits and vegetables (F&V) each day.[9]

In a study of over 1200 older Canadian men, those consuming higher amounts of F&V were three times more likely to rate life satisfaction as high.[10] In an Australian study, examining food diaries of over 12,000 randomly selected adults, increased F&V consumption was associated with increased happiness, well-being, and life satisfaction.[11] A study of 405 young adults, median age 19.9, found that those eating greater amounts of F&V felt happier, more creative, and had greater curiosity than those eating lesser amounts.[12] In a study of 541 Iranian university students, those who ate breakfast every day and ate eight or more servings of F&V were the happiest.[13] In a study of over a thousand young people, those who ate more F&V were found to have greater intellect, curiosity, and social engagement.[14]

A study of 422 young adults in the U.S. and New Zealand found that those eating 6 to 7 servings of fruits and vegetables a day had higher mood, greater life satisfaction, and "flourishing" (feeling that life has meaning, purpose, and fulfillment), and had fewer depressive symptoms. Notably, this study found that raw F&V predicted higher positive mood, life satisfaction, and flourishing; and reduced depressive symptoms, while processed F&V only helped with positive mood. The study also found that greater depressive symptoms and lower life satisfaction were associated with the consumption of soda pop. The raw vegetables significantly associated with flourishing included carrots, dark green leafy vegetables, lettuce, cucumber, celery, red onions, and bell peppers. Pretty much all commonly eaten raw fruit was associated with flourishing, and included frozen, but not cooked, berries. Canned peaches and pineapple also increased flourishing. The processed vegetables that promoted flourishing included mixed frozen vegetables, broccoli, green beans, and dark leafy vegetables.[15]

These studies were all retrospective. It may be that healthier, more affluent, more mobile, less stressed individuals eat more F&V because of better access to them. Also, the selection of fresh F&V rather than processed ones is dependent on F&V availability according to season and culture. Only those F&V that are commonly consumed would be included in the study and have sufficient statistical power to determine their effect. Vegetables such as broccoli might be much more effective when consumed raw, but most people eat them cooked. Processed apples came close to statistical significance in the study above, but may not be consumed frequently enough to show this. Perhaps fresh okra may have excellent effects, but it is rarely available on the shelf. Thus, these retrospective studies have weaknesses.

Intervention studies can provide greater confidence that the outcome is the result of the "intervention" being studied. In a study of university students, aged 18 to 25, study intervention group participants were given a two-week supply of F&V, enough to add two extra servings of fresh fruits and vegetables each day (apples, carrots, and oranges or kiwifruit, depending on the season). The daily intake of F&V was reported using a smartphone in the intervention and non-supplemented groups. Over the two weeks of the study, there were no significant changes in depression or anxiety scores. Those given the fruit supplements had progressive improvement in flourishing, vitality (feeling full of life), and motivation across the 14 days relative to the other groups.[16]

The mechanism of action for the improvement in well-being from the consumption of F&V has not yet been established. The intervention study measured serum vitamin C and carotene and determined that the levels of these vitamins did not explain the benefits of F&V. It seems likely that phenolic compounds and fiber participate in promoting the well-being observed in these studies of the consumption of F&V, particularly unprocessed F&V. It may be as simple as better hydration or replacing unhealthy snacks with ones that are not unhealthy.

Axioms

- A healthy diet should not promote dysbiosis and should be healthy. It should be pleasant and make one feel good.
- Trade up! Whenever possible, substitute a low-rated fruit or vegetable with one with a higher score. Prioritize higher-rated foods. Choose the better bean and the greater grain.
- Consuming a serving of a food rated two (★★) does not balance out the consumption of one rated B (⛈ ⛈). Foods with positive (numbered) ratings do not offset harm from the consumption of lettered ones. The scale is not symmetrical; a B is considerably more detrimental for the microbiome than a two is beneficial.
- The scientific basis for the restrictions and recommendations of the diet is generally left to the later parts of each chapter and chapters later in the book; however, they are also explained along the way. DAD ratings, and in later chapters, the HAR scores, are the author's research-based assessment of the impact of the foods based primarily on review of scientific literature, but also taking clinical observation, testing, and feedback into account. They are proprietary metrics devised by the author.
- Nothing wants to be eaten or to be on your menu, and everything protects itself from being eaten. Every plant defends itself, mostly from insects, worms, bacteria, and fungi, usually by trying to be

inedible. Most food needs at least some preparation to counter these defensive mechanisms.

An exception is that some plants use animals and their digestive systems to disperse their seeds. Some edible fruits have evolved that entice animals to consume the fruit, swallowing the seeds whole. The animal then disperses the seeds in its feces, often far from the plant. Even these plants have protective mechanisms to prevent injury to the fruit before the seeds are ripe. Some examples of fruits that rely on passing through an animal's digestive system for seed dispersal include tomatoes, raspberries, blackberries, cherries, cucumbers, and guavas. Is it coincidental that these are rated a 4 on the DAD scale? Watermelon seeds are also adapted to be dispersed in the stool, but they only get a rating of 3. Mangoes and dates are not usually swallowed, but birds will carry them a distance from the tree to feed on them, helping with dispersal.

- Don't allow the pursuit of perfection to become a pitfall to progress. The SANA program's goal is to improve people's lives, not to make them difficult. Each time one moves towards health and each time one steps away from harmful habits, progress is made. Except for addictions – those need to be completely cut off.
- While the book tries to point towards the optimal, so that it can be best understood and be used in commercial settings, the program will fail if making changes is too difficult, burdensome, unaffordable, or unpleasant. You may enjoy making soy milk and tofu from dried beans at home, and perhaps that provides the pinnacle of quality and flavor, but mixing soy milk powder in water is sufficient to get a very healthy milk substitute, and is much easier. If you don't relish its somewhat beany flavor and can't get it down without a bit of sweetener and vanilla, add them. Optimal soaking conditions for brown rice may be to maintain a constant temperature of 32° C for 8 hours, but starting the soak with hot water and letting the temperature slowly fall to room temperature for 6 hours without special equipment will provide most of the benefit. Don't let perfection be the enemy of the good.
- Avoid getting too hungry. When we are ravenous, we make poor food choices.
- Don't go hungry. It can be a mistake to simply eliminate a food, such as wheat, from the diet without replacing it with higher-rated alternatives. Simply eliminating animal products from the diet does not make for a healthy vegan diet.
- If you don't feel better after eating a meal, think twice about eating those foods again. You should feel satisfied, not stuffed and overburdened. You should be able to think, "I enjoyed that, I'd like to do that again on another occasion".
- A poor-quality vegan diet may not be any healthier than a medium-quality omnivorous diet.

In the Nurses' Health Study, with 4.8 million years of follow-up data, a healthful plant-based diet was associated with a 25% decreased risk of heart disease, but an unhealthful plant-based diet was associated with a 32% increase in heart disease risk as compared to a typical omnivorous diet.[17] While there is evidence that vegan diets can lower the risk of multiple chronic diseases, there is no guarantee. French fries, moon cakes, lemon tarts, and doughnuts are all vegan. Additionally, it can be difficult to get enough protein and other nutrients on a vegan diet. A vegan diet can be a healthy diet, but it takes dedication.

- Use common sense. This diet is not an excuse to make bad choices or to abandon one's doctor's advice. If a person has food allergies, a high rating of a food does not allow them to consume it. Just because a food has a positive score, it does not mean that one can pig out on it.
- The nine most common food allergies are to milk, eggs, fish, shellfish, tree nuts, peanuts, wheat, soybeans, and sesame seeds. One reason for them being common allergens is that these are foods that are commonly eaten, so more people are frequently exposed to them. Nevertheless, many of these foods are also difficult to digest, and thus likely to reach the distal small intestine only partially digested. This can leave protein fragments that may be absorbed by immune cells and processed as foreign proteins, especially for those with leaky gut and in the presence of toxic and immunogenic bacterial compounds. Both careful, appropriate food preparation and avoidance of dysbiosis can help prevent the development of food allergies and food sensitivities. Once food allergies develop, some can last a lifetime.
- This book discusses multiple risk factors for dementia. It is unlikely that exposure to any single risk factor results in dementia. It is far more likely that these factors participate in a series of unfortunate circumstances in which toxins, infections, antibiotics, poor diet, emotional and physical stress, and epigenetics contribute to dysbiosis, altered intestinal permeability, and toxicity. Together, these can sufficiently alter

intestinal function and absorption, giving rise to neurologic disease. Lifestyle changes that eliminate multiple "risk factors" are more likely to succeed in restoring intestinal function than the elimination of a single adverse agent.

- I am a medical doctor, but I am not your doctor. Nothing in this book should be construed as medical advice.

Equipment:

1. It really helps to have a home, a kitchen with a stove, and a refrigerator.
2. If you don't have one, it is recommended that you purchase a stainless steel pressure cooker. The stainless steel ones are a bit more expensive, but worth the difference. They should last for decades. Avoid aluminum ones.
3. A digital kettle is highly recommended. Get one that you can set the exact temperature (preferably in Celsius and Fahrenheit), not just to a few presets. I recommend ones designed with the kettle that can be removed from its base, where the base controls the temperature. It needs to have a "stay warm" setting that will maintain the temperature.
4. Get a pair of stainless steel kitchen scissor-tongs for cooking eggs in water.
5. Ceramic non-stick skillets with clear glass lids are nice.
6. A digital timer is helpful. A smartphone works well.
7. Measuring cups and spoons.
8. A potato peeler.
9. A digital food thermometer. For under $10, this one works nicely: https://www.amazon.com/dp/B0BQ782XNW
10. A digital scale that can measure to at least one-tenth of a gram.
11. Microwave-safe glass coffee mugs.
12. A slow cooker with a temperature probe comes in handy. It can be used to make yogurt and control the soaking and cooking temperature of food. Here is an example: https://www.amazon.com/s?k=hamilton+beach+slow+cooker+33866&crid=JJ6OVWN4596A

Cooking in Water

Most foods in this diet are cooked in water. Water is an excellent medium for heat transfer, it acts as a solvent, and it limits the temperature that the food is exposed to during cooking, which prevents the formation of most of the carcinogenic compounds that can be created by cooking food at high temperatures.

Water boils at 100° C (212° F) at sea level, but at slightly lower temperatures with increasing altitude. Pressure cookers allow cooking at somewhat higher temperatures, generally at 121° C (250° F), which cuts down on cooking time and saves energy as less heat is lost into the room as steam.

One of the laws of physics is that one cannot exceed the boiling temperature of water by increasing the temperature of the burner on a stove. One can get a more vigorous boil, get more splatter, overflow the pot, and make a mess, but one can't speed the cooking with a more vigorous boil. Physics sets the temperature. You can lose moisture faster if that is your goal. High heat can be used to bring water to a boil more quickly, but once it reaches temperature, lower the heat to a point that is just enough to keep a low boil. Using a lid will help retain heat and thus require less power, and keep your house cooler and less humid. A vigorous boil will also cause the food to fall apart more as it is churned in the water. When using a first-generation pressure cooker, the heat should be set so that once the pot comes to pressure, only a tiny amount of steam escapes. Otherwise, you may run low on water and burn the contents, or even melt the pot if you run out of water.

This is in contrast to a "simmer," which is cooking in water at a temperature just below the boiling point (81 – 99 C)

Poaching is cooking in water at an even lower temperature, in the range of about 70–80 °C (158–176 °F). Shallow poaching uses little water and uses a cover to retain the steam in the pan to cook the food. With shallow poaching, most of the food is above the level of the water.

Steaming is cooking in hot water vapor. In the West, it is generally used to lightly cook vegetables and help retain their nutritional value. Steaming is also used to prepare tamales. It is generally done in a pot with the food placed in a steamer tray, with just a half-inch of water or less, and the pot covered with a lid to retain the steam.

When cooking, it is better to use a back burner when possible. Always use the vent fan when cooking on a gas stove. Set the vent fan on low (as it is generally more effective) when cooking to avoid exposure to carbon monoxide and nitrous oxide. If your stove hood does not vent to the outside and you have a gas stove, get this fixed. If you cook with gas, get a high-sensitivity digital carbon monoxide detector.

Carbon Monoxide Detectors

Normal carbon monoxide (CO) detectors are set to give an alarm when dangerously high levels of CO accumulate in the home: 70 ppm for more than 60 minutes, or 40 ppm for 10 hours. When this occurs, the house or apartment should be immediately vacated, 911 called, and the building not reentered until the cause is discovered and the home is declared safe. This is a dangerous situation. CO levels less than this can cause headaches, flu-like symptoms, fatigue, or dizziness.

These alarm levels are too high to protect those with heart and lung conditions. Additionally, we should be preventing exposure to CO before the canary dies. High-sensitivity digital CO detectors (such as the one made by Forensics) display the CO level as low as 10 ppm, allowing one to know if levels are rising and take action well before emergency services are required. One or more UL2034-compliant CO detectors will still additionally be legally required in most homes and garages.

Meta-analyses

Throughout this text, I reference meta-analysis studies. A meta-analysis is a study of studies. When correctly done, it is a statistical review of available pertinent studies on what is usually a narrow topic. By combining the outcome from various studies, with different populations, and typically incorporating various techniques, the meta-analysis offers many advantages; it can be more reliable as it is less likely to be biased; it can combine the strength of several studies to see effects that were too small in smaller studies, and it can be more informative. Thus, findings from meta-analyses are considered to provide stronger evidence that an effect is real. Nevertheless, they can not necessarily be interpreted to mean that the association they document in epidemiologic studies is mechanistically straightforward.

Risk Ratios

When assessing the impact of various exposures, risk, hazard, and odds ratios are used as metrics of the impact. These measure the relative risk, comparing exposure, for example, those who drink alcohol to those who do not. If six of one hundred people aged 65 who live in polluted areas develop Alzheimer's disease over a 5-year follow-up, as compared to only three of one hundred people in otherwise similar but unpolluted areas, that gives a relative risk (RR) of 2.0 for exposure to the pollution. An RR of 0.5 means that the risk is half as much; thus, those with the protective exposure are half as likely to develop the condition. It can also be said that their risk is reduced by 50%. If the risk ratio is 1.0, it means that the exposure was not different for those with and without the study condition.

RRs are generally used in cohort studies where exposures are known at the beginning of the study and the outcomes are assessed after some time. For example, a study that assesses the diet of healthy people and watches to see what diseases develop over several years is a cohort, a.k.a., a follow-up study.

Hazard ratios (HR) are similar, but used in survival analysis, where the time to the outcome is of interest; everyone eventually dies, the HR assesses the difference in survival time until the failure event (heart attack, cancer recurrence, death, etc.).

Odds ratios (OR) are used in case-control studies where exposure and outcome are assessed at the same time. This study design looks at current exposure and subject status. For example, how many bananas are eaten in an average week, and is the subject depressed or taking medications for depression? An OR greater than 1.0 suggests a higher odds of disease among the exposed group, while an OR less than 1.0 suggests a lower odds of the disease in the exposed group.

Case-control studies show association with risk factors, but do not demonstrate causality. If banana consumption is associated with a higher odds of depression, did bananas cause the depression, or did depression cause cravings for bananas? Did suffering from depression create a causal web where only soft, ready-to-eat food was consumed? (I know of no studies linking bananas to depression.)

Animal Studies

We are animals, but we are not mice or rats. Animal studies are useful as researchers can control most of the variables and focus on a single issue at a time, while humans have all kinds of bad habits that make study data noisy. Humans also have significant genetic differences, while genetically similar animals are easily available. Mice and rats have short lifespans and thus age quickly and develop diseases of aging quickly, so studies have outcomes in one to two years rather than decades. While not closely related to humans, rodents (mice, rats, squirrels) and rabbits are genetically more similar to us than are pigs, bears, cats, dogs, sheep, deer, goats, whales, or most other non-primate mammals.

Content Notice

Some sections of this book are drawn from materials from books previously published by the author:

- *Enteroimmunology*
- *Unraveling Cancer*
- *Neurodevelopment and Intelligence*

These sections help provide a foundation for understanding how diet impacts health and describe some of the science supporting the SANA diet. Where appropriate, the material is refocused and enhanced to better align with the topic of dementia and chronic disease prevention.

[1] Loneliness and social isolation as risk factors for mortality: a meta-analytic review. Holt-Lunstad J, Smith TB, Baker M, Harris T, Stephenson D. Perspect Psychol Sci. 2015 Mar;10(2):227-37. doi: 10.1177/1745691614568352. PMID: 25910392

[2] https://www.hrsa.gov/enews/past-issues/2019/january-17/loneliness-epidemic

[3] Loneliness Is Harmful to Our Nation's Health. Claire Pomeroy on March 20, 2019. Scientific American. https://blogs.scientificamerican.com/observations/loneliness-is-harmful-to-our-nations-health/

[4] Psychological language on Twitter predicts county-level heart disease mortality. Eichstaedt JC, Schwartz HA, Kern ML, Park G, Labarthe DR, Merchant RM, Jha S, Agrawal M, Dziurzynski LA, Sap M, Weeg C, Larson EE, Ungar LH, Seligman ME. Psychol Sci. 2015 Feb;26(2):159-69. doi: 10.1177/0956797614557867. Epub 2015 Jan 20. PMID: 25605707

[5] Air Pollution and Alzheimer's Disease: A Systematic Review and Meta-Analysis. Fu P, Yung KKL. J Alzheimers Dis. 2020;77(2):701-714. doi: 10.3233/JAD-200483. PMID: 32741830

[6] Pesticide exposure and risk of Alzheimer's disease: a systematic review and meta-analysis. Yan D, Zhang Y, Liu L, Yan H. Sci Rep. 2016 Sep 1;6:32222. doi: 10.1038/srep32222. PMID: 27581992

[7] Association Between Urinary Glyphosate Exposure and Cognitive Impairment in Older Adults from NHANES 2013-2014. Ren J, Yu Y, Wang Y, Dong Y, Shen X. J Alzheimers Dis. 2024;97(2):609-620. doi: 10.3233/JAD-230782. PMID: 38143355

[8] The association between fruit and vegetable consumption and mental health disorders: evidence from five waves of a national survey of Canadians. McMartin SE, Jacka FN, Colman I. Prev Med. 2013 Mar;56(3-4):225-30. doi: 10.1016/j.ypmed.2012.12.016. PMID: 23295173

[9] Is Psychological Well-Being Linked to the Consumption of Fruit and Vegetables? Blanchflower, D.G., Oswald, A.J. & Stewart-Brown, S. Soc Indic Res 114, 785–801 (2013). https://doi.org/10.1007/s11205-012-0173-y

[10] The relationships between food group consumption, self-rated health, and life satisfaction of community-dwelling canadian older men: the manitoba follow-up study. Lengyel CO, Tate RB, Obirek Blatz AK. J Nutr Elder. 2009 Apr;28(2):158-73. doi: 10.1080/01639360902950182. PMID: 21184363

[11] Evolution of Well-Being and Happiness After Increases in Consumption of Fruit and Vegetables. Mujcic R, J Oswald A. Am J Public Health. 2016 Aug;106(8):1504-10. doi: 10.2105/AJPH.2016.303260. PMID: 27400354

[12] On carrots and curiosity: eating fruit and vegetables is associated with greater flourishing in daily life. Conner TS, Brookie KL, Richardson AC, Polak MA. Br J Health Psychol. 2015 May;20(2):413-27. doi: 10.1111/bjhp.12113. PMID: 25080035

[13] Eating breakfast, fruit and vegetable intake and their relation with happiness in college students. Lesani A, Mohammadpoorasl A, Javadi M, Esfeh JM, Fakhari A. Eat Weight Disord. 2016 Dec;21(4):645-651. doi: 10.1007/s40519-016-0261-0. PMID: 26928281

[14] The Role of Personality Traits in Young Adult Fruit and Vegetable Consumption. Conner TS, Thompson LM, Knight RL, Flett JA, Richardson AC, Brookie KL. Front Psychol. 2017 Feb 7;8:119. doi: 10.3389/fpsyg.2017.00119. PMID: 28223952

[15] Intake of Raw Fruits and Vegetables Is Associated With Better Mental Health Than Intake of Processed Fruits and Vegetables. Brookie KL, Best GI, Conner TS. Front Psychol. 2018 Apr 10;9:487. doi: 10.3389/fpsyg.2018.00487. PMID: 29692750

[16] Let them eat fruit! The effect of fruit and vegetable consumption on psychological well-being in young adults: A randomized controlled trial. Conner TS, Brookie KL, Carr AC, Mainvil LA, Vissers MC. PLoS One. 2017 Feb 3;12(2):e0171206. doi: 10.1371/journal.pone.0171206. PMID: 28158239

[17] Healthful and Unhealthful Plant-Based Diets and the Risk of Coronary Heart Disease in U.S. Adults. Satija A, Bhupathiraju SN, Spiegelman D, Chiuve SE, Manson JE, Willett W, Rexrode KM, Rimm EB, Hu FB. J Am Coll Cardiol. 2017 Jul 25;70(4):411-422. doi: 10.1016/j.jacc.2017.05.047. PMID: 28728684

3: The Intestinal Microbiome

One of the central design criteria for the SANA program is that it mitigates chronic systemic inflammation. There are several dietary and lifestyle factors that promote inflammation, most of which will be addressed in this book.

Lifestyle factors that promote inflammation *include:*

- Smoking
- Sloth, as opposed to physical activity
- Sleep deprivation
- Obesity
- Exposure to certain toxins
- Chronic emotional stress and anger.

Dietary factors that promote inflammation *include,* but are not limited to:

- High-fat diets, especially n-6 and certain saturated fats
- Sugar-sweetened beverages
- Excessive alcohol intake
- Nutrient inadequacies and
- Intestinal dysbiosis, the subject of this chapter.

Several synthetic dietary and lifestyle inflammatory indices have been developed by grouping dietary patterns and assessing the impact of specific foods on blood markers of inflammation in epidemiological studies. While these are coarse measurements that group foods into groups, dietary inflammatory indices (DII) are associated with fatty liver disease, diabetes, all-cause cancer, and cardiovascular disease death.[1] [2] [3] [4] [5]

A healthy, symbiotic microbiome is critical to overall health. Meanwhile, dysbiosis causes intestinal hyperpermeability, leading to systemic inflammation. A central, guiding concept upon which the SANA diet is based is that the intestinal, and to a lesser extent, the oral microbiome play a major role in our health, and that leaky gut is an important cause of inflammation and disease.

Adequate and varied dietary fiber, from legumes, whole grains, vegetables, and fruits, is an essential component of a healthy diet. The industrialized Western diet is heavy in refined grains with limited fiber and refined fats and sugars that are devoid of fiber. The standard American diet is also rich in meat, and thus it is common for poorly digested muscle fiber from the meat to make its way to the colon, where it is fermented, producing toxic and inflammatory compounds. These factors promote dysbiosis and inflammation.

A fundamental concept of the SANA diet is that in health, we have a population of commensal intestinal bacteria with which we have a symbiotic relationship, that act almost as an additional organ. These bacteria ferment soluble fiber from the diet and produce short-chain fatty acids (SCFA) that are absorbed in the colon. Soluble fiber is composed mostly of complex polysaccharides (chains of sugar molecules) that are present in plants, but for which humans do not have intestinal enzymes to separate the bonds between sugars in the molecular chains. The commensal GI bacteria have the enzymes and produce SCFA and other compounds during the fermentation process. These SCFAs supply energy to colonocytes, the main epithelial mucosa cells lining the colon. The SCFAs are also absorbed and help supply energy during fasting. While most of the upper small intestine has relatively very few bacteria, the distal small intestine has some bacteria, including Lactobacilli, and the colon, the large intestine, is heavily populated with trillions of bacteria.

Other bacteria present in the distal small intestine and colon ferment mucous, bile, fats, and protein that escape digestion, but in health, the amount of these substances is low, and the population of bacteria that specialize in their fermentation is limited. Having a healthy diversity of mutualistic bacteria (eubiosis) depends on the consumption of sufficient dietary soluble fiber to support bacterial proliferation.

There are multiple types of chemical bonds between various sugar molecules that make up polysaccharides and other compounds that form dietary fiber. Different bacteria are needed to process these different molecular links. Fiber from a single food may require several species of bacteria to process it.

Dysbiosis and Inflammation

In contrast to healthy eubiosis, dysbiosis is the state of having an unfavorable distribution of intestinal bacteria that harms rather than helps provide health. The overgrowth of certain populations of bacteria can break down the protective mucosal layer in the colon and can form toxic compounds. Together, these and other factors can cause a situation in which toxins from the colon can seep between the colonocytes (the cells lining the colon) into the body, causing inflammation, which can lead to disease. The increased intracellular intestinal permeability, commonly referred to as "leaky gut", allows toxins and immunoreactive compounds from the colon to enter the body, where they promote inflammation and toxicity that injure the brain and other organs. Increased intestinal permeability allows protein fragments (peptides) from foods to leak through the mucosal layer of the intestine. This is an area rich in immune cells; more than half of the body's immune cells reside here to protect us from intestinal pathobionts, fungi, and parasites. Some food peptides that make their way past the mucosal barrier can trigger immunoreactivity, causing food allergies and sensitivities.

Our immune system makes antibodies to recognize diseases that we are exposed to. That is part of the adaptive immune system. We also have an innate immune response to certain compounds in the environment. The innate immune system reacts to Pathogen-Associated Molecular Pattern (PAMP compounds). Two such compounds are LPS (lipopolysaccharide) and flagellin. LPS is a structural compound in the cell wall of gram-negative bacteria that inhabit the colon. Flagellin is a protein in the flagella, a whip-like structure that many bacteria use to swim, including many that are part of our commensal intestinal microbiome. If LPS, flagellin, and certain other PAMPs get past the colonocyte barrier and into the bloodstream, it initiates an innate immune system response. PAMPs act as danger signals for infection and trigger an inflammatory response. In the intestine, the release of inflammatory mediators causes plasma, the liquid part of blood, to leak into the intestine. This leaking can go both ways and can increase the absorption of endotoxins into the body. When the endotoxins get into the bloodstream, they cause inflammation. When they get to the brain, they cause inflammation there (further discussed in Chapter 4).

Dysbiosis, antibiotics, starvation, stress, heat, and toxins can disrupt the mucosal barrier and cause increased permeability of the intestinal barrier; this is often called leaky gut. Leaky gut and injury or damage to the mucosal layer can allow bacteria to enter the body and cause infections such as pneumonia. A principal focus of the SANA diet is to include foods that promote microbiome diversity and balance, and to avoid foods and other substances that harm it or cause dominance of bacteria, which allows them to become pathogenic.

Some food is good for the hundreds of species and trillions of bacteria that live in an individual's colon, and some is not. Antibiotic drugs have low toxicity for humans, but can be devastating to the intestinal microbiome. Antibiotics are made and used to kill, or at least stop the growth, of bacteria, and they do so with surprising alacrity. Some foods have antibiotic effects on the intestinal microbiota. These foods can be a problem and thus should be avoided. Other foods are prebiotic; they feed the intestinal microbiome. The bacteria that thrive are those that are well nourished.

One risk of antibiotics is that they can disrupt the microbiome. Certain antibiotics are prone to causing pseudomembranous colitis. In this disease, the antibiotic kills most of the bacteria, but does not kill the spores of spore-forming bacteria. The inactive spores, which are not harmed by the antibiotic, then later grow after the antibiotic treatment has been completed without competition, and can then dominate the intestinal microbiome, crowding out bacteria that would normally occupy that niche. *Clostridioides difficile (C. diff)*, a principal causative agent in pseudomembranous colitis, not only overgrows, but it also produces toxins.

The Intestinal Microbiome

There are about 3,600 species that live in the human intestine, with the number of species typically present in a single individual generally between 150 and 400.[6] The number of bacteria in the gut of a healthy adult is estimated to be around 38 trillion, far more bacteria than the number of cells in your body. If you think that you are similar to your siblings because of your shared genome, consider that of the about 20 million genes you walk around with, only about 20 – 30 thousand of those are human genes; the rest are microbiome genes, a population that changes with your diet.

Most of these bacteria and other microbes live in the lower intestines (the distal ileum and colon). A quarter to half of the dry mass of the stool is composed of bacteria. While the average person may have several hundred different species living in their gut, there are about 90 core species that are common and in high numbers in the lower intestine of most people. People eating a healthier, more varied diet have a more diverse array of bacteria.[7] This diversity helps maintain a balance of bacteria and lowers the risk of the intestinal microbiome being dominated by pathobionts. Pathobionts are bacteria or other organisms that live as a normal part of the microbiome but, under disrupted conditions (mucosal injury, use of antibiotics, poor diet), may become pathogenic and induce disease.

The SANA diet is designed to support a healthful enteric microbiome through the cultivation of commensal bacteria by supplying them with the types of fiber that support their growth, while minimizing the fermentation of proteins and fats which, when present in high amounts, can promote the overgrowth of bacteria in the lower intestine that become pathogenic when they dominate the microbiome.

The bacteria that are most beneficial in large numbers are those that digest complex carbohydrates that we are unable to digest. These are known as soluble fiber. The *fibrolytic* bacteria consume the soluble fiber and produce short-chain fatty acids such as butyric acid, which the colonocytes lining the colon need to function properly. Butyric acid is also absorbed, and the brain can use it for energy during fasting, for example, at night.

Among the core species of bacteria in the human microbiome are the well-known Lactobacilli and Bifidobacteria that are present in yogurt and included in probiotic supplements. A few examples of other important core species include:[8]

***Akkermansia muciniphila*:** Helps maintain the integrity of the intestinal barrier and thus reduces inflammation. It appears to help prevent insulin resistance, metabolic syndrome, obesity, aging, and cancer, and lower complication risk among those with cystic fibrosis.[9] [10] [11]*A. muciniphila* feeds on fiber from polyphenol-rich foods. Thus, a diet low in polyphenols is unlikely to maintain a healthy population of these bacteria. Polyphenol-rich foods include fruits and vegetables, seeds, nuts, herbs, and spices.

Although normally a beneficial bacterium, overgrowth of *A. muciniphila* can promote disease. *A. muciniphila* feeds on the mucin adherent to the colon cells. If the colonocytes are not getting sufficient butyrate, A. *muciniphila* can compromise mucosal integrity by depleting the mucus that isolates the colonocytes from the contents of the colon. This causes a reduction in the mucus layer depth, compromising the intestinal barrier. *A. muciniphila* over-dominance in the colon is associated with multiple sclerosis, inflammatory bowel disease, perhaps autism, and psychosis.[12] [13]

Ruminococcus bromii breaks down resistant starch in the diet, which leads to the production of short-chain fatty acids (SCFAs), such as butyrate, by other bacteria. These SCFAs are essential for gut health, as they nourish the gut lining, reduce inflammation, support immune function, and reduce the activation of IBD. Foods high in resistant starch include legumes, whole grains, and green bananas and plantains.

Faecalibacterium prausnitzii is a fermenter that provides the short-chain fatty acid butyrate in the colon, which is required for the health of the colonocytes, the cells that line the colon. An enterobiome with a paucity of F. prausnitzii is often observed in individuals with inflammatory bowel disease, irritable bowel syndrome (IBS), and obesity.[14] Pectins and pectin oligosaccharides support the growth of *F. prausnitzii.* Foods high in pectins and pectin oligosaccharides include citrus fruits, plums, guavas, carrots, apples, pears, beets, and broccoli.

Anaerobutyricum hallii is another producer of the SCFAs butyrate and propionate. That in itself is important as it protects against leaky gut, but A. hallii also detoxifies the carcinogenic heterocyclic amine (HCA) PhIP. PHIP is the most abundant HCA formed during the cooking of meat and fish at high temperatures by Maillard reactions between glucose, phenylalanine, and creatinine.[15] A. hallii growth is supported by the consumption of fiber-rich cruciferous vegetables.

Roseburia intestinalis is another colonic butyrate producer; it thrives on arabinoxylan polysaccharides found in whole grains. Like other bacteria that produce butyrate, it lowers the risk of obesity, colon cancer, and atherosclerosis. Butyrate acts directly on CD8+ T cells, enhancing their immune activity against tumor cells.[16]

Butyrate provides energy to the brain during fasting, such as at night and between meals, helping to reduce hunger and drive to eat during the night. Propionate improves pancreatic beta-cell function and prevents beta-cell death.[17] These are the cells that produce insulin. Butyrate is the principal fuel for the colonocytes that line the colon and is essential for the production of the mucous layer that protects these cells from bacteria in the gut. The majority of human intestinal bacteria are saccharolytic (sugar consumers) that rely on non-digestible polysaccharides (soluble fiber) as their energy source.[18]

These bacteria provide a healthy symbiotic relationship, eubiosis, where the enteric microbiome provides needed nutrients for our body. Nevertheless, if the microbiome gets out of balance, it can cause dysbiosis, which can lead to inflammation and disease. The bacteria that live in the colon depend mostly upon the food we feed them; the fiber in our diet and other food that we eat, but that is not digested. Poor dietary choices can starve some bacteria and cause overgrowth of other bacteria and other microbes, causing them to become pathogenic. Certain components of an industrialized diet can cause injury that causes the bacteria to become pathogenic.

The gastrointestinal (GI) tract is lined with a single layer of cells called enterocytes in the small intestine, with enterocytes in the colon being called colonocytes. The enterocytes have the job of absorbing nutrients. The colonocytes also absorb water and a few specific nutrients, but one of their critical functions is to make a mucous layer that separates us from the bacteria in the colon. Many of these bacteria are harmless when in the lumen of the colon, but can cause disease and even death if they get into the body.

A healthy intestinal microbiome has numerous species, living in different communities, occupying different areas of the colon. This is correct, but it could be more elegant: Different bacterial species ferment various substrates, resulting in a stepwise breakdown of fiber. Thus, one species of bacteria partially digests the available materials that were not absorbed into the body in the small intestine, and then a different species that produces different enzymes digests some of what is left, on and on. There are many different molecular linkages in fiber, and the bacteria may be specialists for certain ones. We need a diverse population to do the job well, and the job changes with the food we eat. Consuming a diet that is composed of a variety of foods helps promote a diverse microbiome population that has the capacity to break down different types of fiber.

There are nearly 3,600 different species of bacteria that are common residents of the intestinal microbiome. There are also viruses, fungi, and archaea living in the gut. There are lots of different viruses; at least 140,000. These are bacteriophages, a type of virus that infects bacteria and that can move genes around from one bacterium to another.[19] Things get complicated fast. There are about 250 fungi that have been found living in the human gut microbiome, but only about a dozen that are common. About 80% of people have at least one species of Candida living in their gut. Another fungus, *Malassezia restricta,* is found in the microbiome of about a quarter of adults.[20] *M. restricta* may not be benign, as it is associated with inflammatory bowel disease.[21] There are about a dozen Archaea, including Methanobrevibacter smithii, which consume hydrogen gas and produce methane gas. We sometimes also have critters (amoeba and worms) that take up residence in our bowels.

Dietary fiber is the feedstuff of the commensal microbiome, and it requires a healthy diet. When the commensal bacteria starve, we get sick. This is easy to see in hospitalized patients on total parenteral feeding, who are easily susceptible to pneumonia and sepsis.

Fiber is primarily undigestible food polysaccharides (literally "many sugars") that are connected into chains. Animals lack the digestive enzymes required to separate many of the varied covalent bonds binding these sugars. Thus, we cannot digest, absorb, or utilize those sugar molecules. Various bacteria have the ability to cut these sugar linkages in the polysaccharide chain, breaking it down so that the sugars can be used as their food. In the process, they produce some short-chain fatty acids that the colonocytes and our brains rely on for energy.

1. Diversity in the fiber sources helps maintain diversity in the population of bacteria in the colon. Different bacteria feed on different molecules found in dietary fiber. Thus, eating a variety of fruits, vegetables, and whole grains helps support a diverse and healthy commensal microbiome.

2. The commensal bacteria produce short-chain fatty acids (SCFA) that the cells lining the colon need for energy; without those SCFA, the colonocytes suffer, and the gut gets leaky. SCFA also supplies the brain with energy during fasting. This can help keep us from getting hungry between meals and at night during sleep.

3. Most processed foods are low in fiber. Sugar, vegetable oil, shortening, and lard are dense in calories but contain no fiber.

4. Not all fiber is helpful to the microbiome: "Soluble fiber" is fiber that the commensal bacteria and archaea can ferment and use for their nutrition, and from which they supply short-chain fatty acids to the cells lining the colon. Insoluble fiber does not help and may cause harm.

5. Not all soluble fiber is appropriate for those with dysbiosis and leaky gut. Consumption of food fiber high in β-fructans can increase gastrointestinal inflammation[22] and can cause gas, bloating, belching, and constipation or diarrhea.[23] Thus, several foods high in fructans are kept out of the SANA diet; some examples include artichokes, asparagus, Brussels sprouts, cabbage, and some grains.

The short-chain fatty acids butyric acid, propionic acid, and, to a lesser extent, valeric acid are among the essential end products of this fermentation. These SCFAs are the principal food source for the colonocytes that line the large intestine. Without sufficient butyric acid (butyrate), the colonocytes become weak, can't produce mucin, which is essential for enteric integrity; without sufficient mucin, the colonocyte barrier becomes leaky, and toxins from disintegrating bacteria can leak into the body. The SCFA butyrate also helps feed the brain between meals, and thus, its production from dietary fiber helps keep us from overeating and may help us sleep better.

Short-chain fatty acids (SCFA) have been identified as key mediators of the efficacy of the Mediterranean diet by strengthening intestinal barrier function. A greater production of propionate and butyrate is associated with adherence to the diet, and inversely associated with plasma lipopolysaccharide binding protein (LBP) and zonulin, a fecal marker of leaky gut.[24] Valeric acid is another SCFA that can be produced by bacteria in the gut from carbohydrates. Valerate promotes intestinal stem cell development of serotonergic neurons in the gut[25] and supports intestinal barrier function.[26] Higher valeric acid levels are associated with better renal function,[27] and have anti-inflammatory effects, lowering NF-κB, enhancing IL-10, leading to better bone density.[28]

These SCFAs are mostly formed from the fermentation of plant fiber in the lower intestine, but are also formed from some carbohydrates present, for example, in mother's milk. As a rule of thumb, the beneficial SCFAs are formed from the bacterial fermentation of non-digestible carbohydrates.

Protein Fermentation

In contrast to fibrolytic bacteria, *proteolytic* bacteria ferment amino acids; many of the byproducts of amino fermentation have toxic or noxious effects. See Table 3A below. The SANA diet supports a symbiotic enteric microbiome. It does this by avoiding foods with anti-nutritive properties, foods that have poorly digestible proteins, and other foods that have adverse effects on the commensal microbiome. Protein that is not digested ends up feeding proteolytic bacteria that have evolved to digest protein. Although small numbers of proteolytic and lipolytic bacteria are normal and helpful, they should not dominate the microbiome. Even when fasting or consuming a very low-protein diet, some protein reaches the colon and is fermented. Normally, this is mostly endogenous proteins from the normal replacement of mucosal cells lining the GI tract which have a turnover rate of about 7 days, mucin that sloughs off the surface of the intestine, some digestive enzymes, IgA antibodies that neutralize bacteria by keeping them from being able to adhere to the mucosa, and as well protein from the bacteria. Physiological amounts of protein in the colon are normal and are mostly broken down by fermentation into amino acids that are used by bacteria. Thus, it is normal and helpful to have a small resident population of proteolytic bacteria in the colon.

However, excess undigested protein can cause these bacteria to proliferate and can dominate the lower intestine. The situation is exacerbated by a deficit in dietary soluble fiber. Proteolytic bacteria can consume available SCFA, starving the colonocytes of butyrate, which prevents them from producing adequate mucus to isolate the colonocytes from the bacteria in the lumen. Bacteria can then attach to the cells. When bacteria attach to a surface, they are much more likely to form colonies (biofilms), which causes a phenotypic change in behavior and a large shift in the genes expressed by the bacteria. They begin producing a slimy extracellular matrix capable of producing toxins that the same species does not when it is in its free-floating (planktonic) form. Many bacteria only become pathogenic when they form biofilms. These bacteria may then be able to cross the lining of the intestine and enter the body. This often occurs in hospitalized patients who are not eating, and thus not feeding the colonocytes. The bacteria cross the mucosal barrier and can enter the bloodstream, get caught in the lungs, and cause gram-negative pneumonia.

When these proteolytic bacteria dominate and the mucosal layer is compromised, lipopolysaccharides (LPS) molecules, common in the cell wall of gram-negative bacteria, and flagellin, a protein from the gram-negative bacteria, may leak into the body. LPS and flagellin are recognized by the innate immune system as danger-associated molecular patterns (DAMPs) and trigger an inflammatory response as the body recognizes these molecules as a sign of infection. LPS from the gut bacteria *Bacteroides fragilis* not only can impair the integrity of the intestinal barrier and cause leaky gut, but can also impair the integrity of the blood-brain barrier and thus expose the brain to toxic and inflammatory compounds that it is normally protected from.[29] LPS may also impair the placental barrier; thus, leaky gut during pregnancy may harm the fetus. Some strains of *B. fragilis* also produce *B. fragilis*-toxin (BFT, also known as fragilysin) and other neurotoxins that have been demonstrated to cause neurodegeneration in mice. *B. fragilis*-LPS and fragilysin are strongly pro-inflammatory and extremely neurotoxic to human neuronal-glial cells in culture.[30] A central role of glial cells is to protect the brain from infections. Elevated levels of LPS have been found in the brains of patients dying with AD in comparison to levels found in the brains of people of the same age dying without dementia. Some AD patients had LPS levels in the hippocampus, that area of the brain most affected by AD, 26 times higher than found in non-AD brains.[31] LPS arising in the gut can cause neuroinflammation, disrupt neuronal synaptic signaling, and prevent the development of neuronal branching required for learning and developing memory.[32] LPS is also found in association with damaged white matter in the brains of patients with AD.[33]

Table 3A: Amino acid fermentation products in the colon

Amino Acid Group	Products	Potential Health Risks
Amino Acids: (Alanine, Arginine, Asparagine, Aspartate, Citrulline, Glutamine, Glutamate, Glycine, Histidine, Lysine, Proline, Serine, Threonine)	Ammonia Short-chain fatty acids (SCFA) (acetate, propionate, butyrate)	Generally Beneficial: Short-chain fatty acids (acetate, propionate, butyrate) produced from these amino acids are crucial for colonic health, providing energy for colonocytes and regulating various physiological functions. Ammonia ($NH4^+$) is typically further metabolized by gut bacteria or processed by the liver for excretion. $NH4^+$ can be a problem for children or those with liver disease and can cause neurologic disorders. Colorectal Cancer Risk: In alkaline colonic environments (which can occur with diets low in fermentable fiber and low SCFA production), ammonia ($NH4^+$) becomes NH3, which is easily absorbable and may cause toxicity to the colonocytes. Promotes intestinal permeability and is absorbed into the bloodstream.[34]
Arginine	Putrescine	Considered beneficial, promotes autophagy. (Chapter 19)
Branched-Chain Amino Acids (Leucine, Isoleucine, Valine)	Branched-chain fatty acids (Isobutyrate, Isovalerate)	Emerging Research: Limited but ongoing research suggests potential links between elevated levels of branched-chain fatty acids and insulin resistance, a risk factor for type 2 diabetes. Depression: Isovaleric acid levels are associated with depression.[35] Fecal transplant lowers isovaleric acid levels and is associated with improvement in depression.[36] Colon: Increased inflammation, tissue permeability, and colitis severity.[37] Body: Implicated in metabolic diseases such as obesity, diabetes, and non-alcoholic fatty liver disease (NAFLD).[38]
Sulfur-Containing Amino Acids (Cysteine, Methionine)	Hydrogen sulfide, methanethiol, various sulfur-containing compounds, butyrate, and acetate	Gut Irritation: Excessive production of hydrogen sulfide and methanethiol can contribute to bloating, gas, and gut discomfort. Limited Evidence: Some studies suggest a possible link between high levels of sulfate-reducing bacteria (which produce hydrogen sulfide) and inflammatory bowel disease, but more research is needed.
Phenylalanine	Phenylacetate	Cardiovascular Risk: Phenylacetate is converted to phenylacetylglutamine (PAGln), a risk factor for myocardial infarction, congestive heart failure, stroke, and death.[39] [40] PAGln promotes inflammation, platelet activation, and thrombosis.[41]
Tyrosine	p-Cresol	Colonocytes: Genotoxic to colonocytes. Increases oxidative stress and impairs mitochondrial activity.[42] May increase intestinal permeability and the risk of colon cancer. Endothelial Function: Absorbed and excreted into the urine. May promote atherosclerosis and thrombosis in patients with uremia,[43] and increase mortality in dialysis patients.[44] May impair white blood cell function.[45]
Tryptophan	Indole and skatole	Genotoxicity Concerns: Indole and skatole, at high concentrations, may have genotoxic properties (damaging DNA), but the relevance to human health needs further study. Neurodevelopmental or psychiatric diseases.
Aromatic Amino Acids (Phenylalanine, Tyrosine, Tryptophan)	p-Cresyl sulfate (PCS)	Kidney: PCS is a uremic toxin that can cause kidney dysfunction and injury, damaging renal tubular cells and causing oxidative stress and increasing inflammatory cytokines, and TGF-B1. It can promote insulin resistance.

Some of the amino acids are fermented by bacteria for energy, and the bacteria release the by-products. These by-products contain SCFA and ammonium. Ammonium (NH_4^+) is poorly absorbed and typically further metabolized by other gut bacteria or processed by the liver for excretion.

High amounts of protein entering the colon, however, cause problems. In alkaline colonic environments, which can occur with diets low in fermentable carbohydrates and low SCFA production, ammonium (NH_4^+) becomes NH_3 (ammonia). Ammonia can cause toxicity to the colonocytes and is easily absorbed across the mucosal membrane. Ammonia is toxic to the colonocytes and promotes intestinal permeability. Ammonia is also easily absorbed into the bloodstream.[46] In health, the adult liver readily metabolizes ammonia, but in infants and those with liver disease, toxic levels of ammonia can injure the brain and other organs.

There are several additional metabolites formed from amino acids that are toxic when levels become elevated. Some of these products cause leaky gut, and some are associated with inflammation, obesity, heart disease, depression, and cancer. The amount of *dietary protein* that reaches the colon and is fermented should be minimal. Malabsorption, pancreatic dysfunction, and diets high in meat, especially in edentulous individuals or those who do not chew meat sufficiently, can cause excessive amounts of undigested dietary proteins to make their way to the colon.

Avoiding excess protein fermentation in the colon is one of the fundamental goals of the SANA diet.

Fat Fermentation

Fat entering the lower intestine increases Firmicutes and decreases Bacteroides proliferation. Fat that evades digestion and absorption, and thus enters the lower intestine, causes chronic, low-grade inflammation, increases intestinal permeability, and increases the amount of toxins, such as LPS from the cell walls of bacteria, entering the bloodstream.[47] Fat entering the colon generally has inflammatory impacts and increases the risk for obesity and diabetes.[48] A high-fat diet is associated with reduced microbiome diversity, with smaller populations of beneficial commensal bacteria such as *Bifidobacteria, Lactobacillus,* and *Akkermansia*.[49] Of course, a high-fat diet generally also supplies an excess of calories.[50]

The SANA diet is a low-fat diet. High-fat diets promote dysbiosis and chronic inflammation.

Sugar Fermentation

For most people, table sugar (sucrose) is easily absorbed and thus does not induce intestinal dysbiosis. This should not be taken as a recommendation for high sugar intake. Sucrose, especially in beverages, can cause hyperglycemia even in those without diabetes. Hyperglycemia is a risk factor for vascular and other chronic diseases, even when it is transient.

In healthy persons, sucrose is easily absorbed, and under normal conditions, it does not get into the lower small intestine or colon, and thus does not cause intestinal dysbiosis. It does cause overgrowth of Streptococcus. mutans in the mouth, which causes dental caries and can cause oral dysbiosis if constantly present. Sucrose intolerance is a malabsorption syndrome caused by sucrase-isomaltase deficiency. It can be hereditary, but that is rare, other than among Inuit people. Much more commonly, sucrose intolerance is caused by disease or injury to the intestinal brush border. The mucosal injury causing the loss of sucrase-isomaltase enzymatic activity may be caused by Celiac disease, Crohn's disease, viral enteritis, or chemical compounds in food that injure the mucosa. Sucrose intolerance causes bloating, cramping, gas, and diarrhea after a meal or beverage high in sucrose.[51] Thus, if sugar does reach the lower intestine, it promotes fermentation and dysbiosis and GI symptoms.

Much more common than sucrose entering the colon and fermenting are the sugars lactose from dairy products and sorbitol from fruits or sugarless gum and diabetic treats. They, too, can cause dysbiosis and similar symptoms if they are not absorbed. Fructose malabsorption is less common. Consumption of large amounts of fruit juice, containing fructose and sorbitol, can overload small intestinal absorption and cause symptoms.

- The SANA diet restricts added sugar intake. These empty calories displace real food and thus nutrients from the diet.
- The SANA diet prohibits the consumption of sugar-sweetened beverages, considering them to be deadly.
- The SANA diet is rich in fiber. There is no fiber in sugar or vegetable oil. Most processed foods are low in fiber. Restricting or eliminating nutritionally deficient, fibreless, and over-processed foods encourages the replacement of those calories with real food, substantially increasing the amount of fiber in the diet.

Probiotics

A healthy microbiome is essential for health. Probiotics (encapsulated commensal bacteria) can help, but are not much more than a band-aid. A typical dose has 10 to 15 species and a total dose of 50 billion bacteria. A healthy gut has at least 150 entrenched species and nearly 1000 times the population of bacteria. Probiotics can be helpful when used properly, but they are not enough. Fecal transplant can have life-saving effects in certain situations, but it is not a panacea or a permanent fix. The key to a healthy microbiome and intestinal integrity is a healthy diet, with a rich and diverse source of soluble fiber.

Consider also that the tests of the microbiome are stool tests, and thus mostly test the transient mass of the stool moving through the colon. It is like a rural highway with lots of cars passing through. During the summer, tourists may pass through, and on weekdays, commuters pass by. The local residents are always present. They are entrenched, living in crypts, adhering to or embedded in the mucosa. The tourists just zoom through.

The diet is the principal driver of the microbiome. With a change in diet, dramatic changes in microbiome populations become evident within 24 hours, but things change back just as quickly when the dietary changes reverse.[52] [53] Long-term, sustained modifications in the diet are required to have a long-term change in which bacteria are the "permanent residents" of the colon.[54] In a mouse model, it took 12 weeks to reach a new equilibrium when they were placed on a human Western diet.[55] In a diet trial in patients with type 2 diabetes, changes were seen after one month, more changes after 3 months, and further changes after 6 months of a new diet.[56]

Summary

The SANA diet is designed to overcome dysbiosis by providing a healthy nutritional balance for the microbiome and thus has an anti-inflammatory impact. Adequate fiber from diverse sources is a fundamental need for a diverse, healthy, commensal intestinal microbiome that prevents leaky gut and the systemic inflammation that it causes. The foods recommended on the SANA diet, the fruits, vegetables, legumes, and whole grains, are rich in fiber and act as prebiotics. They contain adequate fiber to support a healthy microbiome. Consuming a wide range of these foods, rather than sticking to just a few, will create a microbiome with greater diversity and which has higher resilience to challenges.

This is in contrast to refined foods, filtered fruit juices, refined grains, processed sugars, vegetable oils, and meat. Consider that adults consuming the standard Western diet consume over 6 Tbsp. of vegetable oil (714 calories), and the average American consumes 34 teaspoons of sugar a day (680 calories).[57] More than half of the calories consumed in the Western diet come from these two dangerous, nutritionally deficient sources. Since so many American adults have insufficient fiber intake, the prevalence of overweight and obesity, and compromised health that is so common, is to be expected.

[1] Development and Validation of Novel Dietary and Lifestyle Inflammation Scores. Byrd DA, Judd SE, Flanders WD, Hartman TJ, Fedirko V, Bostick RM. J Nutr. 2019 Dec 1;149(12):2206-2218. doi: 10.1093/jn/nxz165. PMID: 31373368

[2] Novel Dietary and Lifestyle Inflammation Scores Directly Associated with All-Cause, All-Cancer, and All-Cardiovascular Disease Mortality Risks Among Women. Li Z, Gao Y, Byrd DA, Gibbs DC, Prizment AE, Lazovich D, Bostick RM. J Nutr. 2021 Apr 8;151(4):930-939. doi: 10.1093/jn/nxaa388. PMID: 33693725

[3] Association between pro-inflammatory diet and liver cancer risk: a systematic review and meta-analysis. Chen K, Yang F, Zhu X, Qiao G, Zhang C, Tao J, Gao X, Xiao M. Public Health Nutr. 2023 Dec;26(12):2780-2789. doi: 10.1017/S1368980023002574. Epub 2023 Nov 22. PMID: 37990536

[4] Dietary and Lifestyle Inflammation Scores Are Inversely Associated with Metabolic-Associated Fatty Liver Disease among Iranian Adults: A Nested Case-Control Study. Taheri E, Bostick RM, Hatami B, Pourhoseingholi MA, Asadzadeh Aghdaei H, Moslem A, Mousavi Jarrahi A, Zali MR. J Nutr. 2022 Feb 8;152(2):559-567. doi: 10.1093/jn/nxab391. PMID: 34791370

[5] Dietary and lifestyle inflammatory scores and risk of incident diabetes: a prospective cohort among participants of Tehran lipid and glucose study. Teymoori F, Farhadnejad H, Mokhtari E, Sohouli MH, Moslehi N, Mirmiran P, Azizi F. BMC Public Health. 2021 Jul 2;21(1):1293. doi: 10.1186/s12889-021-11327-1. PMID: 34215245

[6] An expanded reference map of the human gut microbiome reveals hundreds of previously unknown species. Leviatan S, Shoer S, Rothschild D, Gorodetski M, Segal E. Nat Commun. 2022 Jul 5;13(1):3863. doi: 10.1038/s41467-022-31502-1. PMID: 35790781

[7] A healthy gastrointestinal microbiome is dependent on dietary diversity. Heiman ML, Greenway FL. Mol Metab. 2016 Mar 5;5(5):317-320. doi: 10.1016/j.molmet.2016.02.005. eCollection 2016 May. PMID: 27110483

[8] Fostering next-generation probiotics in human gut by targeted dietary modulation: An emerging perspective. Kumari M, Singh P, Nataraj BH, Kokkiligadda A, Naithani H, Azmal Ali S, Behare PV, Nagpal R. Food Res Int. 2021 Dec;150(Pt A):110716. doi: 10.1016/j.foodres.2021.110716. Epub 2021 Sep 30. PMID: 34865747

[9] Akkermansia muciniphila as a novel powerful bacterial player in the treatment of metabolic disorders. Kobyliak N, Falalyeyeva T, Kyriachenko Y, Tseyslyer Y, Kovalchuk O, Hadiliia O, Eslami M, Yousefi B, Abenavoli L, Fagoonee S, Pellicano R. Minerva Endocrinol (Torino). 2022 Jun;47(2):242-252. doi: 10.23736/S2724-6507.22.03752-6. Epub 2022 Feb 1. PMID: 35103461

[10] The influence of Akkermansia muciniphila on intestinal barrier function. Mo C, Lou X, Xue J, Shi Z, Zhao Y, Wang F, Chen G. Gut Pathog. 2024 Aug 3;16(1):41. doi: 10.1186/s13099-024-00635-7. PMID: 39097746; PMCID: PMC11297771.

[11] Disease-associated dysbiosis and potential therapeutic role of Akkermansia muciniphila, a mucus degrading bacteria of gut microbiome. Aggarwal V, Sunder S, Verma SR. Folia Microbiol (Praha). 2022 Dec;67(6):811-824. doi: 10.1007/s12223-022-00973-6. Epub 2022 May 20. PMID: 35596115

[12] The Gut Microbiota's Role in Neurological, Psychiatric, and Neurodevelopmental Disorders. Charitos IA, Inchingolo AM, Ferrante L, Inchingolo F, Inchingolo AD, Castellaneta F, Cotoia A, Palermo A, Scacco S, Dipalma G. Nutrients. 2024 Dec 22;16(24):4404. doi: 10.3390/nu16244404. PMID: 39771025

[13] Excessive consumption of mucin by over-colonized *Akkermansia muciniphila* promotes intestinal barrier damage during malignant intestinal environment. Qu S, Zheng Y, Huang Y, Feng Y, Xu K, Zhang W, Wang Y, Nie K, Qin M. Front Microbiol. 2023 Mar 2;14:1111911. doi: 10.3389/fmicb.2023.1111911. eCollection 2023. PMID: 36937258

[14] Faecalibacterium prausnitzii treatment improves hepatic health and reduces adipose tissue inflammation in high-fat fed mice. Munukka E, Rintala A, Toivonen R, Nylund M, Yang B, Takanen A, Hänninen A, Vuopio J, Huovinen P, Jalkanen S, Pekkala S. ISME J. 2017 Jul;11(7):1667-1679. doi: 10.1038/ismej.2017.24. Epub 2017 Apr 4. PMID: 28375212

[15] Anaerobutyricum hallii promotes the functional depletion of a food carcinogen in diverse healthy fecal microbiota. Ramirez Garcia, Alejandro et al. Frontiers in Microbiomes (2023): https://www.frontiersin.org/journals/microbiomes/articles/10.3389/frmbi.2023.1194516.

[16] *Roseburia intestinalis* generated butyrate boosts anti-PD-1 efficacy in colorectal cancer by activating cytotoxic CD8+ T cells. Kang X, Liu C, Ding Y, Ni Y, Ji F, Lau HCH, Jiang L, Sung JJ, Wong SH, Yu J. Gut. 2023 Nov;72(11):2112-2122. doi: 10.1136/gutjnl-2023-330291. Epub 2023 Jul 25. PMID: 37491158

[17] The fermentable fibre inulin increases postprandial serum short-chain fatty acids and reduces free-fatty acids and ghrelin in healthy subjects. Tarini J, Wolever TM. Appl Physiol Nutr Metab. 2010 Feb;35(1):9-16. doi: 10.1139/H09-119. PMID: 20130660

[18] Composition and metabolic activities of bacterial biofilms colonizing food residues in the human gut. Macfarlane S, Macfarlane GT. Appl Environ Microbiol. 2006 Sep;72(9):6204-11. doi: 10.1128/AEM.00754-06. PMID: 16957247

[19] https://www.medicalnewstoday.com/articles/more-than-140000-different-viruses-live-in-the-human-gut

[20] Fungi in the healthy human gastrointestinal tract. Hallen-Adams HE, Suhr MJ. Virulence. 2017 Apr 3;8(3):352-358. doi: 10.1080/21505594.2016.1247140. Epub 2016 Oct 13. PMID: 27736307

[21] Malassezia Is Associated with Crohn's Disease and Exacerbates Colitis in Mouse Models. Limon JJ, Tang J, Li D, Wolf AJ, Michelsen KS, Funari V, Gargus M, Nguyen C,

Sharma P, Maymi VI, Iliev ID, Skalski JH, Brown J, Landers C, Borneman J, Braun J, Targan SR, McGovern DPB, Underhill DM. Cell Host Microbe. 2019 Mar 13;25(3):377-388.e6. doi: 10.1016/j.chom.2019.01.007. Epub 2019 Mar 5. PMID: 30850233

[22] Unfermented β-fructan Fibers Fuel Inflammation in Select Inflammatory Bowel Disease Patients. Armstrong HK, Bording-Jorgensen M, Santer DM, Dieleman LA, Wine E, et al. Gastroenterology. 2023 Feb;164(2):228-240. doi: 10.1053/j.gastro.2022.09.034. Epub 2022 Sep 29. PMID: 36183751

[23] Could You Have a Fructan Intolerance? (Cleveland Clinic health essentials. https://health.clevelandclinic.org/fructans

[24] Short-chain fatty acids are key mediators of the favorable effects of the Mediterranean diet on intestinal barrier integrity: data from the randomized controlled LIBRE trial. Seethaler B, Nguyen NK, Basrai M, Kiechle M, Walter J, Delzenne NM, Bischoff SC. Am J Clin Nutr. 2022 Oct 6;116(4):928-942. doi: 10.1093/ajcn/nqac175. PMID: 36055959

[25] Gut microbiota drives macrophage-dependent self-renewal of intestinal stem cells via niche enteric serotonergic neurons. Zhu P, Lu T, Wu J, Fan D, Liu B, Zhu X, Guo H, Du Y, Liu F, Tian Y, Fan Z. Cell Res. 2022 Jun;32(6):555-569. doi: 10.1038/s41422-022-00645-7. Epub 2022 Apr 4. PMID: 35379903

[26] Effects of valerate on intestinal barrier function in cultured Caco-2 epithelial cell monolayers. Gao G, Zhou J, Wang H, Ding Y, Zhou J, Chong PH, Zhu L, Ke L, Wang X, Rao P, Wang Q, Zhang L. Mol Biol Rep. 2022 Mar;49(3):1817-1825. doi: 10.1007/s11033-021-06991-w. Epub 2021 Nov 27. PMID: 34837149

[27] Higher Plasma Levels of Valerate Produced by Gut Microbiota May Have a Beneficial Impact on Renal Function. Mazidi M, Katsiki N, Banach M. J Am Nutr Assoc. 2023 Aug;42(6):534-540. doi: 10.1080/07315724.2019.1664955. Epub 2023 Feb 14. PMID: 36786830

[28] Gut microbiota impacts bone via Bacteroides vulgatus-valeric acid-related pathways. Lin X, Xiao HM, Liu HM, Lv WQ, Greenbaum J, Gong R, Zhang Q, Chen YC, Peng C, Xu XJ, Pan DY, Chen Z, Li ZF, Zhou R, Wang XF, Lu JM, Ao ZX, Song YQ, Zhang YH, Su KJ, Meng XH, Ge CL, Lv FY, Luo Z, Shi XM, Zhao Q, Guo BY, Yi NJ, Shen H, Papasian CJ, Shen J, Deng HW. Nat Commun. 2023 Oct 27;14(1):6853. doi: 10.1038/s41467-023-42005-y. PMID: 37891329

[29] Aluminum-induced generation of lipopolysaccharide (LPS) from the human gastrointestinal (GI)-tract microbiome-resident Bacteroides fragilis. Alexandrov PN, Hill JM, Zhao Y, Bond T, Taylor CM, Percy ME, Li W, Lukiw WJ. J Inorg Biochem. 2020 Feb;203:110886. doi: 10.1016/j.jinorgbio.2019.110886. Epub 2019 Oct 22. PMID: 31707334

[30] Gastrointestinal (GI)-Tract Microbiome Derived Neurotoxins and their Potential Contribution to Inflammatory Neurodegeneration in Alzheimer's Disease (AD). Lukiw WJ, Arceneaux L, Li W, Bond T, Zhao Y. J Alzheimers Dis Parkinsonism. 2021;11(6):525. Epub 2021 May 25. PMID: 34457996

[31] Secretory Products of the Human GI Tract Microbiome and Their Potential Impact on Alzheimer's Disease (AD): Detection of Lipopolysaccharide (LPS) in AD Hippocampus. Zhao Y, Jaber V, Lukiw WJ. Front Cell Infect Microbiol. 2017 Jul 11;7:318. doi: 10.3389/fcimb.2017.00318. eCollection 2017. PMID: 28744452

[32] Lipopolysaccharides (LPSs) as Potent Neurotoxic Glycolipids in Alzheimer's Disease (AD). Zhao Y, Jaber VR, Pogue AI, Sharfman NM, Taylor C, Lukiw WJ. Int J Mol Sci. 2022 Oct 21;23(20):12671. doi: 10.3390/ijms232012671. PMID: 36293528

[33] Lipopolysaccharide, Identified Using an Antibody and by PAS Staining, Is Associated With *Corpora amylacea* and White Matter Injury in Alzheimer's Disease and Aging Brain. Zhan X, Hakoupian M, Jin LW, Sharp FR. Front Aging Neurosci. 2021 Nov 24;13:705594. doi: 10.3389/fnagi.2021.705594. eCollection 2021. PMID: 34899263

[34] Colorectal carcinogenesis: a cellular response to sustained risk environment. Fung KY, Ooi CC, Zucker MH, Lockett T, Williams DB, Cosgrove LJ, Topping DL. Int J Mol Sci. 2013 Jun 27;14(7):13525-41. doi: 10.3390/ijms140713525. PMID: 23807509

[35] Isovaleric acid in stool correlates with human depression. Szczesniak O, Hestad KA, Hanssen JF, Rudi K. Nutr Neurosci. 2016 Sep;19(7):279-83. doi: 10.1179/1476830515Y.0000000007. Epub 2015 Feb 24. PMID: 25710209

[36] The multiple effects of fecal microbiota transplantation on diarrhea-predominant irritable bowel syndrome (IBS-D) patients with anxiety and depression behaviors. Lin H, Guo Q, Wen Z, Tan S, Chen J, Lin L, Chen P, He J, Wen J, Chen Y. Microb Cell Fact. 2021 Dec 28;20(1):233. doi: 10.1186/s12934-021-01720-1. PMID: 34963452

[37] Microbial Fermentation of Dietary Protein: An Important Factor in Diet–Microbe–Host Interaction. https://www.mdpi.com/2076-2607/7/1/19

[38] Certain Fermented Foods and Their Possible Health Effects with a Focus on Bioactive Compounds and Microorganisms. https://www.mdpi.com/2311-5637/9/11/923

[39] Gut microbiota-dependent phenylacetylglutamine in cardiovascular disease: current knowledge and new insights. Song Y, Wei H, Zhou Z, Wang H, Hang W, Wu J, Wang DW. Front Med. 2024 Feb;18(1):31-45. doi: 10.1007/s11684-024-1055-9. Epub 2024 Mar 1. PMID: 38424375

[40] Gut Microbiota-Generated Phenylacetylglutamine and Heart Failure. Romano KA, Nemet I, Prasad Saha P, Haghikia A, et al. Circ Heart Fail. 2023 Jan;16(1):e009972. doi: 10.1161/CIRCHEARTFAILURE.122.009972. Epub 2022 Dec 16. PMID: 36524472

[41] Platelets get gutted by PAG. Parra-Izquierdo I, Bradley R, Aslan JE. Platelets. 2020 Jul 3;31(5):618-620. doi:

10.1080/09537104.2020.1759793. Epub 2020 Apr 29. PMID: 32348162

42 Modelling the role of microbial p-cresol in colorectal genotoxicity. Al Hinai EA, Kullamethee P, Rowland IR, Swann J, Walton GE, Commane DM. Gut Microbes. 2019;10(3):398-411. doi: 10.1080/19490976.2018.1534514. Epub 2018 Oct 25. PMID: 30359553

43 p-Cresol affects reactive oxygen species generation, cell cycle arrest, cytotoxicity and inflammation/atherosclerosis-related modulators production in endothelial cells and mononuclear cells. Chang MC, Chang HH, Chan CP, Yeung SY, Hsien HC, Lin BR, Yeh CY, Tseng WY, Tseng SK, Jeng JH. PLoS One. 2014 Dec 17;9(12):e114446. doi: 10.1371/journal.pone.0114446. eCollection 2014. PMID: 25517907

44 Free serum concentrations of the protein-bound retention solute p-cresol predict mortality in hemodialysis patients. Bammens B, Evenepoel P, Keuleers H, Verbeke K, Vanrenterghem Y. Kidney Int. 2006 Mar;69(6):1081-7. doi: 10.1038/sj.ki.5000115. PMID: 16421516

45 Toxicity of free p-cresol: a prospective and cross-sectional analysis. De Smet R, Van Kaer J, Van Vlem B, De Cubber A, Brunet P, Lameire N, Vanholder R. Clin Chem. 2003 Mar;49(3):470-8. doi: 10.1373/49.3.470. PMID: 12600960

46 Colorectal carcinogenesis: a cellular response to sustained risk environment. Fung KY, Ooi CC, Zucker MH, Lockett T, Williams DB, Cosgrove LJ, Topping DL. Int J Mol Sci. 2013 Jun 27;14(7):13525-41. doi: 10.3390/ijms140713525. PMID: 23807509

47 Influence of high-fat diet on gut microbiota: a driving force for chronic disease risk. Murphy EA, Velazquez KT, Herbert KM. Curr Opin Clin Nutr Metab Care. 2015 Sep;18(5):515-20. doi: 10.1097/MCO.0000000000000209. PMID: 26154278

48 Impact of dietary fat on gut microbiota and low-grade systemic inflammation: mechanisms and clinical implications on obesity. Cândido FG, Valente FX, Grześkowiak ŁM, Moreira APB, Rocha DMUP, Alfenas RCG. Int J Food Sci Nutr. 2018 Mar;69(2):125-143. doi: 10.1080/09637486.2017.1343286. Epub 2017 Jul 4. PMID: 28675945

49 Microbial dysbiosis-induced obesity: role of gut microbiota in homoeostasis of energy metabolism. Amabebe E, Robert FO, Agbalalah T, Orubu ESF. Br J Nutr. 2020 May 28;123(10):1127-1137. doi: 10.1017/S0007114520000380. Epub 2020 Feb 3. PMID: 32008579

50 Dysbiosis and metabolic endotoxemia induced by high-fat diet. Netto Candido TL, Bressan J, Alfenas RCG. Nutr Hosp. 2018 Dec 3;35(6):1432-1440. doi: 10.20960/nh.1792. PMID: 30525859

51 Sucrose intolerance in adults with common functional gastrointestinal symptoms. Frissora CL, Rao SSC. Proc (Bayl Univ Med Cent). 2022 Aug 23;35(6):790-793. doi: 10.1080/08998280.2022.2114070. eCollection 2022. PMID: 36304608

52 Diet and the development of the human intestinal microbiome. Voreades N, Kozil A, Weir TL. Front Microbiol. 2014 Sep 22;5:494. doi: 10.3389/fmicb.2014.00494. eCollection 2014. PMID: 25295033

53 Temporal Dynamics of the Intestinal Microbiome Following Short-Term Dietary Restriction. Anderson EM, Rozowsky JM, Fazzone BJ, Schmidt EA, Stevens BR, O'Malley KA, Scali ST, Berceli SA. Nutrients. 2022 Jul 6;14(14):2785. doi: 10.3390/nu14142785. PMID: 35889742

54 Dietary changes in nutritional studies shape the structural and functional composition of the pigs' fecal microbiome-from days to weeks. Tilocca B, Burbach K, Heyer CME, Hoelzle LE, Mosenthin R, Stefanski V, Camarinha-Silva A, Seifert J. Microbiome. 2017 Oct 27;5(1):144. doi: 10.1186/s40168-017-0362-7. PMID: 29078812

55 Integrative Longitudinal Analysis of Metabolic Phenotype and Microbiota Changes During the Development of Obesity. Higgins KV, Woodie LN, Hallowell H, Greene MW, Schwartz EH. Front Cell Infect Microbiol. 2021 Aug 3;11:671926. doi: 10.3389/fcimb.2021.671926. eCollection 2021. PMID: 34414128

56 Changes in intestinal flora in patients with type 2 diabetes on a low-fat diet during 6 months of follow-up. Liu C, Shao W, Gao M, Liu J, Guo Q, Jin J, Meng F. Exp Ther Med. 2020 Nov;20(5):40. doi: 10.3892/etm.2020.9167. Epub 2020 Sep 1. PMID: 32952631

57 https://www.ars.usda.gov/plains-area/gfnd/gfhnrc/docs/news-articles/2012/the-question-of-sugar/

4: Inflammation and the Brain

The SANA Program provides a "user's manual" for avoiding the underlying cause of many of the most common chronic diseases prevalent in our society, and it is relevant to the prevention of most of the non-infectious chronic morbidity. The primary focus of this book is maintaining health and extending the health span, but in particular, this book focuses on the prevention of Alzheimer's disease (AD) and other forms of dementia.

The stats are a bit frightening. About one in eight men and one in six women develop dementia during their lifetime. Sixty to eighty percent of those who develop dementia will have Alzheimer's disease as the cause. One in nine Americans over the age of 65 is living with AD. One in three elderly Americans over the age of 85 has AD. Two-thirds of those with AD, perhaps the curse of longevity, are women. African Americans are nearly twice as likely to carry the ApoE4 gene, an important risk factor for AD, and they are twice as likely to develop the disease.

About 1% of AD is "early-onset" disease, which has strong genetic influences. Although late-onset AD (LOAD) has genetic influences, it is strongly influenced by environmental factors. This discussion is directed at LOAD.

The dietary inflammatory (DII) score is a metric used to describe the inflammatory potential of different dietary patterns. In an analysis of data from the 2011 to 2014 National Health and Nutrition Examination Survey (NHANES) study, cognitive scores of participants over the age of 60 were assessed for their association with the DII. The three cognitive tests were the Consortium to Establish a Registry for Alzheimer's Disease (CERAD), Animal Fluency Test (AFT), and Digit Symbol Substitution Test (DSST). When compared to those in the lowest quartile of DII, those with the highest DII quartile scores were 89% more likely to score poorly on the AFT test and 430% more likely to score poorly on the DSST test. Poor CERAD test scores were more frequent in those with higher dietary inflammatory scores, but the association was not significant in this study.[1] The DII is a rather imprecise, general metric of the inflammatory impact of diet. The SANA diet gives clear guidance on which foods are pro- or anti-inflammatory and on how their preparation impacts their effect. The SANA diet provides a much more informative assessment of which foods help prevent disease.

Diet and lifestyle have major impacts on the risk of developing Alzheimer's disease (AD); The degree of impact is not dissimilar to the impact that lifestyle and diet have on type 2 diabetes. It is not a coincidence that the SANA diet helps prevent both T2D and AD; these diseases have overlapping causation, and T2D is a major risk factor for AD. In fact, many Alzheimer's disease researchers refer to AD as "Type 3 Diabetes".

This chapter introduces some vocabulary and concepts to help the reader understand some of the causal mechanisms of AD, and thus the reasoning for the SANA dietary and lifestyle recommendations. The pathological mechanisms that cause AD are highly complex. This chapter attempts to provide a "primer" to introduce some AD pathological pathways that are impacted by diet and nutrition. Please be aware that it is a simplified and incomplete picture of what is known about a disease that is incompletely understood.

In Alzheimer's disease, there is dysregulation of immunoregulatory processes. The disease process is set off by immune activation and interaction with compensatory mechanisms. Some of the inflammatory mediators that are activated to protect the brain cause dysfunction in the brain, leading to a sustained inflammatory response and a buildup of toxic compounds within the brain. This sets up a very vicious cycle of toxicity, causing cell death that then produces toxic polymers, such as amyloid beta (Aβ) plaques and fragments, that lead to further dysfunction and further cell death. It appears likely that by some point in the disease's progression, even if the underlying inflammatory stressors causing Alzheimer's disease are completely abated, the disease would continue to progress on its own.[2]

First, some background.

Brain Cells 101

Various brain cells will be discussed, so here is a cartoon showing the principal cell types of the brain. There will be a test, so pay attention.

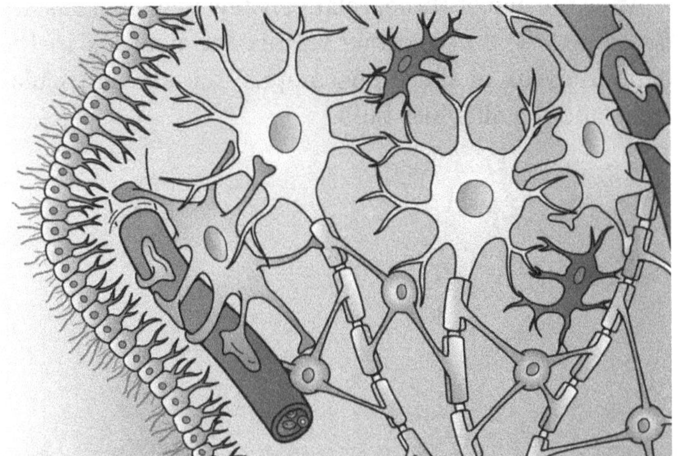

Figure 4A: Cartoon illustrating some classes of brain cells.[3]

Along the left side of Figure 2A, in contact with the ventricle filled with cerebrospinal fluid (CSF), are the ependymal cells (pink). These glial cells produce and regulate CSF. The astrocytes are shown with foot processes on the capillaries entering the brain. A more accurate drawing would show several astrocytes and the foot processes providing near-continuous paving over the capillaries. This layer of foot processes is part of the blood-brain barrier (BBB) that protects the brain by limiting the passage of many blood-borne compounds into the brain.

Astrocytes are the main metabolic managers of the brain. Astrocytes are metabolically and functionally complex, and thus, in a way, have more "metabolic intelligence" than do the neurons. The yellow cells with the large nuclei are the neurons. The short dendritic branches can be seen, as well as the single axon that is wrapped in the myelin sheath by the (light blue) oligodendrocytes. The myelin sheath acts as electrical insulation that prevents interference between nerve transmissions and provides for faster signal transfer. In the peripheral nervous system, Schwann cells do the job of wrapping the axons. The smaller brown cells are microglia. The microglia are multifunctional immune cells in the CNS, and behave like immune dendrocytes, doing immune surveillance, but can easily transform and act as various forms of macrophages, becoming phagocytic. With injury, infection, and in most people, with aging, the microglia, which are normally quiescent, can become chronically activated. They act as if there is always an infection to fight, and they become phagocytic, similar to macrophages in other parts of the body. Think of this activation like PTSD; once traumatized, they stay on high alert and react to trivial or non-dangerous stimuli.

The ependymal cells and microglia arise separately during embryogenesis, and the neuroblasts arise from the ependymal layer. The neuroblasts give rise to the radial glial cells, which give rise to the oligodendrocyte precursor cells, which give rise to neurons and astrocytes.[4] Neural stem cells in adults also give rise to oligodendrocytes, astrocytes, and neurons.

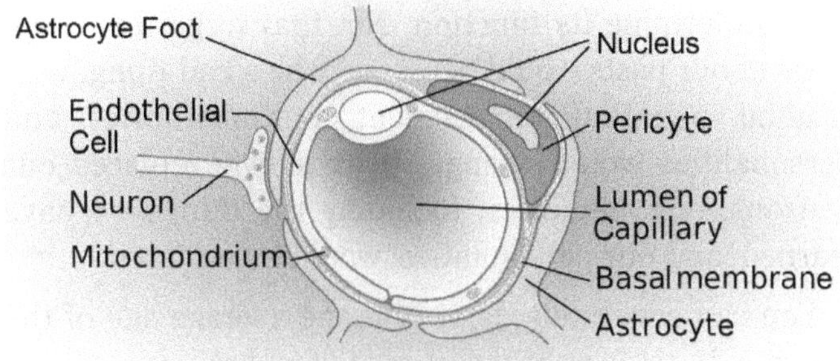

Figure 4B: Cartoon illustrating the cells of the blood-brain barrier.[5]

In addition to astrocyte foot processes surrounding the capillaries, the BBB contains pericytes that help maintain capillary and BBB function.

Some cells of the body have great potential for replacement, but others do not. The blood cells and cells lining the intestine regularly turn over and are replaced frequently throughout our lives. Other cells are replaced more slowly and heal easily after injuries, such as the skin or liver. Some cell types have very limited potential for growth and replacement after development. These cells form while we are young, and are irreplaceable. Some cell types are pretty much done reproducing by the time we are three years old. These cells are sometimes called "immortal cells," not because they live forever, but because they are adapted to last a lifetime. The immortal cells we develop during childhood and adolescence account for most of those we ever have.

Our hearts and minds are not replaceable. Cardiac muscle cells, neurons, and retinal cells only sparsely reproduce after their growth period has been completed. These "immortal" cells include the neurons in our brains; our large muscles, including the heart; and most of the cells of the retina and cochlear hair cells in the ear. If these cells are damaged, there is minimal, if any, recovery. We can grow a modest number of new heart and muscle cells from stem cells as we grow into adulthood; however, this process is quite limited. If we suffer noise-induced hearing loss because of damage to the hair cells, they do not recover. The reproduction of these immortal cells is extremely constrained. The genesis of new neurons in the brain is even more limited than it is for heart cells. It is not that the body cannot develop new neurons or cardiac myocytes, but rather that it would usually be maladaptive. We should not need new heart cells. Cardiac hypertrophy (thickening of the walls of the heart) decreases the ability of the heart to pump blood efficiently, and new cardiac cells might cause dysrhythmias. Replacing old cells with new cells in the brain would likely disrupt learning and memory and thus undermine its function. Not that forgetting some parts of our pasts would necessarily be a bad thing, with gradual neuronal replacement, our memories and personalities would change. If we slowly replaced our neurons, our memories, including the things we have learned, and our personalities, would be replaced.

You can accurately determine the average age of the neurons in the cerebral cortex of your brain by looking at your driver's license,[6] as about half of those neurons were formed before your birth, and the other half were formed after. It is estimated that by 5 months of age, 14 months from conception, around 85 percent of the number of adult neurons have been developed. By a person's first birthday, 95 percent of all neurogenesis for the adult brain has been developed. By the age of three, the human brain has achieved 90 to 95% of its adult mass and then grows more slowly into the early 20s. At the age of three, the brain has its peak synaptic density, about 50% higher than an adult brain.[7]

Myelination increases throughout childhood and then continues at a slower rate into early adulthood. From about the age of four until puberty, there is maturation and specialization of neural networks in the prefrontal cortex. Gray matter volume peaks during adolescence, but white matter volume and connectivity increase in volume into the late twenties.

During adolescence, only a small amount of neurogenesis takes place. The most prominent activity is maturation, involving synaptic pruning and neuroplasticity through the development of dendritic spines. Adolescence is an important time in the development of the brain for adaptation to the current environment. This is a period in which the learning of new skills is relatively easy. Health during adolescence is an important determinant of adult intelligence. There is an increase in both grey and white matter volume. The brain continues to mature at a slower pace, usually until the age of about 28, when the brain can be considered to be fully adult.

Neuronal plasticity, learning, and memory involve the development and pruning of dendritic spines. These spines can emerge or regress quickly, within a day, or overnight. They are the sites for interconnection with synapses from other neurons.

After the age of three, relatively few new neurons are developed. The exceptions to this are neurons in the dentate gyrus of the hippocampus, the subventricular zone, and the olfactory bulb.

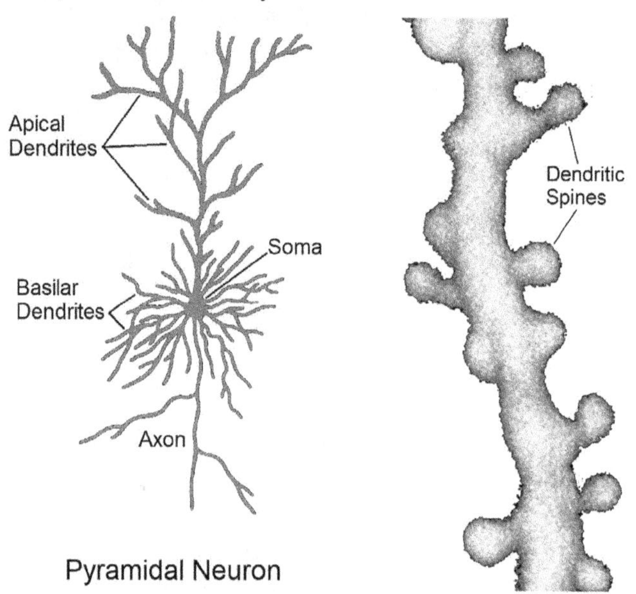

Figure 4C and D: Left: Image of a pyramidal neuron showing basilar dendrites (branches) emerging from the soma (body) of the nerve, as well as apical branching of the dendrites. Right: A close-up image of a dendrite showing the multiple dendritic spines. [8] These spines are points at which interneuronal connections can form. A decrease in the daily formation of these spines indicates a loss of neuronal plasticity, as it limits the ability of the neurons to interconnect. Atrophy of the dendrites indicates a loss of length or number of dendritic branches.

Adult Neurogenesis

The hippocampus is the area of the brain that helps promote new memories. In Alzheimer's disease (AD), the hippocampus is one of the first areas to be damaged, explaining the difficulty in forming new memories.

The anterior (ventral) hippocampus functions in fear conditioning and emotion, while the posterior (dorsal) hippocampus, especially on the right side, helps build spatial memory maps. The posterior hippocampus allows animals to remember where food has been found so that they can return to those areas at the right time of the year to find the food and their way home again, and fear and emotions help them remember the dangerous things and places. The hippocampus helps us sort out what is salient to put into memory (the novel and meaningful) and to discard information not worth remembering, such as the faces of people in the cars passing by us in the other direction as we drive to work. Memory may not be of much use if it is not organized in a way that we can access it easily. The dentate gyrus helps with that organization. The dentate gyrus is an area in the hippocampus where various sensory inputs merge to form a representation of our experience. The dentate gyrus consolidates the sensory modalities to form memories with salience to the experience.

The olfactory bulb, which is responsible for the sense of smell, has a capacity for neurogenesis after injury; however, this diminishes with age.[9] Olfactory stimuli play a significant role in triggering memory.

The subventricular zone (SVZ) is another site in the adult mammalian brain where neurogenesis is known to occur.[10] The subventricular zone is located at the lateral fluid-filled ventricles in the brain. The SVZ contains neural stem cells and continuously produces new neurons, mainly for the olfactory bulb, but neurons from the SVZ respond to brain injury and can migrate to other parts of the brain to replace damaged cells.

Notably, and in contrast to the central nervous system, neurons in the enteric nervous system (ENS) in the intestines are readily replaced from neuronal stem cells after injury. This is adaptive as the neurons in the intestine are frequently exposed to and injured by toxins. Plus, there is no penalty for the gut losing its memories from childhood.

Neurotoxic chemicals should be expected to be far more injurious to the enteric nervous system than the CNS, due to the high exposure of the ENS from toxins in contaminated food and from alcohol. The ENS is not protected by the BBB. The damage to the CNS is often mirrored in the ENS. Autism spectrum disorder, amyotrophic lateral sclerosis, Parkinson's disease, and Alzheimer's disease (AD) all have ENS co-morbidity. Patients with AD have a progressive accumulation of β-amyloid protein in the enteric neurons. This is associated with a decline in the population of ENS neurons, dysmotility, and vulnerability to intestinal inflammation in AD. Constipation is nearly universal and typically a presenting symptom in Parkinson's disease. Herpes zoster, which causes shingles by infecting a peripheral nerve, can cause pseudo-obstruction of the bowel. Animal models of CNS disease are often accompanied by gastrointestinal injury or dysfunction.

Brain Areas Damaged in Dementia

Different types of dementia may impact different parts of the brain. While the hippocampus is not the only area of the brain affected by AD, since it is important for new memory, its injury becomes a central feature of the disease. Parkinson's disease (PD) is characterized by damage to the substantia nigra, an area in the brain that produces the neurotransmitter dopamine, which is crucial for regulating motor functions and coordination of muscle tone, thus explaining the tremors and difficulty with movement. Loss of the sense of smell and constipation are early comorbidities of PD, often manifesting 10 or more years before the movement disorders. Injury to the neurons in the ENS is common and explains the constipation; loss of new neurons from the SVZ explains the anosmia.

The frontal lobe controls executive functions such as judgment, planning, impulse control, and emotional regulation. These abilities are damaged in frontotemporal dementia (FTD). FTD is principally a genetic disease, but head trauma and thyroid dysfunction contribute to the risk.

Vascular dementia can affect any part of the brain and thus nearly any function controlled by the impacted area of injury. Small vessel disease, however, is particularly likely to damage the white matter of the brain, composed of long nerve fibers that carry signals from one area of the brain to another. Frontal lobe (executive) dysfunction is common in vascular dementia, along with slowed thinking and difficulty concentrating. With frontal lobe dementia, the person may function normally but may make faulty decisions and lack normal inhibitions. Midbrain small vessel injury causes a gradual decline in cognitive function, and if the hippocampus is affected, it damages memory. Strokes can affect any part of the brain.

Injury to the cerebellum can cause difficulty with coordination, balance, speech, swallowing, visuospatial and verbal memory, and executive tasks.[11] Cerebellar degeneration commonly contributes to cognitive and motor dysfunction in AD and PD.[12] [13] Difficulty with eating and swallowing, common in mid- to late-stage AD, is a result of cerebellar degeneration and contributes to AD mortality. [14]

Immunology 101

For the non-initiated, there will be a few basic terms that will be helpful to understand some of the discussions ahead.

Inflammation is an important cause of injury. When we get sick from a viral infection, it is rarely the infection that causes what we perceive to be the illness; the runny nose, congestion, fever, and aches and pains of the flu are not caused by the virus, but rather our immune reaction to the infection. The inflammatory response allows the mounting of immune defenses, causing vasodilation in the infected area. This induces redness, leaking of serum, the liquid part of blood, into the tissue, which causes swelling. In a severe allergic reaction, this leaking of serum into the tissue and resultant swelling can cause wheezing and difficulty in breathing. The inflammatory response causes the production of cytokines that draw white blood cells into the area to fight the infection. For intracellular infections such as viruses, the inflammation can cause signaling to the cell, telling the cell to shut down and die, through a process called *apoptosis*. Even though the inflammation causes injury, it would be much worse without it. Bacteria that get into a wound would be free to digest our flesh, just as occurs with a rotting piece of meat, and parasitic worms would roam freely, eating their way through our tissues. It is devastating when it happens in the brain.

If you are pleased to have an immune system, then you should be tickled to know that you have two classes of immunity: the innate immune system and the adaptive immune system.

Adaptive Immunity

In the adaptive immune system, special immune dendritic cells in the tissues, especially the skin and gastrointestinal submucosa, act as sentries sampling for *antigens* – molecules that the body recognizes as a piece of a foreign life form (non-self). The dendritic cells process and present the antigens to T lymphocytes, a class of white blood cells. The T cells then determine if the molecule represents danger or not. If it is a molecule that is a piece of our own cells or a peptide (a short string of amino acids) from an endogenous protein, it is best not to react to it, as doing so would cause autoimmune disease. Similarly, small peptides from the digestion of protein in food should not be recognized as dangerous, as this can cause allergic reactions. Generally, the body is good at telling the difference between self and dangerous pathogens, but we all make mistakes.

The dendritic cells can activate Natural Killer cells that can kill infected cells, and the T cells can activate B cells. The B cells then become either plasma cells that produce *antibodies* to the offending molecule or become B Memory cells that can become plasma cells in the future if the antigen comes back. That way, we can react to the antigen much more quickly, without even getting sick the next time the pathogen is encountered. Antibodies are generally very specific, like a key to a lock; there can be millions of different antibodies for millions of different possible antigenic molecules. But once you figure out the code and commit it to cellular memory, it is much quicker the next go around.

Antibodies are ligands that bind to the antigen. That is often enough. If bacteria can stick to a cell, they can grow and multiply, forming a *biofilm* and causing disease. Single bacteria rarely cause disease, but when they form colonies, they can produce proteins that allow them to become invasive and produce toxins. It is not individual bacteria that are dangerous, but rather colonies of bacteria that form sticky biofilms, produce toxins, and become invasive. The bacteria actually change their form and the proteins they produce when they form a colony, often becoming pathogens as a part of quorum sensing. Thus, bacteria that are commensal when free-floating can become pathogenic when they stick to the cell surface and are present in high density.

If antibodies bind to the bacteria's binding sites, they can prevent the bacteria from binding to the cell and forming a biofilm colony. This is what *immunoglobulin A (IgA)* does in the intestine and tears. Other immunoglobulins, such as IgE and IgG, are sticky on both ends. One end binds to the antigen (peptide, bacterium, virus). If enough antibody sticks to the surface of bacteria or parasites, the other end of the antibody will bind to a white blood cell (WBC) that either uses the antibodies to pull the bacteria inside of the WBC (*phagocytosis*), where the WBC can digest the bacteria, or can attack the bound antigen if it is too big for single cells to swallow.

Vaccines work by introducing antigens to the body, sometimes from dead viruses, from viruses too weakened to cause disease, or from viral spike proteins, so that the body can make antibodies to prevent infection. IgE antibodies are more specific to helminths (worms), play a key role in mediating allergic reactions, and anaphylaxis. IgG is formed against bacteria, viruses, amoebas, and almost any molecules that the T cells recognize as non-self, including cancer cells.

Innate Immunity

The other class of immunity is the innate immune system. Since it is innate, we don't need prior experience with the pathogen to attack it, which is of great advantage. Nevertheless, unlike the precision targeting of adaptive immunity, the innate immune system is less targeted and can be messier.

The innate immune system responds to molecular patterns that it has evolved to recognize over millions of years. Many of these are *Pathogen-Associated Molecular Patterns (PAMPs).* The PAMPS are molecules such as specific types of chains of sugars and lipids from the cell wall of bacteria, or the pili or fimbriae, tiny hair-like structures on the outside of certain bacteria. One of the important PAMPs is lipopolysaccharide (LPS), a molecule that is present in the wall of Gram-negative bacteria. When the bacteria die and fall apart, LPS is released. If released in or absorbed into the body, LPS is recognized as a PAMP. Another PAMP is lipoteichoic acid (LTA), a component of the cell wall of Gram-positive bacteria.

Many families of bacteria are Gram-negative rods. This includes most of the bacteria that live in the lower intestine and many of the bacteria that cause hospital-acquired infections. (Gram-negative simply means that when they are stained with two specific dyes and washed with alcohol, one of the stains does not stay, thus allowing Gram-negative and Gram-positive bacteria to look different under a microscope.

The PAMPs are recognized by immune cell surface receptors called *Toll-Like Receptors (TLRs).* There are several different TLRs, and different ones respond to different arrays of PAMPs. This allows the innate immune system to respond to various PAMPs more appropriately. The TLRs also respond to *DAMPs: Damage-Associated Molecular Patterns.* The recognition of DAMPs acts as a way for the innate immune system to respond to a pathogen-induced injury that it does not recognize as a PAMP, but is still causing injury. Thus, DAMPs are materials from our own cells that have been damaged. It also helps with the clean-up of injured cells.

Toll-like Receptor-2 (TLR2) recognizes lipoteichoic acid from the cell wall of Gram-positive bacteria, the porin protein from *Neisseria meningitidis* and *Haemophilus influenzae,* and several other PAMPS from the microbes and viruses that cause such diseases as tuberculosis, the Black Death, measles, herpes, and certain fungi and parasites, including *Candida* and malaria. It recognizes antigens from the bacteria *Cutibacterium acnes,* and thus, TLR2 activation underlies the inflammatory reaction that causes acne.

Highly relevant to neuroinflammation, TLR4 recognizes and is activated by LPS from Gram-negative bacteria. Interestingly, TLR4 is also activated by morphine and several other opiates. This recognition of opiates by TLR4 plays a role in the loss of pain relief and increased inflammation associated with these drugs. TLR4 can also be activated by certain damage-associated molecular patterns (DAMPs) that may be released from injured or dying cells. One such DAMP is Amyloid Beta Peptide (Aβ), which participates in the development of Alzheimer's disease. Aβ has antibacterial properties, which likely help pick off an occasional rogue bacterium that makes its way into the brain; nevertheless, overproduction of Aβ participates in the inflammatory loss of neurons in Alzheimer's disease. The tendency of Aβ fragments to stick to each other causes the formation of Aβ plaques, which are typically found in the brains of AD patients. Although the plaques are diagnostic of AD, they may not be a principal cause of injury.

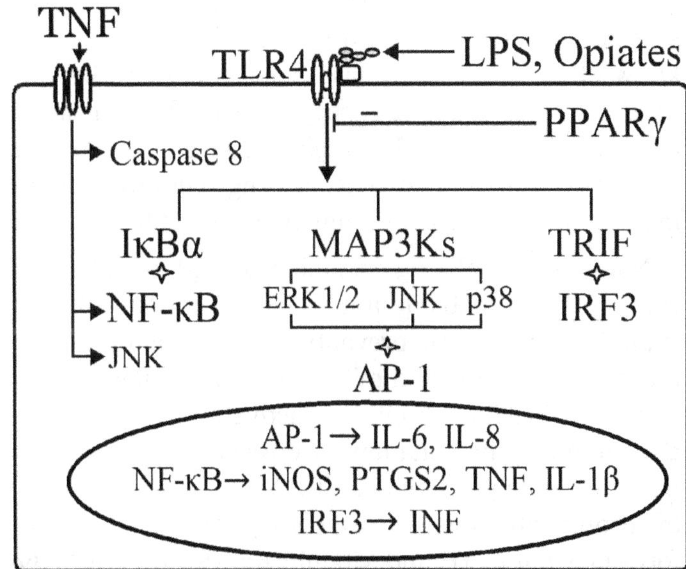

Figure 4E: Toll-like receptor-4 inflammatory cascade. TNF (tumor necrosis factor) can promote cell death by apoptosis via Caspase 8. NF-κB promotes the expression of several inflammatory cytokines, and with sufficient stimulation, can cause cell death. Note that activation of TLR4 increases the expression of TNF.

TLR4 (on the surface of, and embedded in, the cell membrane) initiates a cascade of reactions in the cytosol of the cell, which result in the release of *Nuclear Factor κB (NF-κB),* AP-1, and IRF3, which then migrate through pores in the nuclear membrane into the nucleus of the cell (shown as an oval in Figure 2C). These are transcription factors that promote the expression of messenger RNA for proteins involved in the inflammatory response. NF-κB is shown in Figure 2E to induce the transcription of iNOS, which produces the vasodilator nitric oxide (NO), PTGS2, which produces the inflammatory prostaglandin PGE2, and the pro-inflammatory cytokines TNF (Tumor Necrosis Factor) and Interleukin-1β (IL-1β). AP-1 induces the pro-inflammatory cytokines IL-6 and IL-8. IRF3 induces the transcription of type I interferons, which help fight viral infections but also cause flu-like malaise. Nitric oxide not only increases blood flow to the area of injury but also increases wound healing.

As can also be seen in the diagram, TNF, which is induced by NF-κB, can cause a positive feedback loop, increasing the inflammatory response or sharing it with neighboring cells. TNF also stimulates JNK, which induces AP-1 transcription and Caspase 8, which can induce apoptosis if the signaling is sufficiently robust.

Other inflammatory cytokines and chemokines are also activated, but not shown. *Cytokines* are small proteins that have local signaling action; they often have immune-regulatory signaling effects on cells, especially on cells near where they were produced. This gives nearby cells a warning when there is an infection, sort of like a neighborhood watch to let the neighbors know that someone has been burgled in the neighborhood and that they should be on alert. *Chemokines* are small proteins that act as homing signals for white blood cells, causing them to settle or migrate to the area of inflammation and get to work.

Not shown in the figure is that several polyphenolic compounds in foods inhibit the release of NF-κB from IκBα in the cytosol, preventing its migration to the nucleus, and thus diminishing the inflammatory response. PPARγ inhibits the activation of TLR4 and thus inhibits the inflammatory response, or perhaps more accurately, low levels of PPARγ increase the risk of chronic inflammatory response. Calcitriol (the active form of vitamin D) and vitamin K2 also diminish the inflammatory response by inhibiting the production of some of the transcription factors involved in inflammation.

Alzheimer's Disease

Amyloid precursor Protein (APP) is a multifunctional protein made by neurons. APP is folded in the endoplasmic reticulum, and then becomes a membrane protein with an extension of the protein on the cell's surface that can be processed by extracellular enzymes. Depending on the extracellular conditions, APP can be processed into different peptides and three different intracellular proteins, which have various metabolic effects, depending on where the protein is enzymatically cut. The cleavage of APP is illustrated in Figure 2F. Amyloid beta (A.K.A. Aβ or Abeta), a peptide fragment of APP that accumulates in the brain of patients with Alzheimer's disease (AD), is one of the possible extracellular cleavage products of APP.

In the normal, healthy state, APP is cleaved instead by α-secretase, forming the sAPPα fragment. sAPPα promotes learning and the formation of synapses.[15] Since α-secretase cuts APP in the middle of the Aβ fragment, it prevents the formation of Aβ.

In contrast to the sAPPα support of learning, Aβ acts to protect the brain from infection. The brain produces APP and Aβ as part of an antibacterial innate immune response to help capture bacteria and prevent the development of biofilm in the brain. Aβ is thought to protect against infectious microbes by sticking to them and thus preventing them from forming bacterial colonies that can develop into biofilms in the brain.

When the enzyme BACE1 is highly expressed in the neuron's cell membrane, it promotes β-cleavage of APP, and extracellular soluble-APPβ is formed, leaving an extracellular stub that then undergoes γ-cleavage by γ-secretase, forming extracellular Aβ and intracellular CTFβ (a 99-amino acid fragment), as opposed to CTFα (an 88-amino acid fragment) formed as a result of α-cleavage.

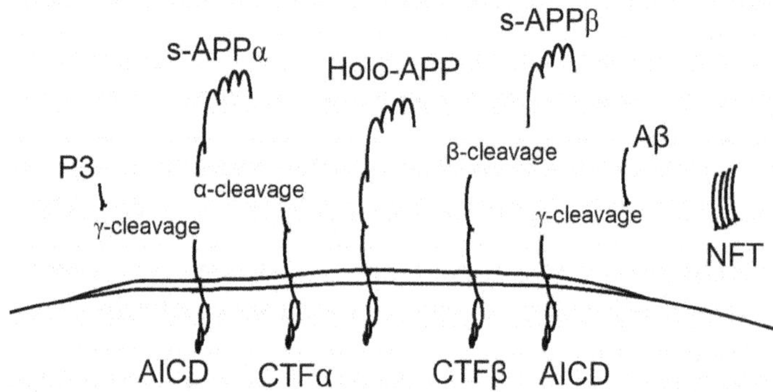

Figure 4F: A cartoon showing APP in a lipid raft on the neuronal cell surface. β-cleavage by BACE1 (beta-site amyloid precursor protein cleaving enzyme 1) forms the small, soluble-APPβ fragment, which allows γ-cleavage to produce Aβ, which can be taken into cells where it interferes with mitochondrial function. It can alternatively polymerize and form neurofibrillary tangles (NFT). In contrast, the protein ADAM10 is thought to act as an α-secretase, which creates soluble-APPα. With alpha cleavage, a fragment forms, but the remaining protein fragment in the lipid raft cannot form Aβ, as it is already cut; γ-cleavage forms P3. Chronic hypoxia downregulates ADAM10.[16]

A key feature in Alzheimer's disease, which is also present in Down syndrome, is impaired mitochondrial oxidative phosphorylation. Aβ can be taken up by neurons (by both the neuron it was produced by and as well, by neighboring neurons). Both Aβ and CTFβ and their AICD (amyloid precursor protein intracellular domain) fragments are taken into the mitochondria, where they inhibit oxidative phosphorylation and mitochondrial DNA (mtDNA) transcription. Aβ impairs

OXPHOS, especially at Complexes I and IV. In AD, where Complex IV is most highly inhibited, not only is there decreased ATP production, but there is also an increase in the leaking of reactive oxygen species (ROS) as electrons get backed up in the OXPHOS pathway. ROS lead to lipid peroxidation, protein oxidation and dysfunction, and DNA damage in the cell and mitochondria. These and other amyloid-β-related processes damage the mitochondrial membranes and impair the generation of new mitochondria.[17] The cells become energy-depleted. This damage can lead to the death of the neuron.

When bacteria form biofilms, it is accompanied by a change in the proteins that the bacteria express. Aβ likely acts to impede biofilm formation. Aβ also appears to promote inflammation and may even promote apoptosis. By sacrificing a few infected neurons early on in infection, apoptosis may protect the brain from bacterial or viral intracellular infection by preventing its spread to other cells.[18] [19] Nevertheless, while preventing brain infection is a very good thing, chronic upregulation of Aβ formation and the sustained destruction of neurons can be devastating. With the accumulation of Aβ, it tends to polymerize to form the neurofibrillary tangles of the sticky protein that are the hallmark of AD.

When APP is cleaved into Aβ, it can be variously cut into peptides from 39 to 43 amino acids long, depending on where it is enzymatically cut from the rest of the protein. The two dominant fragments are one with 40 amino acids and another with 2 extra amino acids at the end. Under physiologic conditions, more than 90% is cleaved into a peptide with 40 amino acids, simply known as Aβ40.[20] Aβ42 is the next most common form of Aβ. This fragment (Aβ42) is thought to protect the brain from infection. If a virus or bacteria gets into the brain and then into a neuron, Aβ42 elicits an immune response, which promotes an inflammatory response. When the ratio of Aβ40 to Aβ42 is high enough, it appears to act as a signal for the brain's immune cells, the microglia, to rest and "deactivate". While excess Aβ40 forms plaques, Aβ42 is more likely to enter neurons, accumulate inside, where it impedes mitochondrial function, and promotes mitochondrial fission. This is thought to promote an increase in APP expression, creating a positive feedback loop that accelerates with disease progression.[21] A lower ratio of Aβ40 to Aβ42 is associated with greater disease progression.

What Goes Wrong

Several things can cause overactivity of beta-secretase and an increase in the production of $Aβ_{42}$, firing up the immune response in the brain.

Lipopolysaccharides

One that the SANA diet seeks to address is the absorption of LPS from the intestine. While by far the major source of LPS in the body, the intestine is not the only source of LPS that ends up in the brain. LPS and other toxins from *P. gingivalis*, a keystone species in periodontal disease, are associated with AD.[22] In a study of post-mortem brain tissues, 40% of AD patients had evidence of LPS from *P. gingivalis*, while none of the age-matched controls without AD did.[23] Periodontal disease is thus another risk factor for AD. Good dental hygiene and a healthy diet can reduce the risk of periodontal disease. Periodontal health will be discussed in Chapter 23. Other chronic or repeated infections may also increase AD risk if they increase levels of LPS in the blood. I see no reason that chronic or repeated urinary tract, vaginal, lung, or skin infections would not increase AD risk.

Leaky gut allows LPS (lipopolysaccharides) from the cell walls of dead gram-negative bacteria in the lumen of the intestine to seep into the wall of the intestine and into the body. The body's immune system recognizes the toxin and responds as if there were a local infection. We have trillions of gram-negative bacteria living in the distal small intestine and colon, and most produce LPS. There are several layers of defense against this, but when this shield fails, LPS and other bacterial compounds can cross the intestinal barrier and get into the bloodstream. LPS impairs the blood-brain barrier, allowing LPS and other toxins to get into the brain. The immune cells in the brain respond to LPS and other bacterial compounds as they signal the presence of infection, even when there is not one; this can start an inflammatory response that progressively damages the brain.

When there is a disruption in the balance of commensal bacteria in the gut or compounds that disrupt the mucous layer that protects and separates the cells lining the colon from bacteria in the colon, it can cause cell injury, membrane dysfunction, and leakage, allowing for toxins, such as LPS, to enter the body and bloodstream. LPS can cross the blood-brain barrier and is recognized as a PAMP, and is thought to cause an inflammatory cascade in the brain, resulting in upregulation of APP and Aβ42 production.

Thus, intestinal dysbiosis, leading to leaky gut, allows for a chronic, sterile inflammatory state that promotes the production of Aβ. Aβ42 causes weak, poorly-functioning mitochondria that deprive the neurons of energy and that promote the formation of reactive oxygen species (ROS) that damage the cell's proteins and lipids.

Glycation

A second mechanism that is thought to amplify the formation/deposition of toxic Aβ is glycation. Protein glycation is a spontaneous reaction in which either a reducing sugar or an α-hydroxy aldehyde binds to either lysine or arginine in an exposed protein. Protein glycation accelerates with hypoglycemia and oxidative stress. The formation of α-hydroxy aldehydes greatly increases during glycolysis, which occurs during hypoxia or mitochondrial dysfunction. These reactions yield the formation of a diverse set of compounds called Advanced Glycation End-products (AGEs). AGEs bind to the RAGE (receptor for AGEs) receptors and trigger inflammation. Glycation is generally only a problem for long-lasting proteins, as most proteins are recycled in less than 24 hours. Glycation, however, can interfere with protein ubiquitination and thus impede protein recycling.

In the case of Aβ, AGEs decrease plaque formation but increase the toxicity of the Aβ fragments. This may be due to an increase in the formation of Aβ42 over Aβ40 as a result of the glycation of APP or γ-secretase, which promotes a change in APP or γ-secretase conformation that promotes greater formation of Aβ42. Glycation of Aβ42 may make it more toxic or immunogenic.[24]

The major cause of toxic AGEs in the body is hyperglycemia, mostly from glucose, but they can also be formed from fructose and aldehydes formed from it. Hypoxia drives the formation of AGEs by promoting a switch from oxidative phosphorylation by the mitochondria to glycolysis for energy production, which is not dependent upon mitochondria or the presence of oxygen. Glycolysis favors the production of MGO and other α-hydroxy aldehydes, which form AGEs.

Diabetes is a major risk factor for AD. Nevertheless, a diabetes diagnosis is not required for one to experience postprandial hyperglycemia or hyperfructosemia and accelerated glycation. Dietary AGEs from glycated proteins in foods may add to the risk of dementia, but most of the evidence points to endogenous AGEs as being the problem.

Kynurenine

A third important mechanism that promotes neurodegeneration is the kynurenine pathway, which is activated by LPS and inflammatory cytokines.

The kynurenine pathway (KP) is an important regulatory nervous system pathway, which impacts sickness and other behaviors, and which is also involved in the pathogenesis of multiple neurodegenerative diseases, including AD, PD, ALS, Lewy body dementia, and schizophrenia.[25] The kynurenine pathway is also important in the enteric nervous system.

Kynurenine is formed from the amino acid tryptophan. Tryptophan also forms the calming neurotransmitter serotonin and the sleep cycle-regulating antioxidant melatonin. In the KP, however, tryptophan is diverted away from serotonin production when the enzyme indoleamine 2,3-dioxygenase 1 (IDO1) is activated by inflammatory cytokines INFγ, IL-1β, IL-6, or TNF. LPS from gram-negative bacteria stimulates IDO1 activity in both the CNS and the ENS via its promotion of these cytokines, as illustrated in Figure 2E (above). With the proinflammatory diversion of tryptophan, there is less calming impact from serotonin and decreased diurnal sleep drive from melatonin. Simultaneously, the kynurenine pathway (KP) promotes inflammatory and toxic processes. Additionally, the KP product quinolinic acid acts as an excitogen that inhibits sleep.

While the KP is active in the brain, peripherally produced kynurenine is also transported across the BBB into the brain. Thus, peripheral activation of IDO1 by LPS or inflammatory cytokines, as in the case of an infected wound or intestinal infection, can promote sickness behavior. Aβ42 induces the expression of IDO1 in microglia and astrocytes.,

A feature of the KP in the brain is that different cells respond differently. Astrocytes lack the enzyme kynurenine monooxygenase (KMO) and, therefore, do not produce 3-hydroxykynurenine (3-HK) from kynurenine (Kyn). Instead, they produce the enzyme KYAT1, which converts kynurenine to kynurenic acid (KA). KA acts to inhibit glutamate excitatory ionotropic receptors. This gives a calming effect. KA also has antioxidant properties. These effects are part of the sickness behavior that promotes sedentary behavior and rest. In chronic disease, such as AD, this calming may present as slow mentation.

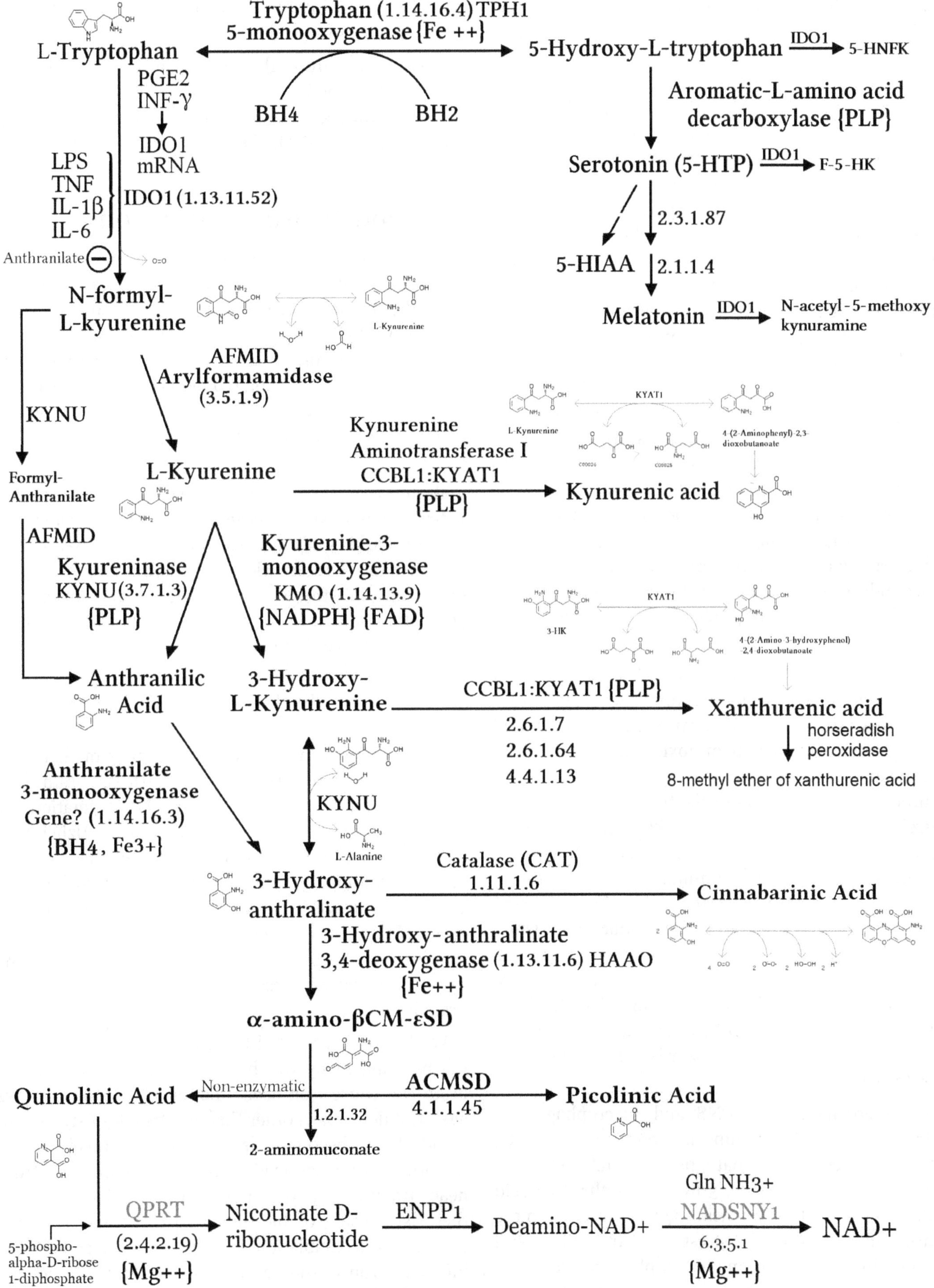
L-Tryptophan
Tryptophan (1.14.16.4) TPH1
5-monooxygenase {Fe ++}
5-Hydroxy-L-tryptophan
IDO1
5-HNFK
BH4
BH2
PGE2
INF-γ
IDO1
mRNA
LPS
TNF
IL-1β
IL-6
IDO1 (1.13.11.52)
Anthranilate
Aromatic-L-amino acid
decarboxylase {PLP}
Serotonin (5-HTP)
IDO1
F-5-HK
2.3.1.87
5-HIAA
2.1.1.4
Melatonin
IDO1
N-acetyl-5-methoxy
kynuramine
N-formyl-
L-kyurenine
L-Kynurenine
AFMID
Arylformamidase
(3.5.1.9)
KYNU
Formyl-
Anthranilate
L-Kyurenine
Kynurenine
Aminotransferase I
CCBL1:KYAT1
{PLP}
KYAT1
L-Kynurenine
4-(2-Aminophenyl)-2,3-
dioxobutanoate
Kynurenic acid
AFMID
Kyureninase
KYNU(3.7.1.3)
{PLP}
Kyurenine-3-
monooxygenase
KMO (1.14.13.9)
{NADPH} {FAD}
KYAT1
3-HK
4-(2-Amino-3-hydroxyphenol)
-2,4-dioxobutanoate
Anthranilic
Acid
3-Hydroxy-
L-Kynurenine
CCBL1:KYAT1 {PLP}
2.6.1.7
2.6.1.64
4.4.1.13
Xanthurenic acid
horseradish
peroxidase
8-methyl ether of xanthurenic acid
Anthranilate
3-monooxygenase
Gene? (1.14.16.3)
{BH4, Fe3+}
KYNU
L-Alanine
3-Hydroxy-
anthralinate
Catalase (CAT)
1.11.1.6
Cinnabarinic Acid
3-Hydroxy-anthralinate
3,4-deoxygenase (1.13.11.6) HAAO
{Fe++}
α-amino-βCM-εSD
Quinolinic Acid
Non-enzymatic
1.2.1.32
ACMSD
4.1.1.45
Picolinic Acid
2-aminomuconate
QPRT
(2.4.2.19)
{Mg++}
5-phospho-
alpha-D-ribose
1-diphosphate
Nicotinate D-
ribonucleotide
ENPP1
Deamino-NAD+
Gln NH3+
NADSNY1
6.3.5.1
{Mg++}
NAD+

Figure 19D-2: The Kynurenine Pathway and tryptophan metabolism (Previous page)

Lactate and glucose are the preferred fuels of neurons and other cells in the brain. Lactate additionally acts as a signaling molecule that may be required for the formation of long-term memory. During intense exercise, the muscles don't get sufficient oxygen for the mitochondria to fully perform oxidative phosphorylation; a portion of the glucose undergoes glycolysis in the cytoplasm of muscle cells, and excess lactate is released into the bloodstream. The brain can utilize the lactate, which is handy since both glucose and oxygen become limited during intense exercise.

In the brain, astrocytes also convert glucose into lactate, which is secreted for the benefit of the neurons and oligodendrocytes. Lactate facilitates neuronal signal transmission, appears to have anti-inflammatory activity, and acts as a neuroprotectant.[26] KA also decreases the production of lactate by astrocytes. While the neurons can use glucose, the lack of lactate can curtail the energy supply of the neuron, especially if O2 is limited, with insulin resistance, or when the mitochondria are ill. In cell cultures, inhibiting IDO1 restored astrocyte lactate production and lactate uptake by neurons.[27]

Kynurenic acid (KA) is an NMDA antagonist and protects the brain from excitotoxicity, but other metabolites, such as 3-OH-kynurenine (3OHK) and quinolinic acid QA), are neurotoxic. Patients with AD have been found to have a shift towards increased kynurenic acid production in the brain as compared to control patients.[28] Vitamin B6 (pyridoxal-l-5-phosphate; PLP, P5P) is a cofactor for the conversion of kynurenine products into non-inflammatory products. PLP deficiency is rare; nevertheless, various stressors deplete PLP. PLP is involved in the production of white blood cells, antibodies, and the production of calming neurotransmitters, including serotonin and GABA. Thus, stress and inflammation can deplete PLP, impeding the production of kynurenic acid and driving the kynurenine pathway towards excitotoxic and neurotoxic metabolites.

The microglia in the CNS and macrophages, in contrast, produce kynurenine monooxygenase (KMO) and other enzymes that process KA into 3-hydroxykynurenine (3-HK), 3-hydroxy anthranilic acid (3-HAA), and quinolinic acid (QA), which promote excitotoxicity, oxidative stress, glucotoxicity, and neuronal injury. They promote the phosphorylation of tau, another protein disrupted in AD. pTau, then form oligomers that increase Kyn production by activating IDO1, in a positive feedback loop.

Aβ promotes microglial activation. In addition to the inflammatory mediators released via TLR4 activation, it indirectly induces the expression of indoleamine 2,3-dioxygenase 1 (IDO1), the rate-limiting enzyme in the kynurenine pathway.

Iron and Neurodegeneration

While not a central theme of this book, excess iron, copper, or manganese in the brain can promote neurodegeneration. Iron will be briefly mentioned here as it helps explain the impact of concussions and mini-hemorrhagic strokes. Even minor concussions can bruise the brain, releasing red blood cells into the brain, and along with them, the iron in hemoglobin. The iron gets cleaned up by microglial cells, but it can activate them.

Brain iron dysregulation is seen in several neurodegenerative diseases, including Alzheimer's disease, Parkinson's disease, Huntington's disease, and amyotrophic lateral sclerosis.[29] Some of the injury occurring in these conditions results from the generation of ROS (H_2O_2 and superoxide anions), which causes oxidative injury. The brains of patients with Alzheimer's disease have been found to have elevated iron concentrations in the hippocampus and parietal cortex.[30]

Iron transport into the brain is in part mediated by amyloid precursor protein (APP); excess brain iron promotes oxidative stress and the formation of neurofibrillary tangles that are typical of Alzheimer's disease. The presence of iron exacerbates the synthesis of the inflammatory cytokine IL-1β by microglial cells exposed to amyloid-beta (Aβ).[31] An increase in iron accumulation in the substantia nigra is typical in Parkinson's disease.[32] Elevated brain iron may be the result of oxidative stress, ischemic injury, or traumatic brain injury.[33 34]

While iron is essential for neurological development, the mechanism by which iron is transported into the brain can cause iron accumulation in later life. As we age, iron deficiency, other than as a result of significant blood loss, becomes less common. Likely more important, iron overload in the brain may arise from head trauma, micro-hemorrhages, or stroke, where there is bruising or bleeding into the brain. The iron may be an accumulation of ferric iron associated with injury or iron dyshomeostasis rather than physiologic iron. This free iron in the brain can be taken up by microglia, causing these immune cells to become activated; a situation in which they can promote inflammatory injury in the brain. Iron participates in the formation of H_2O_2 and reactive oxygen species. These injuries are not uncommon in the elderly and are part of the pathology of dementia and neurodegenerative diseases.

[1] Association between dietary inflammatory index and cognitive impairment among American elderly: a cross-sectional study. Zhang Y, Peng Y, Deng W, Xiang Q, Zhang W, Liu M. Front Aging Neurosci. 2024 Mar 14;16:1371873. doi: 10.3389/fnagi.2024.1371873. PMID: 38550747; PMCID: PMC10976944.

[2] Alzheimer's Disease is Driven by Intraneuronally Retained Beta-Amyloid Produced in the AD-Specific, βAPP-Independent Pathway: Current Perspective and Experimental Models for Tomorrow. Volloch V, Olsen B, Rits S. Ann Integr Mol Med. 2020;2(1):90-114. doi: 10.33597/aimm.02-1007. PMID: 32617536

[3] Image by Holly Fischer

[4] Computational Basis of Neural Elements. Arslan OE. Artificial Neural Network for Drug Design, Delivery and Disposition 2016, Pages 29-82 https://www.sciencedirect.com/science/article/pii/B9780128015599000003X

[5] Schematic sketch showing the blood-brain barrier. https://commons.wikimedia.org/wiki/File:Blood-brain_barrier_02.png Image by Armin Kübelbeck

[6] Retrospective birth dating of cells in humans. Spalding KL, Bhardwaj RD, Buchholz BA, Druid H, Frisén J. Cell. 2005 Jul 15;122(1):133-43. PMID:16009139

[7] Brain development in rodents and humans: Identifying benchmarks of maturation and vulnerability to injury across species. Semple BD, Blomgren K, Gimlin K, Ferriero DM, Noble-Haeusslein LJ. Prog Neurobiol. 2013 Jul-Aug;106-107:1-16. PMID:23583307 doi: 10.1016 /j.pneurobio.2013.04.001

[8] Image modified from Wikimeida commons images.

[9] Age-related impairment of olfactory bulb neurogenesis in the Ts65Dn mouse model of Down syndrome. Bianchi P, Bettini S, Guidi S, Ciani E, Trazzi S, Stagni F, Ragazzi E, Franceschini V, Bartesaghi R. Exp Neurol. 2014 Jan;251:1-11. doi: 10.1016/j.expneurol.2013.10.018. Epub PMID: 24192151

[10] Adult neurogenesis in the mammalian brain: significant answers and significant questions. Ming GL, Song H. Neuron. 2011 May 26;70(4):687-702. doi: 10.1016/j.neuron.2011.05.001. PMID: 21609825

[11] Structural cerebellar correlates of cognitive functions in spinocerebellar ataxia type 2. Olivito G, Lupo M, Iacobacci C, Clausi S, Romano S, Masciullo M, Molinari M, Cercignani M, Bozzali M, Leggio M. J Neurol. 2018 Mar;265(3):597-606. doi: 10.1007/s00415-018-8738-6. Epub 2018 Jan 22. PMID: 29356974

[12] Novel insights into the relationship between cerebellum and dementia: A narrative review as a toolkit for clinicians. Devita M, Alberti F, Fagnani M, Masina F, Ara E, Sergi G, Mapelli D, Coin A. Ageing Res Rev. 2021 Sep;70:101389. doi: 10.1016/j.arr.2021.101389. Epub 2021 Jun 8. PMID: 34111569

[13] Cerebellar involvement in Parkinson's disease: Pathophysiology and neuroimaging. Qiu T, Liu M, Qiu X, Li T, Le W. Chin Med J (Engl). 2024 Oct 20;137(20):2395-2403. doi: 10.1097/CM9.0000000000003248. Epub 2024 Sep 3. PMID: 39227357

[14] Advanced Dementia. Mitchell SL. N Engl J Med. 2015 Sep 24;373(13):1276-7. doi: 10.1056/NEJMc1509349. PMID: 26398084

[15] ADAM-10 over-expression increases cortical synaptogenesis. Bell KF, Zheng L, Fahrenholz F, Cuello AC. Neurobiol Aging. 2008 Apr;29(4):554-65. PMID:17187903

[16] Amyloid precursor protein-mediated mitochondrial regulation and Alzheimer's disease. Lopez Sanchez MIG, van Wijngaarden P, Trounce IA. Br J Pharmacol. 2019 Sep;176(18):3464-3474. doi: 10.1111/bph.14554. PMID: 30471088

[17] Amyloid precursor protein-mediated mitochondrial regulation and Alzheimer's disease. Lopez Sanchez MIG, van Wijngaarden P, Trounce IA. Br J Pharmacol. 2019 Sep;176(18):3464-3474. doi: 10.1111/bph.14554. PMID: 30471088

[18] Amyloid, tau, pathogen infection and antimicrobial protection in Alzheimer's disease -conformist, nonconformist, and realistic prospects for AD pathogenesis. Li H, Liu CC, Zheng H, Huang TY. Transl Neurodegener. 2018 Dec 24;7:34. doi: 10.1186/s40035-018-0139-3. eCollection 2018. PMID:30603085

[19] The antimicrobial protection hypothesis of Alzheimer's disease. Moir RD, Lathe R, Tanzi RE. Alzheimers Dement. 2018 Dec;14(12):1602-1614. doi: 10.1016/j.jalz.2018.06.3040. PMID:30314800

[20] β-Amyloid: the key peptide in the pathogenesis of Alzheimer's disease. Sun X, Chen WD, Wang YD. Front Pharmacol. 2015 Sep 30;6:221. doi: 10.3389/fphar.2015.00221. eCollection 2015. PMID: 26483691

[21] Alzheimer's Disease is Driven by Intraneuronally Retained Beta-Amyloid Produced in the AD-Specific, βAPP-Independent Pathway: Current Perspective and Experimental Models for Tomorrow. Volloch V, Olsen B, Rits S. Ann Integr Mol Med. 2020;2(1):90-114. doi: 10.33597/aimm.02-1007. PMID: 32617536

[22] Analysis the Link between Periodontal Diseases and Alzheimer's Disease: A Systematic Review. Borsa L, et al. Int J Environ Res Public Health. 2021 Sep 3;18(17):9312. doi: 10.3390/ijerph18179312. PMID: 34501899

[23] Determining the presence of periodontopathic virulence factors in short-term postmortem Alzheimer's disease brain tissue. Poole Set et al. J Alzheimers Dis. 2013;36(4):665-77. doi: 10.3233/JAD-121918. PMID: 23666172

[24] An overview on glycation: molecular mechanisms, impact on proteins, pathogenesis, and inhibition. Uceda AB, Mariño L, Casasnovas R, Adrover M. Biophys Rev. 2024 Apr 12;16(2):189-218. doi: 10.1007/s12551-024-01188-4. PMID: 38737201; PMCID: PMC11078917.

[25] The Involvement of Kynurenine Pathway in Neurodegenerative Diseases. Martins LB, Silveira ALM, Teixeira AL. Curr Neuropharmacol. 2023;21(2):260-272. doi: 10.2174/1570159X20666220922153221. PMID: 36154606

[26] Lactate Metabolism, Signaling, and Function in Brain Development, Synaptic Plasticity, Angiogenesis, and

Neurodegenerative Diseases. Wu A, Lee D, Xiong WC. Int J Mol Sci. 2023 Aug 29;24(17):13398. doi: 10.3390/ijms241713398. PMID: 37686202; PMCID: PMC10487923.

[27] Restoring hippocampal glucose metabolism rescues cognition across Alzheimer's disease pathologies. Minhas PS, Jones JR, Latif-Hernandez A, Sugiura Y, Durairaj AS, Wang Q, Mhatre SD, Uenaka T, Crapser J, Conley T, Ennerfelt H, Jung YJ, Liu L, Prasad P, Jenkins BC, Ay YA, Matrongolo M, Goodman R, Newmeyer T, Heard K, Kang A, Wilson EN, Yang T, Ullian EM, Serrano GE, Beach TG, Wernig M, Rabinowitz JD, Suematsu M, Longo FM, McReynolds MR, Gage FH, Andreasson KI. Science. 2024 Aug 23;385(6711):eabm6131. doi: 10.1126/science.abm6131. Aug 23. PMID: 39172838

[28] An overview on glycation: molecular mechanisms, impact on proteins, pathogenesis, and inhibition. Uceda AB, Mariño L, Casasnovas R, Adrover M. Biophys Rev. 2024 Apr 12;16(2):189-218. doi: 10.1007/s12551-024-01188-4. PMID: 38737201; PMCID: PMC11078917.

[29] The Contribution of Iron to Protein Aggregation Disorders in the Central Nervous System. Joppe K, Roser AE, Maass F, Lingor P. Front Neurosci. 2019 Jan 22;13:15. doi: 10.3389/fnins.2019.00015. PMID: 30723395

[30] Investigation on positive correlation of increased brain iron deposition with cognitive impairment in Alzheimer disease by using quantitative MR R2' mapping. Qin Y, Zhu W, Zhan C, Zhao L, Wang J, Tian Q, Wang W. J Huazhong Univ Sci Technolog Med Sci. 2011 Aug;31(4):578. doi: 10.1007/s11596-011-0493-1. PMID: 21823025

[31] Iron potentiates microglial interleukin-1β secretion induced by amyloid-β. Nnah IC, Lee CH, Wessling-Resnick M. J Neurochem. 2020 Jul;154(2):177-189. doi: 10.1111/jnc.14906. PMID: 31693761

[32] Brain iron homeostasis: from molecular mechanisms to clinical significance and therapeutic opportunities. Singh N, Haldar S, Tripathi AK, Horback K, Wong J, Sharma D, Beserra A, Suda S, Anbalagan C, Dev S, Mukhopadhyay CK, Singh A. Antioxid Redox Signal. 2014 Mar 10;20(8):1324-63. PMID:23815406

[33] Characterizing brain iron deposition in subcortical ischemic vascular dementia using susceptibility-weighted imaging: An in vivo MR study. Liu C, Li C, Yang J, Gui L, Zhao L, Evans AC, Yin X, Wang J. Behav Brain Res. 2015 Jul 15;288:33-8. doi: 10.1016/j.bbr.2015.04.003. PMID: 25862942

[34] Increased iron and free radical generation in preclinical Alzheimer disease and mild cognitive impairment. Smith MA, Zhu X, Tabaton M, Liu G, McKeel DW Jr, Cohen ML, Wang X, Siedlak SL, Dwyer BE, Hayashi T, Nakamura M, Nunomura A, Perry G. J Alzheimers Dis. 2010;19(1):363-72. doi: 10.3233/JAD-2010-1239. PMID: 20061651

5: The Other Brain

The gastrointestinal system may not be good at folding a map or at Platonic discourse. It cannot speak, other than some growling and grumbling. We would not call the GI tract highly intelligent, but it does have a semi-independent nervous system that could be considered a second brain. This other brain, the Enteric Nervous System (ENS), uses many of the same neurotransmitters and signaling pathways as the central nervous system (CNS). In fact, the ENS should not be referred to as a second brain; it was the first brain, having evolved much earlier. The ENS is present in all animals with a gut, including those that lack a CNS.[1] The human ENS contains about 500 million neurons; that is a pittance compared to the human brain, but this is more neurons than there are in the CNS of a Nile crocodile or a hamster.

> If we're going to talk numbers, the average adult human brain has 86 billion neurons, about 3 times that of a chimpanzee, but only about one-third of that of an African elephant. Humans have the highest encephalization level (EL) of any animal. The EL adjusts for the brain-to-body size and is a better predictor of intelligence than simple brain mass or neuron count. Dolphins come in second after humans in encephalization. Ravens have about the same EL as chimpanzees, and dogs have levels just above squirrels; squirrels have higher scores than cats, and cats have a higher EL than horses.[2] Chinchillas have EL levels similar to those of dogs. There are two species of chinchillas, and one has been hunted to the brink of extinction for its fur. Social animals, such as chinchillas and prairie dogs, tend to be more intelligent than solitary ones, such as gators. Alternatively, higher intelligence may allow the benefits provided by social behavior. Relationships are complicated, and this complexity necessitates a high level of cognitive processing and intelligence.

The ENS is the largest component of the autonomic nervous system. It functions mostly independently of the CNS, coordinating gastrointestinal functions, including peristalsis of the stomach and intestines. The ENS controls the duration of food's residence in the stomach and its periodic emptying into the jejunum. The ENS controls secretions and helps control pH, electrolytes, and digestive enzyme production and release from the pancreas and cells of the intestine. The ENS responds to taste and other chemosensory cells in the gut. I don't know of a way to discern if the ENS is self-aware, but the ENS is a reliable system that is necessary to extract nutrition from food and help protect us from disease.

The neurotransmitter dopamine is well known for promoting motivation and salience (reward) in the CNS; the ENS produces as much dopamine as does the CNS. The neurotransmitter serotonin affects mood, appetite, learning, and sleep in the CNS; ninety-five percent of the body's serotonin is formed in intestinal enterochromaffin cells as a part of the ENS. Here, it affects intestinal motility and secretions, as well as regulating pancreatic secretions. GI serotonin also modulates pain perception.[3] Impressively, ninety percent of the body's melatonin is formed in the ENS. As in the brain, melatonin in the ENS affects diurnal cycling and acts as an antioxidant.

The ENS regulates all sensory and motor functions within the gut. The ENS protects us by causing nausea and vomiting if it is disgusted by the contents of the stomach, and can rapidly evacuate the small intestine if irritated by its contents, causing diarrhea. The ENS controls the permeability of the mucosa and modulates the development of neuroendocrine cells within the mucous membrane.[4]

The ENS sends and receives information from the CNS through the vagus nerve, the largest and longest of the 12 cranial nerves. Ten times more afferent fibers go from the gut to the CNS than efferent fibers go from the CNS to the gut. Thus, the ENS likely has a greater impact on the brain than the brain has on the gut.

Sickness behavioral changes begin in animals within hours of exposure to the bacterial toxin LPS or after inoculation with the intestinal pathogen *Campylobacter jejuni*. These acute behavioral changes can be mitigated by cutting the vagus nerve. *Lactobacillus rhamnosus* (JB-1) and *Bifidobacterium longum* have anxiolytic effects in certain rat and mouse disease models; however, the effect is lost in animals when the vagus nerve has been severed.[5] The *L. rhamnosus* anti-anxiety effect is accompanied by increased levels of the inhibitory neurotransmitter GABA in various areas of the brain, but only in animals with an intact vagus nerve.[6] While the CNS and ENS communicate with each other, the ENS continues to function independently if the vagus nerve is severed, cutting the inter-communication.

The ENS is made up of two networks: the outer myenteric plexus (also called Auerbach's plexus) and the inner submucosal plexus (also called Meissner's plexus). The myenteric plexus lies between two thin layers of muscle in the intestinal wall and controls GI motility and peristalsis. About 30% of the nerves in the myenteric plexus are sensory. About 16% of the neurons in the submucosal plexus are sensory nerves, which help control epithelial functions and secretion. The ENS regulates neuro-immune function in the mucosa via secretions of hormones and by the release of epithelial cell growth and differentiation factors.[7]

In health, gastrointestinal transit of food takes about an average of 3 days, with a normal range of 2 to 5 days. A meal is slowly digested in the stomach, and small boluses are released over about 4 to 5 hours. It takes another five to six hours to traverse the small intestine and then about 40 hours to pass through the colon. The ENS controls digestive contractions and intestinal transit. There are two principal movements: mixing and propulsion. Similar to a clothes washer, there is an agitation phase where the bolus of food remains in one area and is mixed with enzymes and other digestive juices, followed by a propulsion phase where it is moved forward through the GI tract. If there are noxious stimuli, the small intestine can propel the contents forward quickly to get rid of the GI contents.

Neurotoxic chemicals that injure or impair the central nervous system are likely more injurious to the enteric nervous system, as the ENS is more exposed and lacks the protection of a blood-brain barrier-like system.

ENS comorbidity is observed in amyotrophic lateral sclerosis (ALS), Parkinson's disease (PD), Alzheimer's disease (AD), and autism spectrum disorder (ASD). Patients with AD have a progressive accumulation of β-amyloid protein in the enteric neurons; this is associated with a decline in the population of neurons, impaired gastrointestinal motility, and vulnerability to intestinal inflammation. Constipation is nearly universal and typically a presenting symptom in Parkinson's disease. Herpes zoster, which causes shingles by infecting a peripheral nerve, can cause pseudo-obstruction of the bowel. In animal disease models, pathological mechanisms that cause neurological injury often cause gastrointestinal injury. The damage to the CNS is often mirrored in the ENS.[8]

By the age of three, the CNS has developed most of the neurons it ever will. Neurons are considered immortal cells. That doesn't mean they are guaranteed to live forever, but rather that they can last a lifetime. If neurons are killed, the capacity to replace them is very limited, and the loss of CNS neurons due to injury is generally permanent. One reason for this is that if there were a turnover in neurons, with the replacement of new neurons and new connections, there would be a loss of memory, learning, and personality.

The ENS is far more highly exposed to toxins and mechanical stressors than is the CNS. The proximal small intestine may be exposed to high concentrations of alcohol and other neurotoxins present in food. As we age, there is a shift from anti-inflammatory (M2) to pro-inflammatory (M1) macrophages and an increase in cytokines in the ENS that promote inflammation and aging.[9] And then, there are those dietary indiscretions and overindulgences that the intestine is exposed to, barbequed beef on the weekend, a bit too many fries. The greater exposure of the neurons of the ENS has them facing more stress than those in the CNS.

The epithelial cells lining the mucosa of the intestine have a constant and rapid turnover – the cells are replaced about every four to ten days, depending on the area of the intestine. Thus, the mucosal cells are quickly replaced. The ENS can also generate new glial cells[10] and neurons. The intestine contains enteric neural precursor cells that act as stem cells, which give rise to new enteric neurons. This capacity does not seem to even wait for an injury to occur. In the small intestine of adult mice, about four to five percent of the neurons in the ENS enter apoptosis each day, and there is neurogenesis of new ENS neurons to replace them. This suggests a complete turnover in the enteric neurons in the mouse small intestine about every three weeks throughout adult life.[11]

Birds can replace the sensory cells in the ear, but we cannot. And we are not mice, so a mouse study is not proof that our ENS has rapid turnover. Nevertheless, there is evidence that neurons in the human ENS can regenerate, and given our exposure to alcohol, food with fungal neurotoxins, exposure to glucosepane from barbeque, chemotherapy, and other toxins from which the ENS appears to recover, it is likely that humans similarly replace ENS neurons. If recovery from GI dysmotility after completing chemotherapy can be used as a guide, the turnover rate is likely several months.

If ENS neurons can continually renew themselves in adult humans, this suggests that at least some gastrointestinal dysfunction that is associated with neurological diseases, such as Parkinson's disease and ASD, may recover once the disease-causing processes have been eliminated. It also provides evidence of continued ENS pathological processes indicative of continuing damage to the ENS and CNS. Thus, for diseases that affect both, successful treatments that halt ongoing CNS injury may be revealed by improvements in ENS function within several weeks. If a treatment allows for the recovery of ENS function, it may provide some rapid evidence that the treatment may halt ongoing injury to the CNS.

The leaky gut theory posits that toxins, such as bacterial lipopolysaccharide (LPS) from the gut bacteria that are normally excluded from absorption by the healthy intestinal mucosal barrier, can be absorbed if there is a pathological increase in mucosal permeability. LPS or other toxins that are normally kept out of the body can then affect the ENS, enter the bloodstream, and affect the liver, brain, and other organs. In the case of LPS, the body recognizes the compound as a bacterial PAMP (pathogen-associated molecular pattern) and responds by mounting an inflammatory reaction; this inflammatory reaction can affect brain function and may cause brain injury. Neurodevelopmental delay or injury from "leaky gut" may occur during gestation, or anytime during brain development in childhood or adolescence, and contribute to the development of Parkinson's disease, Alzheimer's dementia, and other neurodegenerative diseases.

The Intestinal Barrier

The mucosa is a continuous and sealed barrier that extends from the lips to the anus. Yet, this surface needs to digest and absorb nutrients. While many cell types make up the intestinal epithelium, about 95 percent of the epithelial cells lining the internal surface of the intestine are enterocytes. Enterocytes specialized for the colon are called colonocytes. The total mucosal surface of the intestine is about 250 square meters (2700 sq. ft.). The intestinal mucosa is our largest interface with our environment, and as a result, more than half of all immune cells in the body reside just below this surface in the lamina propria.

There are six layers of protection guarding the inside against the outside, separating all the nasty things in the lumen of the intestine from the bloodstream and access to the brain and other organs.

1. Luminal intestinal alkaline phosphatase.
2. A mucous layer that adheres to the mucosa.
3. The tight junctions lock the enterocytes together and limit the entry of large molecules or bacteria from reaching the inside of the body.
4. The secretion of antibacterial proteins.
5. Immune defenses, including the secretion of immunoglobulin A.
6. The symbiotic commensal microbiome.

The bacteria that live in the intestine are generally not dangerous as long as they stay in the colon, but many of them can easily become deadly in the bloodstream, lungs, brain, or other organs. Since we carry these bugs with us wherever we go, we need a means of recognizing and dealing with them. Most gram-negative enteric bacteria have lipopolysaccharide (LPS) as a cell wall component. Some types of bacteria produce much more LPS than others. When these bacteria die, the LPS can be released into the colon and distal small intestine. We can also be exposed to LPS from wounds, pneumonia, dental disease, or other infections caused by these gram-negative bacteria.

Toll-like receptors (TLRs) on immune cells recognize pathogen-associated molecular patterns (PAMPs) of molecules that are commonly present in pathogens and thus, can respond by producing cytokines and chemokines, which promote an inflammatory reaction that draws white blood cells to the area to put down the infection. For example, the TLR4 complex recognizes LPS, which is common in Gram-negative bacteria, TLR2 recognizes the PAMP lipoteichoic acid, which is common in Gram-positive bacteria, and TLR9 is activated by bacterial CpG DNA.[12] Each has additional PAMPs or DAMPs (damage-associated molecular patterns) that bind with and activate the TLR. This is part of the innate immune system; we react to these PAMPs innately without having had prior exposure to them. Thus, newborn infants can respond to infections they have never experienced and can respond before developing specific antibodies to the pathogen. These represent the innate immune response in contrast to the adaptive immune response. It would be detrimental to be in a constant state of inflammation from bacterial LPS present in the intestine. Thus, we have an antidote.

The first line of mucosal defense is the enzyme intestinal alkaline phosphatase (IAP), which is produced and secreted by the enterocytes. IAP largely inactivates LPS by clipping off the phosphate groups from LPS that allow it to bind and activate the TLR4 complex. IAP also inactivates flagellin, bacterial CpG DNA,[13] and some other PAMPs. IAP further removes phosphate groups from ATP and ADP, which may be present in the intestinal lumen, which can promote Gram-positive pathogen overgrowth and disrupt bacterial homeostasis. The ATP and ADP can come from sloughing enterocytes and bacteria, but under-digested meat can be a potent source. IAP does not appear to affect bacterial growth directly or harm living bacteria, but rather prevents conditions that allow the overgrowth of pathogens. Thus, IAP not only detoxifies inflammatory antigens but also helps shape the microbiome population, suppressing the growth of predatory bacteria[14] and helping to prevent the translocation of pathogens across the intestinal mucosa.[15] [16] IAP also regulates fatty acid absorption, bicarbonate secretion, and pH in the duodenum. Higher levels of IAP are protective against metabolic syndrome.[17]

IAP is secreted by the enterocytes at the apex of the cells; it remains bound to the apex but is also secreted into the mucous layer. IAP is also secreted from the basal membrane of the enterocyte into the lamina propria and taken up into the bloodstream, where it can inactivate LPS. The apically secreted IAP remains active when it is sloughed off into the lumen. IAP is most highly expressed in the proximal small intestine, but IAP has its greatest activity in the lumen of the terminal ileum, as it accumulates within the lumen of the small intestine. Intestinal alkaline phosphatase works best in an alkaline environment (at pH 9.7), so the activity of IAP that arrives downstream from the small intestine into the lower pH of the colon has considerably less activity. The colon produces a different form of alkaline phosphatase (ALPL) that has substantial activity.[18]

The second line of barrier defense is the mucous layer. Functionally, it is a double layer; the newer inner layer is firmly attached to the cells and is denser, while the more superficial, older mucus, in contact with the lumen, is thicker and more gelatinous. The mucous layer is composed mostly of water and the glycoprotein mucin-2 (MUC2) secreted by goblet cells; it is about 95% water.

The mucus contains digestive enzymes and creates a density gradient that allows for the uptake of nutrients by the enterocytes. The dense inner MUC2 layer in the colon, in health, is devoid of bacteria.[19] This limits the bacteria from having direct contact with the cells or adhering to the epithelium. In contrast, the less dense outer layer harbors commensal bacteria and promotes their colonization. In the small intestine, there may be some adhesion of bacteria to the mucosal cell, as certain commensal bacteria can adhere to both MUC2 and the epithelium.

Damage or depletion of the mucous layer can allow the colonization of pathogenic bacteria and may allow bacteria to access and adhere to the epithelium. This may allow colonization, biofilm formation, toxin production, and even transmigration of bacteria into the lamina propria, and thus into the body.

The third layer of defense is the binding of epithelial cells to each other. Each cell is ringed by adherens junctions and desmosomes that attach the cells to each other. Additionally, there are tight junctions that seal the gap between the cells.

Most nutrients enter the body through the apical enterocyte membranes by transcellular uptake. Some lipid-soluble compounds can diffuse across the membranes, but most nutrients enter by gated channels or active transport. The luminal (apical) surface of the enterocytes is covered with microvilli, which give them a large surface area for absorption. The nutrients, many of which are first processed by these cells, are transported into the lamina propria at the basal pole of the enterocyte, where they can be absorbed into the portal bloodstream. The portal vein collects blood from the intestine and carries it to the liver for the processing of nutrients.

The enterocyte brush border membrane has a peptide transporter (SLC15A1) that transports di- and tri-peptides into the cell, where some are digested into amino acids, and others are released from the basal membrane for uptake into the portal circulation. These di- and tripeptides are enzymatically digested in the liver into simple amino acids, so that they should not reach the general circulation, and thus not have systemic or neurologic effects. However, some peptides may make their way into the circulation via the lymphatic system. The enterocytes do not take in luminal contents through endocytosis, although the immune M cells in the intestinal mucosa do.

The tightness of the tight junctions is controlled by actin within the enterocytes. When actin contracts, it pulls the tight junctions open slightly to increase the gap between the cells, while when actin is at rest, only very small molecules and electrolytes are small enough to squeeze between the tight junctions for paracellular uptake at rest. This generally means small amounts of water and ions such as sodium and chloride can pass in either direction, in or out.

When actin is contracted and the tight junctions are relaxed, molecules up to about 400 Daltons may penetrate the lamina propria.[20] Generally, orally available medications have a practical molecular size limit of about 500 Daltons, as unless they are very lipid-soluble and can pass through the cell membrane, molecules larger than this are difficult to absorb. Activation of actin in the intestinal epithelium is under the control of the enteric nervous system and responds to various stimuli. For example, the bile acid deoxycholate stimulates the ENS to increase local permeability,[21] allowing transient increased paracellular absorption through the mucosa as the bolus of food containing bile excreted with the meal courses its way through the small intestine. This allows many medications to be better absorbed when taken with a meal. The food bolus, already treated with stomach acid and multiple digestive enzymes, hopefully, has a low pathogen and toxin content. During the resting periods, the membrane is more tightly sealed, and large molecules are less likely to be absorbed.

Dysfunction or disruption of the epithelial barrier, which increases paracellular permeability, may allow uptake of peptides, bacterial toxins, and even translocation of bacteria into the lamina propria.

The fourth layer of defense is biochemical. Paneth cells in the epithelial crypts secrete a blend of antibacterial proteins when they sense LPS or other bacterial PAMPs. Among these are α- and β-defensins, phospholipase A2, cathelicidins, and lysozyme.[22] These proteins are thus part of the innate immune response.

The fifth line of defense is the adaptive immune response. Along the small intestine, but particularly in the distal ileum, there are around 100 Peyer's patches. These are ovoid patches, a few centimeters long, in which lymphoid cells are abundant, mostly B lymphocytes, but also T cells and dendritic cells within the lamina propria. The Peyer's patches have immune functions similar to lymph nodes. The intestinal epithelium over the Peyer's patches contains fewer goblet cells, and thus the mucus layer is thinner here. The epithelium also contains microfold cells (M cells). M cells differ considerably from enterocytes, as they lack microvilli for the absorption of nutrients and are capable of endocytosis and transcytosis of content from the intestinal lumen. The job of the M cells is to sample antigens and bacteria present in the lumen and then present them to the dendritic cells for immune processing. The dendrites present processed antigens to the B lymphocytes (plasma cells) in the lamina propria that produce IgA that can bind specific antigens, which are secreted into the lamina propria.

IgA (immunoglobulin A) provides an adaptive immune response that allows specific binding to antigens, including lipopolysaccharides and other bacterial antigens. Some of the IgA is formed as single units (IgA1) and others as dimer pairs (IgA2). IgA does not activate the immune system in the way IgG does. Mostly, IgA just binds to bacteria, toxins, and immune complexes, disabling them and preventing them from doing harm.[23] IgA can bind LPS and prevent it from promoting an inflammatory response. IgA binding to bacterial fimbriae (pili) can prevent the bacteria from attaching to enterocytes or each other. Single bacteria are generally not pathogenic, but rather have to form colonies on a surface (biofilms) before they begin producing toxins and become invasive. IgA can help prevent this.

IgA acts locally in the lamina propria. More importantly, the IgA is additionally taken into the lymphatic system and then into the bloodstream. From here, it is redistributed to the intestine and is also secreted into the saliva, tears, and vagina.[24] Receptors on the base of the enterocytes and other mucosal epithelial cells bind IgA2 and bring it inside the cell. A secretory component protein is added to the IgA2 by the enterocyte and other mucosal cells, and it is then translocated and secreted as secretory IgA (sIgA). Adults secrete about 3 to 5 grams of sIgA into the intestinal lumen each day.[25] It binds to the mucous layer, preventing the growth of pathogenic bacteria, and it binds to antigens, thus preventing them from affecting the enterocytes or from being absorbed. As the luminal surface layer of the mucus ages and disintegrates, the sIgA continues to function, binding to bacteria and other antigens, and carries them into the stool.

At the onset of lactation, IgA2 is avidly taken up by mammary glands and secreted in concentrated amounts into the colostrum. Thus, early mother's milk can transfer protective adaptive immune sIgA to the infant's intestine. The sIgA can bind to the infant's intestinal mucous layer, where it helps prevent pathogenic bacteria from gaining dominance, allowing commensal bacteria to gain a foothold and colonize the infant's mucus layer. sIgA in colostrum is not absorbed into the infant's bloodstream. Colostrum also contains multiple enzymes, antibacterial agents such as lysozyme and lactoferrin and exosomes.

The sixth line of defense is the commensal enteric microbiome, which helps with digestion, prevents overgrowth of noxious species and toxins they produce, and provides energy and nutrients to the cells lining the intestine and to the body.

The GI microbiome is diverse and functions differently in different areas of the intestine. One component of the mucosal defense is the commensal bacteria that reside in the looser, gelatinous layer of the mucus facing the lumen; they help process nutrients and help prevent the colonization of the mucus by potential pathogens. Different areas of the intestinal mucosa have different commensal bacteria; the small intestine is more likely to have *Lactobacillaceae,* while the colon mucous layer is more likely to have *Bifidobacteria* and many other commensal genera. For example, *B. bifidum* bind and reside in the mucous layer, crowding out other bacteria, while *B. infantis* do not.[26] [27] *Lactobacillaceae* have fimbriae that give them the ability to bind to and colonize the mucus glycoprotein layer in the small intestine, but additionally, these bacteria have fimbriae that allow them to bind directly to mucosal cells. Some *Lactobacilli* strains have many cell-binding fimbriae, while others have little cell-binding capacity.[28] The cell-binding helps crowd out other potentially pathogenic bacteria.

In small animals with thin intestinal mucus layers, *Lactobacillaceae* with an intermediate level of cell-binding give the most protection from pathogenic bacteria, presumably crowding them out, blocking adhesion, preventing biofilm formation, and competing with potential pathogens for nutritional resources.[29] Additionally, the cell-binding stimulates the host immune defense. Nevertheless, *Lactobacillaceae* that have very high enterocyte-binding, such as *L. rhamnosus* GG, cause mucosal injury in these small animals.[30] Rarely, *L. rhamnosus* GG can become pathogenic in severely immunocompromised persons[31] [32] or cause bacteremia in those with severe inflammatory bowel disease and mucosal disruption, [33] [34] as a result of its avid binding to the cell surface.

The colon has a large and diverse microbial population containing numerous genera of bacteria. Most of these either reside in the periphery of the lumen within the degrading superficial layer of mucus, while others live free in the lumen of the cecum and colon, where they ferment nutrients that have not been absorbed by the small intestine. These luminal microbiomes are not directly part of the mucosal defense but serve in digestion, nutrient production, and in health, help prevent the overgrowth of noxious species. *B. infantis*, for example, produces bacteriocins – antibiotic proteins that help prevent the dominance by potentially pathogenic species. [35] Most of the potentially pathogenic bacteria living in the colon are normal commensal residents and don't cause harm unless the system gets out of whack.

Antibiotics can easily disrupt the microbiome, as can toxins, unhealthy diets, stress, nondigestible emulsifiers, and sleep deprivation.

In a strict sense, increased paracellular permeability refers only to the third line of defense, and dysbiosis to unhealthy changes in the microbiome, while "leaky gut" refers to any combination of deficits that allow a pathological increase in transmembrane transport across the intestinal mucosal barrier.

Intestinal Alkaline Phosphatase and Diet

As described above, luminal intestinal alkaline phosphatase (IAP) is the first line of defense against LPS toxicity, dysbiosis, and leaky gut, and thus a critical defense against inflammatory and neurodegenerative diseases.

Any injury to the enterocytes in the small intestine may cause a loss of IAP production. This can occur from a viral gastroenteritis or other disease. Celiac disease, caused by an immune reaction triggered by gluten, is associated with a loss in the production of intestinal alkaline phosphatase and increased risk for dysbiosis and LPS exposure.[36] Wheat, barley, and rye contain enzymes that reduce the formation of IAP (Chapter 7).

Diet and bacteria greatly modulate IAP production. IAP secretion falls during fasting and increases after high-fat meals. Nevertheless, a high-fat diet, such as the Western diet, is associated with lower IAP levels.[37] N-3 PUFA enhanced the production of intestinal alkaline phosphatase (IAP) by the enterocytes;[38] however, very high intake of n-3 fatty acids resulted in lower IAP levels and a higher risk of gut-related sepsis in experimental animals.[39]

Having some dietary fat is clearly required for the production of IAP. Vitamin D3, [40] as well as vitamin K1 (phylloquinone)[41] and K2 (menaquinone),[42] upregulate the transcription of IAP, while vitamin D deficiency suppresses IAP expression and activity.[43] Some dietary fat is needed for the absorption of these fat-soluble vitamins. Additionally, the n-3 fatty acid, eicosapentaenoic acid (EPA), is the substrate for resolvin E1, an eicosanoid that down-regulates inflammation in the gut, in part by inducing the IAP.[44] Thus, deficits in vitamin D, vitamin K, or the n-3 fatty acid EPA are associated with impaired IAP production.

The enzyme IAP includes and requires both zinc and magnesium. Secretion of IAP is increased with dietary calcium but decreased by free phosphorus.[45]

The medications levamisole, aspirin, theophylline, and imipenem inhibit IAP.[46] The artificial sweetener aspartame appears to inhibit IAP activity and may contribute to the development of metabolic syndrome. This may help explain why diet soda does not help in weight reduction.[47]

The production of colonic alkaline phosphatase (IAPL) is greatly influenced by certain dietary fibers. IAPL production in the colon appears to be mediated by butyric acid. Butyrate production in the colon depends on dietary fiber and the bacteria that ferment it. Fructooligosaccharides (FOS), galactooligosaccharides (GOS), raffinose, and lactulose (but not isomaltose oligosaccharides [IMO]) have been demonstrated (in rats) to increase both butyrate production and colonic alkaline phosphatase expression and activity. Of these fibers, only GOS was found to have any effect on small intestinal IAP production, and that effect was small. IMOS is partially digested in the small intestine and is not found to increase alkaline phosphatase activity.[48] Another fiber, wheat arabinoxylan, has been found to promote intestinal barrier function and colonic alkaline phosphatase activity in piglets.[49]

Butyrate increases mucin production and colonocyte turnover rate in the colon. GOS, FOS, raffinose, and lactulose are not the only prebiotics that increase IAP production, but rather represent several that were tested and compared in the study cited; so it does not negate the function of other fiber sources. In addition to butyrate, the fermentation of these prebiotics also produces lactic acid. Lactic acid is not absorbed as readily from the colon; thus, it causes more acidification than does butyric acid. The more acidic milieu favors Bifidobacteria, which help ferment these prebiotics. A significant correlation was found between IALP activity, mucin production, butyrate, and *Bifidobacterium* abundance in this study.

Wheat contains the polysaccharide arabinoxylan that promotes intestinal barrier function as a prebiotic that favors butyrate production, but if there is a compromise of the barrier, there may be insufficient butyrate production to prevent dysbiosis from taking hold. One slice of whole-grain wheat bread contains about one gram of soluble arabinoxylan. White bread contains about one-fifth as much fiber as that in whole wheat bread.[50] Wheat, and particularly typically processed whole wheat, however, causes other problems and should be avoided on the SANA diet. A sanctioned source of arabinoxylan is nixtamalized corn.

What Goes Wrong

The mucin layer is dependent on the health of the mucosal epithelial cells, and particularly of the mucin-2-producing goblet cells. In the proximal small intestine, there is generally sufficient nutrition for these cells, but in the distal small intestine and colon, areas of the highest bacterial load, the nutritional requirements of the cells may be unmet in malnutrition, dysbiosis, or constipation, where transit time is excessive.

Total parenteral nutrition (TPN: intravenous (I.V.) feeding in hospitalized patients, for example) results in a dysfunctional mucosal barrier, with the loss of IAP, mucin-2, and lysozyme; promotes dysbiosis, and allows bacterial translocation into the submucosa.[51] This is one reason that hospitalized patients easily develop Gram-negative pneumonia; it is not from pathogenic bacteria in the hospital, but from those bacteria that live harmoniously in the gut until we stop eating. This can be prevented by partial oral feeding. This is also why the SANA program discourages fasting and suggests modified fasting for those who wish to fast (Chapter 21).

In the distal small intestine, the epithelium requires the amino acid glutamine for normal function, as normally there is little or any sugar to feed the enterocytes this far down the intestines. In mice, even when added to TPN, the addition of glutamine to the I.V. feeding increases mucin-2 and lysozyme production in the small intestine as compared to standard TPN. Glutamine (perhaps after conversion to citrulline by enterocytes) [52] stimulates lamina propria lymphocytes to produce the anti-inflammatory cytokines IL-4, IL-10, and IL-13. This promotes the production of IgA. IL-4 also induces the differentiation of secretory progenitor cells in the mucosal crypts into goblet cells, and IL-10 induces their growth. IL-4 and IL-13 induce increased mucin-2 production.[53] Deficient IL-10 is a common pathogenic mechanism in inflammatory bowel disease (IBD).

The addition of glutamine to TPN prevents the invasion of bacteria into the lamina propria of the animals.[54] Long-term glutamine supplementation helps repair injury to the intestine and maintains intestinal mass into old age in rats.[55] Glutamine is a precursor to citrulline, and its supplementation can augment citrulline production by the enterocyte. Citrulline increases blood flow in the splanchnic (intestinal) circulation to the intestine and helps prevent hypo-perfusion during intense exercise.[56] Citrulline levels increase during exercise if the person is adequately hydrated and has adequate glutamine.[57]

Butyrate helps regulate the expression of the tight junction proteins, improving mucosal barrier function. Butyrate is needed for adequate cell energy for the production of mucin by the colonocytes. Thus, prebiotic fiber and a healthy commensal microbiome are essential for adequate colonocyte nutrition and mucin production. Some butyrate is also present in mother's milk, butter, and Parmesan cheese.

A small number of commensal bacteria are responsible for the majority of butyrate production in the colon; *Faecalibacterium prausnitzii, Roseburia intestinalis, Agathobaculum rectale, Anaerobutyricum hallii, Intestinibacterium symbiosum, and Blautia bromii* are the major butyrate producers. A low-fat, high-fiber diet supports butyrate production. Resistant starch is an important feedstock for butyrate production.[58]

A high-fat Western diet impairs mucosal health; however, the addition of fiber to a high-fat diet improves mucosal function, decreases plasma LPS and circulating macrophages and neutrophils, suggesting reduced systemic inflammation.[59] In mice, a methionine/choline-deficient diet promoted dysbiosis and mucosal inflammation.[60] Rice bran, pea fiber, and many other forms of dietary fiber promote eubiosis and serve to maintain intestinal barrier function.

Eubiosis and avoidance of inflammation help maintain enterocyte tight junctions. The 33-mer α-gliadin peptide formed during the digestion of wheat can disrupt the tight junctions, as can the fungal toxin ochratoxin (Chapter 29) and other dietary or microbial toxins.

Inflammation causes increased permeability of the tight junction. Colonocytes exposed to LPS have decreased production of occludin and ZO-1. This may be in part due to the production of the pro-inflammatory cytokine IL-1β; IL-1β downregulates occludin protein production in colonocytes via its induction of microRNA-200C-3p, which stops occludin-mRNA from forming the occludin protein.[61] MiRNA 200C-3p also suppresses PTEN protein production.[62] Thus, LPS uptake stimulates TLR4 → → IL-1β → miR 200C-3 → ↓occludin and ↓PTEN. Lower production of the protein occludin would be expected to increase exposure to LPS from the colon.

PTEN insufficiency causes mitochondrial dysfunction and oxidative stress. In mice with haploinsufficiency of PTEN (in which the PTEN gene from one parent was defective), there is a 50% decrease in Cytochrome C Oxidase activity in the mitochondria. These mice have normal behavior at 8 to 13 weeks of age, but by 20 to 29 weeks, they exhibit autism-like behaviors, including social avoidance, failure to recognize familiar mice, and repetitive self-grooming. The mice also developed brain overgrowth and macrocephaly. PTEN mutations in humans can result in autism associated with microcephaly.[63] [64] [65] Additionally, defects in cytochrome c oxidase have been reported in both ASD and Alzheimer's disease.

Environmental Toxins and Dysbiosis

The herbicide glyphosate not only kills many plants but also kills many bacteria. *Clostridioides* species and some strains of *Salmonella* are resistant to glyphosate, and thus exposure to this compound can alter the GI microbiome, favoring the dominance of pathogenic bacteria.[66] When mice were exposed to glyphosate, it shifted the abundance of the gut microbiome, decreasing the abundance of *Corynebacterium, Firmicutes, Bacteroidota,* and *Lactobacillus,* and caused anxiety and depression-like behaviors.[67] The disruption of the gut microbiome from glyphosate is not limited to mice; it has been observed in bees, crabs, and turtles.[68] [69] [70] While glyphosate-induced dysbiosis is possible in humans, it is likely rare other than those who work with this chemical.

Ethanol increases paracellular permeability by causing the dislocation of the tight junction proteins zonulin, occludin-1 (ZO-1), and claudin.[71] Yeast can cause the tight junctions to reversibly open by activating actin within the enterocytes.[72] The toxic metal cadmium, even in low amounts, induces an inflammatory response in the intestine that damages tight junctions and increases paracellular activity. Cadmium also causes perturbations in the GI microbiome that are accompanied by increased production of LPS, a decrease in short-chain fatty acid (SCFA) producing species, inhibited glutathione metabolism and glutathione conjugation, and removal of toxins.[73]

As previously mentioned, antibiotics can also cause dysbiosis by killing commensal bacteria and selecting for a much reduced diversity of antibiotic-resistant bacterial species.

Diet

To briefly recap and add to the discussion of the impact of diet on dysbiosis discussed in Chapter 3:

- Lack of fermentable fiber can cause the depletion of bacteria that process that fiber and a loss in the production of short-chain fatty acids, which the colonocytes rely on. When the colonocytes are deprived of sufficient butyrate, the production of mucin slows, but the bacteria consuming it continue to feed on it. This causes a depletion of the mucus layer, allowing for bacteria to adhere to the cell surface. This promotes leaky gut and migration of bacteria across the mucosal membrane.
- Bactericidal compounds in food may cause the loss of subsets of bacteria.
- Non-nutrient emulsifiers can break down the mucus, allowing for biofilm growth.
- The incomplete digestion of protein can allow undigested protein to enter the cecum and colon, where it is fermented and can produce toxic compounds such as *p*-cresol, hydrogen sulfide, branched-chain fatty acids, and phenylacetate.

Some things that may increase the fermentation of protein/ amino acids in the colon include:

- SIBO (Small intestinal bacterial overgrowth), dumping syndrome, and malabsorption of sugars (for example, lactose intolerance) can cause rapid transit of the food from a meal to the cecum before it has time to fully digest and allow absorption of amino acids, dipeptides, and tripeptides.
- Lack of stomach acid, or proteolytic digestive enzymes and intestinal peptidases can interfere with the digestion of protein. Pancreatic insufficiency can limit the production of pancreatic enzymes. A lack

of intestinal peptidases can occur from injury to the mucosa, which might result from viral infection, Celiac disease, or inflammatory injury to the small intestine.

- Swallowing food pieces large enough to resist digestion or consumption of a very high-protein diet. This can happen in those with poor dentition and those who eat hurriedly.
- Slow colonic transit. Slower colonic transit is associated with reduced amounts of *Faecalibacterium prausnitzii* and increased abundance of *Methanobrevibacter*, accompanied by elevated production of *p*-cresol, indoles, and other microbial products of protein catabolism. The bacteria want to eat, and those deprived of carbohydrate-based fiber may adapt to the fermentation of proteins.[74]

[1] The first brain: Species comparisons and evolutionary implications for the enteric and central nervous systems. Furness JB, Stebbing MJ. Neurogastroenterol Motil. 2018 Feb;30(2). doi: 10.1111/nmo.13234. PMID: 29024273

[2] https://en.wikipedia.org/wiki/Encephalization_quotient

[3] The expanded biology of serotonin. Berger M, Gray JA, Roth BL. Annu Rev Med. 2009;60:355-66. doi: 10.1146/annurev.med.60.042307.110802. PMID: 19630576

[4] Enteric Nervous System Regulation of Intestinal Stem Cell Differentiation and Epithelial Monolayer Function. Puzan, M., Hosic, S., Ghio, C. *et al. Sci Rep* **8**, 6313 (2018). https://doi.org/10.1038/s41598-018-24768-3 https://www.nature.com/articles/s41598-018-24768-3

[5] The Microbiota-Gut-Brain Axis in Neuropsychiatric Disorders: Pathophysiological Mechanisms and Novel Treatments. Kim YK, Shin C. Curr Neuropharmacol. 2018;16(5):559-573. doi: 10.2174/1570159X15666170915141036. PMID: 28925886

[6] Ingestion of Lactobacillus strain regulates emotional behavior and central GABA receptor expression in a mouse via the vagus nerve. Bravo JA, Forsythe P, Chew MV, Escaravage E, Savignac HM, Dinan TG, Bienenstock J, Cryan JF. Proc Natl Acad Sci U S A. 2011 Sep 20;108(38):16050-5. doi: 10.1073/pnas.1102999108. PMID: 21876150

[7] Nutritional Regulation of Gut Barrier Integrity in Weaning Piglets. Modina SC, Polito U, Rossi R, Corino C, Di Giancamillo A. Animals (Basel). 2019 Nov 29;9(12):1045. doi: 10.3390/ani9121045. PMID: 31795348

[8] The bowel and beyond: the enteric nervous system in neurological disorders. Rao M, Gershon MD. Nat Rev Gastroenterol Hepatol. 2016 Sep;13(9):517-28. doi: 10.1038/nrgastro.2016.107. PMID: 27435372

[9] Age-dependent shift in macrophage polarisation causes inflammation-mediated degeneration of enteric nervous system. Becker L, Nguyen L, Gill J, Kulkarni S, Pasricha PJ, Habtezion A. Gut. 2018 May;67(5):827-836. doi: 10.1136/gutjnl-2016-312940. PMID: 28228489

[10] Glial cells in the mouse enteric nervous system can undergo neurogenesis in response to injury. Laranjeira C, Sandgren K, Kessaris N, et al. J Clin Invest. 2011 Sep;121 (9):3412-24. doi: 10.1172/JCI58200PMID: 21865647

[11] Adult enteric nervous system in health is maintained by a dynamic balance between neuronal apoptosis and neurogenesis. Kulkarni S, Micci MA, Leser J, Shin C, Tang SC, Fu YY, Liu L, Li Q, Saha M, Li C, Enikolopov G, Becker L, Rakhilin N, Anderson M, Shen X, Dong X, Butte MJ, Song H, Southard-Smith EM, Kapur RP, Bogunovic M, Pasricha PJ. Proc Natl Acad Sci U S A. 2017 May 2;114(18):E3709-E3718. doi: 10.1073/pnas.1619406114. PMID: 28420791

[12] CpG motifs in bacterial DNA and their immune effects. Krieg AM. Annu Rev Immunol. 2002;20:709-60. doi: 10.1146/annurev.immunol.20.100301.064842. PMID: 11861616

[13] Identification of specific targets for the gut mucosal defense factor intestinal alkaline phosphatase. Chen KT, Malo MS, Moss AK, Zeller S, Johnson P, Ebrahimi F, Mostafa G, Alam SN, Ramasamy S, Warren HS, Hohmann EL, Hodin RA. Am J Physiol Gastrointest Liver Physiol. 2010 Aug;299(2):G467-75. doi: 10.1152/ajpgi.00364.2009. PMID: 20489044

[14] Intestinal Barrier Dysfunction, LPS Translocation, and Disease Development. Ghosh SS, Wang J, Yannie PJ, Ghosh S. J Endocr Soc. 2020 Feb 20;4(2):bvz039. doi: 10.1210/jendso/bvz039. PMID: 32099951

[15] A role for intestinal alkaline phosphatase in the maintenance of local gut immunity. Chen KT, Malo MS, Beasley-Topliffe LK, Poelstra K, Millan JL, Mostafa G, Alam SN, Ramasamy S, Warren HS, Hohmann EL, Hodin RA. Dig Dis Sci. 2011 Apr;56(4):1020-7. doi: 10.1007/s10620-010-1396-x. PMID: 20844955

[16] Microbiota-host interplay at the gut epithelial level, health and nutrition. Lallès JP. J Anim Sci Biotechnol. 2016 Nov 8;7:66. doi: 10.1186/s40104-016-0123-7. PMID: 27833747

[17] Alkaline Phosphatase, an Unconventional Immune Protein. Rader BA. Front Immunol. 2017 Aug 3;8:897. doi: 10.3389/fimmu.2017.00897. PMID: 28824625

[18] Consumption of non-digestible oligosaccharides elevates colonic alkaline phosphatase activity by up-regulating the expression of IAP-I, with increased mucins and microbial fermentation in rats fed a high-fat diet. Okazaki Y, Katayama T. Br J Nutr. 2019 Jan;121(2):146-154. doi: 10.1017/S0007114518003082. PMID: 30400998

[19] The inner of the two Muc2 mucin-dependent mucus layers in colon is devoid of bacteria. Hansson GC, Johansson ME. Gut Microbes. 2010 Jan;1(1):51-54. doi: 10.4161/gmic.1.1.10470. PMID: 21327117

[20] Role of Corticotropin-releasing Factor in Gastrointestinal Permeability. Rodiño-Janeiro BK, Alonso-Cotoner C, Pigrau M, Lobo B, Vicario M, Santos J. J Neurogastroenterol Motil. 2015 Jan 1;21(1):33-50. doi: 10.5056/jnm14084. PMID: 25537677

[21] Involvement of enteric nerves in permeability changes due to deoxycholic acid in rat jejunum in vivo. Fihn BM, Sjöqvist A, Jodal M. Acta Physiol Scand. 2003 Jul;178(3):241-50. doi: 10.1046/j.1365-201X.2003.01144.x. PMID: 12823182

[22] Microbiota and gut neuropeptides: a dual action of antimicrobial activity and neuroimmune response. Aresti Sanz J, El Aidy S. Psychopharmacology (Berl). 2019 May;236(5):1597-1609. doi: 10.1007/s00213-019-05224-0. PMID: 30997526

[23] Let's go mucosal: communication on slippery ground. Brandtzaeg P, Pabst R. Trends Immunol. 2004 Nov;25(11):570-7. doi: 10.1016/j.it.2004.09.005. PMID: 15489184

[24] Routes of immunization and antigen delivery systems for optimal mucosal immune responses in humans. Mestecky J, Michalek SM, Moldoveanu Z, Russell MW. Behring Inst Mitt. 1997 Feb;(98):33-43. PMID: 9382757

[25] Let's go mucosal: communication on slippery ground. Brandtzaeg P, Pabst R. Trends Immunol. 2004 Nov;25(11):570-7. doi: 10.1016/j.it.2004.09.005. PMID: 15489184

[26] Selection of bifidobacteria based on adhesion and anti-inflammatory capacity in vitro for amelioration of murine colitis. Preising J, Philippe D, Gleinser M, Wei H, Blum S, Eikmanns BJ, Niess JH, Riedel CU. Appl Environ Microbiol. 2010 May;76(9):3048-51. doi: 10.1128/AEM.03127-09. PMID:20228095

[27] Lactobacillus rhamnosus GG Outcompetes Enterococcus faecium via Mucus-Binding Pili: Evidence for a Novel and Heterospecific Probiotic Mechanism. Tytgat HL, Douillard FP, Reunanen J, Rasinkangas P, Hendrickx AP, Laine PK, Paulin L, Satokari R, de Vos WM. Appl Environ Microbiol. 2016 Sep 16;82(19):5756-62. doi: 10.1128/AEM.01243-16. PMID:27422834

[28] Comparative genomic and functional analysis of 100 Lactobacillus rhamnosus strains and their comparison with strain GG. Douillard FP, Ribbera A, Kant R, Pietilä TE, Järvinen HM, Messing M, Randazzo CL, Paulin L, Laine P, Ritari J, Caggia C, Lähteinen T, Brouns SJ, Satokari R, von Ossowski I, Reunanen J, Palva A, de Vos WM. PLoS Genet. 2013;9(8):e1003683. doi: 10.1371/journal.pgen.1003683. PMID: 23966868

[29] Antifungal defense of probiotic Lactobacillus rhamnosus GG is mediated by blocking adhesion and nutrient depletion. Mailänder-Sánchez D, Braunsdorf C, Grumaz C, Müller C, Lorenz S, Stevens P, Wagener J, Hebecker B, Hube B, Bracher F, Sohn K, Schaller M. PLoS One. 2017 Oct 12;12(10):e0184438. doi: 10.1371/journal.pone.0184438. PMID: 29023454

[30] Anti-Infective Effect of Adhesive Probiotic Lactobacillus in Fish is Correlated with Their Spatial Distribution in the Intestinal Tissue. He S, Ran C, Qin C, Li S, Zhang H, de Vos WM, Ringø E, Zhou Z. Sci Rep. 2017 Oct 16;7(1):13195. doi: 10.1038/s41598-017-13466-1. PMID: 29038557

[31] Lactobacillus probiotic use in cardiothoracic transplant recipients: a link to invasive Lactobacillus infection? Luong ML, Sareyyupoglu B, Nguyen MH, Silveira FP, Shields RK, Potoski BA, Pasculle WA, Clancy CJ, Toyoda Y. Transpl Infect Dis. 2010 Dec;12(6):561-4. doi: 10.1111/j.1399-3062.2010.00580.x. PMID: 21040283

[32] Lactobacillus rhamnosus meningitis following recurrent episodes of bacteremia in a child undergoing allogeneic hematopoietic stem cell transplantation. Robin F, Paillard C, Marchandin H, Demeocq F, Bonnet R, Hennequin C. J Clin Microbiol. 2010 Nov;48(11):4317-9. doi: 10.1128/JCM.00250-10. PMID: 20844225

[33] Breakthrough Lactobacillus rhamnosus GG bacteremia associated with probiotic use in an adult patient with severe active ulcerative colitis: case report and review of the literature. Meini S, Laureano R, Fani L, Tascini C, Galano A, Antonelli A, Rossolini GM. Infection. 2015 Dec;43(6):777-81. doi: 10.1007/s15010-015-0798-2. PMID: 26024568

[34] Lactobacillus bacteremia associated with probiotic use in a pediatric patient with ulcerative colitis. Vahabnezhad E, Mochon AB, Wozniak LJ, Ziring DA. J Clin Gastroenterol. 2013 May-Jun;47(5):437-9. doi: 10.1097/MCG.0b013e318279abf0. PMID: 23426446

[35] Bifidobacteria-Insight into clinical outcomes and mechanisms of its probiotic action. Sarkar A, Mandal S. Microbiol Res. 2016 Nov;192:159-171. doi: 10.1016/j.micres.2016.07.001. PMID:27664734

[36] The Role of Intestinal Alkaline Phosphatase in Inflammatory Disorders of Gastrointestinal Tract. Bilski J, Mazur-Bialy A, Wojcik D, Zahradnik-Bilska J, Brzozowski B, Magierowski M, Mach T, Magierowska K, Brzozowski T. Mediators Inflamm. 2017;2017:9074601. doi: 10.1155/2017/9074601. PMID: 28316376

[37] Intestine-specific expression of human chimeric intestinal alkaline phosphatase attenuates Western diet-induced barrier dysfunction and glucose intolerance. Ghosh SS, He H, Wang J, Korzun W, Yannie PJ, Ghosh S. Physiol Rep. 2018 Jul;6(14):e13790. doi: 10.14814/phy2.13790. PMID: 30058275

[38] A host-microbiome interaction mediates the opposing effects of omega-6 and omega-3 fatty acids on metabolic endotoxemia. Kaliannan K, Wang B, Li XY, Kim KJ, Kang JX. Sci Rep. 2015 Jun 11;5:11276. doi: 10.1038/srep11276. PMID: 26062993

[39] Interplay between intestinal alkaline phosphatase, diet, gut microbes and immunity. Estaki M, DeCoffe D, Gibson DL. World J Gastroenterol. 2014 Nov 14;20(42):15650-6. doi: 10.3748/wjg.v20.i42.15650. PMID: 25400448

[40] 1-alpha,25-Dihydroxyvitamin D_3 up-regulates the expression of 2 types of human intestinal alkaline phosphatase alternative splicing variants in Caco-2 cells and may be an important regulator of their expression in gut homeostasis. Noda S, Yamada A, Nakaoka K, Goseki-Sone M. Nutr Res. 2017 Oct;46:59-67. doi: 10.1016/j.nutres.2017.07.005. PMID: 28931466

[41] Vitamin K1 (phylloquinone) or vitamin K2 (menaquinone-4) induces intestinal alkaline phosphatase gene expression. Haraikawa M, Sogabe N, Tanabe R, Hosoi T, Goseki-Sone M. J Nutr Sci Vitaminol (Tokyo). 2011;57(4):274-9. doi: 10.3177/jnsv.57.274. PMID: 22041909

[42] Menaquinone-4 (vitamin K_2) up-regulates expression of human intestinal alkaline phosphatase in Caco-2 cells. Noda S, Yamada A, Tanabe R, Nakaoka K, Hosoi T, Goseki-Sone M. Nutr Res. 2016 Nov;36(11):1269-1276. doi: 10.1016/j.nutres.2016.10.001. PMID: 27865621

[43] Vitamin D-restricted high-fat diet down-regulates expression of intestinal alkaline phosphatase isozymes in ovariectomized rats. Nakaoka K, Yamada A, Noda S, Goseki-Sone M. Nutr Res. 2018 May;53:23-31. doi: 10.1016/j.nutres.2018.03.001. PMID: 29804586

[44] Resolvin E1-induced intestinal alkaline phosphatase promotes resolution of inflammation through LPS detoxification. Campbell EL, MacManus CF, Kominsky DJ, Keely S, Glover LE, Bowers BE, Scully M, Bruyninckx WJ, Colgan SP. Proc Natl Acad Sci U S A. 2010 Aug 10;107(32):14298-303. doi: 10.1073/pnas.0914730107. PMID: 20660763

[45] Microbiota-host interplay at the gut epithelial level, health and nutrition. Lallès JP. J Anim Sci Biotechnol. 2016 Nov 8;7:66. doi: 10.1186/s40104-016-0123-7. PMID: 27833747

[46] https://brenda-enzymes.org/enzyme.php?ecno=3.1.3.1#

[47] Inhibition of the gut enzyme intestinal alkaline phosphatase may explain how aspartame promotes glucose intolerance and obesity in mice. Gul SS, Hamilton AR, Munoz AR, Phupitakphol T, Liu W, Hyoju SK, Economopoulos KP, Morrison S, Hu D, Zhang W, Gharedaghi MH, Huo H, Hamarneh SR, Hodin RA. Appl Physiol Nutr Metab. 2017 Jan;42(1):77-83. doi: 10.1139/apnm-2016-0346. Epub 2016 Nov 18. PMID: 27997218

[48] Consumption of non-digestible oligosaccharides elevates colonic alkaline phosphatase activity by up-regulating the expression of IAP-I, with increased mucins and microbial fermentation in rats fed a high-fat diet. Okazaki Y, Katayama T. Br J Nutr. 2019 Jan;121(2):146-154. doi: 10.1017/S0007114518003082. PMID: 30400998

[49] Arabinoxylan in wheat is more responsible than cellulose for promoting intestinal barrier function in weaned male piglets. Chen H, Wang W, Degroote J, Possemiers S, Chen D, De Smet S, Michiels J. J Nutr. 2015 Jan;145(1):51-8. doi: 10.3945/jn.114.201772. PMID: 25378684

[50] Authorised EU health claim for arabinoxylan. Nicole J. Kellow, Karen Z. Walker, in Foods, Nutrients and Food Ingredients with Authorised EU Health Claims, 2018 https://www.sciencedirect.com/topics/agricultural-and-biological-sciences/arabinoxylan

[51] Partial Enteral Nutrition Preserves Elements of Gut Barrier Function, Including Innate Immunity, Intestinal Alkaline Phosphatase (IAP) Level, and Intestinal Microbiota in Mice. Wan X, Bi J, Gao X, Tian F, Wang X, Li N, Li J. Nutrients. 2015 Aug 3;7(8):6294-312. doi: 10.3390/nu7085288. PMID: 26247961

[52] Reciprocal regulation of Th2 and Th17 cells by PAD2-mediated citrullination. Sun B, Chang HH, Salinger A, Tomita B, Bawadekar M, Holmes CL, Shelef MA, Weerapana E, Thompson PR, Ho IC. JCI Insight. 2019 Nov 14;4(22):e129687. doi: 10.1172/jci.insight.129687. PMID: 31723060

[53] Intestinal development and differentiation. Noah TK, Donahue B, Shroyer NF. Exp Cell Res. 2011 Nov 15;317(19):2702-10. doi: 10.1016/j.yexcr.2011.09.006. PMID: 21978911

[54] Glutamine Improves Innate Immunity and Prevents Bacterial Enteroinvasion During Parenteral Nutrition. Wang X, Pierre JF, Heneghan AF, Busch RA, Kudsk KA. JPEN J Parenter Enteral Nutr. 2015 Aug;39(6):688-97. doi: 10.1177/0148607114535265. PMID: 24836948

[55] Long-term intermittent glutamine supplementation repairs intestinal damage (structure and functional mass) with advanced age: assessment with plasma citrulline in a rodent model. Beaufrère AM, Neveux N, Patureau Mirand P, Buffière C, Marceau G, Sapin V, Cynober L, Meydinal-Denis D. J Nutr Health Aging. 2014 Nov;18(9):814-9. doi: 10.1007/s12603-014-0554-9. PMID: 25389959

[56] L-citrulline improves splanchnic perfusion and reduces gut injury during exercise. van Wijck K, Wijnands KA, Meesters DM, Boonen B, van Loon LJ, Buurman WA, Dejong CH, Lenaerts K, Poeze M. Med Sci Sports Exerc. 2014 Nov;46(11):2039-46. doi: 10.1249/MSS.0000000000000332. PMID: 24621960

[57] Plasma citrulline concentration, a marker for intestinal functionality, reflects exercise intensity in healthy young men. Kartaram S, Mensink M, Teunis M, Schoen E, Witte G, Janssen Duijghuijsen L, Verschuren M, Mohrmann K, M'Rabet L, Knipping K, Wittink H, van Helvoort A, Garssen J, Witkamp R, Pieters R, van Norren K. Clin Nutr. 2019 Oct;38(5):2251-2258. doi: 10.1016/j.clnu.2018.09.029. PMID: 30340895

[58] Formation of short chain fatty acids by the gut microbiota and their impact on human metabolism. Morrison DJ, Preston T. Gut Microbes. 2016 May 3;7(3):189-200. doi: 10.1080/19490976.2015.1134082. PMID: 26963409

[59] Dietary Supplementation with Galactooligosaccharides Attenuates High-Fat, High-Cholesterol Diet-Induced Glucose Intolerance and Disruption of Colonic Mucin Layer in C57BL/6 Mice and Reduces Atherosclerosis in Ldlr-/- Mice. Ghosh SS, Wang J, Yannie PJ, Sandhu YK, Korzun WJ, Ghosh S. J Nutr. 2020 Feb 1;150(2):285-293. doi: 10.1093/jn/nxz233. PMID: 31586202

[60] Fructo-oligosaccharides and intestinal barrier function in a methionine-choline-deficient mouse model of nonalcoholic steatohepatitis. Matsumoto K, Ichimura M, Tsuneyama K, Moritoki Y, Tsunashima H, Omagari K, Hara M, Yasuda I, Miyakawa H, Kikuchi K. PLoS One. 2017 Jun 20;12(6):e0175406. doi: 10.1371/journal.pone.0175406. PMID: 28632732

[61] IL1B Increases Intestinal Tight Junction Permeability by Upregulation of MIR200C-3p, Which Degrades Occludin mRNA. Rawat M, Nighot M, Al-Sadi R, Gupta Y, Viszwapriya D, Yochum G, Koltun W, Ma TY. Gastroenterology. 2020 Jun 19:S0016-5085(20)34838-1. doi: 10.1053/j.gastro.2020.06.038. PMID: 32569770

[62] Ferulic Acid Ameliorates Lipopolysaccharide-Induced Barrier Dysfunction via MicroRNA-**200c**-3p-Mediated Activation of PI3K/AKT Pathway in Caco-2 Cells. He S, Guo Y, Zhao J, Xu X, Wang N, Liu Q. Front Pharmacol. 2020 Apr 3;11:376. doi: 10.3389/fphar.2020.00376. PMID: 32308620

[63] Pten haploinsufficient mice show broad brain overgrowth but selective impairments in autism-relevant behavioral tests. Clipperton-Allen AE, Page DT. Hum Mol Genet. 2014 Jul 1;23(13):3490-505. doi: 10.1093/hmg/ddu057. PMID: 24497577

[64] Mitochondrial dysfunction in Pten haplo-insufficient mice with social deficits and repetitive behavior: interplay between Pten and p53. Napoli E, Ross-Inta C, Wong S, Hung C, Fujisawa Y, Sakaguchi D, Angelastro J, Omanska-Klusek A, Schoenfeld R, Giulivi C. PLoS One. 2012;7(8):e42504. doi: 10.1371/journal.pone.0042504. PMID: 22900024

[65] Balancing Proliferation and Connectivity in PTEN-associated Autism Spectrum Disorder. Tilot AK, Frazier TW 2nd, Eng C. Neurotherapeutics. 2015 Jul;12(3):609-19. doi: 10.1007/s13311-015-0356-8. PMID: 25916396

[66] Gut microbiota and neurological effects of glyphosate. Rueda-Ruzafa L, Cruz F, Roman P, Cardona D. Neurotoxicology. 2019 Dec;75:1-8. doi: 10.1016/j.neuro.2019.08.006. PMID: 31442459

[67] Glyphosate based- herbicide exposure affects gut microbiota, anxiety and depression-like behaviors in mice. Aitbali Y, Ba-M'hamed S, Elhidar N, Nafis A, Soraa N, Bennis M. Neurotoxicol Teratol. 2018 May-Jun;67:44-49. doi: 10.1016/j.ntt.2018.04.002. PMID: 29635013

[68] Glyphosate perturbs the gut microbiota of honey bees. Motta EVS, Raymann K, Moran NA. Proc Natl Acad Sci U S A. 2018 Oct 9;115(41):10305-10310. doi: 10.1073/pnas.1803880115. PMID: 30249635

[69] Effects of the glyphosate-based herbicide roundup on the survival, immune response, digestive activities and gut microbiota of the Chinese mitten crab, Eriocheir sinensis. Yang X, Song Y, Zhang C, Pang Y, Song X, Wu M, Cheng Y. Aquat Toxicol. 2019 Sep;214:105243. doi: 10.1016/j.aquatox.2019.105243. PMID: 31319294

[70] Effects of glyphosate herbicide on the gastrointestinal microflora of Hawaiian green turtles (Chelonia mydas) Linnaeus. Kittle RP, McDermid KJ, Muehlstein L, Balazs GH. Mar Pollut Bull. 2018 Feb;127:170-174. doi: 10.1016/j.marpolbul.2017.11.030. PMID: 29475651

[71] Flavonoid composition of orange peel extract ameliorates alcohol-induced tight junction dysfunction in Caco-2 monolayer. Chen XM, Kitts DD. Food Chem Toxicol. 2017 Jul;105:398-406. doi: 10.1016/j.fct. 2017.04.009. PMID: 28412402

[72] Disruption of epithelial tight junctions by yeast enhances the paracellular delivery of a model protein. Fuller E, Duckham C, Wood E. Pharm Res. 2007 Jan;24(1):37-47. doi: 10.1007/s11095-006-9124-0. PMID: 16969693

[73] Gut as a target for cadmium toxicity. Tinkov AA, Gritsenko VA, Skalnaya MG, Cherkasov SV, Aaseth J, Skalny AV. Environ Pollut. 2018 Apr;235:429-434. doi: 10.1016/j.envpol.2017.12.114. PMID: 29310086

[74] Gastrointestinal Transit Time, Glucose Homeostasis and Metabolic Health: Modulation by Dietary Fibers. Müller M, Canfora EE, Blaak EE. Nutrients. 2018 Feb 28;10(3):275. doi: 10.3390/nu10030275. PMID: 29495569

6: Fruit

The Plums

Recall from Chapter 2 that those eating at least 6 to 7 servings of fruits and vegetables per day had higher mood, greater life satisfaction than those eating less. The goal of the SANA diet is to make people happier by providing them with better health and mental function. Thus, the diet recommends enjoying 6 to 8 servings of fruits each day. Nevertheless, not all fruits and vegetables promote vitality and a sense of flourishing.

This chapter provides recommendations on which fruits provide the most benefit to gastrointestinal and overall health, and which the least.

- ☹ Many of the most popular fruits get poor marks: Strawberries, apples, bananas, and pears.
- The skin of most types of fruit should not be eaten.
- Some of the highest rated fruits include:
    - Stone fruit: cherries, peaches, apricots, and plums
    - Citrus fruit, especially tangerines and oranges
    - Melons, such as honeydew and watermelons
    - Tropical fruit including pineapples, mangoes, papayas, and guavas
    - Berries such as blackberries, raspberries, and mulberries
    - Fig and dates.
- While fresh fruits are the best bet, frozen and canned fruit can provide servings of fruit when fresh fruit is not available.

Why Fruit Fails

Most epidemiologic studies and clinical trials have failed to find that the consumption of fruit lowers the risk or slows the progression of Alzheimer's Disease (AD). In a meta-analysis (combining the results) of 16 dietary consumption studies, no significant decrease in the incidence of AD was found with higher levels of fruit consumption; however, an inverse association with risk of AD and the consumption of vegetables has been documented.[1] In a review of eleven cross-sectional studies, including the Mediterranean, DASH, and MIND diets, fruit consumption was associated with better cognitive function in only one study, but in another, more reliable longitudinal study, fruit consumption was associated with a higher prevalence of mild cognitive impairment. In a 12-year longitudinal study, higher consumption of berries was not found to be protective.[2]

In a study of the British population, people were asked the number of pieces of fresh fruit and dried fruit they consumed per day, and this data was later analyzed to assess any correlation with the diagnosis of AD. There was no association between fresh fruit consumption and later diagnosis of AD. The odds ratio was 0.97 with a confidence interval of 0.50 to 1.91 (half to about double risk), where 1.0 shows no relationship. This is as close to a null result as you would expect from something known to have no effect. Dried fruit consumption, however, was found to be strongly associated with AD risk. People at the 66th percentile for dried fruit consumption were found to be 3 times more likely to develop AD.[3]

While the Mediterranean and DASH diets are high in fruits, the MIND diet only recommends berries, as they are the only fruits found with any population-based evidence for a lower risk of AD.

While ample studies are showing a lack of effect of fruit consumption in reducing the risk of AD or other forms of dementia in the population data, I contend that the problem is not that fruit cannot help prevent dementia, but rather stems from which fruits are eaten.

The SANA diet takes a granular approach to assessing the impact of each fruit individually, rather than lumping all fruits in one (fruit) or two (berries vs. other fruit) baskets, as do most population studies. Some fruits are helpful, others have minimal impact, and some may have an adverse impact on the GI microbiome.

> Imagine a classroom full of 3rd graders; some are sweet, most are terrors, and if any are like I was, they sit quietly and act like vegetables. Some are tiny, and others weigh more than the teacher. Despite being about the same age and in the same class, they are not all alike.
>
> (Thinking about elementary school makes me shudder! I spent most of my third grade staring at the sky through the large classroom windows, daydreaming. In fourth grade, I was white-knuckled, holding the edges of my desk, terrorized by Mrs. Wilson. By 5th grade, I learned how to malinger and stay home with my mother, creating memories I treasure.)

As discussed in Chapter 2, the SANA diet rates individual fruits and other foods on a ten-level scale. The scores assess the food's overall impact on the microbiome, gastrointestinal integrity, and inflammation. Thus, foods that are considered to promote dysbiosis, leaky gut, and systemic inflammation are rated low, and those that promote a symbiotic, anti-inflammatory nourishment are rated higher.

5: Foods with outstanding benefits on the intestinal microbiome and gastrointestinal integrity

4: Foods that provide excellent antiinflammatory activity. And support gastrointestinal (GI) and general health.

3: Foods that strongly promote intestinal and general health.

2: Foods that promote GI and general health.

1: Foods that mildly favor a healthy microbiome.

0: Foods that have little net impact.

A: Avoid: Foods that have mildly adverse impacts on GI and general health.

B: Beware: Foods that have significant adverse impacts on GI and general health.

C: Condemned: Foods that have strongly adverse impacts on GI and general health.

D: Disastrous: Foods that disrupt GI and general health.

Fruit consumption, as a whole, fails to prevent dementia. This is likely the result of which fruits are and are not being eaten.

Bananas are the most consumed fresh fruit in the U.S., with more than a quarter (26 – 27%) of all fruit being consumed being bananas. Technically, bananas are berries, but that is not what the MIND diet has in mind when it recommends berries. The SANA diet gives bananas a DAD score of zero; they are not meaningfully helpful or harmful to the microbiome of GI integrity and are neither inflammatory nor anti-inflammatory. They are a pleasant snack but should likely be avoided by diabetics.

The next most commonly eaten fruit is apples, comprising 15 – 16% of the total mass of fresh fruits consumed. Apples receive a rating of A, indicating that they are non-beneficial and have a mild dysbiotic effect. The main problem with apples is their skin, but even when the skin is removed, apples just barely rate a score of one. Thus, peeled apples can be used on the SANA diet, but are one of the least beneficial fruits for health.

The Red Delicious, Macintosh, Fuji, and other modern apples are highly selected strains chosen for their large size and sweetness. They are quite different from wild apples or the apples planted by Johnathan Chapman (Johnny Appleseed), which were used for making cider, and were tart.

The third most commonly consumed fresh fruit is grapes, which account for about 8 – 9% of the consumption of fresh fruit. Grapes earn an acceptable score of 1 on the DAD rankings. When eating grapes, black grapes are better than red ones, which are better than green grapes for the prevention of AD, from the higher amounts of phenolic compounds in the darker ones. Thus, when there is a choice, choose the black ones. They still only earn a DAD score of one.

The fourth most commonly consumed fruit is strawberries, comprising about 5% of all fresh fruit consumption. Strawberries — not actually a berry — earn a B on the DAD ranking scale, meaning they should be avoided.

Moreover, strawberries have the highest level of pesticide contamination among fruits and vegetables, followed by spinach, kale, and collard greens.[4] The pesticide does not wash off, and strawberries are not peeled. With many fruits, the pesticide cannot be discarded with the peel. Strawberries grown for processing — freezing, jams, and manufactured foods — were found to have high levels of pesticide contamination.

Pesticide Risks

Testing performed by the U.S. Department of Agriculture analyzed pesticide levels in nearly 30,000 samples of produce covering 25 fruits and 34 vegetables. When pesticide is properly used, the amounts of pesticide residue on food should be low, but about 8% of samples had excessive levels. That is approximately one in 12 samples. Of the 100 samples of produce with the highest levels of pesticide contamination, 52 originated in Mexico, mostly strawberries and green beans.

Some of the foods with the highest risk of dangerous levels of pesticide contamination were bell peppers, blueberries, celery, collard greens, green beans, potatoes, and strawberries. Most potatoes are treated after harvesting with chlorpropham to prevent them from sprouting. Mustard greens, kale, and spinach frequently have levels of pesticide residues.

Apples, pears, grapes, and peaches have a moderate risk of pesticide contamination. Grapes should be washed, and these other fruits washed and peeled. While some produce is more likely to be contaminated with pesticides than others, it is important to consider overall pesticide exposure. All fresh produce should be thoroughly washed.

Washing grapes: Soak the grapes for 5 – 10 minutes in cool water, with 1 – 2 teaspoons of baking soda. Then swirl the water and let the baking soda water drain off, and rinse the grapes with fresh water in a colander. Let them air dry before placing them in a ventilated bag in a cool section of the refrigerator. If they are too moist, they are likely to mold.

Watermelons are at moderately high risk of contamination, and it is not just the outside of the melon at risk. About 3% of domestically grown watermelon samples had high pesticide levels on the inside of the melon. Cantaloupes are a safer bet.[5] [6]

Bananas, apples, and strawberries comprise nearly half of all fresh fruit consumed, and they are rated by the SANA diet as being among the poorest choices of available fruits. On average, these three fruits earn a neutral to negative DAD score, especially if the skin of apples is eaten.

There are, however, great fruits that do help promote a healthy GI microbiome and general health, have anti-inflammatory effects, and help prevent diseases associated with dysbiosis. These include stone fruit (peaches, nectarines, plums, prunes, cherries), some citrus fruits, pineapple, blueberries, raspberries, mangoes, and kiwi fruit.

Table 6A shows DAD scores for the 22 most commonly consumed fresh fruits in the U.S. in descending order of total tonnage of fresh fruit consumption, plus a few less commonly consumed fruits. Note that the scores represent a typical rating for mature, fully-ripe fruit in good condition. Unripe and overripe fruit do not score as well.

Health Heroes

The term "superfoods" as it is generally used describes the latest fad in pseudoscience that some blogger wants to pitch or make a buck from. Some foods touted as being superfoods include sea moss, black garlic, bone broth, goji leaf tea, coconut oil, noni juice, bee pollen, wheatgrass, detox tea, and apple cider vinegar. I have no idea what criteria are set to make a food a superfood. If I were choosing a superfood, it might be rice. Billions of people around the world depend on rice as a staple in their diet. The Food and Agriculture Organization (FAO) estimates that rice provides more than one-fifth of the global caloric intake for humans. Now, that is a superfood.

While not "superfoods," there are several fruits that have outstanding health benefits. Tangerines and other mandarin oranges, fresh ripe pineapple, cherries, mulberries, blackberries, raspberries, and dates are among the fruits earning DAD scores of 4.

Table 6A. Fruit ranked by total amount consumed in the U.S.

Rank	Fruit	Score
1	Bananas	0
2	Apples (with skin)	A
	Apples (without skin)	1★
3	Grapes (Black > red > green)	1★
4	Strawberries	B
5	Melon: Cantaloupe	2★★
	Melon: Watermelon	3★★★
	Melon: Honeydew	4★★★★
6	Avocados	2★★
7	Blueberries	3★★★
8	Mandarins (tangerines, clementines, etc.)	5★★★★★
9	Oranges (navel)	2★★
	Oranges (Cara Cara)	3★★★
10	Peaches, nectarines, apricots, or plums	4★★★★
11	Pineapple (canned)	3★★★
	Pineapple (fresh, ripe)	4★★★★
12	Raspberries	4★★★★
13	Cherries	5★★★★★
14	Blackberries	4★★★★
15	Pears (without skin)	1★
16	Lemons	0
17	Limes	0
18	Kiwis (no skin)	3★★★
19	Grapefruit (ruby red), avoiding pith*	3★★★
20	Mangoes	4★★★★
21	Papaya (fully ripe)	4★★★★
22	Cranberries (fresh or dried)	2★★
	Mulberries	5★★★★★
	Dates^	5★★★★★
	Figs (with skin)	2★★
	Figs (without skin)	4★★★★
	Guavas	4★★★★
	Guanabana	3★★★

^ Dates are further discussed in Chapter 20.

* If taking prescription medications, ask your pharmacist before consuming grapefruit or its juice, as they can interfere with the metabolism of several commonly used medications.

Tangerine is a general name used in the U.S. for mandarin hybrids, while Clementine and Satsuma are specific cultivars. Most tangerine cultivars are particularly high in the flavones tangeretin and nobiletin, although the clementine cultivar only has tangeretin and nobiletin levels slightly higher than those of oranges.[7]

If choosing between grapefruit varieties, select pink-fleshed ones. If eating grapefruit out of hand, remove as much of the white, bitter pith as possible. The pith has a ranking score of D.

Tomatoes, pink-fleshed guavas and watermelons, pink grapefruit, Cara Cara oranges, and to a lesser extent, apricots and papayas are rich in lycopene, a bright red, antioxidant carotenoid. Dietary lycopene appears to help lower the risk of dementia and AD.[8 9]

Take-home message: There are much better choices of fruit than apples, bananas, strawberries, and grapes. Stone fruits are a great choice; these include peaches, plums, nectarines, apricots, and cherries. Who doesn't want a date? Tangerines are a terrific, tangy snack.

Farty Fruit:

Cherries and prunes have high levels of sorbitol, a sugar that is poorly absorbed. More than approximately 3 ounces of cherries (90 grams, about a dozen) can cause flatulence as the sorbitol ferments in the cecum of the large intestine; higher amounts can cause diarrhea. Apples, pears, grapes, and watermelon are high in fructose; some individuals absorb it poorly, causing it to end up in the cecum, where it ferments. Small amounts of these sugars entering the colon should not be a problem, but larger amounts that cause discomfort and especially if they cause diarrhea, should be considered to cause dysbiosis. This should be avoided. The microbiome can generally adapt to higher amounts of these sugars if their consumption is increased gradually.

Fruit Skin

The only fruits on this list for which it is not a bad idea to eat the skin are raspberries and blackberries (not true berries) and similar *Rubus* berries; stone fruits (but it is OK to peel stone fruits, such as peaches fruit but not necessary), blueberries, grapes, and tomatoes. Grapes would be better without the skin, but unless you're a pharaoh with slaves to peel the grapes for you, it is not worth the effort. The same is true for cranberries.

Not all skins are equally problematic. Apple peel is rated a C, pear peel a B, and kiwi peel a D. Olives are ranked as an A (avoid) food because of their skin, and strawberries are ranked as a B. Cucumbers are rated a 4, and their skin is a zero.

For some fruits, the skin would be better avoided, but this is difficult. For example, figs and cranberries get lower scores because of their skin. The skin of some fruits, such as stone fruit (cherries, peaches, plums), some berries, and cucumbers, is neutral and thus can be consumed, but cucumbers are generally treated with wax to improve shelf life. The wax and the possibility of pesticides on cucumbers, in addition to it not being especially pleasant, are sufficient reasons to avoid consuming the skin. Pesticide residues are another reason to avoid consuming the skin of certain fruits and vegetables.

Mango skin contains urushiol (the same chemical that causes poison ivy rash) and can cause a poison ivy-like reaction. One of my all-time favorite diagnoses was for a 5-year-old girl with an itchy rash with tiny blisters around her mouth. Straight off, I said to the child, "You like eating mangoes, don't you?" She had a big grin and nodded yes. Her mother was shocked! How did I know she had been eating mangoes?! She related that her husband had just returned from a business trip in South Florida and returned with a box of mangos as a special treat. It was like pleasing an audience with an amazing magic trick. I told her that the child could eat the mango flesh, but should not touch the skin.

Processed Fruit

Table 6B: U.S. Consumption of Processed Fruit (Ranked highest first)

	Fruit	Most Common Uses
1	Oranges	Primarily for orange juice
2	Apples	Used in various juices, applesauce, pies
3	Cranberries	Mostly consumed dried or as juice
4	Grapes	Used in raisins, juice, jams, and wine
5	Cherries	Used in pies, jams, and dried fruit
6	Pineapples	Used in juices, jams, and canned fruit
7	Blueberries	Used in yogurt, cereals, jams, juices
8	Peaches	Used in pies, jams, and canned fruit
9	Bananas	Used in some breads, muffins, and smoothies
10	Mangoes	Used in juices, smoothies, dried fruit
11	Lemons & Limes	Used in juices, lemonades, and desserts
12	Pears	Used in canned fruit, jams
13	Apricots	Used in jams, dried fruit
14	Dates	Used in baked goods, trail mixes
15	Figs	Used in jams, dried fruit, and cookies

Another difficulty in assessing the impact of fruit in the diet is that nearly half of all fruit is consumed as processed food. When a study is done, what qualifies as fruit? In 2021, the U.S. produced 45.9 pounds of apples per person; 23.7 pounds of that went into making apple juice or apple cider. Another 14% of apples were processed, being canned, dried, or frozen, for use in applesauce, apple pies, apple crisp, and other uses. Only a third of all apples are sold as fresh fruit.[10] A large majority of orange production is consumed as orange juice. Here is a list of the fruits most consumed as processed fruits.

Fresh, Frozen, Canned

Fully ripe fresh fruit, as a general rule, is going to be a better health choice than canned fruit or processed fruit. Canned fruit, however, can be a great choice. Canned fruit is available year-round, and is generally harvested at peak ripeness (unlike many fruits that are harvested early so that they can be shipped easily, and may never ripen fully). Canned fruit generally already has the skin removed, and is likely more affordable than fresh fruit.

Canned peaches in their juice still get a rating of 4. Fresh, ripe pineapple gets a score of 4; canned pineapple (in pineapple juice) gets a score of 3. These can be eaten without further preparation. The juice from canned pineapple and peaches is pleasant, but it gets a score of zero. Avoid fruit packed in syrup. The cherries in canned cherry pie filling do not score nearly as well as fresh cherries, but still get a 4. Nevertheless, the "gel," composed mostly of corn starch and sugar, gets a zero, and the sugar needs to be counted as added sugar in the diet. (See Chapter 10 for details.)

Freezing changes the texture of fruit, so they are not like eating fresh fruit; thus, thawing them and eating them as if they were fresh is a disappointment. Frozen blackberries, raspberries, blueberries, mangos, and papaya can be used for making smoothies, ice cream, or other home-processed foods, such as baking. They can be put on cereal or cooked with oatmeal.

Fruit Spreads

These processed fruits are typically spread on toast or used to make a sandwich with peanut butter. They are generally loaded with sugar or high-fructose corn syrup. Jams, jellies, and preserves are all made with about 50% sugar, as this preserves them, lowering their water activity (Aw) to a point that microbes don't grow.

Water Activity (Aw)

Water activity is a concept worth understanding. It is a measurement of how easily water vapor will be released from food as compared to distilled water and vice versa. If dry cereal is exposed to humid air, it will absorb the moisture from the air and lose its crunch if the a_w rises to over about 0.65.

The Aw is essential for food preservation, as it can also be thought of as water availability. Most bacteria cannot grow in food if the water activity is less than 0.90, though some can go as low as 0.85. Most molds cannot grow if the A_w is less than 0.70.[11] There is no microbial growth if the Aw is less than 0.585, even for extremophiles. Honey has an Aw of 0.50 – 0.70, so it does not need refrigeration, but if it is in an open container, it will absorb water vapor from the air in a humid environment, and the Aw can rise. Dried fruit has an A_w of about 0.60.[12] Fructose lowers the Aw more than glucose or sucrose, and is thus preferred by manufacturers as a sweetener in breads and baked goods, in part because it helps lower the Aw and thus provides a longer and more stable shelf life.

Fruit spreads were invented as a way to preserve fruit long before refrigeration was available. Jams were prepared as early as the 11th century in the Middle East, using honey. A cookbook, "*De Re Coquinaria*" (The Art of Cooking), dating from around the 4th or 5th century CE, contained a recipe for cooking fruit with honey, which may have been an early form of jam.

The Mason Jar with a threaded lid, invented by John Landis Mason in 1858, provided access to a simple method for home canning. Making jams and preserves became a common practice in the late 19th and early 20th centuries, before refrigeration, allowing families to preserve the short-term abundance of fruits from their gardens, so that they had access to them throughout the year. My grandparents did, my mother made jams and jellies with us when I was a kid, and we did it with our children.

When properly prepared, jams and preserves do not require refrigeration after opening. Nevertheless, keeping these fruit spreads refrigerated after opening is still advised (and may be required after opening fruit butters) as it will help maintain their quantity and provide a longer shelf life.

Jellies are made from strained fruit juice and don't have a significant amount of fiber. They should generally be avoided as they are similar to fruit juice. They may be appropriate when they are a source of specific phenolic compounds that have a desirable effect; cyanidin is an example.

Jam is made from mashed fruit, while *preserves* are made from whole fruit (for small fruit) or large chunks of fruit. Since raspberries and blackberries usually break up in the process, it may be difficult to tell the difference between jams and preserves. Healthwise, jams and preserves are about the same.

Fruit spreads (no added sugar) generally have added white grape or apple juice and are cooked long enough to remove enough water that they have a low enough water activity level to prevent microbial growth. *Fruit butters* are similar, but without added fruit juice. They are cooked for a much longer time and turn brown.

Diabetics, of course, need to limit their sugar intake, so they should avoid fruit spreads. Among fruits that can be used as a topping, those ranked at level 4 are a good choice. Some that are readily available include blackberry, raspberry, and apricot preserves.

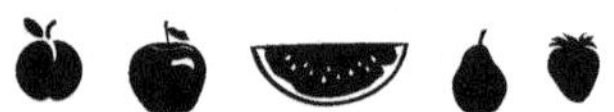

Where Apples Shine

Apples have a low ranking, and there are many better fruit choices. Despite this, applesauce can be a great healthy choice when it is used as a replacement for oil or butter and for eggs in baking. Applesauce can also be used to substitute for some oil in sauces. See Chapter 11 for details.

Bananas and apples can also be used as an egg substitute for making vegan, low-fat, low-cholesterol pancakes. Like apples, bananas can be used to add moisture and richness that would otherwise be provided by vegetable oil and eggs in baked goods. Bananas can be used to make vegan ice cream, but my preference is to use ripe plantains. (See Chapter 10 on dairy and not-so-dairy products.)

Sweet potato and winter squash (such as butternut squash and pumpkin puree) can also be used for this purpose, and have much higher DAD ranking scores, but have stronger flavors.

Fruit Juice

There is a clear scientific consensus that sugar-sweetened beverages, such as soda pop, coolaide, and sweet tea, are damaging to health. Frequent consumption of sugar-sweetened beverages has been found to increase the risk of Type 2 Diabetes (T2D) by 38%, increase the risk of hypertension, heart disease, and stroke, and increase all-cause mortality by 13%.[13] The most effective weight loss programs are those that ban sweet drinks. The consumption of sugar-sweetened beverages is associated with obesity, T2D, fatty liver disease, cardiovascular disease, periodontal disease, and tooth decay. Fruit juice in a baby bottle or sippy cup can cause rampant dental decay.

Table sugar is a disaccharide composed of the monosaccharides glucose and fructose. Soda pop is usually made with high fructose corn syrup that contains both fructose and glucose. Fruits contain various combinations of sugars, depending on the fruit, but those mostly include fructose, sucrose, and sorbitol.

The sugars in beverages are quickly absorbed, and especially on an empty stomach, they cause a spike in blood glucose and blood fructose levels. In a healthy person without diabetes or insulin resistance, excess blood glucose can be stored as glycogen in the muscles, liver, and kidneys. Every cell in the body can use glucose. In contrast, the liver is the only organ that can dispose of fructose. The liver converts fructose into glucose, but when there is too much (as with a big spike from fructose-laden beverages), fructose is converted to fat and glyceraldehyde. Additionally, the metabolism of fructose in the liver depletes ATP and results in the generation of uric acid; high uric acid levels are associated with metabolic syndrome. Thus, high levels of fructose in the diet, particularly when served as a beverage, promote fatty liver, insulin resistance, and metabolic syndrome. Thus, sugar-sweetened and high-fructose-sweetened beverages are black-listed by the SANA diet. The reasons are further discussed in Chapter 10.

A poison is in the dose. A modest 12-ounce serving of soda has between about 125 and 180 calories, which is equivalent to 8 to 11 teaspoons. (or 33 to 47 g) of sugar. A single small-sized (12 oz.) soda might thus provide 10% of the daily caloric needs of a woman, but as empty calories. Fruit juice has a similar amount of sugar per ounce as soda pop.

Consumption of large amounts of fruit juice has also been found to be associated with considerably higher risk of heart disease and death. A study of 13,000 American adults found that the consumption of more than 10% of total dietary caloric intake as fruit juice or other sugar sweetened beverage is associated with a 44% increase risk in coronary heart disease (CHD) deaths and a 14% increase in all-cause mortality, mostly from heart disease, as compared to those consuming less than 5% of calories from fruit juice. Risk was linearly increased with the consumption of these beverages. It did not matter whether the sugar came from soda pop or fruit juice. The risk from sweet beverages was no different.[14] A meta-analysis found that consuming more than 250 ml (8.4 oz.) of fruit juice per day was associated with a 30% increase in the hazard of death, and a 49% increased risk of death from heart disease. Replacing 5% of the daily calorie intake from whole fruit with fruit juice increased mortality by 9%.[15]

In a cross-over study of apple and apple juice consumption where in which subjects consumed 550 grams of whole apples (about three medium apples), or 500 ml (17 oz) apple juice per day for a month, eating apples lowered LDL cholesterol levels by 6.7% (there are better ways!), and cloudy apple juice lowered LDL levels by 2.2%. Meanwhile, 500 ml of filtered, clear apple juice raised LDL levels by 6.9%.[16] The point being that unfiltered juice is less destructive than filtered juice.

These studies looked at high volumes of juice intake. How about more moderate consumption? The following data are from a large meta-analysis. Consumption of 75 ml of fruit juice per day, adults had a slightly (but not statistically significantly lower risk of developing diabetes. The risk of stroke was significantly lower for those drinking 25 to 200 ml of juice per day, with 75 to 100 ml (about 3 – 4 oz) being the sweet spot for the lowest risk. The risk of cardiovascular events was significantly lower for those drinking about 25 to 175 ml of 100% fruit juice per day. Risk was lowest for those drinking 78 ml (about 3 ounces) of fruit juice per day, but juice still provided significant protection as long as the volume was less than around 150 ml, about 5 ounces.[17]

It is easy to overconsume apple juice. It takes about 3 apples to make a cup of juice, more apples than most people would eat in one serving. When one eats an apple, it takes time for the pulp of the apple to leave the stomach, while apple juice will readily enter the duodenum. Apple juice contains sorbitol and fructose. Sorbitol is poorly absorbed. When there is too much non-absorbed sugar, it has an osmotic effect and pulls water into the intestine. It can cause the chyme, including other partially digested foods, to quickly move through the intestine. Once in the colon, the sugar ferments and pulls water into the lumen, resulting in bloating, cramping, and gas. When some people drink enough apple juice to cause borborygmi, foul winds, diarrhea, signs of dumping syndrome, and dysbiotic fermentation

A review of multiple studies of children did not find an increase in weight among children drinking 100% fruit juice.[18] However, a more in-depth, formal meta-analysis found a 4% increase in BMI among children aged 1 to 6 consuming 100% fruit juices, but no association with increased BMI in children aged 7 to 18.[19] Children who drank 100% fruit juice consistently at age 2 were shorter and heavier at the age of four to five than those who infrequently consumed fruit juice.[20] Children who often drink apple juice have been found to, on average, be shorter and heavier than would be expected for their age;[21] however, no detrimental effects on height and weight have been found in a review of studies on the consumption of 100% orange juice in children. While apple juice contains non-digestible, fermentable sorbitol, filtered apple juice contains little pectin or polyphenolic compounds.

Whole fruits are higher in fiber, which benefits the microbiome. A fruit juice that is made by blending the fruit is much preferable to one where the juicing process removes most of the pulp and fiber. An appropriate serving size for fruit juice is the amount that can be produced from the fruit that the person would consume as a serving; a few ounces, rather than replacing their water needs. One orange produces 2 to 3 ounces of juice, which is an appropriate-sized serving for an adult.

- *When fruit juice comprises 10% or more of the dietary caloric intake, it may be just as destructive to health as soda pop.*
- *Whole fruits offer greater health benefits than the same fruit as juice.*
- *Less refined juice is better (less harmful?) than refined ones that remove the fiber*
- *Thus, smoothies made of fresh fruit, while not as good as whole fruit because of their quicker digestion, are better than juice, where the pulp is removed. Smoothies should use fruits with a good DAD rating and avoid those that don't.*
- *Fruit juice from fruit with lower DAD scores (such as apples, bananas, pears, and strawberries) is likely to have a more detrimental impact than that from higher-ranking fruit.*
- *Four ounces of fruit juice per day is allowed on the SANA diet for those without diabetes.*

Allowed Fruit Juices

Some fruit juice is OK. Fruit that has a high rating may, but does not necessarily, provide benefit, as in the case of filtered peach and pineapple juice. Orange, Mango, and Guava juices have positive ratings; however, the total daily portion size is small, and the appropriate upper limit for diabetics is even smaller. In general, the recommended total daily portion size for fruit juice is about 4 ounces, equivalent to 120 ml. It is better to eat the fruit and get the fiber. A ripe mango has a DAD score of four; its juice gets a score of 2. Guava fruit gets a score of 4, its juice a one.

- When purchasing orange juice, get full or high pulp, unfiltered OJ.
- The SANA diet allows 4 oz. of OJ per day, but a maximum of 3 ounces for those with *well-controlled* T2D.

There are exceptions where a fruit juice gets a higher ranking than the fruit. This occurs in some cases where the skin of the fruit is consumed with the fruit. These are cases in small fruits where the fruit skin lowers the rating of an otherwise beneficial fruit.

- Dried cranberries get a rating of one. If you could remove the skin from a cranberry, it would get a score of three. Cranberry cocktail gets a rating of three. Nevertheless, the recommended adult portion size for cranberry cocktail is small, 2 ounces. Cranberry mixes with raspberry, or other fruits with good DAD ratings, are fine; avoid apple juice mixes.
- Concord grape juice gets a rating of three, while table grapes get a rating of one. Concord grapes are rich in polyphenols, and the juice does not contain the grape skin. This is for 100% Concord grape juice and certain wines, but not for most other grape "beverages". It only takes about one to two ounces of Concord grape juice to get its phenolic health benefits.

Recommendation: Purchase some 3-ounce "shot glasses". (Link to find them: [22]) They are also useful for controlling the serving size of fruit juice, wine, and ice cream.

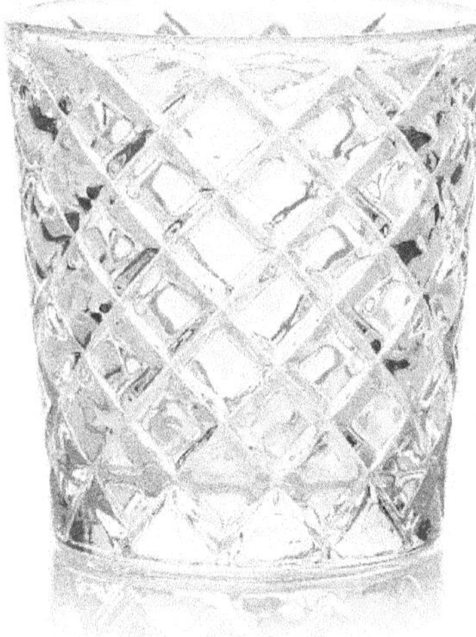

A 3-ounce shot glass

Juice can be watered down to improve hydration and give a sense of having had enough. A 2:1 Concord grape juice dilution, using 6 oz of water and 3 oz of juice, gives a pleasant, flavorful beverage that is not too watered down.

Smoothies

The SANA program does not encourage drinking smoothies. While having more fiber than fruit juices, smoothies remain a means of consuming a large number of calories quickly, and then having them be digested quickly. As with fruit juices, this facilitates rapid absorption of calories that can cause a spike in blood sugar, followed by a surge in insulin demand. Since the food is not chewed, amylase that acts on carbohydrates and lingual lipase that acts on fats are not utilized. While this does not prevent the foods' eventual digestion, it likely delays satiety and thus the decision point of when to stop eating.

When the purpose of a smoothie is to accommodate the consumption of nutritional supplements, it is recommended that it be part of a meal rather than replacing the meal. This should help slow its digestion. Additionally, several nutrients, including carotenoids (lutein, lycopene, β-carotene) and vitamins A, D, E, and K, are fat-soluble and thus best absorbed when consumed with a meal containing some fat.

Dried Fruit

Data from the USDA shows that the per capita availability of dried fruit, which should be similar to the average consumption, is about 2.4 pounds per year, for the most recent year with full data. That includes 1.3 pounds of raisins, 4 ounces of dates, 3 ounces of prunes, and about 1.6 ounces of dried apples, apricots, figs, and even lower amounts of dried peaches and pears. The consumption of raisins has declined to about half of what it was in the 1980s, with lower acreage dedicated to grapes for raisins. The FDA does not provide data for cranberries, cherries, and berries; however, these have partially replaced the consumption of raisins, so that a guesstimate is that, on average, Americans consume about 3 ounces of dried cranberries and smaller amounts of dried cherries and blueberries.

Dried fruit consumption generally appears to be associated with decreased risk of cardiovascular disease, with a lower odds of heart failure (OR = 0.60, ischemic stroke (OR = 0.45), and small vessel stroke (OR = 0.35).[23] Small vessel brain infarcts are an important cause of vascular dementia and white matter lesions in the brain. An OR of 0.35 suggests a 65% decrease in risk. The study counted one dried prune as a serving, for example, but did not describe the number of servings required for protection.

Dried fruit consumption appears to be protective against some forms of cancer (breast and squamous cell lung cancers), but not against other cancers.[24] Some dried fruits are likely more effective than others. Dried fruit consumption appears to be associated with decreased risk of developing type 2 diabetes,[25] and those who commonly consume dried fruit had more than 50% lower odds of low back pain.[26] Unfortunately, the kind, frequency, and amount of dried fruit consumed were not given in the study.

The desert dessert, date fruit (DAD score = 4), is a healthy sweet, which, when considering its sugar content, has a surprisingly modest glycemic index.[27] Dried dates, the ones generally sold in the market, have a lower glycemic index than do fresh dates.[28] In experimental animals and one human trial, dried dates in reasonable amounts did not promote hyperglycemia.[29] In a study, diabetic patients were assigned to eat 30 grams (about one ounce) of dried dates or 30 grams of raisins (DAD score = 2), twice a day, as a midmorning and midafternoon snack for 12 weeks. These snacks had no impact on insulin resistance, hemoglobin A1c (HbA1c), blood pressure, or C-reactive protein, a marker of inflammation.[30] Thus, no benefit or harm. In another study, when raisins were compared to other snack foods, raisins lowered the fasting blood sugar by 19% and did not significantly impact HbA1c. When compared with an equal amount of available carbohydrates, including sugars, raisins had considerably less impact on raising the post-meal blood sugar than did white bread.[31] As an after-school snack, raisins or grapes decreased cumulative food intake in children compared to other snacks,[32] and thus may help prevent childhood obesity. Dates and raisins have a low glycemic index. Dates may even improve glycemic control,[33] likely by displacing foods with higher glycemic indices.

Dates have additional health benefits that are discussed in Chapter 20. When selecting between dates and raisins, dates are the far better choice.

Raisins, dried cranberries, and other dried fruit are generally sweet and often tart. The combination of sucrose and acid is hard on the dental enamel. Thus, there is concern that "Nature's candy" can act like candy when it comes to tooth decay. It appears that raisins do not stick to the teeth and do not drop the pH in the mouth enough to cause caries. Additionally, the antioxidant compounds in raisins inhibit *Streptococcus mutans*, the bacteria that are the primary cause of dental caries.[34] Additionally, the chewing of dried fruit encourages salivary flow, helping to protect the teeth.[35] Mature dates are high in polyphenols and have little sucrose, so they are unlikely to promote dental caries.

Risks: As mentioned in the introduction to this chapter previously, dried fruit is a concern as a potential risk for AD. This data came from a study of people in Great Britain and is in disagreement with other studies. A likely explanation for the health risks associated with dried fruit is that it can easily mold during the drying process or later, during storage. Ochratoxin A, a toxin common in food mold, is neurotoxic and a risk for dementia. Ochratoxin A (OTA) is just one of the mycotoxins found in moldy food that are discussed in Chapter 27, which are not exclusive to dried fruits. Aflatoxins are another class of fungal toxins found in food; they are a risk factor for cancer, especially liver cancer, but are not known to be associated with AD risk.

Sun-dried fruit has the highest risk of ochratoxin A contamination, as the drying time can be slow, and weather may not cooperate. Additionally, spores can be carried in the breeze, especially in agricultural areas where there may be plowing of the soil; these are soil fungi. Growing conditions, location, climate, and post-drying storage can all affect the risk of fungal growth. Closed solar dryers (using glass or plastic sheets) greatly lower the risk of mold growing during drying. Fruits with low "water activity" are at lower risk of mycotoxin contamination, as the fungi don't grow without access to water. Fruit with a high concentration of sugars has lower water activity. Molds, yeasts, and bacteria cannot grow at low water activity (A_W) below about 0.65. One of the reasons that high fructose corn syrup is used in processed foods is that it lowers the food's water activity, giving it a longer shelf life. Some raisins are sun-dried on the vine. These are at higher risk of OTA contamination, as it is harder to control drying in an open environment.

Raisins are one of the foods that are subject to high levels of OTA contamination. One survey study found that raisins, the most highly consumed dried fruit, were contaminated by OTA in 46.2% of samples in France, 54.9% in Greece, 94.3% in Germany, and 91.1% in the United Kingdom, with levels up to 4.3, 16.5, 21.4, and 53.6 μg/kg, respectively. Levels vary by growing conditions and thus, by year.[36]

Apricots, dates, and raisins are highly susceptible to molds with form OTA; figs and prunes are less so. Blueberries and cherries generally do not have much problem, and cranberries have a low susceptibility. Dried fruit from less developed countries is at higher risk, as they generally have less stringent control and less developed infrastructure for processing. The FDA does spot-check mycotoxin levels and limits permissible levels, but this is likely limited to U.S. production facilities and may not include smaller batches of imported fruit.

Even if the fruit has minimal OTA levels when purchased by the consumer, it does not guarantee that levels will still be low by the time it is consumed. If improperly stored, the dried fruit can grow mold. Dry fruits should be stored in a dry and well-ventilated area to prevent moisture condensation on the fruit. Cold-stored dry fruit repeatedly exposed to humid, warm air will gather condensate, and this may encourage the growth of mold. The crisper drawer of a refrigerator is designed to trap moisture and maintain humidity, while the main section is drier. I kept some sun-dried tomatoes in the crisper drawer, and the inside of the tomatoes turned black from mold!

To avoid dried fruit that is a risk for OTA and other fungal toxins, purchase from reputable brands known for following strict quality control measures. Keep in mind that the 3X risk of AD from the consumption of dried fruit was in a British population and much of the dried fruit was likely imported from Turkey, Iran, Pakistan, and other countries that may have had less control and monitoring of the drying processes, and was then stored in Britain's cool, humid climate. If you see black mold spores on food, you can be quite certain that it is not fit to eat. Not seeing the spores, however, does not provide any guarantee that the food is not contaminated.

One way to lower the risk of post-purchase mold growth in dried fruits is to buy smaller, hermetically sealed packages that will be consumed within a short time after purchase, rather than buy a year's worth in a large container. If you do not feel that the dried fruit available to you is of high quality, limit your choices of dried fruit to cranberries, cherries, and blueberries.

Dried fruit should be stored in air-tight sealed containers. They can be frozen if they will not be consumed within a few months. The risk of post-harvest molding is highest in warm, humid climates. If refrigerated or frozen, each time the dried fruit container is taken out and opened is an opportunity for moisture condensation on the fruit. Mold should not grow in a freezer, but it will in a refrigerator. It is better to store small amounts of dried fruit that will be used in a month or less at room temperature under dry conditions. Keep frozen dried fruit sealed until it reaches room temperature before opening it to prevent condensation of moisture in the room air from moistening the fruit.

Fresh fruit can also have mold, but it is more often a penicillin species. You still don't want it. When buying a bag of fruit or potatoes, try to check the fruit while you are still in the store to make sure none of it is molding, and recheck the fruit when you get home, and discard the worthless ones before the mold spreads. Use your nose. Remember that the proverb, "The rotten apple injures its neighbors," is more than just a metaphor.

Citrulline

Citrulline is a non-protein-forming amino acid. While it has the molecular structural elements of an amino acid, animals do not use it to build proteins, but rather use it for other purposes. The body produces citrulline exclusively in the enterocytes, the mucosal cells lining the small intestine that absorb nutrients from glutamine. Citrulline is then absorbed. Low circulating citrulline levels are a marker for intestinal injury, disease, or dysfunction, such as with celiac disease, chemotherapy, and short bowel syndrome, as they indicate a loss in the body's ability to form this compound. After absorption, citrulline enters the circulation and is processed by the kidneys into arginine, bypassing the liver. This is thought to be a mechanism by which the body can balance out and support protein building during fasting states, by holding back on arginine, required for protein production during the fed state. Limiting arginine availability holds back protein production. Citrulline also helps maintain a supply of arginine during the fasting state for use in the urea cycle to eliminate ammonia produced by the body and GI microbiome, and also for the production of NO as a vasodilator during the fasting state.[37]

Ammonia is a toxic substance produced by the breakdown of protein. The urea cycle is a metabolic pathway in the liver that helps remove ammonia and excess nitrogen from the body.

Citrulline is present in some foods, and while non-essential, it is still a nutrient. Watermelons, honeydew, and cucumbers have the highest amounts. Other members of the Cucurbita family, such as cantaloupes and other melons, and summer and winter squash, are also rich in citrulline. Chickpeas and onions contain lower amounts.

Citrulline provides vasodilation properties as a precursor of arginine and thus of nitric oxide (NO). Dietary citrulline can help reduce blood pressure in hypertension and improve erectile dysfunction, and may improve cerebral blood flow. It can improve exercise tolerance, decrease arterial stiffness and adiposity, and increase lean body mass. Dietary citrulline attenuates fructose-induced Non-Alcoholic Steatohepatitis (NASH) and reduces lung and liver inflammation caused by lipopolysaccharides (LPS) from gut gram-negative bacteria. It has been found to improve protein synthesis and counteract sarcopenia in the elderly who have muscle wasting. It has antioxidant properties as a hydroxyl radical scavenger, and in animal models, it protects the hippocampus from oxidative stress and helps protect neuronal plasticity in elderly animals. When added to the diet of mice, citrulline improved intestinal barrier function and reduced signs of senescence in mice.[38] [39] [40] [41] [42]

Thus, citrulline-containing fruits and vegetables get high DAD scores and deserve a place in the diet. Winter squash includes butternut squash and pumpkin, and summer squash includes crookneck and zucchini squash.

Citrulline spares and supplements arginine, which can be converted in the body to spermidine, which induces autophagy and mitophagy. Spermidine is considered to have protective effects against cardiovascular disease, NASH, and Alzheimer's disease.[43] Thus, citrulline may help promote autophagy and longevity.

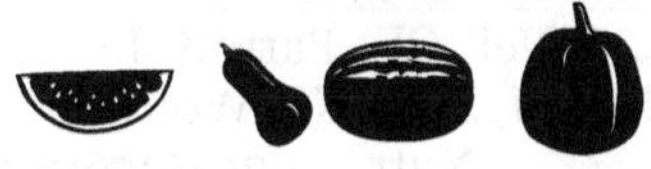

[1] Fruit and Vegetable Consumption and Cognitive Disorders in Older Adults: A Meta-Analysis of Observational Studies. Zhou Y, Wang J, Cao L, Shi M, Liu H, Zhao Y, Xia Y. Front Nutr. 2022 Jun 20;9:871061. doi: 10.3389/fnut.2022.871061. eCollection 2022. PMID: 35795585

[2] The Mediterranean, Dietary Approaches to Stop Hypertension (DASH), and Mediterranean-DASH Intervention for Neurodegenerative Delay (MIND) Diets Are Associated with Less Cognitive Decline and a Lower Risk of Alzheimer's Disease-A Review. van den Brink AC, Brouwer-Brolsma EM, Berendsen AAM, van de Rest O. Adv Nutr. 2019 Nov 1;10(6):1040-1065. doi: 10.1093/advances/nmz054. PMID: 31209456

[3] Fruit Intake and Alzheimer's Disease: Results from Mendelian Randomization. Liao WZ, Zhu XF, Xin Q, Mo YT, Wang LL, He XP, Guo XG. J Prev Alzheimers Dis. 2024;11(2):445-452. doi: 10.14283/jpad.2024.31. PMID: 38374751

[4] https://www.webmd.com/diet/news/20240320/strawberries-spinach-top-annual-dirty-dozen-produce-list

[5] Produce Without Pesticides. Catherine Roberts. Consumer Reports, April 18, 2024 https://www.consumerreports.org/health/food-contaminants/produce-without-pesticides-a5260230325/

[6] https://www.consumerreports.org/health/food-contaminants/fruits-and-vegetables-loaded-with-pesticides-a2508510840/

[7] https://en.wikipedia.org/wiki/Mandarin_orange

[8] Lycopene and cognitive function. Crowe-White KM, Phillips TA, Ellis AC. J Nutr Sci. 2019 May 29;8:e20. doi: 10.1017/jns.2019.16. eCollection 2019. PMID: 31217968

[9] Lycopene: Sojourn from kitchen to an effective therapy in Alzheimer's disease. Kapoor B, Gulati M, Rani P, Kochhar RS, Atanasov AG, Gupta R, Sharma D, Kapoor D. Biofactors. 2023 Mar;49(2):208-227. doi: 10.1002/biof.1910. Epub 2022 Nov 1. PMID: 36318372

[10] https://www.ers.usda.gov/data-products/chart-gallery/gallery/chart-detail/?chartId=107383

[11] MINIMUM WATER ACTIVITIES FOR THE GROWTH OF YEASTS ISOLATED FROM HIGH-SUGAR FOODS. Keito Tokuoka. https://www.jstage.jst.go.jp/article/jgam1955/37/1/37_1_111/_pdf

[12] https://en.wikipedia.org/wiki/Water_activity

[13] Consumption of sugar sweetened beverages, artificially sweetened beverages and fruit juices and risk of type 2 diabetes, hypertension, cardiovascular disease, and mortality: A meta-analysis. Li B, Yan N, Jiang H, Cui M, Wu M, Wang L, Mi B, Li Z, Shi J, Fan Y, Azalati MM, Li C, Chen F, Ma M, Wang D, Ma L. Front Nutr. 2023 Mar 15;10:1019534. doi: 10.3389/fnut.2023.1019534. eCollection 2023. PMID: 37006931

[14] Association of Sugary Beverage Consumption with Mortality Risk in US Adults: A Secondary Analysis of Data From the REGARDS Study. Collin LJ, Judd S, Safford M, Vaccarino V, Welsh JA. JAMA Netw Open. 2019 May 3;2(5):e193121. doi: 10.1001/jamanetworkopen.2019.3121. PMID: 31099861

[15] A Prospective Study of Fruit Juice Consumption and the Risk of Overall and Cardiovascular Disease Mortality. Zhang Z, Zeng X, Li M, Zhang T, Li H, Yang H, Huang Y, Zhu Y, Li X, Yang W. Nutrients. 2022 May 19;14(10):2127. doi: 10.3390/nu14102127. PMID: 35631268

[16] Intake of whole apples or clear apple juice has contrasting effects on plasma lipids in healthy volunteers. Ravn-Haren G, Dragsted LO, Buch-Andersen T, Jensen EN, Jensen RI, Németh-Balogh M, Paulovicsová B, Bergström A, Wilcks A, Licht TR, Markowski J, Bügel S. Eur J Nutr. 2013 Dec;52(8):1875-89. doi: 10.1007/s00394-012-0489-z. Epub 2012 Dec 28. PMID: 23271615

[17] 100% Fruit juice intake and cardiovascular risk: a systematic review and meta-analysis of prospective and randomised controlled studies. D'Elia L, Dinu M, Sofi F, Volpe M, Strazzullo P; SINU Working Group, Endorsed by SIPREC. Eur J Nutr. 2021 Aug;60(5):2449-2467. doi: 10.1007/s00394-020-02426-7. Epub 2020 Nov 4. PMID: 33150530

[18] Impact of 100% Fruit Juice Consumption on Diet and Weight Status of Children: An Evidence-based Review. Crowe-White K, O'Neil CE, Parrott JS, Benson-Davies S, Droke E, Gutschall M, Stote KS, Wolfram T, Ziegler P. Crit Rev Food Sci Nutr. 2016;56(5):871-84. doi: 10.1080/10408398.2015.1061475. PMID: 26091353

[19] Fruit Juice and Change in BMI: A Meta-analysis. Auerbach BJ, Wolf FM, Hikida A, Vallila-Buchman P, Littman A, Thompson D, Louden D, Taber DR, Krieger J. Pediatrics. 2017 Apr;139(4):e20162454. doi: 10.1542/peds.2016-2454. PMID: 28336576

[20] Longitudinal evaluation of 100% fruit juice consumption on BMI status in 2-5-year-old children. Shefferly A, Scharf RJ, DeBoer MD. Pediatr Obes. 2016 Jun;11(3):221-7. doi: 10.1111/ijpo.12048. PMID: 26110996

[21] Children's growth parameters vary by type of fruit juice consumed. Dennison BA, Rockwell HL, Nichols MJ, Jenkins P. J Am Coll Nutr. 1999 Aug;18(4):346-52. doi: 10.1080/07315724.1999.10718874. PMID: 12038478

[22] https://www.walmart.com/ip/Better-Homes-Gardens-Clear-Diamond-Cut-Glass-Shot-Glass-6-Pack/150425762?athbdg=L1100&from=/search

[23] Causal associations between dried fruit intake and cardiovascular disease: A Mendelian randomization study. Zeng Y, Cao S, Yang H. Front Cardiovasc Med. 2023 Feb 6;10:1080252. doi: 10.3389/fcvm.2023.1080252. eCollection 2023. PMID: 36815021

[24] Association between dried fruit intake and pan-cancers incidence risk: A two-sample Mendelian randomization study. Jin C, Li R, Deng T, Lin Z, Li H, Yang Y, Su Q, Wang J, Yang Y, Wang J, Chen G, Wang Y. Front Nutr. 2022 Jul 18;9:899137. doi: 10.3389/fnut.2022.899137. eCollection 2022. PMID: 35923199

[25] Dried fruit intake and lower risk of type 2 diabetes: a two-sample mendelian randomization study. Guan J, Liu T, Yang K, Chen H. Nutr Metab (Lond). 2024 Jul 10;21(1):46. doi: 10.1186/s12986-024-00813-z. PMID: 38987806

26 Dried fruit intake causally protects against low back pain: A Mendelian randomization study. Huang J, Xie ZF. Front Nutr. 2023 Mar 23;10:1027481. doi: 10.3389/fnut.2023.1027481. PMID: 37032770; PMCID: PMC10076586.

27 Effect of dates on blood glucose and other metabolic variables: A narrative review. Meenakshi S, Misra A. Diabetes Metab Syndr. 2023 Feb;17(2):102705. doi: 10.1016/j.dsx.2023.102705. Epub 2023 Jan 9. PMID: 36702045

28 Influence of Date Ripeness on Glycemic Index, Glycemic Load, and Glycemic Response in Various Saudi Arabian Date Varieties. Alzahrani AM, Alghamdi K, Bagasi A, Alrashed OA, Alqifari AF, Barakat H, Algeffari M. Cureus. 2023 Nov 7;15(11):e48433. doi: 10.7759/cureus.48433. eCollection 2023 Nov. PMID: 38074068

29 Investigating Majhool date (Phoenix dactylifera) consumption effects on fasting blood glucose in animals and humans. Jarrar Y, Balasmeh R, Naser W, Mosleh R, Al-Doaiss AA, AlShehri MA. J Basic Clin Physiol Pharmacol. 2024 Apr 29;35(3):175-179. doi: 10.1515/jbcpp-2024-0049. eCollection 2024 May 1. PMID: 38677327

30 Effect of Date Fruit Consumption on the Glycemic Control of Patients with Type 2 Diabetes: A Randomized Clinical Trial. Butler AE, Obaid J, Wasif P, Varghese JV, Abdulrahman R, Alromaihi D, Atkin SL, Alamuddin N. Nutrients. 2022 Aug 25;14(17):3491. doi: 10.3390/nu14173491. PMID: 36079749

31 Acute effects of raisin consumption on glucose and insulin reponses in healthy individuals. Esfahani A, Lam J, Kendall CW. J Nutr Sci. 2014 Jan 7;3:e1. doi: 10.1017/jns.2013.33. eCollection 2014. PMID: 25191601

32 An after-school snack of raisins lowers cumulative food intake in young children. Patel BP, Bellissimo N, Luhovyy B, Bennett LJ, Hurton E, Painter JE, Anderson GH. J Food Sci. 2013 Jun;78 Suppl 1:A5-A10. doi: 10.1111/1750-3841.12070. PMID: 23789934

33 Dates fruits effects on blood glucose among patients with diabetes mellitus: A review and meta-analysis. Mirghani HO. Pak J Med Sci. 2021 Jul-Aug;37(4):1230-1236. doi: 10.12669/pjms.37.4.4112. PMID: 34290813

34 Raisins and oral health. Wong A, Young DA, Emmanouil DE, Wong LM, Waters AR, Booth MT. J Food Sci. 2013 Jun;78 Suppl 1:A26-9. doi: 10.1111/1750-3841.12152. PMID: 23789933

35 Dried fruit and dental health. Sadler MJ. Int J Food Sci Nutr. 2016 Dec;67(8):944-59. doi: 10.1080/09637486.2016.1207061. Epub 2016 Jul 14. PMID: 27415591

36 Occurrence of Mycotoxins in Dried Fruits Worldwide, with a Focus on Aflatoxins and Ochratoxin A: A Review. González-Curbelo MÁ, Kabak B. Toxins (Basel). 2023 Sep 18;15(9):576. doi: 10.3390/toxins15090576. PMID: 37756002

37 Almost all about citrulline in mammals. Curis E, Nicolis I, Moinard C, Osowska S, Zerrouk N, Bénazeth S, Cynober L. Amino Acids. 2005 Nov;29(3):177-205. doi: 10.1007/s00726-005-0235-4. Epub 2005 Aug 8. PMID: 16082501

38 L-citrulline attenuates lipopolysaccharide-induced inflammatory lung injury in neonatal rats. Ivanovski N, Wang H, Tran H, Ivanovska J, Pan J, Miraglia E, Leung S, Posiewko M, Li D, Mohammadi A, Higazy R, Nagy A, Kim P, Santyr G, Belik J, Palaniyar N, Gauda EB. Pediatr Res. 2023 Nov;94(5):1684-1695. doi: 10.1038/s41390-023-02684-1. Epub 2023 Jun 22. PMID: 37349511

39 Citrulline prevents age-related LTP decline in old rats. Ginguay A, Regazzetti A, Laprevote O, Moinard C, De Bandt JP, Cynober L, Billard JM, Allinquant B, Dutar P. Sci Rep. 2019 Dec 27;9(1):20138. doi: 10.1038/s41598-019-56598-2. PMID: 31882891

40 Citrulline, Biomarker of Enterocyte Functional Mass and Dietary Supplement. Metabolism, Transport, and Current Evidence for Clinical Use. Maric S, Restin T, Muff JL, Camargo SM, Guglielmetti LC, Holland-Cunz SG, Crenn P, Vuille-Dit-Bille RN. Nutrients. 2021 Aug 15;13(8):2794. doi: 10.3390/nu13082794. PMID: 34444954

41 Supplementing L-Citrulline Can Extend Lifespan in *C. elegans* and Attenuate the Development of Aging-Related Impairments of Glucose Tolerance and Intestinal Barrier in Mice. Rajcic D, Kromm F, Hernández-Arriaga A, Brandt A, Baumann A, Staltner R, Camarinha-Silva A, Bergheim I. Biomolecules. 2023 Oct 26;13(11):1579. doi: 10.3390/biom13111579. PMID: 38002262

42 Effects of L-Citrulline Supplementation and Aerobic Training on Vascular Function in Individuals with Obesity across the Lifespan. Flores-Ramírez AG, Tovar-Villegas VI, Maharaj A, Garay-Sevilla ME, Figueroa A. Nutrients. 2021 Aug 27;13(9):2991. doi: 10.3390/nu13092991. PMID: 34578869

43 High-Dose Spermidine Supplementation Does Not Increase Spermidine Levels in Blood Plasma and Saliva of Healthy Adults: A Randomized Placebo-Controlled Pharmacokinetic and Metabolomic Study. Senekowitsch S, Wietkamp E, Grimm M, Schmelter F, Schick P, Kordowski A, Sina C, Otzen H, Weitschies W, Smollich M. Nutrients. 2023 Apr 12;15(8):1852. doi: 10.3390/nu15081852. PMID: 37111071

7: Vegetables

In contrast to fruits, multiple population studies provide evidence that the consumption of vegetables helps prevent Alzheimer's disease. Vegetables provide essential nutrients for the body and fiber and nutrients for the microbiome that promote GI health and prevent systemic and neurologic inflammation. Several vegetables provide antioxidant effects.

As with fruits, the ability of vegetables (as a class) to promote microbiome health depends on the weighing of which vegetables are consumed, with some vegetables helping and others not. Some of the most helpful of the vegetables, however, turn out to be fruits that are consumed as vegetables.

Technically, fruits are fleshy, seed-containing parts of a plant that develop from the ovary of a flower. It is widely accepted that tomatoes are actually a fruit. If cantaloupes (*Cucumis melo*) are fruit, then how are cucumbers (*Cucumis sativus)* not? Cucumbers are typically eaten raw, as are most fruits. Butternut squash is a fruit, but needs to be cooked, and is used as a vegetable. Why are pumpkins considered to be vegetables? They are used to make delicious pies as a dessert. In the tropics, bananas and plantains are cooked green and used as a starchy vegetable, and when allowed to ripen, are eaten as fruits.

The division of edible plant materials into classes of fruits and vegetables is an artificial distinction that does not capture their impact on the microbiome. It only tells which basket the food is placed in. The category tells nothing about the food's impact on inflammation or its capacity to reduce disease risk.

Despite this, it is convenient to list foods by how they are used to readily make substitution choices, a design goal for the SANA diet. It makes it easier to contrast and choose the better option for health. As typically prepared, a baked sweet potato gets a considerably higher score than a baked Idaho potato. Spinach gets a considerably better score than does cabbage. Knowing which foods are most or least beneficial helps people choose between food items to make better choices. A tangerine is a better choice than an apple. Separating foods into use categories can help facilitate better choices.

Table 7A: Ranking of the most commonly consumed fresh vegetables (for the U.S.) by amounts consumed, and their Defense Against Dysbiosis ratings.

Rank	Vegetable	Rating
1	Potatoes (with peel)	0
	Potato peel	D
	Potatoes (no peel), boiled or baked	1★
2	Tomatoes	5★★★★★
3	Onions raw	0
	Onions - cooked	2★★
4	Carrots (no skin)	0
5	Lettuce (Iceberg)	
	Lettuce (red Leaf)	0
	Lettuce (Romaine)	0
6	Bell peppers (green, red, orange)	2★★
7	Cucumbers	5★★★★★
8	Mushrooms (white, bottled)	1★
	Mushrooms, Baby Bella, brown	2★★
9	Celery, stalk or leaf	0
10	Corn (sweet)	B
11	Broccoli*	1★
12	Spinach	2★★
13	Garlic*	2★★
14	Green beans	1
15	Cabbage	D
16	Sweet potatoes (skin)	D
	Sweet potatoes (cooked, without skin)	4★★★★
17	Green onions	A
18	Cauliflower*	1★
19	Asparagus	D
20	Brussels sprouts	D
21	Zucchini	2★★
22	Summer squash (yellow)	3★★★
23	Eggplant	D
24	Artichokes	D
25	Avocados	2★★
26	Peas (fresh or frozen)	3★★★
27	Radishes	1★
28	Beets	3★★★
29	Bok choy	
30	Kale	1★

* The health benefits of broccoli, cauliflower, and garlic go beyond their impact on the gastrointestinal microbiome and their nutrient content. Thus, the DAD rating does not capture their impact on health. This will be discussed in a separate chapter.

Table 7B: Vegetables ranked high to low.
About the same for any rating number

Vegetable	Rating
Tomatoes, stewed	5
Tomato Ketchup	5
Tomato (slicing)	5
Squash, Butternut,	5
Cucumber (peeled)	5
Sweet potato, baked (without skin)	5
Pumpkin (fresh)	5
Squash, Acorn	5
Pumpkin (canned)	4
Watercress (raw)	4
Green peas	3
Beets (peeled)	3
Okra	3
Carrots, peeled, sliced, boiled 6 min.	3
Chanterelle mushrooms (fresh)	3
Yellow Summer Squash	3
Sweet corn with BS presoak*	3-
Zucchini Squash	2
Garlic, raw ^	2
Mushrooms, Baby Bella (brown)	2 - 4
Bell Pepper (green, red, or orange)	2
Edamame (soybean)	2
Spinach Greens	2
Hominy Corn (canned, white)	2
Onions cooked	2
Capers ^	1+
Green Beans	1+
Broccoli leaf	1+
Cauliflower (raw)	1+
Turnip Greens	1+
Mushrooms (bottled)	1+
Radish greens	1+
Broccoli (raw) ^	1+

^ Broccoli, garlic. Onions and capers should not be judged on their DAD score alone. These vegetables have important antioxidant, anti-inflammatory, and anti-cancer effects. Their proper preparation and important dietary use are discussed in Chapter 19. Fresh, crushed garlic gets a score of 5.

* See Sweet Corn below.

Vegetable	Rating
Cauliflower (frozen and cooked)	1+
Potato, freshly mashed (no skin)	1
Collard Greens	1
French fries (seasoned frozen) baked	1
Snow peas	1
Radish (root)	1-
Grape leaf, immature	1-
Lima Beans	1-
Carrot (peeled), raw to boiled 4 min.	0
Potatoes, boiled with skin	0
Plantain, ripe, cooked in the microwave	0
Chives (dry)	0
Lettuce Romaine	0
Onion, red raw ^	0
Onion, white raw	0
Red leaf lettuce	0
Celery, stalk or leaf	0
Onion greens, raw	A
Olives (green or black)	A
Dried porcini mushrooms	A
Carrots, raw, washed, unpeeled	B
Corn, sweet (typical preparation) *	B*
Edamame pod	C
Cabbage	D
Radish Skin	D
Asparagus, cooked, tip or stem	D
Sweet potato skin	D
Brussels sprouts, cooked	D
Potato skin (Idaho)	D
Yuca (manioc)	D
Artichoke Hearts creamy center	D
Artichoke Hearts with sepals	D
Jerusalem artichoke	D
Eggplant	D

Tomatoes are listed thrice in Table 7B. This serves to emphasize that tomatoes are helpful, fresh in a salad, cooked into spaghetti sauce, or even when rendered into ketchup. The high score tomatoes receive is likely in large part due to their high content of lycopene. A systematic literature review found that lycopene consumption was associated with better cognitive function, and one study found higher AD mortality in those with lower blood lycopene levels.[1]

Green tomatoes do not get this high a rating. Lycopene is best absorbed when it is consumed with part of a meal that includes a little bit of fat. This can be some cheese or a bit of oil in spaghetti sauce. Other foods high in lycopene include pink or red guavas, watermelon, apricots, and pink grapefruit.

DAD (Defense Against Dysbiosis/ Dietary Antiinflammatory Degree) Scores

A: Mildly dysbiotic
B: Moderately dysbiotic
C: Strongly dysbiotic
D: Profoundly dysbiotic

0: Foods that have little net impact on the microbiome
1: Foods that mildly favor a healthy microbiome
2: Foods that promote a healthy microbiome
3: Foods that strongly promote intestinal and general health
4. Excellent foods for GI and general health
5. Outstanding foods for GI and general health

Table 5C: The most commonly consumed processed vegetables.

Rank	Vegetable	Major Use Examples
1	Potatoes	French fries, hash browns, instant mashed potatoes
2	Corn	Canned corn, frozen corn kernels
3	Tomatoes	Canned diced tomatoes, tomato sauce, salsa, and ketchup
4	Peas	Frozen peas
5	Green beans	Canned green beans
6	Carrots	Baby carrots, canned carrots
7	Broccoli	Frozen broccoli florets
8	Cauliflower	Frozen cauliflower florets
9	Onions	Dehydrated onions, onion rings
10	Spinach	Frozen spinach
11	Mixed vegetables	Frozen or canned combinations
12	Beets	Canned beets, pickled beets
13	Mushrooms	Canned mushrooms, spaghetti sauces
14	Asparagus	Frozen asparagus spears
15	Green peppers	Canned peppers
16	Brussels sprouts	Frozen Brussels sprouts
17	Corn kernels	Used in pizza toppings, salads
18	Pumpkin	Canned pumpkin puree
19	Celery	Used in dehydrated soup mixes
20	Leeks	Used in soups and stews

Skin

A novel and notable feature of the SANA diet is its general prohibition of the consumption of skin. This is not limited to animal skin (pork rind, boot leather, chicken skin, and fish skin) but includes the skin of tubers and roots, and that of most fruits and vegetables.

Animal skin is treyf (not kosher), haram (forbidden by Islamic law), and verboten (forbidden in general)! Animal skin ranks a rating of D (dread) on the DAD scale, meaning it should never be consumed. Consuming the skin of tubers and underground vegetables is also prohibited on the SANA diet.

The reason for this prohibition can be most easily understood by considering the function of skin, which is to keep the inside safe from the outside. Consider a sweet potato growing in a moist tropical area. The soil is abundant with fungi, bacteria, and nematodes, and the sweet, starchy, swollen underground stem is just a millimeter away. As long as the skin is intact, bacteria and fungi, which would otherwise rapidly consume the sweet flesh of the sweet potato, are kept out. What is the greatest danger from a superficial laceration or abrasion of your skin? Infection.

The skin of fruits and vegetables may contain anti-nutritional and antibiotic compounds and may be poorly digestible; thus, it commonly reaches the lower intestine. Antimicrobial substances in the skin disturb the commensal microbiome. Skin is thought to act sort of like an antibiotic, making life difficult for favorable bacteria and promoting overgrowth of unfavorable ones. One of the ways that antibiotics cause dysbiosis is that they kill most of the bacteria, but spores from spore-forming bacteria survive. When the antibiotic is discontinued, the spores activate and spore-forming bacteria dominate the microbiome, often causing disease.

Seed coats are another type of "skin" that protects the seed germ and its endosperm from microbial degradation while the seed is dormant, awaiting germination in the soil. The seed coat of many seeds contains antinutritional compounds that prevent the digestion and utilization of nutrients. These nutrients may thus fail to be absorbed. This is a mechanism that evolved in plants to deter insects and animals from eating large amounts of their seeds. Some will simply move through the animal's gut without being digested. Others will make the animal feel sick and thus dissuade them from grazing on the seed. Humans can eat large quantities of seeds only because we cook or otherwise process them.

As explained in Chapter 3, proteins that are not digested and absorbed due to anti-nutritive compounds in food may cause the overgrowth of proteolytic bacteria in the colon, causing dysbiosis and the generation of toxic compounds. The consumption of animal skin, as well as that of tubers and most fruits and seeds, has a strong negative impact on the microbiome.

Zucchinis and yellow squash are exceptions where the skin is the most favorable part of the fruit. This may be a result of high concentrations of citrulline in the skin of these squashes. The fiber in tomato skin has a beneficial prebiotic effect as a result of an uncommon set of sugar molecule links. The skin is removed when tomatoes are processed for canning, which may be just as well, as it removes most pesticide residues from the fruit.

Potatoes and sweet potatoes may be baked with the skin on, but the skin should be left on the plate. Sweet potato and potato skin get a D, but sweet potato skin is worse, as it has considerably more mass. Carrots, parsnips, and other underground vegetables should be peeled before cooking. The seed coat of many seeds contains antinutritive properties, including saponins, tannins, lectins, and phytates. The SANA program recommends cooking methods that remove the bulk of these compounds.

Fresh, Frozen, Canned

As a general rule, fresh vegetables in good condition are best, followed by frozen ones. Canned tomatoes may be better than fresh ones, as they are harvested ripe for canning, rather than fresh tomatoes that are usually picked early so that they withstand machine harvesting better. For the most part, frozen or canned vegetables have a similar DAD rating when frozen or canned as when fresh, if they were processed at peak quality. Canned pumpkin has a slightly lower rating than freshly cooked pumpkin.

The canning process overcooks many vegetables, and then they need to be reheated to cooking temperatures again before serving; this degrades their quality. Frozen green beans and peas have far better flavor than canned ones. Canned green beans and peas are yucky. (That may just be a childhood observation; I have refused to try them since being compelled to eat bean casserole one Thanksgiving long ago, a dish served once a year too often.)

When buying a bag of frozen vegetables or fruits, the contents should be loose in the bag. If they are frozen into a hard block, it indicates that the fruits or veggies have thawed and then refrozen into the block. You don't know how long they were thawed for, or how hot they got. If they don't separate into individual pieces with just a bit of pressure, don't purchase them. Frozen spinach is generally packed into a rectangular box, so this test does not apply.

Don't buy any vegetables with any signs of molding. If buying a bag of potatoes or onions, try to see if any are bad; however, this may be difficult to tell in the bag. You may have to do a sniff test to discern whether they have a musty or moldy odor. In any case, open the bag on arriving home and check the vegetables, and discard any bad ones. See Chapter 27 for the topic on mold.

Green Leafy Vegetables

As a general rule, when it comes to preserving vitamins and the overall quality of green, leafy vegetables:

Raw > brief microwave, brief blanching or steaming > boiling.

Most vegetables, however, should not be eaten raw, as they have compounds meant to deter digestion or to deter their consumption by animals, mostly the small buggy kind. Broccoli and cauliflower, garlic and onions can be eaten raw if thoroughly chewed, as the maceration causes the formation of compounds (such as sulforaphane and allicin) which are intended to deter insects that attempt to chew on these veggies. In humans, these compounds stimulate the production of anti-inflammatory and anti-cancer proteins in the body. Boiling temperatures destroy these beneficial compounds. Thus, broccoli and cauliflower provide the best benefit when consumed in small amounts raw, or in more typical portions, very lightly steamed. This will be discussed in Chapter 20.

Yellow-Orange Vegetables

You will notice the orange vegetables (winter squash and sweet potatoes) take the top ratings. This is likely because they have a high content of non-beta-carotene carotenoids. In a study of participants in the MIND diet intervention study, participants with higher blood α-carotene (but not β-carotene) levels had better global cognitive function than participants with lower α-carotene levels. Semantic (word) memory scores were better in those with higher circulating levels of α-carotene and with higher levels of lutein and zeaxanthin. Perceptual speed memory was most closely associated with higher lycopene levels.[2] In a meta-analysis of several studies, higher circulating levels of α-carotene, β-carotene, and lutein/zeaxanthin were associated with a lower risk of T2D.[3] Most available studies indicate that lower blood levels of lutein and zeaxanthin are associated with AD risk. Others additionally show benefit from β-cryptoxanthin. Not all studies are consistent. People might take vitamin supplements with individual carotenoids, but foods are complex, and these compounds come jumbled together; this makes it hard to tell in a population study which compounds are beneficial and which are just along for the ride. Lutein, zeaxanthin, and meso-zeaxanthin help prevent age-related macular degeneration; thus, these have the additional benefit of protecting the retina from oxidative injury.[4] Yellow-orange vegetable consumption also appears to be protective against some types of cancer in population studies. Squashes are also high in citrulline.

Carrots, unfortunately, are difficult to digest unless cooked (simmered for 5 - 6 minutes), and should not be eaten raw. Raw carrots (and raw onions) are especially problematic for those with IBD. Avoid overcooking carrots as they lose flavor and texture. Carrots should always be peeled. Raw winter squash and sweet potatoes should also not be eaten raw, but almost no one tries.

Tomatoes

Tomatoes are among the most highly ranked fruits and vegetables, with a DAD score of 5. Tomatoes are one of the fruits that have skin that provides fiber that promotes eubiosis. Tomatoes benefit from being eaten, as their seeds pass the GI tract undigested, helping to disperse the seeds to new locations along with a starter kit of fertilizer. Raw or cooked, they are a gift.

Sweet Corn

Field corn (maize) will be discussed in the next couple of chapters, but it has the same problem as sweet corn: its seed coat. Corn has a large seed coat that gives it a bad score. Sweet corn gets a low B on the DAD scale as a result of its seed coat. Sweet corn, as corn on a cob or as cut corn, is a delicious, enjoyable vegetable, and can be easily prepared in a way that gives it an excellent DAD score. This will be discussed in Chapter 9.

Brassica / Cruciferous Vegetables

Broccoli, cauliflower, watercress, and garlic have special health benefits, and their consumption may lower the risk of cancer and delay aging. The DAD ratings do not reflect these benefits. Broccoli and cauliflower should not be neglected in the diet as a result of their mild benefit to the intestinal microbiome, but rather understood so that the highest benefits can be derived from them. The SANA diet encourages the consumption of broccoli or cauliflower a few times a week. The health benefits of cruciferous vegetables and garlic will be discussed in Chapter 16.

If eaten as a raw vegetable, only a small serving of broccoli, about an ounce, is all that is needed for its antioxidant effect. Excessive consumption of broccoli, cauliflower, and related plants can cause thyroid toxicity, but one has to really work hard, consuming huge amounts, to achieve this effect.

Broccoli and cauliflower only need to be consumed in small amounts to provide their health benefits, and limiting consumption to the flower buds and avoiding larger stems will prevent the noxious outcomes. Getting the health benefits of broccoli or cauliflower only takes a small amount, about an ounce of the flowerhead if eaten raw or not overcooked. Heating broccoli to over 90°C (194°F) destroys the sulforaphane (the beneficial, anti-cancer compound). You can eat a boatload of overcooked broccoli and mostly get GI and thyroid problems.

The woody peel on the stem of broccoli needs to be avoided as it is tough to digest and will ferment and spur the growth of nasty things in the bowel. (DAD score = D). The pale, non-fibrous interior of the stem can be cooked and is similar to kohlrabi, and can be eaten. The fleshy stems of cauliflower leaves are like cabbage and have a DAD rating of D.

Fructans

Several foods that are high in fructans are rated D; however, some, such as onions, have sufficiently redeeming qualities to merit a DAD score of zero. There are various types of fructans, and the response to them differs not just in the molecular bond type, but also in the polysaccharide chain length of the fructans. Short-chain β-fructans increase stool frequency and moisture, while long-chain β-fructans do not. Inulin from chicory contains long fructan chains. Most people do well with up to about 10 grams of fructans per day in the diet, an amount that promotes the growth of *Bifidobacteria* and other commensal bacteria and promotes the production of the short-chain fatty acid butyrate.[5]

It is the long-chained fructans (fructooligo-saccharides - FOS) that have the probiotic effect, as they resist digestion and are fermentable fiber. When large amounts are eaten, they cause gas formation in the bowels. Foods that contain substantial amounts of fructans include chicory root, asparagus, artichokes, yacón, blue agave, wheat, rye, and barley. The king of fructans is the Jerusalem artichoke, also known as the sunchoke, whose dry mass can be 20% fructans, and the consumption of which produces comical levels of gaseous effluent. Fermentation of FOS produces hydrogen and carbon dioxide gases. Granola bars that are sold as fiber supplements often contain chicory to boost the fiber levels. The specific fructans in chicory are called inulin. Inulin gets a DAD score of A. Other foods high in Fructans get DAD ratings of D.

Since the FOS sources we consume in the highest quantities include whole wheat, bananas, and onions, these are the foods that contribute most of the FOS in the Western diet, even though they are not among the foods with the highest FOS content. These get poor DAD scores, but not terrible ones.

The general consensus is that the consumption of long-chain fructans is beneficial. However, the SANA diet does not align with this. In a study of patients with inflammatory bowel disease, β-fructans were found to cause a proinflammatory response mediated by the TLR2 and the NLRP3 inflammasome pathway. This was found to be the result of the patient's microbiota, as the inflammatory response could be seen in vitro when microbes were collected from patients with active disease, but rather had an anti-inflammatory response from cultures of control subjects and in patients with inactive disease. Thus, certain foods high in long-chain fructans are avoided by the SANA diet as they may be mistakenly identified as pathogens as they have similar polysaccharide structures as some fungi, and thus can activate an inflammatory immune response, they may promote the production of acetate which increases ROS production in macrophages, or may foster quorum sensing, promoting more pathogenic behavior of the bacteria in the dysbiotic biome. These foods need to be especially avoided during active disease or dysbiosis, but can promote exacerbation of dysbiosis even during remission.[6]

Fructans in fruits are generally short-chained, largely digestible, and typically mixed polysaccharides with sorbitol and other sugars. Thus, even the fruit fructan polysaccharides that make it to the lower small intestine, when fermented, are less problematic and are usually processed by different bacteria from those that ferment long-chain vegetable β-fructans. The fruit fructans contribute less to promoting commensal bacterial growth.

The FODMAP Diet

The FODMAP diet promotes avoidance of many of the same foods that get negative DAD scores: Artichokes, asparagus, Brussels sprouts, Jerusalem artichokes, leeks, snow peas, and onions.[7] The diet recommends the avoidance of High FODMAP foods, foods high in fermentable carbohydrates, for people suffering from irritable bowel syndrome (IBS). The FODMAP diet correctly identifies many foods that cause GI distress, then limits those and other foods high in fructose and other fermentable carbohydrates. While there is considerable overlap of foods that should be avoided on the SANA and FODMAP diets, there are also several differences.

The FODMAP diet is generally recommended as a short-term bridge diet to give time to normalize the GI microbiome, after which the High FODMAP foods can be gradually reintroduced to the diet. The SANA dietary restrictions are not temporary, and the reality is that many individuals with IBS become symptomatic again if they eat High FODMAP foods.

The SANA diet allows but does not recommend occasional consumption of items ranked A on the DAD score if the person has no evidence of dysbiosis, but strongly recommends complete avoidance of items ranked C of D. While long-chain FOS may contribute to a food's poor digestibility, the DAD score is a holistic assessment of a foods impact on a foods impact on dysbiosis and inflammation. For example, onions are high in FOS, but especially when cooked, allowed on the diet.

Here is a link to a list of FODMAP foods: www.ibsdiets.org/fodmap-diet/fodmap-food-list

Brussel's Sprouts

Even though they are the same species as broccoli, kale, collards, and kohlrabi, which provide GI benefits, Brussels sprouts (BSs) are weird and need to be avoided. Ever see how they grow? Like a neurofibroma along the stem. Even the name is weird. My sister has a more apt name for them: "Fart Bombs".

OK, I get it, they have a sweetness to them; it comes from the sugar raffinose. Raffinose is a trisaccharide (triple sugar) composed of galactose + sucrose. Humans do not have an enzyme to cleave the galactose sucrose bond, so raffinose goes undigested and gets fermented in the lower intestine by bacteria that produce the enzyme α-galactosidase, forming d-galactose and the disaccharide sucrose. You really should not want either sugar in the gut. There are also plenty of sulfur compounds in Brussels sprouts that compound the malodorous effluent. There are positives to BSs; they may increase the production of antioxidant enzymes in the colon wall,[8] likely as a stress response. But in those with dysbiosis, it can greatly exacerbate it.

Raffinose is also present in asparagus, cabbage, and some whole grains. Some is present in broccoli and beans. Brussels sprouts, broccoli, cabbage, asparagus, cauliflower, broccoli, beans, and certain whole grains are known to cause excess gas.

The amino acid cysteine contains sulfur. Cysteine and certain other sulfur-containing compounds, such as those in cabbage and Brussels sprouts, are fermented by *Desulfovibrio* bacteria in the gut, producing hydrogen sulfide (H2S). H2S is a gasotransmitter and has numerous beneficial physiologic actions in multiple organs, including the pancreas and brain. The colonocytes can metabolize H2S produced during fermentation by gut bacteria to use it as a fuel source. H2S is not only a fuel for colonocytes; it helps maintain the integrity of the mucous layer and stimulates the production of glucagon-like peptide 1 (GLP-1) by the neuro-endocrine L-cells in the intestine.[9] GLP-1 regulates postprandial blood glucose and helps control the appetite.

The reader may not be aware of GLP-1, but is likely familiar with the popular medication Ozempic (semaglutide) or one of many biosimilar medications that are used to treat type 2 diabetes and obesity. They have a similar structure to GLP-1 and are GLP-1 mimetics. Thus, the production of H2S and GLP-1 resulting from the fermentation of sulfur compounds in the intestine is beneficial, and in animals has been shown to enhance GLP-1 and insulin secretion, reduce food consumption, and improve oral glucose tolerance.[10]

Nevertheless, H2S is a toxin. At low levels, H2S protects the mucosa and alleviates inflammation; at higher levels, it promotes inflammation and injury. H2S produced by *Desulfovibrio* in the gut can inhibit mitochondrial respiration in the L cells.[11] H2S induces the unfolded protein response that interferes with GLP-1 secretion and inhibits GLP-1 gene expression.[12]

Brussels sprouts and cabbage, and perhaps asparagus are rated D, at least in part because they provoke an over-production of hydrogen sulfide (H2S) during digestion/fermentation. There are better ways to ensure adequate GLP-1 production; short-chain fatty acids such as butyrate increase its production, as do certain indoles and other products of fermentation.[13]

Onions and Garlic

Raw onions are tasty, but get an A for avoid. This is especially a problem for those with active dysbiosis or inflammatory bowel disease (IBD) and IBS. Lightly cooked (boiled) onions are fine, with a score of two. The issue with onions happens when pieces of onions are swallowed with their cells intact, as in contrast, macerated and crushed onions get a score of four, as does crushed garlic. Dried onion bits get a score of one, and thus can be used to add flavoring. The use of garlic powder is encouraged; however, it should be added to food just before serving to give it its most potent health benefits. Garlic has antioxidant effects and lowers the risk of cancer and other chronic diseases. This will also be detailed in a separate chapter.

Mushrooms

White button, cremini (brown button), and portobello mushrooms are all *Agaricus bisporus*, just harvested at different stages of development. The DAD score of mushrooms varied greatly from 4 to 1, depending on freshness and quality.

In a study of healthy aging of older adults in Southeast Asia, those consuming mushrooms more than twice a week had an odds ratio of 0.43 for mild cognitive impairment (MCI), a 57% reduction.[14] In another population study, American adults 60 and older who consumed an average of 13.4 grams/1000 kcal/day (a bit less than an ounce per day) of mushrooms had higher cognitive scores.[15] In a European 18-year follow-up study, the frequency of mushroom consumption was linearly associated with higher cognitive test scores.[16] A study of older Chinese adults also found that those consuming, on average, more than 10 grams of mushrooms a day were 12% less likely to have MCI.[17] Mushroom consumption may also have a positive impact on mood, reducing depression.[18]

Mushrooms are a decent source of vitamin D2, but the impact of mushrooms on cognition can more likely be attributed to their high content of ergothioneine, a nonprotein-forming amino acid that is a cofactor for several enzymes, including the recycling of glutathione, the body's most important antioxidant. Ergothioneine improves exercise tolerance; it is further discussed in Chapter 29 on exercise.

The SANA diet recommends incorporating mushrooms into the diet and consuming a few ounces of mushrooms each week. A button or cremini mushroom with a 1.5 to 2-inch diameter cap should supply a sufficient daily ergothioneine supply. Cooking does not deplete ergothioneine levels. Oyster mushrooms generally contain higher concentrations than do the common *Agaricus bisporus* white button, cremini, and portobello mushrooms typically sold in grocery stores. Other edible mushrooms also contain ergothioneine.

Fresh Legumes

This section covers legumes that are eaten as vegetables, and thus those that are harvested before drying, often before reaching full maturity. This included string beans, snow peas, and green peas that one may find in the fresh vegetable section of your local grocery, and likely an even wider selection in the freezer section or as canned vegetables. In addition to those mentioned, this may include lima beans, black eyed peas, edamame, and many others.

I don't have a whole lot to say other than:

- Fresh is best
- Fresh frozen legumes generally taste much better than canned ones.
- Steaming vegetables helps preserve nutrition.

Steaming over boiling: Many vitamins, minerals, and some amino acids are water-soluble. If vegetables are cooked in water and the water is discarded, some nutrients go with it. Using a steamer or steamer tray above the water maintains most of those nutrients. Excessive steaming does cause loss of vitamin C. Steam only to the extent needed to make the vegetable palatable.

Peas: There are three main types of peas: Garden (or English) peas are grown for shelling; the shell is not eaten. Snow peas (sugar peas) are harvested with small, immature seeds, and snap peas are harvested when the peas have reached full size but have not matured. The peas and pods of snow and snap peas are eaten with the peas inside.

Edamame: Some time ago, I spotted edamame in the freezer section of my grocer, and thought I would give them a try. Edamame are soy beans that are still green. I steamed them for supper. I tried one, and then a second one just to make sure. "Why", I thought, "would anyone ever put these in their mouth?" They were awful! They were woody and unpleasant. You are now likely laughing at me. The way to eat edamame is as a finger food. Steam them, and then when they have cooled, you pop them open and eat the buttery seeds inside the pod, or put the seeds in a salad.

Edamame is like a garden pea in that the pod is discarded. The pods of garden peas and edamame can be eaten, just not on the DAD diet. They get a score of C.

Green beans (*Phaseolus vulgaris*) are immature seed pods from the same species of bean as kidney, pinto, canary, and black beans.

Fresh lima beans (butter beans) are from a different genus from green beans. They contain anti-nutritional compounds, and get a score of 1- on the DAD scale. There are better choices.

Root Vegetables

The "skin" of root vegetables (sweet potatoes, yucca, potatoes, carrots, parsnips, taro, yams, etc.) should not be eaten unless specifically processed for this.

Potatoes

Potatoes are America's most popular vegetable. They are more than that. Although grouped with vegetables, potatoes might be more properly assessed in comparison to grains than being categorized as a vegetable.

They are considered to be the third or fourth most important crop for the total amount of calories provided to humankind after the cereal crops, wheat, rice, and similar to that of maize. Potatoes are grown in the tropics and in Greenland, at sea level and up to 4700 meters (15,420 feet) above sea level. One acre of potatoes can yield about three times as many calories of food as any other crop, and use as little as one seventh as much water as do cereals. [19] While being a lowly starchy tuber, they contain 10% of their calories as protein, slightly higher than that of rice, but lower than that of wheat or corn. Not only that, they are fun to eat. (I'm supposed to say, "They are additionally highly palatable.")

Unfortunately, potatoes barely get a DAD score of one, and then they are bathed in hot oil and showered with salt. In the U.S., about half of all potatoes go into frozen foods – 85% of which are turned into French fries,[20] a high-calorie, starchy, fatty, salty food. Two-thirds of those are sold through fast-food venues. Deep-fried French fries, as served in restaurants, absorb up to 20% of their weight in oil. About 44% of their calories are fat, and not healthy fat. In restaurants, the oil is repeatedly used and forms acrylamide and other oxidized products. Thus, in population studies, eating potatoes is firmly linked to fast and fatty foods, damaging their reputation. Potatoes cooked with their skin get a DAD score of zero. At its best, boiled or baked potatoes, when the skin is discarded, get a DAD score of 1. If they are to be boiled, they should first be peeled. When boiled or baked as usual, potatoes can be eaten on the SANA diet; however, there are much better ways to prepare them.

The long-term impact of potatoes on health was investigated using the NHANES study data, including 24,856 participants and 3433 deaths over an average of 6.4 years. When comparing those in the highest tertile with those in the lowest tertile for potato consumption, blood pressure was minimally higher, waist circumference two centimeters larger, insulin levels higher, and insulin resistance greater. An increased risk of total, cardiovascular, and cancer mortality was found, *but it disappeared* after adjusting for other risk factors. [21] This suggests that high potato consumption is likely associated with a dietary pattern that confers risk, but that potatoes themselves induce minimal if any risk. It also suggests minimal benefit.

While the amino acid profile of potato protein is excellent, the digestibility is not. The protein digestibility-corrected amino acid score (PDCAAS) of Russet potatoes ranged from 0.27 to 0.56. When boiled, 56 percent of the protein is digestible, baked or microwaved about 50%, fried for six minutes, about 36%, and raw, 27%. If fried for a longer amount of time, the digestibility falls.[22] Anti-nutritional factors in potatoes, such as lectins, likely limit their PDCAAS. The low digestibility not only means that much of the nutritional value is lost, but it also indicates that more protein is available for fermentation in the colon, which can promote inflammation and dysbiosis.

Potatoes that are green should not be eaten as they may be toxic. Greening in potatoes comes from improper storage. Potatoes need to be stored in a cool, dry, dark area, but in the grocery store, they are on display under light. If they sit long enough in the light, they will green. The green color in and just below the potato skin is from chlorophyll, which is harmless, but the exposure to light (and injury of the tuber) promotes the production of glycoalkaloid toxins such as α-chaconine and α-solanine. These bitter toxins act as a defense against the tuber being eaten by animals. They are also present in the stems and leaves of healthy potato plants.[23] Solaine irritates the GI tract and causes nausea and vomiting if eaten in large amounts. It is teratogenic, meaning that it can cause birth defects. Insect, disease, or mechanical damage to the potato also causes an increase in the production of these toxins. Potatoes should be cooked soon after cutting them to prevent the formation of these toxins. About 50% of these toxins are in the skin, so peeling greatly reduces the content of these toxins. Boiling only lowers the alkaloid content by a few percentage points. Blanching also lowers alkaloid levels.[24]

To keep your potatoes fresh and delicious, store them in a cool, dark place. They should be kept at temperatures between 45-50°F (7-10°C) and in the dark. Nevertheless, they need some ventilation. They should not be stored with onions or fruits that produce ethylene, as it can induce sprouting. A mesh or paper bag that allows for air circulation helps prevent spoilage. Keeping them in the dark prevents greening. Most of the toxins are close to the skin, so if there is just a small bit of greening, cut any green parts away. A more reliable test for the presence of the toxin may be to taste a small piece of the potato peel to test for bitterness; if the peel is bitter, discard the potato. If the potato has a high amount of toxins, more than 0.2 mg/g of solanine, the peel will cause an immediate burning sensation in the mouth; then, of course, the entire potato should be discarded.[25]

As with grains and legumes, the SANA program has developed a method for increasing the digestibility of potatoes.

SANA Method of Potato Preparation: 5 ★★★★★: **1.** First, inspect and gently clean the potatoes, removing any bad parts or wounds; however, it is best to use potatoes without defects and avoid those that are beginning to sprout.

2A. Soak the potatoes in the warm bath, maintaining a temperature of 35°C (95°F) for 11 hours. Soaking needs to be done in the dark, so soak in a container with a lid that excludes light to avoid the formation of glycoalkaloids. Temperatures of 96°F and higher or below freezing and excessive soak time will cause the inside of the potato to get "blackheart," which is ugly, but not toxic.[26] Potatoes that have started sprouting are more subject to blackheart. Blackheart results from hypoxia (a lack of oxygen) and a buildup of carbon dioxide. Oxygen demand increases with temperature, and additionally, warmer water holds less dissolved oxygen. Higher temperatures lower the amount of soak time needed but increase the oxygen demand of the potato, increasing the risk of blackheart developing. Aerating the water, for example, using an aquarium bubbler and airstone during soaking, helps avoid blackheart and can allow the use of a slightly higher temperature and shorter soak time. Using more water and avoiding crowding the potatoes, for example, soaking only a single layer of potatoes in the vessel allows better aeration of the water. There are several potato diseases besides blackheart injury that will cause the interior of the potato to turn black; thus, potatoes that are black inside should not be eaten. Different potato varieties have varying susceptibility to blackheart injury; thus, some may be injured at a lower temperature than others.

2B. Potatoes can be soaked at 38°C (100°F) for 8 to 10 hours if soaked in sufficient water and using sufficient aeration.

3. If you would like to eat the potato skin, the potato can be "blanched". This can be done by adding one teaspoon (5 grams) of baking soda per liter to the cooking water when boiling the potatoes. The potatoes can then be cut and air-fried if desired.

Alternatively, the same concentration of baking soda can be added to the soaking water during the *last hour* of soaking. This method may be preferred if the potatoes will be baked. Note that excessive alkalinization of the water, a pH of 8.5 or higher, will cause ionization of CO2 and prevent its release from the water, which may contribute to blackheart.

4. After soaking the potatoes, prepare them in the usual manner. Boiling gives the highest digestibility score, as compared to baking or microwaving, which is considerably better than frying. Remember that if not treated, the skin should be discarded. The soaked potatoes take a bit longer to cook.

The potatoes can be baked after blanching, microwaved, and then air-fried, or used in other ways. Boiling whole potatoes so that they are mostly cooked before cutting them for air-frying helps give a soft center and crispy exterior.

Yuca (Manioc, Cassava)

Cassava is a staple in many tropical countries, where it is the third largest source of carbohydrates, after rice and maize. Yuca is a tropical tuber that can contain high amounts of cyanogenic compounds, especially when grown under stress conditions. The compounds form cyanide during their metabolism by the liver. It is toxic enough to cause permanent paralysis in children who are malnourished and have little else to eat. Bitter yuca should never be consumed; it has 8 times as much cyanogenic compounds as sweet yuca, and it is poisonous. About half of the toxic cyanide-forming compounds are in the skin of the tuber. Boiling with water changes lowers the cyanogenic glycoside content of cassava. Even after boiling or pressure cooking, "sweet" yuca still gets a D. Yuca is not allowed on the SANA diet.

Cassava is the source of tapioca (starch, flour, pudding, bubble tea balls). It has been processed sufficiently that it retains minimal amounts of the cyanide precursors. Tapioca has minimal nutritional value beyond being a starch.

Sweet Potatoes

Sweet potatoes are another starchy tuber. Orange-fleshed sweet potatoes are high in carotenoids, and purple ones are high in anthocyanins. Okinawa sweet potatoes are buff colored on the outside and deep purple on the inside. These purple ones are common in the diet of the people of Okinawa, a Blue Zone. Sweet potatoes contain about 9% of their calories as protein, about the same as rice, but it is low in lysine, methionine, and tryptophan, and thus are an incomplete protein. It can be paired with legumes, tofu, quinoa, or brown rice to improve its protein utilization.

The major soluble protein in sweet potatoes, sporamin, is a Kunitz-type trypsin inhibitor,[27] with the Okinawan variety having higher levels than most other types. There are several studies showing beneficial effects of sporamin against inflammation, cancer, and obesity in cell cultures,[28] and when injected into mice, but there is a distinct absence of studies on sporamin's impact on humans (and animals) as a dietary element. Sporamin functions as a trypsin inhibitor that prevents protein digestion in insects, birds, and mammals that try to eat the tuber. Injury to the sweet potato plant increases sporamin production, to increases protection from being eaten.[29] Cooking at a temperature of over 90°C dramatically decreases trypsin inhibitor activity in sweet potatoes.[30] Sporamin is also metabolized into other proteins during the sprouting of the tuber.[31]

As per their name, trypsin inhibitors inhibit trypsin. Trypsin is a protease that activates other digestive enzymes, including chymotrypsin and elastase. These are needed for the digestion of protein. Soybeans also contain an unusually high content of a Kunitz-type trypsin inhibitor, which limits the amount that can be used in animal feed. Cooking can partially or entirely inactivate trypsin inhibitors in foods. Higher temperature, longer cooking times, and greater cooking water volume promote the denaturing of these proteins. Even so, soy-based infant formulas may retain 20 to 28% of the trypsin-inhibiting activity of soy. [32] High levels of dietary trypsin inhibitors can lower the digestion of proteins by as much as 50%; however, this degree of inhibition is unlikely outside of experimental conditions. Soy trypsin inhibitors have been extensively studied because of their economic impact on animal feed and the ease of studying animals. Feeding unprocessed soy to animals causes pancreatic hypertrophy and hyperplasia and slows growth. Don't eat sweet potatoes or soy beans undercooked or raw.

Using normal cooking procedures (boiling and baking), sweet potatoes get a DAD score of 4. Nevertheless, the digestibility can be improved considerably.

SANA Recommended Method: 5 ★★★★★: Presoak the sweet potato as for potatoes, but at a water temperature of 41°C (102°F) for 10 hours with a bubbler using aeration, and then cook as usual. The highest digestibility for sweet potatoes is when they are boiled; however, baking and other methods give high scores. The tubers can be partially boiled (and blanched) and then baked, or air-fried for quicker cooking time and better results. The skin gets a D if not "blanched". Blanching is as for potatoes, above, but note that if the sweet potato is cut before blanching, the alkalinity from the baking soda will cause the exposed anthocyanins of the sweet potato to turn bluish green. Thus, blanching of the intact tuber is recommended. Blanching can also be done by adding baking soda (5 g/L) to the warm water presoak for the last hour.

[1] Lycopene and cognitive function. Crowe-White KM, Phillips TA, Ellis AC. J Nutr Sci. 2019 May 29;8:e20. doi: 10.1017/jns.2019.16. eCollection 2019. PMID: 31217968

[2] Higher circulating α-carotene was associated with better cognitive function: an evaluation among the MIND trial participants. Liu X, Dhana K, Furtado JD, Agarwal P, Aggarwal NT, Tangney C, Laranjo N, Carey V, Barnes LL, Sacks FM. J Nutr Sci. 2021 Aug 16;10:e64. doi: 10.1017/jns.2021.56. eCollection 2021. PMID: 34527222

[3] Dietary Intake and Circulating Concentrations of Carotenoids and Risk of Type 2 Diabetes: A Dose-Response Meta-Analysis of Prospective Observational Studies. Jiang YW, Sun ZH, Tong WW, Yang K, Guo KQ, Liu G, Pan A. Adv Nutr. 2021 Oct 1;12(5):1723-1733. doi: 10.1093/advances/nmab048. PMID: 33979433

[4] Non-Enzymatic Antioxidants against Alzheimer's Disease: Prevention, Diagnosis and Therapy. Varesi A, Campagnoli LIM, Carrara A, Pola I, Floris E, Ricevuti G, Chirumbolo S, Pascale A. Antioxidants (Basel). 2023 Jan 12;12(1):180. doi: 10.3390/antiox12010180. PMID: 36671042

[5] Effects of β-Fructans Fiber on Bowel Function: A Systematic Review and Meta-Analysis. de Vries J, Le Bourgot C, Calame W, Respondek F. Nutrients. 2019 Jan 4;11(1):91. doi: 10.3390/nu11010091. PMID: 30621208

[6] Unfermented β-fructan Fibers Fuel Inflammation in Select Inflammatory Bowel Disease Patients. Armstrong HK, Bording-Jorgensen M, Santer DM, et al Dieleman LA, Wine E. Gastroenterology. 2023 Feb;164(2):228-240. doi: 10.1053/j.gastro.2022.09.034. Epub 2022 Sep 29. PMID: 36183751

[7] https://www.ibsdiets.org/fodmap-diet/fodmap-food-list (Accessed Jan 2021)

[8] Effects of consumption of Brussels sprouts on intestinal and lymphocytic glutathione S-transferases in humans. Nijhoff WA, Grubben MJ, Nagengast FM, Jansen JB, Verhagen H, van Poppel G, Peters WH. Carcinogenesis. 1995 Sep;16(9):2125-8. doi: 10.1093/carcin/16.9.2125. PMID: 7554064

[9] Cysteine-derived hydrogen sulfide and gut health: a matter of endogenous or bacterial origin. Blachier F, Beaumont M, Kim E. Curr Opin Clin Nutr Metab Care. 2019 Jan;22(1):68-75. doi: 10.1097/MCO.0000000000000526. PMID: 30461448

[10] Hydrogen Sulfide and Sulfate Prebiotic Stimulates the Secretion of GLP-1 and Improves Glycemia in Male Mice. Pichette J, Fynn-Sackey N, Gagnon J. Endocrinology. 2017 Oct 1;158(10):3416-3425. doi: 10.1210/en.2017-00391. PMID: 28977605

[11] Cysteine-derived hydrogen sulfide and gut health: a matter of endogenous or bacterial origin. Blachier F, Beaumont M, Kim E. Curr Opin Clin Nutr Metab Care. 2019 Jan;22(1):68-75. doi: 10.1097/MCO.0000000000000526. PMID: 30461448

[12] Hydrogen sulfide produced by the gut microbiota impairs host metabolism via reducing GLP-1 levels in male mice. Qi Q, Zhang H, Jin Z, Wang C, Xia M, Chen B, Lv B, Peres Diaz L, Li X, Feng R, Qiu M, Li Y, Meseguer D, Zheng X, Wang W, Song W, Huang H, Wu H, Chen L, Schneeberger M, Yu X. Nat Metab. 2024 Aug;6(8):1601-1615. doi: 10.1038/s42255-024-01068-x. Epub 2024 Jul 19. PMID: 39030389

[13] Crosstalk between glucagon-like peptide 1 and gut microbiota in metabolic diseases. Zeng Y, Wu Y, Zhang Q, Xiao X. mBio. 2024 Jan 16;15(1):e0203223. doi: 10.1128/mbio.02032-23. Epub 2023 Dec 6. PMID: 38055342

[14] The Association between Mushroom Consumption and Mild Cognitive Impairment: A Community-Based Cross-Sectional Study in Singapore. Feng L, Cheah IK, Ng MM, Li J, Chan SM, Lim SL, Mahendran R, Kua EH, Halliwell B. J Alzheimers Dis. 2019;68(1):197-203. doi: 10.3233/JAD-180959. PMID: 30775990

[15] Mushroom intake and cognitive performance among US older adults: the National Health and Nutrition Examination Survey, 2011-2014. Ba DM, Gao X, Al-Shaar L, Muscat J, Chinchilli VM, Ssentongo P, Beelman RB, Richie J. Br J Nutr. 2022 Dec 14;128(11):2241-2248. doi: 10.1017/S0007114521005195. Epub 2022 Feb 4. PMID: 35115063

[16] The Relationship between Mushroom Intake and Cognitive Performance: An Epidemiological Study in the European Investigation of Cancer-Norfolk Cohort (EPIC-Norfolk). Cha S, Bell L, Williams CM. Nutrients. 2024 Jan 25;16(3):353. doi: 10.3390/nu16030353. PMID: 38337638

[17] The relationship between mushroom consumption and cognitive performance among middle-aged and older adults: a cross-sectional study. Yan Y, Li B, Li F, Zhou X, Li T, Li Y, Liu C, Wang S, Cong Y, Deng Y, Wang Z, Zhou J, Rong S. Food Funct. 2023 Aug 14;14(16):7663-7671. doi: 10.1039/d3fo01101a. PMID: 37540100

[18] A review of the effects of mushrooms on mood and neurocognitive health across the lifespan. Cha S, Bell L, Shukitt-Hale B, Williams CM. Neurosci Biobehav Rev. 2024 Mar;158:105548. doi: 10.1016/j.neubiorev.2024.105548. Epub 2024 Jan 19. PMID: 38246232

[19] https://cipotato.org/potato/potato-facts-and-figures/

[20] https://www.ers.usda.gov/data-products/chart-gallery/gallery/chart-detail/?chartId=107266

[21] Potato consumption is associated with total and cause-specific mortality: a population-based cohort study and pooling of prospective studies with 98,569 participants. Mazidi M, Katsiki N, Mikhailidis DP, Pella D, Banach M. Arch Med Sci. 2020 Feb 11;16(2):260-272. doi: 10.5114/aoms.2020.92890. eCollection 2020. PMID: 32190135

[22] Impact of cooking on the protein quality of Russet potatoes. Bailey T, Franczyk AJ, Goldberg EM, House JD. Food Sci Nutr. 2023 Oct 3;11(12):8131-8142. doi: 10.1002/fsn3.3734. eCollection 2023 Dec. PMID: 38107092

[23] Potato steroidal glycoalkaloids: properties, biosynthesis, regulation and genetic manipulation. Liu Y, Liu X, Li Y, Pei Y, Jaleel A, Ren M. Mol Hortic. 2024 Dec 13;4(1):43. doi: 10.1186/s43897-024-00118-y. PMID: 39668379

[24] Rytel Elżbieta, The effect of industrial potato processing on the concentrations of glycoalkaloids and nitrates in potato granules. Food Control, Volume 28, Issue 2, 2012, Pages 380-384, ISSN 0956-7135, https://doi.org/10.1016/j.foodcont.2012.04.049.

[25] https://en.wikipedia.org/wiki/Solanine#In_potatoes

[26] Detection of Potato Tuber Diseases and Defects https://www.vegetables.cornell.edu/pest-management/disease-factsheets/detection-of-potato-tuber-diseases-defects/

[27] Multiple biological functions of sporamin related to stress tolerance in sweet potato (Ipomoea batatas Lam). Senthilkumar R, Yeh KW. Biotechnol Adv. 2012 Nov-Dec;30(6):1309-17. doi: 10.1016/j.biotechadv.2012.01.022 PMID: 22306516

[28] Sporamin induces apoptosis and inhibits NF-κB activation in human pancreatic cancer cells. Qian C, Chen X, Qi Y, Zhong S, Gao X, Zheng W, Mao Z, Yao J. Tumour Biol. 2017 Jul;39(7):1010428317706917. doi: 10.1177/1010428317706917. PMID: 28714369

[29] Sweet potato NAC transcription factor, IbNAC1, upregulates sporamin gene expression by binding the SWRE motif against mechanical wounding and herbivore attack. Chen SP, Lin IW, Chen X, Huang YH, Chang SC, Lo HS, Lu HH, Yeh KW. Plant J. 2016 May;86(3):234-48. doi: 10.1111/tpj.13171. PMID: 26996980

[30] Purification and Trypsin Inhibitor Activity of a Sporamin B from Sweet Potato (Ipomoea batatas Lam. 55-2). Yan-li SUN, Jun-mao SUN, Qing-peng LI, Agricultural Sciences in China, 8(7) 808-820. 2009 https://doi.org/10.1016/S1671-2927(08)60282-5.

[31] Characterization of major proteins in sweet potato tuberous roots. Masayoshi Maeshima, Takuji Sasaki, Tadashi Asahi, Phytochemistry, 24(9) 1899-1902, 1985 https://doi.org/10.1016/S0031-9422(00)83088-5. https://www.sciencedirect.com/science/article/pii/S0031942200830885

[32] Effects of antinutritional factors on protein digestibility and amino acid availability in foods. Gilani GS, Cockell KA, Sepehr E. J AOAC Int. 2005 May-Jun;88(3):967-87. PMID: 16001874

8: Anti-Nutritive Agents

The Dementia Diet

The dementia diet is just what it says. There was a diet that was common among the poor in parts of the United States and Southern Europe that caused dementia, even in children. Originally, it was known as "Asturian leprosy", after a region of Spain where it was prevalent. By 1880, it had become epidemic, with over 100,000 people affected. The disease was associated with the consumption of a diet high in maize (corn) and manifested with the "Four Ds".

- Dermatitis, especially in sun-exposed areas
- Diarrhea, often dysentery (bloody diarrhea)
- Depression, disorientation, delirium, dementia
- Death if untreated.

The disease and the dementia did not spare children, and even if the person recovered, the brain injury did not, which bodes poorly for the treatment of established Alzheimer's disease. The disease spread to the rural south of the United States in the early 1900s, as subsistence farmers (sharecroppers) were compelled to grow cotton and were not allowed to grow their own food on their land. It was also known as "Spring Disease", as it typically appeared in the spring months when sharecroppers had the least to eat as their funds from the previous harvest were depleted.

We may not hear about this disease, now known as pellagra, nowadays; however, there were over three million cases and over 100,000 deaths from pellagra in the U.S. between 1906 and 1940.

Pellagra was a new disease in the US in the early 20th century, although there had been outbreaks in Italy, Egypt, and other areas. It was particularly prevalent in the South, and it particularly targeted poor African American women,[1] prisoners, and institutionalized (orphan) children, institutionalized adults, and the rural poor. Pellagra is caused by nutritional deficiencies of the amino acid tryptophan and the B vitamin, niacin. The body can convert tryptophan into niacin, so an adequate supply of either prevents pellagra. Gastroenteritis and diarrhea from the disease exacerbate the victim's nutritional deficiencies. Pellagra causes depression, and when severe, causes progressive encephalopathy. It is still occasionally seen in the US among individuals experiencing homelessness and those with poor nutrition who are struggling with alcohol dependence or living with HIV/AIDS.[2] Outbreaks of pellagra continue to occur in developing nations during times of food insecurity. Pellagra remains common during the "hungry season" in parts of Africa and in refugee camps. The number of individuals with subclinical niacin-tryptophan deficiency far exceeds the number diagnosed with pellagra.

The onset of this disease in the American rural south in the early 1900s was the result of a diet principally composed of the least expensive foods available: cornmeal, used to prepare porridge (grits) or cornbread, salt pork from the belly or fatback from the back, both including skin and mostly fat or lard, and molasses. Cornmeal was a cheap food. In contrast to whole corn, cornmeal is degermed to increase its shelf life. Cornmeal is low in niacin and available tryptophan. Since the 1940s, cornmeal and other grains in the U.S. have been fortified with niacin and other vitamins to prevent pellagra and other micronutrient deficiencies. The seed coat of corn has anti-nutritional properties.

Hominy is made from corn that has been treated in a process called nixtamalization that uses an alkali (such as lime - calcium hydroxide) that liberates niacin from hemicellulose, making it available to the body. Nixtamalization increases protein availability and softens the grain so that the starches hydrate more easily, allowing it to be made into masa for making tamales and tortillas. Nixtamalization further deactivates over 90% of mycotoxins produced by Fusarium molds that commonly infest the grain. These mycotoxins include carcinogens, neurotoxins, and enterotoxins.[3]

Pellagra is highly associated with a diet based on corn or its close relative, sorghum. While corn was the staple of the native peoples of America, pellagra was unknown, as its traditional method of preparation with lime or wood ash (nixtamalization) increases the bioavailability of tryptophan. However, when corn was introduced to the Old World around 1530, the traditional methods for its preparation were left behind. Pellagra was first described among the poor by a physician in Spain in 1763. The name pellagra comes from the Italian "pelle agra", meaning "rough skin," and got the moniker during a large outbreak in Italy in 1771.[4]

While suckling infants of mothers with pellagra often suffered from the disease,[5] the medical literature says little about the intellectual sequela of infants born to women with pellagra during pregnancy. In rats, niacin deficiency during pregnancy causes a high fetal fatality rate. It is also associated with multiple birth defects, including skeletal abnormalities, retarded brain development, malformations of the brain, eyes, and urinary system,[6] cleft palate,[7] and hydrocephalus.[8]

Processed Foods

The SANA diet promotes the consumption of processed foods! Nixtamalization of corn is a method of processing this grain. It greatly improves the nutritional value of corn and changes the DAD rating of corn from a C to a 3. Proper processing of many foods, including most grains, is required to improve their nutritional content.

Without processing our food, we would not have a civilization, and the human population, if it had survived, would be tiny. Humans get almost no nutritional value from unprocessed grains. More than half of all calories consumed by the world's human population come from just three species of grain: maize (field corn), wheat, and rice. All of that is processed. We mill it, grind it into flour, bake it into bread, boil it, and ferment it. Humans can eat meat, but it is dangerous unless processed by drying it over heat or cooking it.

Raw leaves and fruit are the near-exclusive diet of mountain gorillas; they feed on nearly 200 species of plants within the range of one national park in Rwanda.[9] But they are better adapted to that diet than are humans, having a longer intestine and a larger cecum, which allows for a more massive fermentation. Our diets are further restricted by what foods are available in commerce. Of the 300,000 known edible plants around the globe, there are only about 200 that enter regular commerce.[10] Most people likely consume fewer than 100 species of plants in any given year. The plants we grow for food are ones that are easily and economically grown, and generally ones that store well so that they can be shipped to market. This may limit the fruits, vegetables, and seeds that can be eaten without the need for processing.

Of the 200 plants in commerce, 15 species account for 75 percent of all caloric intake, with three grains (rice, corn, and wheat) making up about half of all calories consumed by humans. Just three animal species provide 95% of all meat consumed by the human population. (Pork 39%, Chicken 33%, and Beef 23%).[11]

As with corn, most seeds contain anti-nutritional compounds that limit the seeds' nutritional benefits. Several classes of compounds present in seeds, such as lectins, tannins, phytates, and saponins, can interfere with nutrient absorption or cause other health risks. Some compounds in edible seeds are toxic if not properly cooked. Anti-nutritional compounds can cause nausea, bloating, nutritional deficiencies, rashes, and headaches. Tannins, large polyphenols, form complexes with minerals and proteins, inhibiting protein utilization sufficiently that they can cause a severe protein deficiency syndrome in children in Sub-Saharan Africa called Kwashiorkor. Proper preparation of seeds is fundamental to their nutritional value.

Lectins

Lectins are an important class of anti-nutritional proteins. Lectins are proteins that bind to carbohydrates. Many plants produce lectin, especially in their seeds and tubers, as defense agents against herbivorous predators and parasites. The lectins present in kidney beans are toxic enough to cause acute gastroenteritis toxicity from the consumption of five undercooked beans. This lectin damages the enterocytes lining the small intestine. Cooking beans at a boiling temperature denatures the lectin in kidney beans, rendering it harmless.[12] Some lectins, such as abrin in rosary peas and ricin in castor beans, are deadly in microgram doses.

Several lectins interfere with the digestion of proteins. Some lectins can trigger an immune response if they are not denatured during cooking. Lectins are present in soybeans, wheat, barley, winter squash, beans, rice, corn, tomatoes, bananas, chickpeas, sunflower seeds, pineapple, buckwheat, spinach, mustard, cabbage, and many other food plants. Some are innocuous, a few are beneficial, and some are toxic if not cooked sufficiently to denature them. Many interfere with digestion.[13] Lectins bind to glycoproteins on the surface of cells. In the intestine, many lectins adhere to the enterocytes that line the intestine and interfere with membrane repair and potently inhibit mucous secretion, thus acting as toxins that damage the intestinal membrane.[14]

Some lectins can disrupt the intestinal mucous layer, promoting bacterial adhesion, injury, brush-border enzyme production, and thus decreased nutrient absorption. Injury by lectins to the small intestine can promote Crohn's disease, Sprue, and colitis, and increase intestinal permeability. Lectins can decrease the secretion of immunoglobulin A in the small intestine, and thus promote bacterial overgrowth. Interestingly, a low-lectin diet was found to improve impulsivity, hyperactivity, and anxiety symptoms in children with ADHD. Some of the "high-lectin foods excluded from the diet were: Wheat, flour, oats, quinoa, brown rice, wild rice, barley, buckwheat, corn/corn products, tomatoes, eggplants, potatoes, all leguminous plants, including bean sprouts and soy products, cucumbers and gourds, pumpkin seeds, sunflower seeds, chia seeds, peanuts, and cashews. Additionally, meat and eggs from animals raised on feed grain were excluded.[15] Thus, while it may be effective, it is an overly restrictive diet.

Lectins are a diverse class of proteins; it should not be assumed that all lectins have adverse effects on health or intestinal permeability.

Some lectins do not degrade easily at typical cooking temperatures, but not all lectins are harmful. Wheat germ lectins and those in peanuts are extremely heat-stable.[16] Many lectins that are resistant to degradation with dry heat can be inactivated when heated with sufficient moisture.[17] [18] Pressure cooking, which increases the cooking temperature, helps denature some lectins that are otherwise heat-resistant. Thus, cooking methods need to be appropriate to the food, and some foods are better avoided.

Protease Inhibitors

There are several types of protease inhibitors. These are enzyme inhibitors that prevent the activity of enzymes that cut proteins into smaller pieces or that trim single or pairs of amino acids from the protein fragments. One of the common family of protease inhibitors in seeds are the trypsin inhibitors, many of which also inhibit chymotrypsin.

Trypsin inhibitors can act as storage proteins for plants. For example, the storage protein sporamin in sweet potatoes is a trypsin inhibitor that keeps pests from being able to digest protein, and thus keeps the insects from eating the tuber. When the plant needs amino acids for growth, it can sap those from this protein. Animals have adipose tissue and glycogen to store fat and carbohydrates for later use, but we don't have storage proteins. When we have an immediate need for amino acids to build new proteins, we use autophagy to recycle proteins within the cell, but that is a story for another time.

Trypsin inhibitors in human diets can impair growth in children by reducing protein digestion and amino acid availability. When feed with high levels of trypsin inhibitors is given to animals, it causes pancreatic hyperplasia and hypertrophy.

Cholecystokinin (CCK) is released from the special I cells in the mucosa of the small intestine in the presence of fats and proteins. It acts to slow gastric emptying, which prolongs the feeling of fullness after a meal, and reduces the urge to eat more. CCK also enters the bloodstream and acts on receptors in the brain, providing satiety, decreasing hunger. Thus, trypsin inhibitors can reduce appetite and suppress overeating.[19] Wheat, rye, and barley contain α-amylase/trypsin inhibitors that promote intestinal inflammation when gluten is present.[20] Protease inhibitors prevent the digestion of dietary protein, and thus increase the amount of dietary protein that is fermented in the colon, and thus, may provoke dysbiosis and leaky gut. This inhibition may extend beyond the proteins present in the plant being consumed and may impact the digestion of protein present in other foods that are consumed.

Tannins

Tannins, large polyphenols, form complexes with minerals and proteins, inhibiting protein utilization sufficiently that they are often a contributing cause of the severe protein deficiency syndrome, Kwashiorkor, in children in Sub-Saharan Africa.[21] Tannins bind certain minerals and form complexes with proteins, which impairs their digestion and thus decreases the availability of their amino acids.

Tannins can be removed from seeds by leaching (soaking), especially in heated, alkalized water. Cooking, and especially pressure cooking, further reduces tannins. Sprouting also lowers tannin and phytate levels.[22] [23] [24]

Saponins

Saponins are small molecules that resemble steroids or triterpenes that contain a sugar moiety in their structure. There are 11 main classes of saponins and thousands of different ones in various plants.[25] Saponins serve plants as defensive agents against fungal and bacterial pathogens, and as toxins protecting them from insect pests. They are widely distributed among plant species, and since they protect plants, they are important to successful agriculture.[26]

Some saponins have medicinal value, but many have anti-nutritional effects. When boiling legumes, oats, and quinoa, it is common for a foam to suds up; this is caused by saponins. Triterpenoid saponins are found in such foods as legumes (lentils, peas, chickpeas, soybeans, peanuts, and broad beans) and quinoa, sunflower seeds, spinach, sugar beets, onions, and tea. Steroid saponins are found in oats, yucca, yams, tomato seeds, eggplants, fenugreek seed, and asparagus. Saponins are often bitter.

The human digestive system does not break down saponins readily; thus, these can impair digestion. Saponins can inhibit digestive enzymes, including amylase and glucosidase, which break down carbohydrates and sugars, lipase, trypsin, and chymotrypsin, and can cause maldigestion-related health disorders. Saponins also decrease the absorption of fat-soluble vitamins (A, E, D) and other lipids. Saponins can damage the integrity of the enterocytes of the intestine.[27] Some saponins increase the permeability of the small intestinal mucosa, inhibiting active transport of nutrients into the cells and allowing the uptake of substances that would normally be excluded.[28]

Saponins can be leached with soaking and blanching, with higher amounts removed with longer soak times, greater water volume, and warmer water temperatures.[29] Saponins are further degraded by boiling.[30] [31] [32] Soyasaponin VI is a saponin found in beans that is not water-soluble. Blanching degrades some of the soyasaponin VI into soyasaponin I, which is water-soluble, and thus helps it get leached with soaking.[33]

Proteins that cannot be digested as a result of protease inhibitors, tannins, and saponins and that are not digested, are lost into the feces, although some may be fermented in the colon.

Alpha-Amylase Inhibitors

Alpha-amylase inhibitors are another anti-nutritional compound that protects seeds against microorganisms and other pests that would consume them. Alpha-amylase helps break down starches. Although technically anti-nutritional, the impact of α-amylase inhibitors is usually trivial or beneficial. They are generally unstable in the GI tract. By preventing salivary amylase function, they prevent the formation of sugar in the mouth, and thus protect the teeth from cariogenic bacteria, and they slow rather than prevent carbohydrate digestion, lowering the peaks in blood sugar after meals, and helping maintain satiety between meals.

Phytic Acid

Phytic acid (a.k.a. phytate) is a phosphorus storage molecule present in most seeds and in some other plant materials, and is important for the seeds' germination. Phytic acid passes unabsorbed through the human digestive system. It is antinutritional as it binds iron, zinc, calcium, and other minerals, and prevents their absorption as well. Thus, it can cause a deficiency of these minerals, especially for children eating low-quality diets.

> There is enough phytate in the animal feed (based on corn, soy, and other seed or seed meal) that animal (and human) dung is a major cause of phosphate pollution; almost all from phytic acid. This is a major contributor to the 5,000 square mile dead zone in the Gulf of Mexico. The phosphorus, as well as nitrogen runoff, causes algal overgrowth; then, when the plants die, they are fermented by bacteria, consuming the dissolved oxygen in the water. Fish and other animals then suffocate if they swim into these waters.

Phytate content is high in the seed coats of many seeds, including grains and legumes. Phytate is composed of an alcohol sugar (inositol, a.k.a. myoinositol) with six phosphate groups; thus, it is inositol hexakisphosphate (IP6).

In contrast, myoinositol is an important nutrient that was considered a vitamin before it was understood that the kidneys make a couple of grams of it each day from glucose. The highest concentrations of inositol are in the brain, where it is used to make certain neurotransmitters, hormones, and growth factors. Myoinositol increases insulin sensitivity with similar efficacy as the drug metformin.[34] In meta-analyses, myoinositol is useful in the treatment of polycystic ovary syndrome in women (PCOS),[35] and helps lower LDL cholesterol and triglyceride levels, without lowering HDL levels.[36] It lowers the risk of metabolic syndrome and is important for the synthesis of thyroid hormones, insulin signaling, nerve guidance, the metabolism of fats, and other physiologic processes. It has also been found to be helpful in the treatment of depression, panic disorder, and obsessive-compulsive disorder.[37]

Sprouting greatly reduces the amount of phytate in seeds, including grains and legumes, by promoting the activity of phytase enzymes present in the seeds. [38] Soaking seeds and discarding the soaking water also significantly reduces levels. Phytate is water-soluble, and thus soaking helps remove phytate from the bran or seed coat, the area of highest phytate concentration.

Phytate is heat-stable, and thus, boiling and other forms of cooking do not remove it or break it down. Fermentation with bacteria that produce the enzyme phytase also lowers levels. The advantage of the enzymatic dephosphorylation of phytate by phytases is that complete removal of the phosphate groups leaves myoinositol as a nutrient.

Warm water soaking allows activation of phytase enzymes in the seed. As shown in Table 8A, below, soaking temperatures below around 60° C down to about 35° C generally provide optimal phytase activity. A pH value between 4.5 and 6.0 also improves the enzymatic activity of phytase. Studies have found that soaking grains in acidified water (adding vinegar to the soaking water) and soaking at around 60° C is effective for reducing phytate levels. Some phytate from the seed coat diffuses into the soaking water, and inositol availability increases with the warm water soaking.[39] Since the range of activity is fairly wide, starting with hot water and allowing the soak water to slowly cool over several hours is a simple method to degrade phytate. Alternatively, the ideal soak temperature can be maintained in a digital slow cooker that can maintain these temperatures. Note that excessive temperatures degrade the phytase enzyme.

The SANA program does not promote the acidification of soak water or the use of such high temperatures during soaking. More moderate temperatures, between 30 and 45° C, give better overall results for soaking grains, as multiple enzymes are involved and other enzymes have lower optimal temperatures and, as a whole, function better at a more neutral pH.

Table 6A: Phytate is one of several anti-nutritional compounds present in seeds that break down during germination with the activation of an enzyme present in the seed. Phytase (3-phytase – EC 3.1.3.8 and 4-phytase – EC 3.1.3.26) and optimum pH and temperatures are shown.[40 41]

Plant	ISO enzyme	Optimum pH	Optimum Temp° C/F	pH Min	pH Max	Low Temp	High Temp
Avena sativa - **Oats**	3.1.3.26	5.0	38/100	3.5	7.5		40
Glycine max - **Soy**	3.1.3.26	4.5 - 5.0	58/136	3.8	5.8	34	62
Glycine max	3.1.3.8	4.5	58/136	3.8	5.8	34	62
Hordeum vulgare - **Barley**	3.1.3.26	5.5	55/131			35	60
Hordeum vulgare	3.1.3.8	5.2					
Oryza sativa - **Rice**	3.1.3.8	4.3 -4.6	45/113	3.5	5.5	20	60
Phaseolus vulgaris -**Beans**	3.1.3.26	5.5	37/99				
Phaseolus vulgaris	3.1.3.8	5.5	37/99	4.5	6		50
Secale cereale - **Rye**	3.1.3.26	6.0	45/113	4	6		55
Triticum aestivum - **Wheat**	3.1.3.26	5.5	45/113	4.7	6.5	30	55
Triticum aestivum	3.1.3.8	5.0	36/97				
Vicia faba – **Faba Beans**	3.1.3.26	5.0	50/122				
Vigna radiata - **Mung Bean**	3.1.3.8	7.5	57/135				
Zea mays - **Corn**	3.1.3.26	4.8	55/131	4	5.7	45	60
Zea mays	3.1.3.8	5.0	36/97				

Note: Data from various sources differ; when available, more recent and more complete data were used. Especially for older data, the isoforms were not always identified.

Oxalates

Oxalates are another anti-nutritional compound present in some vegetables. Oxalic acid binds Ca2+, Fe2+, and Mg2+, and thus, binding with them prevents the absorption of these minerals. While a diet high in oxalates can cause mineral deficiency and intestinal irritation, a much more common problem with oxalate in foods is that it can cause kidney stones.

The ionized form, oxalic acid, can be absorbed. But once absorbed, it can form insoluble salts during the concentration of urine that precipitate in the kidney, forming kidney stones. The vast majority of kidney stones (85 – 90%) are calcium oxalate stones. Some vegetables high in oxalate include raw spinach, rhubarb, cruciferous vegetables (kale, broccoli), parsley, nuts, chocolate, beets, blueberries, and some beans, such as soybeans.

Some people are highly sensitive to oxalates and may experience bloating and gas from oxalates. It does not appear that oxalate causes dysbiosis, but rather, dysbiosis and SIBO (small intestinal bacterial overgrowth) tremendously increase the absorption of dietary oxalates from a typical 1 to 2% to 40 to 50% of dietary intake.[42] Kidney stones occur in as many as 28% of individuals with irritable bowel syndrome, as compared to 8% of the population as a whole. High oxalate levels and prevalence of kidney stones are seen in Crohn's disease and ulcerative colitis. The high oxalate absorption is associated with decolonization of beneficial bacteria, *Oxalobacter formigenes* in particular, that normally metabolizes oxalate in the gut, leaving the oxalate to be absorbed into the bloodstream.[43] Individuals who form kidney stones should stay well hydrated and may benefit from lowering their dietary intake of foods very high in oxalate, but should also work to improve their enteric microbiome health.

Non-Digestible Sugars

Many plants, beans, and cruciferous vegetables, for example, contain sugars, often tri- and tetra-saccharides composed of three or four simpler sugar molecules, that are linked together by a chemical bond that is not cut by human digestive enzymes. These sugars are not digested and thus ferment in the lower intestine and are responsible for the gas associated with the consumption of these vegetables. As an example, we do not make the enzyme α-galactosidase required to break down the sugars stachyose and raffinose in beans, so they get fermented in the gut, causing the production of flatulent gases, including hydrogen, methane, and CO_2, and often causing cramping and nausea. These sugars are considered to be anti-nutritional compounds as a result of this. Nevertheless, limited quantities of these sugars help maintain a diverse and healthy microbiome.[44]

The quantity of these sugars in beans can be reduced by soaking and blanching, and boiling also promotes the hydrolysis of these sugars into simpler ones that can be digested.[45]

Other Factors

Some foods are goitrogenic and impair thyroid function; some as a result of anti-nutritional factors, but others as thyrotoxins. Many foods contain toxic alkaloids. These are not anti-nutritional compounds, but rather toxins. Certain foods are cyanogenic; cyanogenic glycosides present in foods are absorbed and metabolized into cyanide in the liver. As an example, the tuber yuca (cassava), a staple crop consumed by 700 million people, can have high levels of these compounds, especially when the plants are stressed, as during droughts. Unfortunately, yuca can become one of the few foods available to the poor in rural tropical areas when other crops fail. When bitter yuca, high in cyanogenic glycosides, is consumed as a famine food, it can cause permanent disability or even death in children. This occurs all too frequently in Africa and other impoverished areas, as recently seen during a food crisis in Venezuela.[46] Even at much lower levels, these compounds may impact health and be reflected in the DAD score.

A fundamental part of the SANA diet is the proper processing of food to eliminate anti-nutritional compounds and toxins and to increase nutritional availability. Soaking, cooking, sprouting, and fermentation are some of the “home methods” that can be used to mitigate the levels of anti-nutritional compounds in foods. Milling (removal of the seed coat or bran) also removes or facilitates the removal of some antinutritional compounds. For example, dehulled faba beans have a 70 to 73% decrease in tannin content.[47] Processing of foods will be discussed in the context of the foods or food groups.

[1] Epidemiologists explain pellagra: gender, race, and political economy in the work of Edgar Sydenstricker. Marks HM. J Hist Med Allied Sci. 2003 Jan;58(1):34-55. PMID:12680009

[2] Pellagrous encephalopathy presenting as alcohol withdrawal delirium: a case series and literature review. Oldham MA, Ivkovic A. Addict Sci Clin Pract. 2012 Jul 6;7:12. PMID:23186222

[3] https://en.wikipedia.org/wiki/Nixtamalization and https://en.wikipedia.org/wiki/Hominy

[4] Pellagra and its prevention and control in major emergencies. Prinzo ZW et al. World Health Organization, 2000.

[5] Some Interesting Features Concerning the Study of Pellagra. Jelks,JL. Pacific Medical Journal, Jan. 1916, p.353-358.

[6] Multiple congenital abnormalities in the rat resulting from acute maternal niacin deficiency during pregnancy. Chamberlain JG., Nelson MM. Proc Soc Exp Biol Med. 1963 Apr;112:836-40. PMID:14019937

[7] Effects of acute vitamin replacement therapy on 6-aminonicotinamide induced cleft palate late in rat pregnancy. Chamberlain JG. Proc Soc Exp Biol Med. 1967 Mar;124(3):888-90. PMID:4225749

[8] Early neurovascular abnormalities underlying 6-aminonicotinamide (6-AN)-induced congenital hydrocephalus in rats. Chamberlain JG. Teratology. 1970 Nov;3(4):377-88. PMID:4282424

[9] https://gorillafund.org/uncategorized/learning-more-about-bamboo-a-key-gorilla-food/

[10] https://www.newscientist.com/article/mg22730301-400-the-nature-of-crops-why-do-we-eat-so-few-of-the-edible-plants/

[11] https://www.foodindustry.com/articles/pork-is-the-most-consumed-meat-worldwide/

[12] Dietary Lectin exclusion: The next big food trend? Panacer K, Whorwell PJ. World J Gastroenterol. 2019 Jun 28;25(24):2973-2976. doi: 10.3748/wjg.v25.i24.2973. PMID: 31293334

[13] Peptide-based protease inhibitors from plants. Hellinger R, Gruber CW.Drug Discov Today. 2019 Sep;24(9):1877-1889. doi: 10.1016/j.drudis.2019.05.026. Epub 2019 Jun 3.PMID: 31170506

[14] Lectin-based food poisoning: a new mechanism of protein toxicity. Miyake K, Tanaka T, McNeil PL. PLoS One. 2007 Aug 1;2(8):e687. doi: 10.1371/journal.pone.0000687. PMID: 17668065

[15] The Impact of Integrating a Low-Lectin Diet with Traditional ADHD Treatments on Gut Microbiota Composition and Symptom Improvement in Children - A Cohort Study. Long L, Peng H, Chen X, Wang F, Long W, Cheng M, Ma J. Neuropsychiatr Dis Treat. 2024 Mar 9;20:535-549. doi: 10.2147/NDT.S449186. eCollection 2024. PMID: 38482022 (see supplemental materials.

[16] Assessment of lectin inactivation by heat and digestion.Pusztai A, Grant G. Methods Mol Med. 1998;9:505-14. doi: 10.1385/0-89603-396-1:505.PMID : 21374488

[17] Assessment of lectin inactivation by heat and digestion. Arpad Pusztai, George Grant 31 Dec 1997 - Methods in molecular medicine. (Humana Press) Vol. 9, pp 505-514

[18] Thermal inactivation of lectins and trypsin inhibitor activity during steam processing of dry beans (Phaseolus vulgaris) and effects on protein quality. Vanderpool TB et al. J. Sci. of Food and Agriculture. 1990. https://doi.org/10.1002/jsfa.2740530209

[19] Samtiya, M., Aluko, R.E. & Dhewa, T. Plant food anti-nutritional factors and their reduction strategies: an overview. *Food Prod Process and Nutr* **2**, 6 (2020). https://doi.org/10.1186/s43014-020-0020-5

[20] Nutritional Wheat Amylase-Trypsin Inhibitors Promote Intestinal Inflammation via Activation of Myeloid Cells. Zevallos VF, Raker V, Tenzer S, Jimenez-Calvente C, Ashfaq-Khan M, Rüssel N, Pickert G, Schild H, Steinbrink K, Schuppan D. Gastroenterology. 2017 Apr;152(5):1100-1113.e12. doi: 10.1053/j.gastro.2016.12.006. PMID: 27993525

[21] Screening of traditional South African leafy vegetables for specific anti-nutritional factors before and after processing. Odhav B, Mellon J. July 2017 Food Science and Technology DOI:10.1590/1678-457x.20416 https://www.researchgate.net/publication/317602068

[22] Removal of tannin and improvement of in vitro protein digestibility of sorghum seed by soaking in alkali. Chavin JK, Kadoma S, Salunkhe K. Journal of Food Science. 44(5):1319 – 1322 DOI:10.1111/j.1365-2621.1979.tb06429.x

[23] Effects of processing methods on phytate and tannin content of black small common beans (Phaseolus vulgaris L.) cultivated in Mozambique. Nagessa WB, et al. Cogent Food & Agriculture 9(2), 2023 - Issue 2 https://doi.org/10.1080/23311932.2023.2289713

[24] Comparative evaluation of the effect of boiling and autoclaving of legume grains on tannin concentration. Chisowa DM. Magna Scientia Advanced Biology and Pharmacy, 2022, 07(01), 009–017 DOI url: https://doi.org/10.30574/msabp.2022.7.1.0080

[25] Saponins, classification and occurrence in the plant kingdom. Vincken JP, Heng L, de Groot A, Gruppen H. Phytochemistry. 2007 Feb;68(3):275-97. doi: 10.1016/j.phytochem.2006.10.008. Epub 2006 Dec 4. PMID: 17141815

[26] Saponin toxicity as key player in plant defense against pathogens. Zaynab M, Sharif Y, Abbas S, Afzal MZ, Qasim M, Khalofah A, Ansari MJ, Khan KA, Tao L, Li S. Toxicon. 2021 Apr 15;193:21-27. doi: 10.1016/j.toxicon.2021.01.009. Epub 2021 Jan 26. PMID: 33508310

[27] Samtiya, M., Aluko, R.E. & Dhewa, T. Plant food anti-nutritional factors and their reduction strategies: an overview. *Food Prod Process and Nutr* **2**, 6 (2020). https://doi.org/10.1186/s43014-020-0020-5

[28] Influence of saponins on gut permeability and active nutrient transport in vitro. Johnson IT, Gee JM, Price K, Curl C, Fenwick GR. J Nutr. 1986 Nov;116(11):2270-7. doi: 10.1093/jn/116.11.2270. PMID: 3794833

[29] Saponins from edible legumes: chemistry, processing, and health benefits. Shi J, Arunasalam K, Yeung D, Kakuda Y, Mittal G, Jiang Y. J Med Food. 2004 Spring;7(1):67-78. doi: 10.1089/109662004322984734. PMID: 15117556

[30] Kinetic study of saponins B stability in navy beans under different processing conditions. John Shi, et al. Journal of Food Engineering 93(1)59-65 July 2009. https://doi.org/10.1016/j.jfoodeng.2008.12.035

[31] A KINETIC APPROACH TO SAPONIN EXTRACTION DURING WASHING OF QUINOA (CHENOPODIUM QUINOA WILLD.) SEEDS. ISSIS QUISPE-FUENTES, et al. Journal of Food Process Engineering 36(2)202-210. 28 March 2012, https://doi.org/10.1111/j.1745-4530.2012.00673.x

[32] Exploring the effect of boiling processing on the metabolic components of black beans through in vitro simulated digestion. Wu T, Shen YN, Tian Y, et al. Volume 184, 15 July 2023, 114987 https://doi.org/10.1016/j.lwt.2023.114987

[33] Effect of Soaking and Cooking on the Saponin Content and Composition of Chickpeas (Cicer arietinum) and Lentils (Lens culinaris) Raquel G. Ruiz, Keith R. Price, A. Eddie Arthur, Malcolm E. Rose, Michael J. C. Rhodes, and Roger G. Fenwick Journal of Agricultural and Food Chemistry 1996 44 (6), 1526-1530 DOI: 10.1021/jf950721v https://doi.org/10.1021/jf950721v

[34] Inositol is an effective and safe treatment in polycystic ovary syndrome: a systematic review and meta-analysis of randomized controlled trials. Greff D, Juhász AE, Váncsa S, Váradi A, Sipos Z, Szinte J, Park S, Hegyi P, Nyirády P, Ács N, Várbíró S, Horváth EM. Reprod Biol Endocrinol. 2023 Jan 26;21(1):10. doi: 10.1186/s12958-023-01055-z. PMID: 36703143

[35] Comparative efficacy of oral insulin sensitizers metformin, thiazolidinediones, inositol, and berberine in improving endocrine and metabolic profiles in women with PCOS: a network meta-analysis. Zhao H, Xing C, Zhang J, He B. Reprod Health. 2021 Aug 18;18(1):171. doi: 10.1186/s12978-021-01207-7. PMID: 34407851

[36] The effects of inositol supplementation on lipid profiles among patients with metabolic diseases: a systematic review and meta-analysis of randomized controlled trials. Tabrizi R, Ostadmohammadi V, Lankarani KB, Peymani P, Akbari M, Kolahdooz F, Asemi Z. Lipids Health Dis. 2018 May 24;17(1):123. doi: 10.1186/s12944-018-0779-4. PMID: 29793496

[37] https://en.wikipedia.org/wiki/Inositol

[38] Reduction of phytic acid and enhancement of bioavailable micronutrients in food grains. Gupta RK, Gangoliya SS, Singh NK. J Food Sci Technol. 2015 Feb;52(2):676-84. doi: 10.1007/s13197-013-0978-y. Epub 2013 Apr 24. PMID: 25694676

[39] Phytase for Food Application. R. GREINER and U. KONIETZNY: Phytase for Food Application, Food Technol. Biotechnol. 44 (2) 125–140 (2006) https://www.researchgate.net/profile/Ralf-Greiner/publication/228337756

[40] https://brenda-enzymes.org/enzyme.php?ecno=3.1.3.8

[41] https://brenda-enzymes.org/enzyme.php?ecno=3.1.3.26

[42] Microbial contributions to oxalate metabolism in health and disease. Liu M, Devlin JC, Hu J. January 2020 DOI:10.1101/2020.01.27.20018770

[43] Lin, E., Xu, J., Liu, M. *et al.* Enteric Hyperoxaluria and Kidney Stone Management in Inflammatory Bowel Disease. *Curr Treat Options Gastro* **18**, 384–393 (2020). https://doi.org/10.1007/s11938-020-00295-x

[44] Raffinose Family Oligosaccharides: Friend or Foe for Human and Plant Health? Elango D, Rajendran K, Van der Laan L, Sebastiar S, Raigne J, Thaiparambil NA, El Haddad N, Raja B, Wang W, Ferela A, Chiteri KO, Thudi M, Varshney RK, Chopra S, Singh A, Singh AK. Front Plant Sci. 2022 Feb 17;13:829118. doi: 10.3389/fpls.2022.829118. eCollection 2022. PMID: 35251100

[45] Exploring the effect of boiling processing on the metabolic components of black beans through in vitro simulated digestion. Wu T, Shen YN, Tian Y, et al. Volume 184, 15 July 2023, 114987 https://doi.org/10.1016/j.lwt.2023.114987

[46] https://www.theguardian.com/science/blog/2017/jun/22/cassava-deadly-food-venezuela

[47] Sharma, A., Sehgal, S. Effect of domestic processing, cooking and germination on the trypsin inhibitor activity and tannin content of faba bean (Vicia faba). Plant Food Hum Nutr 42, 127–133 (1992). https://doi.org/10.1007/BF02196465

Chapter 9: Cereals and Bread

Going Against the Grain – All Spelt Out

Cereals need to be properly prepared prior to their consumption; otherwise, they are mostly inedible.

Humans can utilize grains because we process them by milling, fermentation, and cooking. Most cereals consumed within the Western diet, however, are processed in a manner that not only does not optimize their nutritional value but also frequently causes them to be proinflammatory and to promote dysbiosis. Most cereals are prepared in ways that get DAD scores of A or below. This is tragic in terms of the cost to human health, as with proper processing, most grains can get a 5★★★★★ score.

The SANA diet recommends the avoidance of most commercially available wheat products, including whole wheat and wheat bran products. Similarly, most corn products are not permitted on the SANA diet. While the diet encourages the consumption of rice and oats, they receive low DAD scores when typically prepared.

This chapter describes why grains promote inflammation and dysbiosis, and describes how they can be prepared so that they prevent inflammation and provide high nutritional benefits. The processes described here for grains and later for legumes are not limited to benefiting human nutrition. It also applies to the use of feeding seed materials to other animals.

Cereals

A cereal is a grass that is cultivated for its seed, which is also called a grain. Grains are the human population's largest food source. Grasses and grains are also the largest food source for cattle and poultry, and thus, grain is the predominant food source for meat and egg production. Cereals have been fundamental to the development of most civilizations, in part because they are the basis for brewing beer. In the Lord's Prayer, "daily bread" serves as a metaphor for the basic needs of life.

Most bread in Palestine at the beginning of the first century was made from barley, as wheat (*Triticum aestivum*) bread was considered a luxury food. Milled lentil flour was often added to bread. Both unleavened bread and sourdough bread were common in Palestine at that time.[1]

Cereals are starchy, with about 2/3rds of the dry weight of grains being carbohydrates. They generally supply moderate amounts of protein and fiber. Just three grains, rice, corn, and wheat, directly supply more than half of all the caloric energy consumed by the human population. Maize, as feed corn, accounts for more than 95% of grain used as animal feed, with the remainder being oats, barley, and sorghum. There are over 90 million acres of land corn cultivated in the U.S. Corn is everywhere in the diet; tortillas, cornbread, hominy grits, corn flakes, cornmeal on pizza crust, not to mention corn syrup and corn oil, which are ubiquitous in processed and fast foods. (Soy oil is actually used more than corn oil.) We even use corn to feed our cars in the form of alcohol added to gasoline.

Wheat is the second most abundantly produced and consumed grain worldwide. Wheat provides 19% of humanity's daily caloric intake and 21% of all dietary protein consumption, making it the top protein source of any food.[2]

Wheat is used in breads, pastries, pasta, and cereal. Six different classes of wheat are grown in the U.S.: Hard red winter, hard red spring, soft white, soft red winter, hard white, and durum. Soft wheat has less protein and gluten and more starch; it is used for pastries, desserts, and sauces. Hard wheat is higher in gluten and is used in making bread. Durum wheat is especially hard and high in gluten, and is used to make pasta and couscous.

Rice is the next most consumed grain. In much of Asia, China, India, and Southeast Asia, the per capita consumption of rice is about one pound a day![3] Americans only consume about 2 ounces of rice per day on average.

The big three grains are distantly followed by barley, sorghum, millet, oats, and rye. Additionally, there are several grains called millet, although they are not any more closely related to each other than rice is to wheat or oats. Additionally, there are several pseudocereals which are not grasses but whose seeds are used like a cereal; these include but are not limited to buckwheat, quinoa, and related amaranths, and chia.

Americans consume a lot of grain. The "2015-2020 Dietary Guidelines for Americans" suggests that people requiring 2,000 calories per day consume 6 ounce-equivalents of grains, half of which should be whole grains. An ounce serving is about one slice of bread. By 2014, in a rising trend, Americans were eating 5 ounces of wheat a day. There has been a 35% increase in grain consumption from 1970 to 2014, and during this time, there was a decline in the consumption of rye, oats, and barley. People barely eat barley anymore.[4] Most of the barley consumed in the U.S. diet is in the form of beer. The annual per capita consumption of grains is about 170 pounds; this includes about 20 pounds of rice and less than 5 pounds of oats.[5]

Wheat

We will begin with wheat, as it presents the best worst-case of grains causing enteric disorders.

Just as fruit and tuber skins are a problem for the enterobiome and cause dysbiosis, the seed coats protecting the seeds are a skin that protects the seed from premature germination and destruction by soil fungi and bacteria. Consumption of wheat bran increases the losses of endogenous protein from the small intestine, increasing the amount of protein that enters the colon.[6] Seeds also often contain lectins and other anti-nutritional compounds to prevent them from being overgrazed by animals and migrating flocks of birds. The reason that humans can eat large amounts of grains is that we process them by cooking them. However, that does not provide us with full protection.

The SANA diet recommends the avoidance of most wheat products. Most wheat products are rated A's; some are rated B's. Wheat bran is down in the B area – so whole wheat is not better. Wheat products should be avoided by anyone with active dysbiosis and rarely consumed by those who don't.

Gluten

Most grains contain a class of proteins called prolamins that act as a storage protein for when the seed germinates. Gluten is one of these prolamins, and gliadin is one of the proteins that make up gluten. Grains that contain gluten include wheat, barley, and rye and wheat. This includes all forms of wheat, including durum, emmer, spelt, graham, Khorasan, and einkorn.

Gluten is an important protein in wheat and in bread making because they are gluey and stretchy, allowing the dough to hold gas bubbles during baking and making the bread chewy. This is why most bread is made from wheat.

Gluten is composed of two smaller proteins, gliadin and glutenin, that bind to form gluten's stretchy protein. In some individuals, gliadin in wheat causes celiac disease, an autoimmune disorder in which the immune system damages the cells lining the small intestine. This causes malabsorption, bloating, diarrhea, weight loss, and fatigue. About 0.7% of Americans are diagnosed with celiac disease; however, it is suspected that many cases go undiagnosed.

Celiac disease is an autoimmune condition that can result from immune recognition of gliadin, a protein in gluten. Tissue transglutaminase (tTG) is an enzyme that helps crosslink proteins, but that may also have some digestive function in the intestine. tTG acts to partially digest gliadin, but then forms a tTG-gliadin complex, which in some individuals is recognized as a foreign antigen by the immune system. In celiac disease, the immune system forms antibodies to the protein complex and attacks it, and in doing so, damages the intestinal mucosa. About 99% of people with celiac disease have one of two genetic variants of the HLA-D: HLADQ2 or DQ8 alleles. These are proteins that help the immune system recognize self from foreign proteins. People with only one copy of DQ2 or DQ8 have about 3% risk, and those with two copies of either DQ2 or DQ8 have about a 10% risk of developing the disease if they consume wheat. Celiac is a major problem for those with it. The treatment is to avoid the consumption of gluten.

There is a growing body of medical literature, however, that suggests that wheat causes problems, although usually less severe ones, for almost everyone. Some people develop allergies or delayed immune sensitivities to wheat; these immune reactivates may be to gliadin fragments or other proteins in wheat. The underlying problem, however, appears to be that gliadin appears to increase intestinal permeability ("leaky gut") in almost everyone.

In mice (without celiac disease), adding gliadin to a gluten-free diet increases intestinal paracellular permeability (IPP; gut leak) by 4.3 times. Treating the gluten-free mice with indomethacin, an NSAID medication (in the same class as ibuprofen, naproxen, and diclofenac), raised the IPP about 26-fold over untreated animals. The combination of the NSAID with a diet with gliadin raised IPP about 54-fold. When mice on a gluten-free diet were treated with an NSAID alone, it only caused very mild mucosal damage in the small intestine. The cytokine IL-1β is an inflammatory mediator. In these mice, when compared to a gluten-free diet, feed with gluten raised IL-1β levels slightly, while the NSAID alone did not. When the combination of gluten and NSAID was given, it raised IL-1β mRNA levels more than 6-fold.[7] Thus, when using an NSAID, it may be prudent to avoid consuming wheat products.

This combination of gliadin with NSAIDs serves as an example of the potential for additive or synergistic interactions that may occur from agents that may have small effects on their own, but larger effects in combination.

Wheat and other grains contain anti-trypsin inhibitors (ATI), which impede the digestion of the proteins. This curtails complete digestion, resulting in protein fragments (peptides) that the body's innate immune system recognizes as foreign antigens, causing an inflammatory response.[8]

Einkorn wheat, which is genetically similar to wild wheat, has about one-fifth the allergenic potential and one-seventh the amount of ATI as do modern wheats.[9] Einkorn is also more digestible (likely due to the lower amounts of ATI) and thus less likely to be immunogenic.[10] Einkorn contains gluten and is not safe for those with Celiac disease.

Some peptides from particular foods, such as wheat, can have detrimental physiological effects on membrane integrity or can directly affect neurologic function. A small fragment of the gliadin protein, called the "polyQ fragment", binds to a chemokine receptor (CXCR3), which activates zonulin upregulation. Zonulin is a protein that increases intestinal permeability.[11] [12] Another fragment, α-gliadin "33-mer", induces zonulin release by the enterocytes. The release of zonulin from the enterocyte activates a cell signaling pathway that causes a reversible disassembly of the tight junctions between enterocytes that bind the mucosal cells together. This opens the space between the cells, allowing larger molecules to pass between the cells and into the lamina propria layer of the intestine.[13], [14] This not only permits gliadin but also other molecules from the gut, which are normally kept out of the body, to pass through the mucosal layer, and allows some normally excluded compounds, such as LPS and flagellin, to enter the bloodstream. The increased absorption of LPS and other toxins that directly or indirectly cause inflammation can cause neurologic injury.

Gluten-derived peptides, along with antigens from other foods, stimulate the adaptive immune system (IgG and IgE), causing a release of inflammatory cytokines that may indirectly promote neurological injury. The association between gluten and neurologic disease may reflect defects in the gastrointestinal and perhaps the BBB membrane integrity. In a post-mortem case-control study of mostly adults, those with autism were found to have alterations in the expression of various claudin proteins that form the tight junctions of the BBB. These were not considered to be genetic alterations, but rather reactive changes.[15]

α-Amylase/ Trypsin Inhibitors (ATI)

Several grains, including wheat, barley, and rye, contain α-amylase/ trypsin inhibitors (ATI). While celiac disease is rare, affecting only about 1% of the population, about 10% of the population may have non-celiac wheat sensitivity. ATI peptides from certain grains can directly stimulate innate immune reactions, similar to the way the PAMP LPS binds to and activates the TLR4-complex, initiating an inflammatory response. Since this innate immune response is well conserved among animals, the inflammatory effect is not limited to humans.

ATI are non-α-gliadin peptides that evolved to prevent premature seed germination in the spring or during storage, and also serve as pest control, giving the grain a better chance of growing into a plant. Firstly, α-amylase can offset premature germination so that the seeds do not sprout too early in the spring when they are most susceptible to being killed by a hard freeze just as they emerge, or germinate too easily with a bit of moisture before the ground is sufficiently soaked for the plants to establish deep roots. This feature also makes the grain easier to store. More importantly, ATI are digestive enzyme inhibitors that make it more difficult for animals to sustain themselves feeding on the grain; the grain is not an especially nutritious meal if you can't digest it. Thus, this encouraged animals not to graze heavily on these crops in a field, or for a family to lose its store of grain to rats or other animals. These features were important to the success of agriculture and thus selected for use by humans.

α-amylase inhibitors prevent the starches stored in the grain from being converted into sugars, and the trypsin inhibitors interfere with protein digestion, which makes it hard for an animal to derive amino acids from the proteins. Thus, the insects, including mealworms, beetles, and weevils, have a hard time living on wheat, and birds and other grazing animals are likely to eat some but move on without consuming the entire crop. This would be a great advantage if the enzymes were denatured by cooking; thus, humans could eat the grains after cooking them, while animals, lacking opposable thumbs and stoves, could not. While this is true for many plant trypsin inhibitors, unfortunately, wheat ATI resists being denatured during cooking. Recent research suggests that ATI not only inhibits protein digestion, but also that wheat ATI promotes inflammation.

Wheat actually has multiple enzyme inhibitors that affect human amylases and trypsin. ATIs are dual enzyme inhibitors, inhibiting both amylases and trypsin. ATI comprises about two to four percent of the protein in wheat, barley, and rye. For a typical adult who consumes 250 grams of wheat products a day, that is about 0.5 to 1 gram of ATI.[16]

Wheat contains more than a dozen peptides with ATI activity, many of which are antigenic and cause allergic responses. Two of these enzyme-inhibiting peptides (designated as CM3 and 0.19) are strong activators of the innate immune response in humans, and activate an innate immune response via TLR4, similarly to LPS or other PAMPs. Both of these are peptides that are formed from the partial digestion of ω-gliadin. This is a different fraction of gluten from the α-gliadin that promotes celiac disease, and from γ-gliadin. ω-gliadin is the same fraction that has been identified as causing baker's asthma and gastrointestinal hypersensitivity to wheat. These ATIs were found to stimulate monocytes, macrophages, and dendritic cells in vitro to produce inflammatory cytokines, including CXCL8, IL-12, TNF, and MCP-1. While ATI CM3 and 0.19 do not specifically cause celiac disease, ATI participates in the immune reaction by driving the inflammatory response in the disease.[17][18]

Thus, ATI can cause maladaptive, innate immune reactivity to wheat. Not everyone is affected by this. The layered mucosal defenses should protect the immune cells from exposure to ATI. However, when there is a breakdown in the mucosal layer and loss of tight junction integrity, there is a much higher risk of exposure of the immune cells to ATI and thus stimulation of the TLR4 pathway. Additionally, the 33-mer of α-gliadin can cause the release of zonulin and the opening of the tight junctions in anyone. ATI-induced TLR4 activation, which promotes the expression of IL-1β and TNFα, can inhibit IAP activity and increase the risk of bacterial adhesion to the enterocytes and absorption of LPS from the gut.

Why a Gluten-Free Diet Is a Problem

Eliminating a food that makes a major contribution to dietary protein and overall calories, such as wheat, can easily be a problem if those calories are replaced with foods that are more inflammatory or dysbiotic than wheat. A gluten-free diet can worsen metabolic syndrome, dysbiosis, and fatty liver disease if wheat is eliminated and simply replaced with a gluten-free Western diet.[19][20] A gluten-free diet requires more attention and nutritional education.

Wheat Bran

The usual advice for healthy diets, including the Mediterranean diet, DISH, MIND, and Blue Zone diets, is to include significant amounts of whole grains, such as whole wheat bread and pasta. Wheat bran cereal is considered a healthy food. However, wheat bran cereal gets a score of C on the DAD scale. Wheat bran is the seed coat of wheat grain and has typical seed coat issues.

Wheat bran's claim to health benefits is its insoluble fiber. We all know the benefits of insoluble fiber in the diet. It adds bulk to the stool so that poop moves through the digestive tract more quickly. If one is constipated, the insoluble fiber may help keep things moving, which is a benefit, but it does nothing to fix the underlying problems.

Soluble fiber feeds to colonic mucosa and protects it from harm. Insoluble fiber moves the contents of the colon through more quickly. That means that soluble fiber and SCFA postbiotics it creates, which feed the colon, are moved through the colon more quickly. Insoluble fiber does not feed or protect the colon, but rather may rob it of nutrition.

One of the things that causes constipation is a refined diet that has insufficient soluble fiber. Toxins (produced by the fermentation of proteins) can damage the neurons in the intestine and impair peristaltic movement in the gut. Unlike the central nervous system, the enteric nervous system has much more capacity to replace damaged neurons from stem cells, so damaged nerves in the gut can be replaced, and the bowel can recover. Eliminating things in the diet that lead to injury of the enteric nervous system, and thus cause constipation (and intermittent diarrhea), is a far better solution. When adequate soluble fiber is present in the diet, there should be no need for insoluble fiber to push things through.

Sourdough Wheat Bread

Bread choices are limited on the SANA diet as wheat is a concern, plus, you have to read labels.

Freshly baked, white, sourdough wheat flour bread made without preservatives gets a DAD rating of zero, and is thus allowed in limited amounts on the SANA diet. That is the best score you should expect from commercially available bread made with wheat. Most other breads, including whole-grain breads, get scores of B to D. Even commercial white sourdough bread from the bread aisle gets a B.

Sourdough bread is made using a "starter," which is a bacterial culture that allows fermentation of the bread dough as it rises, before it is baked. A starter can be made from bacteria already present in flour, using a technique that favors more desirable bacteria and eliminates others. Since the starter is traditionally a mix of wild bacteria, and the mix evolves with time, as the baker feeds and maintains their starter. No two starters will be exactly the same or produce the exact same results.

The ability of bacteria in sourdough starter to break down alpha-amylase-trypsin inhibitors (ATIs) is fairly universal. Most starter cultures can degrade ATI activity by 40 to 80%. Bacteria in sourdough starter that break down gliadin, the protein that triggers celiac disease, are not universal. It is only in recent years that specific bacterial strains with the ability to break down gliadin have been identified. Some individuals with celiac disease can eat some sourdough bread made with certain sourdough starter cultures. This is not a recommendation for those with celiac to give this a try. Sourdough bread should not be considered gluten-free, nor safe for those with celiac disease, but it does have lower gluten levels, and thus should have less impact on intestinal permeability.

The sourdough fermentation process lowers the amount of ATIs, gluten, and gliadin enough to make sourdough bread easier on the gut and the microbiome.[21] The fermentation process, which occurs in sourdough, also reduces phytic acid and makes magnesium more bioavailable.[22] [23] This is why sourdough bread gets a DAD score of zero.

Sourdough bread can be made without yeast, but some bakers use yeast to make the loaf rise more quickly. Thus, if purchasing it, read the label or ask the baker. Freshly baked sourdough bread is available at many grocery stores and can be purchased from the bakery as a whole loaf or sliced. Freshly made bakery bread may have a lower content of preservatives, dough conditioners, and other additives.

"Daily bread" in the Lord's prayer contains a second spiritual metaphor; it distinguishes freshly made bread from that which was stale, moldy, or otherwise corrupted. Commercially produced bread adds preservatives that are there to prevent the growth of bacteria and mold. No one wants to eat moldy bread, but what stops those biostatic agents from stopping the growth of commensal bacteria in the gut? Commercial bread may also contain other unnatural ingredients that should be avoided.

When you read the ingredient list on commercial baked bread, you are likely to notice that the buns without sesame seeds list sesame seeds in the ingredient list. Looking at a dozen different loaves of bread, almost all of them list sesame seeds as an ingredient.

In an amazing feat of dizzying and counterintuitive logic, most bread manufacturers now add a small amount of sesame seed to all the bread they produce. Does it improve the flavor? No. Does it improve shelf-life, texture, color, fragrance, or have any organoleptic, nutritional, or manufacturing advantage? Nope. So why would bread manufacturers add a significant allergen to their product? Yes, exactly that!

The Federal Government, under the Food Allergy Safety, Treatment, Education, and Research Act (FASTER Act), now mandates that manufacturers have to label major allergens that *may* be present in a food. Previously, sesame seeds were simply listed in the ingredients as a "natural spice or flavoring", but now the law stipulates that the inclusion of sesame seeds in bread needs to be spelled out on the label to protect those with allergies to it.

The problem for manufacturers was that the little seeds used on buns or bread might get into the bread without the seeds; it's difficult and time-consuming, and thus costly to eliminate any traces of sesame seeds that might be present in the dough machines, ovens, or packaging machines, etc., in the factory. It is easier to just add a bit of sesame seed to every loaf, put it on the label, and thus be in compliance with the FASTER Act than it would be to keep the seeds out. The 1.6 million Americans with an allergy to sesame seed, thank you for your concern.[24]

Those with inflammatory bowel disease should avoid sesame seeds, even if they are not allergic to them.

Wheat: Impact of Proper Preparation

Gliadin is a storage protein, and ATI is present to prevent germination. Sprouting wheat changes the balance of proteins in the grain for the development of roots and for the development of leaves and chloroplasts for photosynthesis. Sprouting greatly reduces the amount of anti-nutritional proteins, such as ATI and lectins, and improves digestibility.[25] [26] Sprouting of wheat has been demonstrated to decrease adaptive immune response eliciting gluten peptides by as much as 47% and innate immune response peptides by 46%. Germination also reduced levels of CM3 protein in wheat, which is responsible for provoking baker's asthma and intestinal inflammation, by more than half.[27] Germination increases phytase activity, and thus decreases phytic acid content and increases myoinositol,[28] and increases the bioavailability of zinc and iron.[29] Sprouting wheat triples the amount of soluble fiber and decreases the amount of insoluble fiber by 50%. Germination also increased the amount of vitamin B9 in wheat.[30] Sprouting improves the n-3 to n-6 fatty acid balance of most grains.[31] Germinated wheat flour (GWF) has more antioxidant activity and about 9% more protein than whole wheat flour. [32]

Definitions: Germination and Sprouting are not the same, although they are sometimes used as if they were. There are several stages of germination.

- Germination comes first. Imbibition is the process of the seed absorbing water, swelling, and activation of enzymes and metabolic processes in the seed.
- The enzymatic activity turns on metabolic processes, including the breaking down of proteins and other compounds stored in the cotyledons and endosperm. Starches are converted into simple sugars to use as energy, and amino acids are made available for new protein production for seedling growth.
- Respiration commences with the generation of ATP using the sugars for energy.
- With the emergence of the radicle (the primitive root), the germination phase is drawing to a close.
- Sprouting follows germination and includes the elongation of the roots and the emergence of the shoot and leaves. In dicots, such as legumes, the stem-like hypocotyl elongates, the shoots appear, and the cotyledons unfold and become exposed to air and light. In grasses, the shoot appears first.
- Photosynthesis begins, and minerals and other compounds can be absorbed from the soil.

Sprouted Grain: The sprout is no longer considered to be a whole grain by the Grain Council if the sprout (leaf shoot) is longer than the grain.[33] By this point, the embryonic roots will, however, be longer than the grain. For sprouting flour for bread making, the ideal level of development is considered to be when the embryo is visible, emerging from the seed coat, but the radicle is no longer than the seed. Thus, it is barely a sprout.

Sprouting wheat does not eliminate gluten; thus, sprouted wheat is not recommended for those with celiac disease. Germinated and sprouted wheat should nevertheless be less antigenic than regular wheat.

Sprouted wheat can be dried and made into flour. Sprouted wheat flour is commercially available. Sprouted wheat gets a DAD score of 3 on the SANA diet.

Sprouting of seeds is an important method for removing anti-nutritional compounds and improving the nutritional value of seeds. However, seeds carry risk of microbial contamination. Food safety experts advise that children, the elderly, persons with weakened immune systems, and pregnant women avoid eating *raw sprouts* of any kind. Cooking the sprouts kills the bacteria, but will not eliminate fungal toxins.

Seeds specifically sold for sprouting should be treated to reduce possible microbial contaminants. Seeds not intended for sprouting will not have been treated. Brown rice frequently carries high levels of bacteria, such as *E. coli, Listeria,* and *Salmonella,* and mold spores, which can easily grow during sprouting.

The only common grain that is considered safe to eat as a raw sprout is oat groats, but even they can be contaminated. The sprouts of the pseudo-grains quinoa and buckwheat can be eaten raw as they are considered to have a lower contamination risk. After germination, sprouts should be refrigerated to minimize bacterial growth and discarded if they appear damaged or slimy.

Sprouting Wheat

When wheat is sprouted for commercial flour production, it is first soaked in a 0.5 to 1.0 hypochlorite solution for 5 minutes to sterilize the surface of the grain from bacterial and fungal microbes.

Wheat will germinate at temperatures between 4°and 37°C, but the germination rate is highest a 25°C (77°F). Soaking the wheat in a one-to-one ratio of wheat to water for 16 hours gives the highest germination rate.[34] Thus, for one kilogram of wheat, one liter of water is used; however, there is minimal degradation in germination from using up to twice this much water.

Imbibition, the uptake of water into the seed, is a first step in germination. Enzymes, such as phytase and α-amylase, become activated, as this provides energy for germination and growth. It starts the process of turning the seed into a vegetable. It also begins the degradation of some of the anti-nutritional compounds in the seed. After soaking, the seeds are allowed to air dry for up to an hour so that they don't clump and can get air during germination.

With germination, phenolic compounds bound to lignan and arabinoxylans in the cell walls are cleaved by xylanases, increasing the availability of antioxidant phenolic compounds and making nutrients more bioavailable. Germination activates amylases that convert the starch to sugars and conversion of phytic acid into myoinositol. The impact of germination varies by such factors as time and temperature. This also impacts the cooking characteristics of the flour made from sprouted wheat. The ideal sprouting temperature for vigorous wheat growth is also around 25°C; however, this is not the best temperature from the standpoint of sprouted wheat for preparing flour to make bread, which depends on the presence of gluten. Sprouting wheat at 20°C (68°F) for 18 to 24 hours offers a good balance of gains in nutritional value while preserving gluten proteins that give bread its texture.[35]

(Post-germination blanching of the seed coat in an alkaline solution can further improve digestibility. (5 grams of baking soda per liter of 95°C, 5 volumes of water to grain, for 1 – 2 minutes.)

The sprouted grain is then dried and milled into flour.

Bread made from sprouted wheat flour is firmer and chewier.[36]

Sprouted grain breads (often a mix of wheat and other grains or legumes) generally get good DAD scores (around 4★★★★) and are allowed on the SANA diet. When available, they are often found in the freezer section of the grocery store. Sprouted whole wheat flour can be purchased online, but be ready for sticker shock. At the time of this writing, unless buying wholesale quantities, it is usually considerably less costly to buy sprouted grain bread than to purchase the flour.

Dangerous Bread Additives

Some commercial breads use **potassium-iodate** or **calcium-iodate** as dough conditioners that allow for quicker leavening and a stronger foam. These are used to make "fluffier" breads, such as hot dog and hamburger buns. The amount of iodine in these breads can be excessive and cause thyroid problems, especially in children and pregnant women. These breads are banned from the SANA diet even before the use of iodate. Iodine and thyroid function are further discussed in Chapter 24.

Iodate is not the only halogen baked into bread. Some commercial breads use **brominated flour**, as potassium bromate acts as a foam strengthener and expander. Bromate interferes with thyroid function and has been demonstrated to cause kidney and thyroid cancers in rats.

Yet another carcinogenic foam expander allowed for use in bread in the U.S. but banned in Europe is **azodicarbonamide**.[37] Commercial bread and other manufactured foods may also contain significant amounts (several grams/kg) of the volume expander **sodium stearoyl lactylate (SSL)**. All of these compounds should be avoided and are prohibited from the SANA diet.

Rice

White rice is a pleasant but imperfect food. White rice is easier to cook, more palatable, and has a longer shelf life than whole-grain brown rice. It is less nutritious and has a high glycemic index,[38] which suggests, but does not explain why it causes increased risk for type 2 diabetes. It is suggested that rice may have a more probiotic impact when it is cold and crystallized into resistant starch, but that is hard to eat. Once the rice is reheated, the starch de-crystallizes. Rice has about half as much protein as wheat or oats. White rice, as typically prepared, gets a DAD score of zero to barely one. It is allowed on the SANA diet, but it is just about as low as a beneficial food can be.

Brown rice, as typically prepared, gets a decent rating on the DAD scale as compared to white rice; it gets a 2★★. Brown rice is a more natural product; the rice husk has been removed, but the bran, along with its vitamins and minerals, is still there. Rice bran is high in B vitamins. White rice has a much longer shelf life in part because insects are much less interested in eating white than brown rice. Even when properly stored at less than 15°C or vacuum-packed, rice begins to lose its flavor and begins to degrade after about 6 months.[39] Brown rice may take some getting used to. It has an unrefined presentation. It is something like wearing a wool shirt, not unpleasant, but you know you are wearing it. Brown rice takes a lot longer to cook. It has its own flavor. Still, it is recommended as a healthy grain.

Arsenic in Rice

Like all plants, rice takes up minerals from the soil. Rice, however, is especially adept at taking up arsenic and putting it into its seeds, the part we eat. Rice can contain 10 to 20 times as much arsenic as other grains. Other foods (seafood, poultry, dairy, and meat) also contain some arsenic, but it is in an organic form that is much less toxic than the inorganic form present in rice. Arsenic is a neurotoxin. This is more of a risk for infants and their developing brains than for adults, but even for adults, arsenic is best avoided. It is recommended that infants be fed grains other than rice because of the arsenic, and that wheat be avoided because of its antigenic compounds.

Some areas of the world have high levels of naturally occurring arsenic in the soil. This is a common problem in some parts of Southeast Asia. Since rice bioconcentrates arsenic, the soil content strongly determines the rice's arsenic content. For decades, U.S. farmers used arsenic compounds in chicken feed to control parasites. The manure from those chickens was then spread on the fields as fertilizer. Arsenical pesticides are now banned, but were commonly used to control moths and potato beetles, and used as an herbicide in cotton fields. Since arsenic is an element, it is a true forever chemical that never breaks down; it just stays in the soil. The most efficient way to remove the arsenic from the soil is to grow plants that bioconcentrate it, and then take those plants away. Oh... Rice also bioconcentrates cadmium more than any other cereal.[40]

Consumption of large amounts of white rice is associated with diabetes. This was assumed to be the result of the high glycemic index of polished (white) rice, which has had the bran removed. It turns out that arsenic ($AsO3^{-4}$) can affect insulin secretion, increase insulin resistance, and cause dysfunction of pancreatic beta cells, the cells that make insulin. Arsenic exposure increases the risk of gestational diabetes. Unfortunately, the highest concentration of arsenic in rice is in the bran;[41] thus, brown rice has about 80% more arsenic than white rice.[42] Thus, all rice may increase the risk of diabetes.

There are two major forms of arsenic in rice: inorganic arsenite and organic dimethylarsinic acid (DMA). Arsenite is considerably more toxic than DMA. The arsenic in rice grown in the U.S. has more DMA than arsenite, while the reverse is true in rice from Southeast Asia.[43] On average, rice from Texas has about twice as much arsenic as that grown in California. Rice from the Southern states accounts for about half of the rice sold in the U.S., and it has much higher levels of arsenic as compared to rice from California. Basmati rice and Jasmine rice have lower levels, and rice from India has lower arsenic levels than that from Thailand. Soil and water contamination, soil microbes, and cultivation practices can all impact both the levels of arsenic present in the rice and the form, organic or inorganic, that it is present in.[44]

Arsenic can be mostly removed from rice by rinsing and pre-soaking it. Rinsing the rice well (2 – 4 times) removes about 7% of the inorganic arsenic from the rice.[45] Rinsing the rice also helps remove bacterial and fungal spores from the rice. Soaking the rice overnight in five volumes of water for one volume of rice removes 80% of the arsenic.[46] [47] Changing out the soak water about halfway through will remove more arsenic. Soaking at a warmer temperature is more effective and quicker (i.e., a warm room rather than soaking in the refrigerator). Hot water at 50°C (122°F) and using 5 – 7 volumes of water to rice is an effective method of reducing arsenic in rice. Cooking rice in 6 to 10 volumes of water and then draining the excess water removes about half of the arsenic.

Rice Germination

Even when rice has been polished into white rice and the bran and germ removed, the remaining endosperm still contains intact proteins. Thus, as with wheat, imbibition during soaking activates enzymes such as gibberellic acid (GA) that activate other enzymes and phytase that converts phytic acid in the rice into myoinositol.[48] Soaking brown rice helps remove phytic acid from the bran, but additionally helps convert phytic acid within the seed into the nutrient myoinositol, which improves insulin sensitivity. Sprouting rice increases gamma-aminobutyric acid (GABA) content as much as 10-fold in the rice. GABA is a neurotransmitter that appears to have health benefits when consumed in food, such as the reduction of stress, blood pressure, and inflammation, and may improve insulin sensitivity.[49] [50] Ingestion of GABA may improve cognition and mental health, reduce pain, improve sleep, and increase growth hormone production.[51]

Sprouted rice is a good source of dietary GABA, but there are many other sources. Topping the list in mg/kg is pumpkin seeds, but one is much more likely to eat a pound of rice than a pound of pumpkin seeds. Tomatoes, millet, grapes, cucumbers, potatoes, spinach, buckwheat, corn, and many mushrooms are high in GABA.[52] Adzuki beans have very high levels.[53] Certain strains of lactic acid bacteria produce GABA, and thus, yogurt can have substantial levels; however, this depends upon the strain of lactic acid bacteria used to ferment the milk. *Lactococcus lactis subsp. lactis* and *Streptococcus thermophilus* are species that commonly produce high levels of GABA. [54] [55] Greater levels of GABA are produced when the yogurt is fermented for 24 hours than at 12 hours.[56]

Soaking rice softens that bran, leading to a softer and fluffier texture. It helps to allow the rice to swell without bursting the grain. Pre-soaking rice before cooking also makes the rice more digestible, removes most of the arsenic and pesticide contamination,[57] and may lower the glycemic index,[58] and raise the digestibility, [59] all of which increase the DAD score. The difference between soaking and germination is mostly the temperature, but also the time. If the water is too cold, germination is delayed or even retarded. If the temperature is too hot, germination will not occur.

Germination of seeds before cooking raises the nutritional value and the DAD scores. The optimal soak time and temperature for *germination* of the seed give a very good indication of the optimal conditions for hydration and enzymatic activation of the seed for degradation and utilization of storage proteins, and formation of new proteins in preparation for growth. Thus, optimal soak temperature and time to improve digestibility, nutritional value, and thus DAD score are similar or identical to those for optimal seed germination. These may not be the optimal sprouting conditions, however.

The SANA program encourages germination of most grains and pulses as it improves the nutritional quality, anti-inflammatory impact, and digestively of the rice, while decreasing arsenic exposure.

Rice Germination Protocol

The following is an optimized protocol for germination of brown rice for planting or sprouting. (Old or poor-quality brown rice may fail to germinate.)

1. Wash the rice, rinsing it in clean water.

2. Sterilization: The seed is sterilized with 0.5% sodium hypochlorite, soaking the grain for 5 minutes, then rinsed with distilled water.[60] (This step should not be needed for cooking rice unless it is heavily contaminated with fungal spores, in which case you don't want to eat it anyway.)

3. In a clean vessel, add five to seven volumes of hot water, 50 – 55°C (122 – 130°F) to the volume of rice to be germinated. Stir the rice and allow the temperature to fall to 32 to 34°C (90 – 93°F).[61] This helps soften the seed coat and activates phytase and other enzymes.

4. The optimum rice seed germination temperature is 32°C to 34°C, depending upon the research source and likely the type of rice.[62] Rice imbibition for germination is highly successful between 30°to 40°C with a soak time of 8, but not longer than 12 hours.[63] Thus, soaking the rice in 5 volumes of water to one volume of rice at a target temperature of 33°C (91°F) for 8 hours, but no more than 12 hours, using dechlorinated water, is likely near optimal for germination.

Adding calcium chloride 1% to the soak water may increase the germination rate by removing sodium ions from the starch.[64] A large (5 – 7:1) volume of rice to water ratio used may also help remove sodium as well as arsenic from the rice.

5. Drain the rice and place it in a sprouting container, preferably in the dark, maintaining a temperature of 32°C (90°F) for best results. Rinse the rice every 8 hours. The rice should sprout within 2 to 3 days after the soaking.

Gibberellins (GAs) are plant hormones that modulate germination and other developmental processes. GAs break the seed's dormancy. In the seed embryo, gibberellins stimulate the transcription of α-amylase that converts starch stored in the seed into glucose, which is used for growth. GA is not present in the mature dry grain, but is rather synthesized with seed hydration. GA in most food plants is synthesized via the methylerythritol phosphate (MEP) pathway. The first enzyme in this pathway, ent-copalyl diphosphate synthase (CPS), has optimal activity at a temperature of 30 - 40°C, and at a pH of 7 (pH range 6 to 8) in rice.[65] The second enzyme in the pathway, *ent*-kaurene synthase (KS), has optimal activity at a temperature of 37°C and of pH of 7.[66] The third enzyme, ent-kaurene monooxygenase (KMO), has optimal activity at a temperature of 30°C and a pH of 7.25 in rice.[67] Thus, a neutral pH and a temperature of 30°to 40°C are ideal for breaking seed dormancy in rice.

At lower temperatures, soaking seeds will promote imbibition; however, GA may not be effectively produced, and instead, the plant stress hormone abscisic acid (ABA) is produced, which impedes germination and growth during times of risk. Soaking black beans at room temperature (25°C - 77°C) fails to improve digestibility, while soaking at 38°C (100°C) greatly increases it.

Mild stress during germination, however, can increase the production of phenolic compounds that protect the seedlings from microbial threats and may offer health benefits. Oat germination is highest at around 30°C, and this temperature also provides the highest content of lignans, phenolic acids, and avenanthramides. At 20°C, under mild cold stress, flavonoid and phytosterol levels in the sprouts are highest, but germination falls by a third. At 40°C, germination was most resistant to salinity.[68] [69] The optimal water temperature for high germination rates and the air temperature for rapid sprout growth are not necessarily the same.

Recommended Brown Rice Preparation

(DAD score: 5; without presoak: 2)

1. Rinse the rice in tap water, swirling the rice in a pot of water and draining off the water a few times. Using a sieve to catch the rice makes this step easier. Rinsing lowers the burden of bacteria and mold spores on the rice and removes some arsenic and phytic acid from the rice. Rinse until the water is nearly clear. If the water looks black, it may be

contaminated with mold spores, and that rice is better off not used.

2. Soak the rice in 5 to 7 volumes of water at a temperature of 38 to 45°C (100 to 112°F). A higher volume of water and a higher temperature help remove more arsenic. A yogurt maker, slow cooker, or Instapot, set to about 100°F, works well. At 38°C, soak for 10 – 12 hours; at 45°C, soak for 6 to 9 hours.
3. Discard the soaking water, and rinse the rice three times. The rinse water should be clear. Drain off the rinse water.
4. Cook the rice in a pressure cooker using 1½ volumes of water for each original volume of rice. (1½ cups of water for each cup of dry brown rice). Add ¼ to 1/3 tsp of salt per cup of rice. Pressure-cook (at 15 psi) for 12 to 14 minutes at the minimal heat to maintain pressure, turn off the heat, and allow natural release. Fluff with a fork, and reseal for 15 minutes. Use slightly more water to get a softer rice. Note: You will likely need to adjust the amount of water and cook time according to the type of brown rice used and the texture you are looking for.
5. This should give fully cooked, soft rice. Nicely separated, al dente brown rice. If a softer or stickier rice is wanted, increase the water by 20 percent and increase the time accordingly. If nicely separated, al dente brown rice is desired, decreasing the amount of water slightly.

White Rice Preparation

(DAD score: 5, without presoak: barely a 1)

While not as high in fiber or B vitamins, white rice can be prepared so that it has high digestibility and a high DAD score. Pregnant and lactating women and young children who are at higher risk from arsenic may be better off avoiding brown rice; in this population, white rice is likely a better choice.

1. Rinse and soak the rice as for brown rice; however, the soak time for white rice is shorter. At 38°C, soak white rice for 9 – 12 hours, and at 45°C, soak white rice for 4 to 6 hours. Then rinse the rice.
2. White rice can be cooked in a pressure cooker (4 – 5 minutes) or on the stovetop, about 12 minutes.
3. The amount of water needed to cook rice varies by the type of rice and the style of the dish being prepared. Use at least a 1:1 ratio. Chewy, dense long-grain rice can be made using a 1:1 ratio of water to rice, while a 3:1 ratio of liquid to rice is used to make a creamy risotto. During soaking, the rice will have imbibed some water; thus, slightly less water is needed for cooking. Decrease the amount of water used by 10 – 20 percent, and keep track of your results so that the amount of water used can be adjusted to get the texture you want in the future. More water will give softer and stickier rice.
4. After cooking the rice, let it rest for 10 – 15 minutes to fluff up the grains.

Oats

Compared to other grains, oats are high in protein, with more than twice that of rice or corn. Oats are also very high in soluble fiber, which is good for the gastrointestinal microbiome and for avoiding leaky gut. Consumption of oat (bran), especially hydrolyzed oat bran, lowers cholesterol (a little bit) if you eat enough.

Oats are one of the healthful grains in terms of the way they are typically prepared. Most oats consumed by humans have been mechanically milled into rolled oats that can be cooked quickly. These are used to make oatmeal porridge, oatmeal cookies, granola, and granola bars. Oats are also used to make breakfast cereals such as "Cheerios". Steel-cut oats are sometimes cooked to make porridge, but can also be made into delicious savory dishes. For savory dishes, look for the "traditional" steel-cut oats, not the "quick", "3-minute" ones that turn into mush. Oat bran, present in rolled and steel-cut oats, is high in soluble fiber.

If quick rolled oats are prepared according to the directions provided by Larry, the Quaker gentleman on the Quaker Quick Oats box, the oatmeal gets a rating of 1★. Not bad for a grain.

Those directions (for two servings) are to use 1¾ cups of water for 1 cup of rolled oats, with 1/8th tsp. of salt. Cook it for one minute. Preparing oatmeal in this way gives it a DAD rating of 1. This oatmeal deserves a palatability score of 👎👎👎, which often begs for masking it with brown sugar or other distractors.

Recommended Oatmeal Porridge Preparation:

Using more water better hydrates the starches and the soluble fiber, making them more available. A longer cooking time decreases the content of saponins and other anti-nutritional compounds present in the oats.

★★★Method: For a single serving, use ½ cup of quick-rolled oats and 2 cups of water. (Water to quick oats 4:1). Add a pinch (1/16th tsp.) of salt, to taste. A teaspoon of molasses can be used. Bring the water with the oats to a boil and turn down the heat to maintain a low boil, stirring frequently. Cook for 5 to 6 minutes and turn off the heat; it should thicken as it cools. The oatmeal should be cooked long enough that the fine foam that collects on top with boiling disappears as saponins break down. This results in a creamy, palatable oatmeal with a DAD score of 3. Extras such as chopped pecans or walnuts, raisins, dried cranberries, etc., can be cooked into the cereal.

★★★★★Method: Use three to four volumes of warm water (38 - 43°C) to one volume of quick rolled oats. Soak the rolled oats for at least 30 minutes. This can be done in a yogurt maker. Alternatively, start with water warmed in a digital kettle to 45°C (112°F) and, less ideally, hot tap water, pouring 3 or 4 volumes of hot water over the oatmeal, covering the pot to keep it warm, and soaking the oatmeal for 30 to 60 minutes. <u>Do not drain or rinse</u>. If adding dried fruits (cranberries, raisins, etc.), soak them as well to plump them up. After soaking, add about 1/8th tsp. of salt per cup of oats used and any other ingredients such as nuts or molasses. Bring it to a boil and turn down the heat to maintain a low boil, stirring frequently. A fine foam should form on top for the first minutes, but it will disappear after about 5 minutes. Cook at a low boil for 6 minutes. Turn off the heat. The oatmeal porridge will thicken as it cools. This results in a creamy, pleasant oatmeal with a DAD score of 5. A teaspoon of molasses or a bit of brown sugar can be added before cooking the oatmeal.

Dry breakfast oat "O" cereal has a DAD rating of 3★★★. Toasted O's (the Walmart brand) contains no sugar; those from Cheerios contain less than one gram of added sugar per serving. Honey Nut O's are not prohibited from the SANA diet, but should be considered a dessert as they contain 12 grams of added sugar per serving. The Cheerios brand also contains almonds; the Walmart brand does not. Read labels.

Corn (Maize)

Most corn products are prepared in a way that yields DAD scores of B or lower, and thus, they should not be part of the DAD diet. This includes fresh sweet corn, which is used as a vegetable. But it doesn't have to be this way, and there are readily available corn products that have good DAD scores.

Corn, which is commonly called maize in non-American English-speaking countries, has a large, tough seed coat. Think about popcorn. The reason that it explodes is that when popcorn is heated, steam forms and is compressed within the seed coat of the kernel. When the popcorn reaches a pressure of about 9.2 atmospheres (135 pounds per square inch), a catastrophic rupture occurs, causing a rapid expansion that turns the seed inside out and puffs the starchy interior. That's one tough seed coat. Sweet corn (as a vegetable) and field corn also have tough, hard-to-digest seed coats.

About half the protein mass in corn is zein proteins. Zein proteins are prolamins found in maize; glutens are prolamins found in wheat. Thus, corn has some gluten-like proteins. In intestinal mucosal cells grown in culture, certain zein fragments stimulate the production of IL-8, p38 MAPK, and COX2, and promote the release of zonulin. Further and more telling, when intestinal mucosa biopsies from 5 people with celiac disease were exposed to zein, there was an increase in gamma interferon (INF-γ), an inflammatory cytokine. Zein contains toxic peptides that can have proinflammatory and permeation effects on the intestinal mucosa. While milder than gliadin, zein fragments promote an innate response in intestinal cells that increases permeability.

Chapter 8 discussed how the consumption of corn can cause the disease pellagra, and how nixtamalization prevents this disease by making proteins and other nutrients more accessible for digestion, and that this process also destroys some fungal toxins. Nixtamalization also allows dough to be formed from corn. Nixtamalization is a process in which whole dry corn kernels are cooked in lime (calcium hydroxide). This process dissolves the seed coat of the corn. If one examines whole nixtamalized corn, such as hominy in a can, it can be seen that the seed coat is no longer apparent. During nixtamalization, zein proteins are partially denatured and solubilized. Some zein protein and much of the skin are washed away with the steeping fluid (the nejayote), and the resulting nixtamal (hominy) provides more digestible proteins.

Nixtamalized corn (hominy) and masa, flour made from hominy, get positive DAD scores. Thus, tamales, tortillas, and hominy grits (but not corn grits) can be eaten on the SANA diet.

However, most American tortilla manufacturers (and almost all tortilla chip makers) use regular corn flour.

The "pseudo-tortillas" made from corn flour have a DAD rating of B, while traditional tortillas made from masa get a DAD score of 3. Read the labels. If the label on a pack of tortillas states "lime-treated corn", "corn masa flour", "masa", or nixtamalized corn, the tortillas can be eaten on the SANA diet. If it does not, skip it. Additionally, avoid tortillas made with "cellulose gum" (a.k.a carboxymethylcellulose) and other noxious ingredients that are often added to tortillas.

Masa harina (flour) can be used to make cornbread; it results in a lighter, more flavorful, and a tad sweeter cornbread.

Mission brand corn tortillas are made from masa; La Banda tortillas are made from corn flour. While I have seen no corn chips made of nixtamalized corn, tostadas made with masa are available. Zero net calories and high fiber tortillas get negative ratings on the DAD scoring (A). Flour tortillas made with wheat flour also get negative DAD scores of C.

Cooking Hominy Grits

I lived in the rural South for several decades, and until researching this volume, I had eaten grits about the same number of times. No offence intended, but why bother?

Following the recipe on the box, the hominy grits were unpleasant, gritty, and less than bland. Those grits get between the teeth, and one feels uncomfortable until they floss. The DAD rating was barely one, which is considerably better than corn grits, but still not worth eating.

Soaking the grits in 7 volumes of water for 6 hours, rinsing, and cooking made something worth eating, with a DAD score of two. They even had attractive golden flakes in them that were not previously apparent. They reminded me of the dumplings my mom made with semolina when I was a child.

Recommended Directions for Grits (DAD score 4): Rinse the grits and strain through a fine strainer. Soak the hominy grits in 6 to 8 volumes of water to grits, heated to 50 to 55°C (122 to 131°F) with a tablespoon of vinegar per liter or quart of water, for at least 6 hours. Cover to help retain the heat as it cools to room temperature. As a breakfast cereal, this generally translates to soaking them overnight. Carefully drain off the soaking water using the fine mesh strainer and rinse them again.

Cook the grits in 4 – 5 volumes of water for the original dry grits. Add a pinch (1/16 tsp. salt for one ¼ cup of grits). Flavor as desired, Cook at a low boil for 6 to 7 minutes. More water or time may be needed depending on the desired texture.

Sweet Corn

Sweet corn is a delicious and enjoyable vegetable, but it gets a low B on the DAD scale as a result of its large, tough seed coat. However, sweet corn, as corn on a cob or as cut corn, can be prepared in a way that tastes great and gives a DAD score of four. Here is how:

- Corn on the cob: Cooking the ear of corn at a temperature between 150and 170°F hydrates the starches in corn without breaking down the pectin. This gives a crisp, flavorful corn. If available, use a slow cooker that allows setting and maintaining the temperature of the water at 160°F (71°C). Add and dissolve one teaspoon of baking soda per quart of water, or about a tablespoon for three quarts. There needs to be enough water for the corn to float. Remove the husk and silk before placing the ear of corn into the pot using tongs, and cover the pot. Cook for ten to fifteen minutes and serve right away. The baking soda acts as an alkali treatment that makes the seed coat more digestible.
- If a slow cooker or temperature-controlled cooker is not available, use a large pot with at least 4 quarts of water, add 4 tsp. of baking soda, and bring the water to a boil. Turn off the heat. After the water has stopped boiling, wait about 30 seconds to a minute to let the water cool slightly, and then add up to four ears of corn. Cover and allow the corn to cook for a few minutes before rolling the ears over to cook more evenly. Put the lid back on and let the corn cook in the hot water for a total of 10 to 15 minutes. This should give a cooking temperature of 170 to 150°F for most of the cook time. (Lan Lam method)[70]
- Adding one teaspoon of baking soda to cooking water and cooking for 10 minutes helps break down the seed coat and makes the corn more digestible and nutritious. The same method can be used to cook cut frozen sweet corn, but it should be thawed first. This can be done, rinsing the frozen corn in cool tap water. More simply, place the frozen cut corn in one liter of water with a teaspoon of baking soda and heat it, stirring occasionally, until it reaches a temperature of 170°F. Remove it from the heat and drain it. This raises the DAD score of cut corn from a B to 3.
- An alternative method is to soak frozen sweet corn in water with four tablespoons of baking soda per quart in the refrigerator for 24 hours. At a lower temperature, the process needs a higher concentration of alkali and more time. Rinse the rice twice in cool water to remove the baking soda. Then cook the corn as you usually would; generally, just quickly heating it to a simmer, or microwave it without overcooking it. You may notice that the corn turns a deeper gold color than usual.

Quinoa

The pseudo-grain quinoa (*Chenopodium quinoa*) gets a poor DAD rating of zero with typical preparation (boiling); however, with processing as described below, quinoa gets a rating of three. Like other seeds, it has a seed coat, tannins, phytate, and saponins that are anti-nutritive. Quinoa saponins are bitter and have significant antinutritional effects. Soaking, washing and germination, and fermentation can increase the nutritive value of quinoa.[71]

The optimal germination temperature for quinoa is around 30°C (86°F), but germination rates fall quickly at a temperature of 35°C (95°F) or above in some strains of quinoa and by 40°C in most varieties.[72] The optimal conditions for germination of djulis (*Chenopodium formosanum*) are with soaking for 4 hours at 25°C, followed by germination at 25 to 30°C for 48 hours. Lowering the pH of the soak water to 5.5 to 6.0 increased the GABA content of the sprouts slightly.[73] Optimal soak conditions for the extraction of saponins from quinoa seed are at 50°C (122°F) for 60 – 69 minutes at a 7:1 weight-to-weight ratio (seven milliliters of water per gram of seed).[74]

Recommended Quinoa Preparation

Place the quinoa in a pot and rinse it with tap water, swirling it around, and drain it three times. Use a fine strainer to prevent loss of the seed. Soak the quinoa for 3 hours, using 7 ml of hot water around 33°C (91°F) per gram of seed (about one cup of water for one fluid ounce of seed).

Cook the soaked quinoa with a 1.5:1 ratio of water to the original dry volume of quinoa. Add salt (about ¼ tsp per cup of quinoa) if you like. Bring to a boil and then reduce to a simmer, cover, and allow to cook for 10 minutes, depending on the desired texture, with a longer cook time giving a more tender, fluffier texture. Remove from the heat, fluff it with a fork, and cover it for another 5 – 10 minutes to further cook in its steam.

Unlike rice, which crystallizes and gets hard when cold, cooked quinoa is pleasant served cold after refrigeration, and makes a nice summer dish, and can be used in salads.

Barley

Barley for human consumption is usually "pearled"; the hull and most of the bran are removed. Barley is great in hearty soups and vegan stews and has a chewy texture.

As typically cooked, barley gets a DAD score of zero. A usual method is using 3 parts water to one part barley, and boiling for 25 – 30 minutes.

When properly prepared, barley gets a very nice DAD score of 4. Barley is high in fiber and has a low glycemic index.

As with other grains, the SANA program recommends pseudo-germination of barley before cooking. Soak the barley at 37°C for seven hours, and then cook as usual. It can be pressure-cooked for 18-20 minutes, followed by natural pressure release.

Germination Temperatures For other Grains

Some studies only show ideal germination growth temperatures, but not the ideal soak temperature. Generally, they are similar. When cooking seeds, pre-germination soaking can improve nutritional value.

Optimal sprouting temperature for blue corn for antioxidant activity was found to be 26.9 °C for 208 hours after testing seeds soaked at 25°C for 12 hours.[75]

Chia seeds (Salvia hispanica L.) were optimally sprouted at either 21°C for 157 hours or 33°C for 126 hours with regard to antioxidant activity.[76]

Amaranth seeds were soaked in distilled water at 25°C for 6 hours. The optimal sprouting conditions for antioxidant activity were at a temperature of 30°C and a germination time of 78 hours.[77]

Foxtail millet GABA levels and total phenolic content peaked when the seeds were soaked at 31°C for 4.5 hours and then germinated at 35°C for five days. Interestingly, adding 4.5 grams of sucrose per liter (@ one level teaspoon per quart) to the soak water increased GABA levels and total phenolic content.[78] Adding 3% sucrose to the soaking water of adzuki beans also increases antioxidant activity.[79]

Sprouting temperatures, especially those below about 28°C, may enhance seedling survival as they induce stress and the production of compounds that have antimicrobial activity. For germination for seed consumption, the production of GAs is desired, and thus, sprouting temperatures between 30 and 45°C are most effective. Almost all plants follow this pattern.

Table 9A: Cereal Scores

Cereal	Rating
Barley (Pearled), typical cooking	0
Barley (Pearled): Soaked at 37°C for 7 hours, boiled	4
Corn grits (cooked, gritty) (As per package instructions)	C
Corn grits (cooked as molle with added water, cooked for a long time)	0
Corn, Hominy grits cooked 7 minutes, 4:1 water to corn (as directed on the box)	1
Corn, Hominy grits soaked 6 hours, rinsed, cooked 4:1 water to corn, with a pinch of salt (in the microwave for 3 minutes), little bits of gold skin. Pleasant	2
Corn, Hominy grits soaked in hot water with vinegar for 6+ hours, rinsed, cooked 5:1 water to corn, with a pinch of salt. Pleasant	4
Corn Hominy (nixtamal) canned, white or golden	2
Corn Tortillas (commercial) made from corn flour	B to C
Corn Tortilla, homemade masa, and water	3
Corn Tortilla, commercially made from masa	3
Corn Tostadas, made from Nixtamalized corn masa	3
Moraiyo Jungle rice (boiled with water)	4
Oat bran	2
Oat cereal, Cheerios	2
Oats cereal, Honey-Os	2
Oatmeal: 1-minute oats prepared per instructions on the box. 1 part oats to @2 parts water	1
Oatmeal, Quick oats, 4 to 1 water to oats, cooked 6 minutes	3
Oats, oatmeal 3:1 cooked, cold jelled,	4
Oatmeal, soaked in water at 46°C and covered for 30 minutes, low boil for 7 minutes	5
Quinoa (tricolor) Cooked per instructions (boil for 10 min.)	0
Quinoa (tricolor) rinsed, hot soak 1h, rinse, boil.	3
Rice, white, warm or cold, jasmine, or other type, typical preparation	0 - 1
Rice, white jasmine, rinsed thrice, soaked for 7 hours at 38°C before cooking (see methods)	4
Rice, Brown (typical preparation, rinsed and cooked in a pressure cooker)	2
Rice Brown rice, rinsed thrice, soaked for 8 hours at 38°C before cooking (see methods)	5
Wheat, semolina, cooked as porridge	B
Wheat Bran cereal	C
Wheat Bread Bagels (bleached flour)	A
Wheat Bread Commercial White Sourdough bread with xanthan gum	A
Wheat Bread Commercial whole wheat	B
Sprouted multigrain bread (Ezekiel 4:9)	4
Wheat, Sourdough French bread* (bakery fresh, enriched flour, no preservatives)	0
Wheat, sprouted to the point where > 2 mm root sprout is visible on nearly all grains	3
Wheat flour tortillas, commercial, with vegetable shortening, cellulose gum (CMC), etc.	C
Whole grain wheat, germinated at 38°C and blanched with baking soda	5
Corn Chips	B
Popcorn	B
Oat honey granola bar	1

Constipation

Wheat bran in the form of wheat bran cereal and wheat bran muffins is commonly used to help with mild chronic constipation. While it may be effective, wheat bran in this form is not recommended on the SANA diet. The SANA diet, on its own, should supply sufficient fiber. If chronic constipation is present in adults, it should be a concern.

The onset of constipation during middle age or late middle age, especially when it occurs in men, can be a presenting sign of Parkinson's disease, which may also be present with a diminished sense of smell. These symptoms are caused by loss of neurons in the intestine and olfactory nerve, respectively. Colorectal cancer can also present with constipation. Constipation that does not quickly respond to diet merits a consultation with one's physician.

Guar fiber (Sold as SunFiber) is a treatment for constipation that is beneficial for the gut and its microbiome. It acts as a symbiotic agent and has been found to normalize both diarrhea and constipation in irritable bowel syndrome. The regular daily intake of 5 to 10 grams of guar fiber keeps one regular. [80] At a dose of 2 grams per serving, it helps curb appetite in many people, [81] perhaps as a probiotic that produces short-chain fatty acids.[82] [83] In an animal model, partially hydrolyzed guar gum (PHGG) (guar fiber) inhibited chemically induced colitis and reduced intestinal inflammation.[84] [85]

If one has constipation, guar fiber may be helpful. It may take several days to be effective. One level measuring teaspoon is enough for most people. It dissolves easily in water or other beverages and essentially has no taste.

What is guar? It's a legume that is also called "cluster bean". It is mostly grown in India, but it is also grown in the high plains of Texas.

Guar gum is not so great. It gets a DAD score of D. In an animal study of inflammatory bowel disease, it aggravated colonic inflammation.[86] Guar gum is useful, however, for fracking, and 90% of the production of guar gum produced in India is exported for use in the shale and oil industries.

What's the difference? Guar fiber is made by partially hydrolyzing guar gum. Thus, it is partially broken down into molecules of a size that feeds commensal bacteria in the gut.

Guar fiber is produced by the partial enzymatic hydrolysis of guaran, the galactomannan of the endosperm of guar seeds. This neutral polysaccharide is composed of a mannose backbone chain with single galactose side units decorating nearly two out of every three mannose units. Maybe you didn't need to know that.

Prunes and Kiwi fruit: Prunes are an effective remedy for chronic constipation. The typical dose is 50 grams (about 6 dried prunes) twice daily.[87] Prunes are high in sorbitol, and this explains most of their mode of action, although they also contain other fiber. The sorbitol may cause bloating and flatulence; thus, this may cause problems for those with IBS.[88] Kiwi fruit (one twice a day) is as effective for constipation as prunes, but causes less bloating and was favored over prunes by patients in a clinical trial.[89] A meta-analysis of randomized controlled trials found that kiwi fruit consumption is more effective than psyllium for constipation and has fewer adverse effects.[90]

Psyllium: Psyllium husks are often used for constipation and are promoted as GI-healthy. It gets a DAD score of D and is especially injurious to the gut for those with inflammatory bowel disease and people with Parkinson's disease. Psyllium should be avoided.

Animal Feed

Adding phytase to corn-based feed to chickens increased the distal ileal digestibility of 16 amino acids by as much as 12%, which likely translates to a greater than 50% decline in the amount of protein fermenting in the distal intestine.[91] Soaking and partial germination likely have a similar effect. In young pigs, consumption of sticky rice provided a 7% higher ileal amino acid digestibility coefficient and a 14% higher plasma amino acid level than resistant starch, suggesting that the availability of glucose to the enterocytes spares the conversion of amino acids into fuel energy during digestion.[92]

A broiler chicken consumes about 10 pounds of feed from hatching to slaughter over 6 weeks. About 74 billion chickens are eaten by humans each year. Improving the Feed Conversion Ratio (FCR) in chickens by 10 percent could reduce the amount of feed (mostly soy and corn) required by 74 billion pounds. Seventy-four billion chickens produce a lot of chicken shit, which results in copious nitrogenous wastes and water contamination. As much as half of the nitrogen comes from unabsorbed amino acids. On average, humans eat around 161 eggs per year; thus, nearly 1.3 trillion eggs are consumed. A ballpark estimate puts the required chicken feed for egg production to be around 577 billion pounds. A 10% increase in protein utilization could mean 57.7 billion pounds of feed saved.

Proper processing of the feed, including pre-germination, would likely benefit the animal's health.

Let me recommend red cargo rice as my favorite "brown" rice.

To get a fluffier rice after cooking it, use a fork to gently fluff the rice. This helps separate the grains and prevents them from clumping together.

Table 9B: Pressure cooking times for grains

One cup of grain	Cups of Water	Pressure Cooking Time (minutes)
Brown Rice	1½ cups	12 - 15
White Rice	1½ cups	5 - 6
Quinoa	2 cups	5 - 6
Steel-cut oats	1⅔ cups	10 - 12

Industrial Processing

There are other effective means of treating seeds and grain to remove anti-nutritive compounds that improve digestibility and nutritional value that are not detailed in this book. They are generally more involved, making them less practical for small-batch and daily food preparation, but they can be readily done at a more industrial scale. Herein, hot water soaking (i.e., 50°C), germination, and mild alkali treatment are discussed. There are also more advanced industrial methods, including fermentation and ultrasound.[93]

Some simpler methods of these are described and recommended in this book. Baking soda blanching of beans, for example, is a mild alkali treatment. While the methods used are similar, different seeds and grains require different specific treatments.

Fermentation of seeds and grains is another process that is beyond the scope of this book.

For those interested, the specifics of processing various seeds to improve their nutritive quality can be found in the published scientific literature, such as PubMed or by using Google.

[1] The Seven Plant Species - A Basis of Nutrition of Ancient Israel. Zofia Włodarczyk. Biomed J Sci & Tech Res 25(4)-2020. BJSTR. MS.ID.004239. https://biomedres.us/pdfs/BJSTR.MS.ID.004239.pdf

[2] Shiferaw, B., Smale, M., Braun, HJ. *et al.* Crops that feed the world 10. Past successes and future challenges to the role played by wheat in global food security. *Food Sec.* **5**, 291–317 (2013). https://doi.org/10.1007/s12571-013-0263-y

[3] https://worldpopulationreview.com/country-rankings/rice-consumption-by-country

[4] Consumption of grains by Americans is above recommendations. https://www.ers.usda.gov/data-products/chart-gallery/gallery/chart-detail/?chartId=84153

[5] USDA Food Availability (Per Capita) Data System https://www.ers.usda.gov/data-products/food-availability-per-capita-data-system/

[6] Microbial Fermentation of Dietary Protein: An Important Factor in Diet–Microbe–Host Interaction, Diether, N, Willin PB. Jan. 2019 Microorganisms 7(1):19

[7] Involvement of gliadin, a component of wheat gluten, in increased intestinal permeability leading to non-steroidal anti-inflammatory drug-induced small-intestinal damage. Shimada S, Tanigawa T, Watanabe T, Nakata A, Sugimura N, Itani S, Higashimori A, Nadatani Y, Otani K, Taira K, Hosomi S, Nagami Y, Tanaka F, Kamata N, Yamagami H, Shiba M, Fujiwara Y. PLoS One. 2019 Feb 20;14(2):e0211436. doi: 10.1371/journal.pone.0211436. eCollection 2019. PMID: 30785904

[8] Diploid Wheats: Are They Less Immunogenic for Non-Celiac Wheat Sensitive Consumers? Rotondi Aufiero V, Sapone A, Mazzarella G. Cells. 2022 Aug 3;11(15):2389. doi: 10.3390/cells11152389. PMID: 35954233

[9] Reference proteomes of five wheat species as starting point for future design of cultivars with lower allergenic potential. Afzal M, Sielaff M, Distler U, Schuppan D, Tenzer S, Longin CFH. NPJ Sci Food. 2023 Mar 25;7(1):9. doi: 10.1038/s41538-023-00188-0. PMID: 36966156

[10] Comparative Analysis of *in vitro* Digestibility and Immunogenicity of Gliadin Proteins From Durum and Einkorn Wheat. Di Stasio L, Picascia S, Auricchio R, Vitale S, Gazza L, Picariello G, Gianfrani C, Mamone G. Front Nutr. 2020 May 22;7:56. doi: 10.3389/fnut.2020.00056. eCollection 2020. PMID: 32671087

[11] From celiac disease to coccidia infection and vice-versa: The polyQ peptide CXCR3-interaction axis. Lauxmann MA, Vazquez DS, Schilbert HM, Neubauer PR, Lammers KM, Dodero VI. Bioessays. 2021 Dec;43(12):e2100101. doi: 10.1002/bies.202100101. Epub 2021 Oct 27. PMID: 34705290

[12] Gliadin induces an increase in intestinal permeability and zonulin release by binding to the chemokine receptor CXCR3. Lammers KM, Lu R, Brownley J, Lu B, Gerard C, Thomas K, Rallabhandi P, Shea-Donohue T, Tamiz A, Alkan S, Netzel-Arnett S, Antalis T, Vogel SN, Fasano A. Gastroenterology. 2008 Jul;135(1):194-204.e3. doi: 10.1053/j.gastro.2008.03.023. Epub 2008 Mar 21. PMID: 18485912

[13] Gliadin induces an increase in intestinal permeability and zonulin release by binding to the chemokine receptor CXCR3. Lammers KM, Lu R, Brownley J, Lu B, Gerard C, Thomas K, Rallabhandi P, Shea-Donohue T, Tamiz A, Alkan S, Netzel-Arnett S, Antalis T, Vogel SN, Fasano A. Gastroenterology. 2008 Jul;135(1):194-204.e3. doi: 10.1053/j.gastro.2008.03.023.. PMID: 18485912

[14] Zonulin and its regulation of intestinal barrier function: the biological door to inflammation, autoimmunity, and cancer. Fasano A. Physiol Rev. 2011 Jan;91(1):151-75. doi: 10.1152/physrev.00003.2008. PMID: 21248165

[15] Blood-brain barrier and intestinal epithelial barrier alterations in autism spectrum disorders. Fiorentino M, Sapone A, Senger S, Camhi SS, Kadzielski SM, Buie TM, Kelly DL, Cascella N, Fasano A. Mol Autism. 2016 Nov 29;7:49. doi: 10.1186/s13229-016-0110-z. PMID: 27957319

[16] Plant alpha-amylase inhibitors and their interaction with insect alpha-amylases. Franco OL, Rigden DJ, Melo FR, Grossi-De-Sá MF. Eur J Biochem. 2002 Jan;269(2):397-412. doi: 10.1046/j.0014-2956.2001.02656.x. PMID: 11856298

[17] Wheat amylase trypsin inhibitors drive intestinal inflammation via activation of toll-like receptor 4. Junker Y, Zeissig S, Kim SJ, Barisani D, Wieser H, Leffler DA, Zevallos V, Libermann TA, Dillon S, Freitag TL, Kelly CP, Schuppan D. J Exp Med. 2012 Dec 17;209(13):2395-408. doi: 10.1084/jem.20102660. PMID: 23209313

[18] Wheat ATIs: Characteristics and Role in Human Disease. Geisslitz S, Shewry P, Brouns F, America AHP, Caio GPI, et al. Front Nutr. 2021 May 28;8:667370. doi: 10.3389/fnut.2021.667370. PMID: 34124122

[19] Celiac Disease, Gluten-Free Diet and Metabolic Dysfunction-Associated Steatotic Liver Disease. Cazac GD, Mihai BM, Ştefănescu G, Gîlcă-Blanariu GE, Mihai C, Grigorescu ED, Onofriescu A, Lăcătuşu CM. Nutrients. 2024 Jun 25;16(13):2008. doi: 10.3390/nu16132008. PMID: 38999756

[20] Gluten-Free Diet and Metabolic Syndrome: Could Be a Not Benevolent Encounter? Defeudis G, Massari MC, Terrana G, Coppola L, Napoli N, Migliaccio S. Nutrients. 2023 Jan 26;15(3):627. doi: 10.3390/nu15030627. PMID: 36771334

[21] Bacteria do it better! Proteomics suggests the molecular basis for improved digestibility of sourdough products. Reale A, Di Stasio L, Di Renzo T, De Caro S, Ferranti P, Picariello G, Addeo F, Mamone G. Food Chem. 2021 Oct 15;359:129955. doi: 10.1016/j.foodchem.2021.129955. Epub 2021 Apr 27. PMID: 34010753

[22] Moderate decrease of pH by sourdough fermentation is sufficient to reduce phytate content of whole wheat flour through endogenous phytase activity. Leenhardt F, Levrat-Verny MA, Chanliaud E, Rémésy C. J Agric Food Chem. 2005 Jan 12;53(1):98-102. doi: 10.1021/jf049193q. PMID: 15631515

23 Prolonged fermentation of whole wheat sourdough reduces phytate level and increases soluble magnesium. Lopez HW, Krespine V, Guy C, Messager A, Demigne C, Remesy C. J Agric Food Chem. 2001 May;49(5):2657-62. doi: 10.1021/jf001255z. PMID: 11368651

24 https://www.fastcompany.com/90830854/sesame-seed-allergen-fda-food-law

25 Nutritional and end-use perspectives of sprouted grains: A comprehensive review. Ikram A, Saeed F, Afzaal M, Imran A, Niaz B, Tufail T, Hussain M, Anjum FM. Food Sci Nutr. 2021 Jun 23;9(8):4617-4628. doi: 10.1002/fsn3.2408. eCollection 2021 Aug. PMID: 34401108

26 Improvement in sprouted wheat flour functionality: effect of time, temperature and elicitation. Michał Świeca Food Sci and Tech.Volume50, Issue 9 September 2015 (2135-2142) https://doi.org/10.1111/ijfs.12881

27 Effectiveness of Germination on Protein Hydrolysis as a Way To Reduce Adverse Reactions to Wheat. Boukid F, Prandi B, Buhler S, Sforza S. J Agric Food Chem. 2017 Nov 15;65(45):9854-9860. doi: 10.1021/acs.jafc.7b03175. PMID: 29059515

28 Effect of germination on the phytase activity, phytate and total phosphorus contents of rice (Oryza sativa), maize (Zea mays), millet (Panicum miliaceum), sorghum (Sorghum bicolor) and wheat (Triticum aestivum). Azeke MA, Egielewa SJ, Eigbogbo MU, Ihimire IG. J Food Sci Technol. 2011 Dec;48(6):724-9. doi: 10.1007/s13197-010-0186-y. Epub 2010 Dec 21. PMID: 23572811

29 Sprouted Grains: A Comprehensive Review. Benincasa P, Falcinelli B, Lutts S, Stagnari F, Galieni A. Nutrients. 2019 Feb 17;11(2):421. doi: 10.3390/nu11020421. PMID: 30781547

30 Changes of folates, dietary fiber, and proteins in wheat as affected by germination. Koehler P, Hartmann G, Wieser H, Rychlik M. J Agric Food Chem. 2007 Jun 13;55(12):4678-83. doi: 10.1021/jf0633037. Epub 2007 May 12. PMID: 17497874

31 Analysis of Fatty Acid Composition in Sprouted Grains. Nemzer B, Al-Taher F. Foods. 2023 Apr 29;12(9):1853. doi: 10.3390/foods12091853. PMID: 37174393

32 A study on physicochemical, antioxidant and microbial properties of germinated wheat flour and its utilization in breads. Dhillon B, Choudhary G, Sodhi NS. J Food Sci Technol. 2020 Aug;57(8):2800-2808. doi: 10.1007/s13197-020-04311-x. PMID: 32612297

33 https://wholegrainscouncil.org/whole-grains-101/whats-whole-grain-refined-grain/sprouted-whole-grains/definitions-sprouted-grains

34 Optimization of 'on farm' hydropriming conditions in wheat: Soaking time and water volume have interactive effects on seed performance. Tanwar H, Mor VS, Sharma S, Khan M, Bhuker A, Singh V, et al. (2023). PLoS ONE 18(1): e0280962. https://doi.org/10.1371/journal.pone.0280962

35 Effect of Different Wheat Sprouting Conditions on the Characteristics of Whole-Wheat Flour. Navarro JL, Losano Richard P, Moiraghi M, Bustos M, León AE, Steffolani ME. Food Technol Biotechnol. 2024 Jun;62(2):264-274. doi: 10.17113/ftb.62.02.24.8435. PMID: 39045301

36 Whole wheat flour replaced by sprouted wheat improves phenolic compounds profile, rheological and bread-making properties. Cauduro T, et al. Journal of Cereal Science. Volume 114, November 2023, 103778. https://doi.org/10.1016/j.jcs.2023.103778

37 https://www.theguardian.com/us-news/2019/may/28/bread-additives-chemicals-us-toxic-america

38 Rice: Importance for Global Nutrition. Fukagawa NK, Ziska LH. J Nutr Sci Vitaminol (Tokyo). 2019;65(Supplement):S2-S3. doi: 10.3177/jnsv.65.S2. PMID: 31619630

39 Changes in volatile aroma compounds of organic fragrant rice during storage under different conditions. Tananuwong K, Lertsiri S. J Sci of Food Ag. 18 June 2010 https://doi.org/10.1002/jsfa.3976

40 Identification of cadmium bioaccumulation in rice (Oryza sativa L.) by the soil-plant transfer model and species sensitivity distribution. Li K, Cao C, Ma Y, SuD, LiJ. Science of The Total Environment. 692 (1022-1028) 11-2019. https://doi.org/10.1016/j.scitotenv.2019.07.091

41 The relation between rice consumption, arsenic contamination, and prevalence of diabetes in South Asia. Hassan FI, Niaz K, Khan F, Maqbool F, Abdollahi M. EXCLI J. 2017 Oct 9;16:1132-1143. doi: 10.17179/excli2017-222. eCollection 2017. PMID: 29285009

42 Arsenic in brown rice: do the benefits outweigh the risks? Su LJ, Chiang TC, O'Connor SN. Front Nutr. 2023 Jul 14;10:1209574. doi: 10.3389/fnut.2023.1209574. eCollection 2023. PMID: 37521417

43 Arsenic in rice: II. Arsenic speciation in USA grain and implications for human health. Zavala YJ, Gerads R, Gorleyok H, Duxbury JM. Environ Sci Technol. 2008 May 15;42(10):3861-6. doi: 10.1021/es702748q. PMID: 18546735

44 Arsenic in rice: I. Estimating normal levels of total arsenic in rice grain. Zavala YJ, Duxbury JM. Environ Sci Technol. 2008 May 15;42(10):3856-60. doi: 10.1021/es702747y. PMID: 18546734

45 Cooking rice in a high water to rice ratio reduces inorganic arsenic content. Raab A, Baskaran C, Feldmann J, Meharg AA. J Environ Monit. 2009 Jan;11(1):41-4. doi: 10.1039/b816906c. Epub 2008 Nov 20. PMID: 19137137

46 How to reduce arsenic in rice, and why it matters. Devon Wagner, MS, RD https://health.osu.edu/wellness/exercise-and-nutrition/how-to-reduce-arsenic-in-rice

47 Should I worry about arsenic in my rice? - BBC News https://www.bbc.com/news/health-38910848

48 Effect of several germination conditions on total P, phytate P, phytase, and acid phosphatase activities and inositol phosphate esters in rye and barley. Centeno C,

Viveros A, Brenes A, Canales R, Lozano A, de la Cuadra C. J Agric Food Chem. 2001 Jul;49(7):3208-15. doi: 10.1021/jf010023c. PMID: 11453753

49 Effect of soaking and sprouting treatment on germination rate of paddy (rice). Chatchavanthatri N, et al. E3S Web of Conferences 187, 04016 (2020) https://doi.org/10.1051/e3sconf /202018704016

50 Gamma-aminobutyric acid (GABA): a comprehensive review of dietary sources, enrichment technologies, processing effects, health benefits, and its applications. Hou D, Tang J, Feng Q, Niu Z, Shen Q, Wang L, Zhou S. Crit Rev Food Sci Nutr. 2024;64(24):8852-8874. doi: 10.1080/10408398.2023.2204373. Epub 2023 Apr 25. PMID: 37096548

51 Advances and Perspectives of Gamma-Aminobutyric Acid as a Bioactive Compound in Food Jain, P., Ghodke, M.S. (2021).. In: Pal, D., Nayak, A.K. (eds) Bioactive Natural Products for Pharmaceutical Applications. Advanced Structured Materials, vol 140. Springer, Cham. https://doi.org/10.1007/978-3-030-54027-2_24

52 Gamma-aminobutyric acid (GABA): a comprehensive review of dietary sources, enrichment technologies, processing effects, health benefits, and its applications. Hou D, Tang J, Feng Q, Niu Z, Shen Q, Wang L, Zhou S. Crit Rev Food Sci Nutr. 2024;64(24):8852-8874. doi: 10.1080/10408398.2023.2204373. Epub 2023 Apr 25. PMID: 37096548

53 Isolation, characterization, and evaluation of anxiolytic bioactive compounds from the seed of Vigna radiata (L.) R. Wilczek in mice. Uppalwar SV, Garg V, Joshi S, Dutt R. Nat Prod Res. 2024 Feb-Mar;38(4):706-709. doi: 10.1080/14786419.2023.2189709. Epub 2023 Mar 17. PMID: 36929717

54 Screening of lactic acid bacteria strains isolated from Iranian traditional dairy products for GABA production and optimization by response surface methodology. Edalatian Dovom MR, Habibi Najafi MB, Rahnama Vosough P, Norouzi N, Ebadi Nezhad SJ, Mayo B. Sci Rep. 2023 Jan 9;13(1):440. doi: 10.1038/s41598-023-27658-5. PMID: 36624130

55 Production of γ-aminobutyric acid (GABA) by lactic acid bacteria strains isolated from traditional, starter-free dairy products made of raw milk. Valenzuela JA, Flórez AB, Vázquez L, Vasek OM, Mayo B. Benef Microbes. 2019 May 28;10(5):579-587. doi: 10.3920/BM2018.0176. Epub 2019 May 24. PMID: 31122043

56 Phenotypic, Technological, Safety, and Genomic Profiles of Gamma-Aminobutyric Acid-Producing *Lactococcus lactis* and *Streptococcus thermophilus* Strains Isolated from Cow's Milk. Valenzuela JA, Vázquez L, Rodríguez J, Flórez AB, Vasek OM, Mayo B. Int J Mol Sci. 2024 Feb 16;25(4):2328. doi: 10.3390/ijms25042328. PMID: 38397005

57 Optimization of a rice cooking method using response surface methodology with desirability function approach to minimize pesticide concentration. Medina MB, Resnik SL, Munitz MS. Food Chem. 2021 Aug 1;352:129364. doi: 10.1016/j.foodchem.2021.129364. Epub 2021 Feb 23. PMID: 33657482

58 Pre-soaking treatment can improve cooking quality of high-amylose rice while maintaining its low digestibility. Shen Y, He G, Gong W, Shu X, Wu D, Pellegrini N, Fogliano V. Food Funct. 2022 Nov 28;13(23):12182-12193. doi: 10.1039/d2fo02056d. PMID: 36326288

59 Effect of Presoaking on Textural, Thermal, and Digestive Properties of Cooked Brown Rice. Jung-Ah Han, Seung-Taik Lim. 86(1)100-105. Cereal Chemistry. Jan 19, 2009. https://doi.org/10.1094/CCHEM-86-1-0100

60 https://patents.google.com/patent/CN106561111A/en

61 https://patents.google.com/patent/CN104885621A/en

62 https://patents.google.com/patent/CN106508181A/en

63 Effect of soaking and sprouting treatment on germination rate of paddy (rice). Chatchavanthatri N, et al. E3S Web of Conferences 187, 04016 (2020) https://doi.org/10.1051/e3sconf /202018704016

64 Effect of Soaking Treatments and Temperature During Germination on Germinability and Rice (Oryza sativa L.) Seed Quality. El-Mowafy MR, Kishk MS. J. Plant Production, Mansoura Univ., Vol. 8 (4): 537 – 540. Ap. 2017. DOI: 10.21608/jpp.2017.40062

65 https://www.brenda-enzymes.org/literature.php?e=5.5.1.13&r=691386

66 https://www.brenda-enzymes.org/enzyme.php?ecno=4.2.3.19#TEMPERATURE%20OPTIMUM

67 https://www.brenda-enzymes.org/enzyme.php?ecno=1.14.14.86#TEMPERATURE%20OPTIMUM

68 Germination response of Oat (Avena sativa L.) to temperature and salinity using halothermal time model. Sulaiman., Sami, Ullah., Shah, Saud., Ke, Liu., Matthew, Tom, Harrison., Taufiq, Nawaz., Muhammad, Zeeshan., Jamal, Nasar., Imran, Khan., Muhammad, Adnan., Sunjeet, Kumar., Muhammad, Ishtiaq, Ali., Asif, Jamal., Mo, Zhu., Naushad, Ali., Khaled, M., El-Kahtany., Shah, Fahad. (2023). Plant Stress, doi: 10.1016/j.stress.2023.100263

69 Impact of temperature and humidity conditions as abiotic stressors on the phytochemical fingerprint of oat (Avena sativa L.) sprouts. Marely, G., Figueroa-Pérez., Rosalía, Reynoso-Camacho., Minerva, Ramos-Gomez., Magdalena, Mendoza-Sánchez., Iza, F., Pérez-Ramírez. (2023). Food Chemistry, 439:138173-138173. doi: 10.1016/j.foodchem.2023.138173

70 https://www.americastestkitchen.com/cooksillustrated/articles/315-perfect-boiled-corn

71 A KINETIC APPROACH TO SAPONIN EXTRACTION DURING WASHING OF QUINOA (*CHENOPODIUM QUINOA* WILLD.) SEEDS I QUISPE-FUENTES, A VEGA-GÁLVEZ, M Miranda, R LEMUS-MONDACA, M Lozano. Journal of Food Process Engineering, 2013

[72] Cardinal temperatures for seed germination of three Quinoa (Chenopodium quinoa Willd.) cultivars Mamedi A, Tavakkol Afshari R, Oveisi M. Iranian Journal of Field Crop Science. Special Issue 2017 (89-100) DOI: 10.22059/ijfcs.2017.206204.654106

[73] Effects of different soaking and germinating conditions on γ-aminobutyric acid, antioxidant activity, and chemical composition of djulis (Chenopodium formosanum). Wen-Chien Lu, Yu-Tsung Cheng, Yung-Jia Chan, Jin Yan, Po-Hsien Li, Journal of Agriculture and Food Research. 17,101162, 2024. https://www.sciencedirect.com/science/article/pii/S2666154324001996

[74] Box-Behnken Design: Wet Process Optimization for Saponins Removal From *Chenopodium quinoa* Seeds and the Study of Its Effect on Nutritional Properties. El Hazzam K, Mhada M, Metougui ML, El Kacimi K, Sobeh M, Taourirte M, Yasri A. Front Nutr. 2022 Jul 1;9:906592. doi: 10.3389/fnut.2022.906592. eCollection 2022. PMID: 35845775

[75] Germination in Optimal Conditions as Effective Strategy to Improve Nutritional and Nutraceutical Value of Underutilized Mexican Blue Maize Seeds. Chavarín-Martínez CD, Gutiérrez-Dorado R, Perales-Sánchez JXK, Cuevas-Rodríguez EO, Milán-Carrillo J, Reyes-Moreno C. Plant Foods Hum Nutr. 2019 Jun;74(2):192-199. doi: 10.1007/s11130-019-00717-x. PMID: 30737612

[76] Improvement of Chia Seeds with Antioxidant Activity, GABA, Essential Amino Acids, and Dietary Fiber by Controlled Germination Bioprocess. Gómez-Favela MA, Gutiérrez-Dorado R, Cuevas-Rodríguez EO, Canizalez-Román VA, Del Rosario León-Sicairos C, Milán-Carrillo J, Reyes-Moreno C. Plant Foods Hum Nutr. 2017 Dec;72(4):345-352. doi: 10.1007/s11130-017-0631-4. PMID: 28900797

[77] Increasing the antioxidant activity, total phenolic and flavonoid contents by optimizing the germination conditions of amaranth seeds. Perales-Sánchez JX, Reyes-Moreno C, Gómez-Favela MA, Milán-Carrillo J, Cuevas-Rodríguez EO, Valdez-Ortiz A, Gutiérrez-Dorado R. Plant Foods Hum Nutr. 2014 Sep;69(3):196-202. doi: 10.1007/s11130-014-0430-0. PMID: 24958279

[78] Optimization of Germination Conditions for Enriched γ-Aminobutyric Acid and Phenolic Compounds of Foxtail Millet Sprouts by Response Surface Methodology. Yu S, Li C, Wang X, Herrera-Balandrano DD, Johnson JB, Xiang J. Foods. 2024 Oct 21;13(20):3340. doi: 10.3390/foods13203340. PMID: 39456402

[79] Sucrose-induced abiotic stress improves the phytochemical profiles and bioactivities of mung bean sprouts. Yu J, Lee H, Heo H, Jeong HS, Sung J, Lee J. Food Chem. 2023 Jan 30;400:134069. doi: 10.1016/j.foodchem.2022.134069. Epub 2022 Sep 1. PMID: 36108445

[80] Role of guar fiber in improving digestive health and function. Rao TP, Quartarone G. Nutrition. 2019 Mar;59:158-169. doi: 10.1016/j.nut.2018.07.109. Epub 2018 Aug 23. PMID: 30496956

[81] Role of guar fiber in appetite control. Rao TP. Physiol Behav. 2016 Oct 1;164(Pt A):277-83. doi: 10.1016/j.physbeh.2016.06.014. Epub 2016 Jun 15. PMID: 27317834

[82] Prebiotic Effects of Partially Hydrolyzed Guar Gum on the Composition and Function of the Human Microbiota-Results from the PAGODA Trial. Reider SJ, Moosmang S, Tragust J, Trgovec-Greif L, Tragust S, Perschy L, Przysiecki N, Sturm S, Tilg H, Stuppner H, Rattei T, Moschen AR. Nutrients. 2020 Apr 28;12(5):1257. doi: 10.3390/nu12051257. PMID: 32354152

[83] Effect of Repeated Consumption of Partially Hydrolyzed Guar Gum on Fecal Characteristics and Gut Microbiota: A Randomized, Double-Blind, Placebo-Controlled, and Parallel-Group Clinical Trial. Yasukawa Z, Inoue R, Ozeki M, Okubo T, Takagi T, Honda A, Naito Y. Nutrients. 2019 Sep 10;11(9):2170. doi: 10.3390/nu11092170. PMID: 31509971

[84] Partially hydrolyzed guar gum enhances colonic epithelial wound healing via activation of RhoA and ERK1/2. Horii Y, Uchiyama K, Toyokawa Y, Hotta Y, Tanaka M, Yasukawa Z, Tokunaga M, Okubo T, Mizushima K, Higashimura Y, Dohi O, Okayama T, Yoshida N, Katada K, Kamada K, Handa O, Ishikawa T, Takagi T, Konishi H, Naito Y, Itoh Y. Food Funct. 2016 Jul 13;7(7):3176-83. doi: 10.1039/c6fo00177g. PMID: 27305660

[85] Partially hydrolysed guar gum ameliorates murine intestinal inflammation in association with modulating luminal microbiota and SCFA. Takagi T, Naito Y, Higashimura Y, Ushiroda C, Mizushima K, Ohashi Y, Yasukawa Z, Ozeki M, Tokunaga M, Okubo T, Katada K, Kamada K, Uchiyama K, Handa O, Itoh Y, Yoshikawa T. Br J Nutr. 2016 Oct;116(7):1199-1205. doi: 10.1017/S0007114516003068. Epub 2016 Sep 8. PMID: 27604176

[86] Food Additive Guar Gum Aggravates Colonic Inflammation in Experimental Models of Inflammatory Bowel Disease. Nair DVT, Paudel D, Prakash D, Singh V. Curr Dev Nutr. 2021 Jun 7;5(Suppl 2):1142. doi: 10.1093/cdn/nzab061_026. PMCID: PMC8180737.

[87] Randomised clinical trial: dried plums (prunes) vs. psyllium for constipation. Attaluri A, Donahoe R, Valestin J, Brown K, Rao SS. Aliment Pharmacol Ther. 2011 Apr;33(7):822-8. doi: 10.1111/j.1365-2036.2011.04594.x. Epub 2011 Feb 15. PMID: 21323688

[88] Dried plums, constipation and the irritable bowel syndrome. Halmos EP, Gibson PR. Aliment Pharmacol Ther. 2011 Aug;34(3):396-7; author reply 397-8. doi: 10.1111/j.1365-2036.2011.04719.x. PMID: 21726250

[89] Exploratory Comparative Effectiveness Trial of Green Kiwifruit, Psyllium, or Prunes in US Patients With Chronic Constipation. Chey SW, Chey WD, Jackson K, Eswaran S. Am J Gastroenterol. 2021 Jun 1;116(6):1304-1312. doi: 10.14309/ajg.0000000000001149. PMID: 34074830

[90] Kiwifruit and Kiwifruit Extracts for Treatment of Constipation: A Systematic Review and Meta-Analysis. Eltorki M, Leong R, Ratcliffe EM. Can J Gastroenterol

Hepatol. 2022 Oct 6;2022:7596920. doi: 10.1155/2022/7596920. eCollection 2022. PMID: 36247043

91 The Dynamic Conversion of Dietary Protein and Amino Acids into Chicken-Meat Protein. Macelline SP, Chrystal PV, Liu SY, Selle PH. Animals (Basel). 2021 Aug 3;11(8):2288. doi: 10.3390/ani11082288. PMID: 34438749

92 Digestion rate of dietary starch affects systemic circulation of amino acids in weaned pigs. Yin F, Zhang Z, Huang J, Yin Y. Br J Nutr. 2010 May;103(10):1404-12. doi: 10.1017/S0007114509993321. PMID: 20102672

93 Impact of germination pre-treatments on buckwheat and Quinoa: Mitigation of anti-nutrient content and enhancement of antioxidant properties. Altıkardeş E, Güzel N. Food Chem X. 2024 Feb 5;21:101182. doi: 10.1016/j.fochx.2024.101182. PMID: 38357368

10: Sugar

The Short and Sweet

Perhaps surprisingly, some sugar is allowed on the SANA diet *if it is not restricted for other reasons, such as diabetes.* Sugar gets a DAD score of zero. This means it has little impact on the enteric biome, as long as the amount in the diet is limited and it is normally absorbed.

Added sugars are empty calories that displace nutritious food. More importantly, spikes in the blood sugar cause the formation of advanced glycation end-products (AGEs) that cause oxidative stress and tissue damage. Hyperglycemia and spikes in blood sugar, even in normal adults and children without diabetes, promote fatty liver disease and insulin resistance. Sugar is not a toxic compound; however, large doses of sugar should be considered toxic. The poison is in the dose.

The SANA diet limits the amount of *added sugars* to a maximum of *10% of ideal caloric intake* based on the caloric demand for maintaining the person's ideal body weight. That is not a recommendation or goal, but rather a very liberal cap to make life more pleasant and allow participation in social situations where foods with sugar are served. Thus, for example, if a person's ideal caloric intake is 2000 kcal per day, the added sugar limit would be 50 grams of sugar, equivalent to 200 calories or 11.9 level measuring teaspoons of sugar per day.

There are limitations on how the sugar budget is spent.

- ❖ Added sugar should be almost entirely limited to use in solid foods.
- No more than half of the daily added sugar budget should be consumed within a three-hour period.
- Sugar-sweetened beverages (soda pop, cool-aide, lemonade, sweet tea, etc.) are prohibited from the diet. This includes fruit-flavored drinks.
- Indulgence: Since coffee consumption is encouraged on the SANA diet, one cup of coffee per day can be sweetened with up to 6 grams of sugar, a very slightly rounded measuring teaspoonful. The utility of sugar in coffee is not to create a sweet beverage, but rather to use just enough to mask most of the bitterness.
- ❖ The *added sugar* in jams and jellies and other prepared foods is counted as sugar.
- ❖ Calories from honey, molasses, maple syrup, sweet fruit concentrates, and similar concentrated sweet items are counted as *added sugars.*
- ❖ Any *added sugar* in fruit juice should be counted as sugar. The sugar in 100% fruit juice does not need to be counted; nevertheless, fruit juice should be limited to 4 ounces per day.
- ❖ Dried fruit sugar calories are counted as one-third calories within the sugar budget.
- Whole fruits are not counted as part of the sugar budget.
- Xylitol, Erythritol, and artificial sweeteners get a DAD rating of D ( ) and are prohibited on the SANA diet.
- Creative cheating to get around the sugar budget will not help.

There are no "roll-over" benefits from one day to another.

Sugar and Sweets

Caries

While table sugar gets a DAD score of zero for the enteric microbiome, this is not the case for the *oral* microbiome. Sucrose is a favorite food of *Streptococcus mutans*, the bacteria central to causing dental caries. These bacteria form dental plaque, a sticky biofilm, that sticks to the teeth. When supplied with a variety of sugars, including sucrose, glucose, fructose, lactose, galactose, and sorbitol, *S. mutans* produces lactic acid, which demineralizes the teeth, causing dental caries.[1] Sucrose is more cariogenic than fructose and glucose.[2] Honey is mostly glucose and fructose, and is less cariogenic than sucrose.

Soda pop, even sugar-free soda, causes dental caries as it is acidic. Sodas are especially harmful to the teeth when they are sipped over an extended period, and each sip "refreshes" the oral cavity with an acid bath. Hyperglycemia also provokes dental caries by decreasing salivary flow in the mouth and thus promotes demineralization of the teeth.[3] Sugar-sweetened beverages, whether the sugar is sucrose, high fructose corn syrup, or maple syrup, all promote dental caries.

As discussed elsewhere, sucrose is a disaccharide that is enzymatically cleaved into its component sugars (50% fructose, 50% glucose) during digestion. High fructose corn syrup used in soft drinks is typically HFCS-55, which is 55% fructose and 45% glucose. Glucose and fructose are readily absorbed by the small intestine into the body. Thus, it is unusual for sucrose to get to the lower intestine and ferment, thus providing a DAD score of zero under normal situations. This does not mean it is innocuous. As a rule, the less sugar added to the diet, the better.

The SANA diet allows some added sugar in the diet, not as a recommendation, but rather as a dispensation, which is not expected to cause significant harm to an otherwise healthy diet, when it is incorporated into other solid foods. Accommodating some sugar in the diet makes the diet less restrictive and makes life easier and more pleasant, as it broadens the scope of foods permitted on the diet. Paraphrasing Christ's observation, "The Sabbath was made for man, and not man for the Sabbath", the SANA diet is made for the benefit of people...

Sugar represents empty calories that displace nutritious foods that would otherwise be eaten. If one is consuming 20 percent of their daily calories as added refined sugars, it means that they are consuming 20% less fiber and 20% lower amounts of vitamins, minerals, and other nutrients, such as phenolic compounds, than they would have if they were eating whole foods. The appetite for sweets may be an evolutionarily adaptive drive to seek fruits that supply antioxidants and vitamins. Consuming sugar betrays this mechanism, replacing a drive to derive benefits with one that provokes harm.

Sugar is risky! Diets high in sugar are pro-inflammatory, raising the levels of C-reactive protein, and inflammatory cytokines such as IL-1β and tumor necrosis factor (TNF), which are associated with chronic diseases of aging (T2D, atherosclerosis, dyslipidemia, cancer, and cognitive impairments.[4] [5]

However, to clarify, it is not the sugar, but rather the hyperglycemia and hyperfructosemia that sugars can cause that create pro-inflammatory and injurious metabolic products such as methylglyoxal (MGO). MGO is a reactive compound that is a key precursor to advanced glycation end products (AGEs) (Chapter 16).

Essential Point: The same amount of sugar consumed daily may have little or no negative impact on health or a great deal of negative impact, depending upon how it is consumed. If 200 calories of sugar, 50 grams or 12 level teaspoons of sugar, are consumed on an empty stomach as a 16-ounce serving of soda pop, it will cause a large spike in the blood sugar and wreak havoc, as the body struggles to dispose of the excess fructose and glucose. This increases the formation of AGEs that do nasty things, such as promoting atherosclerosis, and increasing the toxicity of A*β* and α-synuclein fragments; thus promoting the progression of Alzheimer's disease (AD) and Parkinson's disease (PD) respectively.[6] While both fasting and postprandial hyperglycemia are harmful, it appears that a high peak in blood sugar after a meal has a greater impact on promoting disease than does elevated fasting hyperglycemia.[7] [8] Post-prandial hyperglycemia is associated with increased risk of cardiovascular disease even in those without diabetes or fasting hyperglycemia.[9]

Maxims:

1. The maximum daily added sugar allotment is 10% of a person's daily caloric needs required to *maintain their ideal body weight*, for their age and activity level. This amount of sugar, when consumed in <u>*solid foods,*</u> does not increase all-cause mortality. In contrast, added sugar increases mortality risk linearly when consumed as liquid.[10] The more sugar-sweetened beverages consumed, the higher the excess death rate.
2. No more than half of the budget should be consumed within a three-hour period.
3. Soda pop, Cool-Aid, lemonade, Hi-C, sweet tea, and similarly sweet beverages are not allowed on the SANA diet.

Ideal Adult Body Weight Formula:
Male: 50.0 kg + 2.3 kg per inch over 5 feet
Female: 45.5 kg + 2.3 kg per inch over 5 feet
An ideal body weight calculator can be found at: https://www.calculator.net/ideal-weight-calculator.html
Then, using that weight, a calorie calculator for maintaining the ideal body weight can be found at: https://www.calculator.net/calorie-calculator.html.

A healthy woman who needs to consume 1800 calories per day to maintain her ideal body weight would thus have a maximum total sugar allowance of 180 calories. That is equivalent to 45 grams or 11 level teaspoons of sugar. If weight loss is a goal, skimp on added sugars. And this is for you, my sweet-toothed sister; honey, maple syrup, and other concentrated sweet fruit baked into a treat need to be counted as part of the sugar budget.

To be clear, there is no dietary requirement for added sugar, and the SANA diet does not promote it as a healthy addition to the diet. Rather, the insignificant impact of restricted amounts of sugar in an otherwise healthy diet is insufficient to deny it to most of the population. Spare sugar not used on a given day does not roll over to the next day. However, if you inadvertently overconsume, you need to pay down the overdraft you created as quickly as possible.

Hyperglycemia increases intestinal permeability.[11] Elevated blood sugar can occur with high glycemic index meals, such as those composed of easily digestible carbohydrates and sugars. Protein and dietary fiber slow digestion and prevent high peaks of blood sugar after meals.

Fructose appears to be more disruptive to the intestinal mucosal integrity than glucose. When mice were fed a Western-style diet, they had weight gain, but there was no increase in endotoxin (LPS) translocation across the mucosal barrier, as compared to the regular mouse diet. The addition of fructose to the drinking water increased LPS translocation 2.6-fold for animals on the regular diet and 3.8-fold for those on the Western-style diet. The western diet with fructose caused a 46% reduction in the depth of the mucous layer in the colon.[12] A high-fructose corn syrup-sweetened soda pop delivers a large, quickly absorbable bolus of fructose to the bloodstream. A balanced diet of real food should help maintain intestinal mucosal barrier integrity.

A meta-analysis including 12 studies and over 35,000 subjects found that consumption of a single 5 to 7-ounce serving of a sugar-sweetened beverage (150–200 mL, such as soda pop; about 22 grams of sugar) *per week* increases the risk of non-alcoholic fatty liver disease (NAFLD) by 14%. Consumption of between 200 and 1000 ml of sugar-sweetened beverages per week increased the risk of NAFLD by more than a quarter, and consuming one or more sugar-sweetened beverages a day (or more than 1 liter per week) increased the risk of NAFLD by 53% as compared to those consuming one less than once a month.[13] NAFLD is associated with insulin resistance and obesity. These sugar-sweetened beverages should be considered toxic; they have no place in a healthy diet.

A 20-ounce soda has a similar amount of fructose as five bananas. When was the last time you washed a meal down with 5 bananas? Additionally, whole fruits contain carbohydrates and fiber that slow digestion, limiting large spikes in blood-fructose and blood-glucose levels, as occurs with sugar dissolved in water. Sugars dissolved in water are rapidly absorbed, greatly increasing the blood glucose and blood fructose levels. Fiber from the fruit also feeds the microbiome and staves off hunger, and supplies antioxidant compounds, whereas fructose-laden sodas do not. Sipping on soda pop as you go about your day rots the teeth.

In contrast if those same 12 levels teaspoons present in a cola are distributed between meals; a teaspoon in a cup of coffee with breakfast and another as the added sugar in some blackberry jam; some in an oatmeal cookie with lunch, and some more as added sugar in a small serving of ice cream as dessert, the impact of sugar may be negligible (for non-diabetics). When consumed with a meal, the slow release of the food creates a smaller rise in blood sugar.

In studies assessing the "Dietary Inflammatory Indices" of various foods, the high inflammatory index score of sugar has often been limited to sugar-sweetened beverages.[14] The calories consumed from sugar-sweetened beverages are typically calories that are added to a meal beyond those that the consumer would otherwise consume during a meal to satisfy their appetite. Thus, the calories in the soda do not displace other calories; they are added calories that raise the blood sugar spike height and duration, and cause excess insulin release and weight gain. Moreover, the excess fructose favors the deposition of fat in comparison to calories from protein or starches, which are converted to glucose during digestion.

Sweet beverages (such as soda pop, cool-aide, and lemon-aide) are not allowed on the SANA diet.

Whole fruit does not count against the daily sugar allotment, in part because people generally do not overindulge. A 3-inch diameter apple contains around 19 grams of sugar. A medium banana contains about 14 grams of sugar. Two cups of watermelon contain about 18 grams of sugar.

In contrast, apple juice has a similar amount of sugar as soda pop. Apple juice, especially processed apple juice that has had the pectin and starch removed, is not recommended on the diet. It is too easy to consume a large bolus of sugar-laden water in the form of juice in just a few seconds, and keep in mind that apples do not get a great DAD score.

Fruit Juice

Nevertheless, while the human population studies and animal experimental data clearly condemn sugar-sweetened beverages, it is far less clear that 100% fruit juice is harmful. Drinking large volumes of apple juice increases uric acid levels,[15] which is associated with metabolic syndrome, but meta-analyses do not show an increased risk of T2D with the consumption of 100% fruit juices. They do, however, show an increased risk of T2D with the consumption of *fruit beverages with added sugar*.[16] The *added sugar* (listed in the product's Nutrition Facts label) in fruit beverages also counts against the daily sugar budget.

Large servings of fruit juice are discouraged on the SANA diet. Firstly, as a general rule, the serving of fruit juice should not be larger than the amount of juice that would be made from a typical serving of the fruit, and secondly, it is generally healthier to eat the fruit and get the fiber. Try to keep the serving size of fruit juice to 4 ounces. Water and unsweetened tea are healthier methods of hydration.

As stated above, no more than half of the daily added sugar budget should be consumed within a three-hour period. For an adult with a 50-gram daily budget, that limits the amount in a meal to 25 grams of *added sugar*.

A slice of apple pie contains about 15 grams of added sugar, and a slice of commercial pumpkin pie contains about 25 grams of added sugar. A 4-ounce serving of ice cream contains about 17 grams of sugar. Thus, the combination of a slice of pie with plain Greek yogurt would be permitted on the SANA diet for a non-diabetic, but putting pie with ice cream would be over the top. A slice of chocolate cake with icing contains about 44 grams of sugar, which would be too much sugar to be eaten at one time, and is not allowed on the SANA diet. Sugar in jam and fruit preserves gets counted as part of the sugar budget.

Soda Pop, Cool-Aide, Lemonade, Sweet Tea, etc.

The most successful weight loss diets are those that eliminate sugar-sweetened beverages such as soda pop. High consumption of sugar-sweetened beverages increases the risk and severity of obesity, type 2 diabetes, hypertension, inflammatory bowel disease, and cardiovascular disease.

Table 10A: Sugar Content in Various Beverages

Beverage	Volume in ounces	Sugar in Teaspoons	Sugar in Grams
Coca Cola	10	8	34
Root Beer	10	9	38
Mountain Dew	10	9	38
Sweetened Iced Tea	8	6	25
Swiss Mix Hot Chocolate	8 oz pack	5	21
Commercial Lemonade	8	7	29
Kool-Ade	8	6	25
Juice box	6.5	5	21

Mice consuming a high-fat diet become overweight and have mild intestinal inflammation. Mice consuming a high-fat diet and given access to sugar water develop a dramatic increase in gut inflammation and submucosa swelling. Their intestinal microbiome shifts to be dominated by pathogenic bacteria similar to those observed in inflammatory bowel disease (IBD).[17] Soft drink consumption indeed is associated with about a 50% greater risk of IBD.

A DAD rating is not provided for soda pop. They are mostly sugar (sucrose, or glucose/fructose) and water. Water is not a problem. Sugar gets a rating of zero on the DAD scale. It is the high-level consumption and peaks in glucose and fructose blood levels that cause disease.

Table 10B: Sugar scores

Added Sugars	DAD Score
Molasses (unsulfured)	2
Brown sugar	1
Glucose	1
Allulose	1
Maltitol	1
Sucrose (Table sugar)	0
Honey	0
Saccharine	0
Erythritol	D
Xylitol	D
Stevia	D
Sucralose (Splenda)	D
Most Artificial Sweeteners	D

Molasses is a byproduct in the manufacture of sugar, which can be made from sugar cane, sugar beets, or other plants. It provides iron and a lesser amount of other minerals, as well as some vitamin B6. Molasses has a lower glycemic index, promotes less desire to eat, promotes a better sense of fullness, and gives a better metabolic response than sugar. It increases antioxidant capacity and provides fuel for the GI microbiome.[18] Cane sugar molasses contains the phenolic compounds caffeic acid, ferulic acid, and chlorogenic acid.[19] Molasses is used as much as a flavoring agent as a sweetener.

Brown sugar is made by adding some molasses back to refined sucrose, making it resemble raw sugar. Dark brown sugar has more molasses added back than does light brown sugar. Brown sugar gets a DAD score of 1 as a result of its molasses content; nevertheless, brown sugar is mostly sugar and needs to be counted as added sugar. Remember, a DAD score is an assessment of the impact of the food on GI health and inflammation, not on the food's overall nutritional value. It cannot capture the impact of the over-consumption of a food.

Honey can be counted as about 80% sugar as a result of its water content. Occasional use of honey should be fine; however, honey has a proinflammatory effect,[20] and thus should not be used as a primary substitute for sugar. Although a natural food, honey is not a healthier form of sugar.

Honey, corn syrup, and other natural sweeteners can contain the spores of *Clostridium botulinum.* Infants under one year of age should not be given foods made with honey or other such sweeteners, as the spores can colonize and replicate in the large intestine and cause infantile botulism. This can manifest as a "floppy baby" that has muscular weakness, which can result in the infant's death if not promptly recognized and treated correctly.[21]

Sugar Alcohols

Sorbitol, xylitol, and erythritol are natural sugar alcohols. These are poorly absorbed and, if consumed in high amounts, for example, as a replacement for sugar in a sweet food or beverage, often reach the lower intestine where they ferment. This can cause gas, bloating, abdominal distention, pain, borborygmi, diarrhea, and flare-ups of IBS symptoms. This, of course, is discouraged.

Sorbitol is present in many fruits, notably prunes and other stone fruit, pears, apples, coconut, aloe, and cabbage. It is used in some "diabetic" or "sugar-free" treats and gum, and may be listed as glucitol or D-glucitol on the label. Prunes are an old-time remedy for constipation, as they contain sorbitol (and other fiber). The sorbitol has an osmotic effect, which draws water into the colon. Added sorbitol is not recommended as a sugar replacement. Prunes and prune juice are not a first-choice remedy for constipation.

Erythritol

Erythritol is a very low-calorie sugar alcohol that is sold as a "natural sweetener", as it occurs, in tiny amounts, in some fruits, such as grapes, melons, and pears. While it is a natural sugar, the most erythritol one might find in a serving of fruit is less than 10 mg. To put this into perspective, a medium-sized pear, a fruit high in erythritol, contains about 17,000 mg of sugar.

Erythritol is promoted as a low or zero-calorie sweetener. Erythritol is about 60-80% as sweet as sugar. Thus, to get the equivalent sweetness of one teaspoon (5 grams) of sucrose requires about 7 grams. Even when using twice the amount of erythritol as sugar in coffee, it fails to mask coffee's bitterness.

Erythritol gets a rating of D on the DAD scale. In longitudinal studies in three different populations, erythritol has been associated with increased risk of coronary heart disease (CHD). The largest study, which included both an American and a European population, found a hazard ratio of 2.64-fold increased risk of death, non-fatal myocardial infarction, or stroke for those in the highest quartile of plasma erythritol levels. When mechanistic studies were performed using concentrations of erythritol that are sustained in the bloodstream after an amount that would be consumed in an erythritol-sweetened beverage, it caused increased platelet activation in human blood and accelerated clotting in mouse carotid arteries.[22], [23] Thus, erythritol appears to be thrombogenic. Platelet activation is thought to cause micro-emboli in the cerebral circulation; thus, erythritol may be a risk factor for dementia.

It is noteworthy that in one study, those with lower renal function had higher erythritol levels; this was not adjusted for in the data analysis, thus possibly biasing the results. It is possible that, rather than being causal, plasma erythritol is a marker of dysregulation of the Pentose Phosphate Pathway caused by impaired glycemia, rather than a direct causal factor.[24] Thus, more research is needed to clarify the risk. Until then, it gets a rating of D.

Xylitol

Xylitol is also rated a D. It is a sugar substitute loved by dentists as it starves *Streptococcus. mutans*, and thus can prevent dental caries, by starving cariogenic bacteria. It, by the way, can cause hypoglycemic comas in dogs even at a low dose. One piece of xylitol gum can kill a small dog.

Many dentists promote xylitol as a magic bullet that *selectively* targets *Streptococcus mutans* and other periodontopathogens, while preserving beneficial oral bacteria. While xylitol can reduce the oral biofilm that forms plaque, it is not selective in its killing. It also kills *Streptococcus mitis and S. sanguinis*, commensal bacteria that protect the teeth from dental caries. If one starts with a healthy oral microbiome and rarely gets dental caries, using xylitol may make things worse, increasing the risk of caries and other dental diseases.

Chronic chewing of xylitol gum reduces plaque by about a third. Much of the beneficial effects of xylitol gum on plaque, however, may just result from the chewing, which increases the flow of saliva, flushing bacteria and food particles from the mouth.[25], [26] A meta-analysis found that xylitol mints had no anti-caries effect.[27] Evidence that xylitol gum reduces gingival inflammation is very weak.[28] [29] [30] The dose of xylitol that is recommended for dental caries prevention is 6 to 10 grams per day, which can be 20 pieces of xylitol gum. That amount of xylitol often causes constipation.

The same research team that evaluated erythritol as a risk factor for vascular disease found similar risks in longitudinal studies and in vitro testing of the effects of xylitol as they did for erythritol, however, the hazard ratio for xylitol for those in the top third for plasma levels of xylitol was somewhat lower, at 1.57, or a 57% increase risk of death or major vascular event.[31] While not as strong a risk as erythritol is for heart disease, it is still a strong risk factor.

Xylitol doesn't stop working in the mouth; it indiscriminately kills commensal bacteria in the gut. Use of erythritol and xylitol as sweeteners is proscribed from the SANA diet. They should not be used as sugar substitutes. Table sugar is a healthier choice.

Artificial Sweeteners

Both long-term and short-term use of non-caloric artificial sweeteners induce intestinal dysbiosis and glucose intolerance in healthy human subjects.[32] [33] Saccharin and sucralose, as well as the plant-derived sweetener stevia, have been found to disrupt the intestinal microbiome.[34] This is not limited to the colon; non-nutritive sweeteners altered the microbiome of the small intestine as well, increasing levels of potentially pathogenic bacteria and risk of small intestinal bacterial overgrowth (SIBO).[35]

In women, they increase the risk of ectopic pregnancy and placenta previa in pregnancy.[36] Maternal ingestion of non-nutritive sweeteners (sucralose, acesulfame-K) by mice, at human-relevant doses during lactation, causes alteration in the gastrointestinal microbiome of the pups similar to that found in metabolic syndrome and obesity, and suppressed hepatic detoxification mechanisms.[37] One-year-old infants of mothers who consumed artificially sweetened beverages daily during pregnancy were more than twice as likely to be overweight.[38]

While the use of the artificial sweetener aspartame may decrease caloric intake, adding aspartame to a high-fat diet actually promotes glucose intolerance, weight gain, and inflammatory markers in mice. Aspartame inhibits intestinal alkaline phosphatase (IAP) activity, thus increasing the risk of leaky gut.[39] In a follow-up study including over 100,000 people for 9 years, the use of artificial sweeteners was found to be associated with increased risk of cardiovascular events and strokes. Sucralose and acesulfame K were associated with a 32 percent and 40 percent increased risk of heart attacks, respectively. Aspartame intake was associated with a 17% increased risk of stroke.[40] Use of aspartame or acesulfame-K was associated with increased risk of cancer, particularly breast cancer.[41] Sucralose, aspartame, and acesulfame-K were associated with a 34%, 63%, and 70% increased risk, respectively, of developing type 2 diabetes over the 9 years of the study.[42]

You can't outsmart Mother Nature. When we eat something sweet, it induces the release of insulin in preparation for the rise in blood glucose. This is a neurologically mediated response. This appears to result from the activation of sweet-taste receptors in the duodenum, which induce parasympathetic activation of the vagus nerve that increases pancreatic insulin secretion. This surge of insulin has no work to do if the sweet food or beverage does not raise blood sugar. Inappropriately high insulin levels are atherosclerotic. Artificial sweeteners increase insulin resistance and thereby increase inflammation.[43] Thus, the problems with artificial sweeteners may be inherent in them.

The SANA diet strongly recommends avoiding most artificial and non-nutritive sweeteners. This includes the use of stevia and monk fruit. Saccharine appears to be less offensive than most other artificial sweeteners and thus appears to be the least noxious among the artificial sweeteners for those with diabetes.

Allulose and Maltitol: Allulose is a synthetically produced, but naturally occurring, isomer of fructose that is used as a sugar substitute. Maltitol is produced from maltose, derived from starch. Allulose does not raise insulin levels, and maltitol similarly has a low impact on blood sugars. Neither promotes tooth decay nor periodontal disease.[44] [45] They are not absorbed but are rather fermented by intestinal bacteria. Excessive intake of allulose or maltitol (more than about half a gram per kg of body mass per day) can cause flatulence, abdominal discomfort, and diarrhea.[46] Maltitol can even be used as a laxative. At low levels, both have some prebiotic effect.

Allulose and maltitol are about 70% as sweet as sugar. The maximum daily tolerable intake of these sugars for a 60 kg adult would be about 30 grams, thus equivalent to the sweetening of 21 grams or 5 teaspoons of sugar.

Limited amounts of allulose and maltitol appear to be safe to use as sweeteners, and thus, limited amounts are permitted on the SANA diet.

Thus, for diabetics, especially insulin-dependent diabetics, the use of allulose, maltitol, and saccharine appears to be a reasonable means for broadening food choices while avoiding sugar. The amounts of sweet foods consumed, however, still need to be restricted, preferably to about 30 grams of allulose and/or maltitol daily, and occasional use of a small amount of saccharine.

Allulose and maltitol are likely less cariogenic than sucrose. Thus, another use case for them may be for use in in-between-meal snacks to avoid the development of dental plaque.

Sweet-tooth Disorder

A sweet tooth, frequent craving for sweets, is often a sign of increased ghrelin levels. Ghrelin is a hunger hormone. This may be the result of a diet with a high glycemic index and low in soluble fiber. This type of diet promotes insulin overshoot and has deficient butyrate production in the colon, and thus promotes hunger between meals. Sugar gives a fast boost in blood sugar, which feels good and is addictive, but is bad for health. The remedy is to eat better and avoid refined carbohydrates so that one meal carries through to the next. Getting adequate protein in the diet should also help, as it is digested more slowly and releases energy more evenly between meals.

Stress can cause a fall in serotonin, which also increases sugar seeking. Sleep deprivation is another cause, as the sugar gives a short-term surge of energy that helps overcome fatigue.

FGF21 is a hormonal growth factor produced in the liver that regulates the preference for sweet foods and alcohol. Some people have a genetic variant that causes an increased desire for sweets. Type 2 diabetics often have FGF21 resistance; they make more of it, but the receptors for it become desensitized. The central role of FGF21 is to decrease hunger (especially for sweets), decrease lipolysis (the conversion of fat to energy), and increase glucose uptake into fat cells.[47]

Finally, sweets are simply addictive.

The treatment for a sweet tooth is to undo the causes. Take the time to eat real meals, especially breakfast, and don't skip meals. (See Chapter 28 on time-restricted eating). This may mean going to bed and getting up earlier. Get plenty of sleep. Sufficient soluble fiber and protein in the diet are needed for health. These two steps should help with stress, but dealing with stressors is also recommended.

If one has a craving for sweets, get a glass of water, do a bit of exercise, walk around, and get the blood flowing. It may just be a bit of boredom. Then have a healthy snack, some walnuts, slices of cucumber, or maybe a tangerine.[48]

FGF21 expression may be increased through activation of AMPK, SIRT1, and PGC-1α.[49] (See Chapters 19 - 21, adaptations). Thus, fruits and other foods with polyphenols such as quercetin (onions and berries, tea), fisetin (grapes, onions, kiwi, kale), resveratrol (dark grapes), formononetin (in beans, cauliflower), and naringenin (tangerines) may increase FGF21 and help with sugar cravings. Melatonin, produced during sleep, also increases SIRT1.[50], [51], [52]

Adherence to the SANA program, eating 3 real meals a day, getting the recommended 8 hours of sleep, and getting sufficient exercise should help with the craving for sugar over time.

[1] Metabolic Modeling of Streptococcus mutans Reveals Complex Nutrient Requirements of an Oral Pathogen. Jijakli K, Jensen PA. mSystems. 2019 Oct 29;4(5):e00529-19. doi: 10.1128/mSystems.00529-19. PMID: 31662430

[2] Biochemical composition and cariogenicity of dental plaque formed in the presence of sucrose or glucose and fructose. Cury JA, Rebelo MA, Del Bel Cury AA, Derbyshire MT, Tabchoury CP. Caries Res. 2000 Nov-Dec;34(6):491-7. doi: 10.1159/000016629. PMID: 11093024

[3] Hyperglycemia and xerostomia are key determinants of tooth decay in type 1 diabetic mice. Yeh CK, Harris SE, Mohan S, Horn D, Fajardo R, Chun YH, Jorgensen J, Macdougall M, Abboud-Werner S. Lab Invest. 2012 Jun;92(6):868-82. doi: 10.1038/labinvest.2012.60. Epub 2012 Mar 26. PMID: 22449801

[4] Development and Validation of an Empirical Dietary Inflammatory Index. Tabung FK, Smith-Warner SA, Chavarro JE, Wu K, Fuchs CS, Hu FB, Chan AT, Willett WC, Giovannucci EL. J Nutr. 2016 Aug;146(8):1560-70. doi: 10.3945/jn.115.228718. PMID: 27358416; PMCID: PMC4958288.

[5] The Association Between Inflammatory Dietary Pattern and Risk of Cognitive Impairment Among Older Adults with Chronic Diseases and Its Multimorbidity: A Cross-Sectional Study. Lili Wang, Le Cheng, Chenhui Lv, Jie Kou, Wenjuan Feng, Haoran Xie, Ruolin Yan, Xi Wang, Shuangzhi Chen, Xin Song, Lushan Xue, Cheng Zhang, Xuemin Li, Haifeng Zhao. Clin Interv Aging. 2024; 19: 1685–1701. doi: 10.2147/CIA.S474907 PMC11484775

[6] An overview on glycation: molecular mechanisms, impact on proteins, pathogenesis, and inhibition. Uceda AB, Mariño L, Casasnovas R, Adrover M. Biophys Rev. 2024 Apr 12;16(2):189-218. doi: 10.1007/s12551-024-01188-4. eCollection 2024 Apr. PMID: 38737201

[7] Fasting and postchallenge hyperglycemia and risk of cardiovascular disease in Chinese: the Chin-Shan Community Cardiovascular Cohort study. Chien KL, Hsu HC, Su TC, Chen MF, Lee YT, Hu FB. Am Heart J. 2008 Nov;156(5):996-1002. doi: 10.1016/j.ahj.2008.06.019. Epub 2008 Aug 27. PMID: 19061718

[8] Fasting and 2-hour postchallenge serum glucose measures and risk of incident cardiovascular events in the elderly: the Cardiovascular Health Study. Smith NL, Barzilay JI, Shaffer D, Savage PJ, Heckbert SR, Kuller LH, Kronmal RA, Resnick HE, Psaty BM. Arch Intern Med. 2002 Jan 28;162(2):209-16. doi: 10.1001/archinte.162.2.209. PMID: 11802755

[9] Is nondiabetic hyperglycemia a risk factor for cardiovascular disease? A meta-analysis of prospective studies. Levitan EB, Song Y, Ford ES, Liu S. Arch Intern Med. 2004 Oct 25;164(19):2147-55. doi: 10.1001/archinte.164.19.2147. PMID: 15505129

[10] Are all sugars equal? Role of the food source in physiological responses to sugars with an emphasis on fruit and fruit juice. Gonzalez JT. Eur J Nutr. 2024 Aug;63(5):1435-1451. doi: 10.1007/s00394-024-03365-3. Epub 2024 Mar 16. PMID: 38492022

[11] Hyperglycemia drives intestinal barrier dysfunction and risk for enteric infection. Thaiss CA, Levy M, Grosheva I, Zheng D, Soffer E, Blacher E, Braverman S, Tengeler AC, Barak O, Elazar M, Ben-Zeev R, Lehavi-Regev D, Katz MN, Pevsner-Fischer M, Gertler A, Halpern Z, Harmelin A, Aamar S, Serradas P, Grosfeld A, Shapiro H, Geiger B, Elinav E. Science. 2018 Mar 23;359(6382):1376-1383. doi: 10.1126/science.aar3318. PMID: 29519916

[12] Intestinal Barrier Function and the Gut Microbiome Are Differentially Affected in Mice Fed a Western-Style Diet or Drinking Water Supplemented with Fructose. Volynets V, Louis S, Pretz D, Lang L, Ostaff MJ, Wehkamp J, Bischoff SC. J Nutr. 2017 May;147(5):770-780. doi: 10.3945/jn.116.242859. PMID: 28356436

[13] Consumption of Sugar-Sweetened Beverages Has a Dose-Dependent Effect on the Risk of Non-Alcoholic Fatty Liver Disease: An Updated Systematic Review and Dose-Response Meta-Analysis. Chen H, Wang J, Li Z, Lam CWK, Xiao Y, Wu Q, Zhang W. Int J Environ Res Public Health. 2019 Jun 21;16(12):2192. doi: 10.3390/ijerph16122192. PMID: 31234281

[14] Major dietary patterns and dietary inflammatory index in relation to dyslipidemia using cross-sectional results from the RaNCD cohort study.Pasdar Y, Moradi F, Cheshmeh S, Sedighi M, Saber A, Moradi S, Bonyani M, Najafi F. Sci Rep. 2023 Nov 4;13(1):19075. doi: 10.1038/s41598-023-46447-8. PMID: 37925569.

[15] Uric acid but not apple polyphenols is responsible for the rise of plasma antioxidant activity after apple juice consumption in healthy subjects. Godycki-Cwirko M, Krol M, Krol B, Zwolinska A, Kolodziejczyk K, Kasielski M, Padula G, Grebowski J, Kazmierska P, Miatkowski M, Markowski J, Nowak D. J Am Coll Nutr. 2010 Aug;29(4):397-406. doi: 10.1080/07315724.2010.10719857. PMID: 21041815

[16] Fruit and vegetable consumption and the risk of type 2 diabetes: a systematic review and dose-response meta-analysis of prospective studies. Halvorsen RE, Elvestad M, Molin M, Aune D. BMJ Nutr Prev Health. 2021 Jul 2;4(2):519-531. doi: 10.1136/bmjnph-2020-000218. eCollection 2021. PMID: 35028521

[17] Sugar-sweetened beverages exacerbate high-fat diet-induced inflammatory bowel disease by altering the gut microbiome. Shon WJ, Jung MH, Kim Y, Kang GH, Choi EY, Shin DM. J Nutr Biochem. 2023 Mar;113:109254. doi: 10.1016/j.jnutbio.2022.109254. Epub 2022 Dec 24. PMID: 36572070

[18] Kern, M., Orduna, O. and Roberts, T. (2017), Acute metabolic and satiety responses to ingestion of molasses versus sucrose in healthy adults. The FASEB Journal, 31: 798.11-798.11. https://doi.org/10.1096/fasebj.31.1_supplement.798.11

[19] Kong, F., Yu, S., Zeng, F. et al. Phenolics Content and Inhibitory Effect of Sugarcane Molasses on α-Glucosidase and α-Amylase In Vitro. Sugar Tech 18, 333–339 (2016). https://doi.org/10.1007/s12355-015-0385-y

[20] Are all sugars equal? Role of the food source in physiological responses to sugars with an emphasis on fruit and fruit juice. Gonzalez JT. Eur J Nutr. 2024

Aug;63(5):1435-1451. doi: 10.1007/s00394-024-03365-3. Epub 2024 Mar 16. PMID: 38492022

21 Infantile Botulism. Ngoc L. Van Horn; Megan Street. StatPearls https://www.ncbi.nlm.nih.gov/books/NBK493178

22 Metabolomic Pattern Predicts Incident Coronary Heart Disease. Wang Z, Zhu C, Nambi V, Morrison AC, Folsom AR, Ballantyne CM, Boerwinkle E, Yu B. Arterioscler Thromb Vasc Biol. 2019 Jul;39(7):1475-1482. doi: 10.1161/ATVBAHA.118.312236. Epub 2019 May 16. PMID: 31092011

23 The artificial sweetener erythritol and cardiovascular event risk. Witkowski M, Nemet I, Alamri H, Wilcox J, Gupta N, Nimer N, Haghikia A, Li XS, Wu Y, Saha PP, Demuth I, König M, Steinhagen-Thiessen E, Cajka T, Fiehn O, Landmesser U, Tang WHW, Hazen SL. Nat Med. 2023 Mar;29(3):710-718. doi: 10.1038/s41591-023-02223-9. Epub 2023 Feb 27. PMID: 36849732

24 Elevated Erythritol: A Marker of Metabolic Dysregulation or Contributor to the Pathogenesis of Cardiometabolic Disease? Mazi TA, Stanhope KL. Nutrients. 2023 Sep 16;15(18):4011. doi: 10.3390/nu15184011. PMID: 37764794

25 Xylitol and sorbitol effects on the microbiome of saliva and plaque. Rafeek R, Carrington CVF, Gomez A, Harkins D, Torralba M, Kuelbs C, Addae J, Moustafa A, Nelson KE. J Oral Microbiol. 2018 Oct 23;11(1):1536181. doi: 10.1080/20002297.2018.1536181. eCollection 2019. PMID: 30598728

26 Effects of xylitol-containing chewing gum on the oral microbiota. Takeuchi K, Asakawa M, Hashiba T, Takeshita T, Saeki Y, Yamashita Y. J Oral Sci. 2018 Dec 27;60(4):588-594. doi: 10.2334/josnusd.17-0446. Epub 2018 Nov 15. PMID: 30429438

27 The effect of xylitol chewing gums and candies on caries occurrence in children: a systematic review with special reference to caries level at study baseline. Pienihäkkinen K, Hietala-Lenkkeri A, Arpalahti I, Söderling E. Eur Arch Paediatr Dent. 2024 Apr;25(2):145-160. doi: 10.1007/s40368-024-00875-w. Epub 2024 Mar 2. PMID: 38430364

28 Effects of sugar-free polyol chewing gums on gingival inflammation: a systematic review. Söderling E, Pienihäkkinen K, Gursoy UK. Clin Oral Investig. 2022 Dec;26(12):6881-6891. doi: 10.1007/s00784-022-04729-x. Epub 2022 Oct 14. PMID: 36239787

29 Effect of xylitol on Porphyromonas gingivalis: A systematic review. Chen SY, Delacruz J, Kim Y, Kingston R, Purvis L, Sharma D. Clin Exp Dent Res. 2023 Apr;9(2):265-275. doi: 10.1002/cre2.724. Epub 2023 Mar 9. PMID: 36894516

30 Antiplaque and antigingivitis efficacy of medicated and non-medicated sugar-free chewing gum as adjuncts to toothbrushing: systematic review and network meta-analysis. Muniz FWMG, Zanatta FB, Muñoz MDS, Aguiar LM, Silva FH, Montagner AF. Clin Oral Investig. 2022 Feb;26(2):1155-1172. doi: 10.1007/s00784-021-04264-1. Epub 2022 Jan 24. PMID: 35072769

31 Xylitol is prothrombotic and associated with cardiovascular risk. Witkowski M, Nemet I, Li XS, Wilcox J, Ferrell M, Alamri H, Gupta N, Wang Z, Tang WHW, Hazen SL. Eur Heart J. 2024 Jul 12;45(27):2439-2452. doi: 10.1093/eurheartj/ehae244. PMID: 38842092

32 Artificial sweeteners induce glucose intolerance by altering the gut microbiota. Suez J, Korem T, Zeevi D, Zilberman-Schapira G, Thaiss CA, Maza O, Israeli D, Zmora N, Gilad S, Weinberger A, Kuperman Y, Harmelin A, Kolodkin-Gal I, Shapiro H, Halpern Z, Segal E, Elinav E. Nature. 2014 Oct 9;514(7521):181-6. doi: 10.1038/nature13793. Epub 2014 Sep 17. PMID: 25231862

33 Low-dose aspartame consumption differentially affects gut microbiota-host metabolic interactions in the diet-induced obese rat. Palmnäs MS, Cowan TE, Bomhof MR, Su J, Reimer RA, Vogel HJ, Hittel DS, Shearer J. PLoS One. 2014 Oct 14;9(10):e109841. doi: 10.1371/journal.pone.0109841. eCollection 2014. PMID: 25313461

34 Effects of Sweeteners on the Gut Microbiota: A Review of Experimental Studies and Clinical Trials. Ruiz-Ojeda FJ, Plaza-Díaz J, Sáez-Lara MJ, Gil A. Adv Nutr. 2019 Jan 1;10(suppl_1):S31-S48. doi: 10.1093/advances/nmy037. PMID: 30721958

35 Consuming artificial sweeteners may alter the structure and function of duodenal microbial communities. Hosseini A, Barlow GM, Leite G, Rashid M, Parodi G, Wang J, Morales W, Weitsman S, Rezaie A, Pimentel M, Mathur R. iScience. 2023 Nov 23;26(12):108530. doi: 10.1016/j.isci.2023.108530. eCollection 2023 Dec 15. PMID: 38125028

36 Artificial Sweetener and the Risk of Adverse Pregnancy Outcomes: A Mendelian Randomization Study. Mao D, Lin M, Zeng Z, Mo D, Hu KL, Li R. Nutrients. 2024 Oct 3;16(19):3366. doi: 10.3390/nu16193366. PMID: 39408333

37 Maternal Exposure to Non-nutritive Sweeteners Impacts Progeny's Metabolism and Microbiome. Olivier-Van Stichelen S, Rother KI, Hanover JA. Front Microbiol. 2019 Jun 20;10:1360. doi: 10.3389/fmicb.2019.01360. PMID: 31281295

38 Association Between Artificially Sweetened Beverage Consumption During Pregnancy and Infant Body Mass Index. Azad MB, Sharma AK, de Souza RJ, Dolinsky VW, Becker AB, Mandhane PJ, Turvey SE, Subbarao P, Lefebvre DL, Sears MR; Canadian Healthy Infant Longitudinal Development Study Investigators. JAMA Pediatr. 2016 Jul 1;170(7):662-70. doi: 10.1001/jamapediatrics.2016.0301. PMID: 27159792

39 Inhibition of the gut enzyme intestinal alkaline phosphatase may explain how aspartame promotes glucose intolerance and obesity in mice. Gul SS, Hamilton AR, Munoz AR, Phupitakphol T, Liu W, Hyoju SK, Economopoulos KP, Morrison S, Hu D, Zhang W, Gharedaghi MH, Huo H, Hamarneh SR, Hodin RA. Appl Physiol Nutr Metab. 2017 Jan;42(1):77-83. doi: 10.1139/apnm-2016-0346. PMID: 27997218

40 Artificial sweeteners and risk of cardiovascular diseases: results from the prospective NutriNet-Santé cohort. Debras C, Chazelas E, Sellem L, Porcher R, Druesne-

Pecollo N, Esseddik Y, de Edelenyi FS, Agaësse C, De Sa A, Lutchia R, Fezeu LK, Julia C, Kesse-Guyot E, Allès B, Galan P, Hercberg S, Deschasaux-Tanguy M, Huybrechts I, Srour B, Touvier M. BMJ. 2022 Sep 7;378:e071204. doi: 10.1136/bmj-2022-071204. PMID: 36638072

41 Artificial sweeteners and cancer risk: Results from the NutriNet-Santé population-based cohort study. Debras C, Chazelas E, Srour B, Druesne-Pecollo N, Esseddik Y, Szabo de Edelenyi F, Agaësse C, De Sa A, Lutchia R, Gigandet S, Huybrechts I, Julia C, Kesse-Guyot E, Allès B, Andreeva VA, Galan P, Hercberg S, Deschasaux-Tanguy M, Touvier M. PLoS Med. 2022 Mar 24;19(3):e1003950. doi: 10.1371/journal.pmed.1003950. eCollection 2022 Mar. PMID: 35324894

42 Artificial Sweeteners and Risk of Type 2 Diabetes in the Prospective NutriNet-Santé Cohort. Debras C, Deschasaux-Tanguy M, Chazelas E, Sellem L, Druesne-Pecollo N, Esseddik Y, Szabo de Edelenyi F, Agaësse C, De Sa A, Lutchia R, Julia C, Kesse-Guyot E, Allès B, Galan P, Hercberg S, Huybrechts I, Cosson E, Tatulashvili S, Srour B, Touvier M. Diabetes Care. 2023 Sep 1;46(9):1681-1690. doi: 10.2337/dc23-0206. PMID: 37490630

43 Sweetener aspartame aggravates atherosclerosis through insulin-triggered inflammation. Wu W, et al. Cell Metabolism, Feb 19, 2025 https://www.sciencedirect.com/science/article/pii/S1550413125000063
https://doi.org/10.1016/j.cmet.2025.01.006

44 Antibacterial agent consisting of lactitol and maltitol. JP5710111B2 (Patent, Japan 2009)

45 Maltitol based sugar-free chocolates may not promote dental caries: An open-label clinical study. Mehta A ,et al, F1000Research 2022, 11:417 https://doi.org/10.12688/f1000research.109501.1

46 https://en.wikipedia.org/wiki/Psicose

47 The human sweet tooth. Reed DR, McDaniel AH. BMC Oral Health. 2006 Jun 15;6 Suppl 1(Suppl 1):S17. doi: 10.1186/1472-6831-6-S1-S17. PMID: 16934118

48 https://health.clevelandclinic.org/why-am-i-craving-sweets

49 Human HMGCS2 regulates mitochondrial fatty acid oxidation and FGF21 expression in HepG2 cell line. Vilà-Brau A, De Sousa-Coelho AL, Mayordomo C, Haro D, Marrero PF. J Biol Chem. 2011 Jun 10;286(23):20423-30. doi: 10.1074/jbc.M111.235044. Epub 2011 Apr 18. PMID: 21502324

50 Potential of Polyphenols to Restore SIRT1 and NAD+ Metabolism in Renal Disease. Tovar-Palacio C, Noriega LG, Mercado A. Nutrients. 2022 Feb 3;14(3):653. doi: 10.3390/nu14030653. PMID: 35277012

51 Effects of Resveratrol and other Polyphenols on Sirt1: Relevance to Brain Function During Aging. Sarubbo F, Esteban S, Miralles A, Moranta D. Curr Neuropharmacol. 2018 Jan 30;16(2):126-136. doi: 10.2174/1570159X15666170703113212. PMID: 28676015

52 SIRT1 Activation by Natural Phytochemicals: An Overview. Iside C, Scafuro M, Nebbioso A, Altucci L. Front Pharmacol. 2020 Aug 7;11:1225. doi: 10.3389/fphar.2020.01225. eCollection 2020. PMID: 32848804

11: Pasta, Pizza, Pastries, and Pancakes

Pasta, pizza, pastries, and pies are principal provisions within American and European diets. They are the pillars of Western society and the apex of our cultural cuisine. And for the most part, they are sort of banned from the SANA diet along with wheat.

Fear not! Partial solutions are present. At least for pasta.

Pasta

Rice, lentil, and garbanzo bean pastas are commercially available. These are often made of single ingredients, without additives, which is great. And they get great DAD ratings.

✹ Red lentil pasta is rated 4 (★★★★).

✹ The brown rice corkscrew pasta (ingredient list: brown rice and water) I had for lunch today was delicious. DAD score 4 (★★★★)

✹ Chickpea pasta is also available (★★★★).

✹ Mung bean and rice noodles can be found in Chinese or Asian grocery stores.

💣 Corn pasta is available, but gets a B on the DAD scale; it should be avoided.

💣 Wheat pasta gets an A for avoid.

The chickpea pasta foams during cooking; I suggest cooking it in a larger pot than one might usually use to prevent it from boiling over.

Corn pasta can be made at home using masa harina. A recipe is provided at the end of the chapter. A recipe for delicious tortilla lasagna is also provided. Remember that tortillas made from masa get a DAD rating of 3 (★★★) while those made from corn flour get a B (⛈ ⛈). Mission brand corn tortillas are made from masa, but La Banda tortillas are made from corn flour.

Table 11A: Pasta Scores

Pasta	Score
Rice Brown rice spiral pasta (Tinkysada company)	4
Lentil Red Lentil Pasta	4
Chickpea pasta	4
Mung Bean starch paste	1
Wheat (whole wheat) spaghetti (durum) cooked	A
Wheat spaghetti (durum)	A
Corn Pasta (Barilla)	B
Instant Noodles (wheat)	C

Tortilla Lasagna

This quick dish fills the place for pizza and lasagna and gets a DAD score of 4. Surprisingly good.

Ingredients:

- About 10 – 12 Corn tortillas (must use masa or lime-treated corn tortillas)
- About 2 cups (meatless) tomato-based spaghetti sauce.
- 6 oz of shredded white cheese (can be mixed, i.e., mozzarella and jack cheeses)
- 4 – 6 ounces of mushrooms.
- Extras fillings: Diced red onions, cauliflower, surimi, red or orange bell peppers. Diced tomatoes can be used, but seeds should be removed to keep the lasagna from being too wet.

Using an 8x8" baking dish as an example: Pour and spread a thin layer of spaghetti sauce into the baking dish (1/4 cup) and lay a single layer of corn tortillas in the bottom of the baking dish. Cut the tortillas in half, and place the straight edges along the sides. Pour a half cup of spaghetti sauce over the tortillas to make a 3/16th inch (@ 4 mm) deep layer, followed by adding some sliced mushrooms and/or other "toppings, and then a layer of shredded cheese, using about 2 ounces (60 grams) of cheese. Mozzarella gives a nice stretchy chewiness. Other types of cheese add their own flavors.

Add a second layer of tortillas, sauce, cheese, and fillings.

Add a final thin layer of sauce and a full layer of cheese.

Cover the baking dish with aluminum foil (not touching the contents) to prevent browning of the cheese. Place a few slits in the foil so that moisture can escape.

Bake at 370° F for about 20 – 25 minutes until the cheese is fully melted. Cool for a few minutes before serving, but serve while the cheese is still soft.

Pastries and Pancakes

Most readymade pastries you will find are high in sugar, and usually made of wheat, and often with lard or shortening. Bakery confections, including cakes, fudge, brownies, cookies, and candies, are considerably more cariogenic than foods containing intrinsic sugars, such as fruits and milk.[1] Regular wheat flour is not part of the SANA diet. Thus, mostly, readymade pastries are not allowed on the SANA diet. Fruit is a better dessert, and pastries are a poor substitute for breakfast.

I apologize. I'm certain that, given the time, energy, and interest, recipes for croissants, bear claws, flaky pie crust, and cinnamon rolls can be developed that don't contain prohibited ingredients and get a fine DAD score. I have developed a few recipes as examples, but I am not a pastry person. I will leave these creative endeavors for others.

Sprouted wheat flour is commercially available (but expensive). It contains gluten, but has a good DAD score for those who do not have celiac disease. Sprouted wheat flour appears to be only available as whole wheat flour made from hard wheat, which is fine for making bread; however, pastries generally call for flour made from soft winter wheat, and pasta is generally made from Durum wheat. Thus, while sprouted wheat flour is fine on the SANA diet, pastry and homemade pasta recipes will likely need to be modified if using germinated hard wheat flour.

Non-wheat, gluten-free flour is available, but caution needs to be used. Many of these contain gums that cause dysbiosis and should thus be avoided. Additionally, while allowed with a DAD score of zero, tapioca flour and arrowroot flour are mostly starch, with little nutritional value.

Not a delicacy, honey oat granola bars (wheat-free) get a DAD score of 2. Note that a two-bar serving has 11 grams of added sugar per serving. That comes out of your sugar budget.

I find that dry Cheery-Os (with a DAD score of 3) are a nice crunchy, farinaceous snack, and they are nice on ice cream.

Pumpkin pie (without the crust) gets a good DAD score, and does not need to be excessively sweet to be flavorful, and is just as good when made without the crust.

There is one hankering that is hard to fill, that if kept within the added sugar budget, fits into the SANA diet: oatmeal cookies. While eggs are allowed, a vegan recipe is given below for those who prefer to avoid eggs.

Baking Powders: Baking powder made with sodium acid pyrophosphate (SAPP) and baking soda has DAD scores of zero and can be used in baking without concern. The SANA diet recommends the use of aluminum-free baking powder.

Baking soda containing aluminum sulfate ( ) should be avoided.

Double-acting baking soda reacts twice, releasing CO_2 gas bubbles; some during mixing when it gets wet, and again during heating. In contrast, baking soda releases most of its gas as soon as it mixes with acids such as the vinegar, molasses, yogurt, or applesauce in the recipe.

Reducing Fat from Baked Goods

When baking, for most recipes, applesauce can replace the first ¼ cup of oil, and when the recipe calls for more oil, generally at least half of the oil needed in baking can be replaced with applesauce.

The SANA diet allows the use of eggs in baking, but vegans can substitute them with apple sauce or aqua faba (Chapter 12). Applesauce can be used as an egg substitute when baking, using ¼ cup of applesauce for each egg. This works best when the purpose of the oil and eggs is to maintain richness and moisture in the baked good. Bananas can also be used. Pumpkin puree can be used in place of butter for many baked goods, using ¾ of the purée for each cup of butter called for in the recipe, and for oil, using a one-to-one substitution.

Whole milk Greek yogurt (10% fat) can be used to substitute for butter, using five parts Greek yogurt for four parts of butter. The amount of wet ingredients may need to be lowered a bit.

Oatmeal Cookies

Makes about 16 @ 25 gram cookies, each with @ 3 grams of added sugar

- 1¼ cups (quick) rolled oats)
- 1/2 teaspoon baking soda
- 1/4 teaspoon baking powder
- 1/4 teaspoon salt
- 1/3 cup (unsweetened) applesauce
- 1/4 cup light brown sugar (packed)
- Optional: 1 Tbsp. dried cranberries, chopped walnuts

Blend the applesauce, brown sugar, and coconut oil (as a liquid). The coconut oil may need to be warmed if it is solid. Blend the dry ingredients and add them to the moist ones. The salt and baking soda should be sifted and added, or can be sifted and added to the oatmeal, and then all blended. One of the secrets of good cookies is thoroughly mixing the ingredients.

When cookie dough is thoroughly mixed, it should be dry enough to form a dense ball and pull away from the wall of the bowl, leaving almost no dough. This recipe should form a ball, but is a bit stickier than most cookie doughs are. Place the dough in the refrigerator for a couple of hours to let the oats get moisturized. Divide 4 times, into 16 walnut-sized balls, and place the dough balls on a baking sheet (optional) after wiping a thin layer of coconut oil on the sheet or using baking parchment paper. Note: Applesauce, brown sugar, and molasses are slightly acidic and thus help to activate the baking soda, helping to make the cookies rise.

Bake for 12 minutes in a preheated oven set to 350°F.

Gluten-Free Pancakes

Keep in mind that some acid is needed to activate baking soda to make the pancakes rise. This can be yogurt, applesauce, molasses, and even brown sugar, a bit. Gets DAD score of 3.

- ¾ cup oats – use blended to mill into coarse flour
- 1 egg
- ½ tsp baking soda
- 2 tbsp Greek yogurt
- ¼ cup of unsweetened apple sauce
- 2 Tbsp. water
- Pinch of salt

Use coconut oil on a griddle heated to medium-high heat. If it smokes, the pan is too hot. It is best to cook the pancakes in a pan with a clear glass lid; pour in the batter and cover; when the air bubbles in the pancake stop collapsing, it's time to turn the pancake over, and it only takes a few more seconds of cooking on the flip side to finish cooking.

- ½ cup oatmeal soaked in 1/2 cup of hot water for 30 minutes
- 1 large egg
- 1/4 teaspoon baking powder
- 1.5 tsp. tablespoon brown sugar
- 1 tbsp Greek yogurt
- A pinch of salt
- Butter or oil for cooking

- 1 cup of quick oats
- ½ tsp. of double-acting baking soda
- ¼ cup yogurt
- 2 eggs
- 2 Tbsp brown sugar or honey
- 1 Tbsp. applesauce or 2 tsp. coconut oil or butter

Mill the oats and baking soda into a coarse flour in a food processor or blender. Mix the other ingredients separately, and then blend in the oat flour. Allow the batter to rest for 5 minutes to thicken. Cook as usual for pancakes.

Vegan Banana Pancakes

- 1.5 cups of quick rolled oats
- One large over-ripe banana
- One cup of soy or other non-dairy milk
- A pinch of salt
- ½ tsp. of baking soda

Blend until smooth, and then allow the batter to rest for 5 minutes to thicken. Cook as for regular pancakes.

Waffles

Waffle batter is very similar to pancake batter, but waffle batter has several differences to adapt it to make it fluffy on the inside and crisp on the outside. Waffle batter is a bit thicker to help hold its shape; uses more baking powder to make a fluffier interior, has more sugar to increase caramelization and crispiness, and uses more butter or oil, helping with crispiness and to make it richer. Thus, these adaptations make waffles a less healthy dish, especially if they are bathed in syrup.

Oatmeal Masa Molasses Waffles

- 1 cup precooked oatmeal (Chapter 9, but using a 3:1 water to rolled oats ratio)
- ½ cup of whole milk or non-dairy milk
- ½ cup masa harina (flour)
- One egg
- 1 Tbsp. Butter
- ¼ cup light brown sugar
- 2 tsp. molasses
- 1 Tbsp. Double-acting baking powder
- ¼ cup apple sauce

Blend the egg, melted butter, milk, apple sauce, and molasses, and then blend in the oatmeal until it is smooth. In a mixing bowl, mix the masa flour, brown sugar, and baking powder together. Pour the wet ingredients into the bowl and mix them into the dry ingredients. Let the batter stand for 10 minutes before cooking for 5 minutes in a heated waffle iron. Add a tablespoon of water at a time to thin the batter if it is too thick. Makes about 8 waffles.

Nixtamal Pasta Dough

If you would like to make homemade pasta:

Ingredients:

- 1¾ cups Masa Harina
- ¾ cup tapioca flour (also called tapioca starch)
- 1 teaspoon salt
- 3 large eggs
- 3 tablespoons butter
- Water (as needed)

Instructions:

Combine Dry Ingredients: In the bowl of your bread machine, add the masa harina, tapioca flour, chia seed, and salt. Give it a quick stir to combine.

Add Wet Ingredients: Make a well in the center of the dry ingredients. Crack the eggs into the well and add the softened butter.

Mix and Knead: Using the "dough" setting on your bread machine, start the machine. Let it run through its kneading cycle.

Check Dough Consistency: After the cycle, open the machine and check the dough. It should be slightly crumbly but hold together when pinched. If the dough feels too dry, add a tablespoon of water at a time and knead for another minute until it reaches the desired consistency. If it's too wet, add a tablespoon of tapioca flour at a time and knead until it becomes less sticky.

Rest the Dough: Wrap the dough tightly in plastic wrap and let it rest at room temperature for at least 30 minutes, or up to an hour. This allows the dough to hydrate fully and become more elastic.

Roll and Shape: Lightly dust your work surface with tapioca flour. Divide the dough into two portions. Roll out each portion with a rolling pin to a thin sheet, about 1/16 inch thick. Use a pasta machine if you have one, following its instructions for achieving the desired thickness. Cut the pasta dough into your desired shapes, like fettuccine, tagliatelle, or ravioli.

Cook the Pasta: Bring a large pot of salted water to a boil. Add the pasta and cook for 2-3 minutes, or until it floats to the surface. Drain the pasta and toss with your favorite sauce.

Tips:

- Masa harina dough can be a bit delicate compared to regular pasta dough. Be gentle when handling and rolling it out.
- If the dough cracks while rolling, don't worry! Just patch it up and continue rolling.
- You can use this dough to make filled pasta like ravioli. Just be sure to use a rolling pin to get the dough as thin as possible.
- Leftover dough can be stored in an airtight container in the refrigerator for up to 2 days.

Pie

I have always thought of pie as being a rather benign dessert. OK, so apples only get a DAD score of one, but pumpkin gets a DAD score of four. Blackberries, blueberries, and cherries should be fine, right?

So, when I came across a study that identified ready-made pies as one of the very few food items out of 129 that were associated with increased risk of dementia as a result of its impact on gene expression, I had to ask, "Why pie?" Pie consumption was correlated with a decline in the expression of SLC9A8 (NHE8), a sodium-hydrogen transmembrane transport protein.[2]

Americans love dessert. About 93% of Americans have had dessert within the last week, and half have had dessert in the last day.[3] Pie is the third most common dessert ordered at restaurants. About half of the pies purchased in grocery stores are fresh from the bakery, 30% frozen, and about 8% are snack pies. Cakes, however, are much more widely consumed than pie. Over 260 million ready-to-eat cakes are sold by major cake factories each year, not including snack cakes or coffee cakes, while the number of pies is less than 90 million. But if frozen pies (115 million) are added, the number of factory pies comes close to the number of cakes. If refrigerated cheesecakes (over 55 million) are added to the pie ledger, then the number of pies sold would outpace the number of cakes purchased. Still, the number of pies sold per year by large vendors seems small; it is similar to the number of people in the country, and a pie per year seems trivial. The average American eats only 6 slices of pie a year. Much of that is over the Thanksgiving holiday, with 55 million pumpkin pies being consumed.[4 5]

The question is, what about pies makes them lower the expression of NHE8 that does not occur with other foods? Is it the pie crust or the filling, and if it is the filling or crust, which one? In the USA, apple pie is the most popular, while in England, steak and kidney pie wins that honor. Frequently consumed pies in America are apple, cherry, blueberry, pecan, pumpkin, sweet potato, lemon meringue pie, and chocolate cream pies. There are three common styles of crust: flaky, graham cracker, and shortcake cookie.

While there is not much nice to say about the health impacts of lemon meringue or banana cream, or chocolate cream pies. And pecan pie has 32 grams of sugar from corn syrup per serving. The unique issue with pies, however, is likely attributable to the pie crust. Traditional, homemade, flaky pie crust is made with butter, wheat flour, and sugar. Commercial pie crust is made with lard or vegetable shortening, both of which get DAD scores of D, white wheat flour (B to C), and a small amount of sugar. Commercial pie crust gets a score of D.

Lard and vegetable shortening, perhaps in synergy with gluten and ATI and other anti-nutritional properties from wheat, may impede NHE8 expression, especially for those with a low fiber diet and low levels of vitamin D. Pie crust generally has more than half of its calories from fat. Lard in the diet increases the abundance of *Coriobacteriaceae_UCG-002*, and reduces that of *Akkermansia muciniphila,* thus has a deleterious effect on the mucosal barrier, and this promotes obesity and insulin resistance.[6 7 8]

Other than pie crusts, shortening is used in commercial pastries, cinnamon rolls, croissants, crackers, cookies, doughnuts, chips, popcorn, French fries, fried onions, and in many frozen meals, especially breaded foods. All these are likely worth avoiding. Read labels before you buy food. Most vegetable oils get a DAD score of D, and vegetable shortening is like vegetable oil on steroids.

Commercially made pies that use lard or shortening in their crust are not allowed on the SANA diet.

The mechanism for how the reduction of NHE8 expression increases the metabolic risk of dementia may be that it interferes with mucosal integrity.

NHE8 pumps sodium into and hydrogen protons (H^+) out of the cell. NHE8 is highly expressed in the enterocytes lining the intestine and colon, and is more highly expressed in the mucous-producing goblet cells of the intestine. If down-regulated, the cells tend to retain H^+, and thus the cell becomes more acidic. Mice deficient in NHE8 have increased intestinal bacterial adhesion and inflammation, and decreased mucin and production of protective proteins called defensins, especially in the distal colon.[9] Thus, the loss of NHE8 compromises intestinal mucosal integrity. The mice lacking NHE8 were thus more susceptible to intestinal injury and leaky gut. The exposure to inflammatory cytokines, such as TNF, further reduced the expression of NHE8 during intestinal inflammation.[10] Vitamin D deficiency has been found to induce colitis in animal models by downregulating NHE8. Vitamin D also acts to protect the colon by other pathways.[11 12 13] An acidic environment in the colon also appears to promote the expression of NHE8;[14] a healthy microbiome, rich in bifidobacteria, helps maintain the colon's acidity by the production of short-chain fatty acids.

The phenolic compounds myricetin, apigenin, catechin, and proanthocyanidin, and red wine increased NHE8 expression, but their positive impact was weaker than the negative impact of readymade pies.[15]

Pie Crust

Pie should be an acceptable dessert on the SANA diet if it is made with acceptable ingredients.

Shortbread Style Pie Crust

Prepare white rice (as per Chapter 9) using about 25% more water to get sticky rice. Using a short-grain or glutinous rice also helps.

- 1½ cups sticky white rice
- 1 egg
- 6 Tbsp. butter
- ½ cup whole milk Greek yogurt (10% milk fat) (i.e., Cabot's)
- 3 Tbsp. (packed) light brown sugar (for sweet pies)
- 1 cup coconut flour

Place sticky rice in a food processor (or "rice" using another device) along with the egg, Greek yogurt, and brown sugar. Blend until smooth and then add the warmed butter. The butter needs to be soft, or it will not blend well. A pinch of salt can be used if not using salted butter or if the rice was cooked without salt.

Place the dough into a bowl and mix in the coconut flour ¼ cup at a time. Add enough coconut flour so that the dough becomes dry enough that a walnut-sized mass can be rolled into a ball. Then place the dough in the refrigerator for an hour, both to cool the butter to harden, and to allow the coconut flour to take up moisture.

The dough can be rolled, using fine rice flour, or shaped into place in a pie pan that has been oiled with butter, coconut oil, or coconut oil spray.

Cover the crust with baking parchment or foil to avoid browning. Bake the crust for about 20 minutes at 300°F. The crust should come out a light buff color, like a shortbread cookie. Fill with the desired pie filling and bake.

Nixtamal Pizza Crust

Masa Pizza Dough (Yeast-leavened)

Ingredients:

- 1 cup masa harina (corn flour, not cornmeal)

- ½ cup sticky rice, cooked and mashed
- ½ cup oat flour (or finely blended rolled oats)
- 1 teaspoon salt
- 1 teaspoon sugar (optional, helps with browning)
- 1 ½ teaspoons instant yeast
- ¾ cup warm water (adjust as needed)
- 1 tablespoon coconut oil
- 1 teaspoon apple cider vinegar (helps texture)

Instructions:

1. Prepare white rice as per Chapter 9, using about 25% more water to get sticky rice. Using a short-grain or glutinous rice also helps.
2. Activate the yeast: In a small bowl, mix warm water, yeast, and sugar. Let it sit for 5–10 minutes until foamy.
3. Mash the rice: In a large bowl, mash the cooked sticky rice well to create a smooth paste.
4. Combine dry ingredients: Add masa harina, oat flour, and salt to the bowl with rice. Mix well.
5. Mix wet and dry: Pour in the yeast mixture, olive oil, and vinegar. Stir until a soft dough forms.
6. Knead: Lightly knead for about 3–5 minutes until smooth. The dough will feel soft but should hold together.
7. Rise: Cover and let rise for 45–60 minutes in a warm place.

Baking

- Preheat oven: Set to 425°F (220°C).
- Shape the crust: Roll or press the dough onto a greased or parchment-lined pizza pan.
- Prebake: Bake for 8–10 minutes until slightly firm.
- Add toppings: Layer with sauce, cheese, and desired toppings.
- Final bake: Bake another 12–15 minutes until golden and crisp.

Quick-Bread Masa Crust (No-Yeast) Version

Fast, tender, and still delicious.

Adjustments:

- Omit the yeast
- Increase baking powder to 1½ teaspoons
- Reduce water to ½ cup
- Skip the rising step; let the dough rest 10 minutes before rolling out
- Follow the same baking steps as for the yeast-leavened pizza crust.

Here's an adjusted version of the Masa Pizza Dough, replacing sticky rice with cooked oatmeal for a soft, slightly chewy texture.

Masa Pizza Dough (with Cooked Oatmeal) – Yeast Version

Ingredients:

- 1 cup masa harina (corn flour, not cornmeal)
- ½ cup cooked oatmeal (as per Chapter 9, but using 3:1 water to oats, and unsweetened)
- ½ cup oat flour (or finely blended rolled oats)
- 1 teaspoon salt
- 1 teaspoon sugar (optional, helps browning)
- 1 ½ teaspoons instant yeast
- ¾ cup warm water (adjust as needed)
- 1 tablespoon coconut oil
- 1 teaspoon apple cider vinegar (helps texture)

Instructions:

1. Prepare the yeast: In a small bowl, mix warm water, yeast, and sugar. Let it sit for 5–10 minutes until foamy.
2. Mash the oatmeal: In a large bowl, mash the cooked oatmeal until smooth.
3. Combine dry ingredients: Add masa harina, oat flour, and salt to the bowl. Mix well.
4. Mix wet and dry: Pour in the yeast mixture, olive oil, and vinegar. Stir until a soft dough forms.
5. Knead: Lightly knead for about 3–5 minutes until smooth. The dough will be soft but should hold together.
6. Rise: Cover and let rise for 45–60 minutes in a warm place.
7. Preheat oven: Set to 425°F (220°C).
8. Shape the crust: Roll or press the dough onto a greased or parchment-lined pizza pan.
9. Prebake: Bake for 8–10 minutes until slightly firm.
10. Add toppings: Layer with sauce, cheese, and desired toppings.
11. Final bake: Bake another 12–15 minutes until golden and crisp.

Quick-Bread (No-Yeast) Version

For a faster crust, follow these changes:

- Omit yeast.
- Increase baking powder to 1 ½ teaspoons.
- Reduce water to ½ cup.
- Skip the rising step; let the dough rest 10 minutes before rolling out.
- Follow the same baking steps.

This version with oatmeal gives the crust a slightly heartier texture while keeping it gluten-free and wheat-free!

Tortilla Chips

If you must, tortilla chips can be made, baking masa-based tortillas at about 400°F for 6 – 8 minutes. Most recipes call for a light brushing with (coconut) oil or a dusting with coconut oil cooking spray. Sprinkle salt and spices. Tostadas made from masa can be found, and they provide the corn-chip crunch you may be looking for. Tortilla chips made from masa can be found, but I have seen none in the chip aisles from national brands.

[1] The human sweet tooth. Reed DR, McDaniel AH. BMC Oral Health. 2006 Jun 15;6 Suppl 1(Suppl 1):S17. doi: 10.1186/1472-6831-6-S1-S17. PMID: 16934118

[2] Dietary Responses of Dementia-Related Genes Encoding Metabolic Enzymes. Parnell LD, Magadmi R, Zwanger S, Shukitt-Hale B, Lai CQ, Ordovás JM. Nutrients. 2023 Jan 27;15(3):644. doi: 10.3390/nu15030644. PMID: 36771351

[3] https://www.snackandbakery.com/articles/94860-state-of-the-industry-2020-growing-retail-dessert-diversity

[4] https://commercialbaking.com/a-slice-of-perseverance-pies-market-performance/

[5] https://worldmetrics.org/most-popular-pie-statistics/

[6] Comparative Analysis of the Gut Microbiota in Mice under Lard or Vegetable Blend Oil Diet. Qiao B, Li X, Wu Y, Guo T, Tan Z. J Oleo Sci. 2022 Oct 28;71(11):1613-1624. doi: 10.5650/jos.ess22056. Epub 2022 Oct 5. PMID: 36198580

[7] Akkermansia muciniphila inversely correlates with the onset of inflammation, altered adipose tissue metabolism and metabolic disorders during obesity in mice. Schneeberger M, Everard A, Gómez-Valadés AG, Matamoros S, Ramírez S, Delzenne NM, Gomis R, Claret M, Cani PD. Sci Rep. 2015 Nov 13;5:16643. doi: 10.1038/srep16643. PMID: 26563823

[8] Cross-talk between Akkermansia muciniphila and intestinal epithelium controls diet-induced obesity. Everard A, Belzer C, Geurts L, Ouwerkerk JP, Druart C, Bindels LB, Guiot Y, Derrien M, Muccioli GG, Delzenne NM, de Vos WM, Cani PD. Proc Natl Acad Sci U S A. 2013 May 28;110(22):9066-71. doi: 10.1073/pnas.1219451110. PMID: 23671105

[9] Loss of NHE8 expression impairs intestinal mucosal integrity. Wang A, Li J, Zhao Y, Johansson ME, Xu H, Ghishan FK. Am J Physiol Gastrointest Liver Physiol. 2015 Dec 1;309(11):G855-64. doi: 10.1152/ajpgi.00278.2015. Epub 2015 Oct 1. PMID: 26505975

[10] Intestinal NHE8 is highly expressed in goblet cells and its expression is subject to TNF-α regulation. Xu H, Li Q, Zhao Y, Li J, Ghishan FK. Am J Physiol Gastrointest Liver Physiol. 2016 Jan 15;310(2):G64-9. doi: 10.1152/ajpgi.00367.2015.. PMID:26564720

[11] Compromised NHE8 Expression Is Responsible for Vitamin D-Deficiency Induced Intestinal Barrier Dysfunction. Guo Y, Li Y, Tang Z, Geng C, Xie X, Song S, Wang C, Li X. Nutrients. 2023 Nov 19;15(22):4834. doi: 10.3390/nu15224834. PMID: 38004229

[12] 1,25-Dihydroxyvitamin D Protects Intestinal Epithelial Barrier by Regulating the Myosin Light Chain Kinase Signaling Pathway. Du J, Chen Y, Shi Y, Liu T, Cao Y, Tang Y, Ge X, Nie H, Zheng C, Li YC. Inflamm Bowel Dis. 2015 Nov;21(11):2495-506. doi: 10.1097/MIB.0000000000000526. PMID: 26287999

[13] Vitamin D/vitamin D receptor protects intestinal barrier against colitis by positively regulating Notch pathway. Li Y, Guo Y, Geng C, Song S, Yang W, Li X, Wang C. Front Pharmacol. 2024 Jul 26;15:1421577. doi: 10.3389/fphar.2024.1421577. PMID: 39130644

[14] Functional characterization of the sodium/hydrogen exchanger 8 and its role in proliferation of colonic epithelial cells. Zhou K, Amiri M, Salari A, Yu Y, Xu H, Seidler U, Nikolovska K. Am J Physiol Cell Physiol. 2021 Sep 1;321(3):C471-C488. doi: 10.1152/ajpcell.00582.2020. Epub 2021 Jul 21. PMID: 34288721

[15] Dietary Responses of Dementia-Related Genes Encoding Metabolic Enzymes. Parnell LD, Magadmi R, Zwanger S, Shukitt-Hale B, Lai CQ, Ordovás JM. Nutrients. 2023 Jan 27;15(3):644. doi: 10.3390/nu15030644. PMID: 36771351 (supplementary documents.)

12: Legumes: Pulses, and Dals

In much of the world, people consume pulses on a daily basis. When well-prepared, they are delicious. I never get tired of them. When I lived in Costa Rica, they were included in about 20 meals per week. In a single day, one might have black bean paste with sour cream on a gordito (thick tortilla) for breakfast, Gallo Pinto (stir-fried rice dish cooked with black beans, chopped vegetables) for lunch, and casado (white rice with black beans) for supper, and if I stepped out in the evening, I might have patacones (fried plantains) topped with refried beans and cheese as a street food. In contrast, the average American adult consumes legumes/beans about once every 8.3 days.[1] I guess that would be Taco Tuesdays.

Legumes are a great source of plant-based protein and fiber, and have a central place in the SANA diet. One of the Blue Zones described by Dan Buettner, in which people have extremely long lives, is the Nicoya peninsula in Costa Rica, which is reported to have the lowest middle-age mortality rate anywhere on earth. The diet there is largely black beans, nixtamalized corn tortillas, squash, and tropical fruit. Beans are also important components in the diet of the Mediterranean Blue Zones, Sardinia, where men live the longest, and in Ikaria, Greece, where dementia is rare.

This chapter covers "pulses". Pulses are legumes that are harvested as mature seeds, dried, and then cooked for consumption, in contrast to other legumes such as green beans and green peas that are used as vegetables.

The pulses most likely to be available at your local grocer and those of interest in this chapter include *beans, peas, and lentils.* Lupin (lupini) seeds are another pulse. Although some "sweet" cultivars have been developed that do not require special processing, most lupin varieties contain bitter alkaloids that need to be leached out to remove toxins that can otherwise cause poisoning. Lupin allergy cross-reacts with peanut allergy.

Most of the commonly consumed bean varieties are from the species *Phaseolus vulgaris*, a plant native to the Americas. These include back, red, white, pinto, navy, canary, kidney, and many other bean cultivars. Beans have been cultivated for about 8000 years. Lima beans (butter beans; *Phaseolus lunatus*) originated on the west coast of South America, and are closely related. Black-eyed peas (*Vigna unguiculata)*, a cowpea, originated in West Africa. The chickpea (*Cicer arietinum)* is native to the Middle East and has been cultivated for over 10,000 years.

Dal is a term from Indian cuisine that refers to dried pulses that have had their seed coats removed. An example of a dal common in the American market is split peas. Whole dried peas are rarely sold in stores; they take about 3 – 4 times longer to cook. In comparison to whole dried legumes, dal cooks fairly quickly. The word dal also refers to the cooked dal, which can be prepared as a paste that may be thick, like refried beans, or as a watery sauce. Dals are used to make creamed pulses; when served, properly prepared dal does not have intact seeds.

The central emphasis of this chapter is on exploring how to mitigate anti-nutritional compounds and optimize the digestibility of pulses to improve protein availability and the absorption of amino acids.

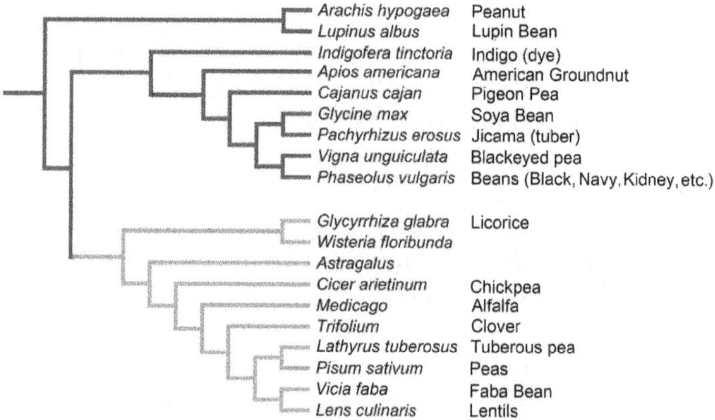

Figure 12A: The phylogenetic tree of edible and some non-edible legumes. Wisteria seeds contain a toxic saponin, and several Lathyrus species seeds contain an array of toxins, including a neurotoxic amino acid. Extracts from the roots of some plants in the *Astragalus* genus are used medicinally, while others, generally referred to as locoweed, contain neurotoxins.

Canned Beans

Let's begin with beans that are simple to prepare. Canned beans are convenient, quick, and easy, and especially practical when cooking for one or two people. When using canned beans, however, the consumer has little control over the preparation process and does not have the option to adequately prepare the beans for optimal nutrition and digestibility.

When purchasing canned beans, the SANA program recommends those that have the highest DAD scores. For the methods of preparation used in commercial canning, some beans get better scores than others. These are generally pulses that are smaller and have thinner seed coats, and that are recognized as hydrating more readily.

- A central tenet of the DAD diet is to select the highest rated items over lower rated ones where possible, to avoid those that are without benefit or harmful (0, A, and B), and never consume those rated C or D.
- The recommended canned pulses are pigeon peas, navy beans, and great northern beans, followed by seasoned/salted black beans and red beans, another small pulse (not to be confused with red kidney beans). See Table 12A below.
- Canned beans that have salt added during the canning process are preferred, as they are cooked longer, helping to soften the beans and the seed coat. Seasoning may also help soften the seed coat. Seasoned beans are also preferable and make the preparation of most dishes easier, although caution is needed to screen the ingredients if one has sensitivities to the spices.
- To reduce flatulence and improve digestibility, gently rinse the beans after removing them from the can to eliminate the aquafaba (bean-water).
- Traditional style refried beans are made with pinto beans, pork lard, salt, and seasonings including onion, chili pepper, cumin, and garlic. Vegan refried beans may be made with vegetable oils. Both should be avoided. Fat-free refried beans are available and come prepared with salt and seasoning. Refried beans contain chili pepper, which can be a problem for some people. Homemade refried beans are likely to be of much higher quality and have much better flavor.
- Note that most brands of canned split pea soup, baked beans, and obviously, pork & beans, are not vegetarian, kosher, or halal, and have lard, bacon, or ham added. Some canned baked beans are vegan. Lard, bacon, and ham are rated D.

Table 12A: DAD Scores for Canned Beans

Canned Beans	Rating
Pigeon Peas, from dry peas, salted	4
Pigeon Peas, from green peas, salted	4
Navy beans, salted	3
Great Northern beans, salted	2
Red Beans, salted	1+
Black beans, salted, seasoned	1+
Black beans, salted	1
Black beans, no salt	1-
Pinto beans, salted	1-
Refried Pinto beans (Vegan), spiced	1-
Light Red Kidney Beans, salted	1-
Light Red Kidney Beans, unsalted	0
Chickpea (Garbanzo bean) salted	0*
Dark Red Kidney Beans, salted	A
Black-eyed peas, salted	A
Cannellini beans, peas, salted	B

Table 9A: Canned beans. Rated high to low. Beans were rinsed, fresh water added, and boiled for 10 minutes, other for the refried beans. The refried beans had sufficient water added to heat them on a stovetop, and were stirred until brought to a boil. All of the canned beans, other than the pigeon peas, were from a single brand, so that processing was likely to be consistent. * See Chickpea salvation in "Notes" below.

Between the green and dry pigeon peas, I prefer the flavor of the green ones. The great northern beans have a creamy texture and mild flavor, while the navy beans are a bit more beany. The seasoned black beans had the best flavor and can be used for quickly prepared, delicious meals. The flavor of the refried beans was not worth repeating. If making refried beans at home, try using the red beans (for a more traditional appearance). The garbanzo beans get a poor rating, but can be rescued by blanching as described below.

Aquafaba (literally, bean-water): Aquafaba, best known from chickpeas, is used in vegan recipes to prepare a vegan whipped cream, mousse, meringues, mayonnaise (recipe below), or as an egg white substitute in many recipes. Many aquafaba recipes, both sweet and savory, are available on the internet. If the bean water is too thin, it can be thickened by heating slowly until it has the consistency of egg whites. If not needed for immediate use, aquafaba can be frozen, i.e., in an ice cube tray, for later use. Unsalted beans are preferred, especially for aquafaba for sweet dishes, although salted bean water can be used.[2] Aquafaba from chickpeas gets a score of 2 on the DAD scale. Great Northern or navy beans, aquafaba has a score of 1, and there is less aquafaba available in the can of beans. Aquafaba from canned pigeon peas scores 2 but is not viscous. Aquafaba from other beans gets poor ratings and should be discarded.

Now Hold On...

As can be seen in Table 12A, most canned beans only get DAD scores of about 1. Beans are supposed to be a healthy source of vegan protein, high in fiber. These DAD scores are highly disappointing for a class of foods widely considered to be a major source of healthy proteins for those on a plant-based diet. What gives?

In an assessment of six large population studies from the U.S., Europe, and Asia, with a total of over 200,000 participants, none of the studies found a statistically significant impact of legume consumption on cardiovascular disease mortality. On overall assessment, the meta-analysis found a non-significant (NS), 4% decrease in CVD mortality risk for those consuming higher amounts of legumes.[3] Another more inclusive meta-analysis of legume consumption that included 32 studies and over 1.1 million participants and 93,000 deaths, put the CVD reduction from legume consumption at 1% (NS). For coronary artery disease mortality, risk was reduced by 7% (NS), cancer mortality by 15% (NS), stroke mortality by 9%, and overall mortality by 6% among those with higher intakes of legumes.[4] Even these small risk reductions are suspect, as the dose-response curves fail to show significant benefits at higher consumption levels, and small studies, which have a higher potential for publication bias for showing positive results, impacted the outcome. (This occurs as researchers are much less likely to publish negative results from small studies than those with positive outcomes.) Another review found that legume consumption was associated with a lower risk of cardiovascular disease (CVD) and coronary heart disease (CHD) but not stroke.[5] The results are thus inconsistent across these meta-analyses.

A major weakness of these studies is that the method of preparation of the legumes was not included in most of the underlying studies, and few participants in the various studies consumed more than 50 grams of legumes per day. A "serving" of beans is generally a half cup of cooked beans (4 oz. or 90 grams); 50 grams of cooked beans supplies about 5 grams of protein. If the 50 grams refer to dry beans, it would supply about 12 grams of protein.

When evaluating the impact of legumes on health, it is important to take into account the correlates of bean consumption. Those eating more legumes generally eat less meat. It is possible that any benefits from legumes may result from the displacement of a harmful food (i.e., red meat) by one with little intrinsic impact on risk.

On the flip side, legume consumption is closely tied to food culture and may thus reflect the overall dietary pattern. Other foods or lifestyle factors among high legume-consuming cultures may overwhelm the impact of legumes on health. Consumption of beans is common among the poor (as they are inexpensive). Some cultures cook animal fat into their beans, an unhealthy practice. Those consuming higher amounts of beans often have a food pattern that is low on choline, folate, magnesium, vitamin E, and the n-3 fatty acid α-linolenic acid, all of which may lead to poorer health.[6] These factors may weaken or mask a positive association between legume consumption and health.

As emphasized in this chapter, legumes contain anti-nutritional factors; this would be expected to minimize their benefits. The DAD ratings for canned beans, which represent typical processing (cooking methods) of beans, show mediocre scores for most beans and negative scores for others. Only canned pigeon peas and navy beans got decent scores. As with grains, proper preparation greatly increases the nutritional and prebiotic benefits of legumes. When pulses are properly prepared, they are an excellent source of protein that is far better for health than meat. With proper processing, most *Phaseolus vulgaris* bean varieties can get a DAD score of 5. Thus, processing can greatly improve pulse digestibility and benefit the intestinal microbiome. Proper processing of pulses provides anti-inflammatory properties that improve GI health.

A Seed's Life

Being a successful seed is not a simple matter. It is a dangerous world when you are a nutritious morsel. Birds, insects, and other animals want to eat you even before you are ripe. Your best chance for success is to somehow get buried in the soil by being trampled by huge hoofed beasts, but at the same time, you have to avoid being squished. Then, you need to avoid germinating until the weather is right. The seed needs enough rain and soil moisture to grow, and once it germinates, it needs to grow quickly to sink its roots deep and grow tall enough to get sunlight to power its survival. If you germinate too soon, a late frost may doom you. All the while, bacteria, fungi, nematodes, and other underground wildlife would love to make a meal of you. The things that help you grow quickly, your store of proteins for growth and sugars for energy, are things that make you such a great meal.

Most seeds, such as pulses, have developed multiple survival mechanisms in order to survive. They store sugars as starches and pectins that dry hard and are indigestible. They have a tough seed coat. The seed coat contains tannins and other phenolic compounds that deter bacterial growth. Even if swallowed, they may pass through an animal's digestive system unharmed. Some beans make toxic proteins. All beans contain lectins (as do many other edible plants) that interfere with starch and protein digestion. Beans also contain digestive enzyme inhibitors and saponins that interfere with digestion, so that even if eaten, the animal gets little nutritional benefit from them. Thus, wild animals have little incentive to seek out mature seeds as food. They may eat some along the way, and may help disperse some of the seeds in their feces. But they get little nutrition from them.

Soy is used as animal feed, but needs to be processed first. Grains such as corn are fed to animals; it is typically minimally processed (cracking or coarsely grinding it), but this is like feeding the animal a Western human diet; it is a proinflammatory diet and causes obesity, insulin resistance, and other chronic diseases in the animals. A diet high in grains causes animal diseases that were not even included in veterinarian textbooks until the late 20th century, as they were just not seen before the introduction of significant amounts of grain into their feeds.[7] This is not a major problem for beef, because these animals are slaughtered at an age of only 18 to 22 months, and obesity in the beef (marbled meat) is an economic benefit for the meat producer. Cattle typically live 15 – 20 years; these feedlot animals are very young when they are harvested. Chickens that live for six or more years under natural conditions are now typically harvested at 7 to 12 weeks, and often as early as 6 weeks after hatching for meat production. These animals just don't have time to develop symptoms of chronic disease caused by their diet and sedentary lifestyle.

Pulses and cereals are important human foods only because we process them before eating them. How they are processed is important. Unfortunately, we mostly don't do a good job of it.

During cooking, water enters the cells of the bean cotyledon, the main body of the bean, and gelatinizes the starch granules. Soaking pulses in water hydrates them and causes the beans to swell, but does not make them digestible. When testing, only 2% of starches from uncooked, soaked chickpeas were digestible. Starches from other beans were more accessible, but still, only a maximum of 7% of starches from any pulse could be digested without cooking. Cooking (in water) promotes starch gelatinization, which increases the starch granules' susceptibility to hydrolysis by the digestive enzyme α-amylase.[8]

Pectin in beans is a tough storage carbohydrate. It is stabilized by the minerals magnesium (Mg^{2+}), calcium (Ca^{2+}), and other divalent cations. With hydration and cooking, some of the minerals dissociate from the pectin and go into the water. Cooking with hard water, high in magnesium and calcium, prevents the cation dissociation and prevents softening of beans during cooking. Thus, cooking with hard water can increase the cooking time and may prevent the beans from ever fully softening. Adding sodium ions to the soaking and cooking water promotes replacement of the divalent cations with monovalent sodium (Na^{+}), which weakens the pectin's bonds and softens the beans and makes them more digestible.

Hydrothermal processing (boiling pulses in water) can denature and hydrolyze much of the pulse's proteins. After the proteins get hydrated, the heat from cooking breaks the hydrogen bonds that maintain the shape of the protein, denaturing the protein. This inactivates the function of some proteins and makes it easier for digestive enzymes to cleave the covalent bonds between the amino acids that make up the protein. Hydrolysis occurs when the protein breaks a covalent bond between two amino acids in the protein, and a water molecule gets bound at the free end of the peptide. The process is quicker at higher temperatures. Many proteins, however, are resistant and do not denature with cooking, especially at low cooking temperatures.

Beans (and many other plant-based foods) contain lectins, which are proteins that bind specific polysaccharides. The lectins in some beans, such as kidney beans, are toxic and can cause severe gastrointestinal distress if it is not denatured by cooking the beans at an adequate temperature. Slow cookers (crock pots) that cook at temperatures less than 90° C do not denature the lectin phytohemagglutinin in kidney beans, and just eating several undercooked ones can cause poisoning.

Lectins in legumes can stimulate immune responses in the gastrointestinal mucosa, causing inflammation. They can increase intestinal permeability, bacterial overgrowth, and bacterial translocation from the lumen into the body.[9] It is thus important that they are cooked sufficiently and at a sufficiently high temperature. Lectins are not only present in beans, lentils, and peas; they are also present in cereals, such as wheat, barley, and rice; and in quinoa, bananas, mushrooms, and tubers such as potatoes. Not all lectins are nefarious, but the ones in legumes bind metal ions, and if not digested, have an affinity for the intestinal epithelial cells. Here, they can disrupt mucosal integrity and cause inflammation, intestinal disease, and autoimmune disease. Proper cooking can reduce lectin activity by 94 to over 99 percent.[10]

Beans also contain enzyme inhibitors, saponins, and tannins, which are antinutritional and inhibit protein and starch digestion.

Saponins have antifungal, antiviral, and antibacterial activity, and are toxic to insects, worms, and mollusks, which helps prevent the seeds from being eaten. (Good for the survival of the legumes; not good to eat.) Soy saponins increase intestinal permeability and induce distal intestinal inflammation in farmed salmon.[11] Fortunately, they don't seem to bother mammals as much. Many of the plants we eat contain saponins; lentils and some beans have high amounts. So do quinoa, licorice, and spinach. Some saponins have medicinal effects, some of which are beneficial and others not. Saponins have a soap-like property – they cause the formation of foam during cooking. Saponins in chickpea aquafaba are what allow it to form foam (see below), and this one is fine to eat. Most saponins are cleaved in the human digestive system into other molecules; some of these products may also be bioactive. The flavor of saponins is often bitter, astringent, or metallic,[12] [13] and thus often not desirable.

After cooking, the mechanical pressure (grinding the beans between one's molars or mashing the bean against the roof of one's mouth with the tongue) disintegrates the cotyledon; however, the cells remain intact and enter the digestive system as intact cells containing the nutrients. This hinders access to the nutrients. This turns out to be a feature rather than a bug, as it slows digestion and gives the pulses prolonged satiation and a low glycemic index. Surprisingly, the cell walls of the cotyledon cells remain intact during digestion. Gastric enzymes begin the digestion, and the process continues with pancreatic enzymes in the small intestine. Amylase and proteolytic enzymes permeate the legume's cell walls.[14] This allows small protein fragments (peptides) and sugars from the starches to be released from the cotyledon cells over several hours.

Tannins (polyphenols) in the seed coats of pulses can form complexes with proteins, slowing or preventing their digestion. These tannins can be leached out during processing. The seed coat of the pulse can also interfere with starch digestion.[15]

The percentage of starch and protein that is digestible is increased with longer and more intense hydrothermal processing. As might be expected, digestibility is inversely proportional to how hard and intact the legume is. Digestibility increases with cooking, up to a point where the effect plateaus; this is the full cooking time. Adequate cooking times make more protein available to the body,[16] and thus leave less protein to enter the colon and be fermented. More processing makes for a softer bean.

Mitigation of Anti-Nutritional Compounds in Pulses

Lectins are denatured by hydrolysis with soaking and boiling, as well with fermentation. Protease inhibitors are reduced by soaking, boiling, and sprouting.[17] Cooking legumes at a boiling temperature reduces lectin content by over 90%.[18] In lentils, as an example, cooking increased soluble protein content by 17% and reduced lectins by 94%, while pressure cooking resulted in complete destruction of the lectins.[19] Saponins, trypsin inhibitors, and the lectin phytohemagglutinin are heat sensitive and are nearly completely destroyed by autoclaving (cooking in a pressure cooker at 121°C (249°F).[20]

Many of the antinutritional compounds in seeds, including beans and other pulses, are in the seed coat. Phytate and tannins are reduced by soaking (leaching) and discarding the water. Beans contain α-galactosides. These small molecules consist of one molecule of galactose attached to one of an assortment of other small molecules. These α-galactosides are not digested and are fermented in the colon, inducing foul vapors and causing intestinal and social discomfort. Soaking helps by leaching out a large portion of these problematic molecules.

With soaking and boiling, a small portion of the water-soluble vitamins, minerals, sugars, and free amino acids are lost, along with the phytate, saponins, and tannins. It is a trade, but it is a trade-up. By soaking and cooking in a larger volume of water and rinsing after soaking, more water-soluble molecules are lost from the pulses, both the undesirable and the desirable. It is a beneficial trade; thus, larger volumes of soak water are better than smaller ones. Soaking also helps to convert some of the insoluble fiber into soluble fiber.[21]

Phytate levels in beans can be reduced by soaking, especially with hot water (55°C; 131°F) and long soak times;[22] however, phytate is not destroyed by cooking temperatures. Phytate is also reduced by gemination.[23]

Phytate (a.k.a. phytic acid) has long been considered

to be antinutritional. Nevertheless, phytate acts as an antioxidant and has anti-cancer effects. It inhibits the crystallization of biological calcium, and in doing so lowers the risk of cardiovascular calcification, osteoporosis, and kidney stones.[24] Women with higher dietary phytate intake have been found to have higher bone mineral density.[25] Phytate is anti-nutritional in that it binds to zinc and iron in the diet, lowering the amount available for absorption. Phytate is a concern for growing children and adolescents, and during pregnancy; even then, the concern is mostly for populations that are consuming a restricted, low-quality diet. Thus, complete avoidance of phytate is not a goal of pulse preparation.

Sprouting and Germinating Legumes

Notice: Germination can be used as a primary step in processing in most legumes, as long as the legumes are adequately cooked. Germination and sprouting increase protein availability and help diminish anti-nutritional compounds. Sprouting lowers lectin levels, but does not lower them sufficiently in some beans to make them safe to eat. Sprouting does not eliminate some toxic lectins, and thus, *most legume sprouts are not safe to eat raw*. The legume sprouts that are considered safe to eat raw are mung bean, alfalfa, lentil, and chickpea sprouts.

While most edible seeds can be sprouted and are safe to eat after adequate cooking, others are not. Lima (butter) beans and flax plants produce the toxin linamarin in their roots, which is converted into cyanide by the body. Sprouting them, thus, causes the formation of this cyanogenic toxin.

Another caution for raw seed sprouts is that they may carry bacteria (such as *E. coli* and *Salmonella*) and act as a growth medium for bacteria; thus, raw sprouts should be avoided by young children, pregnant women, and those otherwise immunocompromised.

Ideal Sprouting Conditions for Legumes

The ideal sprouting conditions for various legumes vary; higher temperatures are generally needed for those that originated in warmer climates. The soak time is longer for larger legumes and those with thicker or tougher seed coats. Older, harder legumes often take longer than fresher ones.

The optimal *sprouting* conditions for black soybeans, in terms of the development of GABA and enzymatic activation, occur with soaking the beans at 38°C for 5 hours, and then sprouting them at 28°C for 6 days.[26]

Mung beans have an optimal imbibition temperature of 30 – 35°C, soaking for 6 to 8 hours, and then germinating at 25 – 30°C, and rinsing or spraying the seeds every 12 hours on the first day and more frequently as the sprouts germinate.[27]

Chickpea germination in terms of antioxidant activity is optimized when soaked and germinated at 30°C with a soaking time of 6 hours and germination for 6 days.[28]

Several studies provide the best sprouting temperatures, but do not provide the best imbibition temperatures. These studies mostly focus on the best sprouting temperatures for seedling survival for growing crops. In an assessment for the maximum antioxidant activity of sprouted chickpeas, the optimal sprouting temperature was 33.7°C and a germination time of 171 hours; however, soaking temperature was not assessed; the legumes were soaked at 25°C for 8 hours in this study.[29] The optimal germination temperature is between 24.0 and 24.4°C for lentils and between 30 to 35°C for cowpeas.[30] [31] The peak germination temperature for peas (*Pisum sativum L.*) is at 25°C.[32]

Table 12B: Impact of Bean Preparation on DAD score

Bean Cooking Method Examples	
Canned, salted, dark red kidney beans, rinsed, water added, and cooked for 10 minutes.	A
Canned pinto beans, prepared as above	1-
Canned black beans, salted, prepared as above	1
Dry pinto beans, soaked 8 hours in water at room temperature, boiled for 50 minutes.	0
Dry pinto beans, soaked with baking soda for 8 hours at room temperature, cooked with salt for 50 minutes	2-
Dry pinto beans, blanched in boiling water with baking soda for 10 minutes, soaked in water at room temperature for 8 hours, and cooked in a pressure cooker.	3+
Dry pinto beans, "germinated" at 40°C for 8 hours, blanched in water with baking soda for 15 minutes, and cooked in a pressure cooker.	5
Dry black beans, "germinated" at 36°C for 7 hours, blanched with baking soda for 15 minutes, and cooked in a pressure cooker for 15 minutes.	5

When cooking legume seeds for the highest digestibility, we want to begin the *germination* process by increasing the production of gibberellin in the seed. Thus, our goal is to soak the seed in warm water until the seed completes the imbibition process. For most legumes, this can be done by soaking the seeds at temperatures between 30 and 40°C. Additionally, the seeds should be treated to reduce anti-nutritive saponins and tannins before cooking them to improve digestibility and protein absorption.

Method Section: Preparing Pulses

Standard home cooking methods for pulses give very unimpressive DAD scores similar to those from canned beans. Soaking provides slightly better scores. Using the SANA cooking and blanching method, most (not all) pulses can get a score of 5, as shown in Table 12B.

Cooking dry beans is more economical than canned ones and allows much more control over the processing, allowing for healthier, more digestible beans with higher ratings. Proper preparation gives outstanding results.

The SANA Method for Preparing Pulses

The SANA method is designed to optimize the digestibility and nutrient absorption of amino acids and other nutrients, and increase fiber solubility for feeding the commensal microbiome. This maximizes the DAD scores for the pulses. Most beans will get a DAD score of 5 using this method.

Step 0: Check the dry beans and cull broken and damaged ones, and eliminate any trash. I have found dirt clods and even tooth-breaking pebbles in bags of dry beans. Spread the dry legumes out and look for foreign objects and broken beans, and discard them. If your source of beans has consistently clean beans, you may be able to skip this step. In any case, rinse the dry pulses in a pot of clean water as many times as needed for the water to be clear.

Step 1: Soak (germinate) the pulses in water at 35 to 40°C (95 to 104°F) for 7 – 12 hours. This can be done in a yogurt maker or slow cooker with a yogurt setting. The maximum recommended temperature for soaking is 40°C (104°F); above this, the temperature impedes the germination process. With warmer temperatures, slightly less time is required. After soaking, rinse the pulses. Black beans take about 7 hours; lentils need about 11 hours.

While not required, aeration of the soak water helps optimize germination, improving digestibility. This can be done by bubbling fine air bubbles into the water using an aquarium aerator using food-safe silicone tubing. This is especially helpful when using warmer temperatures, as warmer water holds less oxygen. Aeration reduces the soak time required and improves digestibility further.

Note that aeration of pulses during soaking helps remove saponins but causes the formation of foam that can overflow and cause a mess. If using aeration, use a sufficiently sized vessel to accommodate the foam.

At completion of the germination step, drain the soaking water and rinse the legumes twice.

Step 2: Blanching. Boil a minimum of four volumes of water with 5 g of sodium bicarbonate (SB; a.k.a. baking soda) per liter (1 tsp./quart) for each volume of dry legumes that were soaked. Once the solution boils, remove it from the heat. When boiling has stopped, add the pulses and cover them. Allow them to steep at least ten minutes but no more than 20 minutes. Drain the pulses and then rinse them. Alternatively, SB (5 grams/liter) can be added to the soak/germination water for the final 1 – 2 hours of soaking. Blanching is described below.

Step 3: Cook the pulses as typical for that type of legume. Salt (¼ to ½ tsp.) per cup of dry legumes can be added to improve the flavor and firmness of the bean. Use of a stainless steel pressure cooker is recommended.

An example of best practices for preparing black beans is to soak clean, rinsed beans for 8 hours at 36° C (97° F) with aeration, followed by blanching by adding SB to the warm soak solution for the final hour. The beans are rinsed and then pressure-cooked for 15 minutes with natural pressure release.

Seed Coat Processing (Blanching)

Sodium bicarbonate (SB) (baking soda) or other agents are sometimes used in the soaking water for beans to decrease the required soaking time to hydrate beans. The principal purpose of its use is to reduce cooking time and energy cost for commercial food processors. Kidney bean hydration at 30°C with a 1.5% concentration of sodium bicarbonate decreases the required soak time to hydrate beans considerably. Sodium bicarbonate helps to replace calcium ions in the pectin, which weakens it, and makes the seed coat more permeable to water. The increased pH from SB causes ionization of amino acid side chains in the seed coat proteins, weakening their structure.[33] The alkalinity of the soak water also promotes the release of tannins from the seed coat.

Using a weaker 0.5% SB solution to soak legumes has been found not only to increase hydration, but to increase protein and fiber, while reducing carbohydrates, including starch, stachyose, and raffinose. Stachyose and raffinose are non-digestible sugars that ferment in the colon GI discomfort and "foul winds". The SB treatment also reduces anti-nutritional factors such as trypsin inhibitor and hemagglutinin activity, and phytic acid and tannin levels.[34] In a study of velvet beans, soaking the beans in an SB solution followed by pressure cooking increased protein digestibility by 187 to 201%, while lowering raffinose by 76–82%, stachyose by 77%, verbascose by 75–76%, and tannins by 74–84%.[35] In an assessment of sodium hydroxide, sodium carbonate, and sodium bicarbonate, SB was most effective at extracting tannins and in denaturing trypsin inhibitors, while sodium carbonate was more effective in promoting the breakdown of phytates in beans.[36]

Blanching

Blanching the seed coats of pulses is an important step in preparing them to provide the most favorable health benefits. Most of the research on processing pulses, including the use of sodium bicarbonate, has not been concerned with digestibility, but has rather focused on processing time for commercial canning operations to save on energy costs. These processes typically use 1 to 2% sodium bicarbonate (SB; baking soda), which is 10 to 20 grams per liter, or about 1 to 2 tsp. per quart. When chefs use baking soda for soaking or cooking beans, their concern is to have tasty, attractive, intact beans with a buttery consistency. They generally recommend ¼ tsp per quart of water and often also add salt. Cooking beans with too much baking soda can give them a soapy taste.

For the SANA diet, blanching with baking soda is recommended as an alkali treatment to improve digestibility and nutrition, but also takes organoleptics (flavor and aroma), texture, and ease of preparation into consideration. The purpose is to blanch the seed coat, removing tannins, saponins, and other anti-nutritive elements to make the beans more digestible. Beans with a tougher seed coat may take a longer blanching time. The goal of the blanching is to blanch the seed coat but leave the cotyledons alone. This explains why blanching is not needed for dal, as there is no seed coat to treat.

Legumes can be "Cold blanched" by soaking them at room temperature with baking soda. The seed coat (outer shell) and the cotyledon (the fleshy part inside the bean) will be softened if soaking is done with baking soda. SB creates an alkaline environment that weakens pectin in the legume by exchanging calcium and magnesium ions in the pectin that resist hydration with sodium ions. Baking soda is alkaline, while beans are naturally acidic. The baking soda raises the pH of the soaking water, which helps break down the cell walls of the beans, making them softer faster. This allows water to penetrate the bean more easily, further aiding softening. Adding baking soda to the soaking water for beans helps soften the beans and makes them creamier. Some cooks add about 1.25 grams of baking soda per liter of water, or about ¼ tsp. per quart of the soaking water, but cooking or soaking with too much baking soda can give a soapy flavor to the beans.

A preferred *non-germination* blanching method is to use 6 volumes of water for each volume of dry pulses. Add one level teaspoon of baking soda per quart of water (5 mg/L) to prepare a 0.5% solution. Bring the water with the baking soda to a boil and turn off the heat. When the boiling stops, add the pulses to the pot of hot water and cover the pot to retain the heat, and set a timer for 15 minutes. Since the pulses are not boiling, the saponins will not foam, and there should not be any risk of the water boiling over. There will be no boiling motion to break or disintegrate the beans. Blanching can also be done in a boiling SB-solution with but this can cause foaming and break the seed coat, resulting in beans that may cook unevenly.

During blanching, the legumes may float to the top of the hot water. For many legumes, the seed coat will expand and get wrinkly, and especially for pigmented legumes, the blanching water will darken considerably. When done, if you take a seed, let it cool for several seconds, and then squeeze it, the cotyledon should slip out easily, and may even "shoot out" like shooting a watermelon seed. When ready, the seed coat will be softer and tear easily. When the seed coat slips, the water is dark, but the cotyledon has little or no swelling, the blanching is complete. Drain off the water and rinse the legumes at least twice so that the rinse water is clear; the legumes are then ready to be soaked and cooked.

While blanching can be effectively done during or before soaking pulses, the use of high-temperature water kills the germ and denatures enzymes in the seed, thus preventing the germination effects on the seed. Soaking in an alkaline environment also impedes germination. Thus, neither hot nor cold pre-soak blanching are preferred method for the SANA diet.

Recommended Blanching Methods: The SANA preferred time for blanching pulses is after germination of the seeds in warm water, rather than before soaking.

The preferred SANA method is to blanch the seed coats at the end of the germination process. This can be done by either adding SB (1 tsp. /quart, 5 g/L) to make a 0.5% SB solution for the germination soak for the last hour, or by blanching the germinated legumes in a very hot SB solution. This method is the same as for hot blanching before soaking: Boil 6 volumes of water for each volume of dry pulses. Add one level teaspoon of baking soda per quart of water (5 mg/L) to prepare a 0.5% solution. Bring the water with the baking soda to a boil and turn off the heat. When the boiling stops, add the germinated and rinsed pulses to the pot of hot water and cover the pot to retain the heat, and set a timer for 15 minutes. After blanching, discard the blanching water and rinse the legumes two to three times so that the rinse water is clear.

Cooking Beans:

The cooking time of beans depends on multiple factors, including the growing environment, storage conditions and time, and genetics of the strain of bean. Generally, smaller beans have a shorter cooking time, but even beans of the same size can be easy (fast) or hard to cook (requiring long cooking times. The thickness of the seed coat and the degree of insolubility of the cell walls of this are genetically determined. Soaking beans has its greatest impact on the seed coat, with less impact on impact on the cooking time of the cotyledon.[37]

- If you don't already own one, consider getting a stainless steel pressure cooker. It will help save time, generally lowering the cooking time by two-thirds. A typical pressure cooker cooks at a pressure of 15 psi and a temperature around 250°F (121°C), which is hotter than boiling water (212°F or 100°C); however, less heat is lost to steam escaping into the room. This higher temperature helps hydrolyze proteins, making them more digestible. Using a pressure cooker is also much quicker, uses less energy, and keeps your house cooler and less humid in the summer. When using the pressure cooker, after getting to temperature, the heat should be lowered so that the heat just maintains the pressure and limited venting of steam. "Natural release" is preferred, meaning turning the heat off at the end of the cooking time and allowing the pot to cool on its own until the pressure seal relaxes.
- The lower cooking time on the time chart (Table 12D) should give denser, more intact legumes, while the upper bound will give softer and often broken beans, which are fine for making pureed, creamed, or refried beans.
- If one is going to cook dry pulses, one might as well cook a few meals' worth at a time. They keep for several days refrigerated, and alternatively can be frozen after cooking for later use.
- Properly prepared pulses will have a buttery texture and digest better.
- Beans should absorb enough water during soaking and germination to reach about 80% of their final cooked mass.[38 39 40]
- Pulses are likely to foam up, especially at the onset of cooking. This can cause the pot to overflow, creating a mess, and can clog the pressure release vent on the pressure cooker, which can cause a mess and even injury. This is especially a problem if cooking a large amount of dal. Don't overfill the pressure cooker (above the 2/3rds line). The foam is caused by saponins and proteins in the pulses. Foaming can be managed by keeping the boiling on the minimal heat level needed to maintain a boil. This also has a slower release of the proteins and saponins. When boiling in a cooking pot, the foam can be skimmed off and removed. Soaking and blanching with baking soda helps reduce saponins and thus decreases foaming during cooking. Pulses will foam up during soaking if a bubbler is used for aeration. (Make sure the pot is large enough not to overflow.) Pressure cooking is more effective for breaking down saponins than regular boiling.
- Avoid old beans or those with many seeds with broken seed coats, as they may be hard to cook, and you can end up with a mix of hard and mushy beans in the same pot. It's better to buy smaller bags of beans from a store with a high turnover and use them over the next few months than to be a prepper and buy large bags to last a year or more. If the bag does not look fresh in the store, the beans may have sat for a long time. Old beans (more than several months since harvest) may need longer soak times.[41]
- Cooking the legumes with salt and spices will bring those flavors into the beans.[42] Cooking with salt helps keep the legume more solid. If making bean paste or lentil soup, for example, add salt and seasoning after cooking the legumes. Salt can be added before or after cooking, but adding salt to the cooking water will increase cooking time.
- Foul Winds: Both soaking and pressure cooking beans lower the amounts of raffinose, α-galactosides, and other large sugars moderately. These sugars are not digested, but rather fermented in the lower intestine, and cause farting.
- Introducing small amounts of pulses to the diet multiple times a week, and slowly increasing the

amount consumed, will help train your gut and microbiome to deal with them and allay unpleasantness.[43] Begin with the beans that are the gentlest on the gut before trying the more challenging ones. (Dals, pigeon peas, navy, great northern beans), In most people, flatulence improves after 3 – 4 weeks of a change in diet to include beans.[44]

- Not all legumes earn the same DAD rating as others. Some are easier to digest than others. Additional aspects likely impact their ratings, including the toughness of the seed coat or if it is removed, as it is for dal. Some beans have thicker, more resilient seed coats (skin) than others. Some pulse cotyledons are more gut-friendly and nutritious than others. Pre-germination and blanching greatly improve the digestibility of these legumes.
- Kidney beans, and to a lesser extent, white beans, contain a toxin (phytohemagglutinin) that is broken down at cooking temperatures over 90°C. Eating kidney beans that have been slow-cooked in a crockpot at lower temperatures can cause poisoning.
- Note: If you have very hard water, high in minerals, it may take more soaking time, or the beans may never soften.
- Longer soaking and cooking times increase digestibility and make for a softer bean. Note that it is not difficult to overprocess beans so that they begin to disintegrate. This is fine for some dishes, but not for others.

Notes

- Take notes when you cook pulses, so that you can perfect the cooking time for the type of bean you are cooking and the outcome you are looking for. The table should get you close, but it should be considered a rough guideline.
- If the pulses are hard or gritty at the end of cooking, they are improperly cooked.
- When properly processing pulses to increase their digestibility and health benefits, a lot of color may go down the drain with the soaking, cooking, or blanching water. Expect this. The color from red kidney beans can be used to dye cotton a ruddy brown.
- There are a lot of different pulses. Some beans are "Hard-to-Cook" (HTC) using the academic lingo of bean experts. Any bean type can be HTC depending on its genetics, growing, and storage conditions. Some kidney beans are HTC, while others are not. Thus, the soaking and cooking times can vary considerably, even from one batch of kidney beans to another. Longer soak times will generally be more reliable. The downside to pressure cookers is that one cannot easily tell how well-cooked the beans are during the cooking process. Undercooked beans can be reheated to cook longer, but overcooked ones don't turn around.
- Chickpea salvation: Canned chickpeas get a DAD rating of zero. This legume, however, is dense enough to withstand post-processing. They can be blanched. After draining the aquafaba, bring the chickpeas to a boil in a saucepan with 1 tsp. of baking soda per quart of water. Cook them at a low boil for five minutes. Discard the water, and rinse the peas. The chickpeas will now get a rating of 2. This can be tried with other canned beans, and it should improve their score somewhat. Using a low boil will help keep the beans intact as compared to a vigorous boil.
- Bitter beans: If lima (butter) beans are bitter, do not eat them. They may contain the cyanide-producing compound linamarin.
- Lima beans (fresh or dry) get a poor DAD score (barely a one) even after best practice processing. There are better choices, and thus, are not recommended on the DAD diet.
- Properly processed pulses will taste very similar to traditionally prepared ones. If testing them side-by-side, the main difference will be that the properly prepared pulses may have a softer and more friable seed coat. They are also likely to have a smoother, creamier texture.
- Most pulses can get a DAD score of 5 if properly prepared. Lima beans do not.
- Table 12C provides suggested cooking times for several common pulses, using a pressure cooker. All times are for pre-soaked pulses, using 15 lbs. PSI, and "natural release". Natural release means that the heat is turned off and the vessel is allowed to cool on its own until the pressure drops. For "quick release" (where the pot is put under cool water to drop the pressure more quickly, for example), add about 3 to 4 minutes to the cooking time. The water volume is the recommended volume of water per 1 cup, or ½ pound of pulses.

As a rule of thumb:

- One pound of dried beans = 2 cups of dried beans = yields about 6 cups of cooked beans.

✹ These cooking times are intended as general starting points; understand that the times will likely need to be adapted to the beans, your cooking situation, and your preferences. If the beans are older or your water is hard, cooking times may be longer. If you want to have intact, firm beans, you should select the lower end of the cooking time range; if you want to make a bean paste, use a longer cooking time and a bit more water.

Dal

"Pease porridge hot, pease porridge cold, Pease porridge in the pot, nine days old."

Dals are pulses whose seed coats have been mechanically processed to remove the seed coat, and the two cotyledons are generally split from the other. Since the seed coat is gone, there is no need for blanching, and most types of dal do not *require* soaking. Even so, soaking is advised, especially for chana dal (split chickpeas), as it will both speed up cooking time and give a creamier result. After soaking, rinse the dal; this will decrease foaming and lower the content of saponins. The soaking time required is shorter for dals than for the intact pulse, but the cotyledon should still be translucent all the way through when breaking one at the end of the soak time. Most importantly, soaking can increase the DAD score.

Dals, including split peas, mostly get scores of 4 with typical cooking, as their seed coat has been removed and they are fully cooked into a paste, helping them to be more easily digested.

Table 12C: Typical Dal cooking and soaking times

Indian Name	English Name	Soak Time	Pressure Cooking Time minutes	Boiling Time minutes
Toor Dal (Arhar Dal)	Pigeon Pea	0 – 2 hours	10 – 12 minutes	25 – 30
Chana Dal (soaked)	Split Chickpeas	6 – 24 hours	10 – 12 minutes	40 – 45
Moong Dal (Yellow)	Yellow Mung Beans	0 – 1 hour	6 – 8 minutes	20 – 25
Urad Dal (Black Gram)	Black Lentils	0 – 1 hour	10 – 12 minutes	25 – 30
Masoor Dal	Red Lentils	0 – 1 hour	6 – 8 minutes	20 – 25
Split Peas	Split Peas	0 – 1 hour	10 – 12 minutes	40 – 45

Since the dal turns into "pease porridge," it can be salted and spiced to taste after the main cooking is done, in contrast to whole legumes, in which flavorings are best cooked into the legume. Adding salt to cooking water delays cooking and keeps the cotyledons intact, which is undesirable for dal, as the goal is to make them into a paste. The cooking of dal is sped up with a pressure cooker, but there is less difference in cooking time as compared to whole pulses.

If presoaked, try 1 2/3 cups of water to each 1 cup of chana dal or toor dal. Soaking chana dal for 4 – 6 hours is considered to help with digestion, but overlong soaking, more than 12 hours, will cause them to lose flavor. Start the soak with hot (50°C/122°F) water. Soaking may decrease the foaming of dal during cooking.

The SANA method: Even though dal cannot be sprouted, the cotyledons still contain the enzymes for germination. Thus, "germination" in warm water, using the same methods as for intact pulses, is recommended. Blanching is, however, not needed. If aeration is used during soaking, it will cause considerable foaming. Thus, use an adequately sized vessel. Foaming can also be diminished by changing out the soaking water during the germination process. Rinse the dal after soaking to further reduce saponins before cooking it.

Split peas are sometimes cooked for use in salad by boiling them for just 20 minutes so that they remain intact. This is not recommended, as they remain undercooked and harder to digest. A better choice is to use fresh peas or frozen peas that have been lightly steamed.

Other Processes for Pulses

There are several methods beyond soaking and cooking for processing pulses to remove antinutritional and toxic compounds and make them more digestible. These include sprouting, fermentation, ultrasound, chemical, and mechanical treatments.

Mechanical Processing: Textured Vegetable Protein, which is used to make veggie-burgers, is mechanically processed from defatted soy flour.

Fermentation is a traditional method of processing pulses. In Japan, soy is fermented and made into miso, tempeh, and natto.

Tofu

Tofu is coagulated soy milk, with the resulting curds pressed into a solid block. It is something like bean cheese. Tofu gets a score of 4 on the DAD scale and is a great source of vegan protein, and its consumption is associated with a lower incidence of breast cancer. Yogurt made from soy milk is discussed in Chapter 16.

Recommendations:

- Extra-dense tofu has more structure and is more fun to eat. It is made by putting more pressure on the block of tofu as it is made, which eliminates more water. Although a bit more expensive, it has a higher protein content, so that the actual cost per gram of protein is typically lower than for regular tofu.
- Tofu has a DAD score of 4; nonetheless, its digestibility can be further increased and its antigenicity decreased by steaming it in a pressure cooker for 15 minutes (with natural release). This also increases the density a bit more. Place it on a stainless steel steamer tray in the pressure cooker with water beneath.

Recipes

Split Pea Soup

Recommended Pease Porridge Preparation (DAD score 4)

1. Rinse the split peas in cool tap water three or four times and drain off the water.
2. Soak the split peas in 5 volumes of water (Five cups of water for each cup of rice). Use ½ tsp. of salt per quart. The salt will help keep the grains from becoming mushy later when the peas are cooked. Soak for at least 6 hours. When fully hydrated, if you break a cotyledon, you can see that it is soaked through.
3. Discard the soaking water, and rinse the peas three times. The rinse water should be clear. Drain off the rinse water.
4. Cooking: Cook the soaked split peas with 2 cups of water for every cup of peas you started with. Add ¼ tsp. of salt for each two cups of water.
   a. If you want intact cotyledons, bring the split peas to a boil. Skim off the foam and discard it. Cook for 20 – 25 minutes until they are the consistency you want. (These peas barely have a score of 3.) If using a pressure cooker, try 7 minutes of cook time with natural release.
   b. For soup, pease porridge, or sauce, pressure cook the peas for 16 minutes, with natural release. The peas should be creamy like soft pudding and flavorful without any grit. There may be some water on top, in the pressure cooker, but it should blend in with adding condiments and thicken. (DADA score of 4)
5. Add sautéed onions and garlic, and season to taste. Grated or shredded aged Parmesan cheese can be used as a topping when served.

Sauteed Tofu with Mushrooms

Begin by steaming extra-dense tofu in a pressure cooker for 15 minutes. After it cools, lay the tofu on its side and slice it in both directions in 1 cm sections so that it forms rectangular cubes that are about 1 x 1 x 4 cm.

Dice a quarter of a red onion and finely chop half of a clove of garlic, and then gently sauté them in one to two tsp. of coconut oil. Coconut oil has a low smoke temperature, so keep the heat low. Green onions and plum tomatoes can also be sautéed. When the onions are nearly ready, add about 1/3 cup of sliced baby bella mushrooms and sauté them. Then sauté the tofu. A pinch of salt can be added.

Mock Tuna Salad

Mock tuna salad, made from chickpeas, is tasty. Adding nori (seaweed sheets used for sushi) gives it a hint of sea. Nice as a summer dish or in a sandwich.

- 1 cup cooked or sprouted chickpeas (garbanzo beans)
- 1 tablespoon mayonnaise or mayo substitute
- 1 finely chopped scallion
- 1 sheet of nori
- 2 small sweet pickles
- salt to taste

If using canned garbanzos, drain them; the aquafaba can be set aside for other uses. Mash the chickpeas or use a food processor. I suggest leaving some of the chickpeas "chunky".

Vegan Mayonnaise

Ingredients:

- ¼ cup chickpea aquafaba (from a can of chickpeas)
- 1 tablespoon lemon juice
- 1 tablespoon apple cider vinegar
- ¼ teaspoon salt
- ¼ teaspoon ground turmeric (for a subtle yellow color, optional)
- ½ cup to ¾ cup coconut oil

Instructions: Whisk the chickpea aquafaba, lemon juice, apple cider vinegar, salt, and turmeric (if using) together. The aquafaba should be at room temperature before using to help with emulsification.

Slowly blend the oil in at low speed. Start at the bottom of the container if using an immersion blender. Slowly drizzle in the chosen oil, a very thin stream at first, then gradually increasing to a thin stream as the mixture thickens. Be patient, and drizzle slowly, as it is key to creating a stable emulsion. Adding it too quickly can prevent the mixture from emulsifying properly. Keep blending until the mixture becomes thick and creamy. This can take 1-2 minutes, depending on your blender's power.

Coconut oil will solidify slightly when chilled, making a firmer mayonnaise. Soy oil will create a lighter and more spreadable consistency. Choose or mix, based on your preference.

Taste the vegan mayo and adjust seasonings as needed. You can add a pinch more salt or a touch more vinegar for a brighter flavor. Store your mayonnaise in an airtight container in the refrigerator for up to two weeks. Since the vegan mayo does not contain uncooked egg yolks, it is less likely to spoil and from salmonella than regular homemade mayonnaise, but it does not contain preservatives, and thus has a limited refrigerated shelf life. Thus, it is best to make small batches that will be used within a short time. Aquafaba can be frozen and used when needed.

Table 12D: Suggested Cook Times. (Please refer to the text) Water volume is per cup of pulses.

Pulse	Methods 1 /2 Blanche Time Est. (Minutes)	Cooking Water per Cup	Soak Time (Hours)	Natural Release minutes (Lower)	Natural Release minutes (Upper)	Traditional Boiling Method (Minutes)
Aduki/Adzuki beans	6	4	4 to 6	6	8	50 to 60
Anasazi beans	5	3	4 to 8	5	7	50 to 60
Appaloosa beans	8	3	4 to 8	8	12	60 to 90
Black beans	4	4	6 to 8	4	7	75 to 90
Borlotti beans	7	3	6 to 8	7	10	45 to 60
Butter beans (Avoid)	3	4	10 to 12	3	5	60 to 90
Calypso beans	6	3	6 to 8	6	8	60 to 90
Cannellini beans	6	3	6 to 8	6	9	60 to 90
Chickpeas (garbanzo bean)	5	4	12 to 24	14	19	120 to 240
Corona runner	9	4	6 to 8	9	12	60 to 90
Cranberry beans	7	3	6 to 9	7	10	45 to 60
European Soldier beans	8	3	6 to 8	8	11	60 to 90
Flageolet beans	10	3	4 to 8	10	14	120 to 150
Great Northern beans	6	4	6 to 8	8	11	90 to 120
Kidney beans	9	3	6 to 8	9	14	60 to 90
Lentils, brown	5	4	NR	1	2	20 to 30
Lima, baby	6	4	8 to 10	2	3	50 to 60
Lima, Christmas	6	4	8 to 10	7	10	60 to 90
Lima, large	6	4	8 to 10	3	4	45 to 60
Mayocoba, Canary beans	8	4	8 to 24	8	12	60 to 90
Navy beans (white, haricot)	6	3	8 to 10	7	10	90 to 120
Peas, whole (dried)	4	6	12 24	4	6	60 to 90
Pigeon peas, Guandules (Dry)	7 / 20	3	8 to 10	7	11	30 to 45
Pink beans	6	3	6 to 8	6	10	50 to 90
Pinto beans	6	3	6 to 8	6	8	60 to 90
Red beans, small	4	2	6 to 8	4	6	60 to 90
Romano beans	7	3	4 to 8	7	10	45 to 60
Scarlet runner beans	9	4	10 to 24	9	12	180 to 240
Small red beans	4	2	6 to 8	4	6	60 to 90
Soy beans (black)	15	4	12 to 24	16	24	180 to 240
Soy beans (yellow)	10	4	12 to 24	10	14	120 to 180

NR: not required.

[1] Dietary Intake Among US Adults, 1999-2012. Rehm CD, Peñalvo JL, Afshin A, Mozaffarian D. JAMA. 2016 Jun 21;315(23):2542-53. doi: 10.1001/jama.2016.7491. PMID: 27327801

[2] Evaluation of Textural and Microstructural Properties of Vegan Aquafaba Whipped Cream from Chickpeas, Nguyen T.M.N., Quoc L.P.T., Tran G.B., 2021, Chemical Engineering Transactions, 83, 421-426.

[3] Legume Consumption and All-Cause and Cardiovascular Disease Mortality. Li H, Li J, Shen Y, Wang J, Zhou D. Biomed Res Int. 2017;2017:8450618. doi: 10.1155/2017/8450618. Epub 2017 Nov 2. PMID: 29230416

[4] Legume Consumption and Risk of All-Cause and Cause-Specific Mortality: A Systematic Review and Dose-Response Meta-Analysis of Prospective Studies. Zargarzadeh N, Mousavi SM, Santos HO, Aune D, Hasani-Ranjbar S, Larijani B, Esmaillzadeh A. Adv Nutr. 2023 Jan;14(1):64-76. doi: 10.1016/j.advnut.2022.10.009. Epub 2023 Jan 5. PMID: 36811595

[5] Intake of legumes and cardiovascular disease: A systematic review and dose-response meta-analysis. Mendes V, Niforou A, Kasdagli MI, Ververis E, Naska A. Nutr Metab Cardiovasc Dis. 2023 Jan;33(1):22-37. doi: 10.1016/j.numecd.2022.10.006. Epub 2022 Oct 21. PMID: 36411221

[6] Adult dietary patterns with increased bean consumption are associated with greater overall shortfall nutrient intakes, lower added sugar, improved weight-related outcomes and better diet quality. Papanikolaou Y, Slavin J, Fulgoni VL 3rd. Nutr J. 2024 Mar 20;23(1):36. doi: 10.1186/s12937-024-00937-1. PMID: 38504300

[7] https://theequinepractice.com/why-horses-should-not-be-fed-grain/

[8] Effects of Hydrothermal Processing Duration on the Texture, Starch and Protein In Vitro Digestibility of Cowpeas, Chickpeas and Kidney Beans. Khrisanapant P, Leong SY, Kebede B, Oey I. Foods. 2021 Jun 18;10(6):1415. doi: 10.3390/foods10061415. PMID: 34207291

[9] Sucrose co-administration reduces the toxic effect of lectin on gut permeability and intestinal bacterial colonization. Ramadass B, Dokladny K, Moseley PL, Patel YR, Lin HC. Dig Dis Sci. 2010 Oct;55(10):2778-84. doi: 10.1007/s10620-010-1359-2. Epub 2010 Aug 5. PMID: 20686845

[10] Naturally Occurring Plant Food Toxicants and the Role of Food Processing Methods in Their Detoxification. Urugo MM, Tringo TT. Int J Food Sci. 2023 Apr 27;2023:9947841. doi: 10.1155/2023/9947841. eCollection 2023. PMID: 37153649

[11] Dietary soya saponins increase gut permeability and play a key role in the onset of soyabean-induced enteritis in Atlantic salmon (Salmo salar L.). Knudsen D, Jutfelt F, Sundh H, Sundell K, Koppe W, Frøkiaer H. Br J Nutr. 2008 Jul;100(1):120-9. doi: 10.1017/S0007114507886338. Epub 2008 Jan 2. PMID: 18167174

[12] Saponins: A concise review on food related aspects, applications and health implications. Sharma K, et al. Food Chemistry Advances, Vol 2, 2023. https://doi.org/10.1016/j.focha.2023.100191.

[13] Perspectives on Saponins: Food Functionality and Applications. Timilsena YP, Phosanam A, Stockmann R. Int J Mol Sci. 2023 Aug 31;24(17):13538. doi: 10.3390/ijms241713538. PMID: 37686341; PMCID: PMC10487995.

[14] A mechanistic model to study the effect of the cell wall on starch digestion in intact cotyledon cells. Rovalino-Córdova AM, Aguirre Montesdeoca V, Capuano E. Carbohydr Polym. 2021 Feb 1;253:117351. doi: 10.1016/j.carbpol.2020.117351. Epub 2020 Nov 5. PMID: 33278961

[15] How Cooking Time Affects In Vitro Starch and Protein Digestibility of Whole Cooked Lentil Seeds versus Isolated Cotyledon Cells. Duijsens D, Verkempinck SHE, De Coster A, Pälchen K, Hendrickx M, Grauwet T. Foods. 2023 Jan 24;12(3):525. doi: 10.3390/foods12030525. PMID: 36766054

[16] The Effect of Processing on Digestion of Legume Proteins. Drulyte D, Orlien V. Foods. 2019 Jun 24;8(6):224. doi: 10.3390/foods8060224. PMID: 31238515

[17] https://www.healthline.com/nutrition/how-to-reduce-antinutrients#TOC_TITLE_HDR_8

[18] Effect of Soaking and Cooking on Dietary Fibre, Protein and Lectins of Rajmash (Phaseolus vulgaris) Beans Hina Vasishtha, RP Srivastava, 31 Dec 2013. Indian Journal of Agricultural Biochem. Vol. 27, Iss: 2, pp 219-222

[19] Srivastava, Rp and Hina Vasishtha. "Dietary fiber, protein and lectin contents of lentils (Lens culinaris) with soaking and cooking." Current Advances in Agricultural Sciences 5 (2013): 238-241.

[20] Effect of processing on antinutrients and in vitro protein digestibility of kidney bean (Phaseolus vulgaris L.) varieties grown in East Africa. Emire Admassu Shimelis, Sudip Kumar Rakshit. Food Chemistry 103(1)161-172, 2007, https://doi.org/10.1016/j.foodchem.2006.08.005

[21] Soaking and cooking modify the alpha-galacto-oligosaccharide and dietary fibre content in five Mediterranean legumes. Njoumi S, Josephe Amiot M, Rochette I, Bellagha S, Mouquet-Rivier C. Int J Food Sci Nutr. 2019 Aug;70(5):551-561. doi: 10.1080/09637486.2018.1544229. Epub 2019 Jan 7. PMID: 30614326

[22] Phytate Reduction in Brown Beans (Phaseolus vulgaris L.) E-L. GUSTAFSSON, A-S. SANDBERG, Food Science, 60(1)149-152, Jan. 1995. https://doi.org/10.1111/j.1365-2621.1995.tb05626.x

[23] Phytic acid, in vitro protein digestibility, dietary fiber, and minerals of pulses as influenced by processing methods. Chitra U, Singh U, Rao PV. Plant Foods Hum Nutr. 1996 Jun;49(4):307-16. doi: 10.1007/BF01091980. PMID: 8983057

[24] Phytates as a natural source for health promotion: A critical evaluation of clinical trials. Pires SMG, Reis RS, Cardoso SM, Pezzani R, Paredes-Osses E, Seilkhan A, Ydyrys A, Martorell M, Sönmez Gürer E, Setzer WN, Abdull Razis AF, Modu B, Calina D, Sharifi-Rad J. Front

Chem. 2023 Apr 14;11:1174109. doi: 10.3389/fchem.2023.1174109. eCollection 2023. PMID: 37123871

25 Estimated Phytate Intake Is Associated with Bone Mineral Density in Mediterranean Postmenopausal Women. Sanchis P, Prieto RM, Konieczna J, Grases F, Abete I, Salas-Salvadó J, Martín V, Ruiz-Canela M, Babio N, García-Gavilán JF, Goday A, Costa-Bauza A, Martínez JA, Romaguera D. Nutrients. 2023 Apr 6;15(7):1791. doi: 10.3390/nu15071791. PMID: 37049631

26 Sprouting Condition Optimization Based on Protease Activity and GABA of Black Soybean. Yu-zhi, J. (2009). Food Science.

27 Method for producing mung bean sprout. Hua Yefeng, 23 Feb 2016, Chinese patent: CN101731133A

28 Kim Sung Mi, Aung Thinzar, Kim Mi Jeong. Optimization of germination conditions to enhance the antioxidant activity in chickpea (Cicer arietimum L.) using response surface methodology. Korean J. Food Preserv. 2022;29(4):632-644. https://doi.org/10.11002/kjfp.2022.29.4.632

29 Optimal germination condition impacts on the antioxidant activity and phenolic acids profile in pigmented desi chickpea (*Cicer arietinum* L.) seeds. Domínguez-Arispuro DM, Cuevas-Rodríguez EO, Milán-Carrillo J, León-López L, Gutiérrez-Dorado R, Reyes-Moreno C. J Food Sci Technol. 2018 Feb;55(2):638-647. doi: 10.1007/s13197-017-2973-1. Epub 2017 Nov 25. PMID: 29391628

30 The Influence of Temperature on Seed Germination Rate in Grain Legumes: I. A COMPARISON OF CHICKPEA, LENTIL, SOYABEAN AND COWPEA AT CONSTANT TEMPERATURES S. COVELL, R. H. ELLIS, E. H. ROBERTS and R. J. SUMMERFIELD Journal of Experimental Botany. Vol. 37, No. 178 (May 1986), pp. 705-715 https://www.jstor.org/stable/23691498.

31 Optimal temperature for germination and seedling development of cowpea seeds. Juliane, Rafaele, Alves, Barros., Francislene, Angelotti., Jéssica, de, Oliveira, Santos., Rodrigo, Moura, e, Silva., Bárbara, França, Dantas., Natoniel, Franklin, de, Melo. 14 (2020).:231-239. doi: 10.17584/RCCH.2020V14I2.10339

32 Optimizing Water, Temperature, and Density Conditions for In Vitro Pea (Pisum sativum L.) Germination. Zoltán, Kende., Petra, Piroska., Gabriella, Erzsébet, Szemők., Hussein, M., Khaeim., Asma, Haj, Sghaier., Csaba, Gyuricza., Ákos, Tarnawa. Plants, 13 (2024).:2776-2776. doi: 10.3390/plants13192776

33 Modelling the Hydration kinetics of kidney beans (Phaseolus vulgaris) in sodium salts using Response surface methodology. Agarwal, N. et al. (2020). Journal of Applied and Natural Science, 12 (1): 42 – 52 https://doi.org/10.31018/jans.v12i1.2234

34 Effect of soaking process on nutritional quality and protein solubility of some legume seeds. T., A., El-Adawy., E., H., Rahma., A., A., El-Bedawy., T., Y., Sobihah. Nahrung-food, 44 (2000).:339-343. doi: 10.1002/1521-3803(20001001)44:5<339::AID-FOOD339>3.0.CO;2-T

35 Effect of soaking in sodium bicarbonate solution followed by autoclaving on the nutritional and antinutritional properties of velvet bean seeds. Vadivel V, Pugalenthi M. (2009). Journal of Food Processing and Preservation, 33(1):60-73. doi: 10.1111/J.1745-4549.2008.00237.X

36 Effect of alkali treatments on the nutritive value of common bean (Phaseolus vulgaris). Jyothi V, Sumathi S. Plant Foods Hum Nutr. 1995 Oct;48(3):193-200. doi: 10.1007/BF01088440. PMID: 8833425

37 Genetic variability of cooking time in dry beans (Phaseolus vulgaris L.) related to seed coat thickness and the cotyledon cell wall. Bassett A, Hooper S, Cichy K. Food Res Int. 2021 Mar;141:109886. doi: 10.1016/j.foodres.2020.109886. Epub 2020 Nov 10. PMID: 33641942

38 Effect of Soaking and Cooking on Nutritional and Quality Properties of Faba Bean Waleed Mohamed Abdel-Aleem et al, Nutri Food Sci Int J 9(3): NFSIJ.MS.ID.555765 (2019)

39 Modelling the Hydration kinetics of kidney beans (Phaseolus vulgaris) in sodium salts using Response surface methodology. Nisha Agarwi et al. Journal of Applied and Natural Science, 12(1), 42-52. https://doi.org/10.31018/jans.v12i1.2234

40 Ultrasound-assisted hydration with sodium bicarbonate solution enhances hydration-cooking of pigeon pea. Upa;I Vasquez, et al. LWT Volume 144, June 2021, 111191. https://doi.org/10.1016/j.lwt.2021.111191

41 https://www.seriouseats.com/how-to-cook-dried-beans

42 https://www.seriouseats.com/salt-beans-cooking-soaking-water-good-or-bad

43 https://www.eatingwell.com/article/8051018/why-do-beans-make-you-fart/

44 Perceptions of flatulence from bean consumption among adults in 3 feeding studies. Winham DM, Hutchins AM. Nutr J. 2011 Nov 21;10:128. doi: 10.1186/1475-2891-10-128. PMID: 22104320

13: Protein Requirements

The Basic Components

We are protein machines. Every enzymatic process in metabolism is a function of proteins. Every movement, every breath, every thought is a process run by proteins. These proteins are built from amino acids we get in our diet from the digestion of proteins.

A healthy diet for a healthy young adult requires a considerable amount of protein. The needs are actually higher in older, less healthy adults. If the quality or quantity of protein is insufficient, age-associated muscle loss accelerates, and people become frail with age.

This chapter discusses the difficulty of getting sufficient quality protein in the diets of older adults and the nutritional hurdles present for vegans of any age. It is difficult for vegans to get sufficient protein if not consuming processed soy-based products. Vegans need nutritional supplements to maintain their health.

Recommendation: The SANA diet recommends that older adults include at 30 grams of protein into at least two meals a day, or alternatively, concentrating high amounts of protein into one a single meal, in order to provide sufficient dietary leucine (about 2.5 grams for most older adults) for the induction of muscle protein synthesis, and to prevent muscle loss, sarcopenia, disability, and frailty. High-protein meals should be within an hour of exercise on days when moderate to vigorous exercise is done.

Little protein should be eaten between breakfast and lunch and between lunch and dinner, so as to help reset muscle synthesis signaling. Dairy, for example, is high in leucine, the amino acid that helps trigger signaling for muscle protein synthesis, and thus, is best consumed with a meal, rather than as an in-between-meal snack. Exercise should be scheduled just before or soon following high-protein meals to take advantage of the post-exercise increase in muscle protein synthesis.

It is essential to recognize, however, that not all proteins in the diet deliver a balanced amount of amino acids needed for muscle synthesis. Animal proteins (dairy, eggs, fish, and meat) more closely align with the balance of amino acids needed for the growth and maintenance of our cells and their metabolism. Additionally, as discussed in Chapter 6, plant proteins often come bundled with anti-nutrition factors that limit protein utilization.

How Much Protein?

The recommended dietary allowance (RDA) for protein is 0.83 g of protein per kg of body weight for adults. The RDA is designed to provide a level at which 97% of the population gets sufficient nutrients. For a 70 kg (154) man, that would amount to 58.1 grams of protein, which provides 232 calories. For a 40-year-old man weighing 70 kg doing moderate exercise a few times a week, and thus requiring about 2300 calories per day, that works out to be about 10% of caloric intake.

This chapter and most of this book refer to diets for adults, particularly older adults. Growing children and especially toddlers and infants, require a diet with a higher percentage of protein than is needed by adults, and small children may need higher-quality protein than adults.

The recommendation of 0.83 grams of protein per kg was made for omnivorous humans who get most of their protein from animal sources. Although animals evolved to adapt to mostly consume plant-based proteins, the plants did not evolve to feed us. As one would expect, plant protein has a less favorable amino acid profile for building animal proteins than do animal proteins. Additionally, the secondary structure of plant proteins is dominated by β-sheet protein conformation with a relatively low α-helix protein content as compared to animal proteins. The β-sheet proteins are hydrophobic and more resistant to proteolytic digestive enzymes in the GI tract. As discussed in previous chapters, plant materials also contain antinutritive factors that impede proteolytic enzymes or otherwise impede digestion. Trypsin inhibitors from legumes can reduce amino acid digestibility by up to 50% in rats and pigs.[1] [2] Dietary protein requirement may thus be 50 to 100% higher for lower quality proteins.[3]

Most animal protein has a high "digestible indispensable amino acid score" (DIAAS), which is a composite estimate of the percent digestive absorption and utilization of a food protein. For example, milk has an ileal indispensable amino acid score of 114, and eggs get a score of 113. Soy protein isolate gets a score of 100, white rice gets a score of 57, peanut butter 46, black beans 59, and white bread 29.[4] The typical DIASS score of an omnivorous diet is 90, but it is about 70 for a vegan diet. Thus, to achieve the protein intake utilization of an omnivore, a vegan needs about 129% as much plant protein (90/70 = 1.29). Thus, a minimum target protein for a vegan should likely be closer to 1.07 grams of protein per kg (or about 0.5 grams per pound) of body weight. Furthermore, the DIAAS rating may not adequately take into account the impact of anti-nutritive factors present in plant-based proteins; thus, the DIAAS rating may overestimate the amount of protein available in plant-based diets.[5]

The DIAAS rating is based on the ratio of essential amino acid (AA) distribution of the food, and determines which amino acid has the lowest ratio as compared to the ideal distribution for protein building. This AA thus acts as a limiting factor for protein synthesis. If there are insufficient amounts of any of the nine essential amino acids needed to build a protein within a cell, the production of that protein cannot continue until the amino acid is found. It is like a production line in a factory that comes to a halt if a part is unavailable. The cell will then recycle other proteins to get the amino acids it needs through autophagy. This is not a bad thing as it refreshes old, worn-out proteins, but if there are continuous amino acid deficits, it is more like tearing down the wall of one room in a house to get materials to build a different wall.

Another metric to assess the *optimal protein intake*, rather than the minimum needed to maintain protein balance, is the indicator amino acid oxidation (IAAO) method. This metric estimates the minimum protein needed to fully utilize protein-building mechanisms by the body. Beyond this, excess dietary amino acids are oxidized as fuel. The IAAO method estimates that 1.2 grams of dietary protein are needed per kilogram of body weight per day.[6] For the 70 kg man consuming 2300 calories, that would be 84 grams of protein and 336 calories, and thus 14.6% of the caloric intake as protein. Again, this assumes a proper balance of amino acids in the food and protein absorption that is not hindered by anti-nutritional factors or other impediments.

Lysine is commonly the limiting amino acid in plant-based diets. Furthermore, lysine can be damaged during food preparation, further decreasing its availability but also producing toxic AGEs (Advanced Glycation End-products).

Lysine and arginine form AGEs during the browning of food. Arginine can form acrylamide, and lysine carboxymethyl lysine (CML); both are toxins. A more severe example of this is the formation of glucosepane, a toxic and proinflammatory compound produced during the cooking of meats containing creatine at high temperatures. Glucosepane is readily formed, especially when cooking ground meat, such as hamburger.

Acrylamide inhibits autophagy, the recycling of proteins in the cell, meaning that the cell will have more difficulty repairing damaged proteins as well, and will not function as well, causing aging of the cells. CML impairs the function of cells that rebuild bone (osteoblasts and osteocytes), which may lead to lower bone mineral density.[7] Higher CML levels are associated with neurodegenerative disease, insulin resistance, type 2 diabetes (T2D), heart disease, kidney damage, and oxidative stress.[8] [9] [10] Older adults in the top quartile for AGEs (measured by skin autofluorescence) were 2.4 times more likely to have sarcopenia (loss of muscle mass and loss of strength).[11]

Antinutritional factors can also form during food processing. For example, D-amino acids, lysinoalanine, and oxidized sulfur amino acids can form during Maillard reactions in both animal and vegetable proteins, causing them to be poorly digestible and potentially noxious.[12]

Sufficient dietary protein, exercise, and prevention of chronic inflammation are required to maintain muscle mass. After the age of 40, most adults begin to lose muscle mass at a rate of about 1 percent each year. This **sarcopenia** is the result of several factors, which include a decline in physical activity, hormonal changes (a decline in testosterone or menopause), chronic inflammation, insulin resistance, and inadequate protein intake. The International Society of Sports Nutrition (ISSN) recommends a daily protein intake in the range of 1.4 – 2.0 g of protein/kg body weight/day (g/kg/d) to build and maintain muscle mass.[13] A high protein diet (1.25–1.5 g/kg/d) is recommended just for the prevention of pressure sores in the bed-bound elderly. The European Union Geriatric Medicine Society recommends a daily intake of 1.0 – 1.2 g protein/kg/d for those over age 65 to prevent sarcopenia, and recommends 1.2 – 1.5 g protein/kg/d for those with acute illness or injury.[14]

Sarcopenia is a risk factor for dementia. A meta-analysis including 77 studies found that sarcopenia was associated with a 58% higher odds of mild cognitive impairment (MCI), a 68% higher odds of non-Alzheimer's disease dementia, and triple the risk (298% higher odds) of Alzheimer's disease.[15] Sarcopenia increases the risk of cancer mortality, dysphagia (difficulty swallowing), fractures, falls, hospitalizations, and all-cause mortality in the elderly.[16]

The most common reason for an older adult to be placed in a nursing home is that they cannot get up off a toilet on their own, and thus cannot self-care.[17] This is usually the result of sarcopenia. Sarcopenia and loss of balance, rather than osteoporosis, are the most common causes of hip fracture. Sarcopenia makes people feeble. Exercise is an important component of the SANA program for the prevention of dementia and other chronic diseases of aging. Sarcopenia gets in the way of exercise. Lack of exercise promotes sarcopenia.

Sarcopenia is associated with lower progression-free survival and higher cancer mortality rates.[18] [19] A considerable portion of this risk is due to the greater toxicity of chemotherapy and other cancer treatments among those with sarcopenia.[20] Sarcopenia is associated with longer hospitalizations, poorer recovery, and more frequent infections during cancer treatment. Cancer causes sarcopenia, with some cancers having a greater effect than others; thus, some of the mortality risk may have to do with the sarcopenic potency of the cancer.

In a meta-analysis of studies on hip fractures in the elderly, a high-protein diet lowers fracture risk.[21] This is likely the result of poorer musculature and increased risk of falling.

Myosteatosis is the infiltration of fat into skeletal muscle. Myosteatosis is epidemic in Western society and is a strong predictor of cancer mortality. It increases the risk of disease progression and death by about 50% as compared to those with cancer but without myosteatosis.[22] [23] [24] [25] In some studies, sarcopenia and myosteatosis were found to be independent risk factors for poorer cancer survival.[26] Thus, each adds to the risk.

Like NASH (Non-Alcoholic Steato-Hepatitis), myosteatosis (muscle-fat accumulation) is caused by excessive fat deposition resulting from a high-fat diet and elevated glucocorticoid levels resulting from chronic inflammation and mitochondrial dysfunction. Myosteatosis can be thought of as fatty muscle disease, akin to NASH, being a severe form of fatty liver disease. Some of the fat infiltration may be the effect of dietary trans fats, as the body lacks a mechanism for their utilization as energy. Once trans fats are absorbed into the body, there is no way to get rid of them. NASH and myosteatosis are epidemic; 37% of American adults have NASH, and one in four have the more severe form, Non-alcoholic Fatty Liver Disease (NAFLD). Well over half of American adults meet the diagnostic criteria for myosteatosis.

When the capacity of the subcutaneous adipose tissue (fat layer beneath the skin) to take up fat is exceeded, the fat tissue secretes the hormone resistin that promotes fat storage in the muscle.[27] Resistin levels are associated with obesity, especially central (abdominal) obesity. Resistin is pro-inflammatory and associated with chronic inflammation. It should be noted that LPS, a bacterial compound that is absorbed into the bloodstream with leaky gut, promotes the expression of resistin.[28] Blood resistin levels are associated with, but not necessarily causal of, insulin resistance.[29]

Lipid infiltration into the muscles increases with age, even when weight and subcutaneous fat levels are stable over time. Age-related lack of exercise contributes to the decline in lean muscle mass. Fortunately, myosteatosis can be reversed by exercise regardless of age.[30]

Cancer patients consuming higher amounts of protein have increased overall survival and a better quality of life than those consuming lower levels.[31] Women with ovarian cancer consuming more than 20% of total calories from protein, and those consuming more than one gram of protein per kg had lower cancer recurrence and better survival than those consuming less, with a slightly greater benefit for those consuming around 1.5 g/kg/day. Dairy-sourced protein appeared particularly beneficial.[32] In the Nurses' Health Study, women with breast cancer who consumed around 81 grams of protein per day had the lowest risk of recurrence and breast cancer death as compared to women in the lowest quintile of protein intake, at an average of around 62 grams per day, but the body mass of the study participants was not described. Here, too, dairy protein appeared helpful.[33] Branched-chain amino acids (such as those found in whey), however, did not reduce cancer risk.[34] Protein intake of around 1.2–1.5 g protein/kg of body mass per day thus appears to be appropriate for those with cancer.

A 60 kg (132-pound) 45-year-old woman, who does moderate exercise 1 to 3 times a week, needs about 1655 calories to maintain their weight. To get 1.5 g/kg of protein, that woman would need to consume 90 grams (360 calories of protein) per day, 22% of all caloric intake, or around 30 grams per meal. Consumption of 22% of calories as protein, however, may be associated with increased mTOR signaling and cardiovascular risk as a result of blocking autophagy in immune cells.[35]

There are 6 grams of protein in ½ cup (@ 50 grams) of dried rolled oats, the amount to make a typical serving of oatmeal; to get 30 grams would require 5 large bowls of cooked oatmeal and be 700 calories for breakfast, if nothing but water and salt were added. Let's try eggs; there are 6 grams of high-quality protein in one large egg, so 5 large eggs will give 30 grams of protein for breakfast. Lunch would be easier. It will take 16-oz. (4 servings) of cooked black beans to get 30 grams of protein for lunch. To make it easier, it would only take two veggie-burgers to get 28 grams of protein. For supper, two 3-oz servings of salmon at supper would give 34 grams. Two 3-oz servings of extra-dense tofu only contain 18 grams of protein. It is thus difficult to get 90 grams of protein, even of low-quality protein, on a 1655-calorie, mostly plant-based diet.

Prevention and recovery from myosteatosis require avoiding or reversing its underlying causes: high-fat diets, leaky gut, chronic inflammation, impaired autophagy, mitochondrial dysfunction, and sloth. Adult protein requirements may be lower when there is a lower inflammatory load, when the mitochondria are healthy, and autophagy is efficiently recycling protein. For example, an analysis of data from six NHANES studies from 2003 to 2018 found that the composite-dietary-antioxidant-index and the healthy eating index were inversely associated with the risk of sarcopenia.[36]

For a slightly different perspective of protein requirements, a meta-analysis including 31 prospective studies, including 715,128 persons and 113,039 deaths, over follow-up periods from 3.5 to 31 years assessed overall, cardiovascular disease (CVD), and cancer mortality with dietary protein intake, and provided a diet response curve (Figures 9A - 9C). Higher levels of total protein intake were associated with a lower overall mortality, but animal protein intake was not associated with a lower risk of CVD or cancer death. This may in part be due to the inclusion of red meat, which increases risk. Plant protein intake was associated with a lower risk of all-cause and CVD mortality. Diets with around 17 – 19 percent of total energy as protein had the lowest overall mortality, with an effect size of about 8% lower mortality for those consuming around 18% of calories as protein, as compared to those only consuming 8% of calories as protein. All-cause mortality was lowest when *animal protein* comprised about 6.5% of total energy as compared to 4%, but this only lowered overall mortality by about 2%. Consumption of over 9% of total calories from animal proteins was associated with increased all-cause mortality, with levels over 12% of calories from animal protein having a statistically significant increased risk. Protein from red meat is special. It increases mortality risk. Plant-based protein intake was highly associated with lower overall mortality, with diets containing around 7.5 to 9% plant protein having the lowest relative risk. At around 8.5% of caloric intake from plant protein, all-cause mortality was about 13.5% lower compared to those consuming only 3% plant-based proteins. Most of the risk reduction was for CVD. There was about a 25% lower risk of CVD mortality when 8.5% of energy came from plant proteins as compared to 3% of the energy from vegetable proteins in the diet.[37]

For a 60 kg (132-pound) 45-year-old woman, consuming 1655 calories, the 1.2 grams of protein per kg from the IAAO estimate for minimal adequate protein would give an optimal protein intake of 72 grams or 17.4 percent of calories. This is very close to the amount suggested by the overall and CVD survival data.

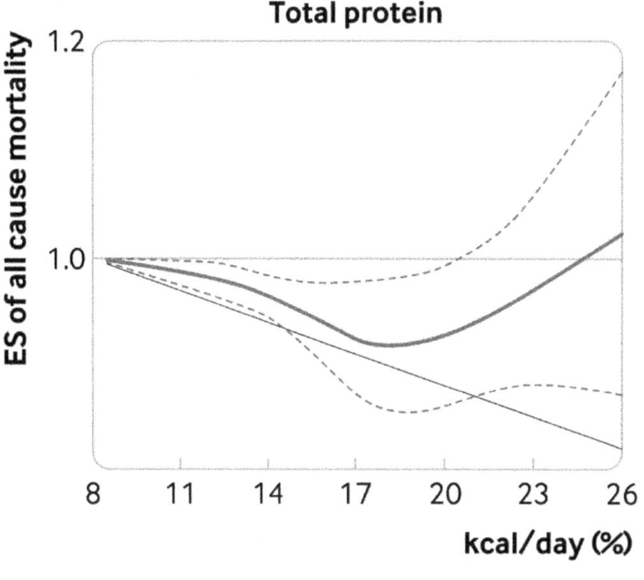

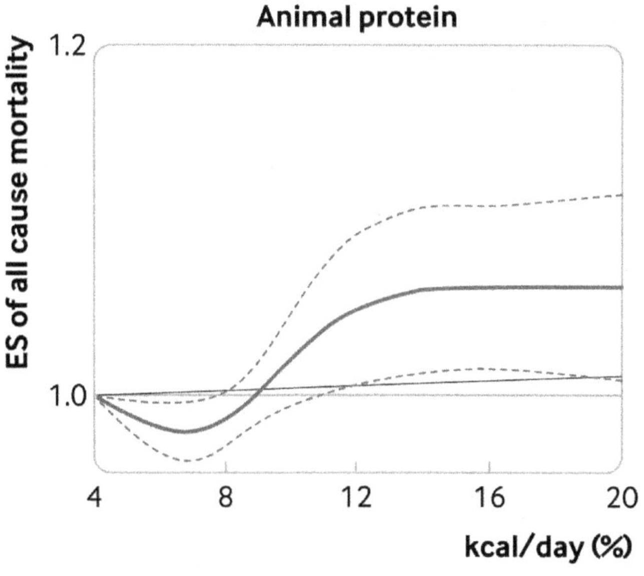

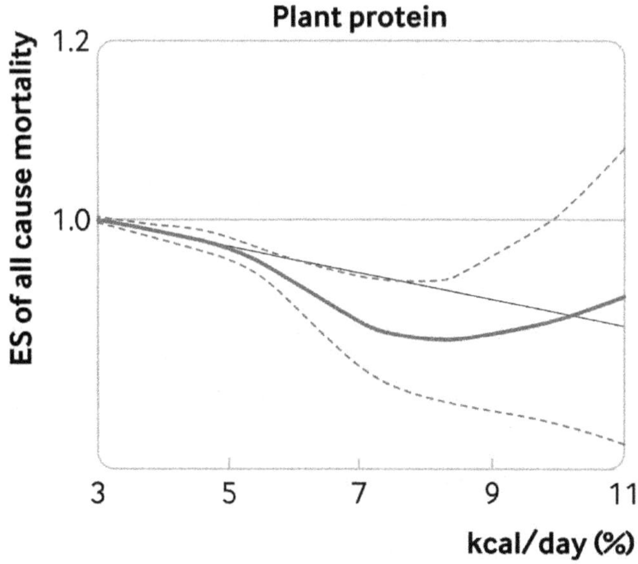

Figure 13 A-C: Effect size (ES) of protein intake as a percent of total energy intake from protein. Note that the scale of each graph is different. (Nagashi et al. PMID: 32699048)

These data suggest that animal protein intake should be limited to about 6% of daily energy consumption, and about one-third of all protein intake. Nevertheless, this should not be taken as a prescriptive without further studies in appropriate populations consuming a healthy diet of properly prepared foods. The results of this study are almost certainly skewed by the consumption of red meat, which is known to increase mortality risk. Future studies should separate sources of animal proteins rather than lump dairy, fish, eggs, and beef into one category.

Note: This data is presented to better understand optimal nutrition. Please note that a 2% or 8% difference in mortality, while important, is relatively small when compared to many other dietary risk factors. The RDA for protein is set so that it covers the nutritional needs of 97% of the population. Some individuals require less protein than others to maintain health and muscle mass. I suspect that myosteatosis increases the dietary requirement for protein. This data was generated from a population study principally made up of omnivores. A closer to ideal study would look at the protein intake and mortality risk for vegans, lacto-ovo-vegetarians, and omnivores separately, to better understand ideal protein intake in adults for optimal health.

While dietary protein needs during growth and development may be different than those for healthy adults, it is interesting to compare the protein requirements of growing animals. Efficiency in feeding farm animals is essential for farmers who want to keep farming; thus, this has been an area with substantial controlled experimental data. Meat production (typically growth into adolescence) is most efficient in rabbits and pigs when their diets contain 16 to 18% of their total energy intake as protein. Hens produce eggs, and dairy cows produce milk most efficiently when their diets also contain 16 to 18% of their calories as protein. Broiler chickens, from hatching to 42 to 49 days before going to slaughter, get fed a ration with 22 to 24% protein. Grazing ruminants have a much lower protein requirement, closer to about 7% protein, but grow slowly, making range-fed beef more costly. For feedlot beef, the dietary recommendation is 12 to 16% protein.

Of further interest is that the recommended diet for pigs contains 65 to 75% carbohydrates but only 5 to 10% fat. Between 5% to 10% of their recommended diet is fiber.[38]

In a study comparing the amount and ratio of animal to vegetable-sourced protein, older adults consuming a lower percentage of total dietary protein from animal sources had a lower risk of hip fracture than did those consuming a higher percentage of animal-sourced proteins. The hazard ratio for time to hip fracture was 3.7 times lower for those in the lowest tertile for animal source protein as compared to those in the top third for proportion of protein intake from animal sources. It should be noted that even those in the lowest animal protein group still had more than half of their dietary protein from animal sources. In the highest animal protein intake group, the median intake of animal protein was over 4 times that of vegetable protein intake.[39] The typical Western diet has an animal-to-vegetable protein ratio of about 55 to 45.[40]

Leucine and Other Amino Acids

There are 21 protein-forming amino acids. These amino acids are strung together in specific sequences to form proteins. This is sort of like letters in the alphabet being strung one after another to form words, sentences, and paragraphs to express a myriad of ideas. These strings form the primary structure of protein; they are then folded and combined with other proteins to form functional proteins.

Nine amino acids are considered to be essential amino acids in adult humans. These are amino acids that we cannot synthesize or be made from other amino acids by the body. There are 14 amino acids that infants cannot synthesize. The essential amino acids for adults are: histidine, isoleucine, leucine, lysine, methionine, phenylalanine, threonine, tryptophan, and valine. While we use the other amino acids to build protein and form neurotransmitters and other signaling molecules, these are critical elements in the diet, as a deficit of any one of them can hinder or stop the production of protein.

Certain amino acids have additional regulatory activity on protein production. If there are not sufficient amounts of each required amino acid, protein production by the ribosome gets stuck without being able to complete the string. The amino acids leucine, arginine, and methionine are potent activators of mTORC1, a protein complex that activates protein synthesis and inhibits autophagy, setting the stage for growth.

S-adenosylmethionine (SAMe) is needed for activation of mTORC1. If there is a deficiency of methionine, and thus inadequate SAMe, mTORC1 activation is inhibited, and protein production is hindered. Inadequate SAMe also acts as a signal for the breakdown and recycling of older proteins (autophagy), to mine for essential amino acids needed to keep essential housekeeping protein production going. If the production of these proteins stops, the cell dies. Autophagy occurs in the lysosomes within the cell.

Leucine has an even more direct role in the activation of mTORC1, and thus, protein synthesis, inhibition of autophagy, and cell growth. In leucine-starved conditions, mTORC1 is inhibited. Arginine also plays a role in mTORC1 activation, in part by facilitating the transport of leucine from the lysosome into the cytosol, where mTORC1 resides. In a study in rats, a diet replete with leucine increased muscle protein synthesis (MPS), and in a parallel experiment, adding arginine to that diet increased muscle mass by an additional 15%.[41] Dietary citrulline can be converted into arginine, thus helping to assure an adequate supply. Glutamine also helps with leucine transport on the Golgi membrane, which is a slower mechanism for mTORC1 activation.[42]

Thus, leucine, methionine, arginine, and glutamine sufficiency act to regulate protein synthesis. Since leucine and methionine are essential amino acids, they are the most limiting among these.

To build muscle and to avoid sarcopenia, we need a diet with sufficient dietary leucine, methionine, as well as other proteins, and sufficient exercise to trigger muscle protein synthesis (MPS). Building muscle mass is not an essential daily survival function, and thus not a top survival priority, but rather occurs when the conditions are right; when there is an abundance of raw materials and stimulus from exercise.

Leucine comprises about 8 percent of the protein in the human body. Leucine signals protein formation in the muscles and some other cells by activating mTOR when a meal contains a sufficient amount to ensure adequate protein availability for muscle building.[43] If there is inadequate leucine available, it acts as a signal that the materials (amino acids) needed to build muscle mass are inadequate, so it would be futile and possibly harmful to try. If levels of leucine are very low, as during starvation, it allows the breakdown of muscle into amino acids so that the body can make the housekeeping proteins needed for survival.

Leucine additionally helps increase muscular response to insulin, increasing uptake of glucose into the muscle cells, and either utilization of glucose for energy by glycolysis or the storage of energy in the form of glycogen or triglycerides. Insulin facilitates MPS in the presence of high amino acid availability, inhibits muscle protein breakdown independent of amino acid levels, and thus has a sparing effect on muscle protein.[44] Insulin resistance not only impedes muscle protein synthesis but also promotes sarcopenia.[45]

A substantial amount of leucine needs to be present and remain present for MPS. In healthy, active young men, 2 grams of leucine in a meal proximal to exercise is sufficient to double muscular protein synthesis, but in this population, exercise alone increases MPS. Acting together, exercise and high protein availability help maximize MPS. The amount of leucine needed *in a meal* for older adults to double muscle protein synthesis is about 3 grams of leucine, and without it, there is little MPS even with exercise. While some older studies suggested an all-or-nothing effect, with a threshold level of leucine required to permit MPS, this does not appear to occur. In older adults, MPS is linearly associated with higher leucine content in meals consumed about an hour before or after exercise.[46] The more MPS-stimulating amino acids present, the higher the MPS, up to perhaps four grams of leucine. The amount of leucine required to stimulate MPS may be higher for sedentary adults in poorer physical condition.[47]

Digestion and absorption of amino acids from food appear to be slower in older adults. This gives a slower rise and lower peak, but also a longer delivery of MPS-stimulating amino acids in older individuals. This slow release may be the result of natural aging or diseases of aging, including a decline in stomach acid from chronic *H. pylori* infection, declines in pancreatic enzymes, poorer perfusion of the intestine from vascular disease, or other factors that slow uptake. Additionally, older individuals typically have anabolic resistance resulting from myosteatosis, insulin resistance, and poorer muscular perfusion. Thus, older adults need more protein intake to maintain and build muscle mass.

Muscle protein synthesis begins about 45 minutes after the meal, and continues for about 45 to 90 minutes. After this, leucine-induced mTOR signaling in muscle will not recur until the levels of branched-chain amino acids in the bloodstream fall below a certain level, and "reset" the muscle protein generation signal for another cycle for the next meal with sufficient leucine.

The anabolic resistance that occurs with aging, and which creates a higher threshold for leucine-induced muscle protein synthesis, results from insulin resistance and lack of muscular activity.[48] Exercise can restore a more normal leucine threshold for muscle synthesis. While the exercise helps induce protein synthesis for about the next 24 hours, the maximum effect appears to occur for high-protein meals within two hours of exercise, and perhaps even greater when consumed within one hour before or after the exercise.

Understanding the leucine threshold for building (and retaining) muscle mass provides critical information about how we should eat. In a young adult, 20 grams of protein at breakfast may be sufficient, but with age, 25 to 30 grams may be required at each meal to trigger protein synthesis for muscle mass maintenance, largely as a result of insulin resistance and myosteatosis.

Thus, it becomes more important to either distribute protein consumption evenly into three daily meals, if sufficient leucine is included in the diet, or alternatively to concentrate leucine into fewer meals so that at least some meals promote protein synthesis. The amount of leucine required to suppress muscle protein breakdown is lower than that needed to promote its synthesis. Additionally, these data show that protein fasting between meals, with a drop in circulating branched-chain amino acids (leucine, isoleucine, and valine), is needed to reset the leucine-mTOR protein building trigger.

Bearing this in mind, it can be easily understood that women with ovarian cancer may benefit from a very high protein intake dietary pattern (1.5 g/kg/day, or 90 grams per day for a 60 kg woman) to avoid sarcopenia.

As alluded to above, it is not easy to get 25 grams of protein into breakfast and lunch on a plant-based diet. Furthermore, while the typical Western diet contains about 8 to 10% of its amino acid content as leucine, a well-planned healthy vegan diet generally contains 7 to 8% leucine. If the goal is to get 2.5 grams of leucine into a meal for an older adult, at 9% leucine, it takes 27.7 grams; at 7.5% leucine, it takes 33.3 grams of protein.

- Vegetarian breakfast: 3 large eggs + ½ cup Greek yogurt: @ **30 grams protein**, 2.3 grams leucine.
- Vegan breakfast: 1¼ cups cooked quinoa, 1 cup tofu: @**30 grams of protein**, 2.1 grams of leucine.
- Oatmeal made using ½ cup of rolled oats: **5 grams of protein**, 0.3 grams of leucine.

The higher protein requirements for muscle protein synthesis with aging result from insulin resistance, but likely also result from a high-fat, pro-inflammatory diet, leaky gut, and a lack of physical activity. If there is no insulin resistance and the older person is physically active, the leucine/SAMe requirements for muscle protein synthesis should be no greater in the old than in the young. Nevertheless, as people age, sufficient protein should be included in each meal in order to maintain muscle mass.

There are additional dietary factors that impact muscle protein synthesis. Consumption of balanced proteins, those with an essential amino acid profile close to that of muscle of the body, is more efficient in building muscle and providing overall health. Plant protein can be used more effectively when complementary proteins are consumed in a meal, such as eating a combination of grains and legumes in the same meal. Proteins with a high DIAAS score and improved digestibility provide better protein utilization.

Whole foods provide greater MPS than partial foods. When 30 grams of protein were ingested by healthy young men following exercise as either whey protein (high in leucine) or cheddar cheese, there was no difference in MPS.[49] After exercise, whole eggs and whole milk, both high in fat, had a greater anabolic response than egg whites or skim milk in healthy adults. Free amino acid supplements give a rapid, high level of serum amino acids and give a short-lived increase in MPS as compared to whole foods that have a more prolonged effect.[50] Real food should be used to build muscle mass. Amino acid supplements are likely to be quickly absorbed and used to fuel metabolism, rather than remain at an appropriate circulation level for efficient MPS.

It should be noted that exercise, at least resistance exercise, promotes muscle protein turnover. Thus, exercise that is performed when sufficient circulating amino acids are unavailable, such as when fasting, can contribute to muscle protein breakdown and loss of muscle mass as the amino acids are catabolized for energy and building of housekeeping proteins.

Consumption of carbohydrates *with* a meal with protein increases the release of insulin, which has an inhibitory effect on muscle protein breakdown, and thus decreases the amount of protein required to maintain a positive muscle protein balance. With sufficient levels of protein, including sufficient leucine in the meal, carbohydrates provide no additive effect on MPS.[51] But since getting sufficient protein into a meal can be difficult, whole foods and avoiding insulin resistance become an important strategy for avoiding sarcopenia and fragility.

Proper preparation of grains, legumes, and other foods can increase their DIAAS score and improve protein and carbohydrate availability, allowing for better protein utilization from vegan foods.

In a clinical trial of healthy but overweight young men (average age 23, BMI 24.2, fat mass 22.8%), two grams of either leucine or dileucine were administered with a meal. Dileucine is a peptide composed of two leucine molecules. In this trial, 2 grams of dileucine raised muscle protein synthesis over the baseline meal, but 2 grams of leucine did not. This is an interesting finding, but it needs replication. It is likely the result of slower and more sustained release of leucine from dileucine into the bloodstream, rather than any special activity of the leucine dipeptide.[52]

It would be of interest if dileucine has a direct effect on MPS. Milk proteins are high in leucine pairs, which promote muscle growth in infants and children. Peas and mung beans have high levels of dileucine, and rice and egg whites have moderate levels. Hemp protein, which is high in leucine, is low in dileucine.[53] More research on this is needed, as this data comes from a single study, and the list of foods assessing dileucine content is very small. Additionally, germination and sprouting may have little impact on the amino acid content of a grain or pulse, but amino acids can get rearranged during sprouting and growth, altering the dileucine content as new proteins are formed. It would be of interest to know if sprouting seeds altered the dileucine content of various seeds.

♠

Ketogenic diets are not recommended as part of the SANA program. They are no more effective for weight loss than other isocaloric diets, and are associated with loss of lean body mass (loss of muscle) as compared to a high-carbohydrate diet.[54] Ketogenic diets are also associated with increased intestinal permeability, arterial stiffening, decreased coronary artery blood flow, and insulin resistance.[55, 56]

Recommendation: The SANA diet recommends that older adults consume 1.2 grams of high DIAAS protein per kilogram of body mass daily. Exercising should precede or follow a high-protein meal with sufficient dietary leucine to induce muscle protein synthesis. The meal should be within an hour of exercise on days when moderate to vigorous exercise is done.

Little protein should be eaten between breakfast and lunch and between lunch and dinner, to help reset the leucine-mTOR protein synthesis signal. Dairy is high in leucine and dileucine, and is best consumed with a meal to increase MPS. Exercise should be scheduled just before or soon following high-protein meals to take advantage of the post-exercise increase in muscle protein synthesis. If one wanted to limit egg consumption, for example, if doing vigorous exercise every other day, one might have eggs on mornings when vigorous exercise was done and then have oatmeal on off days.

Proper Processing of Plant Protein

As outlined at the beginning of this chapter and in other chapters, several factors cause plant proteins to be poorly digested, making their amino acids less nutritionally available. Poor digestibility also potentially provides fodder for protein fermentation in the colon; however, plant protein does not appear to generally promote dysbiosis to the extent that animal protein, such as beef, does.

The digestibility of both plant and animal protein can be improved by proper preparation. For seeds such as grains and legumes, soaking, germination, cooking, and milling can increase the digestibility and bioavailability of amino acids, carbohydrates, and lipids. Proper processing of seeds increases the solubility of fiber and makes it more available for utilization by the commensal intestinal microbiome. Soaking and heating grains and pulses can improve protein digestibility.[57] Processing legume protein can greatly diminish anti-trypsin proteins that inhibit proteolytic enzymes.[58] Pairing vegetable proteins in a meal can improve protein utilization. For example, pairing corn with beans; corn is low in lysine but high in methionine, while beans are high in lysine but low in methionine. Thus, when paired, they improve the DIAAS score.

Whole Grains

Excluding alcohol, calories come from carbohydrates, proteins, and fats. As a proportion of calories, brown rice has about 9% protein, oats about 17%, and whole grain wheat about 15.5% protein. Boiled potatoes have about 11% of their caloric content as protein, but have only about 3% of their calories as protein when consumed as French fries, as a result of added fats.

Diets high in whole grains are associated with a lower risk of all-cause mortality, CVD, stroke, diabetes, respiratory disease, infectious disease, and cancer mortality. Consumption of 100 grams of whole grains a day is associated with a 20% decrease in all-cause mortality and more than a 50% reduction in risk of death from diabetes, compared to the consumption of none. Consumption of *less than 100* grams of whole grains a day is associated with as much as a 20% increase in the risk of mortality from diseases of the nervous system. Consumption of 200 grams of whole grains a day offers additional reductions in risk.[59] A bowl of oatmeal made from ½ cup of rolled oats has 40 grams of whole grain. A cup of cooked brown rice has about 60 grams of whole grain. Note that the all-cause risk reduction from a diet with sufficient *whole grains* is greater than that from differences in protein intake. There is minimal difference in the protein content of white flour and whole grain flour or white rice and brown rice, but there is a significant difference in the health impact.

Lentils have about 31% of their calories as protein, black beans have 27%, and great northern beans have 28% of their calories as protein. Soybeans have 42% of their calories as protein.

Rather than focusing on very high-protein diets (greater than 1.4 g/kg/day or over 20 percent of caloric intake) for protection against sarcopenia, I suggest a low-fat diet with minimal empty carbohydrates and adequate plant-based protein. Protein availability can be enhanced by preparing the foods using the methods described in this book. The SANA diet imparts low risk for fatty liver disease, fatty muscle disease, obesity, insulin resistance, type 2 diabetes, cardiovascular disease, and cancer. A mostly plant-based diet can provide sufficient protein if nutritionally empty calories, and especially proinflammatory polyunsaturated and trans fats, and excess sugar and other refined foods, are avoided. (See Chapter 17.)

Recommendation: The SANA diet recommends a diet with about 18 percent of calories as protein, or about 1.25 grams/kg/d (0.563 grams/pound) of body mass. The SANA diet recommends that most of the protein, about two-thirds, be plant-based. Ideally, about a third of the protein should be in each of the three meals. Nevertheless, if the diet is lower in protein intake, it is better to concentrate the protein into two or even one daily meal so that enough leucine is present to promote the development of muscle protein.

At least 100 grams (about two servings) and preferably 3 to 4 servings of whole grains should be included in the diet daily. If this includes wheat, it should be germinated or sprouted wheat.

Back to the subject of diet and cancer: Most of the studies on diet and cancer are prospective studies; they look at diet and see the outcome after some years to see who does and who doesn't develop, and later succumb to different diseases. While this helps us understand what may cause or prevent the disease, it does not guarantee that the same things help improve survival for those already diagnosed with the disease.

Soy protein lowers the risk of breast cancer, especially postmenopausal breast cancer, with a 12% reduction in breast cancer risk for every 5 grams of soy protein consumed.[60] Soy isoflavones also reduce risk. Alcohol use is associated with a higher risk of breast cancer,[61] but does not impact survival in most studies. Fruit and vegetable intake is associated with a lower risk of breast cancer. Those consuming higher levels of fruits and vegetables had an 11% and 26% lower risk of hormone-positive and hormone-negative breast cancers, respectively. Fruit juice, however, was associated with a slightly greater risk.[62] Yogurt consumption is associated with a lower risk of developing breast cancer. Red meat consumption is associated with a higher breast cancer risk.[63]

After the diagnosis of breast cancer, consumption of soy products increases overall and breast cancer-specific survival.[64] In a comprehensive review and meta-analysis that assessed various diets and dietary components, the diet *after the diagnosis* has a significant impact on survival. Adherence to the "Prudent diet", "Healthy Eating Index", DASH, Mediterranean, and "Chinese Healthy Food Pagoda" (CHFP) all improved cancer survival, generally by about 25%, while the Western diet was associated with an about 40% increased mortality risk. Individual elements in the diet associated with better survival were *vitamin D, dietary fiber, and isoflavones*. While other beans, including black beans and chickpeas, are high in isoflavones, soy has the most. Kidney beans, peas, and lentils are not good sources of isoflavones.[65] The CHFP diet was reported to lower breast cancer mortality risk more than the other healthy diets, likely because it emphasizes low-fat and high soy intake. Dietary isoflavones were also found to decrease breast cancer recurrence.[66]

The most significant dietary factor associated with reductions in breast cancer mortality is dietary fiber. A 13 percent reduction in mortality was found for every 10 grams of daily fiber intake. A 7% reduction in mortality was observed per 10 nmol/L of serum vitamin D3 levels, although it would be more correct to say that low vitamin D levels, less than 50 nmol/L of 25(OH)D3, were associated with elevated risk.[67] Recreational exercise was also associated with improved post-diagnosis survival.[68] The isoflavone protection in breast cancer is likely limited to estrogen-sensitive cancers.

Vegans

Vegans need to have a better diet than non-vegans to get enough protein. There is little room in a vegan diet for empty calories from vegetable oil and sugar. Consumption of processed soy, in the form of tofu, veggie burgers, or other soy protein products, can help vegans get enough protein.

In a study that assessed the actual intake of protein by Danish vegans for three days, only 60% of them met the recommended minimal overall protein requirement on all three days, and only half met the lysine requirement on each day. One in six vegans did not meet the daily protein requirement on any of the three days.[69]

Note: While the primary focus of this book is on the prevention of dementia, and thus diet and lifestyle for mid-life and older adults; nonetheless, the SANA diet is appropriate for most people. While encouraging a mostly plant-based diet, a vegan diet has several nutritional constraints as outlined below. The SANA diet is appropriate during pregnancy, lactation, and throughout childhood. Nevertheless, I do not encourage pregnant or lactating women to adhere to vegan diets, nor for small children. Too much is at risk during these critical periods. It is not that it is impossible to have a healthy vegan diet during early life, but rather that it requires a level of commitment and care that is difficult to maintain in a busy lifestyle.

Healthy vegans *may* require a lower amount of leucine in a meal to trigger the generation of muscle proteins as compared to older adults with myosteatosis. It is not an easy task to cram 30 grams into vegan meals without the consumption of processed soy or other ultra-processed high-protein vegan products.

Rather than trying to get 30 grams of protein into a 600 to 700-calorie meal, it may be more practical to restore a normal threshold for leucine-induced muscle protein synthesis. Thus, I recommend that those interested in becoming vegan transition to it over time. My concern is that if a person has myosteatosis (most American adults), they will likely lose muscle as a result of "leucine resistance" if the diet is not replete in protein and if they are not physically active. Thus, by first transitioning to a low-fat, low-added-sugar, vegetarian diet, containing egg and dairy for added protein (as per the SANA diet), and by engaging in an active exercise regimen, a person can recover from myosteatosis without the loss of muscle mass. At that point, a transition to a vegan diet can be done with less risk of loss of muscle mass.

Nutritional Concerns for Vegans

Vitamin B12: There is no vitamin B12 in a vegan diet. *Vegans have to supplement it.* It should be taken as a chewable tablet or lozenge, as mixing the vitamin B12 with the saliva protects the vitamin from gastric degradation. As we age, vitamin B12 absorption generally declines. Most people, over the age of 60, vegan or not, benefit from a vitamin B12 supplement. B12 as a component of a multi-vitamin is not helpful. Vitamin B12 supplementation is discussed in Chapter 25 (Micronutrients).

Vegan women are often low in vitamin B12, and their infants and breast milk may also be low in vitamin B12.

B12 deficiency can cause infants to be small for gestational age, fail to thrive, and have low birth weight, hypotonia, developmental delays, and microcephaly.[70] [71] About one in six of *all women* have low-B12 breastmilk, most often a result of maternal B12 malabsorption, rather than from a vegan diet.[72]

Vitamin B2 (riboflavin): Vegans and vegetarians who avoid dairy products may have deficient riboflavin intake, especially those who engage in vigorous athletic activities.[73] The RDA for adults is 1.1 mg for women and 1.3 mg for men.

Taurine: Vegans have difficulty getting sufficient amounts of the non-protein amino acid taurine in their diets. Taurine is a neuromodulator that helps activate $GABA_A$ receptors and thus helps protect the brain.[74] Taurine is the only nutrient known to increase the expression of Ubiquinol-Cytochrome C Reductase Core Protein 1 (UQCRC1), an essential component of the electron transport chain needed to produce ATP in the mitochondria.[75] Lower levels of this UQCRC1 are associated with dementia. Lower levels of taurine are also associated with insulin resistance and vascular disease.[76] Vegan mothers often have low taurine levels in their breastmilk, putting the infant at risk.

Our bodies can make taurine from cysteine and methionine, but then a higher intake of those amino acids is also needed, along with the cofactors needed to convert them into taurine (vitamins B6, B9, B12, and choline). Seafood, including shellfish and fish, is high in taurine, as is red meat. Fish get their taurine from algae; red seaweed has an appreciable amount, but it would be hard to get 300 mg of taurine a day, a typical amount present in a non-vegan diet, from eating seaweed. Taurine supplements should be considered for those wishing to maintain a vegan diet.

Carnitine is another non-essential nutrient found exclusively in animal products. The typical non-vegan intake is 50 to 150 mg per day. Carnitine is required for the utilization of fat for energy by the mitochondria. There are only negligible amounts of carnitine present in vegan foods. The body is normally capable of producing sufficient carnitine, about 14 mg a day, from dietary lysine and methionine.[77]

Carnitine deficiency is unusual, but it can occur as a genetic disorder, with very poor nutrition, or as a result of renal disease. Carnitine supplementation may help in the treatment of depression.[78] In many children and some adults, carnitine supplementation is an effective prophylaxis for chronic migraine.[79] [80]

Carnitine supplementation may be helpful in dementia, cardiovascular disease (CVD), diabetes, insulin resistance, and peripheral artery disease. It has also shown benefit in treating infertility in women with polycystic ovary disease (PCOS). Carnitine is used to enhance athletic performance and for weight loss, but while trials show positive benefits from carnitine supplements in the short term, longer-term studies fail to show benefits for athletic performance or weight loss. This lack of benefit may result from high doses of carnitine use, causing a shift in the colonic microbiota to increasingly ferment it.

Excessively high doses of carnitine cause abdominal cramps, nausea, vomiting, diarrhea, and a fishy body odor as a result of TMA production from its fermentation in the colon and subsequent TMAO formation by the liver. TMAO is associated with an increased risk of renal and cardiovascular disease.[81] Dietary carnitine has a bioavailability of around 55 to 85%, while only 5 to 25% of supplemental forms are absorbed, increasing the risk of TMAO formation. Acetyl-L-carnitine may be better absorbed than other forms, and it is the form that best crosses the blood-brain barrier. It is better absorbed (and less of it ends up in the colon where it is fermented) if it is taken with meals that contain fat. TMAO and the risk of kidney and heart disease are discussed in Chapter 33.

If carnitine supplements are used, use of acetyl-L-carnitine is recommended, keeping the dose low, less than 250 mg per day, to be taken with a meal that contains some fat to help with absorption. If 45% is absorbed and 100 mg is needed, 225 mg should be sufficient. If more is taken, it should be divided between meals.

Speculation: A high-fat diet may create the need for supranormal carnitine levels for the processing of fats by the mitochondria. That is, a high-fat diet may necessitate more carnitine than the body can produce on its own. A primeval diet that was high in fat would usually be limited to the consumption of meat, and such a diet would also supply carnitine. More importantly, the main circumstance under which the body is designed to switch from using glucose as its main fuel to burning high amounts of fat is during starvation, and under this situation, the muscle is also being catabolized, and thus provides carnitine for the processing of fat into energy. Thus, I hypothesize that the metabolic demand for carnitine is lower and can be met by endogenous production of carnitine when high-fat diets are avoided. Consumption of vegetable fats that are not associated with carnitine intake, however, would be expected to create a carnitine deficit.

Creatine is another non-essential dietary compound that is present in animal-based diets and completely lacking in vegan diets. Creatine formation by the body is a two-step process that uses three amino acids. The first step occurs in the kidney or pancreas, and requires glycine and arginine; the second step happens in the liver, and uses methionine. About 1.7% of the body's pool of creatine is spontaneously converted into creatinine daily and is lost in the urine, thus requiring the replacement of creatine.[82] [83] Between one and three grams of creatine need to be replaced each day. Inborn errors of creatine metabolism can cause speech delays, autism, epilepsy, and other neurologic disorders.[84]

Creatine forms phosphocreatine, which is used to regenerate ATP from ADP. We have high levels in the brain and muscles, as these are high-energy-demand tissues. When taken as a supplement, creatine is preferentially absorbed into the muscles (and likely the brain).[85] The best time to take the supplement for increasing muscle mass is after exercise. Although it can help with weight loss, weight gain can be expected for the first several days, perhaps from the accumulation of glycogen in the muscles.

A meta-analysis found that creatine doses between 7 and 10 grams per day were most helpful, and that the effect worked best for about 3 months. Thus, creatine may be most helpful in the recovery from myosteatosis over this time frame.[86] Using 7 grams of creatine per day during resistance training (weight lifting) increased lean body mass by one kilogram and reduced fat mass by 0.7 kg.[87] Creatine supplementation may be helpful for recovery from myosteatosis, but there is not sufficient evidence to recommend its long-term use.

More relevant to dementia, in a placebo-controlled double-blinded clinical trial of vegetarian young adults, supplementation with 5 grams of creatine (monohydrate) daily for 18 weeks progressively improved scores on memory and intelligence tests.[88] One meta-analysis found that creatine had positive effects on memory, attention time, and processing speed, but another meta-analysis found the evidence to be weak. Vegetarians have lower levels of creatine in their muscles than do omnivores.[89] In one (very brief) study that compared omnivores with vegetarians, the benefit of carnitine on cognition was only seen in vegetarians.[90] [91] These data suggest that vegetarians may neither consume nor synthesize optimal amounts of creatine. If true for vegetarians, this situation is likely worse for vegans. Studies need to be performed among vegans and vegetarians consuming a healthy low-fat diet, to determine if more creatine is actually needed or if it is rather that a low-quality, nutritionally deficient vegetarian diet causes deficits in creatine and energy metabolism.

β-Alanine and Carnosine: Carnosine is a dipeptide composed of two amino acids, the essential amino acid L-histidine, and beta-alanine, a nonproteinogenic amino acid. Excitable tissues are those that are highest in carnosine: cardiac and skeletal muscle, and the brain. It has several functions, including protecting against oxidative stress, inflammation, protein glycation, and the formation of advanced glycation end (AGE) products. It acts as a buffer to maintain acid-base balance in muscle cells and chelates certain metals. Carnosine reduces muscular fatigue, slows cellular senescence, improves mitochondrial activity, and may help prevent cancer proliferation. Carnosine appears to help prevent amyloid-induced toxicity and protect against cognitive decline in ApoE4-positive subjects with mild cognitive impairment. [92] Carnosine helps build muscle mass, helps prevent sarcopenia, and is used as a supplement by bodybuilders. Higher muscle carnosine levels provide for sustained muscular activity.[93]

Dietary carnosine is broken down into β-alanine and histidine by carnosinase in the enterocytes lining the small intestine, which are then absorbed. Carnosine is then formed from these nutrients within the muscles, brain, and other tissues.

Neither carnosine nor β-alanine is present in plants; thus, it is not present in a vegan diet. Women, younger adults, and vegetarians have lower carnosine levels in their muscles than do men, older adults, and omnivores, respectively.[94] There are trivial amounts present in dairy products.

Obviously, vegans (including elephants and gorillas) and vegetarians get by without dietary carnosine and β-alanine. The level of carnosine in the muscles is increased in vegetarians by high-intensity interval exercise training (HIIT).[95] Some β-alanine is formed in the gut by microbes fermenting L-aspartate, and some is created when L-alanine is catabolized to form pyruvate and during the breakdown of pantothenic acid (vitamin B5).

While carnosine supplements can be used, β-alanine supplements appear to be equally effective in increasing carnosine levels.

Choline: Most people eating a Western diet consume less choline than the recommended "adequate intake" for choline,[96] and vegans get considerably less in their diets. While the body can make some choline, the amounts produced are less than those needed for health. Choline is needed for neurodevelopment and brain health. Inadequate choline very likely increases the risk of Alzheimer's disease among those who carry the ApoE4 allele.

Excess choline and betaine, which are not absorbed, ferment in the colon and form TMA, which is converted to TMAO in the liver. The use of large-dose supplements of choline should be avoided. Choline is discussed in Chapter 25 (Nutritional Supplements).

Fatty Acids: There are a few fatty acids that are important nutrients that are not found in a vegan diet. Pentadecanoic acid (C15:0, a product of fermentation) is not found in plants, but is found in cow's milk and some fish, and its intake is associated with a lower risk of diabetes, heart disease, and liver disease. It is discussed in Chapter 15 – Dairy.

EPA and DHA, anti-inflammatory fatty acids, are found in fish. While the body can make these fatty acids from the essential fatty acid, α-linolenic acid, the capacity is limited. Vegan, algae-based EPA and DHA supplements are available.

Vitamin D and Calcium: Vegan children aged 5 - 10 tend to have low vitamin D levels, low calcium intake, and as a result, have lower bone mass and shorter stature. Most children, but particularly vegan children, benefit from vitamin D3 supplementation at least in the winter months.[97]

The SANA program recommends that those who wish to adopt a vegan diet first transition to a low-fat, no-added polyunsaturated fat, low-sugar, vegetarian diet, in which the consumption of dairy, eggs, and fish help maintain a high protein intake, until they have recovered from myosteatosis and insulin (and leucine) resistance, to avoid loss of (lean) muscle mass.

Along with a low-fat diet, use of a carnitine (monohydride) supplement may help with the recovery from fatty liver [98] [99] and myosteatosis, especially when moving to a diet that has less abundant protein levels.

The paucity of endogenous carnitine production suggests that a vegan diet should be (and perhaps needs to be) a low-fat diet. As a rule of thumb, calories from fat should not exceed those from protein in a vegan diet, unless carnitine is supplemented. In health, glucose is the preferred fuel source for muscles and the liver. A high-fat diet forces the body to use fat instead. This increases the need for carnitine to process fat, and also increases insulin resistance.

The *minimum* recommended protein intake required for muscle mass maintenance in healthy young adults is 0.83 grams per kg of body mass. For a 60 kg woman burning 1,655 calories a day, a diet supplying 0.83 grams of protein per kg requires 49.8 grams of protein with high availability. Fifty grams of protein supplies 200 calories, 12% of total calories. Two hundred calories of fat is about 22 grams. Carbohydrates and fiber would make up the remainder, about 76% of calories in a minimal protein diet.

Table 9A. Leucine content in some foods: (grams leucine per serving)[100] [101]

Turkey breast (no skin)	2.07 g/ 3 oz.
Trout	1.44 g/ 3 oz.
Tuna:	1.9 g/ 100 g
Salmon:	1.6 g/ 100 g
Lentils:	1.8 g/ 100 g
Black beans:	1.7 g/ 100 g
Chickpeas:	1.5 g/ 100 g
Oats:	1 g/ 100 g
Yogurt (plain, skim milk):	0.54 g/ 100 g
Greek Yogurt, nonfat:	1.03 g/ 100 g
Cottage Cheese, 1% milk fat:	2.88 g/ cup
Cheddar Cheese:	0.682 g/ 1 ounce
Chicken breast, no skin:	2.25 g/ 3 ounces
Brown rice (cooked):	0.216 g/ 1/2 cup
Soy milk:	0.26 g/ cup
Tofu, extra firm:	0.73 g/ 3 ounces
Corn tortilla, 6":	0.109 g
Black beans:	0.61 g/ half cup cooked
Pinto beans:	0.11 g/ half cup cooked
Red beans:	0.54 g/ half cup cooked
Chickpeas:	0.42 g/ half cup cooked
Lentils:	0.69 g/ half cup cooked
Split peas:	0.58 g/ half cup cooked
Potatoes:	0.22 g/ half cup cooked
Sweet potatoes:	0.19 g/ half cup cooked
Cashews:	0.417 g/ 1 ounce raw
Walnuts:	0.332 g/ 1 ounce raw
One large egg:	0.525 g

[1] The Role of the Anabolic Properties of Plant- versus Animal-Based Protein Sources in Supporting Muscle Mass Maintenance: A Critical Review. Berrazaga I, Micard V, Gueugneau M, Walrand S. Nutrients. 2019 Aug 7;11(8):1825. doi: 10.3390/nu11081825. PMID: 31394788

[2] Effects of antinutritional factors on protein digestibility and amino acid availability in foods. Gilani GS, Cockell KA, Sepehr E. J AOAC Int. 2005 May-Jun;88(3):967-87. PMID: 16001874

[3] Protein quality and the food matrix: defining optimal versus maximal meal-based protein intakes for stimulating muscle protein synthesis. Barnes TM, Deutz MT, Zupančič Ž, Askow AT, Moore DR, Burd NA. Appl Physiol Nutr Metab. 2023 Apr 1;48(4):340-344. doi: 10.1139/apnm-2022-0373. Epub 2022 Feb 3. PMID: 36735923

[4] The Role of the Anabolic Properties of Plant- versus Animal-Based Protein Sources in Supporting Muscle Mass Maintenance: A Critical Review. Berrazaga I, Micard V, Gueugneau M, Walrand S. Nutrients. 2019 Aug 7;11(8):1825. doi: 10.3390/nu11081825. PMID: 31394788

[5] Digestible indispensable amino acid score (DIAAS): 10 years on. Moughan PJ, Lim WXJ. Front Nutr. 2024 Jul 3;11:1389719. doi: 10.3389/fnut.2024.1389719. eCollection 2024. PMID: 39021594

[6] Defining meal requirements for protein to optimize metabolic roles of amino acids.

Layman DK, Anthony TG, Rasmussen BB, Adams SH, Lynch CJ, Brinkworth GD, Davis TA. Am J Clin Nutr. 2015 Jun;101(6):1330S-1338S. doi: 10.3945/ajcn.114.084053. Epub 2015 Apr 29. PMID: 25926513

[7] Pentosidine and carboxymethyl-lysine associate differently with prevalent osteoporotic vertebral fracture and various bone markers. Nakano M, Nakamura Y, Suzuki T, Miyazaki A, Takahashi J, Saito M, Shiraki M. Sci Rep. 2020 Dec 16;10(1):22090. doi: 10.1038/s41598-020-78993-w. PMID: 33328494

[8] The neurotoxicity of Nε-(carboxymethyl)lysine in food processing by a study based on animal and organotypic cell culture. Wu Y, Li Y, Zheng L, Wang P, Liu Y, Wu Y, Gong Z. Ecotoxicol Environ Saf. 2020 Mar 1;190:110077. doi: 10.1016/j.ecoenv.2019.110077. Epub 2019 Dec 18. PMID: 31864122

[9] Studies on mechanism of free Nε-(carboxymethyl)lysine-induced toxic injury in mice. Wang YX, Xu H, Liu X, Liu L, Wu YN, Gong ZY. J Biochem Mol Toxicol. 2019 Jul;33(7):e22322. doi: 10.1002/jbt.22322. Epub 2019 Mar 29. PMID: 30924232

[10] Serum Carboxy Methyl Lysine, Insulin Resistance and Sensitivity in Type 2 Diabetes Mellitus and Diabetic Nephropathy Cases; an Observational Study. Deepika SR et al. Biomed Pharmacol J 2020;13(4). DOI : https://dx.doi.org/10.13005/bpj/2077

[11] Association Between Advanced Glycation End Products and Sarcopenia: The Mediating Role of Osteoporosis. Zhang X, Chen X, Li S, Gao M, Han P, Cao L, Gao J, Tao Q, Zhai J, Liang D, Qin L, Guo Q. J Clin Endocrinol Metab. 2024 Feb 20;109(3):e1105-e1116. doi: 10.1210/clinem/dgad640. PMID: 37925684

[12] Effects of antinutritional factors on protein digestibility and amino acid availability in foods. Gilani GS, Cockell KA, Sepehr E. J AOAC Int. 2005 May-Jun;88(3):967-87. PMID: 16001874

[13] International Society of Sports Nutrition Position Stand: protein and exercise. Jäger R, Kerksick CM, Campbell BI, Antonio J. J, et al. Int Soc Sports Nutr. 2017 Jun 20;14:20. doi: 10.1186/s12970-017-0177-8. 2017. PMID: 28642676

[14] Protein Requirements for Older Adults: What Are the Current Recommendations for Intake? Phyllis Famularo. J Caring for the Ages. 24(4)9, may 2023. DOI: https://doi.org/10.1016/j.carage.2023.04.015

[15] Meta-analysis on the interrelationship between sarcopenia and mild cognitive impairment, Alzheimer's disease and other forms of dementia. Amini N, Ibn Hach M, Lapauw L, Dupont J, Vercauteren L, Verschueren S, Tournoy J, Gielen E. J Cachexia Sarcopenia Muscle. 2024 Aug;15(4):1240-1253. doi: 10.1002/jcsm.13485. Epub 2024 May 7. PMID: 38715252

[16] Sarcopenia and adverse health-related outcomes: An umbrella review of meta-analyses of observational studies. Xia L, Zhao R, Wan Q, Wu Y, Zhou Y, Wang Y, Cui Y, Shen X, Wu X. Cancer Med. 2020 Nov;9(21):7964-7978. doi: 10.1002/cam4.3428. Epub 2020 Sep 13. PMID: 32924316

[17] Comparing associations of handgrip strength and chair stand performance with all-cause mortality-implications for defining probable sarcopenia: the Tromsø Study 2015-2020. Johansson J, Grimsgaard S, Strand BH, Sayer AA, Cooper R. BMC Med. 2023 Nov 20;21(1):451. doi: 10.1186/s12916-023-03172-3. PMID: 37981689

[18] Association of possible sarcopenia with all-cause mortality in patients with solid cancer: A nationwide multicenter cohort study. Yin L, Song C, Cui J, Lin X, Li N, Fan Y, Zhang L, Liu J, Chong F, Cong M, Li Z, Li S, Guo Z, Li W, Shi H, Xu H; Investigation on Nutrition Status and Clinical Outcome of Common Cancers (INSCOC) Group. J Nutr Health Aging. 2024 Jan;28(1):100023. doi: 10.1016/j.jnha.2023.100023. Epub 2024 Jan 11. PMID: 38216426

[19] Sarcopenia and prognosis of advanced cancer patients receiving immune checkpoint inhibitors: A comprehensive systematic review and meta-analysis. Deng HY, Chen ZJ, Qiu XM, Zhu DX, Tang XJ, Zhou Q. Nutrition. 2021 Oct;90:111345. doi: 10.1016/j.nut.2021.111345. Epub 2021 May 21. PMID: 34166897

[20] Sarcopenia in Breast Cancer Patients: A Systematic Review and Meta-Analysis. Roberto M, Barchiesi G, Resuli B, Verrico M, Speranza I, Cristofani L, Pediconi F, Tomao F, Botticelli A, Santini D. Cancers (Basel). 2024 Jan 31;16(3):596. doi: 10.3390/cancers16030596. PMID: 38339347

[21] High Versus low Dietary Protein Intake and Bone Health in Older Adults: a Systematic Review and Meta-Analysis. Groenendijk I, den Boeft L, van Loon LJC, de Groot LCPGM. Comput Struct Biotechnol J. 2019 Jul 22;17:1101-1112. doi: 10.1016/j.csbj.2019.07.005. eCollection 2019. PMID: 31462966

[22] The influence of sarcopenia and myosteatosis on severe laboratory toxicity and overall mortality in older adults

with cancer receiving chemotherapy. Papadopoulous E, et al. Journal of Clinical Oncology. 42(6) https://doi.org/10.1200/JCO.2024.42.16_suppl.1213

[23] Evaluating the influence of sarcopenia and myosteatosis on clinical outcomes in gastric cancer patients undergoing immune checkpoint inhibitor. Deng GM, Song HB, Du ZZ, Xue YW, Song HJ, Li YZ. World J Gastroenterol. 2024 Feb 28;30(8):863-880. doi: 10.3748/wjg.v30.i8.863. PMID: 38516238

[24] Prognostic impact of myosteatosis in patients with colorectal cancer undergoing curative surgery: an updated systematic review and meta-analysis. Chang YY, Cheng B. Front Oncol. 2024 Jun 19;14:1388001. doi: 10.3389/fonc.2024.1388001. eCollection 2024. PMID: 38962266

[25] The prognostic impact of myosteatosis on overall survival in gynecological cancer patients: A meta-analysis and trial sequential analysis. Cao H, Gong Y, Wang Y. Int J Cancer. 2022 Dec 1;151(11):1997-2003. doi: 10.1002/ijc.34179. Epub 2022 Jun 30. PMID: 35723079

[26] The Impact of Sarcopenia and Low Muscle Attenuation on Overall Survival in Epithelial Ovarian Cancer: A Systematic Review and Meta-analysis. McSharry V, Mullee A, McCann L, Rogers AC, McKiernan M, Brennan DJ. Ann Surg Oncol. 2020 Sep;27(9):3553-3564. doi: 10.1245/s10434-020-08382-0. Epub 2020 Mar 27. PMID: 32221737

[27] Updated systematic review and meta-analysis on diagnostic issues and the prognostic impact of myosteatosis: A new paradigm beyond sarcopenia. Ahn H, Kim DW, Ko Y, Ha J, Shin YB, Lee J, Sung YS, Kim KW. Ageing Res Rev. 2021 Sep;70:101398. doi: 10.1016/j.arr.2021.101398. Epub 2021 Jun 29. PMID: 34214642

[28] Lipopolysaccharide increases resistin gene expression in vivo and in vitro. Lu SC, Shieh WY, Chen CY, Hsu SC, Chen HL. FEBS Lett. 2002 Oct 23;530(1-3):158-62. doi: 10.1016/s0014-5793(02)03450-6. PMID: 12387885

[29] https://en.wikipedia.org/wiki/Resistin

[30] Effect of exercise on myosteatosis in adults: a systematic review and meta-analysis. Ramírez-Vélez R, Ezzatvar Y, Izquierdo M, García-Hermoso A. J Appl Physiol (1985). 2021 Jan 1;130(1):245-255. doi: 10.1152/japplphysiol.00738.2020. Epub 2020 Nov 12. PMID: 33180646

[31] High-protein home parenteral nutrition in malnourished oncology patients: a systematic literature review. Cotogni P, Shaw C, Jimenez-Fonseca P, Partridge D, Pritchett D, Webb N, Crompton A, Garcia-Lorda P, Shepelev J. Support Care Cancer. 2023 Dec 22;32(1):52. doi: 10.1007/s00520-023-08218-z. PMID: 38129578

[32] Association of Protein Intake with Recurrence and Survival Following Primary Treatment of Ovarian Cancer. Johnston EA, Ibiebele TI, Friedlander ML, Grant PT, van der Pols JC, Webb PM; Ovarian cancer Prognosis And Lifestyle (OPAL) Study Group. Am J Clin Nutr. 2023 Jul;118(1):50-58. doi: 10.1016/j.ajcnut.2023.05.002. Epub 2023 May 3. PMID: 37146759

[33] Protein Intake and Breast Cancer Survival in the Nurses' Health Study. Holmes MD, Wang J, Hankinson SE, Tamimi RM, Chen WY. J Clin Oncol. 2017 Jan 20;35(3):325-333. doi: 10.1200/JCO.2016.68.3292. Epub 2016 Nov 7. PMID: 28095274

[34] Dietary Intake of Branched Chain Amino Acids and Breast Cancer Risk in the NHS and NHS II Prospective Cohorts. Tobias DK, Chai B, Tamimi RM, Manson JE, Hu FB, Willett WC, Eliassen AH. JNCI Cancer Spectr. 2021 Apr 12;5(3):pkab032. doi: 10.1093/jncics/pkab032. eCollection 2021 Jun. PMID: 34632269

[35] Identification of a leucine-mediated threshold effect governing macrophage mTOR signalling and cardiovascular risk. Zhang X, Kapoor D, Jeong SJ, Fappi A, Stitham J, Shabrish V, Sergin I, Yousif E, Rodriguez-Velez A, Yeh YS, Park A, Yurdagul A Jr, Rom O, Epelman S, Schilling JD, Sardiello M, Diwan A, Cho J, Stitziel NO, Javaheri A, Lodhi IJ, Mittendorfer B, Razani B. Nat Metab. 2024 Feb;6(2):359-377. doi: 10.1038/s42255-024-00984-2. Epub 2024 Feb 19. PMID: 38409323

[36] The inverse associations between composite-dietary-antioxidant-index and sarcopenia risk in US adults. Wang K, Zhou Q, Jiang Z, Liu S, Tang H. Front Endocrinol (Lausanne). 2024 Sep 17;15:1442586. doi: 10.3389/fendo.2024.1442586. PMID: 39355616

[37] Dietary intake of total, animal, and plant proteins and risk of all cause, cardiovascular, and cancer mortality: systematic review and dose-response meta-analysis of prospective cohort studies. Naghshi S, Sadeghi O, Willett WC, Esmaillzadeh A. BMJ. 2020 Jul 22;370:m2412. doi: 10.1136/bmj.m2412. PMID: 32699048

[38] Data from the National Research *Council. Nutrient Requirements of Dairy Cattle, Nutrient Requirements of Swine, Nutrient Requirements of Beef Cattle, Nutrient Requirements of Poultry, etc.* Washington, DC: The National Academies Press. https://nap.nationalacademies.org/topic/296/agriculture/animal-health-and-nutrition

[39] A high ratio of dietary animal to vegetable protein increases the rate of bone loss and the risk of fracture in postmenopausal women. Study of Osteoporotic Fractures Research Group. Sellmeyer DE, Stone KL, Sebastian A, Cummings SR. Am J Clin Nutr. 2001 Jan;73(1):118-22. doi: 10.1093/ajcn/73.1.118. PMID: 11124760

[40] The Role of the Anabolic Properties of Plant- versus Animal-Based Protein Sources in Supporting Muscle Mass Maintenance: A Critical Review. Berrazaga I, Micard V, Gueugneau M, Walrand S. Nutrients. 2019 Aug 7;11(8):1825. doi: 10.3390/nu11081825. PMID: 31394788

[41] Egg White Protein Promotes Developmental Growth in Rodent Muscle Independently of Leucine Content. Kido K, Koshinaka K, Iizawa H, Honda H, Hirota A, Nakamura T, Arikawa M, Ra SG, Kawanaka K. J Nutr. 2022 Jan 11;152(1):117-129. doi: 10.1093/jn/nxab353. PMID: 34610138

[42] Amino acid-dependent control of mTORC1 signaling: a variety of regulatory modes. Takahara T, Amemiya Y, Sugiyama R, Maki M, Shibata H. J Biomed Sci. 2020 Aug 17;27(1):87. doi: 10.1186/s12929-020-00679-2. PMID: 32799865

43 Where to Find Leucine in Food and How to Feed Elderly With Sarcopenia in Order to Counteract Loss of Muscle Mass: Practical Advice. Rondanelli M, Nichetti M, Peroni G, Faliva MA, Naso M, Gasparri C, Perna S, Oberto L, Di Paolo E, Riva A, Petrangolini G, Guerreschi G, Tartara A. Front Nutr. 2021 Jan 26;7:622391. doi: 10.3389/fnut.2020.622391. eCollection 2020. PMID: 33585538

44 Role of insulin in the regulation of human skeletal muscle protein synthesis and breakdown: a systematic review and meta-analysis. Abdulla H, Smith K, Atherton PJ, Idris I. Diabetologia. 2016 Jan;59(1):44-55. doi: 10.1007/s00125-015-3751-0. Epub 2015 Sep 24. PMID: 26404065

45 Causal relationship between insulin resistance and sarcopenia. Liu ZJ, Zhu CF. Diabetol Metab Syndr. 2023 Mar 15;15(1):46. doi: 10.1186/s13098-023-01022-z. PMID: 36918975

46 Association of postprandial postexercise muscle protein synthesis rates with dietary leucine: A systematic review. Wilkinson K, Koscien CP, Monteyne AJ, Wall BT, Stephens FB. Physiol Rep. 2023 Aug;11(15):e15775. doi: 10.14814/phy2.15775. PMID: 37537134

47 Leucine supplementation enhances integrative myofibrillar protein synthesis in free-living older men consuming lower- and higher-protein diets: a parallel-group crossover study. Murphy CH, Saddler NI, Devries MC, McGlory C, Baker SK, Phillips SM. Am J Clin Nutr. 2016 Dec;104(6):1594-1606. doi: 10.3945/ajcn.116.136424. Epub 2016 Nov 9. PMID: 27935521

48 Defining meal requirements for protein to optimize metabolic roles of amino acids. Layman DK, Anthony TG, Rasmussen BB, Adams SH, Lynch CJ, Brinkworth GD, Davis TA. Am J Clin Nutr. 2015 Jun;101(6):1330S-1338S. doi: 10.3945/ajcn.114.084053. Epub 2015 Apr 29. PMID: 25926513

49 Cheese Ingestion Increases Muscle Protein Synthesis Rates Both at Rest and During Recovery from Exercise in Healthy, Young Males: A Randomized Parallel-Group Trial. Hermans WJH, Fuchs CJ, Hendriks FK, Houben LHP, Senden JM, Verdijk LB, van Loon LJC. J Nutr. 2022 Apr 1;152(4):1022-1030. doi: 10.1093/jn/nxac007. PMID: 35020907

50 Protein quality and the food matrix: defining optimal versus maximal meal-based protein intakes for stimulating muscle protein synthesis. Barnes TM, Deutz MT, Zupančič Ž, Askow AT, Moore DR, Burd NA. Appl Physiol Nutr Metab. 2023 Apr 1;48(4):340-344. doi: 10.1139/apnm-2022-0373. Epub 2022 Feb 3. PMID: 36735923

51 utritional regulation of muscle protein synthesis with resistance exercise: strategies to enhance anabolism. Churchward-Venne TA, Burd NA, Phillips SM. Nutr Metab (Lond). 2012 May 17;9(1):40. doi: 10.1186/1743-7075-9-40. PMID: 22594765

52 Dileucine ingestion is more effective than leucine in stimulating muscle protein turnover in young males: a double blind randomized controlled trial. Paulussen KJM, Alamilla RA, Salvador AF, McKenna CF, Askow AT, Fang HY, Li Z, Ulanov AV, Paluska SA, Rathmacher JA, Jäger R, Purpura M, Burd NA. J Appl Physiol (1985). 2021 Sep 1;131(3):1111-1122. doi: 10.1152/japplphysiol.00295.2021. Epub 2021 Jul 29. PMID: 34323596

53 https://fdc.nal.usda.gov/fdc-app.html#/food-details/170148/nutrients

54 Energy expenditure and body composition changes after an isocaloric ketogenic diet in overweight and obese men. Hall KD, Chen KY, Guo J, Lam YY, Leibel RL, Mayer LE, Reitman ML, Rosenbaum M, Smith SR, Walsh BT, Ravussin E. Am J Clin Nutr. 2016 Aug;104(2):324-33. doi: 10.3945/ajcn.116.133561. Epub 2016 Jul 6. PMID: 27385608

55 The Effects of a Very-Low-Calorie Ketogenic Diet on the Intestinal Barrier Integrity and Function in Patients with Obesity: A Pilot Study. Linsalata M, Russo F, Riezzo G, D'Attoma B, Prospero L, Orlando A, Ignazzi A, Di Chito M, Sila A, De Nucci S, Rinaldi R, Giannelli G, De Pergola G. Nutrients. 2023 May 30;15(11):2561. doi: 10.3390/nu15112561. PMID: 37299524

56 The effect of high-protein diets on coronary blood flow. Fleming RM. Angiology. 2000 Oct;51(10):817-26. doi: 10.1177/000331970005101003. PMID: 11108325

57 The Role of the Anabolic Properties of Plant- versus Animal-Based Protein Sources in Supporting Muscle Mass Maintenance: A Critical Review. Berrazaga I, Micard V, Gueugneau M, Walrand S. Nutrients. 2019 Aug 7;11(8):1825. doi: 10.3390/nu11081825. PMID: 31394788

58 Effects of antinutritional factors on protein digestibility and amino acid availability in foods. Gilani GS, Cockell KA, Sepehr E. J AOAC Int. 2005 May-Jun;88(3):967-87. PMID: 16001874

59 Whole grain consumption and risk of cardiovascular disease, cancer, and all cause and cause specific mortality: systematic review and dose-response meta-analysis of prospective studies. Aune D, Keum N, Giovannucci E, Fadnes LT, Boffetta P, Greenwood DC, Tonstad S, Vatten LJ, Riboli E, Norat T. BMJ. 2016 Jun 14;353:i2716. doi: 10.1136/bmj.i2716. PMID: 27301975

60 Soy, Soy Isoflavones, and Protein Intake in Relation to Mortality from All Causes, Cancers, and Cardiovascular Diseases: A Systematic Review and Dose-Response Meta-Analysis of Prospective Cohort Studies. Nachvak SM, Moradi S, Anjom-Shoae J, Rahmani J, Nasiri M, Maleki V, Sadeghi O. J Acad Nutr Diet. 2019 Sep;119(9):1483-1500.e17. doi: 10.1016/j.jand.2019.04.011. Epub 2019 Jul 2. PMID: 31278047

61 Association of food groups and dietary pattern with breast cancer risk: A systematic review and meta-analysis. Shin S, Fu J, Shin WK, Huang D, Min S, Kang D. Clin Nutr. 2023 Mar;42(3):282-297. doi: 10.1016/j.clnu.2023.01.003. Epub 2023 Jan 12. PMID: 36731160

62 Fruit and vegetable consumption and incident breast cancer: a systematic review and meta-analysis of prospective studies. Farvid MS, Barnett JB, Spence ND. Br J Cancer. 2021 Jul;125(2):284-298. doi: 10.1038/s41416-021-01373-2. Epub 2021 May 18. PMID: 34006925

63 Dietary Protein Sources and Incidence of Breast Cancer: A Dose-Response Meta-Analysis of Prospective Studies. Wu J, Zeng R, Huang J, Li X, Zhang J, Ho JC, Zheng Y. Nutrients. 2016 Nov 17;8(11):730. doi: 10.3390/nu8110730. PMID: 27869663

64 Soy and isoflavones consumption and breast cancer survival and recurrence: a systematic review and meta-analysis. Qiu S, Jiang C. Eur J Nutr. 2019 Dec;58(8):3079-3090. doi: 10.1007/s00394-018-1853-4. Epub 2018 Oct 31. PMID: 30382332

65 Soy and other legumes: 'Bean' around a long time but are they the 'superfoods' of the millennium and what are the safety issues for their constituent phytoestrogens? Setchell KD, Radd S. Asia Pac J Clin Nutr. 2000 Sep;9 Suppl 1:S13-22. doi: 10.1046/j.1440-6047.2000.009s13.x. PMID: 24398273

66 Review of Nutrition Guidelines and Evidence on Diet and Survival Outcomes for Cancer Survivors: Call for Integrating Nutrition into Oncology Care. Li Z, Ding X, Chen Y, Keaver L, Champ CE, Fink CL, Lebovits SC, Corroto M, Zhang FF. J Nutr. 2024 Aug;154(8):2346-2362. doi: 10.1016/j.tjnut.2024.05.024. Epub 2024 May 24. PMID: 38797479

67 Postdiagnosis dietary factors, supplement use and breast cancer prognosis: Global Cancer Update Programme (CUP Global) systematic literature review and meta-analysis. Becerra-Tomás N, Balducci K, Abar L, Aune D, Cariolou M, Greenwood DC, Markozannes G, Nanu N, Vieira R, Giovannucci EL, Gunter MJ, Jackson AA, Kampman E, Lund V, Allen K, Brockton NT, Croker H, Katsikioti D, McGinley-Gieser D, Mitrou P, Wiseman M, Cross AJ, Riboli E, Clinton SK, McTiernan A, Norat T, Tsilidis KK, Chan DSM. Int J Cancer. 2023 Feb 15;152(4):616-634. doi: 10.1002/ijc.34321. Epub 2022 Oct 24. PMID: 36279902

68 Postdiagnosis body fatness, recreational physical activity, dietary factors and breast cancer prognosis: Global Cancer Update Programme (CUP Global) summary of evidence grading. Tsilidis KK, Cariolou M, Becerra-Tomás N, Balducci K, Vieira R, Abar L, Aune D, Markozannes G, Nanu N, Greenwood DC, Giovannucci EL, Gunter MJ, Jackson AA, Kampman E, Lund V, Allen K, Brockton NT, Croker H, Katsikioti D, McGinley-Gieser D, Mitrou P, Wiseman M, Cross AJ, Riboli E, Clinton SK, McTiernan A, Norat T, Chan DSM. Int J Cancer. 2023 Feb 15;152(4):635-644. doi: 10.1002/ijc.34320. Epub 2022 Oct 24. PMID: 36279885

69 Protein content and amino acid composition in the diet of Danish vegans: a cross-sectional study. Aaslyng MD, Dam AB, Petersen IL, Christoffersen T. BMC Nutr. 2023 Nov 15;9(1):131. doi: 10.1186/s40795-023-00793-y. PMID: 37968717

70 Clinical presentation and metabolic consequences in 40 breastfed infants with nutritional vitamin B12 deficiency--what have we learned? Honzik T, Adamovicova M, Smolka V, et al. Eur J Paediatr Neurol. 2010 Nov;14(6):488-95. doi: 10.1016/j.ejpn.2009.12.003. PMID: 20089427

71 Vitamin B-12 supplementation during pregnancy and early lactation increases maternal, breast milk, and infant measures of vitamin B-12 status. Duggan C, Srinivasan K, Thomas T, et al. J Nutr. 2014 May;144(5):758-64. doi: 10.3945/jn.113.187278. PMID: 24598885

72 Vitamin B-12 content in breast milk of vegan, vegetarian, and nonvegetarian lactating women in the United States. Pawlak R, Vos P, Shahab-Ferdows S, Hampel D, et al. Am J Clin Nutr. 2018 Sep 1;108(3):525-531. doi: 10.1093/ajcn/nqy104. PMID: 29931273

73 https://ods.od.nih.gov/factsheets/Riboflavin-HealthProfessional/

74 Taurine and GABA neurotransmitter receptors, a relationship with therapeutic potential? Ochoa-de la Paz L, Zenteno E, Gulias-Cañizo R, Quiroz-Mercado H. Expert Rev Neurother. 2019 Apr;19(4):289-291. doi: 10.1080/14737175.2019.1593827. Epub 2019 Mar 20. PMID: 30892104

75 Dietary Responses of Dementia-Related Genes Encoding Metabolic Enzymes. Parnell LD, Magadmi R, Zwanger S, Shukitt-Hale B, Lai CQ, Ordovás JM. Nutrients. 2023 Jan 27;15(3):644. doi: 10.3390/nu15030644. PMID: 36771351

76 The potential protective effects of taurine on coronary heart disease. Wójcik OP, Koenig KL, Zeleniuch-Jacquotte A, Costa M, Chen Y. Atherosclerosis. 2010 Jan;208(1):19-25. doi: 10.1016/j.atherosclerosis.2009.06.002. Epub 2009 Jun 11. PMID: 19592001

77 https://ods.od.nih.gov/factsheets/Carnitine-HealthProfessional/

78 https://lpi.oregonstate.edu/mic/dietary-factors/L-carnitine

79 L-carnitine versus Propranolol for pediatric migraine prophylaxis. Amini L, Yaghini O, Ghazavi M, Aslani N. Iran J Child Neurol. 2021 Spring;15(2):77-86. doi: 10.22037/ijcn.v15i2.25558. Epub 2021 Mar 1. PMID: 36213159

80 Carnitine Responsive Migraine Headache Syndrome: Case Report and Review of the Literature. Charleston L 4th, Khalil S, Young WB. Curr Pain Headache Rep. 2021 Mar 23;25(4):26. doi: 10.1007/s11916-021-00936-5. PMID: 33755806

81 Carnitine: Fact Sheet for Health Professionals https://ods.od.nih.gov/factsheets/carnitine-HealthProfessional/ (accessed Sept. 2024)

82 Creatine synthesis: hepatic metabolism of guanidinoacetate and creatine in the rat in vitro and in vivo. da Silva RP, Nissim I, Brosnan ME, Brosnan JT. Am J Physiol Endocrinol Metab. 2009 Feb;296(2):E256-61. doi: 10.1152/ajpendo.90547.2008. Epub 2008 Nov 18. PMID: 19017728

83 Synthesis of guanidinoacetate and creatine from amino acids by rat pancreas. da Silva RP, Clow K, Brosnan JT, Brosnan ME. Br J Nutr. 2014 Feb;111(4):571-7. doi: 10.1017/S0007114513003012 PMID: 24103317

84 Cerebral creatine deficiencies: a group of treatable intellectual developmental disorders. Stockler-Ipsiroglu S, van Karnebeek CD. Semin Neurol. 2014 Jul;34(3):350-6. doi: 10.1055/s-0034-1386772. Epub 2014 Sep 5. PMID: 25192512

85 Carbohydrate ingestion augments skeletal muscle creatine accumulation during creatine supplementation in humans. Green AL, Hultman E, Macdonald IA, Sewell DA, Greenhaff PL. Am J Physiol. 1996 Nov;271(5 Pt 1):E821-6. doi: 10.1152/ajpendo.1996.271.5.E821. PMID: 8944667

86 Creatine supplementation protocols with or without training interventions on body composition: a GRADE-assessed systematic review and dose-response meta-analysis. Pashayee-Khamene F, Heidari Z, Asbaghi O, Ashtary-Larky D, Goudarzi K, Forbes SC, Candow DG, Bagheri R, Ghanavati M, Dutheil F. J Int Soc Sports Nutr. 2024 Dec;21(1):2380058. doi: 10.1080/15502783.2024.2380058. Epub 2024 Jul 23. PMID: 39042054

87 The Effect of Creatine Supplementation on Resistance Training-Based Changes to Body Composition: A Systematic Review and Meta-analysis. Desai I, Wewege MA, Jones MD, Clifford BK, Pandit A, Kaakoush NO, Simar D, Hagstrom AD. J Strength Cond Res. 2024 Jul 23. doi: 10.1519/JSC.0000000000004862. Online ahead of print. PMID: 39074168

88 Oral creatine monohydrate supplementation improves brain performance: a double-blind, placebo-controlled, cross-over trial. Rae C, Digney AL, McEwan SR, Bates TC. Proc Biol Sci. 2003 Oct 22;270(1529):2147-50. doi: 10.1098/rspb.2003.2492. PMID: 14561278; PMCID: PMC1691485.

89 Effect of creatine and weight training on muscle creatine and performance in vegetarians. Burke DG, Chilibeck PD, Parise G, Candow DG, Mahoney D, Tarnopolsky M. Med Sci Sports Exerc. 2003 Nov;35(11):1946-55. doi: 10.1249/01.MSS.0000093614.17517.79. PMID: 14600563

90 The influence of creatine supplementation on the cognitive functioning of vegetarians and omnivores. Benton D, Donohoe R. Br J Nutr. 2011 Apr;105(7):1100-5. doi: 10.1017/S0007114510004733. Epub 2010 Dec 1. PMID: 21118604

91 Creatine supplementation research fails to support the theoretical basis for an effect on cognition: Evidence from a systematic review. McMorris T, Hale BJ, Pine BS, Williams TB. Behav Brain Res. 2024 May 28;466:114982. doi: 10.1016/j.bbr.2024.114982. Epub 2024 Apr 4. PMID: 38582412

92 Carnosine and Beta-Alanine Supplementation in Human Medicine: Narrative Review and Critical Assessment. Cesak O, Vostalova J, Vidlar A, Bastlova P, Student V Jr. Nutrients. 2023 Apr 5;15(7):1770. doi: 10.3390/nu15071770. PMID: 37049610

93 High level of skeletal muscle carnosine contributes to the latter half of exercise performance during 30-s maximal cycle ergometer sprinting. Suzuki Y, Ito O, Mukai N, Takahashi H, Takamatsu K. Jpn J Physiol. 2002 Apr;52(2):199-205. doi: 10.2170/jjphysiol.52.199. PMID: 12139778

94 Vegetarianism, female gender and increasing age, but not CNDP1 genotype, are associated with reduced muscle carnosine levels in humans. Everaert I, Mooyaart A, Baguet A, Zutinic A, Baelde H, Achten E, Taes Y, De Heer E, Derave W. Amino Acids. 2011 Apr;40(4):1221-9. doi: 10.1007/s00726-010-0749-2. Epub 2010 Sep 24. PMID: 20865290

95 High-Intensity Interval Training Augments Muscle Carnosine in the Absence of Dietary Beta-alanine Intake. DE Salles Painelli V, Nemezio KM, Pinto AJ, Franchi M, Andrade I, Riani LA, Saunders B, Sale C, Harris RC, Gualano B, Artioli GG. Med Sci Sports Exerc. 2018 Nov;50(11):2242-2252. doi: 10.1249/MSS.0000000000001697. PMID: 30334920

96 https://ods.od.nih.gov/factsheets/Choline-HealthProfessional/

97 Growth, body composition, and cardiovascular and nutritional risk of 5- to 10-y-old children consuming vegetarian, vegan, or omnivore diets. Desmond MA, Sobiecki JG, Jaworski M, Płudowski P, Antoniewicz J, Shirley MK, Eaton S, Książyk J, Cortina-Borja M, De Stavola B, Fewtrell M, Wells JCK. Am J Clin Nutr. 2021 Jun 1;113(6):1565-1577. doi: 10.1093/ajcn/nqaa445. PMID: 33740036

98 The efficacy of L-carnitine in patients with nonalcoholic steatohepatitis and concomitant obesity. Zakharova N, Luo C, Aringazina R, Samusenkov V. Lipids Health Dis. 2023 Jul 12;22(1):101. doi: 10.1186/s12944-023-01867-3. PMID: 37438785; PMCID: PMC10337194.

99 L-carnitine supplementation to diet: a new tool in treatment of nonalcoholic steatohepatitis--a randomized and controlled clinical trial. Malaguarnera M, Gargante MP, Russo C, Antic T, Vacante M, Malaguarnera M, Avitabile T, Li Volti G, Galvano F. Am J Gastroenterol. 2010 Jun;105(6):1338-45. doi: 10.1038/ajg.2009.719. PMID: 20068559

100 https://nutritionheartbeat.com/sports-nutrition/leucine-diet-muscle

101 https://fdc.nal.usda.gov/fdc-app.html#/food-search?query=&type=Foundation

14: Fish, Poultry, Meat

The Meat

Briefly, mammalian meat (a.k.a. red meat) gets a DAD score of D (for dreadful – do not consume) and is proscribed from the SANA diet. For those interested, Chapter 33 details additional health risks associated with meat, especially red meat consumption.

Consumption of the skin of any animal, mammal, fowl, fish, or frog is prohibited on the SANA diet.

A principal problem is that meat from mammals is insufficiently degraded by the human digestive system, and undigested remnants ferment in the lower intestine, promoting dysbiosis and toxic metabolites. Mammalian meat is banned from the SANA diet. No pork, no beef, no goat, no venison, no lamb. No "Great green gobs of greasy, grimy gopher guts, mutilated monkey meat, dirty little rabbit feet or French-fried eyeballs rolling down a dirty street."

White meat from healthy, free-range chicken and turkey, if properly prepared, can be occasionally consumed as part of the SANA diet. Even when properly prepared, it typically gets a DAD score of zero. Most chicken meat gets a DAD score of A or lower.

Several commercially available fish are excellent sources of omega-3 fatty acids that provide health benefits and can be consumed as part of the SANA program when they are properly prepared. Other fish are not. In general, these are "oily" fish. Other fish, mostly "white" fish and fish that are top predators, are not recommended in the diet. Fried and breaded fish is not allowed on the SANA diet.

Meat and Health

Elephants have a fairly long lifespan of 60 to 70 years. Although they can suffer from parasitic disease, respiratory infections, anthrax, and predation by humans, they don't succumb to chronic inflammatory diseases of aging as do humans. While we get one set of primary and one set of adult teeth, elephants get their last of six sets of molars at the age of 30 to 40. Elephants are large animals that eat enormous amounts of vegetation; grass, leaves, twigs, and tree bark. The constant grinding from eating wears down their molars over time, and most elephants in the wild eventually die of starvation as they can no longer process sufficient food. Elephants rarely get cancer, but they also have the advantage of having 15 – 20 copies of the tumor suppressor gene TP53.[1]

Gorillas are another vegan in which cancer is extremely rare; a single case of melanoma has been reported in gorillas. Like elephants, gorillas suffer from parasites, respiratory infections, malaria, and human predation. While the mountain gorillas rarely get dental caries, they can develop periodontitis, leading to tooth loss,[2] but this is mostly when eating a captive diet with fruits cultivated for human consumption. Ebola is a great risk to the about 1000 mountain gorillas remaining in the wild.[3] The common chronic diseases of aging in humans, diabetes, atherosclerotic heart disease, stroke, and cancer, are not evident in gorillas in the wild. In contrast, cardiovascular disease is common in primates in captivity, and in zoos, cardiovascular disease is the cause of death of nearly 40% of chimpanzees and 45% of bonobos. Gorillas do suffer from myocardial fibrosis in the wild, but that is a result of viral infections.[4]

Cancer appears to cause death in all families of animals, including fish and invertebrates. Although cancer risk increases with age, small animals with a shorter lifespan do not escape this risk. In an assessment of 191 species of non-domesticated animals, kowari, a small ravenous marsupial predator in Australia that feeds on mice, rats, and almost any other animal it can catch, has the highest incidence of cancer mortality (ICM) of any animal; 57% of kowari die of cancer, mostly malignant oral squamous cell carcinoma. Animals in the order *Perissodactyla* (zebras, giraffes, tapirs, rhinos), and *Artiodactyla* (mostly hoofed ungulates such as camels, pigs, deer, bison, hippos, and moose) have the lowest ICM: 2.4 and 3.2% respectively. In contrast, *Carnivora* (jackals, wolves, seals, raccoons, lions, tigers, and bears have an ICM of 11.2%. Overall, non-human primates have an ICM of 5.5%. Notably, the animals that have the lowest cancer risk are vegans; the high-risk *Carnivora* are carnivorous. When assessed by class, the various species of fish, reptiles, birds, and mammals that consume flesh as a primary or secondary food source are more than twice as likely to die of cancer as are other animals in their class that infrequently or never eat meat. Mammals that eat mammals were found to be at significantly higher risk of cancer mortality. Interestingly, the consumption of invertebrate prey (such as mollusks) was not found to be associated with increased ICM.[5] To be fair, some cancers associated with the consumption of meat by carnivorous animals may be transmitted via viral vectors. Adequate cooking, which most carnivores neglect to do, should inactivate viral vectors in meat.

Islam forbids the consumption of predators with canine teeth and birds with talons, which is a good idea health-wise, as predators tend to bioaccumulate toxins;

this hazard has become much more severe in the last century. The Bible considers reptiles (lizards), all amphibians (frogs), worms, centipedes, and insects (cockroaches), except for four types of locusts, unclean. Four-footed animals with paws (dogs, bears, and cats, including lions and tigers, predators, are also unclean). Carrion eaters are definitely unclean, as are birds of prey, as well, ostriches, storks, herons, and bats. Camels and rabbits are also unclean in Judaism. The list of "clean" animals is much smaller than the unclean list. Please consider these animals prohibited by the SANA diet as well.

The SANA diet differs from the Biblical prohibitions, as it allows the consumption of invertebrate seafood, including oysters, crabs, clams, shrimp, and young lobsters after cooking.

Skin from poultry and fish also gets a D and is prohibited on the SANA diet. The consumption of chicken skin, fish skin, turkey skin, shrimp shells, and all other animal skin is banned from the diet.

Basic rules, easy to follow. No mammalian flesh, no skin of poultry or fish, don't eat weird stuff.

The central goal of the SANA program is to provide dietary guidance that helps people live healthier, happier lives. There are some things that people who want to consume flesh can eat on the SANA diet, but the recommendations are narrow. The list limits consumption to those foods that provide the most health benefits, or at least, the lowest adverse impacts on health. The consumption of animal flesh is not a requirement for human health; however, it is a concentrated source of protein and other nutrients.

The DAD scores for fish and poultry shown in Table 14 are near optimal scores, meaning that the scores reflect the use of high-quality products and proper preparation.

Meat as a Protein Source

We need adequate protein in our diets, and need substantial amounts to build muscle mass. Meat is a rich source of protein; nevertheless, not all sources are equally healthy.

A meta-analysis of studies that examined the risk of type 2 diabetes (T2D) and protein source found that higher levels of dietary protein intake were associated with an about 12% increased risk of T2D. However, when stratified by the source and amount of protein intake, animal protein was associated with a 14% increase in T2D risk, red meat was associated with a 22% increase in risk, and processed meat with a 37% increase in risk of T2D. Protein consumption from fish and eggs did not impact T2D risk, and dairy protein intake was associated with a significantly lower risk of T2D. Higher intake of plant proteins, including soy, was associated with a decreased risk of T2D in women but did not reach statistical significance in men.[6]

Table 14A: Fish. Poultry, Meat Scoreboard

Herring, pickled, without skin	4
Mackerel (without skin) (in water)	4
Mullet fresh, baked	4
Herring (smoked in oil), skin removed	3
"Steelhead Trout (farmed) (poached)	3
Spotted seatrout (speckled trout) baked	3
Oysters, steamed	3
Salmon, fresh (poached)	2
Salmon, from pouch (Alaskan pink)	2
Swai, from Vietnam	2
Herring (smoked in oil) with skin	2
Sardines (Chicken of the Sea) (with or without skin)	2
Clams (canned, chopped)	1+
Surimi, Artificial Crab	1+
Seafood, Bay scallop	1+
Grouper	1
Tilapia	1
Yellowfin tuna, wild caught, Vietnam	1
Shrimp (steamed)	1
Tuna, albacore canned	1
Chicken breast, free range, cooked 1.5 hours at 145° F	1
Chicken breast, canned (Swanson brand)	1
Tuna, light, canned in water	0
Tuna, light, in pouch	0
Chicken Liver (boiled)	0
Chicken breast, free range, boiled	0
Chicken (light meat from the breast) boiled	A
Turkey cold cut, no preservatives, smoked	A
Fish, Cod	A
Chicken (dark meat from the thigh)	A-
Chicken Gizzard	B
Beef	D
Chicken Skin	D
Fish Skin: Trout, Salmon, Herring	D
Pork, ground	D
Pork, baked ham off the bone	D
Sausage	D
Shrimp shell	D

In a meta-analysis of the association of animal protein intake and neurodegenerative disease, those consuming higher amounts of fish were 25% less likely to develop Alzheimer's disease (AD) and 16% less likely to develop any form of dementia. The risk of Parkinson's disease (PD) was significantly (40%) higher for those in the top quartile of milk consumption as compared to those in the lowest quartile. Total dietary protein intake was associated with a lower risk of cognitive impairment. Interestingly, dairy consumption was associated with a lower risk of dementia but a higher risk of PD.[7] In a mouse model of PD, if casein protein from milk entered the lower intestine, it decreased the alpha diversity of the microbiome, induced inflammation, and reactivated dopaminergic nerve injury that underlies PD.[8] Casein should not reach the lower intestine, but it may if there is malabsorption or dumping syndrome. This may happen in lactose intolerance.

The risk of inflammatory bowel disease (IBD) is also impacted by the sources of dietary protein. A meta-analysis of prospective follow-up studies with over 4.3 million participants and over 8,000 cases of IBD found that dairy consumption was associated with a lower risk of IBD. Among those consuming higher amounts of dairy products, the risk of ulcerative colitis was 18% lower, and the risk of Crohn's disease was 31% lower. Fish consumption was associated with a non-significant decrease in risk, while meat consumption increased risk.[9]

A central tenet of the SANA program is that dietary protein that is not digested and absorbed, and thus ends up in the lower intestine, where it ferments, promoting dysbiosis, leaky gut, and inflammation. This is reflected in the DAD scores of foods with poorly digested proteins.

Some cuts of chicken have a less-detrimental (still not great) DAD score than others, and some fish have better scores than others. The preparation of fish and meat also has an impact on their digestibility and on the formation of toxins. Some people batter, fry, and eat the skin of fish and chicken; this is prohibited on the SANA diet as a result of its detrimental impact on health.

While the SANA diet proscribes red meat, restricts the intake of poultry, and limits which fish are consumed, it does not advocate a low-protein diet, as discussed in the previous chapter. If meat is removed from the diet, it needs to be replaced with high-quality protein from other sources. Legumes, eggs, and dairy can be excellent sources when properly prepared. The amount of dietary protein required for health on the SANA diet may be somewhat lower than in other diets, as this diet focuses on preparing proteins so that they are easily and nearly completely digested and absorbed.

Fatty Acids

The balance of polyunsaturated fatty acids in the diet can impact health and promote chronic inflammation. If the balance of n-6 to n-3 fatty acids is high, it promotes inflammation. Ideally, the dietary n-6 to n-3 ratio is less than 2:1. For Americans, who typically have a n-6 to n-3 ratio of about 15 to one or higher, an aspirational goal of less than four to one has been recommended.

One of the many negative aspects of red meat is that cattle are fed a diet high in corn, and thus their muscle has an n-6 to n-3 ratio that reflects that of their diet. This is true for chicken as well. Grass-fed beef, dairy cows, and free-range chicken may have healthier n-6 to n-3 ratios, depending on what other feed they are given.

Wild fish feed on a food chain based on algae, which is high in n-3 fats. Thus, wild-caught fish are high in n-3 fats, including EPA and DHA. Catfish raised commercially are generally given feed containing soybean and cottonseed meal, corn, and corn and wheat by-products, and thus have a polyunsaturated fat ratio reflecting that.

Poultry

Chickens that spend their life cooped up in crowded conditions are going to be less healthy than free-range birds. Free-range animals have more opportunity for exercise and are generally leaner. They will have the opportunity to eat some bugs, various seeds, and leaves. When cooped up, their diet is mostly corn, resulting in meat high in n-6 fats.

While eating poultry is not encouraged on the DAD diet, its occasional consumption is allowed. For the most part, chicken and turkey get scores of A, for avoid. It is recommended that if poultry is eaten, it be limited to no more than once a week. Eating healthy, free-range poultry is a better choice than eating those from cooped conditions.

Although limited amounts of poultry are permitted, there are some caveats:

- ❖ If the person has active dysbiotic disease, such as a flare of inflammatory bowel disease, it is advised not to eat any A – D rated foods, including poultry.
- ❖ Processed poultry meat containing preservatives (such as nitrates) or fillers is not permitted on the SANA diet.
- ❖ The meat should not be cooked at high temperatures; it should not be fried or braised.

The meat should not have its surface dry or charred during cooking. A better method of preparation is to remove the skin and simmer the meat in water. Even cooking chicken in a pressure cooker raises the temperature enough to encourage the formation of advanced glycation end-products (AGEs), which are detrimental to health.

❖ Chicken skin has a score of D and should never be eaten.

The *light meat* (for example, breast and wings) from *free-range chickens and turkeys*, properly prepared, gets a rating of zero to one, meaning that it has little impact on dysbiosis. Chicken liver (boiled, not fried) is a source of easily accessible iron; it also gets a zero. Consumption of chicken liver can be helpful for women with iron deficiency. Thus, although not encouraged for daily consumption, free-range chicken breast cooked in water can be eaten as a part of the DAD diet.

The drumsticks and thighs are dark meat, while the breast and wings are white in these flightless birds. The dark meat has more heme (as myoglobin) and more fat, as these muscles have a more sustained workload. Ducks are not flightless and do not have light meat; duck meat is very fatty, and if fed corn, will have a high n-6 to n-3 ratio. It should be avoided.

Properly prepared *white meat* from free-range chickens and turkeys, and breasts from typically raised birds get an A+, while dark meat from typically raised chickens and turkeys gets an A-. Gizzards, which are a tougher meat, rate a B. Chicken wing-tips, unless carefully dissected to remove the skin, get a D. Fried chicken is not permitted on the SANA diet.

Preparation: Select free-range chicken breast that has had the skin removed and the fat trimmed off. The breast should be stewed, simmering it at a temperature of 63°C to 75°C (144°F to 167°F) for at least one hour to improve flavor, digestibility, and satiation.[10] Check this reference for a discussion of the best methods.

Note: I have concerns about the long-term health risks from cooking in plastic bags (sous vide), and thus, rather recommend cooking in water of the appropriate temperature.

Thus, the best selection of poultry is the breasts of free-range chicken or turkeys that are cooked at below a boiling temperature. For those who do not have an active problem with dysbiosis, who are otherwise compliant with the DAD diet, an *occasional* serving of white meat from chicken or turkey that is not free-range, and is not fried or cooked at excessive temperatures should not cause dysbiosis.

Fast food in a pinch: Subway Sandwiches will serve any sandwich as a salad. Oven-roasted turkey or Rotisserie-style chicken, [11] served as a salad with tomatoes, cucumbers, spinach, and avocado, but without the bread, sauces, or dressing or other contraband items, is a reasonable choice for those who choose to eat meat when choices are limited. As of the time of this writing, Subway has unfortunately discontinued serving gluten-free or sourdough bread.

Alternatively, the Swanson brand premium canned chicken breast gets a score of one and can be used in salads or sandwiches. Even properly prepared chicken is not a highly recommended food on the SANA diet, but it is allowed in limited amounts.

Fish Frets

1. Preparation and Selection
2. Fish Oil
3. Methylmercury and forever chemicals
4. Digestibility
5. Mislabeled Fish
6. Farming practices.
7. Sustainability

Preparation

While seafood is generally allowed on the SANA diet, it should not be assumed that eating fish is necessarily healthy. In fact, on the whole, fish consumption does not lower mortality rates. In follow-up studies such as the Nurses' Health Study, fish consumption does not lower mortality risk. It just gets kudos for being less damaging than red meat. Similarly, beans, as generally prepared and consumed, have a minimal beneficial impact on health. Proper preparation is essential.

Fish's failure to improve health is in part the way it is consumed. Some of the most frequent fish meals are things such as a McDonald's Filet-O-Fish sandwich, served on an iodinated bleached wheat flour bun, with (un)-American cheese, and tartar sauce. The fish is breaded, and the sandwich contains 19 grams of fat. This is commonly washed down with a medium (21-ounce) cola and a serving of French fries. Fried fish is part of the deadly, high-fat Southern Diet. Fried fish, especially when breaded, is not permitted on the SANA diet.

Another fishy meal is a tuna fish sandwich made with mayonnaise and white bread. This would likely get a DAD score of B. Thus, while on the whole, fish consumption does not reduce overall mortality, it is not because it can't, but rather because of which fish are eaten and how the fish is prepared.

Omega-3 Fats

As a rule of thumb, oily fish have a beneficial dietary effect on chronic disease prevention, in large part due to the high content of omega-3 fatty acids in their muscle tissue. The fillets of oily fish may contain as much as 30% oil, while non-oily fish (whitefish) generally have about 2% fat in their fillets. Consumption of oily fish can thus provide health benefits. The fish oil includes linolenic acid, but more importantly, it contains DHA (docosahexaenoic acid), which is important for brain health, and EPA (eicosapentaenoic acid), which is a precursor to anti-inflammatory metabolites.

A simple categorization divides commonly consumed fish into two groups, whitefish and oily fish. Whitefish generally have white flesh, while oily fish have darker or reddish flesh. Oily fish are generally "pelagic", meaning that they live in the water column, as opposed to living near the shore or along the seafloor or bottom of lakes, as do "demersal" fish, which generally are whitefish. If one is consuming fish for its healthy n-3 oil content, whitefish is a poor source of n-3 fats as compared to oily fish. Many of the oily fish are forage fish that live in large schools, while white fish are often predators.

Oily fish ranked by their approximate n-3 fat per 100-gram serving include:

- Mackerel
- Herring
- Salmon
- Mullet
- Trout
- Sablefish
- Sardines

The name sardines is a catch-term for small fish that include at least 4 different genera of small oily fish. Sardines, sprats, and anchovies are oily fish that have high levels of n-3 fats.

Albacore tuna has low levels of n-3 fats, and skipjack tuna has insignificant amounts. Demersal fish that are common in the seafood trade include flounder, halibut, sole, cod, redfish, sea bass, hake, haddock, pollock, and fish called confusingly named whitefish (*Coregonidae*), which is a freshwater fish found in the Great Lakes and other lakes. If you are eating fish for their n-3 fats, eating beans would likely be a more effective choice than eating most white fish. Skipjack tuna gets a DAD score of zero. Albacore at twice the cost gets a 1. If you are going to eat fish for its health benefits, you might as well choose fish that provides the most benefit.

Forage fish are smaller, oily fish that live in large schools and feed on plankton. They are at the bottom of the food chain and are consumed by larger fish. They are also referred to as bait fish. These are generally oily fish and include herring (sardines), mullet, anchovies, and menhaden. One of the best oily fish in terms of n-3 fats is menhaden, but it is so bony and oily that no one eats it. It is harvested and made into fish oil capsules and animal feed, including feed for fish.

Eating fried, and especially breaded-fried, fish gets a negative DAD score, as the added n-6 fats overwhelm the n-3 fatty acids. One can take fish-oil capsules, but they are ineffective for disease prevention unless the person's diet is low enough in n-6 fats that the fish oil content nearly matches the amount of n-6 fats consumed. This likely explains why fish oil supplements work well for disease prevention in animal (rat) models but rarely show any benefit in human studies.[12]

It may come as a surprise, but some studies of dietary habits have shown that fish consumption was associated with the risk of diabetes. It is speculation on my part, but this may have resulted from the selection of fish eaten at the time of these studies. In the U.S., the most consumed "fish" is shrimp, with an average consumption of around 4 pounds per year. Until 2011, the next-most consumed fish was tuna, with a consumption of about 2.8 pounds a year, followed by salmon. In recent years, salmon consumption has overtaken tuna consumption, with the average consumption in the U.S. being nearly 4 pounds per year.[13]

The studies that showed an increased risk of diabetes collected data in the early 2000s. Those consuming fish several times a week were probably mostly eating tuna. Tuna salad sandwiches were widely available in cafeterias, sandwich and fast food outlets, and even vending machines; shrimp and salmon were not. Tuna consumed as salad in sandwiches contained mayonnaise made with vegetable oil. Frequent fish consumption may also have been breaded, fatty fish burgers from fast food franchises.

Mercury >((((°≥ >(((°≥ >(((°≥

Little fish are eaten by bigger fish that are eaten by still larger fish. Along the way, mercury and some other nasty chemical pollutants can build up in the top predators, accumulated from all the little fishies' diets along the food chain. Top predator fish accumulate methylmercury in their flesh; these fish should be avoided. Fish from polluted areas also accumulate forever-chemicals. The Baltic Sea in Northern Europe is heavily polluted, and fish from it have high levels of PCBs and dioxin, *especially in oily fish.* Avoid fish from this and other polluted areas.

Fish with Low Mercury Levels[14]

Anchovy	Atlantic croaker	Black sea bass
Butterfish	Catfish	Clam
Cod	Crab	Crawfish
Flounder	Haddock	Hake
Herring	Lobster	Mackerel
Mullet (American and spiny)		Oyster
Pacific chub	Perch	Pickerel
Plaice	Pollock	Salmon
Sardine	Scallops	Shad
Shrimp	Skate	Smelt
Sole	Squid	Tilapia
Tuna canned light (skipjack)		Whitefish
Trout (freshwater)		Whiting

Predator fish spend most of their time chasing and snacking on small and medium-sized fish every day. Fish can live a long time. Slimehead (sold under the name "orange roughy") can live over 200 years before it lands on your plate. That is a long time to build up mercury and forever chemicals. Long-lived top predator fish accumulate methylmercury and should not be consumed. Some of the fish with the highest mercury levels include tilefish, bigeye tuna, king mackerel, marlin, orange roughy, shark, bluefin tuna, and swordfish. Sharks are top predators and accumulate mercury. Albacore and yellowfin tuna have somewhat lower levels of mercury and should only be eaten occasionally. Mercury is a neurotoxin that gets trapped in the brain and accumulates there over one's lifetime. The consumption of these fish should be avoided.

Canned and Pouched Fish

Canned tuna: Albacore *Thunnus alalunga*) has whiter flesh and is usually labeled "white" tuna. It contains some n-3 fats, but not much. Canned tuna labelled "light tuna" is typically Yellowfin (*Thunnus albacares*), Bigeye (*Thunnus obesus*), Skipjack (*Katsuwonus pelamis*), or a combination of these. Skipjack is the tuna lowest in mercury, but also very low in n-3 fatty acids.

Pouch tuna generally has a better flavor and texture than canned tuna. For prepping and camping, canned tuna in oil is packed with extra calories, and the oil can be used to help get a cooking fire going. Other than that, it should be avoided. Canned sardines, mackerel, and herring come packed in vegetable oil. The oil can be used to help start a campfire, but eating the oil is not recommended except as a survival food. Fish packed in oil get lower DAD scores than those packed in brine, even after discarding the oil.

Pouch tuna appears to be about twice as expensive per ounce as canned tuna, but this is usually an illusion. Checking a common brand, a 5-ounce can of light tuna containing a single serving had 17 grams of protein, while the similarly priced 2.6-ounce pouch from the same brand contained 19 grams of protein. For the amount of protein, and therefore the quantity of fish, the pouch was less expensive than the can.

A healthier choice than canned or pouched tuna is skinless, boneless, pouched wild-caught, Alaskan pink salmon. It is about 50% more expensive per serving than tuna pouches, but the salmon contains much more n-3 fat and gets a DAD rating of 2, while the tuna gets a zero. Mackerel and herring can also be found sold in pouches. Avoid those packed in oil; they get a lower DAD score and introduce undesirable fats that interfere with the benefits of the n-3 fats in the fish.

Wild-caught Alaskan salmon is also sold canned. It is generally made from smaller fish, may occasionally have soft vertebral bones, and may contain skin that needs to be removed. It is overcooked for many uses, but can still be used to make salmon salad (as per tuna salad), and with some creativity, it can be used to prepare tasty meals. Here are some ideas: salmon and potato chowder, pasta with a salmon cream sauce, and salmon with crushed pineapple salad. Some recipes for pouched and canned fish are given below.

Finally, if you have a hankering for a tuna salad sandwich and would like a vegan version, consider a mock-tuna salad sandwich made with properly prepared chickpeas. A recipe is included in the legume section, and it is quite tasty.

Fatfood Fish

At the time of this writing, McDonald's, Dairy Queen, Burger King, and Wendy's fish sandwiches all use wild-caught Alaskan Pollock in their fish burgers. All of these are breaded and contain substantial amounts of fat (with very little fat coming from the fish). Burger King's fish sandwich contains more than 1.5 ounces (45.7 grams, 411 calories) of fat! Quiznos Small Tuna Melt is a less-terrible choice with *only* 11 grams of fat and is served with tomatoes and pickles.[15] Subway also serves tuna. All of these are best avoided.

Digestibility

Some fish are easier to digest than others. Thus, some fish are tougher to digest and get worse scores, while others get better DAD ratings. Cod, a white fish, gets an A, while swai (pangasius), a freshwater white fish, gets a DAD score of 2. Swai is a low-cost fish imported as fillets from Vietnam with a mild taste and firm texture. It is not a premium fish, but with the right preparation, it is presentable. Swai may get its unexpectedly high score for a white fish, as it provides a digestible protein.

Surimi, a.k.a. "crab sticks", "imitation crab", or "kani", is made of pulverized whitefish, most commonly from Alaskan pollock in the U.S. Although it usually does not, it may contain wheat and egg white, so read the label, especially if you have allergies. Surimi gets a DAD score of 1. The processing may help make the protein especially easy to digest.

Farming Practices and Sustainability

>((((°> >((((°> >((((°>

Let me preface the following section by saying that the dietary recommendations provided for the SANA diet are based on medical science as I understand it, and not on moral or value judgments. Some people may avoid eating meat or may be vegan out of concern for animal welfare, the environmental impact, or based on religious values. I leave these decisions to the individual. The concerns expressed in this section are practical. Dietary recommendations need to be based on foods that are available, thus foods that can be sustainably provided. The SANA diet recommends the consumption of oily fish that are low in mercury for their health benefits. These are, by their nature, generally smaller fish that have short reproductive cycles and thus can be more sustainably harvested.

Salmon famously hatch in rivers and migrate into the ocean during their adult lives. Twelve species of *Oncorhynchus* live along the Pacific coast and rivers of North America; half of these are salmon and half are considered trout. After the eggs are laid in streams, the babies (parr) live in the streams for up to 3 years, and then their metabolism changes so that the smolts can live in salt water. They move into estuaries where their bodies can gradually adapt to the higher salinity before migrating out into the open ocean. Most salmon then live in the ocean for 3 to 5 years before they reach sexual maturity. The fish then return to where they hatched to mate, lay eggs, and then die. Before the building of dams in the Pacific Northwest, some chinook and sockeye salmon would swim up the Columbia River into British Columbia, and up the Snake River as far as Wyoming. Still, some swim over 900 miles (1,400 km) with an increase in elevation of over 7,000 feet (2.1 km).

There are 150 hydropower dams on the Columbia River and its tributaries, with 18 dams on the main river.[16] The salmon are amazing jumpers, and even their name comes from the Latin "salire," which means "to leap". But jumping over dams and up the fish ladders is too much. So, the U.S. government, in the 1930s, built hatcheries to move the parr upriver as the adult salmon could not make it. It is not working so well. In the last 20 years, the Federal Government has spent $2.2 billion trying to maintain a poorly conceived hatchery system while the salmon population continues to collapse. It is estimated that it costs between $250 and $650 for each salmon that makes it back to the river to spawn. Habitat restoration and the removal of many small, obsolete dams would be a better use of funds.[17]

Most of the salmon sold in the U.S. is imported from Chile and Canada, and is labeled Atlantic Salmon. Atlantic salmon are endangered, so commercial catching of wild Atlantic Salmon is illegal; wild Atlantic Salmon is not legally sold in the U.S.

Most farmed salmon are grown in feedlots in bays and fjords. Fish farming practices destroy the local environment. There is so much salmon poop that it kills everything on the seafloor and causes algal blooms that deplete oxygen from the water, causing a dead zone. Some of the salmon in the pens suffocate from swimming in their own feces. The crowding causes the spread of disease and parasites. These are not healthy conditions, and not healthy fish.

If you take the global salmon harvests (most of which are farmed) and divide them by the human populations, your share would be less than a pound a year: 3 to 4 servings per year. And even at that consumption rate, it is unsustainable and destroys the wild salmon population through the spread of disease and the harvest of smaller fish as feed for the farmed fish. Meanwhile, you may be eating a diseased animal that spent its life in horrid, filthy conditions.

(Pounds of salmon produced) 6,363,377,802/ (World population in January 2024) 8,019,876,189 = 0.787 pounds per person = 12.6 oz per person per year.

Salmon is not a dietary requirement. Until we humans fix this situation, I suggest leaving most salmon off the menu. If you do purchase salmon, I recommend wild-caught Alaskan salmon or Coho salmon farmed on shore.

A better alternative to farmed salmon is inland farmed steelhead from the Pacific Northwest, which are sustainably produced. Since these farmed fish never go out to sea, it is inaccurate to call them "steelhead," which is what the fish is called after it goes out to sea during its adult life. They are technically large rainbow or Columbia River Redband trout that are marketed as steelhead.

Herring is generally harvested sustainably and has a very good DAD rating if the skin is removed.

Fresh mullet does not keep well and is usually only available locally. It is usually smoked to preserve it. It, too, has a good DAD score.

While "sustainably harvested" indicates that the industry is managing the fishery to avoid overfishing and declines in the wild population, unfortunately, it doesn't mean that current populations are anywhere close to what they were in 1950 or earlier. The goal of fish management should be to rebuild fish stocks over time for long-term sustainability.

When purchasing fish, look for labels from organizations like the Marine Stewardship Council (MSC), Fishery Improvement Projects (FIP), or the Marine Conservation Society (MCS) to support sustainable fishing practices. Avoid tuna labeled as "ocean-caught" as this doesn't guarantee sustainable practices. By making informed choices, you can help promote sustainable fishing practices and healthy oceans, and the availability of fish into the future.

As of this writing, among "Chicken of the Sea", "Bumble Bee", "Starkist", and the Walmart tuna, only "Chicken of the Sea" and the Walmart brand are MSC labeled.

Fraudulent Fish

Fish fakery flourishes in the U.S. Using DNA fingerprinting, it has been determined that about one-third of fish purchases in the U.S. were not "as labeled". In Sushi restaurants, 74% of fish were misrepresented; 38% of fish in restaurants, and 18% at grocers were also mislabeled. Red snapper was severely overfished, and while still popular, the fish is hard to come by. Sushi represented as having red snapper is usually tilapia on the East coast and rockfish on the West coast, but it is rarely red snapper.[18] Restaurants commonly misrepresent fish and serve less expensive fish or less sustainable fish in their place. The "wild-caught Alaskan salmon" served in restaurants is often actually farm-raised Atlantic salmon, which costs the restaurant half as much. Swai, as a result of its low cost, is often served in restaurants as catfish or other fish. From talking with people who have worked in the restaurant and bar business, the top-shelf bottles of liquor and wine with premium prices are commonly refilled with a cheaper product at the end of the business day.

White tuna is mislabeled 59% of the time; 84% of that is actually escolar, a fish banned from sale in Japan and Italy because of its high concentration of gempylotoxin. This fish, like oilfish (not to be confused with oily fish), is a snake mackerel that accumulates toxic wax esters in its flesh. If consumed in sufficient quantities, it causes cramping and diarrhea or anal leakage with orange, oily, greasy stools, usually a few hours, but up to 4 days after its consumption.[19] [20] I can attest to this from personal experience, from the consumption of counterfeit tuna on a couple of occasions before I learned my lesson. Tuna served in restaurants should thus be considered a D on the DAD scale.

Proper Preparation

The preparation of the fish impacts its health benefits. Frying fish, and worse, breading and frying fish, may negate much of the benefits of fish consumption from n-3 fats, as well as introducing toxic compounds into the meal. Shallow, steam poaching is the preferred preparation method. The consumption of fish skin is prohibited on the SANA diet. Fish may be carefully baked if covered and not allowed to char.

How to Shallow Poach a Fish Fillet

Choose a wide pan or skillet with a well-fitting lid. Add enough poaching liquid (water, broth, or beer) to barely cover the bottom of the pan. Season the liquid with salt and any herbs you like (lemon slices, parsley sprigs are common options).

Use gentle heat. Bring the poaching liquid to a simmer. Simmering is key – some small bubbles should be breaking the surface gently, and there should not be a rolling boil. The goal is to steam the fish.

Season the fish fillet with salt. Carefully slide the fish fillet into the simmering liquid. Cover the pan with the lid to retain the steam with a lid and gently simmer for 4-6 minutes per ½ inch thickness of the fillet. For thicker fillets, you might need to adjust the cooking time slightly. The temperature should be high enough to steam the fish, low enough that neither the pan nor the fish dries out.

After the estimated time, gently flake the fish with a fork. If it flakes easily and appears opaque throughout, it's cooked through. If not, simmer for another minute or two.

Carefully remove the fish fillet from the pan with a slotted spoon or spatula and transfer it to a plate. You can spoon some of the poaching liquid over the fish for extra flavor, or use it as a base for a sauce.

Fish and seafood should be cooked to a minimum internal temperature of 145°F (63°C) to ensure that any bacteria in the fish are not viable.

What to Do with Pre-Cooked Fish

Canned and pouched fish can be an affordable way of getting sustainable n-3 fats and protein that is reliably available year-round. Where I live, chub mackerel and herring, fish highest in n-3 fats, are only available canned or pouched.

Before fish are canned, they are cleaned, but some fish are still raw when placed into the can. Larger fish, such as tuna, may be precooked. Fish that comes in pouches and cans has been cooked, typically at a temperature of 113–160° C. The fish are cooked long enough for the small bones to soften, and nearly dissolve the bones in smaller fish.

The fish may be soaked in brine, broth, or oil. Avoid those soaked in oil, as it will undo the benefits from the n-3 fats present in the fish. The ratio of n-3 to n-6 fats helps determine the inflammatory impact of the fats, and the n-3 fats are hard to come by.

Canned and pouched fish are overcooked and taste overcooked, but still provide n-3 fatty acids and protein. I find that fish in pouches with trivial amounts of broth or brine generally tastes better and has a better texture than canned fish, but this is not always the case.

What can be done with this overcooked fish to make it taste good?

- Fish can be used to make salad as per tuna salad, but using salmon or other high-scoring fish instead.
- Sardines, herring, mackerel, and salmon can be used to make yellow rice. Smoked fish adds flavor.
- It can be made into a chowder.
- Fish can be used to make fish cakes (as per crab cakes) and fish loaf (as per meatloaf). This may sound unappetizing, but if you give it a try, you may just want to repeat the experience.

Fish cakes are often fried, something excluded from the SANA diet. Here, instead, they can be air-fried or baked. The fish loaf is basically the same recipe, but baked as a loaf rather than individual cakes, and thus, there is less crisping and browning. Here, it is recommended that the fish cakes or loaves be cooked as one would a quiche or flan, with the pan or bowls in water and covered with foil to avoid browning. This improves the quality and flavor. The cakes can be cooked in custard dishes or cupcake tins using cupcake liners, and baked to make individual-sized servings and avoid undesirable browning.

For those who want crispy fish cakes, they can be made in an air-fryer, which gives a different flavor and a lower score.

Fish skin should be removed when possible. For these small pre-cooked fish, if the skin is present, it is usually as a thin layer that one may be able to gently scrape away with the edge of a butter knife and discard.

Fish Cakes and Fish Loaf (DAD score 4)

Ingredients:

- Pre-cooked fish:
  - 1 (14¾ ounce) can of salmon
  - or (14¾ ounce) can of mackerel,
  - or 12 oz pouch of mackerel, undrained
- ¾ cup masa harina or presoaked hominy grits*
- ¾ cup onion, chopped or diced
- 1/3 cup unsweetened applesauce
- ¼ cup medium salsa picante
- ¼ teaspoon salt
- 1 teaspoon garlic powder
- 3 Tbsp grated Parmesan cheese
- 2 eggs, beaten
- 1 tsp baking powder (optional, for a lighter loaf)

Preheat the oven to 350 deg F.

In a medium-sized mixing bowl, combine all ingredients and mix thoroughly. I suggest lightly scraping the fish to remove the thin layer of skin and splitting the fish, and removing the easily accessible bones, although it is not really necessary.

If not using the brine, increase the amount of applesauce to ½ cup.

- Press mixture into a lightly greased 9x5 loaf pan, cover with foil or baking parchment, and bake for 45 minutes or until done, let cool 5 minutes before slicing; <u>or</u>
- Place into custard dishes about 2/3 full, cover with foil, place in a water bath, and bake for 25 – 30 minutes.
- If there is excessive browning of the base, place the loaf pan in a tray of water during baking next time.

Fish cakes: This recipe can be used to make fish cakes. The mix can be formed into patties, and they can be air-fried.

* If using hominy grits, presoak the grits as per the hominy grit recipe in Chapter 9.

Fish Pate

Fish pate can be made with various types of pre-cooked fish, but if available, smoked fish is especially good.

Ingredients:

- 4 - 6 ounces skinless pre-cooked fish
- 1/3 cup plain Greek yogurt
- 1 freshly crushed clove of garlic
- 1 Tbsp salsa
- A pinch of salt

- ½ tsp. lemon juice (to taste)
- 1¼ cup finely chopped broccoli or cauliflower buds
- 1 Tbsp chopped fresh cilantro (optional)
- 2 tsp. nonpareil capers (optional to garnish)

Separate the fish from the brine/broth. Remove and discard any skin on the fish.

Put the fish in a bowl and break it up with a fork. You can remove any bones you find, but they should be soft and not cause any problems. Add the Greek yogurt and crushed garlic, and then add the salt, salsa, and lemon juice to taste and mix until the pate is a consistency of your liking (chunky or smooth). Gently fold in the broccoli/cauliflower and cilantro.

Salmon Salad

Ingredients:

- One 5-ounce pouch of sustainably harvested Pacific/Alaskan salmon
- 1 Tbsp Greek yogurt
- 3 Tbsp pickle relish or drained, crushed pineapple
- 1 Tbsp minced fresh cilantro

Gently mix the ingredients, leaving some chunks of salmon. A sprinkle of salt can be used. If using canned pineapple, it should be sweet and tart (some canned pineapple is bland and thus not helpful). Refrigerate.

Anisakis Seafood Allergy

Although many people have allergies to shellfish and fish, one of the most common causes of IgE-mediated seafood allergy is not an allergy to fish or other shellfish. It is an allergy to *Anisakis*, a parasite that lives in fish, squid, and mollusks.[21] These worms live in the flesh of the fish, and if eaten, can trigger an immune hypersensitivity reaction. The most common reaction is urticaria, but abdominal pain is not uncommon, and anaphylaxis can occur. Fish are variably infested with these nematodes; for example, about 10% of tuna are infested. This may explain why eating one type of fish may cause a reaction on one occasion but not on another; it can depend on whether the fish was infected.

Far grosser than eating well-seasoned and cooked worms hidden in a fish filet is eating live worms and having them eat you back! Allergy to *Anisakis* is most commonly the result of a previous infection by this worm. Consumption of raw (e.g., sushi), pickled (e.g., ceviche), or inadequately cooked fish allows live *Anisakis* larvae to invade the intestinal wall. A few hours after consumption of live *Anisakis* larvae, nausea and abdominal pain, and vomiting may occur. If the larvae are successful at burrowing into the stomach or intestinal wall, an inflammatory granuloma will form over the next several days, which can give symptoms similar to inflammatory bowel disease.[22] In rare cases, this can cause bowel obstruction. In contrast to fish, the human immune system is usually able to rid itself of this parasite, but the immune reaction sets the stage for IgE-mediated allergic reactions to *Anisakis* proteins in the future.

Anisakis larvae live in crustaceans and in the fish and squid that consume these crustaceans. Freezing seafood and storing it at/ or below -4°F (-20°C) for 7 days will kill the *Anisakis* larvae, as well as those of *Pseudoterranova* (cod worm) and *Diphyllobothrium* (fish tapeworms)[23]; some other parasites that humans can get from eating fish. Home freezers that do get this cold may allow survival of these parasites. Cooking fish to an internal temperature of over 160° will also kill the parasites.

Cooking may decrease allergenicity somewhat, but it does not eliminate the allergic reactions.[24] The best way to avoid developing an allergy to *Anisakis* is to avoid the brief infection with this parasite by eating properly prepared seafood. Ceviche, sushi, and other uncooked seafood should only be prepared with fish that have been frozen for at least seven days in a commercial freezer; never fresh.

[1] https://en.wikipedia.org/wiki/Peto%27s_paradox

[2] WHAT ILLNESSES DO GORILLAS SUFFER FROM? https://www.berggorilla.org/en/gorillas/general/everyday-life/what-illnesses-do-gorillas-suffer-from/

[3] https://nationalzoo.si.edu/global-health-program/gorilla-health-wild

[4] Cardiovascular Disease in Great Apes. Rita McManamon, Linda Lowenstine. Verterian Key, Chapter 53, https://veteriankey.com/cardiovascular-disease-in-great-apes/

[5] Cancer risk across mammals. Vincze O, Colchero F, Lemaître JF, Conde DA, Pavard S, Bieuville M, Urrutia AO, Ujvari B, Boddy AM, Maley CC, Thomas F, Giraudeau M. Nature. 2022 Jan;601(7892):263-267. doi: 10.1038/s41586-021-04224-5. Epub 2021 Dec 22. PMID: 34937938

[6] Dietary Protein Consumption and the Risk of Type 2 Diabetes: A Systematic Review and Meta-Analysis of Cohort Studies. Tian S, Xu Q, Jiang R, Han T, Sun C, Na L. Nutrients. 2017 Sep 6;9(9):982. doi: 10.3390/nu9090982. PMID: 28878172

[7] Association between animal protein sources and risk of neurodegenerative diseases: a systematic review and dose-response meta-analysis. Talebi S, Asoudeh F, Naeini F, Sadeghi E, Travica N, Mohammadi H. Nutr Rev. 2023 Aug 10;81(9):1131-1143. doi: 10.1093/nutrit/nuac114. PMID: 36647769

[8] Casein Reactivates Dopaminergic Nerve Injury and Intestinal Inflammation with Disturbing Intestinal Microflora and Fecal Metabolites in a Convalescent Parkinson's Disease Mouse Model. Pu Z, Liu S, Guo Z, Zhang X, Yan J, Tang Y, Xiao H, Gao J, Li Y, Bai Q. Neuroscience. 2023 Aug 1;524:120-136. doi: 10.1016/j.neuroscience.2023.05.014. Epub 2023 Jun 14. PMID: 37321369

[9] The Association between Total Protein, Animal Protein, and Animal Protein Sources with Risk of Inflammatory Bowel Diseases: A Systematic Review and Meta-Analysis of Cohort Studies. Talebi S, Zeraattalab-Motlagh S, Rahimlou M, Naeini F, Ranjbar M, Talebi A, Mohammadi H. Adv Nutr. 2023 Jul;14(4):752-761. doi: 10.1016/j.advnut.2023.05.008. Epub 2023 May 14. PMID: 37187455

[10] https://www.seriouseats.com/the-food-lab-complete-guide-to-sous-vide-chicken-breast

[11] https://www.eatthis.com/healthiest-subway-sandwiches/

[12] Omega-3 fatty acids for the primary and secondary prevention of cardiovascular disease. Abdelhamid AS, Brown TJ, Brainard JS, Biswas P, Thorpe GC, Moore HJ, Deane KH, AlAbdulghafoor FK, Summerbell CD, Worthington HV, Song F, Hooper L.Cochrane Database Syst Rev. 2018 Jul 18;7(7):CD003177. doi: 10.1002/14651858.CD003177.pub3. PMID: 30019766

[13] https://aboutseafood.com/about/top-ten-list-for-seafood-consumption/

[14] https://www.fda.gov/food/consumers/advice-about-eating-fish

[15] https://www.aol.com/5-healthiest-fast-food-fish-153324896.html

[16] https://www.opb.org/article/2024/04/07/power-generated-by-northwest-dams-falls/

[17] https://www.opb.org/article/2022/05/24/pacific-northwest-federal-salmon-hatcheries-declining-returns/

[18] Oceana Study Reveals Seafood Fraud Nationwide. Warner K, Timme T, Lowel B, Hirhsfiled M.

[19] Bad Bug Book: Handbook of Foodborne Pathogenic Microorganisms and Natural Toxins. FDA

[20] *"National Seafood Fraud Testing Results Highlights" (PDF). Oceana Report. 2013-02-21.*

[21] The clinical characteristics of Anisakis allergy in Korea. Choi SJ, Lee JC, Kim MJ, Hur GY, Shin SY, Park HS. Korean J Intern Med. 2009 Jun;24(2):160-3. doi: 10.3904/kjim.2009.24.2.160. PMID: 19543498

[22] Anisakidosis: report of 25 cases and review of the literature. Bouree P, Paugam A, Petithory JC. Comp Immunol Microbiol Infect Dis. 1995 Feb;18(2):75-84. doi: 10.1016/0147-9571(95)98848-c. PMID: 7621671

[23] HACCP: Hazard Analysis Critical Control Point Training Curriculum (Blue) SGR 120 4th Edition. Appendix 3: Hazards Found in Seafood

[24] Immediate and cell-mediated reactions in parasitic infections by Anisakis simplex. Ventura MT, Tummolo RA, Di Leo E, D'Ersasmo M, Arsieni A. J Investig Allergol Clin Immunol. 2008;18(4):253-9. PMID: 18714532

15: Eggs

Easter Egg

Eggs can be an excellent health food or induce a destructive proinflammatory impact depending upon how they are prepared. They have a bad reputation, which is partially deserved. But it is not the fault of the egg, but rather the cook.

When overheated or overcooked, egg proteins become hard to digest. When overheated cholesterol in the eggs becomes oxidized. The DAD score of eggs can range from four ★★★★ to D, depending on how they are prepared.

Eggs are delicate and need to be handled carefully. This includes proper storage and cooking. Eggs are ideally cooked at about 170°F (@ 76°C). They should never be heated to the boiling point; hard-boiled eggs get a score of C. Proper preparation of eggs takes attention, patience, and a gentle hand.

Eggs

Most primates are omnivores, but consume a mostly plant-based diet. There is a great variation between the diets of various primates, but mostly their diets are dominated by fruits, leaves, and other vegetable matter. Marmosets are insectivores (insect-eating) and also consume tree gum. Male chimpanzees will hunt small animals, but meat typically makes up less than 2% of their diets. Female chimps can, but rarely hunt. Other than those that eat insects, the most universal non-vegan food for non-human primates may be eggs. While bird eggs are the most commonly eaten eggs among primates, baboons, chimpanzees, and orangutans will risk their lives robbing crocodile nests for their eggs. There must be something in eggs that makes them worth the risk.

Eggs are a great source of protein and of choline, and for modern humans, they are easily available without any danger from crocs or gators. The proteins in eggs have strong antioxidant activity;[1] however, this may not have much effect after digestion. Eggs have a bad reputation for being a health hazard, which is deserved, however, for the wrong reasons. Perhaps there is no other food that is more commonly consumed and more perniciously prepared.

The principal reason for eggs' nefarious infamy is that they are high in cholesterol (discussed later), and thus, eggs are often maligned as increasing the risk of heart disease.

A meta-analysis looked at the impact that egg consumption has on premature death. It included 32 publications, 2.2 million participants, and more than 232,000 deaths. Overall, eggs did not impact mortality. Egg consumption did not increase the risk of coronary artery or respiratory disease-related death. They were associated with a nearly significant 19% decreased risk of death from stroke (RR: 0.81; 95% CI: 0.64, 1.02), and they were associated with a *20% increase in risk of cancer* (RR: 1.20; 95% CI: 1.04, 1.39). Each egg consumed per week was associated with a 4% decreased risk of stroke mortality but a 4% increased risk of all-cause and cancer mortality.[2] The good and the bad balance out.

But before you stop eating eggs, eggs are not carcinogenic. People created carcinogens by cooking eggs at excessive temperatures. Also note that the result of the meta-analysis conclusively debunks bogus advice about eggs increasing the risk of heart disease that has been bandied about since the 1960s. We have been fed sixty years of misinformation for breakfast.

Eggs can range from being beneficial to being toxic, depending on their preparation. The gentle handling that eggs require before they are used foreshadows how delicately and patiently they need to be prepared if one hopes to retain their health benefits. The term "hard-boiled" refers to a person who is tough and callous and to an egg, one that is tough and hard to digest.

Eggs can have a DAD rating from ★★★★ to D, depending upon their preparation.

A hard-boiled egg that has been overcooked is dense, rubbery, and has a sulfurous odor; the outside of the yolk has a greenish cast, and its consumption results in foul vapors. As a dubious advantage, the loss of water from the egg during overcooking shrinks the egg enough that it makes peeling the egg easier. The shrinking occurs as a result of denaturing various proteins in the egg, followed by cross-linking the proteins. This allows water to be expelled. These tightly cross-linked proteins are not as easily degraded by the pancreatic and intestinal proteolytic enzymes. More of the egg's protein can thus escape digestion and end up in the colon, where it is fermented; thus, the foul vapors.

Egg yolk is a substantial source of choline, an important nutrient. The genetic variant ApoE4, which is a risk factor for Alzheimer's disease, causes astrocytes in the brain to accumulate triglycerides, causing injury to the cells. Having a sufficient supply of choline helps convert the triglycerides into phospholipids, which the cells can get rid of. Thus, adequate choline is thought to decrease astrocyte injury in those with ApoE4.[3]

If there is maldigestion and malabsorption, however, choline can escape digestion and be fermented in the colon, with trimethylamine (TMA) as the product. TMA is absorbed into the body and converted to trimethylamine-N-oxide (TMAO) in the liver. TMAO is at least a marker of risk, if not a direct risk, for cardiovascular disease. This, however, does not seem to be a significant problem from poorly cooked eggs, as typically prepared eggs (which are, for the most part, badly prepared) do not significantly raise TMAO levels in population studies when 2 or fewer eggs are consumed per day. For individuals with dumping syndrome or malabsorption, however, overcooked eggs may increase the risk of TMAO formation.

For a while, it was thought that brown eggs had higher levels of TMA than white eggs.[4] If eggs have enough TMA content, they get a fishy or crabby odor. This is caused by feeding the hens high portions of feed containing sinapine, such as mustard seed and canola (rape) seed. After making canola oil, the seed cake left over is used in animal feed, and when the sinapine ferments in the chicken's lower gut, it forms TMA. Certain breeds of chicken have low expression of the enzyme FMO3 in their livers. This was first observed in chickens that lay brown eggs. Further research found the trait in Rhode Island Red and Light Sussex hens, which lay brown eggs, and in Brown Leghorns, which lay white eggs.[5] The solution to this dilemma was not to stop using canola meal, but rather to eliminate the recessive trait through selective breeding, so that TMA is properly metabolized into TMAO,[6] which obviously does not protect the bird from TMAO, but it keeps the eggs from having a fishy odor. (I love the irony.)

Cholesterol

Eggs are notorious for being high in cholesterol. (Here is one of those "I am not your doctor, I am not a financial advisor" disclaimers: this is not medical advice, consult your physician moments).

Eggs are high in cholesterol. Cholesterol is an essential component in the cell membrane of every cell in your body, and your body produces it all on its own. It is the substrate from which your body forms vitamin D when you are exposed to sunlight. There is no good or bad cholesterol; however, there may be poor cholesterol management, and this can be associated with high levels of apolipoprotein B (ApoB), a protein that helps direct where cholesterol is transported to in the body. Elevated ApoB and triglyceride levels are associated with increased risk of coronary artery calcification (CAC), but after accounting for the impact of ApoB and triglyceride levels, cholesterol is no longer a significant risk factor for CAC.[7]

Dietary cholesterol can impact blood cholesterol levels in some people. Some individuals with elevated LDL cholesterol levels are cholesterol hyperabsorbers. They very efficiently absorb cholesterol from the diet, but their bodies fail to downregulate the normal endogenous cholesterol production mechanism that helps balance cholesterol levels. These people may respond to a diet low in cholesterol. Some people with high LDL cholesterol levels are endogenous cholesterol hyper-producers; their diet may not impact their cholesterol levels significantly.[8] Cholesterol is not made by plants, so vegans don't consume any. Despite this, some vegans have high ApoB levels anyway.

In Chapter 16, the effects of dietary polyunsaturated fats are discussed. Higher amounts of polyunsaturated fats and lower amounts of saturated fats in the diet are associated with lower cholesterol levels, but an increased risk of coronary artery disease. We know that very high cholesterol levels are associated with heart disease. So, for decades, the thought has been that the lower the cholesterol level, the better. But is that correct?

We need cholesterol for normal physiologic function. What then is a healthy, normal level? Since cholesterol levels change with age, it's easier shown than said. The data illustrated in Figures 15A and 15B are from a study that collected routine medical exams from 12.8 million Korean adults from 2001–2004, and then followed the patients through 2013. Over the follow-up period, there were 694,423 fatalities within the cohort. Figure 12A shows normal (median) total cholesterol (TC) levels by age, and 15B shows mortality risk by cholesterol levels. Using the median level rather than the average provides data that is less likely to be impacted by those with pathogenic or extreme TC values.

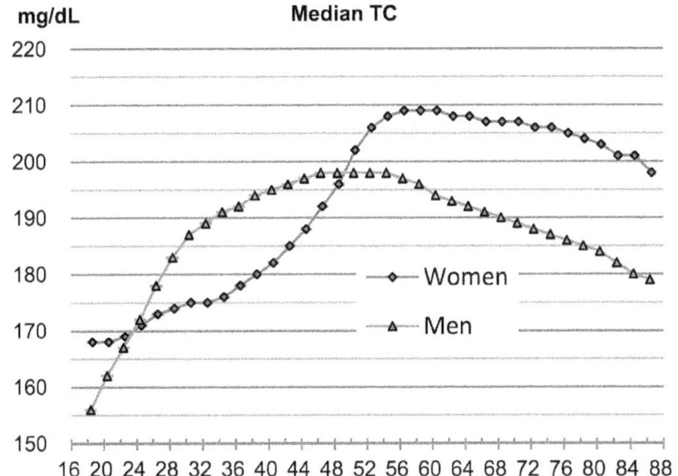

Figure 15A: Median Total Cholesterol by Age. Sang-Wook Yi et al. PMID: 30733566 (Multiply mg/dL by 0.02586 to convert cholesterol to mmol/L)

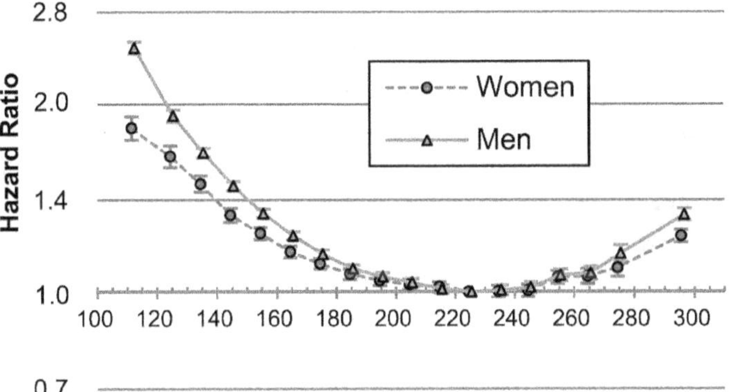

Figure 15B: Total cholesterol (TC) at baseline and risk of death during and approximately 10-year follow-up. Sang-Wook Yi et al. PMID: 30733566

Evident from these data is that low cholesterol is just as, if not more, dangerous than elevated levels. Of note, the median cholesterol levels at various ages differ between men and women, but there is much less difference in the hazard ratios associated with cholesterol levels. Not evident in these grafts is that high cholesterol levels convey more risk in those under 44 years of age. Low cholesterol levels were associated with a significant excess risk, especially in younger men. A TC level of 155 had a similar mortality risk as a total cholesterol (TC) level of 300. The association of low cholesterol levels with increased mortality is likely the result of reverse causality, wherein underlying disease causes low cholesterol levels. Low cholesterol levels, especially in younger to middle-aged men, merit an in-depth investigation to rule out alcohol abuse, liver disease, cancer, or other diseases.

Healthy cholesterol levels have a U-curve distribution, with the lowest mortality at 210–250 mg/dL, except for the youngest young men, aged 18–34 years (nadir: 180–220 mg/dL), and younger women aged 18–34 years (nadir: 160–200 mg/dL) and 35–44 years (nadir: 180–220 mg/dL). Furthermore, the risk flattens with age, so that after the age of 65, when most CVD mortality is expected, the mortality risk for total cholesterol levels between 180 and 250 mg/dL is nearly flat.[9] Using medications to lower cholesterol when levels are under 270 mg/dL likely does more harm than good, especially in the elderly.

Let me point out that the nadir of mortality risk for total cholesterol was at 230 mg/dL. This is higher than the median cholesterol level for any age or gender group (shown in Figure 12A). This suggests that (at least in Koreans) most people *might benefit from dietary modifications that raise their cholesterol levels.* (For example, by avoiding PUFA vegetable oil.)

That's just for total cholesterol. How about LDL cholesterol (LDL-C), which is commonly referred to as "bad cholesterol"? In a meta-analysis of studies including 30 cohorts, including over 68,000 individuals over the age of 60, an *inverse association between LDL-C and all-cause mortality* was found in 16 of the cohorts, representing 92% of all participants, and in the other studies, no significant association between LDL-C and all-cause mortality was found. *Cardiovascular mortality was highest* among those in the *lowest* quartile for LDL-C.[10] Analysis of over 12,000 Americans from the NHANES study found that those with non-HDL cholesterol below 130 mg/dl (total cholesterol minus "good" HDL cholesterol) in *the lowest tertile had the highest overall mortality* rate over the next 7.5 years. The nadir for all-cause mortality was a non-HDL cholesterol level of around 158 mg/dl, a level well above the mean non-HDL cholesterol level for Americans. This suggests that (at least in the U.S.A.) most people *might benefit from dietary modifications that raise their non-HDL cholesterol levels.* Looking only at cardiovascular death, non-HDL cholesterol levels over 190 mg/dl were associated with higher cardiovascular mortality; however, levels less than 220 mg/dl were not associated with higher overall mortality risk.[11] Another study that looked at a larger population of adults over the age of 18 found the nadir for all-cause mortality for non-HDL cholesterol was at 164 mg/dl (4.23 mmol/L).[12]

Diet does affect cholesterol, low-density lipoprotein (LDL) cholesterol, and ApoB levels. In a meta-analysis of 30 dietary intervention studies, switching from an omnivore diet to a vegan or vegetarian one was associated with a 7% decline in cholesterol levels, a 10% decline in LDL cholesterol levels, and a 14% decline in ApoB levels, but the switch did not lower triglyceride levels.[13] The switch was most effective in those who were not overweight or obese. The lack of dietary response in these people can likely be explained by the increased hepatic and intestinal cholesterol synthesis known to occur in obese individuals. The dietary change to a vegan diet did not significantly lower LDL levels among healthy individuals, but only those at elevated coronary vascular disease (CVD) risk, suggesting that high-risk individuals had worse baseline diets. A vegan diet has a more profound impact than a vegetarian one, but both work to lower lipid "risk" markers.

It is noteworthy that the dietary modification studies before 2006 had more than 3 times as much reduction in LDL as compared to studies performed later. Perhaps this is a result of shifts in diet within the community over time. Additionally, smaller studies showed a greater decline in cholesterol and LDL, suggesting publication bias, where negative studies did not get published. Finally, LDL levels came down more in those with above-average LDL levels than in those with less than average LDL levels. In this meta-analysis, being vegetarian implied the consumption of dairy, eggs, and likely fish. The results suggest that going from a low-quality diet to a decent one lowers ApoB, LDL, and cholesterol levels. Not a big surprise.

In a study that looked at the relationship between non-HDL cholesterol and ApoB, mortality risk was isolated to those with non-HDL cholesterol to ApoB ratios of less than 1.4. When the ratio of non-HDL cholesterol to ApoB is low (less than 1.2), it indicates small-dense low-density lipoprotein cholesterol (sdLDL-C) particles, which are depleted of cholesterol and are highly atherogenic. Interestingly, treatment using cholesterol-lowering medications did not change this risk association in this study.[14] Thus, concern and treatment over cholesterol should focus on sdLDL-C and Lipoprotein(a), as this is where the risk lies.

Lowering elevated ApoB levels should lower cardiovascular disease risk. The by far strongest correlates for elevated ApoB in a cross-sectional lifestyle study of 24,984 northern Europeans were elevated body mass index, smoking, and consumption of sugar-sweetened beverages also increased ApoB levels. Diets associated with a high ApoB to ApoA ratios additionally included those high in added sugar and non-fermented milk; the consumption of fermented dairy products, cheese, and alcohol, especially wine, was inversely associated with ApoB to ApoA ratios. Egg consumption was associated with slightly, but significantly, *lower* ApoB to ApoA ratios.[15] Elevated ApoB is likely mechanistically linked to hepatic steatosis. ApoB clearance and repression of secretion by the liver are mediated by insulin. Insulin resistance both impairs the clearance of cholesterol-depleted LDL (sdLDL) and favors the synthesis of ApoB.[16] A sustained exercise program that increased insulin sensitivity in diabetics was found to be associated with a 47% decline in circulating ApoB and a more than halving of ApoB secretion.[17]

The SANA program is well designed to prevent elevated ApoB levels and cardiovascular disease risk. The SANA diet is much less concerned about dietary cholesterol than it is about excess fat, and especially long-chain saturated fats and n-6 fats in the diet. The SANA diet is a low-fat diet; dietary fat has a larger impact on LDL cholesterol for most people than does dietary cholesterol.[18] Not everyone's metabolism is the same, but the SANA diet should help reduce CAD risk as compared to the Western diet in almost everyone, as it should help increase insulin sensitivity and lower inflammation.

I am not proposing that individuals with dyslipidemia may not benefit from treatment, but rather pointing out that most of the concern about eliminating cholesterol from the diet is likely misplaced and misdirected. I am rather offering support for the elimination of polyunsaturated vegetable oils, lard, and sugar-sweetened beverages from the diet, and allaying misguided fears about eggs.

Some people are at elevated risk of coronary artery disease from having high levels of Lp(a) (Lipoprotein-little-a), a type of LDL cholesterol associated with the risk of CVD and stroke. Lp(a) levels are largely influenced by genetics. High Lp(a) levels are particularly common among those of South Asian descent. The standard medical consensus is that dietary interventions do not impact Lp(a).

Nevertheless, when overweight and obese volunteers were placed on a plant-based diet, Lp(a) levels fell by 16% after only 4 weeks. ApoB levels fell by 11%, and small-dense low-density lipoprotein cholesterol (sdLDL-C) fell by 30%. The plant-based diet was essentially a vegan diet with minimal added fat or sugar. The inflammatory marker hsCRP was reduced by 31% and IL-6 by 23%.[19] In another clinical intervention trial, volunteers adopted a non-dairy vegetarian diet for 5 weeks. Lp(a) levels fell by 10%, sdLDL levels fell by 21%, insulin levels fell by 43%, and TMAO levels fell by 42%.[20] (TMAO is discussed in Chapter 33.)

Lp(a) does respond to diet; it just has to be the right diet.

COPs

The concern with dietary cholesterol should likely be with the amount of oxidized cholesterol in the diet.

Where does that come from? Overheating eggs or meat on the stovetop would be one way. Frying eggs so that they sputter and sing, leaving a brown lace, may be an efficient method to oxidize cholesterol. The general consensus among chefs is that light browning of an omelet is desirable. This means a browned surface, with pyrolyzed proteins and cholesterol.

I DON'T LIKE COPs! (Cholesterol Oxidation Products, a.k.a. oxysterols) COPs are biologically active and have various toxic effects, including promotion of neurodegenerative disease, atherogenesis, and carcinogenesis. At least 5 COPs can arise in eggs. 7α-hydroxycholesterol spontaneously forms in egg powder during storage.[21] Avoid powdered eggs. When scientists are looking for an animal model to quickly induce atherosclerosis, they feed powdered egg yolks to rabbits.[22] Other than 7α-hydroxycholesterol, most of the COPs form at higher cooking temperatures, well above the boiling temperature of water. For example, 7-ketocholesterol, one of the most abundant COPs, is not formed when cholesterol is heated at 125°C for 30 min, but production rises quickly at a temperature of 150°C and peaks around 180–200°C,[23 24] which is a typical frying pan temperature. Frying increases the COPs as compared to boiling, as boiling water does not rise to temperatures over 100°C. Fish do not produce high levels of COPs, as fish are fairly low in cholesterol as compared to red meat, poultry, and eggs.[25]

The yolk is the part of the egg containing the cholesterol, thus the portion that creates COPs when overheated or over-exposed to oxygen. Egg yolks are not generally whipped, but it would not be a good idea. Egg yolks contain only small amounts of creatine and thus are not a large risk for the formation of carcinogenic heterocyclic amines (HCA). Polycyclic aromatic hydrocarbons (PAHs) are created when eggs are "toasted" or browned. Overheating the egg also causes the formation of Advanced Glycation End-products (AGEs) (also known as glycotoxins) and acrylamide.

The most common detrimental aspect of egg consumption is that when they are overcooked, they are poorly digested as a result of excessive cross-linking of their proteins during cooking, making them hard to digest, and allowing the proteins to ferment in the lower intestine. This contributes to dysbiosis, leaky gut, and chronic inflammation. A colonic microbiome dominated by proteolytic bacteria is also associated with higher colorectal cancer risk.

Cooking Eggs

The coagulation or gelation of the proteins in eggs occurs during cooking, with different proteins having different gelation temperatures. With adequate temperatures, the various proteins "denature" and unravel. Then, the millions of small individual proteins in the egg stick to each other, forming a 3-dimensional polymer lattice and changing it into a semisolid or solid. If heating continues, the cross-linking increases. As water is driven out with more heat and time, the bonding becomes tighter and denser. Cooking eggs increases protein digestion and absorption;[26 27] however, overcooking, which hardens the egg and lowers its accessibility to digestive proteases, thus impeding protein digestion. Thus, neither raw nor overcooked eggs is good for the gut.

Gelation of egg proteins also occurs from physical means, such as whipping or exposure to alkali. Adding sugar raises the temperature of coagulation, and adding acids lowers it. Adding salt helps the egg retain more water, keeping the egg a bit softer.

Protein Location	Protein Name	Coagu-lation (°C)	Coagu-lation (°F)	Contribution to white or yolk (%)
Albumin (egg white)	Ovalbumin	63.5°	146.5°	54%
Albumin (egg white)	Ovotrans-ferrin	57.3°	135.1°	12.7
Albumin (egg white)	Ovomucoi d	Does not coagulat e	-	3.5
Albumin (egg white)	Lysozyme	81.5°	178.7°	3.5
Yolk	Livetin	70°	158°	30
Yolk	Phosvitin	68°	154.4°	10
Yolk	LDL	62.5°	144.5°	6
Yolk	HDL	>70°	>158°	3.5

Table 15A: The protein contribution percentages listed above represent the percentage contribution by weight of each protein relative to the total protein content in its respective location (egg white or yolk).

Egg whites begin to thicken around 63°C (145°F) and form a soft, tender solid around 65°C (149°F). The yolk begins to thicken at about 65.5°C (150°F) as a result of livetin, the major yolk protein, and sets at 70°C (158°F). This difference in coagulation temperature is why the yolk may stay liquid even when the white is cooked. When the albumin and yolk are blended, eggs will solidify at around 73°C (163.4°F).[28] Eggs come out of the hen's cloaca. The word cloaca is the same as the word for sewer in Spanish, so eggs get poop on them, and that poop has bacteria. Store-bought eggs have been washed, which removes the poop, but it also removes a film that protects the egg from infiltration by bacteria. Thus, washed eggs (like the ones in grocery stores) need to be and stay refrigerated at below 40°C (40°F) until they are cooked. Keep your eggs refrigerated at 4°C (40°F) or colder. Discard cracked eggs, as eggs are an excellent growth medium for *Salmonella*.[29]

Eggs left out in warm weather (85°F) for more than about 30 minutes, for example) should be discarded. On an 80-degree day, the inside of a car can hit 109°F in 20 minutes and 118°F in 40 minutes. This means that if you shop for eggs, you can't leave them in a hot car or trunk for even a few minutes to stop to buy beach toys on your way home, or even drive them home a long distance, if the air conditioning is not used.

Eggs en Cáscara

(That sounds better than eggs cooked in their shell.)

While fresh eggs should not contain bacteria, an adequate cooking temperature is still highly recommended to ensure this. Egg dishes that do not contain meat or poultry should be heated to 65.5°C (150°F) for at least 1 minute or reach a temperature of 71°C (160°F) for at least 10 seconds to completely kill *Salmonella*. If one takes eggs from the refrigerator, the interior temperature will be about 3.3°C (38°F). When the whole egg in its shell is placed in hot water, it takes time for the heat to transfer to the yolk. It takes about 8 minutes for the center of a large egg placed in boiling water to reach 67.8°C (154°F) and 9 minutes to reach a temperature of 71°C (160°F). At 3 minutes, the cooking time for a typically prepared soft-boiled egg, the yolk temperature is about 32°C (90°F).[30]

Thus, pregnant women, children under 5 years old, and those with a compromised immune system should refrain from eating eggs with runny yolks; if the egg is contaminated with Salmonella, the temperature has not gotten high enough to even slow its growth. If the yolk is gelled, it is a pretty good indication that the temperature has gotten high enough to kill *Salmonella*.

Boiling water cooks the periphery of the eggs too hot, too quickly, and the interior does not have time to cook before the white is overcooked. Cooking the eggs at a lower temperature gives a better result and a higher DAD score.

Eggs Cooked in Shell

This method of cooking optimizes the digestibility of eggs cooked in their shell and provides an optimal DAD rating for eggs. It requires a controlled temperature; a digital kettle with temperature control to the single degree will allow it to be easily done at home. A sous vide heater (without plastic bags) or a slow-cooker with a temperature probe can also be used.

Recommended Method: Set the temperature of the water to 170°F (76.67°C) and turn on the "Stay Warm" option on the kettle. If "Stay Warm" is not engaged, the eggs will not cook correctly. Set a timer (on a smartphone, for example) for 17 minutes and 30 seconds. Have the eggs ready. *After the water reaches a temperature of 170°F,* start the timer and then gently place the eggs into the kettle using scissor tongs, avoiding dropping them. Position them so that they do not roll up and touch the thermostat on the bottom of the kettle, as this will interfere with getting correct temperature control. Do not cook more than one layer of eggs at a time.

Prepare a bowl or pot of cool tap water. As soon as the timer goes off, remove the eggs from the kettle using the tongs and place them into the cool tap water. Do not allow them to overcook, as the quality and DAD score will quickly degrade. After being placed in the cool water, the interior of the egg will continue to cook on the inside as it cools from the outside. Allow the eggs to "cook" in the cool water for at least 2 minutes. The eggs will be ready to eat.

Crack the egg and use a spoon to eat the contents. The egg white should be solid, but soft and delicate like flan. The yolk should be gooey and bright yellow-orange, and flavorful.

Temperature and time: Alternatively, the water temperature may be set to Celsius:

76°C (168.8°F) with a cooking time of 18 minutes.
76.7°C (170°F) with a cooking time of 17 minutes, 30 seconds.

Benefits: This is an easy-to-digest, delicious egg that has a DAD score of 4 ★★★★.

Downsides: The egg is neither hard nor boiled. It cannot be easily peeled.

Above or below this narrow time and temperature range, the DAD rating is not as good.

Hard-Cooked Eggs

To get a hard cooked-in-shell egg that is easy to peel is very simple if you are ready to get one rated C. A friend recently told me that they pressure-cooked their eggs

(250°F) to make them easy to peel. That has to get a D, just for deadly farts. A hard-boiled egg, cooked at 100°C (212°F) for 16 minutes, gets a score of C, but is easy to peel after cooling.

In order to get a firm, solid egg white that has a good DAD score, cook it in water at 85°C (185°F). Make sure that the "keep warm" button is on, as the temperature needs to stay hot for the entire cooking time. Preheat the water and add 1 Tbsp of vinegar to it. Set the timer for 15 minutes. After the cooking temperature has been reached, place the eggs in the hot water with tongs. Do not overcook them. As soon as the timer goes off, move the eggs from the hot water into a deep bowl of ice water. Let them cool for 2 – 3 minutes. They can be peeled while they are still warm. These eggs should get a DAD score of 3★★★.

That is the easy part. Peeling the eggs is the hard part. To make the hard-cooked eggs peelable:

- Use eggs that are at least a week old; they are easier to peel.
- Crack them gently, then roll them to crack all around.
- Start peeling from the fat end, where the air pocket is.
- Peel them under water
- Get started, and then use a spoon to separate the peel
- Letting the egg fall into the bowl of ice water so that it cracks may help.

Cooking Eggs in a Pan

If cooking eggs on a stovetop, be gentle. Once one realizes that laced, browned, bubbly eggs are a mistake, the hard part of cooking eggs in a pan is not overshooting the pan temperature on a stovetop.

I recommend cooking eggs in a ceramic-lined pan (non-stick) with a glass lid, and using a small amount of butter. The butter is used as a temperature gauge. Butter browns at 250°F and smokes at higher temperatures. If you are browning the butter when cooking eggs, you are getting the pan way too hot. Butter will boil at around 100°C (212°F). If the butter is making large bubbles, the pan is still too hot to cook eggs. If there is vigorous bubbling and spattering, the pan is far too hot. Stop and start over after cleaning the pan. If you add eggs to a pan that is this hot, they will get a DAD score of less than zero, and the eggs will be detrimental to your health.

You want the pan to be warm enough to melt the butter and begin to see tiny bubbles. These bubbles form from tiny air bubbles trapped in the butter, and begin to expand just around the butter's melting point of 32°C to 35°C (90°F to 95°F). At around 49-60°C (120-140°F), the bubbles are small and evenly distributed, creating a smooth, frothy appearance.

The difficult part is preventing the stove from overshooting the temperature as the pan gets warm. The goal is to get a pan temperature of about 93° C (200° F), but not hotter. At this temperature, the egg will cook quickly.

Start by turning the heat on to medium heat. Use a small pad of butter to make sure the pan is not too hot. A tablespoon of water can alternatively or additionally be used. Put the eggs in the pan as you would like: omelet, scrambled, or with the yolk broken, and cover them. It is likely time to turn off the heat. Vapor will cover the inside of the lid. When the egg white becomes opaque and solid enough, fold or flip it over and cover it again. The egg should be ready soon to slide onto a plate. It is best if the egg is mostly gelled, but still moist and not completely solidified when it is removed from the pan, as it will cook a little more as it settles.

The eggs should be delicate, soft, and have a good flavor. There should not be any browning or lacing. The underside should not be covered with craters like the surface of the moon. If eggs are properly pan-cooked properly they should get a rating of 4. Meanwhile, the way most people prepare eggs gets a rating of C to D.

Cooking an egg that is healthy to eat takes patience and a bit of skill. Having everything prepared before placing the eggs in the pan helps; any condiments, vegetables, mushrooms that will be added, and a plate to receive the cooked eggs should be ready before the eggs are placed in the pan. Getting the timing right is essential to the proper preparation of eggs, and that is difficult if the cook is distracted by other tasks.

Baking with Eggs

Baking: Eggs are used in baking mostly to add "moisture" but also to help hold things together. For baking, eggs can often be substituted with applesauce, bananas, or the puree of pumpkin or winter squash.

Baked goods are generally done while they are still moist inside, but after most of the water has evaporated. This keeps the internal temperature from rising above the boiling temperature. Although you may bake cookies at a temperature of 350 to 375° F (177 – 191°C, as an example, the cookies are done when they reach an internal temperature between 175 and 185°F (79 and 85°C). Thus, eggs in baked goods should not impart a significant digestive risk, as long as the baked good is not pyrolyzed or burned.

Quiche and Flan

Flan, composed mostly of eggs and milk when properly prepared, gets a DAD rating of 4. Flan is baked at 325 to 350° F; however, it is cooked in bowls that sit in a tray of water, which holds the temperature down. The goal is for the flan or quiche to reach a temperature of 165° F (74°C) to 175°F (80°C), with an ideal target temperature of 170° F (76.7°C) while avoiding any browning. If cooked at a higher temperature, the flan will become dense, and at higher temperatures, it will curdle and become grainy.[31] The flan is taken out of the oven as soon as it has set, and continues to firm up more while it cools. Covering the flan (with foil or cooking parchment) reduces the cooking time and prevents the formation of a skin (which has a lower DAD score) and prevents browning. Flan can be made with less sugar than called for in most recipes.

Similarly, quiche, which is sort of a savory flan with vegetables and cheese, can get a similarly high DAD score when prepared at the proper temperature. If baked in a pie tray rather than individual custard dishes, the pie tray should sit in a bath of water and be covered as it bakes. It should be baked at a temperature of 325°F to achieve a cooked temperature of 165° F (74°C) to 175°F (80°C) and removed from the oven when it sets. The quiche should not be allowed to brown on top. Using a cooking thermometer can help determine when the quiche has reached the right temperature.

Quiche can be made without using a pie crust.

Please note that, similar to eggs, toasted cheese that has browned gets a DAD rating of D, and should be avoided.

1 Chicken Egg Proteins and Derived Peptides with Antioxidant Properties. Benedé S, Molina E. Foods. 2020 Jun 3;9(6):735. doi: 10.3390/foods9060735. PMID: 32503187

2 Egg Consumption and Risk of All-Cause and Cause-Specific Mortality: A Systematic Review and Dose-Response Meta-analysis of Prospective Studies. Mousavi SM, Zargarzadeh N, Rigi S, Persad E, Pizarro AB, Hasani-Ranjbar S, Larijani B, Willett WC, Esmaillzadeh A. Adv Nutr. 2022 Oct 2;13(5):1762-1773. doi: 10.1093/advances/nmac040. PMID: 35396834

3 Sienski G., et al. *APOE4* disrupts intracellular lipid homeostasis in human iPSC-derived glia. *Sci Transl Med.* 2021 Mar 3;13(583):eaaz4564. doi: 10.1126/scitranslmed.aaz4564.

4 Arthur, W., Pearson., Neil, M., Greenwood., Edward, J., Butler., Caralyn, L., Curl., G., Roger, Fenwick. (1983). Fish meal and egg taint. Journal of the Science of Food and Agriculture, doi: 10.1002/JSFA.2740340311

5 Edward, J., Butler., Arthur, W., Pearson., Neil, M., Greenwood. (1984). Trimethylamine taint in eggs: the occurrence of the causative metabolic defect in commercial hybrids and pure breeds in relation to shell colour. Journal of the Science of Food and Agriculture, doi: 10.1002/JSFA.2740350305

6 Fishy-egg tainting is recessively inherited when brown-shelled layers are fed canola meal. Ward AK, Classen HL, Buchanan FC. Poult Sci. 2009 Apr;88(4):714-21. doi: 10.3382/ps.2008-00430. PMID: 19276413

7 Apolipoprotein B but not LDL cholesterol is associated with coronary artery calcification in type 2 diabetic whites. Martin SS, Qasim AN, Mehta NN, Wolfe M, Terembula K, Schwartz S, Iqbal N, Schutta M, Bagheri R, Reilly MP. Diabetes. 2009 Aug;58(8):1887-92. doi: 10.2337/db08-1794. Epub 2009 Jun 2. PMID: 19491209

8 Evidence for cholesterol hyperabsorbers and hyperproducers based on comparative low-density lipoprotein reductions achieved by ezetimibe versus statins. Senaratne J, Griffiths J, MacDonald K, Senaratne MP. J Cardiopulm Rehabil Prev. 2012 Sep-Oct;32(5):250-4. doi: 10.1097/HCR.0b013e31825d29ee. PMID: 22785146

9 Total cholesterol and all-cause mortality by sex and age: a prospective cohort study among 12.8 million adults. Yi SW, Yi JJ, Ohrr H.Sci Rep. 2019 Feb 7;9(1):1596. doi: 10.1038/s41598-018-38461-y.PMID: 30733566

10 Lack of an association or an inverse association between low-density-lipoprotein cholesterol and mortality in the elderly: a systematic review. Ravnskov U, Diamond DM, Hama R, Hamazaki T, Hammarskjöld B, Hynes N, Kendrick M, Langsjoen PH, Malhotra A, Mascitelli L, McCully KS, Ogushi Y, Okuyama H, Rosch PJ, Schersten T, Sultan S, Sundberg R.BMJ Open. 2016 Jun 12;6(6):e010401. doi: 10.1136/bmjopen-2015-010401.PMID: 27292972

11 The U-Shaped Association of Non-High-Density Lipoprotein Cholesterol Levels With All-Cause and Cardiovascular Mortality Among Patients With Hypertension. Cheng Q, Liu XC, Chen CL, Huang YQ, Feng YQ, Chen JY. Front Cardiovasc Med. 2021 Jul 14;8:707701. doi: 10.3389/fcvm.2021.707701. eCollection 2021. PMID: 34336961

12 The U-shaped association of non-high-density lipoprotein cholesterol with all-cause and cardiovascular mortality in general adult population. Huang Y, Yan MQ, Zhou D, Chen CL, Feng YQ. Front Cardiovasc Med. 2023 Feb 8;10:1065750. doi: 10.3389/fcvm.2023.1065750.. PMID: 36844732

13 Vegetarian or vegan diets and blood lipids: a meta-analysis of randomized trials. Koch CA, Kjeldsen EW, Frikke-Schmidt R. Eur Heart J. 2023 Jul 21;44(28):2609-2622. doi: 10.1093/eurheartj/ehad211. PMID: 37226630

14 Association of non-HDL-C/apoB ratio with long-term mortality in the general population: A cohort study. Zhang K, Wei C, Shao Y, Wang L, Zhao Z, Yin S, Tang X, Li Y, Gou Z. Heliyon. 2024 Mar 15;10(6):e28155. doi: 10.1016/j.heliyon.2024.e28155. eCollection 2024 Mar 30. PMID: 38545184

15 Lifestyle and Dietary Determinants of Serum Apolipoprotein A1 and Apolipoprotein B Concentrations: Cross-Sectional Analyses within a Swedish Cohort of 24,984 Individuals. Frondelius K, Borg M, Ericson U, Borné Y, Melander O, Sonestedt E. Nutrients. 2017 Feb 28;9(3):211. doi: 10.3390/nu9030211. PMID: 28264492

16 The regulation of ApoB metabolism by insulin. Haas ME, Attie AD, Biddinger SB. Trends Endocrinol Metab. 2013 Aug;24(8):391-7. doi: 10.1016/j.tem.2013.04.001. Epub 2013 May 27. PMID: 23721961

17 The effect of a six-month exercise program on very low-density lipoprotein apolipoprotein B secretion in type 2 diabetes. Alam S, Stolinski M, Pentecost C, Boroujerdi MA, Jones RH, Sonksen PH, Umpleby AM. J Clin Endocrinol Metab. 2004 Feb;89(2):688-94. doi: 10.1210/jc.2003-031036. PMID: 14764782

18 Association of dietary lipid intake with low-density lipoprotein cholesterol levels: analysis of two independent population-based studies. Kwon YJ, Lee HS, Chang HJ, Koh SB, Lee JW. Eur J Nutr. 2020 Sep;59(6):2557-2567. doi: 10.1007/s00394-019-02104-3. Epub 2019 Oct 10. PMID: 31602495

19 Consumption of a defined, plant-based diet reduces lipoprotein(a), inflammation, and other atherogenic lipoproteins and particles within 4 weeks. Najjar RS, Moore CE, Montgomery BD. Clin Cardiol. 2018 Aug;41(8):1062-1068. doi: 10.1002/clc.23027. Epub 2018 Aug 17. PMID: 30014498

20 Nutrition Intervention for Reduction of Cardiovascular Risk in African Americans Using the 2019 American College of Cardiology/American Heart Association Primary Prevention Guidelines. Williams KA, Fughhi I, Fugar S, Mazur M, Gates S, Sawyer S, Patel H, Chambers D, McDaniel R, Reiser JR, Mason T. Nutrients. 2021 Sep 28;13(10):3422. doi: 10.3390/nu13103422. PMID: 34684423

21 Formation of cholesterol oxidation products (COPs) and loss of cholesterol in fresh egg pasta as a function of thermal treatment processing. Stefano Zardetto, Davide Barbanti, Marco Dalla Rosa, Food Research International.

Vol 62 (177-182) 2014 https://doi.org/10.1016/j.foodres.2014.02.028

22 Yinfei, Qiao, Zhu Kejian, Zheng Bo, Yu Zhengke, Han Yuming, Zhao Qi, Wenli Yang, Xia Xiangyi, Zhang Ting and Xia Changjiang. "A method of rapid rabbit atherosclerosis model establishment." Biomedical Research-tokyo 28 (2017): 7614-7618.

23 Monitoring the formation of cholesterol oxidation products in model systems using response surface methodology. Min JS, Lee SO, Khan MI, Yim DG, Seol KH, Lee M, Jo C. Lipids Health Dis. 2015 Jul 23;14:77. doi: 10.1186/s12944-015-0074-6. PMID: 26201850

24 Oxidation of cholesterol by heating. Osada K, Kodama T, Yamada K, Sugano M. J. Agric. Food Chem. 1993, 41, 8, 1198–1202:August 1, 1993 https://doi.org/10.1021/jf00032a006

25 Quantification of Cooking Method Effect on COP Content in Meat Types Using Triple Quadrupole GC-MS/MS. Hashari SZ, Rahim AA, Meng GY, Ramiah SK. Molecules. 2020 Oct 28;25(21):4978. doi: 10.3390/molecules25214978. PMID: 33126403

26 Digestibility of cooked and raw egg protein in humans as assessed by stable isotope echniques. Evenepoel P, Geypens B, Luypaerts A, Hiele M, Ghoos Y, Rutgeerts P. J Nutr. 1998 Oct;128(10):1716-22. doi: 10.1093/jn/128.10.1716. PMID: 9772141

27 The extent of ovalbumin in vitro digestion and the nature of generated peptides are modulated by the morphology of protein aggregates. Nyemb K, Guérin-Dubiard C, Dupont D, Jardin J, Rutherfurd SM, Nau F. Food Chem. 2014 Aug 15;157:429-38. doi: 10.1016/j.foodchem.2014.02.048. PMID: 24679801

28 On Food and Cooking: The Science and Lore of the Kitchen. Harlod McGee. Scribner NY NY 2004

29 https://www.cdc.gov/foodsafety/communication/salmonella-and-eggs.html

30 Destruction of Salmonellae in hard-boiled eggs. Licciardello JJ, Nickerson JT, Goldblith SA. Am J Public Health Nations Health. 1965 Oct;55(10):1622-8. doi: 10.2105/ajph.55.10.1622. PMID: 5890516

31 https://www.seriouseats.com/double-caramel-flan-recipe

16: Dairy and Faux Dairy

The Skinny

- Milk is for kids. By the age of 10, most children don't digest lactose well. 🌩
- Full-fat milk is not terrible for those who are not lactose intolerant. ☁
- Skim and 1% milk (🌩 🌩 🌩 🌩) are worse than whole milk.
- Fermented milk (i.e., yogurt and kefir) is OK. Greek yogurt is a better choice for most adults. ★ - ★★
- Most hard cheeses are fine. ★★
- Processed, "un-American" cheese should be considered dangerous junk food and gets a DAD score of D. ☠☠☠☠
- Butter is an acceptable fat when not used in excess. Margaine, however, should be considered poison ☠☠☠☠ and never consumed.
- Most commercially prepared vegetable milks contain noxious compounds that disrupt the intestinal mucous layer. For those not allergic or intolerant to it, whole cow's milk is a healthier choice than vegetable milks with gums and thickeners. 🌩 🌩 🌩 🌩
- Homemade plant-based milks, however, can get good DAD scores. ★★ – ★★★★
- Certain "ice cream" desserts get good DAD scores. ★ - ★★★★
- Avoid low-calorie dairy products. 💣💣💣💣
- Avoid sheep and goat dairy products as they are very high in Neu5Gc. (See Chapter 32 for explanation.)

Table 15-A ranks various dairy products. This chapter provides recipes for homemade non-dairy milk and "ice-cream" desserts that get good DAD scores. It also lists and describes several noxious food additives that are commonly found in faux-dairy products that should be avoided.

Dairy

A lacto-ovo-vegetarian (LOVe) diet can be a healthy diet, with a lower risk of most chronic diseases than the WMD (Western meal diet). Nevertheless, the health benefits and risks of dairy are controversial and somewhat convoluted.

What is the evidence? A meta-analysis including nine prospective, seven retrospective, and two cross-sectional studies found that dairy consumption was *inversely* associated with the risk of developing breast cancer.[1] Another meta-analysis found that dairy intake was not quite statistically significantly associated with an increased risk of non-advanced prostate cancer, but was associated with decreased risk of fatal prostate cancer.[2] Seeing that all men get prostate cancer if they live long enough, it would suggest that choosing cheese and the non-fatal forms of prostate cancer is the better choice. Other meta-analyses have found that diary consumption is associated with a lower risk of colon cancer, type 2 diabetes (T2D), cardiovascular disease, stroke, and hypertension.[3] Dairy and cheese consumption appear to have a mild protective effect against Alzheimer's disease. This effect was most easily discerned in Asian populations, where dairy consumption is not as common as in the West.[4] In a study of the relationship between dairy product consumption and Parkinson's disease (PD), a *positive* association for increased risk of PD for milk consumption was found, especially in men, for the consumption of milk, but there was no significant risk associated with the intake of yogurt.[5] A 20-year follow-up study found that at low volume, around 100 ml per day, liquid milk was associated with a lower risk of PD in women, but found that PD risk increased linearly with milk intake over about 350 ml (11.8 oz) per day.[6] Liquid milk consumption is associated with higher all-cause and cardiovascular mortality as well as a higher risk of hip fracture and overall mortality in women.[7] However, another large, well-conducted study including over 120,000 participants found decreased risk of hip fracture with the consumption of liquid milk in male and female adults over the age of 50.[8]

A more granular understanding complicates this. In a large French study, the consumption of dairy products was not associated with prostate, breast, or colon cancer risk; however, "formage blanc" (a type of cottage cheese) and sugary dairy desserts were associated with increased risk of colorectal cancer.[9] In a meta-analysis of 12 meta-analyses, milk and dairy consumption were found to be associated with a lower incidence of type 2 diabetes (T2D).[10] Soy products, such as soy milk, are associated with decreased risk of death from breast cancer; soy milk may improve survival in women with, or at high risk of, breast cancer.

Looking at cheese specifically, its consumption is associated with a 5% reduction in all-cause mortality. Cheese consumption was associated with a 7% decrease in type 2 diabetes (T2D) and stroke, an 8% reduction in cardiovascular disease and coronary heart disease, a 10% decrease in fractures, an 11% decrease in estrogen receptor-negative (ER-) breast cancers (the deadliest forms), and a 19% decrease in dementia.[11]

We all have to eat. If a person eats steak and potatoes at supper every day, they are less likely to eat fish and brown rice for supper on those days. Diet is not just what one eats, it is also what one does not. Lacto-ovo-vegetarians are likely to consume more dairy and eggs than omnivores, as these become more important sources of protein. When assessing the epidemiologic studies of the impact of diet, sometimes *what is not eaten is as important as what is.* Eating dairy products generally means eating less of something else. If this is red meat (mammalian meat) being displaced in the diet, it might explain the benefits of dairy without any specific mechanism other than it being less detrimental than meat. Vegans generally have an even lower burden of chronic metabolic disease than do LOVes. Is dairy beneficial or just less harmful than animal-based alternatives? And as with fruits and veggies, clustering dairy foods into a single group obscures the helpful and harmful elements within the group.

Little Miss Muffet, she sat on her tuffet, eating her curds and whey.

During the preparation of cheese, cow's milk is acidified, for example, with a small amount of citric acid, and the milk is treated with rennet, a combination of the enzymes chymosin and pepsin. Rennet cleaves the water-soluble fragment from κ-casein, which allows casein to remain suspended in the whey. With a fall in the pH to 4.6, and heating the milk to 180° F (which also kills bacteria), the milk separates into white clumps, the curd, and yellow fluid; the whey. The milk is cooled and then separated using a cheesecloth that retains the curd, and the whey may be collected and used as a byproduct for other purposes. Since lactose is water-soluble, it drains out with the whey. This is similar to what occurs in the stomach, where the casein forms a clot and is digested slowly, while the whey proteins, remaining water-soluble, exit the stomach more quickly into the duodenum, providing rapid energy, as whey contains the sugar lactose.

The liquid whey contains several proteins that are high in branched-chain amino acids. This is why whey is sometimes used as an anabolic supplement to help build muscle. Most hard cheeses contain very little whey and thus are low in lactose. Butter, hard or aged cheeses such as cheddar, Swiss cheese, Parmesan, brie, and Camembert, contain low amounts of lactose and whey in contrast to cheeses such as ricotta, which is made from whey. High-quality Greek yogurt also has most of the whey removed. Cow's milk contains about 4.8% lactose, and the amount in whey is higher.

The word mammal comes from the same root as mammary gland. Pretty much all adult mammals are "lactase non-persistent," leading to lactose intolerance. This includes dogs and cats. In most humans, lactase expression in the small intestine begins to disappear around the age of six, reducing the ability to cleave the disaccharide lactose into its two component sugars, glucose and galactose, that are transported across the enterocyte membrane by glucose transport proteins (GLUT2 and SGLT-1).

When lactose is not digested, it ends up in the colon, where it is fermented. The symptoms of lactose fermentation include bloating, borborygmi, flatulence, cramping, diarrhea, and sometimes nausea and vomiting after the consumption of milk, which generally occurs 6 to 48 hours after the consumption of milk. If symptoms occur within a few hours of milk consumption, it may be the result of an allergic reaction or the result of small bowel bacterial overgrowth (SIBO), in which case, fermentation occurs in the upper small intestine.

Even those adults who are genetically capable of digesting lactose can develop secondary lactose intolerance if they have injury to the mucosal lining of the small intestine from infection, celiac disease, Crohn's disease, bacterial overgrowth, gastrointestinal infection, or other injury. Thus, an adult who has had no problem digesting milk can suddenly become lactose intolerant, but this generally reverses if they heal.

New onset of lactose intolerance (other than the typical decline during childhood and adolescence) should be considered a sentinel event revealing epithelial injury in the small intestine.

In patients with secondary lactose intolerance, lactose should be avoided until they have recovered. In patients with Celiac disease, recovery of lactose tolerance usually takes between 6 and 12 months.[12]

If small amounts of milk are consumed regularly and slowly increased, the abundance of *Lactobacillaceae* and/or *Bifidobacteria* in the lower intestine, which can digest lactose increases, decreasing or eliminating symptoms of lactose intolerance, enough so that many non-lactase non-persistent (LNP) adolescents and adults can tolerate about 12 grams of lactose (the amount in 8 oz. of milk) a day.[13] [14] The tolerance can disappear, likely within a few weeks, if regular milk consumption stops.

Thus, in limited quantities, lactose may act as a probiotic in those with lactase non-persistence (LNP) but be dysbiotic in higher amounts, similar to the microbiome adaptation to small amounts of raffinose and stachyose in beans and vegetables when frequently consumed. Intermittent milk consumption in those with LPN or secondary lactose intolerance causes the lactose to provoke dysbiosis and bowel symptoms. This should be avoided. Fermentation of lactose can produce toxic metabolites, including alcohols, diols, ketones, acids, and aldehydes, such as methylglyoxal,[15] that cause glycation and are atherogenic if absorbed.[16]

Whole milk may be better tolerated than skim milk, as the fat may help slow gastric emptying and provide a lower lactose load. Lactose may be less of a problem when part of a meal, for the same reasons.

As will be explained towards the end of this chapter, I assess that casein, the major proteins that comprise hard cheese, is a healthy dietary choice, while whey, the yellow liquid that separates when milk curdles during the making of cheese and Greek yogurt, carries risk for adults.

The impact of yogurt and other forms of fermented dairy products, such as kefir, is less controversial. There is considerable evidence that yogurt and other forms of fermented milk lower the risk of cancer and overall mortality. A meta-analysis found that yogurt consumption was associated with a 13% reduction in the risk of colorectal cancer.[17] Another meta-analysis, including 17 studies, with a total study population of nearly 900,000 participants, found that yogurt consumption was associated with an 11% lower hazard of cardiovascular disease death. Overall mortality risk was lowest when about 40 to 50 percent of a serving of yogurt was consumed per day. Since one serving was defined as 244 g of yogurt, just over 8 oz,[18] this seems to be a clumsy way of saying that mortality was lower among those consuming around three 8-oz or four 6-oz servings of yogurt per week. Consumption of higher amounts of yogurt was associated with diminished benefits. Much of the yogurt consumed was sweetened, and this likely impacts the benefits and risks, including the upper limits of intake that were found to be beneficial. A randomly selected national brand of strawberry yogurt (without fruit on the bottom) contained 16 grams of added sugar (four teaspoons) in an 8-ounce serving. Those with fruit on the bottom typically have even more added sugar.

The studies do not mention Greek yogurt, so it can be assumed that the yogurt was largely typical commercial yogurt, which contains full amounts of whey proteins and considerable amounts of lactose and table sugar. There are around 11-17 grams of lactose in a 6 to 8-ounce serving of regular yogurt, about the same as in a cup of milk (@ 13 grams). In contrast, a 6-ounce serving of Greek yogurt contains about 4 grams of lactose. There is nearly 3 times as much protein in Greek yogurt (10 grams per 100 grams) as in regular plain yogurt (3.5 grams per 100 grams). Greek yogurt is more concentrated as a result of the removal of whey.

High-quality Greek yogurt (whole milk, full cream, no flavoring, sugar, gelatin, or additives other than culture media) has a DAD score of 2, while that for regular yogurt barely gets a one. The SANA diet recommends Greek yogurt over regular yogurt for adults. The only study found on the health impact specifically of Greek yogurt for this review found it to be associated with a decreased risk of cardiovascular disease.[19] It is just one man's opinion, but rich, creamy, high-quality, 10% fat yogurt is delicious without sugar or other flavoring. Fermented milk is generally associated with lower disease risk. It should be noted that several types of cheese are made from fermented milk or fermented during the aging process. Some of these included cheddar, mozzarella, Swiss, feta, brie, Gouda, Edam, Gruyere, Parmesan, and Provolone cheeses. It may be that the fermentation process of some of these has an effect on their health impacts.

Milk

Fresh, whole milk gets a DAD score of about zero. UHT (ultra-high temperature) pasteurized milk gets a slightly lower score than fresh milk. While not recommending milk as a beverage, if using liquid milk, the SANA diet recommends using whole milk, and that adults limit the amount used to less than 12 ounces a day. One percent and skim milk get Ds on the DAD scale, and should not be avoided by children and adults.

If milk is consumed, it is better to have small amounts regularly to maintain the intestinal flora that ferments lactose. Lactose-reduced milk and lactase enzyme tablets are available; while they may eliminate the gastrointestinal symptoms associated with milk consumption, they merely split the lactose into glucose and galactose. Galactose has adverse health impacts for adults, as explained later in this chapter. Thus, lactose-reduced milk is not a step-up, but may rather be a step-down. It is better to avoid consuming quantities of milk that provoke symptoms. Even better may be to replace it with something better.

Table 16A: Dairy Scoreboard

Dairy Products	Rating
Soy milk (from powder) ^	4
Cheese, Monterey Jack	3
Cheese, Provolone	3
Cheese, Muenster	3
Cheese, Parmesan, dry, grated	3
Cheese, Parmesan (shredded)	2
Cheese, Swiss	2
Cheese, white Cheddar	2
Cheese, white Sharp Cheddar♣	2
Cheese, white Extra Sharp Cheddar	2
Cheese, Mozzarella, low moisture	2
Cheese, Gouda (with annatto)	2
Cheese, Havarti	2
Cheese, Mexican	2
Greek yogurt (Cabot 10% fat, low-fat)	2
Ice cream (vanilla)	1
Sour cream	1
Soy milk (Silk original with gellan gum)	1
Half and Half (50% milk, 50% cream)	1
Butter	1
Cheese; Cottage (large curd 4% milkfat) *	1
Greek yogurt (Chiboni, plain, nonfat)	1
Whole milk, fresh	0
Milk, whole ultra-high temp. pasteurized	A+
Blue cheese♠	A
Milk, 2% ultra-high temp. pasteurized	B
Oat milk (Silk Original)	C
Whey (from unsweetened Greek yogurt)	C
Whey protein powder	C
Cream Cheese*	C
Milk, pasteurized, 1% milkfat	D
American (processed) "cheese"	D
Oat milk with gellan gum (non-dairy)	D
Almond Milk (with gellan gum)	D
Chocolate milk•	D
Cheese, Ricotta	D

Table 16A Notes:

^ Soy milk, made from powdered soy milk, after heated to 249° F (115° C) in a pressure cooker. See soy milk in the Faux Milk section below.

* The cottage cheese tested contained added whey and whey protein, carrageenan, guar, and locust bean gum. The cream cheese contained guar, carob bean, and xanthan gums. The C rating for cream cheese may be a result of much higher levels of the gum, or that cream cheese is high in aldehydes as a result of its manufacturing processes.

♣ All cheeses, if not otherwise noted, were white cheeses to avoid the potential impact from the use of annatto (Bixin) on testing. Annatto is a colorant often used in cheese and other dairy products.

♠ Blue cheese and similar cheeses, such as gorgonzola, are aged and cultured with specific strains of mold to give them their distinctive flavoring as well as the colored mottling. As a result of this, these cheeses contain modest levels of the mycotoxins Roquefortine C (ROQ C), mycophenolic acid (MPA), penicillic acid (PA), PR toxin, andrastatin A, and penitrem A (PNA). These cheeses also contain biogenic amines, 2-phenylethylamine, histamine, tyramine, putrescine, cadaverine, and tryptamine, some of which can trigger migraine in sensitive persons. Since each batch of blue cheese is different, depending on the conditions and location where it is produced, aging, strain of mold, and other conditions, the amount of these compounds in the cheese may vary. The risks from consumption of blue cheese are considered to be low, other than for persons using MAO-inhibiting medications, migraineurs, toddlers, and the elderly. Most of the concern about potential risk is for the biogenic amine content of blue cheese. [20] Blue cheese gets a rating of A (avoid) on the DAD diet. Since it is used as a condiment, typically in small amounts, occasional use is unlikely to be a problem for most people.

• Chocolate milk: Ingredients: skim milk, sucrose syrup, alkali-processed cocoa, corn starch, salt, carrageenan, guar gum, natural flavor, vitamin A, vitamin D3. This beverage is often served as an option to the 1% milk provided to children in schools.

Cow's Milk

Skim and 1% cow's milk get a score of D; 2% milkfat milk gets a B. Whole milk gets a zero. UHT is made by heating milk to 138–150 °C (280–302 °F) for one or two seconds. This allows it to be packaged in sterile, hermetically sealed containers and have a shelf life of several months without refrigeration until opened. Ultra-high temperature (UHT) pasteurized whole milk just misses getting a zero and gets an A. UHT 2% milk has a slightly lower score, but still gets an A. UHT 1% milk gets a D.

The UHT pasteurization process disrupts most, if not all, exosomes that are present in milk.[21] Exosomes are submicroscopic lipid vesicles that contain nucleic acids, proteins, and metabolites. Milk exosomes are absorbed by the body and contain non-coding RNA that impacts growth and immune function. The exosomes protect these fragile bits of nucleic acid and help them get absorbed into the bloodstream and cells. When the exosomes are disrupted, the RNA is destroyed either before or after consumption, and thus does not impact health. The cow's milk exosomes are present in milk for the benefit of calves, not adult humans.

When making homemade Greek or regular yogurt, UHT milk has the added advantage that it is sterile and thus does not need to be preheated to 180 degrees before adding the yogurt culture.

Yogurt

The consumption of fermented milk such as yogurt, skyr, and kefir is associated with a lower risk of most chronic diseases. The reasons for this are, in part, the beneficial probiotic bacteria that are present in these fermented products, and in part, the breakdown of compounds present in milk, as explained in the science section below. While the bacteria, most commonly *Lactobacilli* and *Bifidobacteria*, are generally helpful, certain strains help with different conditions. Thus, the highest benefit occurs when an individual gets bacterial strains that help their individual situation. Some yogurt brands will be more beneficial for one person and another for another. If you find one that makes you feel better, use that one.

Greek yogurt is made by first making yogurt and then letting the whey separate out using cheesecloth. The SANA diet recommends Greek yogurt for adults, as it recommends the avoidance of whey proteins and galactose, which promote growth. These compounds may be fine for infants and growing children, but they likely increase the risk of cancer proliferation in adults. Children who drink milk throughout adolescence grow taller than those who don't.

Thus, regular yogurt is recommended for growing children and adolescents, and during pregnancy and lactation, while Greek yogurt is favored for other adults after the age of about 27, when development is completed.

Non-Dairy Milks

One can find soy milk, coconut milk, almond milk, oat milk, rice milk, and others in the dairy section of your grocer. Coconut milk for cooking can also be found in cans. Beware: Read the ingredients. These often contain thickeners and emulsifiers (CMC, polysorbate, carrageenan, gums) and other additives that cause intestinal problems. It should not be assumed that commercial non-dairy milks are a healthier substitute for cow's milk, as they may contain compounds that are considerably more detrimental than those being avoided in milk. The SANA program discourages the use of these products; they get DAD scores of Cs and Ds. The noxious compounds in non-dairy milks are discussed in the science section below.

Several forms of non-dairy milk without the noxious compounds are fairly simple to prepare at home. The drawback of these homemade milks is that they are unstable suspensions that settle; thus, they need to be stirred before using.

Soy milk, like tofu, gets a high 4 score if properly prepared without added noxious agents. Recipes for making soy milk "from scratch" using dry soybeans are available on the internet. If cooking the dried soybeans, blanch the beans as per method 1 or 2 in the chapter on pulses before soaking and cooking them, to get the best results.

DAD scores give the overall impact of a foodstuff. Silk brand original soy milk contains gellan gum, which lowers its score considerably. The gum is added to make the milk creamier and to keep it from settling. The gum is bad for the gut. Edensoy makes a ready-to-use soymilk with no other ingredients.

Non-dairy milk powders, including soy milk, oat milk, and coconut milk powders, are available (online) and typically do not contain added emulsifiers or other questionable ingredients. Soy milk powder can be purchased (online) and gets an excellent DAD score, and is highly recommended over the readymade stuff. These can be a convenient way to prepare vegan milk, and allow for small amounts to be made as needed, and the powder can simply be added to smoothies. Soy and coconut milk powders can be used as coffee creamers.

Milk made from these powders will settle and need to be stirred before use. They should be used within 4 – 5 days in the refrigerator after preparation.

Vegan Milks

The following are some simple recipes for making milk at home.

Home-made non-dairy milk needs to be refrigerated, and should keep for about 5 days before degrading. Using 1-2 tsp. of sugar or an alternative natural sweetener (honey or maple syrup) and ½ tsp. of vanilla extract per quart or liter is optional and gives a more dairy milk-like flavor. Shake or stir before use.

There are 51 grams of lactose in a quart of milk, and lactose is about 3/10ths as sweet as sucrose. Thus, 15 grams of table sugar (about one level Tbsp plus one level tsp.) provides a similar sweetness to faux milk as whole milk.

Soy Milk – Using Powdered Soy Milk

Recommended: I find powdered soy milk made by adding water and mixing as per the package directions to be a bit gritty, and the flavor not especially pleasant. The label for Silk brand original soy milk shows that it contains natural flavor and 5 grams of added sugar per cup. Since it smells like vanilla, I assume that the natural flavor they use is vanilla. With this recipe, the flavor comes fairly close to the ready-made stuff without the gellan gum.

- One quart plus ½ cup water (36 oz.)
- 1 cup (@ 75 grams) of soy milk powder
- 1 rounded Tbsp. (22 grams) sugar, brown sugar, honey, or similar sweetener
- A very small pinch of salt
- 1/8th tsp. vanilla extract (about 1 ml or 16 drops)

To avoid lumping of the powder, either make the milk in a blender, starting with the water first and adding the soy powder to the top, or alternatively start with the dry soy powder and sugar mixed in a container and mix in just a bit of water at a time to make a thick "mud," to get all the powder moistened before whisking in more water. Add the salt, but do not add the vanilla yet. Heat the milk in a pressure cooker until it comes to full pressure (15 psi), and then allow the pressure to release naturally. Allow it to cool. Add the vanilla extract at the end; this prevents the vanilla flavor from being boiled off. The first time you make the recipe, add salt at the end to see how much (how little) is needed to "round out" the flavor. It does not take much salt; you should not taste the salt, just the improved flavor.

Stir each time before using, as the milk will settle.

If using soy milk to make yogurt, a thicker yogurt that is more like Greek yogurt can be made by using less water in the milk. Try decreasing the water by 1/3 or slightly more. Unlike with cow's milk, there are no whey proteins or lactose in the soy yogurt, thus no health advantage to eliminating the whey. Soy yogurt may have anti-Alzheimer's properties beyond that of soymilk, as a result of the probiotic bacteria improving the bioavailability of soy isoflavones.[22]

Rice, oat, coconut, almond, and cashew milks are not appropriate for children under the age of 5 because these milks have low protein content. Rice milk also carries the risk of high arsenic levels and should be avoided in children less than 6 years old, as this is a period of rapid brain development. Soy milk may have high levels of aluminum. The SANA program advises that any vegan milk-like beverage containing non-nutritive emulsifiers should be avoided by children or adults as a result of their impacts on the intestinal mucosa.

Oat Milk

- 1 cup quick rolled oats
- 4 - 5 cups water (less water for thicker, creamier milk)
- ⅛ tsp. salt
- 2 tsp. sugar optional
- Blend at high speed for 40 seconds. Filter through a cloth or fine mesh strainer. Presoaking, over-blending, or heating may make oat milk slimy.

DAD score:4

Oat Smoothie Milk. Same recipe as for oat milk, but use 2/3rds cup of rolled oats. After straining, boil for 1 minute. Goes from white to oatmeal color and gets slimy and thick. Works well as a base for fruit smoothies. DAD score: 2

Rice Milk

- One cup of cooked brown rice (cooked as instructed in the chapter on cereals).
- One quart/liter of water
- Salt: none if rice was cooked with salt, otherwise, ⅛ tsp. per quart/liter.
- 2 tsp. sugar
- Blend at high speed for 3 - 5 minutes. Filter through a cloth or fine mesh strainer.

DAD score: 2 using brown rice. (Filtered residue score: 4, can be used in porridge).

For richer, tastier rice milk (optional)

- 1 to 2 tablespoons of coconut oil with 1½ grams of lecithin per tablespoon of oil.

Mix and then blend into seed milk for several seconds at high speed.

Rice-Oak Milk

Recommended: This mix gives a richer mouth feel and less noticeable rice or oat flavor than using either grain alone. It will not fool anyone into thinking it is the real thing, but it gets a DAD score of 4 and tastes pretty good.

- One cup of cooked brown rice (prepared as per the chapter on cereals)
- 2/3 cup quick rolled oats (uncooked)
- 1¾ quarts water
- 2 – 2½ Tablespoons of sugar (optional, depending on use)
- 1/8 tsp. vanilla extract (optional)
- Pinch of salt to taste if needed (may not be needed if rice was cooked with salt.

Blend for 4 minutes, and then filter through a cloth or very fine mesh strainer. If it is not going to be used immediately, warm the milk in a saucepan to @ 76° C (@ 170° F) to pasteurize it, and allow it to cool. When "Pasteurized," it should keep in the refrigerator for several days. Cooking it for a longer time or at a higher temperature will cause it to get slimy (adding water can help), cause it to darken to an oatmeal color, and degrade the DAD score if it is boiled for more than one minute. It can be used in smoothies.

Cashew Milk

- 1 cup raw cashews (soaked for 1-2 hours in hot water or overnight in cold water)
- 4 – 4½ cups water (less for a thicker milk / more for a thinner milk)
- ⅛ tsp. salt

Blend at high speed for one minute.
Coconut and Cashew nut milks get a DAD score of 1.

Cashew Cream

This vegan cream adds a creamy texture and a very subtle nutty flavor that can be used for a cream sauce, chowder, or other dishes:

- Soak 1 cup of raw cashews in hot water for 30 minutes or until softened.
- Drain the cashews and rinse them well.
- Add the soaked cashews to a blender along with 1 cup of water and a pinch of salt. Blend until smooth and creamy. Add a small amount of water if needed to achieve the desired consistency.

Alternatively, unsweetened coconut milk can be used to make cream sauces. If using canned coconut milk, read the label and avoid those with CMC, polysorbate, or carrageenan.

Ice Cream and Similar Desserts

Astonishingly, quality vanilla ice cream gets a DAD score of two (★★), as long as the serving size is limited and does not cause problems with lactose intolerance. Vanilla was tested to avoid having other flavors or colors impact the score. Ice cream is permitted in the SANA diet, however, with several caveats.

Frozen dairy dessert as an evening snack can even get a blessing on the SANA diet if it is within guidelines below, as population data suggests that a dairy snack after dinner is associated with an 18% lower all-cause, and 33% lower cardiovascular mortality. Who would have thunk!? This may be a case of the dairy snack acting by displacing other after-dinner snacks that increase risk, such as starchy after-dinner snacks, which increase overall mortality by 50%![23] Or it may be that those who prefer starchy snacks have an overall less healthy lifestyle. In any case, avoid French fries as a late evening dessert.

Searching for another excuse? Consumption of casein before sleeping increases muscle protein synthesis and metabolic rate.[24] It helps build muscle (if you have been exercising).

A four-ounce serving of ice cream generally contains 14 to 20 grams of added sugar. This is one standard scoop. The SANA diet recommends limiting ice cream to a slightly smaller serving size, between 3 oz (85 grams) and 3.5 oz (100 grams), but accepts that it is practical to use the standard serving scoop. This added sugar comes out of the daily sugar budget limit (Chapter 10).

It takes an average of 50 licks to polish off a four-ounce scoop of ice cream. Seems like a nice serving size.

Ice cream is a dangerously delicious dessert. Controlling serving size is key. Using a small (3 – 4 ounce) juice glass or limiting the serving to one scoop can help control the portion. It also limits the risk of cold-induced sphenopalatine ganglion-neuralgia (A.K.A.: ice cream headaches).

Ice cream is often made with thickeners and emulsifiers that should be avoided as they cause dysbiosis, as detailed below. Read labels and choose wisely. Most brands, including premium, national brands, put emulsifiers and thickening agents in their ice creams.

Häagen-Dazs vanilla ice cream contains cream, milk, eggs, sugar, and Madagascar vanilla. It has 14 grams of added sugar in a 4-ounce serving.

Ingredients labels list contents by weight in descending order, including water. Thus, the first ingredient is present in the highest amount, and the last is the least.

Lower-quality ice cream uses more milk and thus has a higher content of whey. Blue Bunny vanilla ice cream contains milk, cream, skim milk, sugar, egg yolks, natural flavors with vanilla extract and vanilla specks, and has 11 grams of added sugar in a 4 fl. oz. serving. These two are considerably better than most ice creams, including those from premium, national brands that use emulsifiers and thickening agents in their ice creams. If ice cream made with dairy products causes GI distress or flatulence, either it is not for you, or you are consuming too much. With homemade ice cream, frozen yogurt, or sorbets, you can control the ingredients and make delicious frozen desserts with a DAD score of 4.

Fruits and Dairy Combos

Some fruits contain enzymes that will cause milk to curdle and turn bitter as a result of the release or exposure of bitter-tasting amino acids. Citrus fruit will curdle milk due to its acidity, and can cause milk or yogurt to get bitter. These include papaya, pineapple, and kiwi. A pineapple that is not fully ripe is the worst offender. These fruits may be used to make sherbets or sorbets, and avoid this problem.

There are some workarounds. Canned pineapple has been heated, and this denatures the enzymes, decreasing the tendency to make milk or yogurt to get bitter. Also, UHT pasteurized milk or yogurt made from it is partially denatured and somewhat less likely to react. If the fruits are blended before adding, *gently* mixing in the milk, it also decreases the tendency for the blend to get bitter. Non-dairy milks are less likely to become bitter when mixed with these fruits, but may get bitter, especially those with higher protein content.

If you love ice cream and can limit your portion size, it may be best to make homemade ice cream so that you can control what is put into it.

The general formula for vanilla ice cream is:

- 1 quart half and half (not the low-fat substitute).
- ¾ cup sugar
- 1 tablespoon vanilla extract
- 1 pinch salt

To reduce the amount of whey, whole milk Greek yogurt (from a brand that does not use additives) is recommended.

For homemade ice cream, recycled 4-ounce single-serving applesauce containers can be used to store the frozen dessert for later use. Fill the cups with the ice cream that is not going to be eaten immediately, straight out of the ice cream maker, and cover the cups with 4-inch squares of foil to save in the freezer as individual servings.

Carob Fro-yo (DAD score 4)

- ½ cup carob powder (about 7 – 8 grams per 4 oz. final serving)
- 1 cup soy, oat, rice, or coconut milk, or water
- 1/3 cup brown sugar
- 1 Tbsp molasses
- 1/16 tsp. salt
- 3 cups whole milk Greek yogurt

Place the carob powder, brown sugar, and salt in a small saucepan or mixing bowl and mix. Mix in a small amount of the water or faux-milk to make a "mud", get the dry ingredients evenly wet, then slowly stir in the rest of the liquid. This should prevent the formation of lumps of carob. Let this sit for 20 – 30 minutes to help hydrate the carob and make it less grainy. (Alternatively, the mix can be brought to a simmer in a saucepan and allowed to cool.

Add the molasses and Greek yogurt and blend together. Place in an ice cream maker.

Carob should not be thought of as a substitute for chocolate but rather as its own earthy flavor.

Peach Fro-Yo (DAD score 4)

- 1 cup plain, whole-milk Greek yogurt
- One 14.5 oz can of sliced peaches in juice (undrained)
- 2 to 3 Tbsp light brown sugar (packed)

Blend the yogurt, peach juice, brown sugar, and peaches in a blender. If about a third of the peaches are held back, finely diced, and added after blending, then small bits of peaches will appear in the ice cream. Place in the ice-cream maker. Makes about 7 half-cup servings.

Mango Fro-yo (DAD score 4)

- Two cups of ripe mango fruit
- Two cups of Greek yogurt
- Tiny pinch of salt

Blend and place in an ice cream maker. Makes about 7 half-cup servings. If the mangos are not fully ripe, a small amount of honey or another sweetener may be added.

Plantain Fro-yo

Well-ripened bananas can be used to make a single-ingredient sorbet. A bit more exotic frozen dessert uses over-ripe plantains. By the time plantains are fully sweet, their skin is often turning black, and they are getting soft. Plantains are usually eaten cooked, but can be eaten as a fruit when fully ripe, and have a bit of an apricot flavor.

To prepare plantain fro-yo, cut the tips off the ripe plantains and pierce the skin in a few spots (to keep them from bursting during baking). Cover and bake them in a microwave for 3 to 4 minutes. They should be like jelly inside. They are a treat to eat just like this. Let them cool, remove the skin, and blend them with equal amounts of Greek yogurt and a pinch of salt to bring up the flavor. Freeze in an ice cream maker.

Sorbets

By FDA rules, ice cream contains a minimum of 10% milk fat; that's the cream in ice cream. A sherbert (a.k.a. sherbet) is made with fruit and or fruit juice and dairy milk. Sorbets are made without milk and thus are typically vegan.

Guava Sweet Potato Delight (Non-dairy, DAD score 4 - 5)

Two cups of cooked sweet potato (skin removed)

½ of a 14-oz pack of guava paste, cut into 1-cm chunks

2 cups water

Put two cups of water into the blender and add the chunks of guava paste through the hole on the lid. Next, add in the sweet potato, about ¼ cup at a time, and blend until smooth and creamy. You may need to pulse the blender to keep from overheating it until things are smooth.

Freeze in an ice cream maker. That's it! Makes 8 – 9 half-cup servings.

Note: Guava paste has added sugar. Iberia and Conchita brands have sugar as the second ingredient (more fruit than sugar), while some other brands have sugar as the first ingredient.

Papaya Pear Sorbet (Non-dairy, DAD score 3)

- Two cups of ripe papaya fruit
- One 14-oz can of pears in pear juice
- 1 Tbsp of Lemon juice or ¼ tsp of citric acid
- 1 level Tbsp (packed) brown sugar

Blend until smooth and freeze in an ice cream maker. Makes about 6 half-cup servings.

Piña Colada Sorbet

This recipe uses canned unsweetened coconut milk that is used in Thai and Caribbean cooking, not a coconut-based dairy-alternative beverage. When used for cooking, getting coconut milk that is high-fat is generally preferred. Multiply the number of servings on the can's label times the grams of fat per serving; there should be at least 60 grams of fat in the can. For this recipe, however, the "light" coconut milk can be used. With the light coconut milk, they just separate off some of the fat.

Read the label! Reject brands that use carboxymethyl cellulose, guar gum, or other additives! Sadly, this means rejecting most brands. Unfortunately, it's hard to find coconut milk without gum or other thickeners. Jiva Organics coconut milks contain just coconut and water, which is how coconut milk for cooking is traditionally prepared. Trader Joe's Organic coconut milk has no additives and is reasonably priced. Getting a decent DAD score depends on using coconut milk without noxious additives.

- One 13.5 - 14 oz. *can* of coconut milk
- One 20-oz can of pineapple in pineapple juice
- ¼ tsp. of citric acid powder or 1 Tbsp. lemon juice
- Less than 1/8 tsp. of salt
- ¼ cup of brown sugar.
- Optional: 1 Tbsp shredded coconut.

Crushed pineapple, bits, or chunks can be used. If using crushed pineapple, hold back about 1/3 cup of the pineapple to add after blending to give bits of fruit in the sorbet. Blend the coconut milk with the pineapple and citric acid or lemon juice. The sweetness of canned pineapple has a wide variance, and thus, more or less sugar will be needed depending on how sweet the pineapple is. One quarter cup of brown sugar is around the average amount needed, but start with less and add a bit at a time to come up to the desired sweetness. Add a pinch or two of salt to bring up the flavor. Put into the ice cream maker with the pineapple bits that were held back earlier and the shredded coconut.

Hibiscus-Plantain Sorbet

Make a hibiscus tincture using 4 to 5 grams of dried hibiscus sepals, soaking them in one cup of cold water in the refrigerator for 4 to 24 hours. Separate the sepals. Prepare the plantains as for plantain fro-yo above. Blend the hibiscus tincture with one cup of cooked, ripe plantain, and add one Tbsp of sugar, honey, or maple syrup. Freeze in an ice cream maker.

Food Additives in Dairy and Faux Dairy Products

Another major issue with dairy products is the additives that are sometimes found in them.

Annatto

Annatto (bixin) (E160b) is a natural coloring agent derived from the seed of the tropical tree *Bixa orellana*. It is a lake (a food coloring for lipids), and is used to give a red-orange color to fatty foods; it is most notably used in yellow (orange) cheeses. Annatto is a natural coloring and has antioxidant effects; nevertheless, it gets a DAD rating of B. Annatto is allergenic and can cause hives, edema, and even anaphylaxis. In some individuals, it has been reported to provoke IBS.[25] Thus, it is suggested that annatto and foods colored with it, such as yellow (orange) cheese and yellow rice, be avoided; white cheeses are thus preferred. Annatto may also be used, generally in small amounts, in ice cream to give it a "richer" appearance.

Titanium Dioxide

Who would put titanium dioxide in dairy products? Titanium dioxide (TiO2) is a very reflective material that is used in white paint. It is the whitest of all known pigments. Since it reflects light, it is used in sunscreen, and it increases the shelf life of various items, including food. In Europe, it has the food additive designation E171. TiO2 is suspected to be a cause of exacerbations of ulcerative colitis, Crohn's disease, and other inflammatory bowel diseases (IBDs).[26]

If you want white chocolate, TiO2 will make it whiter. It may be in coffee creamer, salad dressing, snacks, sauces, vitamin supplements, and candy. It is also added to some dairy products, including some milk.

If you would like to avoid TiO2, just read the label of the foods before you purchase them, and it will be listed as... oh wait.

The FDA does not require titanium dioxide to be named. It will likely be listed as "color added" or "artificial color" in the ingredient list. The product may contain up to 1% titanium dioxide,[27] which may not be much if the product is a few little white candy sprinkles on a cupcake, but if one percent of 8 servings of milk were TiO2, it would be over two grams, about ½ a teaspoon. Write your congressperson and tell them that TiO2 should be clearly listed on food labels when it is used in a food.

Emulsifiers

Emulsifiers act to suspend polar and nonpolar liquids with each other, keeping them from separating after mixing them. You have likely seen simple oil and vinegar salad dressings separate. Emulsifiers allow oil and water-based liquids to stay in a stable suspension.

Lecithins, mixtures of glycerophospholipids such as phosphatidylcholine, are present in eggs and soybeans. They are important nutrients. Lecithin is used to blend oil and water to make mayonnaise. In the digestive tract, the nutritive emulsifiers are absorbed as nutrients and are generally beneficial. They don't normally pass into the colon. Non-nutritive emulsifiers are not digested and pass through the small intestine into the colon, where they cause trouble.

Non-nutritive emulsifying and thickening agents decrease or degrade the intestinal mucosal layer, and thus facilitate bacterial adhesion to the enterocytes and colonocytes. This increases bacterial translocation into the body. The emulsifiers decrease the population of beneficial bacteria such as *Bifidobacteria*, *Lactobacillus*, and *Akkermansia*, and increase levels of pathogenic *Escherichia, Shigella,* and *Fusobacterium.* They increase the production of LPS and flagellin and decrease the production of short-chain fatty acids, which the colonocytes rely on for energy. LPS and flagellin are PAMPS (pathogen-associated molecular patterns) that the immune system recognizes as danger signals that we have an innate inflammatory response to. As a result, the emulsifiers appear to increase the risk of metabolic syndrome diseases, including cardiovascular disease and type 2 diabetes.[28] Epidemiologic and animal studies link dysbiosis, leaky gut, and inflammatory bowel disease to non-nutritive food emulsifiers. In an experimental model of 20 different food emulsifiers and thickeners, only two, soy lecithin and mono- and diglycerides, did not show strong detrimental effects on the microbiome. Even sunflower lecithin increased the expression of flagellin (a protein on Gram-negative bacteria that the body has an innate inflammatory response to. Sunflower lecithin may also be proinflammatory as a consequence of the high n-6 content of sunflower lecithin's phospholipids.

Carrageenans, xanthan, guar, and locust bean gums all induced flagellin levels several-fold higher than did sunflower lecithin. Maltodextrin, xanthan gum, sorbitan monostearate, and glyceryl stearate all promoted a strong and sustained increase in LPS levels in the bloodstream of test animals. The LPS expression remained after the withdrawal of the emulsifiers. Most of the emulsifiers decreased beta-diversity, the number of species present in the microbiome.[29] Gellan gum is used as a gelling agent and is used in non-dairy milks to keep the plant proteins suspended, to avoid settling. It is an anionic polysaccharide derived from the bacterium *Sphingomonas elodea*. Faux milk products tested using gellan gum received DAD scores of D and thus, should be avoided. Please note that while guar gum is suspected to promote intestinal inflammation, hydrolyzed guar gum (Sunfiber) does not.

Carboxymethylcellulose and Polysorbate-80: Some emulsifiers used in food are not food, and disrupt the mucous lining of the intestine. Look out for *carboxymethylcellulose (CMC)* and *polysorbate-80*, two non-nutritive emulsifiers that are used in dairy and other food products. Polysorbate-80 (P-80) causes an increase in the abundance of bacteria associated with inflammation. While CMC was not found to alter the bacterial microbiome, it decreased the population of viral bacteriophages. Recent studies have found that alterations in the ileal (small intestinal) virome could exacerbate flare-ups of Crohn's disease.[30]

In animal studies, CMC promoted more severe colitis than did P-80.[31] Both of these emulsifiers increased the gene expression of flagellin, a pro-inflammatory molecule, by the microbiota.[32] These emulsifiers act as a detergent to the mucus layer that separates the colonic cells lining the intestine from the bacteria in the colon, and in doing so, may allow translocation of bacteria into the body. Animal studies suggest that these non-nutritive emulsifiers induce low-grade inflammation that promotes obesity and metabolic syndrome.[33] In an animal model, CMC and P-80 exacerbated intestinal tumor development.[34]

Carboxymethylcellulose may be listed as CMC, "cellulose gum," or even just as "dietary fiber" on food labels.

In a study using mice bred to be genetically deficient in the anti-inflammatory cytokine IL-10, mimicking the situation of many patients with IBD, adding CMC to the diet provoked massive bacterial overgrowth, migration of bacteria deep into the mucosa crypts, and migration of white blood cells into the intestinal lumen; pathological changes similar to those of Crohn's disease.[35] This model suggests that CMC is vastly more deleterious to some individuals than others. As discussed in the chapter on cereals, gluten was found to moderately increase intestinal permeability alone, but to have major effects on permeability if used with an over-the-counter anti-inflammatory medication. The risks associated with food additives may be small under ideal conditions, yet easily promote disease under different circumstances.

Maltodextrin: Long-term intake of maltodextrin (MDX) in mice (10 weeks) promoted low-grade inflammation, changes in the structure of the intestinal mucosa, and an increase in the inflammatory proteins Il-1β and lipocalin-2. It caused changes to the intestinal epithelial barrier and caused impairment in the response to infection with Salmonella.[36] [37] MDX exacerbated intestinal inflammation in animals and triggered endoplasmic reticulum stress in goblet cells, provoking a reduction in mucin-2 expression. This increases the risk of the development of IBD.[38]

The DAD diet advises the avoidance of non-nutritive emulsifiers that survive digestion.

Carrageenan

Carrageenan may be found in dairy products such as ice cream. It makes them creamier. It is cheaper to add thickeners than cream, and the manufacturer can label the item as low-fat. Chocolate milk in the dairy section typically contains carrageenan. It may be found in non-dairy milk and other processed foods.

Carrageenan is used in the laboratory setting to create animal models of colitis. It does this by two mechanisms: 1) it activates the NF-κB inflammatory pathway when it comes in contact with the epithelial cells lining the intestine, and 2) carrageenan alters the balance of the colonic microbiota, leading to degradation of the mucosal barrier, and triggers an inflammatory immune response.[39] Carrageenan is especially injurious to animals on high-fat diets.[40] Carrageenan comes in different molecular weights: iota, kappa, and lambda. The risk from carrageenan is impacted by the molecular weight of the carrageenan used.

Sciencey Section

Here is my perspective on dairy: whey and lactose cause problems.

Milk Proteins

Bovine milk contains about 34 grams of protein per liter. The curd contains milk fat and caseins, the dominant protein family in cow's milk; about 82% of the proteins in cow's milk are caseins. About 18% of the proteins in bovine milk are water-soluble proteins that comprise whey proteins. In contrast, in human mother's milk, about 30% of the protein is casein and 70% is whey protein.

The protein in hard cheese is mostly casein and has very little lactose, so hard cheese should not bother those who are lactose intolerant. Whey can be used to make ricotta cheese, and is retained in some soft cheeses. About 65% of the protein in whey is β-lactoglobulin, 25% is α-lactalbumin, 8% is bovine serum albumin, and most of the remaining proteins are immunoglobulin.[41]

Several milk proteins included in the whey, including sIgA (anti-infective), lactoferrin (anti-microbial), and lactalbumin (antioxidant and antiviral), are resistant to digestion and have retained functions. All these proteins are capable of triggering antigenic activation. Non-human dairy products contain the sialic acid Neu5Gc, which may be associated with inflammation. (Neu5Gc is discussed in Chapter 32).

Lactose

Lactose in dairy is a problem. Cow's whey contains about 4.8% lactose. Few adults digest lactose; this is not an evolutionary bug, but rather a feature. When most adults drink milk, the lactose is not absorbed, and the lactose moves through the gut and ends up in the cecum, the first part of the large intestine, where it ferments. This fermentation forms gas, can cause cramping, and acts as an osmotic agent pulling water into the colon, which can cause diarrhea. Most adults limit their milk intake for this reason.

Most adults can tolerate a small amount of milk, mostly as a result of adaptation of the microbiome. Those adults who retain the enzymatic ability to digest lactose are mainly people from areas that historically depended on animal milk for survival; some herders from East Africa, such as the Masai, some people from Nordic countries (Sweden and Finland) who raised reindeer and had depended upon it for survival, and descendants of Bedouins who have relied on camel milk. While a survival advantage over starvation and dehydration (from diarrhea) for the Bedouins, it may not be a great advantage in areas where people could survive without milk.

Lactose, milk sugar, is a disaccharide that is digested into glucose and galactose. Our bodies need galactose. It is used in the formation of certain glycoproteins, and it is used to form galactosylceramide, an essential component of myelin, which wraps nerve fibers. The enzyme galactosylceramide synthase, which forms galactosylceramide from galactose and the lipid ceramide, is found in Schwann cells, oligodendrocytes in the brain, including those cells that do not produce myelin. The enzyme is also present in the kidneys, testes, and intestines. Babies and small children benefit from milk as it supplies large amounts of galactose that are not just used as a caloric energy source, but as a raw material for the developing brain and peripheral nervous system. Some galactose, in the form of galactose oligosaccharides (GOS), is also present in the milk to feed the developing intestinal microbiome. As adults, we make our own galactose; a 70 kg adult male can produce about 2 grams of galactose a day.

Galactose, as D-galactose (D-Gal), has a highly distinctive use in the biological sciences. It is used to accelerate aging and senescence in animals. If you want a mouse to get old more quickly and manifest the diseases of aging, rather than waiting 16 months, you can do it in less than 10 months by feeding the animal galactose. D-Gal shortens the life span in mice by 30 to 50%. The D-Gal induced accelerated aging primarily impacts the brain, heart, lungs, liver, kidneys, and skin. D-Gal induces mitochondrial dysfunction, impedes respiratory chain enzyme activity, and ATP synthesis. It thus increased the production of reactive oxygen species (ROS). In the brain, oxidation of galactose causes the formation of H_2O_2 (hydrogen peroxide), which reacts with and reduces iron, causing the production of ROS. This leads to peroxidation of cell membranes, causing neuronal dysfunction. D-Gal also binds to amino groups, which subsequently form Amadori products that form advanced glycation products (AGEs) that activate RAGE (receptor-advanced glycation end products), causing neuronal injury and promoting cognitive dysfunction. D-Gal further promotes apoptotic cell death (cell suicide) and inflammation as a result of its impact on mitochondria.

Galactose promotes the replication of mitochondrial DNA (mtDNA), which is fine during neurogenesis, but it also increases the risk of mtDNA errors, especially with aging. Galactose induces oxidative stress and deletions in the mtDNA, causing poorly functioning mitochondria. This is likely central to the mechanism by which D-Gal accelerates aging in lab animals.[42]

Galactose does this well enough that D-galactose is the most commonly used agent to accelerate aging in lab animals for the study of diseases of aging.

In experimental mice, D-Gal also causes cardiac hypertrophy, changes in the lung similar to emphysema, liver inflammation, injury, and aging of the kidney. The D-Gal-treated mice have thin, wrinkled skin, as there is a loss in the amount and in the organization of elastin and collagen fibers in the skin. There is destruction of hair follicles. When beagle dogs were given D-Gal at a dose of 50 mg/day (by subcutaneous injection) for 90 days, it resulted in lung injuries in the form of alveolar wall destruction and inflammatory infiltration. Lactobacilli in the gut mitigate D-Gal-induced injury there,[43] but if already absorbed in the small intestine, it is too late. Fermented milk products such as yogurt and kefir with lactobacilli may prevent or mitigate some D-Gal induced injury, if the bacteria digest the lactose and consume the galactose.

Other than hereditary dysfunction of galactose metabolism, the main cause of elevated galactose levels in the body results from the consumption of galactose-rich foods. Is the amount of D-Gal in food sufficient to induce aging in humans? Using a standard dose equivalency, converting 50 mg/kg per day from a 10 kg beagle to a 70 kg man would give an estimated equivalent dose about 2.9 times lower; thus, about 17.2 mg/kg per day. This is about 1.2 grams of galactose for a 70 kg man (if injected) or presumably if completely absorbed from the diet.

Small amounts of galactose in the diet are unlikely to cause a problem. Milk, however, has a lot. An 8-ounce serving of milk has about 12 grams of lactose; thus, 6 grams of that is D-Gal. Using milk that has been treated with enzymes or taking the enzyme lactase to prevent its malabsorption cleaves the galactose from the glucose in lactose, permitting its absorption. This does not appear to be a well-informed choice.

If not digested by the body, lactose is fermented in the colon into glucose and galactose. Here, it is fermented and can cause the formation of gas. With adaptation of the microbiome, bacteria likely digest up to several grams of it.

Some types of cheeses are made from whey, such as ricotta and mizithra. The whey is allowed to ferment and acidify, which causes most of the remaining protein in the whey to flocculate; it can then be filtered with a fine cloth. Ricotta contains less lactose than do most other types of cheese. Mexican fresh cheese and cream cheese are higher in lactose than most hard cheeses.[44] Fresh cheeses often have many times more galactose than do mature cheeses.[45] Mature cheese contains less than 25 mg of galactose per 100 grams, while fresh cheese may contain 3000 mg per 100 grams.[46] Thus, they can be 3% lactose by weight. Cheddar cheese generally has levels less than 5 mg per 100 grams (0.005% lactose).[47] This may explain the increased risk of colorectal cancer among those who frequently consume fromage blanc, a fresh cheese. Cottage cheese has whey added to it. Cheese, which is made using bacterial fermentation, as in the case of Swiss or Emmental cheese, enhances the flavor and causes the formation of carbon dioxide bubbles. The fermentation process decreases the amount of lactose in the cheese.

D-Gal, along with arsenic, fluoride, cobalt, copper, iron, folate deficiency, ochratoxin A, and acrylamide, inhibits glutathione synthetase (GSS) expression.[48] [49] GSS is an enzyme needed for the biosynthesis of glutathione (GSH), the body's principal antioxidant. GSH is also used by the body to bind to excrete unwelcome xenobiotic compounds from the body.

In a seven-day study of eight-year-old boys, consumption of the equivalent casein to 1.5 liters of milk per day increased serum insulin-like growth factor-1 (IGF-1) by 15% but did not affect insulin levels. Inclusion of whey in the diet, equivalent to 1.5 liters of milk per day, increased fasting insulin levels by 21%.[50] The consumption of skimmed milk among adolescents was also found to increase plasma leptin levels, which is associated with obesity.[51]

Milk is intrinsically programmed to promote growth. In addition to the effects of IGF-1 and insulin, milk is higher in leucine, methionine, and glutamine than most other foods. Methionine acts as a gatekeeper, signaling that the cell has sufficient protein for growth; glutamine participates in mTORC1 activation, a critical mechanism for the cell's decision to undergo mitosis, and leucine acts as a secondary gatekeeper for S6K1 downstream of mTORC1, which promote activation of the ribosomes for the generation of new proteins. As discussed in Chapter 13, leucine is critical for the development of muscle protein. S6K1 causes the degradation of PDCD4, which also readies the cell for cell division. Galactose promotes the activation of mTORC1. Galactose is also incorporated into glycoproteins, which may participate in growth signaling.

Both mother's milk and cow's milk contain exosomes containing microRNA. Exosomes are tiny nanoparticle vesicles that can deliver relatively large molecules, such as miRNA, across the lipid cell membrane; miRNA would otherwise be quickly degraded and unable to penetrate the cell membrane. The exosomes protect it and assist with its entry across the cell membrane, allowing cells in distant parts of the body to share information about their status. miRNAs are a component of gene expression that limits the transcription of specific proteins.

Mother's milk contains these exosomes. The principal function of these milk-derived exosomes appears to be in aiding the infant's intestine to adapt to the presence of bacteria and to promote cell growth. The miRNA in milk includes several bioactive miRNAs. MiR-148a in milk increases IGF1, insulin output, insulin resistance, and inhibits AMPK, thus promoting cell growth; great for kids, not great for adults, and terrible for adults with cancer cells. Cow and human miR-148a are identical, and thus, those from cow's milk are active in humans. MiR-21 is regarded as an "oncomir" promoting sustained cell proliferation and cancer growth. MiR-125b and miR-30, which are in cow's milk, inhibit the expression of TP53, a protein that induces apoptosis in aberrant cells; TP53 prevents cancer cells from reproducing. Thus, several of the miRNAs in milk may promote cell proliferation.[52] Nevertheless, exosomes from camel milk are under investigation as an anti-cancer therapy.[53 54]

Mother's milk has several functions in the developing infant beyond simple nutrition. It protects the child from infection and supports their growth. The miRNA-induced adaptation to a cow's microbiome is likely less helpful to infants (and adults) than that from mother's milk. Increased IGF-1 likely explains the increase in stature associated with milk consumption. The increase in insulin likely explains the increase in body mass associated with milk consumption. Activation of mTORC1/S6K1 however, promotes insulin resistance. This promotes obesity and acne during adolescence, and often later, type 2 diabetes. The activation of mTORC1 and degradation of PDCD4 (programmed death protein 4) prevent apoptosis of aberrant cells and increase the risk of cancer. Indeed, high amounts of milk consumption during adulthood are associated with an increased risk of cancer. Milk appears to increase the risk of diffuse large B-cell lymphoma and breast, hepatic, and perhaps prostate cancers. Skim milk is generally associated with a higher hazard ratio than whole milk. Skim milk and 1% milk are associated with a higher risk of obesity and acne than is whole milk. Fermented milk (yogurt), meanwhile, has an inverse risk for cancer.[55]

Most of the exosomes and thus the miRNA will be separated into the whey portion of the milk when cheese and Greek yogurt are made. Fermentation of milk digests the galactose, breaks down, and inactivates the milk exosomes. Fermented milk in the form of Greek yogurt has most of the whey drained off, further removing the content of branched-chain amino acids found in milk that promote mTORC1 and insulin resistance. MiRNAs are highest in raw milk, and are partially degraded by pasteurization, and further degraded during fermentation and processing for making cheese. During fermentation, some proteins are denatured and amino acids are released, degrading some functional proteins. Cheese making coagulates and alters some proteins, and aging has further effects. MiRNA is more abundant in fresh cheeses, such as queso fresco, especially when made with raw milk.[56]

Table 16B: Lactose content in some dairy products[57]

Enfamil Ready to Feed	4 oz.	8.76 g
Low-fat milk; 1% milk fat	8 oz.	12.69 g
Whole milk 3.25% milk fat	8 oz.	12.83 g
Yogurt, unsweetened, whole milk	8 oz.	11.42 g
Ice cream	4 oz.	4.0 g
Dulce de Leche	100 g	4.92 g
Cream, sour, cultured	100 g	3.50 g
Cream cheese	100 g	3.21 g
Cheese, cottage, low-fat, 2%	100 g	2.90 g
Cheese, Cheddar	100 g	0.32 g
Mozzarella, whole milk	100 g	0.07 g
Cheese, Swiss	100 g	0.06 g
Butter	1 Tbsp	0.01g

Humans (some, not all) are the only adult mammal that produces sufficient lactase to be able to consume milk. It is only in the last 6000 years that a point mutation on chromosome 2 occurred, allowing lactase persistence into adulthood to become common in some human populations. This mutation persisted in populations whose survival depended on cattle, and for whom this mutation gave a survival advantage. These populations lived in climates favorable to cattle, reindeer, yaks, sheep, or goat production and unfavorable to a year-round supply of other foods. These areas included northern Europe, northern Asia, and some areas of North Africa and the Middle East, where nomadic herders could survive, and also an area of India.

Lactase *non-persistence* is the normal genetic phenotype. About 12 percent of European-Americans, 75 percent of African Americans and rural Mexicans, about 90 percent of Asian Americans, and nearly 100 percent of Native Americans have lactase non-persistence. Lactase-phlorizin hydrolase (LCT) non-persistence can be tested using genotype testing of the C/T-13910 LCT promoter region.[58]

The American Academy of Pediatrics recommends two servings of milk per day in children, an amount that is associated with increased linear growth but not obesity. The consumption of dairy products is associated with increased adult stature. Children aged 4 and 5 who drank two or more servings of milk per day were about one centimeter taller than those who consumed one or fewer servings of milk.[59] In another population study, 24 to 59-month-old children who consumed milk were about 1.15 cm taller; however, other dairy products were not found to increase stature.[60] Data from the 1999-2002 NHANES study found that adult height was positively associated with milk consumption during adolescence, but not significantly associated with preadolescent milk consumption after controlling for age, birth weight, energy intake, and ethnicity.[61] Children who consume more dairy have greater bone mineralization, fewer fractures during childhood, and less osteoporosis when they reach late adulthood. The peak bone mass is reached at the end of adolescence, about the age of 18 in women and 20 in men. Childhood and adolescence are the best times to develop bone mass.[62] A Chinese study found that children aged 7 to 17 who drank more than 100 ml of milk per month were 1.26 cm taller than children who drank no milk.[63] Consumption of more than three servings of milk per day in children 9 to 14 years of age was associated with an increase in BMI; this association was found for skim and 1% milk-fat milk, but not whole milk. The milk fat does not explain the increase in body fat mass.[64]

Increased IGF-1 likely explains the increase in stature associated with milk consumption during childhood and adolescence. The increase in insulin likely explains the increase in BMI. Activation of mTORC1/S6K1 however, promotes insulin resistance. This promotes obesity and acne during adolescence, and later, can promote type 2 diabetes. The activation of mTORC1 and the degradation of PDCD4 prevent apoptosis of aberrant cells and may increase the risk of cancer. Indeed, consumption of high volumes of liquid milk during adulthood is associated with an increased risk of prostate, breast, and hepatic cancers,[65] but this is not the case for yogurt or cheese, which are associated with lower breast cancer risk. In a meta-analysis including 13 studies and over 47,000 breast cancer cases, consumption of liquid milk had a non-linear association and breast cancer. The risk of breast cancer only became significantly increased among women drinking more than 600 grams (19.7 ounces) of milk per day, which increased the risk by about 5%. Women consuming 1000 grams (32.8 ounces) of milk per day have about an 18% increased risk of breast cancer.[66]

The best-documented association between food and acne is milk. Milk consumption, especially skim and 1% milk, is associated with increased risk for acne in adolescents. Teenage boys who consumed more than two glasses of whole milk a day were about 10 percent more likely to have acne than those who drank less than one glass a day, but 19 percent more likely if they drank skim milk[67]. Data from the Nurses' Health Study similarly found that whole milk consumption was associated with about a 12% increase in the incidence of severe acne, but that skim milk consumption was associated with a 44% increase in risk. Other dairy products, including instant breakfast drinks, cottage cheese, and cream cheese, were also positively associated with acne.[68] Skim milk is two to four times more likely to cause acne than whole milk.

Milk Fat and Reduced Fat Milk

Whole milk gets a DAD score of about zero, while one percent milk gets a D. Half and half gets a DAD score of 1★. Ice cream and cheese can have scores of 2 to 3. Milk fat is encouraged, in reasonable amounts, as a healthy part of the SANA diet.

Contrary to popular opinion, milk fat contains saturated fatty acids that support health and reduce the risk of several chronic diseases. Pentadecanoic acid (C15:0) and perhaps heptadecanoic acid (C17:0) found in milk fat are important nutrients. These are unusual as dietary fatty acid nutrients in that they have an odd number of carbons. Most of the pentadecanoic acid (a.k.a. pentadecylic acid) in the diet comes from dairy, from cheese, ice cream, and butter, and when found in the blood, it is considered a marker of dairy fat intake. Pentadecanoic acid is incorporated into phospholipids and is inversely associated with cardiovascular disease and coronary heart disease.[69]

Milk fat consists of tiny globules along with proteins that allow the fat to be suspended in an aqueous medium. Digestion of milk-fat protein-globule membrane proteins yields peptides that have been found to have antioxidant effects that enhance mitochondrial biogenesis and function.[70]

The consumption of dairy fat has been found to be inversely related to fasting insulin (thus higher insulin sensitivity) and lower systolic blood pressure.[71] In an investigation of over 3300 individuals participating in the Health Professionals Follow-Up Study and the Nurses' Health Study, those with higher plasma C15:0 levels had a 44% lower risk of diabetes mellitus after 15 years of follow-up.[72] In a 16.6-year follow-up of 4,150 Swedish adults, C15:0 and C17:0 fatty acids, both markers of dairy fat intake, were inversely associated with cardiovascular disease.[73] Pentadecanoic acid is also inversely associated with fatty liver disease, fatty liver in children, and nonalcoholic steatohepatitis. Furthermore, penta-decanoic acid levels are inversely associated with several specific types of cancer, including colorectal cancer.[74]

Since they are generally consumed together, although they may have different physiologic effects, it is hard to separate the impact of pentadecanoic and hepta-decanoic acid on disease. Moderate consumption is healthy; nevertheless, some studies show increased risk for very high levels of these fatty acids.[75] Most of the medical research has focused on pentadecanoic acid. Recent research suggests that it may be an essential nutrient that is less toxic and that has a broader beneficial impact than the essential fatty acid eicosapentaenoic acid (EPA).[76]

In cell culture, pentadecanoic acid has been found to decrease the expression of numerous proteins associated with chronic inflammation, autoimmunity, and fibrosis, and decrease the inflammatory impact of LPS in cell culture. It had similar anti-aging effects as metformin and rapamycin.[77] C15:0 appears to prevent peroxidation of cell membranes and thus stabilize cell membranes and prevent ferroptosis-induced cell death, thereby protecting the heart, pancreas, and liver.[78]

Pentadecanoic acid typically constitutes about 1.2% of the fatty acids in cow's milk. The amount of C15:0 in cows' milk is associated with their consumption of grass and fiber, and inversely with the proportion of corn in their diets.[79] Some fish have fair amounts of C15:0, including mullet, catfish, and sea bass.

Pentadecanoic acid from dairy fat forms the metabolite pentadecanoylcarnitine, which is an endogenous cannabinoid with anti-inflammatory properties. It may help with anxiety, stress, and sleep.[80]

Whey and BCAA

Whey Protein Amino Acids: Whey is high in branched chain amino acids (BCAA: Leucine, Isoleucine, Valine). Having higher blood plasma levels of these amino acids is associated with a higher risk of T2D, non-alcoholic fatty liver disease (NAFLD), and heart failure.[81] [82] While BCAA has beneficial effects on young, growing mice, they appear to promote obesity in adult ones. In obese mice consuming a Western diet, reducing the consumption of BCAA was accompanied by weight loss and loss of fat mass until they were a normal weight as a result of an increase in (resting) energy expenditure.[83] Both diabetics and patients with Alzheimer's Disease (AD) have been found to have higher levels of circulating BCAA and their metabolites than did healthy controls. Sotolone, a metabolite of isoleucine, was inversely related to scores on the Mini-Mental State Examination in these patients. In animal models of AD, restricting BCAA delayed the onset of cognitive decline. In cell culture, BCAA increased the expression of the inflammatory markers TNF and IL-6.[84]

If whey protein evades digestion as a result of malabsorption, it ferments in the colon. When the BCAAs are fermented in the gut, they form the branched chain fatty acids (BCFA) isobutyrate and isovalerate, and ammonia in the gut. Isovaleric acid in the plasma and stool is associated with depression.[85] [86] In a study comparing men with and without benign prostatic hypertrophy BPH), those with BPH had significantly higher isobutyric and isovaleric acid levels in their stools.[87] In a study of microbial metabolites in the stools of elderly patients, isovaleric acid levels were considerably higher in those with AD than in healthy controls. Other microbial metabolites that were markedly elevated in AD patients included formic acid and indole-3-pyruvic acid, a product of tryptophan fermentation in the gut.[88]

Milk contains Neu5Gc. Neu5Gc is a sialic acid present in mammalian meat and dairy. Eggs, poultry, and fish do not contain Neu5Gc. Humans are unique among mammals, as we lost the ability to make Neu5Gc millions of years ago, likely as a result of a pathogen that killed all the hominids that made this immune marker. Certain pathogens attach to Neu5Gc as a way to get into the cell to cause infection. The hominids with the genetic defect wherein they did not make Neu5Gc were the only ones that survived.

Neu5Gc can be absorbed from the diet, and the enzymes to incorporate into glycoproteins are still present, so Neu5Gc from the diet gets incorporated into glycoproteins in cell membranes. Consumption of mammalian meat and dairy causes the formation of Neu5Gc sialic acids on red blood cells and other cells in the body, and higher levels of Neu5Gc are associated with increased risk of vascular and autoimmune diseases and cancer. While an association between Neu5Gc levels and disease in humans has been established, it does not necessarily prove a causal relationship. It may be that Neu5Gc is a marker of meat and whey exposure, and that a different component in red meat and whey causes the pathology. For those interested, Neu5Gc is further discussed in Chapter 32 (Chapter 32 - Meat Two). [89] [90] Sheep and goat milks have much higher levels of Neu5Gc than bovine milk, and buffalo milk has considerably lower levels. Yogurt and hard cheeses have lower amounts of Neu5Gc than milk does. Cheese that contains high amounts of whey has higher levels, while cheese making that separates out the whey has lower lactose, D-Gal, branched chain amino acids, and Neu5Gc levels.

Since Neu5Gc is a concern, goat and sheep dairy products, and cheese products containing high amounts of whey should be avoided for those with autoimmune disease and during pregnancy, unless they are needed for other reasons.

[1] The association between breast cancer and consumption of dairy products: a systematic review. Arafat HM, Omar J, Shafii N, Naser IA, Al Laham NA, Muhamad R, Al-Astani TAD, Shaqaliah AJ, Shamallakh OM, Shamallakh KM, Abusalah MAH. Ann Med. 2023 Dec;55(1):2198256. doi: 10.1080/07853890.2023.2198256. PMID: 37078247

[2] The association between dairy products consumption and prostate cancer risk: a systematic review and meta-analysis. Zhao Z, Wu D, Gao S, Zhou D, Zeng X, Yao Y, Xu Y, Zeng G. Br J Nutr. 2023 May 28;129(10):1714-1731. doi: 10.1017/S0007114522002380. Epub 2022 Aug 10. PMID: 35945656

[3] Theoretical attributable risk analysis and Disability Adjusted Life Years (DALYs) based on increased dairy consumption. Cohen SS, Bylsma LC, Movva N, Alexander DD. BMC Public Health. 2022 Aug 27;22(1):1625. doi: 10.1186/s12889-022-14042-7. PMID: 36030208

[4] Dairy Intake and Risk of Cognitive Decline and Dementia: A Systematic Review and Dose-Response Meta-Analysis of Prospective Studies. Villoz F, Filippini T, Ortega N, Kopp-Heim D, Voortman T, Blum MR, Del Giovane C, Vinceti M, Rodondi N, Chocano-Bedoya PO. Adv Nutr. 2024 Jan;15(1):100160. doi: 10.1016/j.advnut.2023.100160. Epub 2023 Dec 1. PMID: 38043604

[5] Milk and Fermented Milk Intake and Parkinson's Disease: Cohort Study. Olsson E, Byberg L, Höijer J, Kilander L, Larsson SC. Nutrients. 2020 Sep 10;12(9):2763. doi: 10.3390/nu12092763. PMID: 32927800

[6] Consumption of milk and other dairy products and incidence of Parkinson's disease: a prospective cohort study in French women. Hajji-Louati M, Portugal B, Correia E, Laouali N, Lee PC, Artaud F, Roze E, Mancini FR, Elbaz A. Eur J Epidemiol. 2024 Sep;39(9):1023-1036. doi: 10.1007/s10654-024-01152-2. PMID: 39294525

[7] Milk intake and risk of mortality and fractures in women and men: cohort studies. Michaëlsson K, Wolk A, Langenskiöld S, Basu S, Warensjö Lemming E, Melhus H, Byberg L. BMJ. 2014 Oct 28;349:g6015. doi: 10.1136/bmj.g6015. PMID: 25352269

[8] Milk and other dairy foods and risk of hip fracture in men and women. Feskanich D, Meyer HE, Fung TT, Bischoff-Ferrari HA, Willett WC. Osteoporos Int. 2018 Feb;29(2):385-396. doi: 10.1007/s00198-017-4285-8. Epub 2017 Oct 27. PMID: 29075804

[9] Dairy product consumption and risk of cancer: A short report from the NutriNet-Santé prospective cohort study. Deschasaux-Tanguy M, Barrubés Piñol L, Sellem L, Debras C, Srour B, Chazelas E, Wendeu-Foyet G, Hercberg S, Galan P, Kesse-Guyot E, Julia C, Babio Sánchez NE, Salas Salvadó J, Touvier M. Int J Cancer. 2022 Jun 15;150(12):1978-1986. doi: 10.1002/ijc.33935. Epub 2022 Jan 29. PMID: 35041764

[10] Effects of Milk and Dairy Product Consumption on Type 2 Diabetes: Overview of Systematic Reviews and Meta-Analyses. Alvarez-Bueno C, Cavero-Redondo I, Martinez-Vizcaino V, Sotos-Prieto M, Ruiz JR, Gil A. Adv Nutr. 2019 May 1;10(suppl_2):S154-S163. doi: 10.1093/advances/nmy107. PMID: 31089734

[11] Cheese consumption and multiple health outcomes: an umbrella review and updated meta-analysis of prospective studies. Zhang M, Dong X, Huang Z, Li X, Zhao Y, Wang Y, Zhu H, Fang A, Giovannucci EL. Adv Nutr. 2023 Sep;14(5):1170-1186. doi: 10.1016/j.advnut.2023.06.007. Epub 2023 Jun 15. PMID: 37328108

[12] Regression of lactose malabsorption in coeliac patients after receiving a gluten-free diet. Ojetti V, Gabrielli M, Migneco A, Lauritano C, Zocco MA, Scarpellini E, Nista EC, Gasbarrini G, Gasbarrini A. Scand J Gastroenterol. 2008;43(2):174-7. doi: 10.1080/00365520701676138. PMID: 17917999

[13] Changes in gut microbiota and lactose intolerance symptoms before and after daily lactose supplementation in individuals with the lactase nonpersistent genotype. JanssenDuijghuijsen L, Looijesteijn E, van den Belt M, Gerhard B, Ziegler M, Ariens R, Tjoelker R, Geurts J. Am J Clin Nutr. 2024 Mar;119(3):702-710. doi: 10.1016/j.ajcnut.2023.12.016. Epub 2023 Dec 28. PMID: 38159728

[14] Association of Estimated Daily Lactose Consumption, Lactase Persistence Genotype (rs4988235), and Gut Microbiota in Healthy Adults in the United States. Kable ME, Chin EL, Huang L, Stephensen CB, Lemay DG. J Nutr. 2023 Aug;153(8):2163-2173. doi: 10.1016/j.tjnut.2023.06.025. Epub 2023 Jun 23. PMID: 37354976

[15] Bacterial metabolic 'toxins': a new mechanism for lactose and food intolerance, and irritable bowel syndrome. Campbell AK, Matthews SB, Vassel N, et al. Toxicology. 2010 Dec 30;278(3):268-76. PMID: 20851732

[16] Glycation of LDL by methylglyoxal increases arterial atherogenicity: a possible contributor to increased risk of cardiovascular disease in diabetes. Rabbani N, Godfrey L, Xue M, et al. Diabetes. 2011 Jul;60(7):1973-80. PMID:21617182

[17] Higher Yogurt Consumption Is Associated With Lower Risk of Colorectal Cancer: A Systematic Review and Meta-Analysis of Observational Studies. Sun J, Song J, Yang J, Chen L, Wang Z, Duan M, Yang S, Hu C, Bi Q. Front Nutr. 2022 Jan 3;8:789006. doi: 10.3389/fnut.2021.789006. eCollection 2021. PMID: 35047546

[18] Yogurt consumption and risk of mortality from all causes, CVD and cancer: a comprehensive systematic review and dose-response meta-analysis of cohort studies. Tutunchi H, Naghshi S, Naemi M, Naeini F, Esmaillzadeh A. Public Health Nutr. 2023 Jun;26(6):1196-1209. doi: 10.1017/S1368980022002385. Epub 2022 Nov 9. PMID: 36349966

[19] An Evidence Base for Heart Disease Prevention using a Mediterranean Diet Comprised Primarily of Vegetarian Food. Gupta UC, Gupta SC, Gupta SS. Recent Adv Food Nutr Agric. 2023;14(3):135-143. doi: 10.2174/2772574X14666230725094910. PMID: 37489789

[20] The Occurrence and Dietary Exposure Assessment of Mycotoxins, Biogenic Amines, and Heavy Metals in Mould-Ripened Blue Cheeses. Reinholds I, Rusko J,

Pugajeva I, Berzina Z, Jansons M, Kirilina-Gutmane O, Tihomirova K, Bartkevics V. Foods. 2020 Jan 16;9(1):93. doi: 10.3390/foods9010093. PMID: 31963130

[21] Regular Industrial Processing of Bovine Milk Impacts the Integrity and Molecular Composition of Extracellular Vesicles. Kleinjan M, van Herwijnen MJ, Libregts SF, van Neerven RJ, Feitsma AL, Wauben MH. J Nutr. 2021 Jun 1;151(6):1416-1425. doi: 10.1093/jn/nxab031. PMID: 33768229

[22] Lactocaseibacillus-deglycosylated isoflavones prevent Aβ 40-induced Alzheimer's disease in a rat model. Liu CF, Young ZY, Shih TW, Pan TM, Lee CL. AMB Express. 2024 Aug 6;14(1):90. doi: 10.1186/s13568-024-01735-y. PMID: 39105988

[23] Association of Meal and Snack Patterns With Mortality of All-Cause, Cardiovascular Disease, and Cancer: The US National Health and Nutrition Examination Survey, 2003 to 2014. Wei W, Jiang W, Huang J, Xu J, Wang X, Jiang X, Wang Y, Li G, Sun C, Li Y, Han T. J Am Heart Assoc. 2021 Jul 6;10(13):e020254. doi: 10.1161/JAHA.120.020254. Epub 2021 Jun 23. PMID: 34157852

[24] International Society of Sports Nutrition Position Stand: protein and exercise. Jäger R, Kerksick CM, Campbell BI, Antonio J. J, et al. Int Soc Sports Nutr. 2017 Jun 20;14:20. doi: 10.1186/s12970-017-0177-8. 2017. PMID: 28642676

[25] Dyes Used in Processed Meat Products in the Polish Market, and Their Possible Risks and Benefits for Consumer Health. Czech-Załubska K, Klich D, Jackowska-Tracz A, Didkowska A, Bogdan J, Anusz K. Foods. 2023 Jul 6;12(13):2610. doi: 10.3390/foods12132610. PMID: 37444348; PMCID: PMC10341050.

[26] Dietary Guidance From the International Organization for the Study of Inflammatory Bowel Diseases. Levine A, Rhodes JM, Lindsay JO, Abreu MT, Kamm MA, Gibson PR, Gasche C, Silverberg MS, Mahadevan U, Boneh RS, Wine E, Damas OM, Syme G, Trakman GL, Yao CK, Stockhamer S, Hammami MB, Garces LC, Rogler G, Koutroubakis IE, Ananthakrishnan AN, McKeever L, Lewis JD. Clin Gastroenterol Hepatol. 2020 May;18(6):1381-1392. doi: 10.1016/j.cgh.2020.01.046. Epub 2020 Feb 15. PMID: 32068150

[27] https://www.webmd.com/diet/titanium-dioxide-in-food

[28] Food Emulsifiers and Metabolic Syndrome: The Role of the Gut Microbiota. De Siena M, Raoul P, Costantini L, Scarpellini E, Cintoni M, Gasbarrini A, Rinninella E, Mele MC. Foods. 2022 Jul 25;11(15):2205. doi: 10.3390/foods11152205. PMID: 35892789

[29] Direct impact of commonly used dietary emulsifiers on human gut microbiota. Naimi S, Viennois E, Gewirtz AT, Chassaing B. Microbiome. 2021 Mar 22;9(1):66. doi: 10.1186/s40168-020-00996-6. PMID: 33752754

[30] The gut ileal mucosal virome is disturbed in patients with Crohn's disease and exacerbates intestinal inflammation in mice. Cao Z, Fan D, Sun Y, Huang Z, Li Y, Su R, Zhang F, Li Q, Yang H, Zhang F, Miao Y, Lan P, Wu X, Zuo T. Nat Commun. 2024 Feb 22;15(1):1638. doi: 10.1038/s41467-024-45794-y. PMID: 38388538

[31] The Emulsifier Carboxymethylcellulose Induces More Aggressive Colitis in Humanized Mice with Inflammatory Bowel Disease Microbiota Than Polysorbate-80. Rousta E, Oka A, Liu B, Herzog J, Bhatt AP, Wang J, Habibi Najafi MB, Sartor RB. Nutrients. 2021 Oct 12;13(10):3565. doi: 10.3390/nu13103565. PMID: 34684567

[32] Dietary emulsifiers directly alter human microbiota composition and gene expression ex vivo potentiating intestinal inflammation. Chassaing B, Van de Wiele T, De Bodt J, Marzorati M, Gewirtz AT. Gut. 2017 Aug;66(8):1414-1427. doi: 10.1136/gutjnl-2016-313099. Epub 2017 Mar 21. PMID: 28325746

[33] Dietary emulsifiers impact the mouse gut microbiota promoting colitis and metabolic syndrome. Chassaing B, Koren O, Goodrich JK, Poole AC, Srinivasan S, Ley RE, Gewirtz AT. Nature. 2015 Mar 5;519(7541):92-6. doi: 10.1038/nature14232. Epub 2015 Feb 25. PMID: 25731162

[34] Consumption of Select Dietary Emulsifiers Exacerbates the Development of Spontaneous Intestinal Adenoma. Viennois E, Chassaing B. Int J Mol Sci. 2021 Mar 5;22(5):2602. doi: 10.3390/ijms22052602. PMID: 33807577

[35] Bacterial overgrowth and inflammation of small intestine after carboxymethylcellulose ingestion in genetically susceptible mice. Swidsinski A, Ung V, Sydora BC, Loening-Baucke V, Doerffel Y, Verstraelen H, Fedorak RN. Inflamm Bowel Dis. 2009 Mar;15(3):359-64. doi: 10.1002/ibd.20763. PMID: 18844217

[36] Impact of Food Additives on Gut Homeostasis. Laudisi F, Stolfi C, Monteleone G. Nutrients. 2019 Oct 1;11(10):2334. doi: 10.3390/nu11102334. PMID: 31581570

[37] The dietary polysaccharide maltodextrin promotes Salmonella survival and mucosal colonization in mice. Nickerson KP, Homer CR, Kessler SP, Dixon LJ, Kabi A, Gordon IO, Johnson EE, de la Motte CA, McDonald C. PLoS One. 2014 Jul 7;9(7):e101789. doi: 10.1371/journal.pone.0101789. eCollection 2014. PMID: 25000398

[38] The Food Additive Maltodextrin Promotes Endoplasmic Reticulum Stress-Driven Mucus Depletion and Exacerbates Intestinal Inflammation. Laudisi F, Di Fusco D, Dinallo V, Stolfi C, Di Grazia A, Marafini I, Colantoni A, Ortenzi A, Alteri C, Guerrieri F, Mavilio M, Ceccherini-Silberstein F, Federici M, MacDonald TT, Monteleone I, Monteleone G. Cell Mol Gastroenterol Hepatol. 2019;7(2):457-473. doi: 10.1016/j.jcmgh.2018.09.002. PMID: 30765332

[39] How does carrageenan cause colitis? A review. Guo J, Shang X, Chen P, Huang X. Carbohydr Polym. 2023 Feb 15;302:120374. doi: 10.1016/j.carbpol.2022.120374. Epub 2022 Nov 21. PMID: 36604052

[40] Native κ-carrageenan induced-colitis is related to host intestinal microecology. Mi Y, Chin YX, Cao WX, Chang YG, Lim PE, Xue CH, Tang QJ. Int J Biol Macromol. 2020 Mar 15;147:284-294. doi: 10.1016/j.ijbiomac.2020.01.072. Epub 2020 Jan 8. PMID: 31926226

[41] Bovine milk in human nutrition--a review. Haug A, Høstmark AT, Harstad OM. Lipids Health Dis. 2007 Sep 25;6:25. doi: 10.1186/1476-511X-6-25. PMID: 17894873

42 Mitochondrial transcription factor A overexpression and base excision repair deficiency in the inner ear of rats with D-galactose-induced aging. Zhong Y, Hu YJ, Chen B, Peng W, Sun Y, Yang Y, Zhao XY, Fan GR, Huang X, Kong WJ. FEBS J. 2011 Jul;278(14):2500-10. doi: 10.1111/j.1742-4658.2011.08176.x. PMID: 21575134

43 Antioxidative potential of Lactobacillus sp. in ameliorating D-galactose-induced aging. Kumar H, Bhardwaj K, Valko M, Alomar SY, Alwasel SH, Cruz-Martins N, Dhanjal DS, Singh R, Kuča K, Verma R, Kumar D. Appl Microbiol Biotechnol. 2022 Aug;106(13-16):4831-4843. doi: 10.1007/s00253-022-12041-7. Epub 2022 Jul 4. PMID: 35781838

44 https://fitaudit.com/categories/chs/sugars

45 Determination of the lactose and galactose content of common foods: Relevance to galactosemia. Shakerdi LA, Wallace L, Smyth G, Madden N, Clark A, Hendroff U, McGovern M, Connellan S, Gillman B, Treacy EP. Food Sci Nutr. 2022 Jul 19;10(11):3789-3800. doi: 10.1002/fsn3.2976. eCollection 2022 Nov. PMID: 36348783

46 Lactose and Galactose Content in Spanish Cheeses: Usefulness in the Dietary Treatment of Patients with Galactosaemia. Vitoria I, Melendreras F, Vázquez-Palazón A, Rausell D, Correcher P, González-Lamuño D, García-Peris M. Nutrients. 2023 Jan 23;15(3):594. doi: 10.3390/nu15030594. PMID: 36771301

47 The Lactose and Galactose Content of Cheese Suitable for Galactosaemia: New Analysis. Portnoi PA, MacDonald A. JIMD Rep. 2016;29:85-87. doi: 10.1007/8904_2015_520. Epub 2015 Dec 19. PMID: 26683467

48 RGD Glutathione synthase. https://rgd.mcw.edu/rgdweb/report/gene/main.html?id=2752

49 Hydrogen sulfide protects SH-SY5Y neuronal cells against d-galactose induced cell injury by suppression of advanced glycation end products formation and oxidative stress. Liu YY, Nagpure BV, Wong PT, Bian JS. Neurochem Int. 2013 Apr;62(5):603-9. doi: 10.1016/j.neuint.2012.12.010. Epub 2012 Dec 26. PMID: 23274001

50 Differential effects of casein versus whey on fasting plasma levels of insulin, IGF-1 and IGF-1/IGFBP-3: results from a randomized 7-day supplementation study in prepubertal boys. Hoppe C, Mølgaard C, Dalum C, Vaag A, Michaelsen KF. Eur J Clin Nutr. 2009 Sep;63(9):1076-83. doi: 10.1038/ejcn.2009.34. PMID: 19471293

51 Effect of increased intake of skimmed milk, casein, whey or water on body composition and leptin in overweight adolescents: a randomized trial. Larnkjaer A, Arnberg K, Michaelsen KF, Jensen SM, Mølgaard C. Pediatr Obes. 2015 Dec;10(6):461-7. doi: 10.1111/ijpo.12007. Epub 2015 Jan 22. PMID: 25612082

52 Mitochondrial transcription factor A overexpression and base excision repair deficiency in the inner ear of rats with D-galactose-induced aging. Zhong Y, Hu YJ, Chen B, Peng W, Sun Y, Yang Y, Zhao XY, Fan GR, Huang X, Kong WJ. FEBS J. 2011 Jul;278(14):2500-10. doi: 10.1111/j.1742-4658.2011.08176.x. PMID: 21575134

53 Prospective Role of Bioactive Molecules and Exosomes in the Therapeutic Potential of Camel Milk against Human Diseases: An Updated Perspective. Khan FB, Ansari MA, Uddin S, Palakott AR, Anwar I, Almatroudi A, Alomary MN, Alrumaihi F, Aba Alkhayl FF, Alghamdi S, Muhammad K, Huang CY, Daddam JR, Khan H, Maqsood S, Ayoub MA. Life (Basel). 2022 Jul 4;12(7):990. doi: 10.3390/life12070990. PMID: 35888080

54 Therapeutic Effect of Camel Milk and Its Exosomes on MCF7 Cells In Vitro and In Vivo. Badawy AA, El-Magd MA, AlSadrah SA. Integr Cancer Ther. 2018 Dec;17(4):1235-1246. doi: 10.1177/1534735418786000. Epub 2018 Jul 10. PMID: 29986606

55 Lifetime Impact of Cow's Milk on Overactivation of mTORC1: From Fetal to Childhood Overgrowth, Acne, Diabetes, Cancers, and Neurodegeneration. Melnik BC. Biomolecules. 2021 Mar 9;11(3):404. doi: 10.3390/biom11030404. PMID: 33803410

56 Effects of Cow's Milk Processing on MicroRNA Levels. Abou El Qassim L, Martínez B, Rodríguez A, Dávalos A, López de Las Hazas MC, Menéndez Miranda M, Royo LJ. Foods. 2023 Aug 4;12(15):2950. doi: 10.3390/foods12152950. PMID: 37569218

57 U.S. Department of Agriculture Nutrient Data Base, Nutrient Data Laboratory, Beltsville MD. Human Nutrition Research Center of the Agricultural Research Service, USDA.

58 Correlation between lactose absorption and the C/T-13910 and G/A-22018 mutations of the lactase-phlorizin hydrolase (LCT) gene in adult-type hypolactasia. Bulhões AC, Goldani HA, Oliveira FS, Matte US, Mazzuca RB, Silveira TR. Braz J Med Biol Res. 2007 Nov;40(11):1441-6. PMID:17934640

59 Milk intake, height and body mass index in preschool children. DeBoer MD, Agard HE, Scharf RJ. Arch Dis Child. 2015 May;100(5):460-5. doi: 10.1136/archdischild-2014-306958. PMID: 25512962

60 Consumption of milk, but not other dairy products, is associated with height among US preschool children in NHANES 1999-2002. Wiley AS. Ann Hum Biol. 2009 Mar-Apr;36(2):125-38. doi: 10.1080/03014460802680466. PMID: 19241191

61 Does milk make children grow? Relationships between milk consumption and height in NHANES 1999-2002. Wiley AS. Am J Hum Biol. 2005 Jul-Aug;17(4):425-41. doi: 10.1002/ajhb.20411. PMID: 15981182

62 Milk and Dairy Products: Good or Bad for Human Bone? Practical Dietary Recommendations for the Prevention and Management of Osteoporosis. Ratajczak AE, Zawada A, Rychter AM, Dobrowolska A, Krela-Kaźmierczak I. Nutrients. 2021 Apr 17;13(4):1329. doi: 10.3390/nu13041329. PMID: 33920532

63 Association between milk intake and childhood growth: results from a nationwide cross-sectional survey. Guo Q, Wang B, Cao S, Jia C, Yu X, Zhao L, Dellarco M, Duan X. Int J Obes (Lond). 2020 Nov;44(11):2194-2202. doi: 10.1038/s41366-020-0625-4. PMID: 32546859

64 Milk, dairy fat, dietary calcium, and weight gain: a longitudinal study of adolescents. Berkey CS, Rockett HR, Willett WC, Colditz GA. Arch Pediatr Adolesc Med. 2005 Jun;159(6):543-50. doi: 10.1001/archpedi.159.6.543. PMID: 15939853

65 Lifetime Impact of Cow's Milk on Overactivation of mTORC1: From Fetal to Childhood Overgrowth, Acne, Diabetes, Cancers, and Neurodegeneration. Melnik BC. Biomolecules. 2021 Mar 9;11(3):404. doi: 10.3390/biom11030404. PMID: 33803410

66 Intake of Various Food Groups and Risk of Breast Cancer: A Systematic Review and Dose-Response Meta-Analysis of Prospective Studies. Kazemi A, Barati-Boldaji R, Soltani S, Mohammadipoor N, Esmaeilinezhad Z, Clark CCT, Babajafari S, Akbarzadeh M. Adv Nutr. 2021 Jun 1;12(3):809-849. doi: 10.1093/advances/nmaa147. PMID: 33271590

67 Milk consumption and acne in teenaged boys. Adebamowo CA, Spiegelman D, Berkey CS, Danby FW, Rockett HH, Colditz GA, Willett WC, Holmes MD. J Am Acad Dermatol. 2008 May;58(5):787-93. doi: 10.1016/j.jaad.2007.08.049. Epub 2008 Jan 14. PMID: 18194824

68 High school dietary dairy intake and teenage acne. Adebamowo CA, Spiegelman D, Danby FW, Frazier AL, Willett WC, Holmes MD. J Am Acad Dermatol. 2005 Feb;52(2):207-14. doi: 10.1016/j.jaad.2004.08.007. PMID: 15692464

69 Biomarkers of dairy fatty acids and risk of cardiovascular disease in the Multi-ethnic Study of Atherosclerosis. de Oliveira Otto MC, Nettleton JA, Lemaitre RN, Steffen LM, Kromhout D, Rich SS, Tsai MY, Jacobs DR, Mozaffarian D. J Am Heart Assoc. 2013 Jul 18;2(4):e000092. doi: 10.1161/JAHA.113.000092. PMID: 23868191

70 Identification and anti-oxidative potential of milk fat globule membrane (MFGM)-derived bioactive peptides released through in vitro gastrointestinal digestion. Li H, Guan K, Liu M, Jiang W, Yan F, Zhu A, Zhou S. Bioorg Chem. 2024 Apr;145:107232. doi: 10.1016/j.bioorg.2024.107232. Epub 2024 Feb 21. PMID: 38437762

71 trans-Palmitoleic acid, other dairy fat biomarkers, and incident diabetes: the Multi-Ethnic Study of Atherosclerosis (MESA). Mozaffarian D, de Oliveira Otto MC, Lemaitre RN, Fretts AM, Hotamisligil G, Tsai MY, Siscovick DS, Nettleton JA. Am J Clin Nutr. 2013 Apr;97(4):854-61. doi: 10.3945/ajcn.112.045468. Epub 2013 Feb 13. PMID: 23407305

72 Circulating Biomarkers of Dairy Fat and Risk of Incident Diabetes Mellitus Among Men and Women in the United States in Two Large Prospective Cohorts. Yakoob MY, Shi P, Willett WC, Rexrode KM, Campos H, Orav EJ, Hu FB, Mozaffarian D. Circulation. 2016 Apr 26;133(17):1645-54. doi: 10.1161/CIRCULATIONAHA.115.018410. Epub 2016 Mar 22. PMID: 27006479

73 Biomarkers of dairy fat intake, incident cardiovascular disease, and all-cause mortality: A cohort study, systematic review, and meta-analysis. Trieu K, Bhat S, Dai Z, Leander K, Gigante B, Qian F, Korat AVA, Sun Q, Pan XF, Laguzzi F, Cederholm T, de Faire U, Hellénius ML, Wu JHY, Risérus U, Marklund M. PLoS Med. 2021 Sep 21;18(9):e1003763. doi: 10.1371/journal.pmed.1003763. eCollection 2021 Sep. PMID: 34547017

74 Pentadecanoic Acid (C15:0), an Essential Fatty Acid, Shares Clinically Relevant Cell-Based Activities with Leading Longevity-Enhancing Compounds. Venn-Watson S, Schork NJ. Nutrients. 2023 Oct 30;15(21):4607. doi: 10.3390/nu15214607. PMID: 37960259

75 Serial measures of circulating biomarkers of dairy fat and total and cause-specific mortality in older adults: the Cardiovascular Health Study. de Oliveira Otto MC, Lemaitre RN, Song X, King IB, Siscovick DS, Mozaffarian D. Am J Clin Nutr. 2018 Sep 1;108(3):476-484. doi: 10.1093/ajcn/nqy117. PMID: 30007304

76 Broader and safer clinically-relevant activities of pentadecanoic acid compared to omega-3: Evaluation of an emerging essential fatty acid across twelve primary human cell-based disease systems. Venn-Watson SK, Butterworth CN. PLoS One. 2022 May 26;17(5):e0268778. doi: 10.1371/journal.pone.0268778. eCollection 2022. PMID: 35617322

77 Ibid 66. PMID: 37960259

78 The Cellular Stability Hypothesis: Evidence of Ferroptosis and Accelerated Aging-Associated Diseases as Newly Identified Nutritional Pentadecanoic Acid (C15:0) Deficiency Syndrome. Venn-Watson S. Metabolites. 2024 Jun 23;14(7):355. doi: 10.3390/metabo14070355. PMID: 39057678

79 Milk Odd- and Branched-Chain Fatty Acids as Biomarkers of Rumen Fermentation. Kupczyński R, Pacyga K, Lewandowska K, Bednarski M, Szumny A. Animals (Basel). 2024 Jun 6;14(11):1706. doi: 10.3390/ani14111706. PMID: 38891752

80 Pentadecanoylcarnitine is a newly discovered endocannabinoid with pleiotropic activities relevant to supporting physical and mental health. Venn-Watson S, Reiner J, Jensen ED. Sci Rep. 2022 Aug 23;12(1):13717. doi: 10.1038/s41598-022-18266-w. PMID: 35999445

81 Non-Alcoholic Fatty Liver Disease and Risk of Incident Type 2 Diabetes: Role of Circulating Branched-Chain Amino Acids. van den Berg EH, Flores-Guerrero JL, Gruppen EG, de Borst MH, Wolak-Dinsmore J, Connelly MA, Bakker SJL, Dullaart RPF. Nutrients. 2019 Mar 26;11(3):705. doi: 10.3390/nu11030705. PMID: 30917546

82 Circulating branched-chain amino acids and incident heart failure in type 2 diabetes: The Hong Kong Diabetes Register. Lim LL, Lau ESH, Fung E, Lee HM, Ma RCW, Tam CHT, Wong WKK, Ng ACW, Chow E, Luk AOY, Jenkins A, Chan JCN, Kong APS. Diabetes Metab Res Rev. 2020 Mar;36(3):e3253. doi: 10.1002/dmrr.3253. Epub 2020 Jan 19. PMID: 31957226

83 Restoration of metabolic health by decreased consumption of branched-chain amino acids. Cummings NE, Williams EM, Kasza I, Konon EN, Schaid MD, Schmidt BA, Poudel C, Sherman DS, Yu D, Arriola Apelo SI, Cottrell SE, Geiger G, Barnes ME, Wisinski JA, Fenske RJ, Matkowskyj KA, Kimple ME, Alexander CM, Merrins MJ, Lamming DW. J Physiol. 2018 Feb 15;596(4):623-

645. doi: 10.1113/JP275075. Epub 2017 Dec 27. PMID: 29266268

84 Branched-Chain Amino Acids Are Linked with Alzheimer's Disease-Related Pathology and Cognitive Deficits. Siddik MAB, Mullins CA, Kramer A, Shah H, Gannaban RB, Zabet-Moghaddam M, Huebinger RM, Hegde VK, MohanKumar SMJ, MohanKumar PS, Shin AC. Cells. 2022 Nov 7;11(21):3523. doi: 10.3390/cells11213523. PMID: 36359919

85 Isovaleric acid in stool correlates with human depression. Szczesniak O, Hestad KA, Hanssen JF, Rudi K. Nutr Neurosci. 2016 Sep;19(7):279-83. doi: 10.1179/1476830515Y.0000000007. PMID: 25710209

86 Associations between fecal short-chain fatty acids, plasma inflammatory cytokines, and dietary markers with depression and anxiety: Post hoc analysis of the ENGAGE-2 pilot trial.

Burton TC, Lv N, Tsai P, Peñalver Bernabé B, Tussing-Humphreys L, Xiao L, Pandey GN, Wu Y, Ajilore OA, Ma J. Am J Clin Nutr. 2023 Apr;117(4):717-730. doi: 10.1016/j.ajcnut.2023.01.018. PMID: 36796440

87 Alterations in fecal short chain fatty acids (SCFAs) and branched short-chain fatty acids (BCFAs) in men with benign prostatic hyperplasia (BPH) and metabolic syndrome (MetS). Ratajczak W, Mizerski A, Rył A, Słojewski M, Sipak O, Piasecka M, Laszczyńska M. Aging (Albany NY). 2021 Apr 13;13(8):10934-10954. doi: 10.18632/aging.202968. PMID: 33847600

88 Altered Gut Microbial Metabolites in Amnestic Mild Cognitive Impairment and Alzheimer's Disease: Signals in Host-Microbe Interplay. Wu L, Han Y, Zheng Z, Peng G, Liu P, Yue S, Zhu S, Chen J, Lv H, Shao L, Sheng Y, Wang Y, Li L, Li L, Wang B. Nutrients. 2021 Jan 14;13(1):228. doi: 10.3390/nu13010228. PMID: 33466861

89 Human species-specific loss of CMP-*N*-acetylneuraminic acid hydroxylase enhances atherosclerosis via intrinsic and extrinsic mechanisms. Kawanishi K, Dhar C, Do R, Varki N, Gordts PLSM, Varki A. Proc Natl Acad Sci U S A. 2019 Aug 6;116(32):16036-16045. doi: 10.1073/pnas.1902902116. PMID: 31332008

90 Challenging the Role of Diet-Induced Anti-Neu5Gc Antibodies in Human Pathologies. Soulillou JP, Cozzi E, Bach JM. Front Immunol. 2020 Jun 9;11:834. doi: 10.3389/fimmu.2020.00834. PMID: 32655538

Chapter 17: Oils and Fats

Summary

There is very little room in a healthy diet for refined seed oils. Although it may say so on the container of corn oil, it is not heart-healthy. Nor are safflower, sunflower, cottonseed, peanut, or other fats high in n-6 saturated fats. What about soy and canola oil, which have more n-3 fats? Olive oil? No, no, and no.

The average American consumes the equivalent of 6 tablespoons (90 ml) of vegetable oil per day, mostly as soy oil, followed by canola, corn, and palm oils, and mostly hidden in processed foods. At about 120 kcal per tablespoon of oil, 6 Tbsp. of oil contain 720 calories, about a third of all calories consumed. That is before any fats from meat, eggs, dairy, nuts, and other foods. That is unhealthy, and frankly, a bit gross. I am having a hard time believing it.

We need certain polyunsaturated fats in our diet: linoleic acid (LA, an n-6 fatty acid) and α-linolenic acid (ALA, a n-3 fatty acid), and we likely need pentadecanoic acid (C15:0). LA and ALA cannot be made by the body, and they are required for numerous metabolic purposes. Thus, they are considered essential, sort of like vitamins. LA is used by the body to form pro-inflammatory compounds that the body uses to fight infectious disease. ALA is used to form anti-inflammatory compounds that quell inflammation and keep it under control to prevent injury from an overactive immune system. We are healthiest when we get enough and when we are in balance. But we don't need large amounts. An adult needs less than 2.5 grams of LA per day, an amount supplied by one teaspoon (5 ml) of most vegetable oils. Since vegetable oil contains far more LA than ALA, vegetable oils promote inflammation and chronic inflammatory diseases. Even if there was a type of vegetable oil that had a healthy balance of LA and ALA, or if one could balance out excess LA in the diet by taking ALA supplements, too much LA would still be harmful, and the excess ALA intake would also increase risks. High n-3 oils also suffer from short shelf lives and quickly become rancid.

The SANA diet recommends something close to a "*no added polyunsaturated fat*" diet. There should be enough natural polyunsaturated fats in the real foods included in the SANA diet without the need to add refined ones. When fats are called for baking, as much oil as possible should be substituted with applesauce, bananas, squash puree, or similar food. *Fried foods are not permitted on the SANA diet.* Butter and coconut oil can be used as added fat on the SANA diet in moderation (no more than 10% of daily calories combined and preferably less than half this much, i.e., at less than 1 Tbsp combined. They are composed mostly of saturated fats, and butter is high in short-chain saturated fats (SCFA) that have health benefits. Grass-fed dairy products are preferred, as they have a better balance of fats.

Fats Against Health

Back in the early 1900s, the Russian physician Nikolay Anichkov fed rabbits a diet high in cholesterol, and they developed fatty deposits in their coronary arteries. It was not a big deal back then, as coronary artery disease (CAD) was rare. By the 1950s, however, CAD had become the leading cause of death in the U.S. President Eisenhower was among those who had heart attacks. His personal physician and cardiologist, Ancel Keys, had noticed that people in southern Europe, eating what we now call the Mediterranean Diet, had lower rates of heart disease than those in Northern Europe. In a feat of incredible insight, he developed the hypothesis that saturated fats increase (and polyunsaturated fats lower) cholesterol levels.

In 1960, the Framingham Heart Study reported that elevated blood pressure, smoking, obesity, lack of exercise, and high cholesterol levels were linked with heart disease risk.[1] In 1961, the advice to avoid dietary saturated fats became the official policy of the American Heart Association, advising people to replace butter with margarine. This may have had nothing to do with Procter and Gamble, a major manufacturer of margarine and vegetable shortening, being among the AMA's top sponsors.

The landmark Minnesota Coronary Experiment (1968 – 73) tested the hypothesis that polyunsaturated fats would lower cholesterol levels. Indeed, they did. Keys was right about the effect of polyunsaturated fats on cholesterol levels. In the study, the treatment group's diet had saturated fats, such as butter, replaced with corn oil and margarines made from vegetable oils high in polyunsaturated fats. Those on the intervention had an average decline in serum cholesterol of 31 mg/dl (13.8%) compared to baseline.

What was not made apparent was the minor detail that in a follow-up study of participants aged 65 or older, those in the *polyunsaturated fat treatment group had a 35% increased risk of death* over the next decade. The greater the decline in cholesterol, the higher the mortality rate.[2] Similarly, the Sydney Heart Study (1966-73) replaced saturated fats with polyunsaturated fats using safflower oil and margarine, in men aged 30 to 59. The intervention lowered cholesterol but *increased* overall mortality by 62% and increased cardiovascular disease (CVD) death by 70%.[3] In yet another study, corn oil also lowered cholesterol and increased mortality risk, but the authors at the time (1965) assumed that the increase in deaths was a failure of randomization.[4] Oopsy. It only took 40 years and the death of the researchers before mortality data from two of these studies would be published.[5]

> Keys was right about fats and cholesterol, but wrong about CAD. He clearly showed that populations such as those consuming the Mediterranean diet and the Japanese who consume *low-fat diets* had less heart disease. If not blinded by his hypotheses, he might have seen that saturated fat in the diet is closely tied to the consumption of animal protein, and that animal protein was even more predictive of CAD than was fat *in his study*. CAD risk was highest in the countries that consumed a lot of meat and few vegetables, and lower in countries where people eat less meat and more of their nutrition comes from vegetables and fish, which are low in saturated fat.[6]

We have nearly 60 years of misguided guidelines that push refined vegetable fats and 1% milk, or worse, chocolate milk, for children, which causes dysbiosis, fatty liver, and raises the risk of metabolic disease as a result of the loss of milk fat as a source of essential fatty acids. (See Chapter 15, Dairy.)

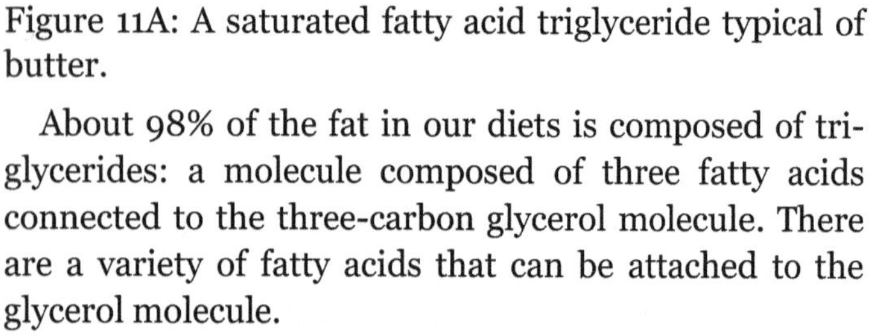

Caprylic Acid 8:0
Lauric Acid 12:0
Glycerol
Capric Acid 10:0

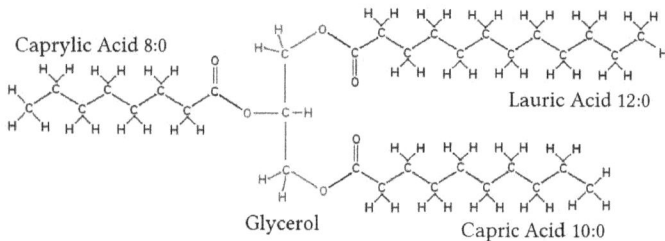

Figure 11A: A saturated fatty acid triglyceride typical of butter.

About 98% of the fat in our diets is composed of triglycerides: a molecule composed of three fatty acids connected to the three-carbon glycerol molecule. There are a variety of fatty acids that can be attached to the glycerol molecule.

Fatty acids are chemical structures made up of chains of carbon atoms with a carboxyl group (the acid) on one end. If they have two hydrogen atoms attached to each carbon, they are considered to be saturated fats, as the molecule is saturated with hydrogen. If they have one double bond between a pair of carbon atoms and thus are missing two hydrogen atoms, they are called monounsaturated, and if there are two or more double bonds, they are called polyunsaturated fats, as shown in Figure 11B. Unsaturated fats have double bonds between the carbon atoms. If the first double bond is 3 carbons from the end of the chain, the fat is called an omega-3 or n-3 fat, and if it is 6 carbons from the end, it is called an omega-6 or n-3 fat. This is because Omega is the last letter of the Greek alphabet, so 3 or 6 carbons from the end. With a double bond in the fatty acid chain, only one hydrogen is bonded to the carbon; hence the name unsaturated. The single hydrogen allows more rotational flexibility, giving the polyunsaturated fats a higher melting temperature, and helps make the lipid membranes more flexible. Fish – cold-blooded animals – especially those living in cold water, need cell membranes that are flexible in a cold environment; thus, cold water fish are rich in n-3 fatty acids.

The body uses different fatty acids to make various metabolically active compounds, so the molecular structure of the fatty acids is important. Some fatty acids are essential in the diet, as they are basic nutrients that our metabolism cannot synthesize. In general, n-3 fatty acids give rise to anti-inflammatory and n-6 fatty acids are precursors for inflammatory compounds. To maintain health, we need both; we need to be able to mount inflammatory responses against infections, parasites, and cancer cells. We also need to be able to stop inflammatory processes. Thus, ideally, our diet, and thus our bodies, should have an about even balance of n-3 and n-6 fats.

LA is a precursor of the proinflammatory fatty acid, arachidonic acid (AA), which we also get from the diet. Eicosapentaenoic and docosahexaenoic acids (EPA and DHA) are anti-inflammatory. EPA and DHA can be found in the diet and also formed in the body from ALA, but this capacity is limited. DHA is essential for brain health. Diets high in n-6 fatty acids and even those high in ALA can impede DHA formation.

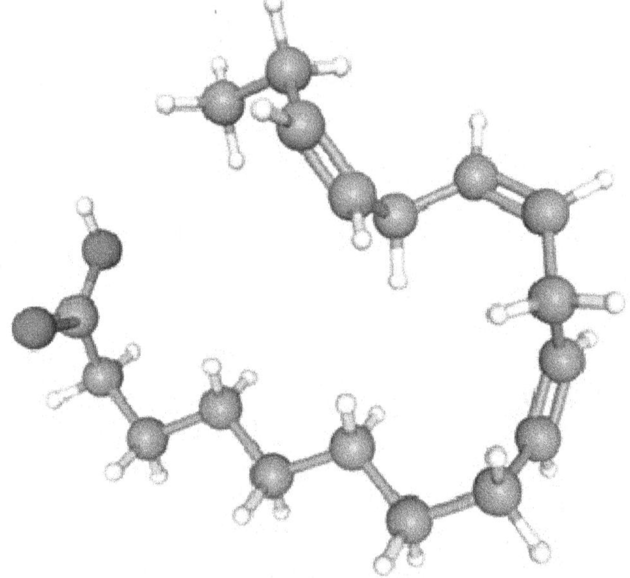

Figure 17B: Essential polyunsaturated fatty acids. Above is linolenic acid (18:3, n-3). Note the 3 double C bonds.

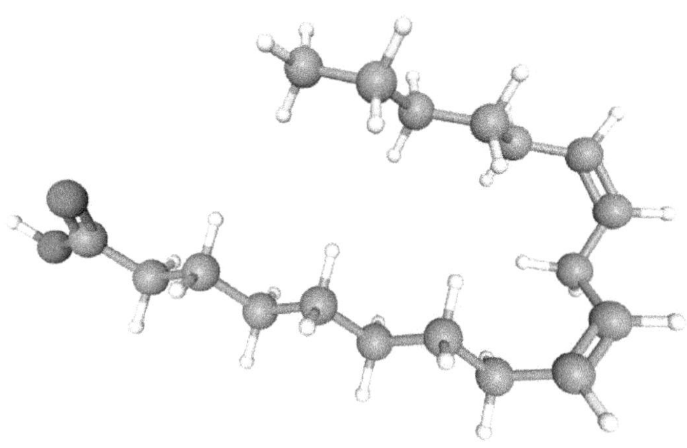

Figure 17C: Linoleic acid (18:2, n-6). Note that the first unsaturated double-bond at the 6th carbon from the (omega) end and a second unsaturated double-bond at the 9th carbon, alpha-linolenic acid has the first double bond at the third carbon from the omega end. The carboxylic acid group (COOH), with two oxygen atoms, can be seen at the alpha end of the fatty acids.

A key takeaway from this chapter is that n-6 fatty acids promote inflammation, whereas n-3 fatty acids, including DHA, which our bodies can synthesize from ALA, are anti-inflammatory. For optimal health, the n-3 and n-6 fats should be in balance, ideally with the diet containing no more than 2 times as much n-6 fat as n-3 fat. Regardless of the balance, excessive LA is harmful (as is excessive) ALA, as excessive amounts can impede the formation of EPA and DHA.

Diseases Associated with High N-6 Fatty Acid Levels

Bipolar disorder and major depression**Error! Bookmark not defined.**[7]
Neuro-oxidative stress[11]
Coronary artery disease[8]
Alzheimer's disease and Parkinson's disease[9]
Rheumatoid arthritis
Learning disorders[10]
Chronic headache[11]
Sleep disorders[12]
Acne vulgaris[13]
Epilepsy[7]
Obesity
Anxiety
Asthma
Cancer
Rage[14]

Cooking oils have an enormous excess of n-6 fats while containing little or no n-3 fatty acids. Corn oil, for example, has a mix of fatty acids bound to glycerol, dominated by linoleic acid (C18:2) (54%) and with 27% monounsaturated oleic acid (C18:1), 11% palmitic acid (C16:0), 2% stearic acid (C18:0), and 1% ALA (C18:3), with small amounts of other fatty acids. The first number in the parentheses shows the number of carbons in the fatty acid chain, and the second number tells the number of unsaturated bonds. The n-6 to n-3 ratio of corn oil is about 46 to 1. Safflower oil has no n-3 fats, so an n-6:n-3 ratio cannot even be calculated.

But why is canola oil banned from the SANA diet? It has a decent n-6 to n-3 ratio of 2.2 with 21.7% LA and 9.6% ALA (and 62% monounsaturated oleic acid). When compared to sunflower oil, canola oil improves "cardiovascular risk factors" more than sunflower oil.[15] [16] As we have seen with other polyunsaturated fats, however, lowering cholesterol levels is no guarantee of heart health nor CAD risk reduction. Canola oil is made from a variety of rape seed, a plant similar to mustard, that has been bred to have a low content of erucic acid. Erucic acid is a fatty acid that, when added to the diet of rats, causes fatty deposits in the heart and skeletal muscles and impaired growth. By FDA regulations, canola oil must contain less than 2% erucic acid. This is thought to be a safe level. Canola oil also contains about 3.6% trans fats. Trans fats are harmful and *accumulate in the body* with time, as we lack the enzymes to break them down. Since canola has less than 0.5 grams per (one tablespoon) serving, it is listed as having zero trans fats on the label. Corn and soy oil also contain trans fats at similar levels. Trans fatty acids should be considered toxic and avoided as such, even at low levels.

The main problem with canola oil, however, is the same as for other vegetable oils. There is too much linoleic acid.

The same enzymes that convert n-6 arachidonic acid into inflammatory eicosanoids can convert LA into LA-derived oxylipins. Those LA-oxylipins formed by cytochrome P450 (CYP) enzymes cause mitochondrial dysfunction and, in animal models, cause vasoconstriction, heart failure, kidney damage, and respiratory distress. CYP oxylipin metabolites of LA and ALA in the liver are highly correlated with obesity and metabolic disease. When compared in animals, high-fat soy and olive oil diets caused marked obesity, fatty liver, and liver dysfunction, while the same caloric intake of coconut oil only promoted mild obesity, which did not progress to metabolic disease.[17] LA oxylipins are associated with atherosclerosis, non-alcoholic liver disease (NASH), and Alzheimer's disease.[18]

LA and the Gut

Linoleic acid appears to have a direct adverse impact on the gut. A diet high in LA encourages intestinal overgrowth of adherent invasive *E. coli* (AIEC) that crowd out beneficial bacteria, promoting dysbiosis. LA further directly impairs the mucosal barrier, increasing permeability. LA is a ligand for a transcription factor (HNF4α) in the intestinal mucosa. LA increases the expression of a form of HNF4α that increases intestinal epithelial barrier permeability. Dietary LA in mice promoted symptoms consistent with inflammatory bowel disease (IBD), immune dysfunction, and leaky gut.[19]

LA impairs oxidative phosphorylation (the production of energy by the mitochondria). It also blunts alkaline phosphatase (ALP) activity.[20] Intestinal ALP (IAP) is an essential enzyme produced by enterocytes for detoxifying LPS and flagellin produced by bacteria in the gut. IAP helps normalize the GI microbiome, impeding the proliferation of many bacteria with pathogenic potential. Impaired IAP is implicated in the causation of IBD.[21] IAP protects the GI tract from permeability and inflammation that is typical during aging. In mice, IAP supplementation decreased age-related leaky gut and its associated inflammation, decreasing frailty and extending lifespan.[22]

The refining process for canola and other oils may cause oxidation of fatty acids. ALA has three unsaturated bonds, making it highly susceptible to autoxidation. This effect is vividly demonstrated by the ability of a cotton rag soaked in linseed oil (flaxseed oil; n-6 to n-3 ratio 0.27) to spontaneously burst into flame! Fatty acids with three unsaturated bonds, such as ALA, and less so those with two, are easily oxidized. Storing oil under refrigeration and in the dark slows this process. Nevertheless, oils with triple unsaturation easily autoxidize. Consumption of oxidized fats can lead to the formation of free radicals that cause a chain reaction of lipid peroxidation in the body, especially in the presence of reduced iron (Fe^{2+}),[23] as might occur in red blood cells in the venous circulation. Heating of vegetable oil during its refinement and when frying foods causes the formation of high levels of advanced glycation end-products (AGEs). AGEs are ligands for RAGEs (Receptor for AGEs), which promote white blood cell activity typical of autoimmune disease.[24] Dietary AGEs increase oxidative stress and inflammation. In animal models, dietary AGEs promote kidney disease, atherosclerosis, and Alzheimer's disease.[25] [26]

An analysis of the NHANES study examined the association of dietary factors with NT-proBNP, a protein fragment released during cardiac stress that is a marker of CVD mortality risk. Dietary intake of monounsaturated fats and polyunsaturated fats was associated with higher levels of NT-proBNP; meanwhile, diets low in saturated fats had higher levels.[27] (Note that all saturated fats are not the same.)

Thus, these vegetable oils promote inflammation and thus need to be banned from the diet.

The Western diet typically has an n-6 to n-3 ratio of about 16 to 1, when the ideal ratio is less than 2:1. The problem is not limited to vegetable oils. Corn has an n-6 to n-3 ratio of 25:1 to 60:1. Corn is the predominant feed for livestock, including chickens, and thus the tissue of these animals has a high n-6 to n-3 fatty acid ratio reflecting this. Free-range animals' triglyceride content reflects their diets. Milk cows generally graze and have much healthier diets than cattle raised in feedlots.

Cooking and Fat

A diet that is considerably more destructive to health than the Standard American Diet (SAD), a variant of the Western diet, is called the Southern diet. This diet is characterized by the consumption of fried chicken (often breaded and with the skin eaten), fried fish, hushpuppies (fried cornmeal dumplings), organ and processed meats, and sugar-sweetened beverages such as sweet tea, Hi-C, and sodas. The Southern Diet is associated with a 56% higher risk of acute coronary heart disease as compared to the SAD diet.[28]

The SANA diet is a low-fat diet, but moreover, it is a minimal "added polyunsaturated fat" diet. The SANA diet limits vegetable oil to coconut oil, which has 92% saturated fatty acids and less than 2% polyunsaturated fatty acids. Other vegetable oils get D rankings; margarine and vegetable shortening deserve a rating lower than never-consume. Butter is also allowed on the SANA diet; it has about 3 to 4% polyunsaturated fatty acids, and an n-6 to n-3 ratio of about 0.64.

While butter and coconut oil are allowed, the goal is not to replace 700 calories of one fat with another. Also, whipped butter is high in AGEs and thus should not be used.

While butter and coconut oil are high in the dreaded saturated fats, not all saturated fats have the same impact on health. Coconut oils are primarily composed (@ 80%) of medium-chain fatty acids (MCFA), with 12 or fewer carbon atoms. The predominant fat in coconut oil is lauric acid (C12:0, at 47%), followed by myristic acid (C14:0 at 19%). It has about 2.5% stearic acid (C18:0), about the same as most vegetable oils, but only about 7% oleic acid (C18:1), far less than most vegetable oils. Corn, soy, and cottonseed oils are higher in palmitic acid (16:0) than coconut oil.

The adverse health impact of saturated fat is mostly from long-chain saturated fat, such as palmitic acid and stearic acid, and from consuming so much beyond the caloric needs that it exceeds the capacity of fat cells to store it. It can then be deposited in other tissues, such as the liver, pancreas, and muscles. It can then promote metabolic syndrome. They are not inherently pro-inflammatory. One just needs to keep the amount down to a reasonable amount.

The two fatty acid species that appear most closely associated with hepatotoxicity are excesses of C16:0 and 18:1. The fatty acids imbalance most strongly associated with muscle toxicity and loss of strength was a *deficit* in phospholipids composed of DHA (docosahexaenoic acid, (C22:6 n-3) (found in fish, but which is also formed in the body from alpha-linolenic acid (C18:3, n-3).[29]

Stearic acid (C18:0) and palmitic acid (C16:0) are not inherently dangerous. Consumption of these fats is associated with increased expression of PINK1,[30] which promotes autophagy of poorly functioning mitochondria, and promotes neurite maintenance and neuronal differentiation in the brain, while PINK1 dysfunction is a cause of Parkinson's disease.[31]

Palmitic acid helps mediate inflammatory processes by microglia in the brain. It promotes TLR4-mediated inflammation, induced by LPS from gram-negative bacteria, while down-regulating TLR2 inflammatory processes induced by lipoteichoic acid (LTA) from gram-positive bacteria. TLR activation is beneficial for eliminating fungal and bacterial infections; nevertheless, palmitic acid becomes detrimental when consumed in excess. Much of the risk is mediated by obesity, insulin resistance, and increased insulin secretion associated with excess overall fat consumption.[32] [33]

It is the excess intake of oleic and palmitic acids, above that which can be used or stored in fat cells, that causes problems. This should not be a problem on a low-fat diet.

Butter is predominantly composed of palmitic acid (C16:0, about 33%) and contains about 17% short and medium-chain fatty acids. It contains about 21% oleic acid and 13% stearic acid (C18:0). Milk fat is the principal source of pentadecanoic acid (C15:0) in the diet, a semi-essential nutrient, which is associated with a lower risk of metabolic syndrome, diabetes, and vascular disease. (Will be discussed in Chapter 15: Dairy)

The amount of fat the body can utilize is limited by the production of creatine, which is dependent upon the dietary intake of arginine, glycine, and especially, methionine. I suggest that calories from dietary fat be kept below those from protein to assure fat utilization.

Naked Salads

Avoid vegetable oils. Feel free to go "au naturel!" Salads do not need lubrication or dressing. They are better naked. If you don't like the taste of lettuce that is not bathed in dressing, perhaps your taste buds get it. Have a salad made of the vegetables you enjoy, and skip the rest. That way, you don't have to dig through the salad bowl to get the gems. Vinegar, such as balsamic vinegar, can be used.

Baking

Baked goods are often made with lard, shortening, butter, and oil. The principal reasons are to make the baked good flakier, moister, more tender, and more flavorful.

For many baked goods, including cakes, muffins, cookies, brownies, and other sweet baked goods, applesauce can replace vegetable oil. Greek yogurt can be used to substitute for butter, using 5 parts Greek yogurt for four parts of butter. The amount of wet ingredients may need to be lowered a bit.

Along with coconut oil, butter, and ghee can be used on the SANA diet. As with other dairy products, those from grass-fed cows are preferred over those from cows on industrial farms.

Vegans

If dairy and eggs or fatty fish are consumed, the SANA diet should provide plenty of fats, including the essential polyunsaturated fats LA and ALA. Vegans may have a hard time getting sufficient essential fatty acids, especially ALA, without supplementation. This supplementation might be in the form of freshly ground flaxseed or hydrated chia seed. Flaxseed should be stored refrigerated to help maintain its freshness. Half an ounce of chia seed provides 2.5 grams of ALA, more than the recommended "adequate intake" (AI) of ALA.[34] Ten walnut halves provide about 80% of the AI for ALA.[35] One quarter ounce of flaxseed provides the AI for ALA.[36]

Fried Foods Cooked in Oil

Different oils tolerate heating to different temperatures. Above an oil's smoke temperature, it will begin to smoke and can burst into flame. Oils with high smoke temperatures are easier to cook with, as they require less care in making sure that the cooking temperature is not excessive; they can get hotter without smoking or igniting. However, cooking food at high temperatures comes with risks. When meat is cooked at high temperatures, several carcinogenic compounds are formed. The amount of the carcinogens formed increases quickly with temperatures between 300°C to 600°C. Heterocyclic amines (HCA)[37] and polycyclic aromatic hydrocarbons (PAH), such as benz(a)pyrenes and nitrosamines, are chemicals that are formed when cooking meats at high temperatures. The formation of HCA accelerates at temperatures over 200°C (392°F). Nitrosamines, which also form at high temperatures, are potent oxidants. These are toxic and carcinogenic compounds.

PAH forms when fat drips onto coals, a burner, or flame, and creates smoke. Many HCAs and PAH are carcinogenic and have been linked to prostate, pancreatic, and colon cancers. They have been found to increase inflammatory cytokines IL-1β and TNF-α in the intestines. They reduce GLP-1 and thus may promote obesity and type 2 diabetes.[38] The highest concentration of these toxic compounds is found in the drippings and oil that remain in the pan. When meat is cooked at high temperatures, the drippings should not be eaten or used for gravy. Charred areas of meat or other proteins should never be eaten.

The generally recommended temperature for frying food is 185°C (365°F). Temperatures lower than this are used for sautéing. Since the SANA diet recommends against eating fried foods, there is little need for fats with high smoke temperatures.

Table 6-9: Smoke Temperature for Some Cooking Oils

Fat	Degrees C	Degrees F
Butter	150	302
Coconut oil	177	351
Virgin olive oil	207	406
Corn oil	236	457
Soy oil	241	466
Canola oil	242	468

Frying fish may undo any benefits imparted by the DHA and EPA content in fish. Fried fish consumption has been associated with an increased risk of stroke in the deep-fried South of the United States.[39] The SANA program advises that if chicken is cooked that it should not be fried.

Acrylamide

Acrylamide is a neurotoxic food pollutant that is formed during high-temperature cooking, especially of starch foods and particularly during frying starchy foods, as is the case for French fries and potato and corn chips. It is also formed during the toasting of bread and other starchy foods.

Acrylamide (ACR) inhibits autophagy (cell organelle renewal) and promotes oxidative stress and apoptosis (cell suicide), promoting neurotoxicity to the brain, peripheral, and enteric (GI) nervous systems. ACR increases intestinal permeability and increases LPS and inflammatory response. It has been shown to promote dysbiosis in rats.[40] ACR also induced circadian disorder by suppressing the expression of proteins associated with day/night cycles, aggravating cognitive dysfunction in animal models.[41]

French fries and potato chips are the largest source of ACR in the Western diet. Levels are higher in fries (and toasted bread) that are overcooked and brown. ACR production is highest for frying, followed by roasting, and then baking. Boiling potatoes or microwaving them with the skin on does not cause the formation of ACR.[42]

If one can't live without crispy French fries, air-frying produces only 10% as much ACR as does frying the potatoes, and further reduction is possible by presoaking the cut potatoes in a 2% salt solution for 30 minutes.[43] (20 grams or 3.5 tsp./liter) Potatoes that are already cooked (boiled or microwaved) can be air-fried to give a crispy surface texture with little browning, and thus lower ACR production.

As will be briefly discussed in Chapter 33 on Indoor Air Quality, the health risks of fried foods, including fried vegetables, are not limited to eating them. Aldehydes, acrylamide, PAH, and numerous other volatile organic compounds and small airborne particles are generated during the frying of foods. Many of these are toxic and are systemically absorbed through the respiratory tract. The frequent exposure to vapors created during the frying of foods increases the risk of lung cancer, even in non-smokers.

1 https://www.mcgill.ca/oss/article/health-nutrition/great-cholesterol-debate

2 Re-evaluation of the traditional diet-heart hypothesis: analysis of recovered data from Minnesota Coronary Experiment (1968-73). Ramsden CE, Zamora D, Majchrzak-Hong S, Faurot KR, Broste SK, Frantz RP, Davis JM, Ringel A, Suchindran CM, Hibbeln JR.BMJ. 2016 Apr 12;353:i1246. doi: 10.1136/bmj.i1246.PMID: 27071971

3 Use of dietary linoleic acid for secondary prevention of coronary heart disease and death: evaluation of recovered data from the Sydney Diet Heart Study and updated meta-analysis. Ramsden CE, Zamora D, Leelarthaepin B, Majchrzak-Hong SF, Faurot KR, Suchindran CM, Ringel A, Davis JM, Hibbeln JR.BMJ. 2013 Feb 4;346:e8707. doi: 10.1136/bmj.e8707.PMID: 23386268

4 CORN OIL IN TREATMENT OF ISCHAEMIC HEART DISEASE. ROSE GA, THOMSON WB, WILLIAMS RT. Br Med J. 1965 Jun 12;1(5449):1531-3. doi: 10.1136/bmj.1.5449.1531. PMID: 14288105

5 Records Found in Dusty Basement Undermine Decades of Dietary Advice Sharon Begley, Sci Am. https://www.scientificamerican.com/article/records-found-in-dusty-basement-undermine-decades-of-dietary-advice/

6 Fat in the diet and mortality from heart disease; a methodologic note. YERUSHALMY J, HILLEBOE HE. N Y State J Med. 1957 Jul 15;57(14):2343-54. PMID: 13441073

7 Omega-3 polyunsaturated essential fatty acids are associated with depression in adolescents with eating disorders and weight loss. Swenne I, Rosling A, Tengblad S, Vessby B. Acta Paediatr. 2011 Jul 6. PMID:21732977

8 Correlation of omega-3 levels in serum phospholipid from 2053 human blood samples with key fatty acid ratios. Holub BJ, Wlodek M, Rowe W, Piekarski J. Nutr J. 2009 Dec 24;8:58. PMID:20034401

9 Omega-3 fatty acids: potential role in the management of early Alzheimer's disease. Jicha GA, Markesbery WR. Clin Interv Aging. 2010 Apr 7;5:45-61. PMID:20396634

10 Supplementation of polyunsaturated fatty acids, magnesium and zinc in children seeking medical advice for attention-deficit/hyperactivity problems. Huss M, Völp A, Stauss-Grabo M. Lipids Health Dis. 2010 Sep 24;9:105. PMID:20868469

11 Low omega-6 vs. low omega-6 plus high omega-3 dietary intervention for chronic daily headache: protocol for a randomized clinical trial. Ramsden CE, Mann JD, Faurot KR, et al. Trials. 2011 Apr 15;12:97. PMID:21496264

12 Omega-3 fatty acids as treatments for mental illness: which disorder and which fatty acid? Ross BM, Seguin J, Sieswerda LE. Lipids Health Dis. 2007 Sep 18;6:21. PMID:17877810

13 The relationship of diet and acne: A review. Pappas A. Dermatoendocrinol. 2009 Sep;1(5):262-7. PMID:20808513

14 Essential fatty acids and their role in conditions characterised by impulsivity. Garland MR, Hallahan B. Int Rev Psychiatry. 2006 Apr;18(2):99-105. PMID: 16777664

15 The effects of Canola oil on cardiovascular risk factors: A systematic review and meta-analysis with dose-response analysis of controlled clinical trials. Amiri M, Raeisi-Dehkordi H, Sarrafzadegan N, Forbes SC, Salehi-Abargouei A. Nutr Metab Cardiovasc Dis. 2020 Nov 27;30(12):2133-2145. doi: 10.1016/j.numecd.2020.06.007. Epub 2020 Jun 18. PMID: 33127255

16 Effects of Canola Oil Consumption on Lipid Profile: A Systematic Review and Meta-Analysis of Randomized Controlled Clinical Trials. Ghobadi S, Hassanzadeh-Rostami Z, Mohammadian F, Zare M, Faghih S. J Am Coll Nutr. 2019 Feb;38(2):185-196. doi: 10.1080/07315724.2018.1475270. Epub 2018 Oct 31. PMID: 30381009

17 Omega-6 and omega-3 oxylipins are implicated in soybean oil-induced obesity in mice. Deol P, Fahrmann J, Yang J, Evans JR, Rizo A, Grapov D, Salemi M, Wanichthanarak K, Fiehn O, Phinney B, Hammock BD, Sladek FM. Sci Rep. 2017 Oct 2;7(1):12488. doi: 10.1038/s41598-017-12624-9. PMID: 28970503

18 Advances in Our Understanding of Oxylipins Derived from Dietary PUFAs. Gabbs M, Leng S, Devassy JG, Monirujjaman M, Aukema HM. Adv Nutr. 2015 Sep 15;6(5):513-40. doi: 10.3945/an.114.007732. Print 2015 Sep. PMID: 26374175

19 Diet high in linoleic acid dysregulates the intestinal endocannabinoid system and increases susceptibility to colitis in Mice. Deol P, Ruegger P, Logan GD, Shawki A, Li J, Mitchell JD, Yu J, Piamthai V, Radi SH, Hasnain S, Borkowski K, Newman JW, McCole DF, Nair MG, Hsiao A, Borneman J, Sladek FM. Gut Microbes. 2023 Jan-Dec;15(1):2229945. doi: 10.1080/19490976.2023.2229945. PMID: 37400966

20 Linoleic acid blunts early osteoblast differentiation and impairs oxidative phosphorylation in vitro. Nesbeth PC, Ziegler TR, Tripathi AK, Dabeer S, Weiss D, Hao L, Smith MR, Jones DP, Maner-Smith KM, Tu CL, Chang W, Weitzmann MN, Alvarez JA. Prostaglandins Leukot Essent Fatty Acids. 2024 Feb;201:102617. doi: 10.1016/j.plefa.2024.102617. Epub 2024 May 9. PMID: 38788347

21 The Role of Intestinal Alkaline Phosphatase in Inflammatory Disorders of Gastrointestinal Tract. Bilski J, Mazur-Bialy A, Wojcik D, Zahradnik-Bilska J, Brzozowski B, Magierowski M, Mach T, Magierowska K, Brzozowski T. Mediators Inflamm. 2017;2017:9074601. doi: 10.1155/2017/9074601. Epub 2017 Feb 21. PMID: 28316376

22 Intestinal alkaline phosphatase targets the gut barrier to prevent aging. Kühn F, Adiliaghdam F, Cavallaro PM, Hamarneh SR, Tsurumi A, Hoda RS, Munoz AR, Dhole Y, Ramirez JM, Liu E, Vasan R, Liu Y, Samarbafzadeh E, Nunez RA, Farber MZ, Chopra V, Malo MS, Rahme LG, Hodin RA. JCI Insight. 2020 Mar 26;5(6):e134049. doi: 10.1172/jci.insight.134049. PMID: 32213701

23 'Lipid Peroxidation: Chemical Mechanism, Biological Implications and Analytical Determination'. Marisa Repetto, Jimena Semprine and Alberto Boveris. Lipid Peroxidation, InTech, 29 Aug. 2012. Crossref,

doi:10.5772/45943. https://www.intechopen.com/chapters/38477

24 Effect of dietary AGEs on the transcriptional profile of peripheral blood lymphocytes Manjot Sudha, Banita, Anil K. Ram, Alka Bhatia. Applied Food Research, 2(1) 2022,100086, ISSN 2772-5022, https://doi.org/10.1016/j.afres.2022.100086.

25 Advanced glycation end products in foods and a practical guide to their reduction in the diet. Uribarri J, Woodruff S, Goodman S, Cai W, Chen X, Pyzik R, Yong A, Striker GE, Vlassara H. J Am Diet Assoc. 2010 Jun;110(6):911-16.e12. doi: 10.1016/j.jada.2010.03.018. PMID: 20497781

26 High dietary advanced glycation end products are associated with poorer spatial learning and accelerated Aβ deposition in an Alzheimer mouse model. Lubitz I, Ricny J, Atrakchi-Baranes D, Shemesh C, Kravitz E, Liraz-Zaltsman S, Maksin-Matveev A, Cooper I, Leibowitz A, Uribarri J, Schmeidler J, Cai W, Kristofikova Z, Ripova D, LeRoith D, Schnaider-Beeri M. Aging Cell. 2016 Apr;15(2):309-16. doi: 10.1111/acel.12436. Epub 2016 Jan 19. PMID: 26781037

27 Role of dietary inflammatory index in the association of NT-proBNP with all-cause and cardiovascular mortality in NHANES 1999-2004. Xie L, Liu J, Wang X, Liu B, Li J, Li J, Wu H. Sci Rep. 2024 Aug 28;14(1):19978. doi: 10.1038/s41598-024-70506-3. PMID: 39198638; PMCID: PMC11358152.

28 Southern Dietary Pattern is Associated With Hazard of Acute Coronary Heart Disease in the Reasons for Geographic and Racial Differences in Stroke (REGARDS) Study. Shikany JM, Safford MM, Newby PK, Durant RW, Brown TM, Judd SE. Circulation. 2015 Sep 1;132(9):804-14. doi: 10.1161/CIRCULATION AHA.114.014421. Epub 2015 Aug 10. PMID: 26260732

29 A comprehensive study of phospholipid fatty acid rearrangements in metabolic syndrome: correlations with organ dysfunction. Bacle A, Kadri L, Khoury S, Ferru-Clément R, Faivre JF, Cognard C, Bescond J, Krzesiak A, Contzler H, Delpech N, Colas J, Vandebrouck C, Sébille S, Ferreira T. Dis Model Mech. 2020 Jun 15;13(6):dmm043927. doi: 10.1242/dmm.043927. PMID: 32303571

30 Dietary Responses of Dementia-Related Genes Encoding Metabolic Enzymes. Parnell LD, Magadmi R, Zwanger S, Shukitt-Hale B, Lai CQ, Ordovás JM. Nutrients. 2023 Jan 27;15(3):644. doi: 10.3390/nu15030644. PMID: 36771351

31 Beyond the mitochondrion: cytosolic PINK1 remodels dendrites through protein kinase A. Dagda RK, Pien I, Wang R, Zhu J, Wang KZ, Callio J, Banerjee TD, Dagda RY, Chu CT. J Neurochem. 2014 Mar;128(6):864-77. doi: 10.1111/jnc.12494. Epub 2013 Nov 13. PMID: 24151868

32 Palmitic Acid and Oleic Acid Differently Modulate TLR2-Mediated Inflammatory Responses in Microglia and Macrophages. Howe AM, Burke S, O'Reilly ME, McGillicuddy FC, Costello DA. Mol Neurobiol. 2022 Apr;59(4):2348-2362. doi: 10.1007/s12035-022-02756-z. Epub 2022 Jan 25. PMID: 35079937

33 A new frontier for fat: dietary palmitic acid induces innate immune memory. Seufert AL, Napier BA. Immunometabolism. 2023 May 15;5(2):e00021. doi: 10.1097/IN9.0000000000000021. PMID: 37197687

34 https://tools.myfooddata.com/nutrition-facts/170554/wt1/1

35 https://tools.myfooddata.com/nutrition-facts/170187/wt6/1

36 https://tools.myfooddata.com/nutrition-facts/169414/wt9/1

37 Screening for heterocyclic amines in chicken cooked in various ways. Solyakov A, Skog K. Food Chem Toxicol. 2002 Aug;40(8):1205-11.PMID: 12067585

38 Polycyclic aromatic hydrocarbons potentiate high-fat diet effects on intestinal inflammation. Khalil A, Villard PH, Dao MA, et al. Toxicol Lett. 2010 Jul 15;196(3):161-7. PMID: 20412841

39 Racial and geographic differences in fish consumption: the REGARDS study. Nahab F, Le A, Judd S, et al. Neurology. 2011 Jan 11;76(2):154-8. PMID:21178096

40 The Mechanism of Acrylamide-Induced Neurotoxicity: Current Status and Future Perspectives. Zhao M, Zhang B, Deng L. Front Nutr. 2022 Mar 25;9:859189. doi: 10.3389/fnut.2022.859189. eCollection 2022. PMID: 35399689

41 Acrylamide aggravates cognitive deficits at night period via the gut-brain axis by reprogramming the brain circadian clock. Tan X, Ye J, Liu W, Zhao B, Shi X, Zhang C, Liu Z, Liu X. Arch Toxicol. 2019 Feb;93(2):467-486. doi: 10.1007/s00204-018-2340-7. Epub 2018 Oct 29. PMID: 30374679

42 https://www.fda.gov/food/process-contaminants-food/acrylamide-and-diet-food-storage-and-food-preparation

43 Effect of pretreatments and air-frying, a novel technology, on acrylamide generation in fried potatoes. Sansano M, Juan-Borrás M, Escriche I, Andrés A, Heredia A. J Food Sci. 2015 May;80(5):T1120-8. doi: 10.1111/1750-3841.12843. PMID: 25872656

Chapter 18: Oh Nuts!

In a Nutshell

Most nuts do not live up to their reputation as being healthy foods. People are better off avoiding most nuts other than walnuts, pecans, Brazil nuts, and cashews. The most beneficial consumption of nuts is to consume 16 grams (about half an ounce) of walnuts or pecans a day. Much of the benefit from the consumption of nuts results from their causing a decrease in appetite. Thus, eating them as an afternoon snack not only decreases the consumption of other afternoon snacks but may also decrease hunger at supper time.

A single Brazil nut can be added to the @ 16 grams of walnuts or pecans. Brazil nuts are so high in selenium that two Brazil nuts a day can risk selenium overdose.

Cashews can also be consumed and have some utility as a base to replace dairy products for vegans, but should not be expected to have much beneficial impact on health other than to perhaps suppress appetite (and taste great when roasted and salted). Cashews are high in fat and are a High FODMAP food, meaning that they can cause gastrointestinal symptoms and diarrhea in individuals with irritable bowel syndrome (IBS). Thus, care should be taken to limit the amount of cashews consumed.

Most other nuts get poor DAD scores and should be avoided. Caution: About 25 to 40% of people with allergies to peanuts have allergic reactions to at least one type of tree nut. There is high allergic cross-reactivity between various nuts, and children who are allergic to peanuts may also react to lentils.[1]

Nuts

Nuts are large edible seeds that have a high fat content, which can be eaten raw and are commonly roasted to enhance their flavor. They have a hard, inedible shell that protects their rich goodness, protecting them from being easily eaten by birds.

Culinary nuts include: almonds, Brazil nuts, cashews, chestnuts, coconuts, hazelnuts, macadamia nuts, peanuts, pecans, pine nuts, pistachio nuts, and walnuts.

Nuts have gained a reputation for being a healthy food associated with a lower risk of heart and other chronic diseases. Most nuts are high in protein and polyunsaturated fats. Daily consumption of an ounce of nuts may help with weight control, contribute to reduced cholesterol levels, and reduce all-cause mortality.

A meta-analysis including 122 studies looked at peanut and tree nut consumption and blood lipids. Frequent consumption of nuts is associated with lower LDL cholesterol and ApoB, and higher HDL cholesterol levels.[2] Impressively, nut consumption among 30,000 Seventh Day Adventists who ate nuts at least 5 days a week had half the risk of myocardial infarction and a 48% reduction in coronary heart disease (CHD) over a 12-year follow-up ending in 1992, as compared to those who ate nuts less than once a week.[3] In a 2014 meta-analysis, each serving of nuts consumed per week decreased coronary artery disease by 5 percent, so that 6 servings lowered risk by 30%.[4] In a 2022 meta-analysis from more recent studies, the consumption of one ounce of nuts a day lowered cardiovascular disease (CVD) risk by 21%, lowered the risk of all-cause mortality by 22%, and the risk of cancer death by 11%. *The lowest risk was for those consuming about 15 grams (0.54 ounces) of nuts per day*, with less risk reduction for those consuming more.[5] A meta-analysis by a different group of researchers found no impact of dietary nuts on the risk for type 2 diabetes, but found a 23% reduction in CVD mortality, and a 25% reduction in CHD mortality. They also found a slight decrease in the risk of stroke mortality. Risk was lowest with a consumption of about 15 grams of nuts per day.[6]

See where this is going? We started with a 48% reduction in death and ended with a 22% decrease associated with the consumption of nuts over 30 years. Still not bad.

How do just 15 grams, half an ounce, of peanuts or tree nuts lower the hazard of death so well? That is about 15 almonds or 9 pecan halves, or less than a tablespoon of chunky peanut butter.

One explanation might be what I will call the “Great Replacement Theory”. Here, the effect is explained by nuts displacing other detrimental foods from the diet. In the Nurses’ Health Study, rather than just looking at nut consumption, the researchers also looked at what it replaced. When nut consumption replaced red meat consumption, it reduced CHD risk by 30%, but nuts replacing fish provided no benefit. Replacing red meat with beans also lowered risk.[7] In the Adventist Study, older men who regularly ate doughnuts had a 40% higher all-cause mortality.[8] The doughnut itself may not be as harmful as the dietary pattern of skipping breakfast and replacing meals with quick, hedonistic, fast food.

With secular trends in the diet, including a shift from red meat to poultry, an increase in folate (Vitamin B9) fortification in processed foods, and a reduction of trans fats in processed foods, heart disease risk has fallen considerably. This may also help explain the decline in the "potency" of nuts.

Furthermore, the distribution of nuts in the diet has also undergone a secular change with time. Almond production and consumption have increased more than tenfold, while walnut and pecan consumption have remained about the same. This may not be ideal.

Nuts are a low-carb snack. The high fat content helps suppress hunger.

Warnings:

- One to two percent of the population is allergic to at least one nut. For these individuals, nuts are dangerous.
- Chewing nuts well is important, as nuts may not be digested well when large pieces are swallowed. This can allow them to be fermented in the gut. The risk here is that protein fragments (peptides) from nuts that are not digested may get absorbed in the lower intestine, especially in those with leaky gut, and be recognized as a foreign protein that triggers an immune response. This may cause the person to develop allergic reactions to the nut in the future.
- Brazil nuts are a rich source of selenium; too rich. A single Brazil nut alone contains twice the recommended daily intake of selenium, and thus limiting intake to one a day is recommended. While an essential nutrient, excessive selenium intake causes toxicity.
- Roasting nuts causes the formation of high levels of advanced glycation end-products (AGEs).[9] [10]
- Nuts get old. Nuts that are in trail mix or packs of mixed nuts can get rancid with time. Avoid pre-packaged nuts that have been sitting on shelves for extended periods. Light, oxygen, and heat degrade the nuts. Nuts should be stored in airtight containers in a dark cabinet for a few weeks, but every time the package is opened, it is exposed to more oxygen. Thus, using smaller containers that are used more quickly will help retain freshness. Nuts can be frozen in an airtight container for long periods. Shelled nuts go bad more quickly than ones in their shells. Whole nuts, or whole halves, sell at a premium over broken ones, but for many uses, one wants pieces anyway. Broken ones have a shorter shelf life before they become oxidized and start getting rancid. Check the "Best if Used by" date on the package.
- Economy nuts, especially in trail mixes, may have been quality control seconds. Nuts are perceived as a healthy snack, so it might be tempting to snatch a serving-sized bag from a display or grab a bag of trail mix in a convenience store when a snack is needed. Warning: These nuts may be factory seconds or worse, which get bought and sold by manufacturers trying to squeeze value where there is none.
- Questionable nuts should be avoided.
- Most nuts are *not* recommended on the SANA diet.

Table 18A: SANA Nut Ratings

Nut	DAD Rating
Walnuts	2*
Pecans	2*
Brazil Nuts (free of seed coat)	1
Pistachio (*green and free of the seed coat*)	1
Nuts, Cashews	1
Coconut	0
Macadamia	B
Almond, blanched (no skin)	C
Doughnuts	C
Peanuts, roasted	C
Almonds (sliced)	C
Peanut butter	C
Almond, roasted	C
Hazel Nuts	D
Peanuts, roasted, with dark spots consistent with published images of peanuts with fungal contamination.	D
Almond seed coat	D
Pistachio (with entire seed coat)	D
Peanut seed skin (seed coat)	D
Peanut butter (crunchy, rapeseed, soy oils)	D

* The score for nuts is highly dependent on quality. The score for nuts shown for walnuts and pecans is for new, high-quality, tasty nuts. The score falls as the nuts get old. Store nuts in a freezer to preserve freshness.

Peanuts

Peanut butter was a staple for me when I was in college. A three-pound jar of peanut butter would, at best, last me a couple of weeks. If only that were among my top regrets...

There are several varieties of peanuts, but here they will be divided into two types: Spanish peanuts and Virginia peanuts. Spanish peanuts are shorter and generally used to make peanut butter and boiled peanuts (of Southern cuisine), while Virginia peanuts have a longer seed and are used in ballpark and ready-to-eat roasted peanuts. Spanish peanuts are generally used with their seed coat, which is more adherent to the seed in Spanish peanuts, while Virginia peanuts, when sold as roasted peanuts, generally have their seed coat removed. Thus, peanut butter is typically made with the seed coat, which is reported as giving a richer, more earthy flavor.

If you have never seen how peanuts grow, it is amazing. I recommend planting some just to see it. Peanuts (also called groundnuts) are a legume that grows as a small bushy herb about a foot tall with pretty yellow pea flowers. But instead of just growing a pod as do other peas, the stem on the pod that develops from the flower hangs down and grows long enough to reach the ground, and keeps going until it is buried. The pea pod then forms the peanut underground. When ready for harvest, the whole plant is pulled up along with one to two dozen peanut pods.

One of the problems with peanuts is that they are exposed to the soil, and the soil contains fungi and their spores. Peanuts are notorious for contamination with fungal toxins. The level of aflatoxin, a carcinogen, mutagen, and immunosuppressive toxin, which is allowed in peanut butter, is set by the F.D.A. at 20 µg/kg, and randomly monitored by the USDA's Agricultural Marketing Service (AMS). For most food companies, it is better to maintain in-house testing to keep levels under 15 µg/kg to avoid having a product recall and thereby destroy their brand name; thus, the risk of encountering peanut butter with aflatoxin levels beyond the legal limits in name-brand peanuts and peanut butter in the U.S. is low.

Nevertheless, U.S. farmers are losing their foreign market to peanut growers in Argentina and China, as they have lower aflatoxin levels, and as Europe, Japan and other countries have considerably more stringent standards for mycotoxins than those in the U.S. Climate change is not helping grower in the Southern states as warmer temperatures and higher humidity encourage the proliferation of the fungus *Aspergillus flavus* that produces aflatoxins.[11]

The greatest risk of exposure to mycotoxins from peanuts may be making homemade peanut butter or, even worse, making it in a grinder at an organic market. Never eat shriveled or green-tinged peanuts, ones with mottled areas, or ones with black spots on their skin. Recently, I bought some raw bulk Spanish peanuts from a grocery store to plant some in the garden for fun. Many of them had black spots on the skin, typical of fungal contamination.

Roasting peanuts, if done properly, can lower aflatoxin levels by as much as 90%.[12] Thus, roasted peanuts should be safer than raw or boiled peanuts.

Highly contaminated peanuts can be identified optically, and mechanized optical sorting machines can sort and eliminate the bad ones at high speed.[13] For this research, I bought a container of roasted peanuts. Unexpectedly, the container has both lightly colored peanuts and darker, splotchy-looking ones, which were consistent with the images from the report on optical sorting of peanuts, showing the aflatoxin-contaminated rejects. These nuts smelled similar to old peanut butter, so they were also getting rancid. The package did not state the country of origin, but it was from a company that imports many of its products from China. Sorting by hand, the *best-looking* peanuts were not fit to eat.

Another issue is that peanuts are high in n-6 fatty acids. Nuts are touted as having heart-healthy fats, likely because polyunsaturated fats lower cholesterol levels. As discussed in Chapter 17, this ain't necessarily so.

And of course, there is the issue of the peanut seed coat. Although it is a thin seed coat with little mass, it should still be avoided.

Peanut butter (on a spoon) is a choking hazard. A high school classmate asphyxiated while in his early 20s when he grabbed a spoonful of peanut butter as a snack upon arriving home from work.

Peanuts are hard to digest. They are high in protein, so undigested particles are fermented by proteolytic bacteria, creating toxic byproducts. Added to that, they often come packed with a fungal toxin (ochratoxin A), which increases intestinal paracellular permeability, allowing protein fragments to be absorbed and presented to dendritic (immune-presenting) cells in the wall of the intestine. This is a recipe for the development of allergies and food sensitivities. Peanuts are highly allergenic.

Peanuts contain very heat-resistant lectins. They can be inactivated, however, by roasting them at 177°C for

30 minutes or boiling the peanuts in a saline solution for one hour.[14]

Most commercial peanut butter is made with added hydrogenated oil and additives to keep the oil from separating. More bad fat.

Consumption of peanuts and peanut products is highly discouraged on the SANA diet.

Almonds

The SANA program also discourages the consumption of almonds. Like peanuts, the seed coat of almonds gets a rating of D. In almonds, however, it is thick and adherent. Blanched almonds with the seed coat removed get a rating of C. So why bother? Commercial Almond butter contains the seed coat.

Healthy Fats?

Nuts are often described as a source of healthy fats. Given that a high n-6 to n-3 ratio promotes inflammation, this does not appear to be the case. Lower is better.

Table 18B: Fats in nuts and seeds

Nut/ Seeds (Raw)	n-6 to n-3 ratio15
Flaxseed	0.26
Chia Seeds	0.33
Walnuts	4.2
Pecans	21
Pinenuts	32
Pistachios	49
Sesame seeds	57
Hazelnuts	90
Cashews	126
Pumpkin/ Winter Squash Seeds	172
Sunflower seeds	384
Brazil nuts	663
Almonds	4107
Peanuts	5185

Mycotoxin Risk

While peanuts are at higher risk of contamination with mycotoxins than tree nuts, other nuts may also be contaminated. In one study, the percentage of almonds, Brazil nuts, hazel nuts, cashews, walnuts, and peanuts contaminated with aflatoxins was 33.3, 40.0, 20.0, 13.3, 26.6, and 53.3% respectively; and for ochratoxin A, the contamination rates were 26.6, 33.3, 13.3, 20.0, 13.3, and 33.3%, respectively. Peanuts have the highest level of aflatoxins, followed by walnuts and Brazil nuts. Peanuts had the highest levels of ochratoxin A, followed by Brazil nuts.[16]

In Europe, the MTL (maximum tolerable limits) for aflatoxin B1 (AFB_1) is set at 2 μg/kg for peanuts and most other tree nuts, and at 8 μg/kg for almonds and pistachio nuts. A recent study did not find any samples exceeding these limits; however, it did report that pistachio nuts are occasionally contaminated with high levels of aflatoxins.[17] While aflatoxin does most of its harm by causing liver cancer, pistachios contaminated with aflatoxin in Africa have been reported to have caused death from acute toxicity.[18]

Pistachio Nuts

Pistachio nuts are the seeds of an inedible fruit that is borne in clusters on trees that grow to about 30 feet tall and can live 300 years. It is native to dry areas of central Asia, where it has been eaten by humans for over 8000 years. It is related to mango, cashews, and poison oak and contains urushiol, an irritant that can cause allergic reactions.

As the pistachio seed matures on the tree, the shell hardens and then splits open, making an audible pop, making it much easier to eat. Although first introduced to California in the 1850s, it was not grown commercially in the U.S. until around 1970, when a combination of political factors in Iran and tax shelters in the U.S. made it economically viable. The U.S. now produces about 40% of the world's supply of pistachios, and Fresno County, California, alone produces 16% of the world's supply.[19]

The SANA program discourages the consumption of pistachio nuts. As with other seeds, the inner seed coat (a testa) is the main problem. The yellow-green seeds that are free of the seed coat get a DAD score of 1. Those with a partial seed coat get a C, and those with a full seed coat, a D. Furthermore, if not harvested and stored properly, they are easily susceptible to molding with aflatoxin-forming fungi. This should not be a problem for those grown in the U.S., where they are produced by a relatively small number of commercial growers who use mechanized harvesting and processing techniques. There is more concern for those grown in Iran and other areas where they are mostly grown on small family farms, where they are harvested in small lots and may not be processed with sufficient care.

Huh?

So then, if the most eaten nuts are not beneficial, how do nuts appear to benefit health? My take after reviewing the literature is that nuts help curb the appetite. It may also be that the people who consume nuts more frequently do it as part of an overall healthy diet, and that it is the dietary pattern rather than the nuts that is responsible for better health.

Let's examine the effect of nuts in clinical trials. In a meta-analysis of health trials of nuts given to children 4 – 17 years of age, the consumption of 15–30 g of hazelnuts (with or without the seed coat for eight weeks was associated with a decrease in carbohydrate intake, and with it a decrease in empty calories. Daily consumption of 15 to 30 grams of almonds was associated with a reduction in constipation, and a change, but no improvement in fecal bacteria. Neither hazelnuts nor almonds were found to improve blood biomarkers of health. Brazil nut consumption was associated with reductions in triglycerides, total and LDL cholesterol, and oxidized LDL.[20] Remember, from the chapter on oils, that a reduction in LDL cholesterol levels should not be assumed to be a marker of health benefits; however, a reduction in oxidized cholesterol likely is.

A meta-analysis of randomized controlled trials assessing the impact of nut consumption on the GI microbiome failed to find any significant benefit.[21]

In yet another meta-analysis of clinical trials, consumption of pistachios was associated with a significant reduction in blood triglyceride levels with 3 months of follow-up. Additionally, the analysis found that the addition of tree nuts (hazelnuts > walnuts > almonds) to the diet was associated with small, non-significant reductions in fasting blood glucose and glycated hemoglobin levels.[22] These might be explained by a reduction in empty carbohydrate calories, as was observed in children.

Peanuts contain trypsin inhibitors, which, as discussed in Chapter 5, impede the digestion of proteins. They also increase the endogenous secretion of cholecystokinin (CCK), which suppresses appetite.[23] For peanuts at least, the trypsin inhibitor was found to be heat stable, and not lose potency when "toasted" at 100° C for 30 minutes.[24] Walnuts have both anti-trypsin and anti-pepsin activity.[25] Cashews contain tannins, trypsin inhibitors, and phytic acid.[26] Thus, the impact of nuts may be explained by anti-nutritional compounds that increase CCK secretion from the pancreas, thereby inhibiting appetite. At low levels of consumption, especially between or just before meals, this may not be harmful and may help reduce weight in those who tend to overeat.

Walnuts or Pecans

When nuts are eaten, the cells in the cotyledons mostly remain intact throughout their transit through at least the small intestine. As they travel through the digestive tract, the lipids are slowly digested from these cells, thus providing a slow release of lipids. Walnuts provide a larger particle size than almonds or pistachio nuts, and thus should provide a longer and more effective slow release. Studies examining the impact of adding nuts to the diet on the diversity of the colonic microbiome have had inconclusive results.

There is some evidence that eating walnuts protects the stomach and perhaps helps heal it after *H. pylori-induced* injury.[27] Animal models suggest that walnuts help protect the colon from chemically induced ulceration and colitis, alleviate intestinal inflammation, and help restore mucosal integrity.[28]

Walnuts and pecans are related trees; walnuts are native to Europe and Asia, while pecans are native to the Southern U.S. and northern Mexico. There is less medical literature on pecans. Nevertheless, trials show promise. In one clinical trial, the consumption of pecans was associated with an increase in the resting metabolic rate, with an increase in oxidation (energy utilization) of fat.[29] In another trial addition of pecans was found to improve the blood lipid profile significantly, lowering LDL cholesterol and ApoB levels.[30] In a different study, the consumption of pecans was associated with an increase in fasting postprandial peptide YY, a satiety hormone that reduces food intake and increases energy expenditure.[31] In mice, supplementation of a high-fat diet with pecans protected the animals from obesity, fatty liver, and insulin resistance. A diet with pecan polyphenol extract had the same effect, thus suggesting the polyphenols in pecans contribute to this health effect. With either treatment, the animals also had considerably lower circulating lipopolysaccharide levels, indicating improved intestinal barrier function.[32] The health impact from walnuts and pecans may be a hormetic effect (see chapter on Adaptive Mechanisms) as a result of phenolic compounds; walnuts and pecans contain the polyphenol ellagic acid.[33] Walnuts are also high in gallic acid. Ellagic and gallic acids are hydroxybenzoic acids that help activate AMPK. (Chapter 19).

Walnuts have an n-6 to n-3 ratio of 4:1, while the ratio is 21:1 for pecans. Thus, walnuts appear to be the healthier choice between the two. Walnuts are generally consumed raw rather than roasted, which avoids the formation of AGEs. The quantity of walnuts and pecans that provides the highest benefits appears to be around 16 grams, just over one-half ounce per day.

Brazil nuts

Brazil nuts have a very high concentration of selenium. Selenium is used in the body to make selenoproteins that reduce inflammation and platelet aggregation, and prevent lipid oxidation. In a study of 130 healthy Brazilian volunteers, eating one Brazil nut a day for 8 weeks lowered fasting glucose levels.[34] In a meta-analysis, Brazil nut consumption increased glutathione peroxidase activity (GPx), thus improving antioxidant activity.[35] In a small trial with 31 older adults, consuming one Brazil nut a day increased selenium levels, GPx activity, and improved cognitive function as compared to the control group.[36]

Brazil nuts can give too much of a good thing; thus, it is recommended that they be limited to a single nut, about 4 grams, per day. The thin brown seed coat contains anti-nutritive properties and should be completely removed.

Cashews

Cashews are weird nuts, as they come on the tree with a sweet, juicy edible fruit, with the nut positioned on the outside of the fruit, rather than on the inside. Furthermore, the seed is encased in a shell that is too toxic to open; it contains urushiol, the same toxin as in poison oak. Before the seed can be harvested, the nut needs to be roasted. Thus, "raw cashews" are not raw but rather once roasted, while roasted cashews are twice roasted, once in the shell and once out of the shell. This means that even "raw" cashews may add to the burden of AGEs in the diet. Cashews, however, have anti-inflammatory and antioxidant activity both systemically and on the GI mucosa. In an animal study of bowel ischemia, consumption of cashews improved intestinal barrier function and mitigated mucosal damage, translocation of bacteria, and toxins.[37] In another study, cashew consumption reduced markers of oxidative injury and microscopic evidence of cell injury in animals with chemically induced colitis.[38] Cashew consumption decreased damage from chemically induced degenerative arthritis in rats, greatly reducing X-ray evidence of joint destruction.[39] They even found a decrease in oxidative stress in the brains of rats treated with the chemotherapy agent cisplatin.[40] When 30 grams (@ 1 oz.) of cashews were consumed a day for 12 weeks, it lowered systolic blood pressure and raised HDL cholesterol level in diabetic adults.[41]

Although cashews have some health benefits, they only get a DAD score of 1 (★). Dry (twice) roasted cashews are far too easy to eat. A one-ounce serving has 13.2 grams of fat, mostly monounsaturated oleic acid (7.6 grams) but also about 2.2 grams of LA and 2.6 grams of saturated fats. It has a trivial amount of n-3 fats. About 73% of the 163 calories in an ounce come from fats.

Cashews are eaten as a nut and are also used to make vegan milk, ice cream, and other sundries for those wishing to avoid dairy. A typical cashew milk recipe uses a cup (130 grams, just over about 4½ ounces) of "raw" cashews with 3 to 4 cups of water; thus, a cup of milk would contain about one ounce of cashews. They can also be used to make nut butter, which can be used to replace peanut butter or almond butter, which are proscribed from the SANA diet. They are being used commercially to make vegan cheese.

Macadamia nuts

Macadamia nuts contain a fatty acid, palmitoleic acid (16:1n-7), an omega-7 fatty acid, which is rare in foods other than macadamia nuts and certain oily fish such as mackerel. Palmitoleic acid has anti-inflammatory, anti-thrombotic properties and improves insulin sensitivity in lab animals.[42] Nevertheless, higher palmitoleic acid blood and fat tissue levels are associated with obesity, fatty liver, and insulin resistance in humans. Thus, the health impact of dietary palmitoleic acid is complex. Palmitic acid (16:0) can be converted into palmitoleic acid in the liver. It seems likely that the elevated levels of palmitoleic acid in obese individuals are the result of obesity and over-consumption of palmitic acid, rather than palmitoleic acid consumption causing insulin resistance.[43] As with other nuts, the consumption of macadamia nuts is associated with decreased appetite and food intake.

Macadamia nuts have a short shelf life and get rancid more easily than most other nuts. They are also costly. Since they go bad easily, it is usually best to purchase unsalted, dry-roasted macadamia nuts, rather than raw ones. Macadamia nuts get a low DAD score and are likely best avoided.

Recommendations

Only a few nuts are health nuts. It appears that the consumption of nuts helps suppress the appetite. Pecans appear to increase the metabolic rate some. Limited data suggest that pecans and walnuts may improve gastrointestinal barrier function, help restore the lining of the stomach, and prevent colitis.

If you enjoy nuts, walnuts are recommended first, followed by pecans, and a Brazil nut a day is fine. They are best consumed raw, rather than roasted.

Posh up your oatmeal, cooking some chopped walnut bits into it. (Cooking them at a boiling temperature for a few minutes does not cause the formation of AGEs.)

Cashews are used to make vegan cheese, or milk can be made at home and used to make ice cream. Cashews can be eaten, and they are fine roasted. Note that cashews can cause GI problems, especially for those with IBS.

How Much Nuts

A meta-analysis indicated that 15 grams of nuts a day is optimal.

It was reported that as president, Barack Obama reportedly snacked on 7 almonds (7 – 8 grams) as he read briefings in the evening.[44] He should have been snacking on walnuts.

For health benefits, have about 16 grams of walnut or pecan halves a day. At around 2 grams per walnut half, that is about eight walnut halves. For pecans, that is about 10 - 11 halves. The health benefits from Brazil nuts are different from those from walnuts and pecans, and thus, a Brazil nut without its seed coat can be added to the walnut/pecan allotment.

Sixteen grams of walnuts contain about 1.45 grams of n-3 (alpha-linolenic acid) and 6.1 grams of n-6 fatty acids for an n-6 to n-3 ratio of 4.2 to 1; more than half of the daily requirement for α-alpha-linolenic acid, and more than twice the daily requirement for linolenic acid.[45] [46]

Sixteen grams of pecans contains only 0.16 grams of n-3 (alpha-linolenic acid) and 3.3 grams of n-6 fatty acids for an n-6 to n-3 ratio of 20.9 to 1, which is quite poor. Most of the fatty acid in pecans is monounsaturated oleic acid (18:1).[47]

One Brazil nut contains about one gram of oleic acid and 1 gram of linoleic acid.[48]

Although they have anti-oxidative properties, cashews don't get a great DAD score and should not be a large component of the diet. Nevertheless, in contrast to the 16-gram (about ½ oz.) "dose" for walnuts and pecans, up to 50 grams (1.7 grams) of cashew products per day are permitted on the SANA diet. A concern with cashews is that one ounce contains far more than the daily requirement for linoleic acid, but contains almost no ALA.

Purchase and Storage of Nuts

As noted above, Walnuts and pecans get DAD scores of 2 when fresh and in good condition, but degrade as they age. Nuts stay fresh best when whole and in their shells. Once broken, they are at increased susceptibility to oxidation, degradation, and rancidity. "Pieces", sliced, and chopped nuts have more exposed surface area and thus are more susceptible to oxidation.

Walnuts, macadamia, pecans, and hazelnuts are among those that go bad most easily, while almonds, pistachios, and cashews are less susceptible.

Dry-roasted nuts are less susceptible to oxidation than are raw ones. Salt can accelerate oxidation, so unsalted dry-roasted nuts are less likely to go bad before you purchase them.

Store nuts in air-tight containers to minimize exposure to oxygen and moisture. Avoid buying nuts from bulk containers, as they have likely been highly exposed to oxidation. Buying smaller packages may allow getting fresher, less exposed nuts.

Store nuts in a cool, dark area. Refrigerators are cool and dark, and freezers are even cooler and darker. Freezing nuts helps prevent their degradation.

[1] Patterns of Clinical Reactivity in a Danish Cohort of Tree Nut Allergic Children, Adolescents, and Young Adults. Juel-Berg N, Larsen LF, Küchen N, Norgil I, Hansen KS, Poulsen LK. Front Allergy. 2022 Mar 28;3:824660. doi: 10.3389/falgy.2022.824660. PMID: 35958942

[2] Tree Nut and Peanut Consumption and Risk of Cardiovascular Disease: A Systematic Review and Meta-Analysis of Randomized Controlled Trials. Houston L, Probst YC, Chandra Singh M, Neale EP. Adv Nutr. 2023 Sep;14(5):1029-1049. doi: 10.1016/j.advnut.2023.05.004. Epub 2023 May 5. PMID: 37149262

[3] A possible protective effect of nut consumption on risk of coronary heart disease. The Adventist Health Study. Fraser GE, Sabaté J, Beeson WL, Strahan TM. Arch Intern Med. 1992 Jul;152(7):1416-24. PMID: 1627021

[4] Nut consumption and the risk of coronary artery disease: a dose-response meta-analysis of 13 prospective studies. Ma L, Wang F, Guo W, Yang H, Liu Y, Zhang W. Thromb Res. 2014 Oct;134(4):790-4. doi: 10.1016/j.thromres.2014.06.017. Epub 2014 Jul 5. PMID: 25047173

[5] Consumption of Nuts and Seeds and Health Outcomes Including Cardiovascular Disease, Diabetes and Metabolic Disease, Cancer, and Mortality: An Umbrella Review. Balakrishna R, Bjørnerud T, Bemanian M, Aune D, Fadnes LT. Adv Nutr. 2022 Dec 22;13(6):2136-2148. doi: 10.1093/advances/nmac077. PMID: 36041171

[6] Nuts and seeds consumption and risk of cardiovascular disease, type 2 diabetes and their risk factors: a systematic review and meta-analysis. Arnesen EK, Thorisdottir B, Bärebring L, Söderlund F, Nwaru BI, Spielau U, Dierkes J, Ramel A, Lamberg-Allardt C, Åkesson A. Food Nutr Res. 2023 Feb 14;67. doi: 10.29219/fnr.v67.8961. eCollection 2023. PMID: 36816545

[7] Major dietary protein sources and risk of coronary heart disease in women. Bernstein AM, Sun Q, Hu FB, Stampfer MJ, Manson JE, Willett WC. Circulation. 2010 Aug 31;122(9):876-83. doi: 10.1161/CIRCULATIONAHA.109.915165. PMID: 20713902

[8] Risk factors for all-cause and coronary heart disease mortality in the oldest-old. The Adventist Health Study. Fraser GE, Shavlik DJ. Arch Intern Med. 1997 Oct 27;157(19):2249-58. PMID: 9343002

[9] Advanced glycation end products in foods and a practical guide to their reduction in the diet. Uribarri J, Woodruff S, Goodman S, Cai W, Chen X, Pyzik R, Yong A, Striker GE, Vlassara H. J Am Diet Assoc. 2010 Jun;110(6):911-16.e12. doi: 10.1016/j.jada.2010.03.018. PMID: 20497781

[10] High dietary advanced glycation end products are associated with poorer spatial learning and accelerated Aβ deposition in an Alzheimer mouse model. Lubitz I, Ricny J, Atrakchi-Baranes D, Shemesh C, Kravitz E, Liraz-Zaltsman S, Maksin-Matveev A, Cooper I, Leibowitz A, Uribarri J, Schmeidler J, Cai W, Kristofikova Z, Ripova D, LeRoith D, Schnaider-Beeri M. Aging Cell. 2016 Apr;15(2):309-16. doi: 10.1111/acel.12436. Epub 2016 Jan 19. PMID: 26781037

[11] https://www.farmprogress.com/harvest/time-to-deal-with-aflatoxin-in-peanuts-and-this-is-why

[12] Kinetics of aflatoxin degradation during peanut roasting. Martin LM, et al. Food Research International. Vol. 97, July 2017, pp 178-183. https://doi.org/10.1016/j.foodres.2017.03.052

[13] Remove Aflatoxin Contaminated Kernals from Peanuts, Kumar, V. Niottck Articles. 2015-04-13. https://www.biotecharticles.com/Agriculture-Article/Remove-Aflatoxin-Contaminated-Kernels-from-Peanuts-3356.html

[14] Lectin Quantitation in Peanut and Soybean Seeds1 E. M. Ahmed. University of Florida. 31 Dec 1985. Peanut Science, (American Peanut Research and Education Society) 13(1)4-7 Florida Agricultural Experiment Station Journal Series No. 6454.

[15] https://tools.myfooddata.com/nutrition-facts

[16] Natural Incidence of Aflatoxins and Ochratoxin A Nuts Collected from Local Market in Tripoli. Essawet, N., H. Abushahma, S. Inbaia1, A. Najii and Amra, H.A. 2017. *Int. J. Curr. Microbiol. App. Sci.* 6(3): 1479-1486. doi: https://doi.org/10.20546/ijcmas.2017.603.170

[17] Public health risk associated with the co-occurrence of aflatoxin B_1 and ochratoxin A in spices, herbs, and nuts in Lebanon. Daou R, Hoteit M, Bookari K, Joubrane K, Khabbaz LR, Ismail A, Maroun RG, El Khoury A. Front Public Health. 2023 Jan 9;10:1072727. doi: 10.3389/fpubh.2022.1072727. eCollection 2022. PMID: 36699892

[18] https://en.wikipedia.org/wiki/Pistachio

[19] https://en.wikipedia.org/wiki/Pistachio

[20] The Effect of Nut Consumption on Diet Quality, Cardiometabolic and Gastrointestinal Health in Children: A Systematic Review of Randomized Controlled Trials. Mead LC, Hill AM, Carter S, Coates AM. Int J Environ Res Public Health. 2021 Jan 8;18(2):454. doi: 10.3390/ijerph18020454. PMID: 33430029

[21] Nuts and their Effect on Gut Microbiota, Gut Function and Symptoms in Adults: A Systematic Review and Meta-Analysis of Randomised Controlled Trials. Creedon AC, Hung ES, Berry SE, Whelan K. Nutrients. 2020 Aug 6;12(8):2347. doi: 10.3390/nu12082347. PMID: 32781516

[22] Effect of tree nuts on glycemic outcomes in adults with type 2 diabetes mellitus: a systematic review. Muley A, Fernandez R, Ellwood L, Muley P, Shah M. JBI Evid Synth. 2021 May;19(5):966-1002. doi: 10.11124/JBISRIR-D-19-00397. PMID: 33141798

[23] Supplementation with a new trypsin inhibitor from peanut is associated with reduced fasting glucose, weight control, and increased plasma CCK secretion in an animal model. Serquiz AC, Machado RJ, Serquiz RP, Lima VC, de Carvalho FM, Carneiro MA, Maciel BL, Uchôa AF, Santos EA, Morais AH. J Enzyme Inhib Med Chem. 2016 Dec;31(6):1261-9. doi: 10.3109/14756366.2015.1103236. Epub 2016 Feb 29. PMID: 26928305

[24] Characterization of novel trypsin inhibitor in raw and toasted peanuts using a simple improved isolation. Amanda Fernandes de Medeiros, et al. Acta Chromatographica, 31(2)79-84. June 2019. https://doi.org/10.1556/1326.2017.00353

25 Wang Y, Cao S, Meng Y, et al. Mechanisms underlying the effect of walnut pellicle extracts and its four representative polyphenols on in vitro digestion of walnut protein isolate Food and Bioproducts Processing. 2024 Mar;144:166-177.

26 Nutritional evaluation of cashew (Anacardium occidentale, l.) nut protein concentrate and isolate. Ogunwolu, Henshaw, Oguntona, Afolabi. 29 Jan 2015. African Journal of Food Science. Vol. 9, Iss: 1, pp 23-30

27 Dietary intake of walnut prevented *Helicobacter pylori*-associated gastric cancer through rejuvenation of chronic atrophic gastritis. Park JM, Han YM, Park YJ, Hahm KB. J Clin Biochem Nutr. 2021 Jan;68(1):37-50. doi: 10.3164/jcbn.20-103. Epub 2020 Oct 13. PMID: 33536711

28 Effect of Nuts on Gastrointestinal Health. Mandalari G, Gervasi T, Rosenberg DW, Lapsley KG, Baer DJ. Nutrients. 2023 Apr 1;15(7):1733. doi: 10.3390/nu15071733. PMID: 37049572

29 Pecan-enriched diets increase energy expenditure and fat oxidation in adults at-risk for cardiovascular disease in a randomised, controlled trial. Guarneiri LL, Paton CM, Cooper JA. J Hum Nutr Diet. 2022 Oct;35(5):774-785. doi: 10.1111/jhn.12966. Epub 2021 Nov 28. PMID: 34841598

30 Pecan-Enriched Diets Alter Cholesterol Profiles and Triglycerides in Adults at Risk for Cardiovascular Disease in a Randomized, Controlled Trial. Guarneiri LL, Paton CM, Cooper JA. J Nutr. 2021 Oct 1;151(10):3091-3101. doi: 10.1093/jn/nxab248. PMID: 34383903

31 A pecan-enriched diet reduced postprandial appetite intensity and enhanced peptide YY secretion: A randomized control trial. Cogan B, Pearson RC, Jenkins NT, Paton CM, Cooper JA. Clin Nutr ESPEN. 2023 Aug;56:25-35. doi: 10.1016/j.clnesp.2023.05.002. Epub 2023 May 8. PMID: 37344080

32 Pecans and Its Polyphenols Prevent Obesity, Hepatic Steatosis and Diabetes by Reducing Dysbiosis, Inflammation, and Increasing Energy Expenditure in Mice Fed a High-Fat Diet. Delgadillo-Puga C, Torre-Villalvazo I, Noriega LG, Rodríguez-López LA, Alemán G, Torre-Anaya EA, Cariño-Cervantes YY, Palacios-Gonzalez B, Furuzawa-Carballeda J, Tovar AR, Cisneros-Zevallos L. Nutrients. 2023 May 31;15(11):2591. doi: 10.3390/nu15112591. PMID: 37299553

33 https://en.wikipedia.org/wiki/Ellagic acid

34 SEPP1 polymorphisms modulate serum glucose and lipid response to Brazil nut supplementation. Donadio JLS, Rogero MM, Guerra-Shinohara EM, Desmarchelier C, Borel P, Cozzolino SMF. Eur J Nutr. 2018 Aug;57(5):1873-1882. doi: 10.1007/s00394-017-1470-7. Epub 2017 May 13. PMID: 28501922

35 Effect of Brazil Nuts on Selenium Status, Blood Lipids, and Biomarkers of Oxidative Stress and Inflammation: A Systematic Review and Meta-Analysis of Randomized Clinical Trials. Godos J, Giampieri F, Micek A, Battino M, Forbes-Hernández TY, Quiles JL, Paladino N, Falzone L, Grosso G. Antioxidants (Basel). 2022 Feb 16;11(2):403. doi: 10.3390/antiox11020403. PMID: 35204285

36 Effects of Brazil nut consumption on selenium status and cognitive performance in older adults with mild cognitive impairment: a randomized controlled pilot trial. Rita Cardoso B, Apolinário D, da Silva Bandeira V, Busse AL, Magaldi RM, Jacob-Filho W, Cozzolino SM. Eur J Nutr. 2016 Feb;55(1):107-16. doi: 10.1007/s00394-014-0829-2. Epub 2015 Jan 8. PMID: 25567069

37 Consumption of *Anacardium Occidentale L.* (Cashew Nuts) Inhibits Oxidative Stress through Modulation of the Nrf2/HO-1 and NF-kB Pathways. Fusco R, Cordaro M, Siracusa R, Peritore AF, Gugliandolo E, Genovese T, D'Amico R, Crupi R, Smeriglio A, Mandalari G, Impellizzeri D, Cuzzocrea S, Di Paola R. Molecules. 2020 Sep 26;25(19):4426. doi: 10.3390/molecules25194426. PMID: 32993187

38 The Antioxidant and Anti-Inflammatory Properties of *Anacardium occidentale* L. Cashew Nuts in a Mouse Model of Colitis. Siracusa R, Fusco R, Peritore AF, Cordaro M, D'Amico R, Genovese T, Gugliandolo E, Crupi R, Smeriglio A, Mandalari G, Cuzzocrea S, Di Paola R, Impellizzeri D. Nutrients. 2020 Mar 20;12(3):834. doi: 10.3390/nu12030834. PMID: 32245085

39 The Role of Cashew (*Anacardium occidentale* L.) Nuts on an Experimental Model of Painful Degenerative Joint Disease. Fusco R, Siracusa R, Peritore AF, Gugliandolo E, Genovese T, D'Amico R, Cordaro M, Crupi R, Mandalari G, Impellizzeri D, Cuzzocrea S, Di Paola R. Antioxidants (Basel). 2020 Jun 10;9(6):511. doi: 10.3390/antiox9060511. PMID: 32532064

40 Roasted cashew (*Anacardium occidentale* L.) nut-enhanced diet forestalls cisplatin-initiated brain harm in rats. Akomolafe SF, Asowata-Ayodele AM. Heliyon. 2022 Oct 12;8(10):e11066. doi: 10.1016/j.heliyon.2022.e11066. eCollection 2022 Oct. PMID: 36276737

41 Cashew Nut Consumption Increases HDL Cholesterol and Reduces Systolic Blood Pressure in Asian Indians with Type 2 Diabetes: A 12-Week Randomized Controlled Trial. Mohan V, Gayathri R, Jaacks LM, Lakshmipriya N, Anjana RM, Spiegelman D, Jeevan RG, Balasubramaniam KK, Shobana S, Jayanthan M, Gopinath V, Divya S, Kavitha V, Vijayalakshmi P, Bai R MR, Unnikrishnan R, Sudha V, Krishnaswamy K, Salas-Salvadó J, Willett WC. J Nutr. 2018 Jan 1;148(1):63-69. doi: 10.1093/jn/nxx001. PMID: 29378038

42 Is Palmitoleic Acid a Plausible Nonpharmacological Strategy to Prevent or Control Chronic Metabolic and Inflammatory Disorders? de Souza CO, Vannice GK, Rosa Neto JC, Calder PC. Mol Nutr Food Res. 2018 Jan;62(1). doi: 10.1002/mnfr.201700504. Epub 2017 Dec 11. PMID: 28980402

43 Roles of Palmitoleic Acid and Its Positional Isomers, Hypogeic and Sapienic Acids, in Inflammation, Metabolic Diseases and Cancer. Bermúdez MA, Pereira L, Fraile C, Valerio L, Balboa MA, Balsinde J. Cells. 2022 Jul 8;11(14):2146. doi: 10.3390/cells11142146. PMID: 35883589

44 https://www.nytimes.com/2016/07/29/us/politics/obama-sets-the-record-straight-on-his-7-almond-habit.html

45 https://tools.myfooddata.com/nutrition-facts/170187/100g/1

46 https://fdc.nal.usda.gov/fdc-app.html#/food-details/170187/nutrients

47 https://fdc.nal.usda.gov/fdc-app.html#/food-details/2346395/nutrients

48 https://tools.myfooddata.com/nutrition-facts/170569/wt3/1

19: Adaptive Mechanisms for Health and Longevity

This chapter introduces some of the mechanisms by which foods lower the risk of chronic disease and the aging process beyond their impacts on macro and micronutrients and the microbiome. Some foods contain phenolic or other compounds that trigger a stress response, which, at low levels of exposure, induce the expression of antioxidants and other defensive proteins. These "hormetic" adaptive mechanisms explain the beneficial contribution of certain foods to health, which are not captured by the DAD score. Some of these include green tea, coffee, broccoli, certain berries, and garlic.

The first section of this chapter gives an overview of this process, and the second section gets into details. Reading the first section will help with understanding the next several chapters. The second section adds detail for those interested.

Aging

Age is the strongest predictor of chronic degenerative disease. It is a major risk factor for most cancers. Age is the strongest risk factor for dementia and is a major risk factor for osteoporosis, cancer, and several other chronic diseases. Clearly, the body wears out with time. While everyone gets a year older each year, not everyone ages at the same rate. An extreme case of accelerated aging is Werner syndrome, which is caused by a genetic mutation in the WRN DNA-repair enzyme. Individuals with this syndrome have short stature. Their hair turns grey, their faces age, they have hearing loss, and they develop diseases of aging during early adulthood. Most people with Werner syndrome die from cardiovascular disease or cancer, with a median survival of 48 years. However, even among the normal population, there is a wide variance in biological age.

Lifestyle generally adds or subtracts about 15 years to or from the average lifespan. The typical life expectancy of an alcoholic man is 47 to 53 years, cutting an average of 24 years of life. Cigarette smokers not only die about 10 years sooner, but they are biologically older and less healthy throughout their lives while they smoke.

There are several methods for assessing biological age, as compared to chronological age. These methods are used in studies to better understand the impact of lifestyle on aging and disease, and are predictive of healthspan, lifespan, and absence of disability. These methods include:

- Phenotypic age: Based on aspects such as wrinkles, muscle mass, and posture. Both people and artificial intelligence, when trained, can give reliable estimates of biological age.
- Fragility: A measurement of physical function and strength among the elderly
- Homeostatic dysregulation: Assesses the body's ability to regulate blood sugar, temperature, sympathetic activity, balance, etc. With aging, there is a weakening of synaptic feedback control, so that there is a loss of dampening after overstimulation.[1]
- Metabolic blood tests: The Klemera-Doubal Method and similar metrics use the results of routine blood tests to predict metabolic age.
- Telomere length: At the end of each chromosome, there is a section called a telomere that is often compared to the aglet at the end of a shoelace that allows the lace to be easily threaded through a small hole, and which keeps the lace from unraveling. Every time a cell divides, the chromosomes need to be replicated, and a small piece of the telomere is consumed in the process. This limits the number of times a cell can divide, which limits lifespan, but also helps prevent aberrant cells from developing into cancers. Examining the telomere length in white blood cells gives an estimate of biological age. The body has some capacity to repair and extend the telomere, and thus can increase the number of times a cell line can replicate.
- DNA methylation age: Likely mostly as a result of random exposure, dirty little specks of carbon (methyl groups) attach to the DNA; this makes the DNA stick to the histone protein more tightly. DNA methylation accumulates with age and exposure to stressors. For example, exposure to tobacco smoke increases DNA methylation.[2] DNA methylation causes the affected gene to become more resistant to transcription, and thus, the protein that the gene codes for will have diminished expression. For many genes, methylation has a beneficial function, but for others, it is detrimental. Random methylation is generally unhelpful and leads to a loss of adaptive gene expression.

Several studies have shown that biological age metrics can be impacted by lifestyle changes. We can lie about our calendar age, but can't change it. It does little good to lie about our biological age; however, it can be changed. Unfortunately, it is easier to change it in the wrong direction. For example, smokers in their 30s typically have a metabolic age similar to non-smokers in their mid-40s.[3] Quitting smoking can reduce phenotypic skin age by 13 years.[4] Women who are survivors of breast cancer were found to have telomere lengths equivalent to those of non-affected women who were 21 years older.[5] Just the stress of the diagnosis is traumatizing; the surgery, chemotherapy, and radiation each take their toll.

Biological age can also respond to improvements in lifestyle and outlook. In a 5-year follow-up study of older men with low-risk prostate cancer, those who participated in a 3-month comprehensive lifestyle change program had their telomeres shorten by less than one-fourth as much as did those of men with the same diagnosis who were non-participants in the intervention. Adherence to the lifestyle protocol did not explain the beneficial effect.[6] These men had a fifteen-month reprieve from aging over 5 years, apparently from gaining a sense of agency and hope provided by the 12-week intervention soon after their diagnosis.

Just eight weeks of diet and lifestyle intervention was demonstrated to lower the Horvath DNAmAge clock (DNA methylation age) by an average of 1.96 years.[7] Lifestyle factors that are associated with lower markers of biologic age to chronologic age (BA: CA) include a healthy diet, leisure time physical activity, adequate sleep, not smoking, and avoiding heavy alcohol consumption.[8] Physical activity and social engagement prevent frailty and frailty-associated adverse events (hospitalization, moving into a nursing home, or worse).[9]

The same lifestyle factors that are associated with younger biological/chronologic age are also associated with lower levels of neuroinflammation and lower risk of neurodegenerative disease and psychiatric disorders. Alzheimer's disease (AD), Parkinson's disease (PD), multiple sclerosis, amyotrophic lateral sclerosis (ALS), schizophrenia, bipolar disorder, and depression are all neuroinflammatory conditions.

Hormesis

Hormesis is an adaptive mechanism by which the body adapts to the exposure of a harmful agent by increasing its defenses against the offensive compound. The body has several of these defensive pathways. An example of a highly important hormetic adaptive mechanism is the NRF2 pathway. NRF2 is a small protein that stays parked in the cytosol of the cell and does absolutely nothing there. But when the cells sense oxidative stress, the NRF2 is released and makes its way into the nucleus of the cell where it acts as a transcription factor that promotes the expression of numerous cytoprotective proteins that protect the cell from oxidative stress and help to detoxify the offensive compounds and transport them out of the cell and out of the body.

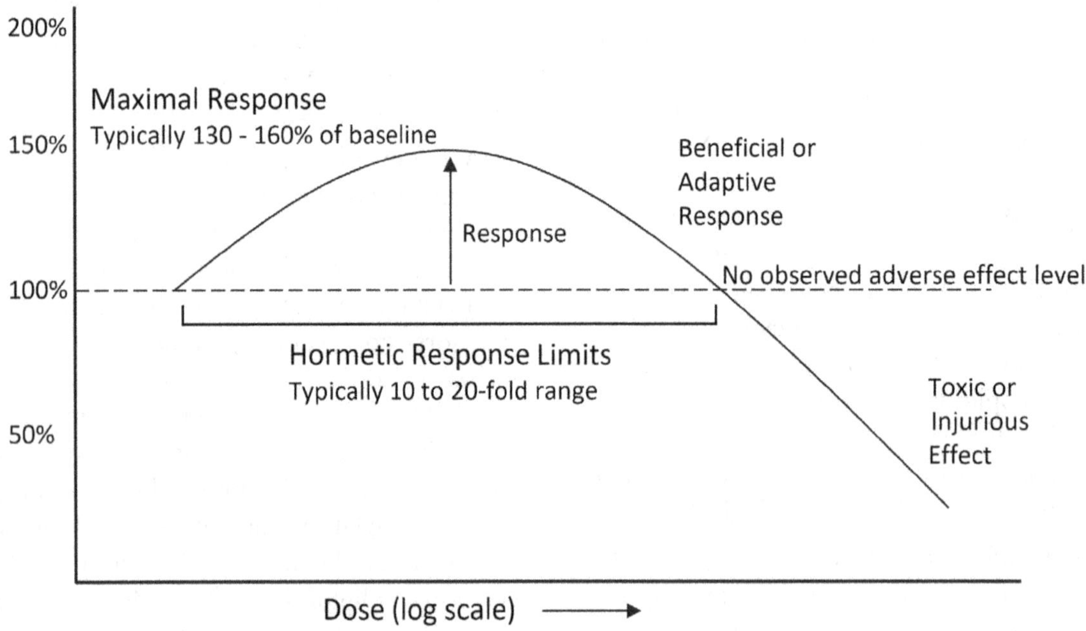

Figure 19A: Diagram illustrating a typical hormetic response. (Image adapted from Calabrese[10])

There is a minimum level of exposure required for a hormetic adaptive response and as well, an upper beneficial level, beyond which the stressor causes injury. The peak adaptive response is generally 130 to 160 percent of the baseline response, but may be as high as 200%. Thus, the expression and activity of certain antioxidant enzymes, for example, may increase 30% to 100% after exposure to certain hormetic agents.

Typically, the maximum dose above the no-observed-adverse-effect level (NOAEL) (horizontal axis) is about 10 to 20 times that of the minimal above-NOAEL dose; this is the no adverse effect range. In contrast, most pharmaceuticals have a much narrower effective dose range. The useful, beneficial hormetic response range, however, is generally narrower, closer to a 5-fold range. Since biologic dose-response is generally logarithmic, the peak response is usually at the geometric mean of the minimum and maximum effective doses.

As illustrated in Figure 19A, hormetic agents are generally active at low doses but have a fairly wide beneficial dose range. Nevertheless, higher doses don't provide more benefits but may rather cause inflammation and injury.

Many dietary hormetic agents are para-hormetic without actually having significant toxicity. Parahormetic means that the adaptive response occurs as if there were a low dose of toxins, even though they have little, if any, toxicity effect, even at several times the hormetic dose. That is, they may, for example, trigger NRF2 release, without actually having significant toxicity to the cell. Many phenolic compounds in fruits and vegetables are parahormetic. The limited hormetic dose range, however, remains. Adding two parahormetic compounds together that act on the same pathway should not be expected to give a greater response, but may move the exposure beyond the ideal response range.

The parahormetic effect is in stark contrast to very low exposure doses of acrolein in food acting as a hormetic agent, and higher doses, which are clearly toxic. X-ray radiation and even arsenic can have hormetic effects at *very low* exposure levels, but don't try them; they are injurious at higher doses. There are many safe hormetic agents found in a healthy diet and lifestyle.

As an example, sulforaphane (SFN), derived from cruciferous vegetables such as broccoli and cauliflower, and allicin in garlic, activate NRF2. Low-dose alcohol can act as a hormetic agent by a different mechanism. Alcohol likely has its beneficial hormetic impact by upregulating the expression of ALDH, an enzyme needed for one step in the metabolism of alcohol, but ALDH also helps metabolize other aldehydes, including those that form advanced glycation end-products (AGEs). Details are discussed in the chapter on alcoholic beverages. Coffee, green tea, and some herbal teas have hormetic effects. While polyphenolic compounds are widely recognized for their antioxidant effects, their principal benefits are mediated as hormetic (stress-inducing) effects. Plants do not make these phenolic and sulfurous compounds for our benefit; they are generated to protect the plant from microbes and insects that would harm them. They often have a bitter taste and may be antimicrobial, anti-nutritional, or even toxic to insects and small animals.

Different compounds promote the upregulation of different pathways; some act on multiple pathways. Exercise benefits health, and the mechanism for this includes the hormetic effects caused by stress and muscle hypoxia during aerobic exercise. It is important to understand that just like other hormetic and adaptive responses, excessive exercise is injurious rather than beneficial. As will be discussed in Chapter 29, vigorous exercise three to four times a week lowers heart disease risk; vigorous exercise seven days a week carries about the same risk as never exercising.

When it comes to hormetic effects, clearly, more is not better. Once the required dose for the maximal response for a given pathway has been met, adding more will not provide a greater hormetic response. Doubling a dose is generally not a problem for most hormetic pathways, but going further than that may diminish effectiveness. Adding more hormetic agents that act on the same pathway is not helpful. For example, if two toxic compounds act as hormetic agents on the same pathway, adding them together will not give an additive effect, but may rather push the stress effect beyond the hormetic level if both are close to the upper dose.

Combinations of hormetic agents may additionally activate, or additively exceed the hormetic window if they act on the same stress response system. Combinations of hormetic agents may give synergistic impacts if they act on different pathways.

The duration of the hormetic effect, and thus the optimal frequency of "dosing interval" in humans, has received a surprising lack of investigation. (I will try to provide some guidance in the following chapters.)

Polyphenolic compounds also interact with the intestinal microbiome; GI bacteria process them, can derive energy from them, and often make polyphenolic compounds more bioavailable. Other polyphenolic compounds have unfavorable antibiotic effects on GI bacteria. The primary effects of phenolic compounds and other hormetic agents on health are not from their impact on the microbiome nor as a nutrient. Therefore, while a food may have a DAD score, the DAD rating does not describe the food's hormetic impact. Thus, coffee (caffeinated) gets a DAD score close to neutral, but can have an excellent "Hormetic Adaptive Response" (HAR) rating. The HAR rating goes from 1 to 10, with 10 being a strong and broad hormetic response.

Many dietary and lifestyle factors induce hormesis. Some of these include:

- Certain Beverages: Coffee, green tea, some herbal tisanes
- Some Vegetables: Broccoli, cauliflower, garlic
- Many Fruits: Phenolic compounds in berries, citrus, and certain other fruits
- Other foods: Phenolic compounds in black beans, some herbs and spices, capers, and chocolate
- Alcohol (in small amounts)
- Exercise

There is not a single, but rather there are multiple, often overlapping hormetic–adaptive pathways. These include:

Hormetic and Adaptive Pathways

- NRF2 Pathway (Oxidative Stress and Antioxidant Defense)
- Aldehyde Dehydrogenase Pathway
- Telomerase Activity
- AMPK Activation and Autophagy
- HMOX1 Pathway
- Sirtuin Pathway
- MAPK Pathway
- Brain-Derived Neurotrophic Factor (BDNF) Pathway
- PGC1α Activation
- DNA Repair Pathways

There are also many anti-adaptive or maladaptive mechanisms, several of which have been discussed in previous chapters. Lifestyle risk factors for neuroinflammation and inflammaging include childhood trauma and distress, environmental toxins (heavy metals, pollution, pesticides, and smoking), sleep deprivation, dysbiosis, and a pro-inflammatory diet.[11] Social isolation is both a cause and a result of neuroinflammation. Exposure to air pollution is associated with an increased risk of fetal neurologic injury and dementia.

Anti-Adaptive or Maladaptive Mechanisms

- Insulin Resistance
  - A high-fat diet
  - Sugar-sweetened beverages
  - High glycemic index diet
  - Sedentary lifestyle
- Enteric Dysbiosis, Leaky-gut
  - Mammalian Flesh
  - Animal Skin
  - Vegetable skin
  - Non-digestible emulsifiers
- Aberrant DNA Methylation
  - Environmental toxins
    - Lead, mercury, pesticides, and bisphenol A (BPA)
  - Aging and disease
    - Obesity and T2D[12]
- Oral dysbiosis– periodontitis, caries
  - Sugary beverages and foods
  - Poor dental hygiene
  - Tobacco use
- Malnutrition
  - Nutrient deficiencies
  - Unbalanced diet
  - Anti-nutritional and toxic compounds
  - Non-nutritional "food" ("empty calories")
  - High-fat diet
  - Sugar-sweetened beverages
  - Lack of soluble fiber
- Exposure to toxins
  - Tobacco
  - Excess alcohol
  - Environmental toxins
    - Pesticides
    - Mycotoxins
    - Toxic metals (arsenic, mercury, lead, cadmium, etc.)
    - Air pollution*

---

* The impact of air pollution is discussed in Chapter 32.

- Sleep Deprivation
- Deadly sins
  - Pride
  - Wrath
  - Gluttony
  - Sloth
  - Tribalism
- Emotional or psychological stress
  - Toxic relationships
  - Trauma (emotional or physical)
  - Isolation and loneliness
  - Toxic news media
  - Exposure to violence and ugliness; (i.e.; TV)
- Addictions
  - Substance abuse
  - Electronic Media stimulus
- Deficiency of:
  - Love
  - Friendship
  - Play
  - Intimacy
  - Recreation (re-creation)
  - Cognitive stimulation
  - Nature, quiet, calm, and darkness and quiet at night

NOTE: *The remainder of this chapter explores the mechanism of action of hormetic agents. It gets pretty nerdy. It is not required reading, but it may be fun for those into this stuff.*

Hormetic Pathways

Nuclear factor erythroid 2-related factor 2 (NRF2, officially NFE2L2) is a transcription factor for a group of proteins that protect the cell from oxidative and metabolic stress. As a group, these are sometimes referred to as the Antioxidant Response Element (ARE). NRF2 increases glutathione metabolism both as an antioxidant mechanism and for cellular detoxification; it increases resistance to ferroptosis, a cell death mechanism; and helps export xenobiotic compounds such as drugs and toxins from the cell.

Either NRF2 or NF-κB may be activated, or neither may be, but rarely both are, as they inhibit each other. AP-1 activation can occur with either NF-κB or NRF2. AP-1 activation with NF-κB promotes cell proliferation, which is good when it rapidly promotes the development of white blood cells for fighting an infection, but a drag when it spurs the growth of cancer cells. When AP-1 is activated and NF-κB is inhibited, AP-1 is more likely to signal apoptosis.

Table 19A: Cellular Stress Responses

Low-Level Oxidative Stress	Moderate Oxidative Stress	High Oxidative Stress
NRF2 →Antiinflammatory Response Element	NF-κB → Inflammatory Response	Activator Protein-1 (AP-1)
Induction of antioxidant enzymes and increased conjugation and elimination of xenobiotics. Increases the expression of antioxidant enzymes and glutathione production. Prevents cancer by helping to eliminate potential mutagens from the body.	Inflammatory mediators can increase the risk of inflammation by inhibiting the ARE response and by increasing the production of ROS and RNS that can damage protein and DNA. It can induce apoptosis.	AP-1 can induce the transcription of Cyclin D1, promoting proliferation, angiogenesis, and tumor growth. Alternatively, AP-1 can signal cellular apoptosis depending on the upstream signaling and other intracellular factors.

Stress Response and Phenolic Compounds

Various food compounds induce NRF2 transcription. Some compounds in food, such as Diallyl sulfide (DAS) in garlic, both induce NRF2 and downregulate NF-κB.[13] In animal models of Alzheimer's disease (AD), DAS inhibited Aβ-induced neuronal death and increased the formation of dendritic spines and synapses in the hippocampus. By promoting antioxidant activity, DAS reverses scopolamine-induced cognitive impairment in rats.[14] Anthocyanins are plant pigments that give purple, blue, or red colors to plants depending on their pH. These pigments also induce NRF2 and downregulate NF-κB. Anthocyanins in purple sweet potatoes,[15] black currants,[16] blueberries, black beans, and blackberries increase NRF2 while inhibiting NF-κB.[17 18]

Ursolic acid and naringenin have been found to prevent hepatotoxicity and fibrosis caused by oxidative stress through the induction of NRF2 → ARE signaling.[19 20] Ursolic acid is present in basil, bilberries, cranberries, peppermint, rosemary, oregano, thyme, and prunes. Naringenin may additionally inhibit NF-κB. Naringenin is present in citrus fruit, especially tangerines. Some flavonoid compounds downregulate NF-κB without affecting NRF2. Dark roasted coffee, chocolate, broccoli, cauliflower, garlic, and berries containing anthocyanins increase NRF2 activation and may decrease NF-κB activation. Diets rich in flavonoid compounds decrease NF-κB activity.

In an assessment of the NHANES study data, including the follow-up of 14,029 participants, cancer mortality was inversely associated with dietary intake of flavonols. Of 29 dietary flavonoids assessed, three were associated with decreased risk of cancer mortality: peonidin (present in wine and berries), naringenin (from citrus), and catechin (from green tea).[21] While this association should not be assumed to represent causation, it does suggest that wine, berry, citrus, and tea consumption are associated with lower cancer risk.

NRF2 protects cells from mutations from DNA adducts and oxidative stress. The protein BRCA1 prevents cancer and helps protect cells from injury in part by inducing NRF2. Mice with deficient BRCA1, similar to those of individuals with BRCA1 mutations, have low levels of NRF2-induced antioxidant enzymes.[22]

Sulforaphane (SPH) and the phenolic compound resveratrol induce NRF2 transcriptional activity, reduce reactive oxygen species (ROS) levels, and reduce DNA damage from benzo[a]pyrene in BRCA1-deficient animals.[23] BRCA1 is a tumor suppressor that helps repair double-stranded breaks in the DNA, and if the DNA cannot be repaired, it promotes the apoptosis of the cell. Thus, one of the reasons that BRCA1 mutations induce cancer is that they impair NRF2 reactivity to oxidative stress and genotoxins. Although they may not restore this activity to normal levels, food compounds that increase NRF2 activity in normal individuals also do so for those with BRCA1 mutations; thus, for aberrant BRCA1 carriers, they provide an even more needed salutary effect for cancer prevention.

Agents that augment NRF2 and inhibit NF-κB not only help prevent oxidative injury and DNA damage, but they can also promote apoptosis of injured and aberrant cells. As examples, dark roasted coffee, chocolate, cruciferous vegetables containing sulforaphane, allium vegetables, and berries and vegetables containing anthocyanins increase NRF2 activation and may decrease NF-κB activation. Diets rich in flavonoid compounds decrease NF-κB activity.

Table 19B: Some of the Many Antioxidant-Response Element (ARE) Proteins[24 25]

ARE Genes	Functions
GCL and GCLM	Glutamate Cysteine Ligase and the glutamate-cysteine ligase regulatory subunit are enzymes that work together on the rate-limiting step in the synthesis of glutathione, the body's most important antioxidant system.
SOD1	Superoxide dismutase converts oxygen radicals into normal O2 and hydrogen peroxide that can then be reduced by glutathione.
TXNRD1 and SRXN1	Thioredoxin and sulfiredoxin reductase repair oxidized disulfide bonds
NQO1	NAD(P)H dehydrogenase (quinone 1) detoxifies reactive quinones that cause oxidative stress and redox cycling.
GST	Glutathione S-transferases create antioxidant conjugates with toxins so that they can be removed from the body, generally into the urine. They also mediate the elimination of many reactive oxygen species.
GR	Glutathione reductase mediates the reduction (recycling) of glutathione.
CAT	Catalase mediates the elimination of reactive oxygen species along with GST and SOD1.
UGT	UDP-glucuronosyltransferase catalyzes glucuronic acid conjugates, to help transport toxins into the bile or urine for elimination from the body.
HMOX1	Heme oxygenase breaks down heme from hemoglobin and produces a molecule of carbon monoxide that acts as an anti-inflammatory signal. HMOX1 is thought to protect the organs from damage from oxidative stress during injury and sepsis. Note, however, that excessive levels of HMOX1 can induce cell death as a protective mechanism against diseased cells.
ABCC2	This ABC protein binds and transports negatively charged metabolic waste across cell membranes into the renal tubule or bile canaliculi for disposal.

Aldehyde Dehydrogenase Pathway

During alcohol metabolism, the toxic compound acetaldehyde is formed. Aldehyde dehydrogenases (ALDHs) are enzymes that break down acetaldehyde, reducing its toxicity. ALDH2 is localized in the mitochondria, while ALDH1 is in the cytosol, especially in the liver.

The consumption of small amounts of alcohol has a hormetic effect as it induces the expression of ALDH, and particularly ALDH2, which helps protect cells from oxidative stress and inflammation caused by AGEs such as methylglyoxal (MGO), which is created in the body as a result of hyperglycemia, and 4-hydroxy-2-nonenal (4-HNE), which is generated from peroxidized fatty acids. ALDH can metabolize these aldehydes before they cause DNA adducts, which can lead to mutations and protein adducts, which can cause protein misfolding or dysfunction, and which can cause cellular inflammation and injury. Methylglyoxal, for example, is converted by ALDH into pyruvate, which can then be used in the generation of ATP.

Many individuals of Asian genetic heritage have a deficiency of ALDH2 activity, and this is associated with an increased risk of late-onset AD.[26] Lab animals bred to overexpress ALDH2 have been found to have a delayed onset of cognitive impairment. Alcohol consumption in small amounts increases ALDH2 expression and protects the brain from 4-HNE and other aldehydes; nevertheless, higher levels of alcohol consumption increase damage to the brain.[27] (Chapter 22)

Telomere Lengthening

Telomere lengthening is one of the ways that the body can adapt to stay in the realm of the living. Each time our cells divide, the leading end of the DNA strand, the telomere, gets a bit shorter; thus, our cells have a limited number of times they can divide. Nevertheless, there is a telomere repair mechanism that can add to the length of the telomere, and thus increase the number of times the cell can divide. In general, however, our telomeres get shorter with age.

In a meta-analysis including 20 studies of the impact of lifestyle interventions on white blood cell telomere length (TL), participants getting physical activity and dietary interventions had increased TLs, while those in the control group had shorter telomeres at the end of the interventions.[28]

Another meta-analysis looked specifically at exercise; aerobic exercise was associated with greater TL, while no change was seen for combined training or resistance exercise. The positive changes in TL from exercise were not observed in short-term trials but were clear in those lasting at least 6 months.[29] Moderate to vigorous intensity aerobic training appears to help preserve TL.[30] These are lifestyle changes, not a quick intervention for a photo opportunity.

In a Spanish study of over 400 people at high risk of cardiovascular disease, a greater adherence to a Mediterranean diet was associated with having a lower risk of shortened white blood cell telomeres. Seventeen dietary groups were assessed for their impact on telomere length. The dietary factors that were significantly associated with a greater telomere length (TL) in this study were: 1) daily servings of fruit or fruit juice, 2) vegetables, pasta, rice, or other dishes seasoned with sofrito (garlic and onions based seasoning, usually with tomatoes), 3) servings of whole grains, and for women, 4) servings of seafood, 5) and *fewer servings of refined grain products* including bread, rice and pasta. Aspects of the Mediterranean diet that were not significantly associated with TL were olive oil, vegetables, red meat, butter/margarine, pastries, nuts, white meat, sugar, white bread, and wine.[31]

One cannot conclude that these items do not affect health; however, they do not appear to impact TL. Cooking with sofrito may extend TL; however, sofrito may serve as a proxy for a more traditional dietary pattern and lifestyle. It is likely associated with cooking meals at home, and may be associated with sitting down for meals as a family, and perhaps a less busy lifestyle.

Living in a neighborhood with green space is associated with longer telomeres in both children and adults. In a study using data from a cross-section of 7827 American adults, living in an area with green space (trees, parks) was associated with greater TL; after adjusting for other factors, the green space effect reduced the biological age by 2.2 to 2.6 years. Green space in neighborhoods is associated with many variables, including safe outdoor space to walk, play, relax, do yard work, less noise and nighttime light pollution; better sleep, lower crime, and less exposure to air pollution (however, air pollution was not a significant factor in this study).[32 33]

Persistent or repeated stress can accelerate telomere shortening.

Many healthy lifestyle activities promote a beneficial impact on the length of telomeres.

Factors that can increase telomere length include:

- A healthful diet.
- Adequate vitamin D levels are associated with longer telomeres. Sun exposure and vitamin D-fortified foods can help.
- Physical activity with regular aerobic exercise
- Lesser amounts of emotional distress
- Positive social engagement with family and friends
- Adequate, regular quality sleep
- Living in an area with green space
- Not smoking, limiting alcohol consumption, avoiding red meat, and avoiding environmental toxins.

Activation of AMPK

Another mechanism that improves health and longevity is the activation of AMPK. AMPK (adenosine monophosphate-activated protein kinase) is a master regulator of the metabolic budget. AMPK acts as an auditor that helps decide whether cells will grow and open a new franchise or hold a fire sale and get rid of some non-essential assets. AMPK is activated in response to low energy levels and acts to promote cellular repair while inhibiting cell division. Activation of AMPK promotes autophagy, a mechanism that has the beneficial side effect of protecting cells from oxidative stress and inflammation. Activation of AMPK also appears to promote immune clearance of senescent cells that accumulate with aging. Senescent cells are old, worn-out cells that secrete inflammatory cytokines that inhibit the development of new cells. They maintain local inflammation and thus promote dysfunction.[34]

AMPK senses the energy status of the cell by the ratio of adenosine monophosphate (AMP) to adenosine tri-phosphate (ATP). When a high-energy phosphate bond in ATP has been used to fuel cell activity, ATP is converted to adenosine diphosphate (ADP) and then, if further depleted, to AMP. AMPK (AMP-activated protein kinase) senses this low energy status by the AMP: ATP ratio; when the ratio is high, it activates cellular processes for energy conservation and production.

When energy levels in the cell are low, AMPK conserves energy by constraining mTOR when energy switches to the use of catabolic processes to generate ATP, and turns off ATP-consuming pathways such as non-essential protein synthesis and cell proliferation. AMPK activation prevents the synthesis of fatty acids and cholesterol, which are needed for the creation of new cell and organelle membranes. It stimulates lipolysis and proteolysis and the uptake of glucose by the cell to generate ATP. This process promotes autophagy and mitophagy, and thus the elimination of old, worn-out proteins, organelles, and mitochondria. Later, when sufficient ATP is restored, new proteins, organelles, and mitochondria will be made. This recycling refreshes the cell.

Muscle activity is one of the main stimulators of AMPK activity. During exercise, ATP is converted to ADP. ADP is not used as an energy source directly, but instead, one phosphate group from ADP can be transferred to ATP, resulting in one ATP molecule and one AMP molecule. The newly formed ATP can then be used for energy.

$$ADP + ADP \rightarrow ATP + AMP$$

which can be written as

$$A2P + A2P \rightarrow A3P + A1P)$$

The effect of exercise may only occur, however, when ATP availability to the muscle is sufficiently depleted that it raises the AMP: ATP ratio to the point that AMPK is stimulated. When an individual is adapted to a moderate exercise routine, this depletion may not occur at moderate exercise workloads. Thus, a variation in exercise routine on different days or vigorous exercise helps maintain the efficacy of exercise in depleting ATP and raising AMP levels.

AMPK is activated about 100-fold by the tumor suppressor protein LKB1 and CaMKKβ in the presence of sufficient AMP. ADP also increases AMPK activity, but only by about 10 times, while AMP increases it by 100 times. While LKB1 is universally present, CaMKKβ can phosphorylate Thr-172 in some cells. This is particularly important in neurons, T lymphocytes, and endothelial cells.[35] AMP can also bind at a second site on the AMPK protein complex, giving a greater than 1000-fold increase in activity of AMPK. Meanwhile, ATP inhibits AMPK activity. The concurrent stimulus of LKB1 and CaMKKβ gives additive AMPK activation.

Downstream from AMPK is mTOR. mTOR regulates protein synthesis and cell division, and is inhibited by p-AMPK (phosphorylated-AMPK), but permitted when AMPK is not activated. Growth depends on having an adequate supply of ATP for energy, amino acids for building new proteins, and lipids for building membranes, and AMPK and mTORC1 act to make sure there are sufficient materials and energy to build new cells both in health and in cancer. Upstream of mTORC1, AMPK determines whether there is a sufficient cellular supply of ATP, lipids, and amino acids for current operations and growth. If supplies are insufficient, p-AMPK prevents growth by inhibiting mTOR activation and promoting autophagy. Autophagy recycles proteins and organelles within the cells to maintain critical operations. P-AMPK causes the cell to recycle lipids from organelle membranes and burn them as fuel. It is like clearing out old food from the freezer and pantry, and having a garage sale to help pay for rent, utilities, and groceries during hard times. For immortal cells such as the neurons, AMPK activation promotes renovation, repairing, or replacing worn out leaking windows, doors, and appliances with new, more energy-efficient ones.

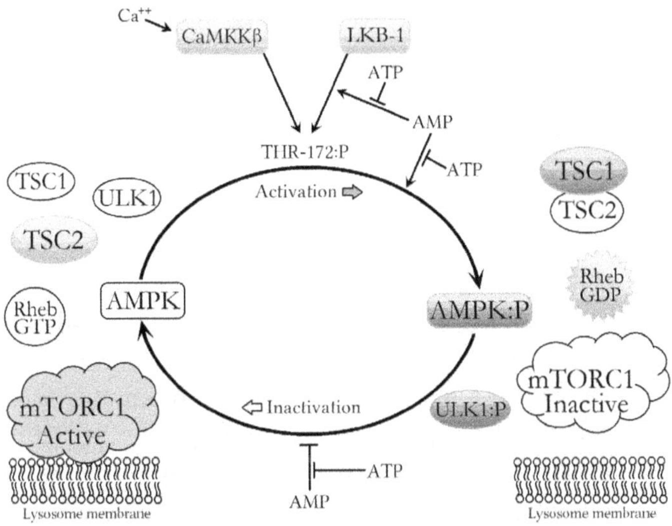

Figure 19B: AMPK activation and deactivation

Autophagy describes the degradation of older components of the cell. Mitophagy is the selective elimination of old, feeble, and poorly functioning mitochondria. Old geezer mitochondria tend to make and leak free radicals, reactive oxygen species (ROS), and reactive nitrogen species (RNS), which damage intracellular proteins and lipids, and can cause DNA damage. Mitophagy allows the culling of weak mitochondria and the reproduction of strong, healthy ones. Autophagy is mediated by the phosphorylation of ULK1. P-AMPK is thought to activate or promote the expression of SIRT1, which promotes PCG-1α expression, which promotes the generation of new mitochondria.

Spermidine is a polyamine present in many foods (green peas, cheddar cheese, some fruits) that promotes autophagy by tagging proteins for recycling and by inhibiting the mTOR pathway.

The mTOR1 complex determines the external support for the growth of the cell through signaling from growth factors and the systemic availability of glucose through sensing of insulin and the availability of amino acids needed for protein construction. The availability of SAMe and leucine (Chapter 13) participates in this. Inflammation creates intracellular signals that overlap with those triggered by external growth factors, and thus, inflammation can support cell survival and impede apoptosis. Inflammation can thus promote cancer cell growth.

AMPK Activators

Various compounds and hormones can activate AMPK:

Mitochondrial inhibitors

These inhibit mitochondrial production of ATP, thus giving the cell less ATP and more AMP and ADP. These inhibitors may act at different steps in ATP production. The anti-diabetic medication metformin inhibits mitochondrial electron chain Complex 1 activity, also decreasing ATP production. Metformin is a medication used to treat diabetes, but also used as an anti-aging drug as a result of its impact on AMK.

Several phenolic compounds have been demonstrated to activate AMPK. These mostly act indirectly, and often through multiple mechanisms. Resveratrol and quercetin inhibit mitochondrial ATP synthase and thus activate AMPK through the formation of ROS by inhibiting mitochondrial function.[36] This can induce mitophagy. These compounds also inhibit the activation of NF-κB, Akt, and ERK. Some of those documented to activate AMPK are listed in Table 19C.

Table 19C: Modifiable AMPK Activity Factors

	Promote AMPK Activity	Impede AMPK Activity
Leptin	Decrease Leptin Levels: Fasting (24 - 72 hours) Exercise training[37]	Increase Leptin Levels: Sleep Deprivation, Sleep Apnea Obesity and Insulin High-fructose, high-fat diet Psychological stress[38] Estrogen
Adiponectin	Increase Adiponectin Levels Exercise training N-3 fatty acids: EPA and DHA Berberine, Curcumin, Capsaicin, Gingerol, Catechins	Decrease Adiponectin Levels The combination of obesity with sleep apnea or sleep hypoxia.[39] Uric acid (when elevated, such as with high-fructose diets)

Fat Cell Hormones:

The satiety hormone leptin is produced by fat cells when they have had plenty to eat. They signal the brain to let it know they feel full, and it's time to stop eating. *Leptin impedes AMPK* activity in most tissues. It may do this by stimulating fatty acid oxidation as an energy source for the cell, thus increasing the supply of ATP.[40] Leptin resistance, a condition associated with obesity, is associated with high leptin levels.

Ghrelin is a hunger hormone that does the opposite; it is produced by the stomach when it is empty and tells the brain that the stomach can handle another meal. Ghrelin does not encourage us to eat more, just more frequently. Although ghrelin does not directly regulate hunger, it increases food intake. Ghrelin activates AMPK.[41]

Adiponectin, like leptin, is secreted by the fat cells. Adiponectin, however, is secreted by the adipocytes when they get hungry, as occurs during caloric restriction. Adiponectin activates AMPK. Adiponectin decreases the utilization of amino acids and favors the use of lipids for energy. It also increases the uptake of triglycerides and glucose into the cell. Adiponectin also has an anti-inflammatory effect, as it suppresses AKT and ERK → NF-κB signaling.[42] Adiponectin has been found to suppress cancer cell growth or induce apoptosis in several cancer cell lines.[43]

Reduction in sleep time, and especially limitations of deep sleep (slow-wave sleep, SWS) time, increases insulin resistance and risk of diabetes, and thus risk of neurodegeneration. Lack of SWS may occur during sleep apnea, in patients in pain, or in those who are stressed and have frequent nighttime arousals.

One reason that sleep insufficiency promotes obesity is its effects on appetite hormones. Sleep restriction increases leptin production and decreases ghrelin levels, both of which increase feeding. Sleep deprivation may also favor the selection of high-caloric, palatable foods.[44]

Patients with sleep apnea have been found to have leptin levels twice as high as control subjects.[45] The combination of sleep deficits and obesity causes low adiponectin levels. Successful treatment of sleep apnea helps normalize both adiponectin and leptin levels. Exercise training, especially vigorous exercise, lowers leptin levels, decreases insulin resistance, and increases adiponectin levels. This effect is especially pronounced in overweight and obese persons and those with high levels of inflammatory markers.[46]

Melatonin can decrease leptin levels.[47] Normally, melatonin lowers appetite during the night and lowers leptin levels. In contrast, however, if insulin levels are elevated, melatonin increases insulin's effect on leptin resistance and raises leptin levels. This effect is amplified by high levels of corticosteroids. Light exposure in the evening or during the night that disrupts melatonin production increases leptin. Circadian disruption likely increases leptin levels. [48] Most of the body's melatonin is made in the gut, where it slows digestion during sleep.

Since insulin raises leptin levels at night, it is recommended that late evening meals, sweet desserts, and bedtime snacks, which raise blood sugar and maintain high insulin output during the sleep period, be avoided, especially for those with insulin resistance. Excessive fructose (more than required for current energy needs) increases leptin production, most likely through its promotion of obesity and insulin resistance.[49]

Individuals who have higher leptin levels are more likely to skip breakfast,[50] a habit that is associated with increased all-cause mortality. Thus, those who don't have an appetite in the morning or are often able to go until lunchtime without feeling hungry may be eating too much too late in the day, causing increased nighttime leptin and decreased adiponectin, and raising the risk of cancer, diabetes, heart disease, and dementia. (This is discussed in Chapter 28).

A high-fat, high-fructose diet can cause leptin resistance within a few weeks. It can also be reversed within a few weeks by a diet containing a limited and healthful fat content and limited fructose content. Fructose is not inherently unhealthy. Fructose consumed in whole fruit, when eaten when feeling hungry, is slowly absorbed and much more likely to be utilized for energy than be stored as fat. Eating whole fruit decreases the risk of type 2 diabetes. Fructose in sweet beverages is a problem.

Direct AMPK Activators

AMPK is activated by a change in the protein's conformation when it is phosphorylated at the threonine situated at the 127th amino acid (THR-127) in the AMPK molecule. Two proteins do this: STK-11 and CaMKKβ, as shown in Figure 19B.

STK11 (also commonly called LKB1 in the medical literature) suppresses cell growth and proliferation when nutrient and energy resources are scarce. STK11 phosphorylates AMPK when there is a low ATP to AMP ratio in the cell. STK11 is known as a tumor suppressor protein, as the activation of AMPK inhibits the growth of tumors. STK11 phosphorylates "THR-127", activating AMPK, forming p-AMPK. Metformin's partial inhibition of ATP production promotes STK11 phosphorylation. STK11 production is inhibited by androgens, so androgens such as testosterone can act as growth promoters.

Myoinositol, present in the diet or as a supplement, increases intracellular phosphatidyl-inositol, which serves as the phosphate donor for LKB1 phosphorylation, which then activates AMPK. Furthermore, myoinositol supplementation has been demonstrated to increase the expression of AMPK mRNA.[51] Myoinositol increases insulin sensitivity by activating AMPK, which increases the expression of GLUT4, increasing glucose uptake by the cells.

Certain compounds directly activate AMPK. Two agents that have been reported to have this activity are salicylic acid and gallic acid. Aspirin is rapidly converted into salicylate in the body. Gallic acid is found in many fruits, black tea, and other plants and vegetables.

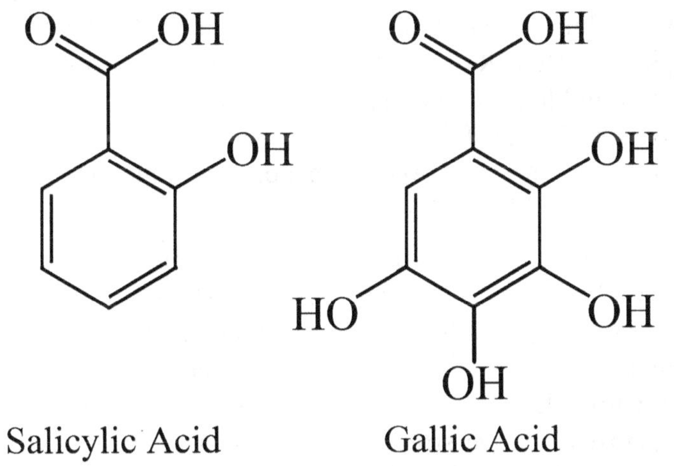

Salicylic Acid   Gallic Acid

Figure 19C: Two of the hydroxybenzoic acids that activate AMPK

Gallic and salicylic acids are hydroxybenzoic acids, a class of phenolic compounds. At least 27 hydroxybenzoic acids have been identified in various foods, and some of these may also activate AMPK. The hydroxybenzoic acids (HBA), such as salicylic acid, are phenolic compounds that appear to act directly or through activation of STK11. Epigallocatechin gallate (EGCG) from green tea breaks down into gallic acid and epigallocatechin, activating LKB1, thereby activating AMPK.[52] Salicylate, from willow bark, activates AMPK [53] after it is metabolized into 4-hydroxybenzoic acid.

Metformin and salicylates activate AMPK by different mechanisms. When used together, they activate AMPK synergistically.[54, 55] This means that a greater AMPK activation occurs than would be expected as an additive effect of the two agents. Thus, combining low doses of agents that stimulate AMPK activity at different points in its activation may allow a stronger effect with less risk of toxicity. Caffeine and myoinositol, both present in foods, also activate AMPK.

The CaMKKβ protein is a separate, AMP: ATP-independent AMPK activation pathway that, like STK11, adds a phosphate group to the "THR-127" segment of AMPK, thus also activating it. CaMKKβ is activated by an elevation in intracellular calcium. Typically, this occurs as the result of an influx through calcium channels. Different cell types have different calcium channel membrane proteins and thus, can respond according to the needs of the cell and its functions. The activation of CaMKKβ requires the protein calmodulin and magnesium.

Several compounds have been demonstrated to activate AMPK via CaMKKβ. These include baicalin (a Chinese herbal medication), the flavone luteolin,[56] lipoic acid,[57] S-allyl cysteine (from garlic),[58] and the thyroid hormone T3 (triiodothyronine).[59] T3 output may be impeded by sleep deprivation. Calcium is required for, and magnesium assists in, CaMKKβ enzymatic activity. CB2 agonists also stimulate CaMKKβ. Certain cannabinoids, such as cannabidiol, have been shown to have anticarcinogenic properties and may partially act through this mechanism.[60]

Lipoic acid is a nutritional supplement. Only the R-isomer is naturally present in nature; the L-isomer appears to partially inhibit the activity of lipoic acid. Thus, only R-lipoic acid (sodium stabilized) is recommended. A dose of 50 to 100 mg appears to be as effective as 600 mg of alpha-lipoic acid. Lipoic acid is an antioxidant.

Table 19D: Compounds that Activate CaMKKβ

CaMKKβ Activators	Foods Containing High Levels of CaMKKβ Activators
Luteolin	Globe artichokes, oregano, thyme, sage, black olives
S-allyl cysteine	Garlic
R-lipoic acid	Small amounts are present in many foods. Therapeutic doses are most easily available from supplements. Avoid the more easily found, racemic, alpha-lipoic acid. Use Sodium R-lipoic acid supplements. Typical therapeutic doses of R-lipoic acid range from 50 – 100 mg for adults.
Minerals	Calcium and magnesium are required for CaMKKβ activation.[61]

Table 19E: Phenolic compounds that activate AMPK

Phenolic Compound[62]	Food Sources
Epigallocatechin gallate[63]	Green tea, oolong tea, pecans, hazelnuts
Quercetin	Chocolate, capers, elderberries, orange juice, cloves, oregano, shallots, red onions,
Genistein	Soy products (tofu, tempeh, etc.)
Resveratrol	Muscadine grape wine, other red wine, cranberries, red currants, loganberries, strawberries
Punicalagin	Pomegranates. This is another hydroxybenzoic acid. [64]
Hispidulin	Oregano, sage, thyme, rosemary
Curcumin	Turmeric (found in curry powder)
Theaflavins	Tea (black, green)
4-hydroxybenzoic acid	Loquat, green olives, red wine, coconut, green tea. It may also be formed during the metabolism of catechins.
Gallic Acid	Very high levels: Chestnuts, chicory, walnuts, cloves, blackberries High levels: Oregano, black tea, red wine, sage, chicory,
Catechin	Chocolate, red wine, drupes (peaches, plums, prunes, apricots, cherries), black grapes, strawberries, broad beans, red beans, pecans.
Capsaicin	Chili peppers
Gingerol	Raw ginger root. Dried ginger.
Nootkatone[65]	Nootkatone, found in grapefruit, activates AMPK.
Berberine	A yellow pigment found in several plants, including goldenseal. Berberine-rich plants are used in traditional Chinese medicine. It is present in barberry but otherwise uncommon in foods. It is allergenic.

When amino acid levels in the cytosol of the cell fall, it triggers an elevation of intracellular calcium and CaMKKβ activation of AMPK. This activation causes the phosphorylation of ULK1 that initiates autophagy.[66] In this way, the cell acts to increase the availability of amino acids to maintain the production of essential proteins required for cell survival. CaMKKβ can activate AMPK even in the presence of ATP levels that inhibit STK-11 activation. Either a lack of energy in the form of ATP or a lack of the amino acids building materials for proteins, perhaps specifically a lack of methionine in the form of SAMe, can activate AMPK and shut down the cell growth cycle. This amino acid depletion occurs with fasting. (Fasting is discussed in Chapter 28).

Caloric restriction and short-term fasting can activate AMPK, promoting autophagy. Caloric restriction also promotes an increase in intracellular NAD+ (nicotinamide adenine dinucleotide) levels. NAD+ is a coenzyme for energy production (ATP) and is essential for cellular repair. Caloric restriction activates sirtuins, particularly SIRT1, SIRT3, and SIRT6, which promote the unfolded protein response (UPR) and autophagy of unfolded or misfolded proteins; promote DNA repair; and promote improved mitochondrial function, thus reducing oxidative stress.

The biogenic polyamine spermidine promotes autophagy and longevity as a caloric restriction mimetic. Spermidine promotes autophagy in animal models of the aging brain. It protects the brain by downregulating inflammatory cytokines, protecting against oxidative stress, and improving mitochondrial function.[67] Animal studies have shown that spermidine and spermine prevent inflammation and neuronal apoptosis, and increase the expression of BDNF, a neurotrophic factor, thus protecting the brain during aging. Spermidine and spermine likely act by phosphorylating AMPK.[68] Several foods are rich in spermidine, and others contain spermine and putrescine, which the body can use to make spermidine. These include wheat germ, soy products, aged cheddar cheese, mushrooms, brown rice, peas, mangos, legumes, pears, and cruciferous vegetables.

Mitochondrial Renewal 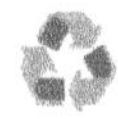

The mitochondria are the powerhouses of the cell, providing ATP as the basic fuel for building proteins, for ion exchange and compound transport, for enzymatic reactions, elimination of toxins, as well as thousands of other activities. The mitochondria live a stressful life and are exposed to high levels of energetic protons and oxidative agents. Think of them as being

like a car engine; they wear out with time. As they get older, they become inefficient and begin to leak free radicals and causing the formation of ROS and NOS.

A sedentary lifestyle allows the old, leaky, geezer mitochondria to hang around, causing cellular dysfunction and senescence. Caloric restriction, vigorous exercise, and certain compounds in food can promote mitochondrial renewal and the culling of poorly functioning mitochondria. Mitophagy is a special type of autophagy that can help recycle old mitochondria.

Following mitophagy, an increase in energy demand by the cell promotes mitochondrial biogenesis. Exercise promotes this. Additionally, SIRT1 activators stimulate mitochondrial biogenesis. AMPK activation also promotes mitophagy.

PGC-1α

Peroxisome proliferator-activated receptor γ coactivator-1α (PGC-1α) promotes mitochondrial renewal and is essential to brain health. PGC-1α promotes autophagy, including mitophagy, in microglia of the nervous system. It is essential for the proliferation and maturation of astrocytes and for the myelination of nerves by oligodendrocytes. PGC-1α is required for synaptogenesis in the developing brain and supports the generation and maintenance of synapses in postnatal life.

Vigorous exercise can promote PGC-1α in the muscles, and fasting increases levels in the heart and liver. Diabetes decreases PGC-1α activity in the muscles, which may contribute to insulin resistance.[69] PGC-1α is activated by phosphorylation of AMPK, as well as by deacetylation by sirtuin 1 (SIRT1).[70] ApoE-ε4 (APOE4), a major risk factor for Alzheimer's disease, hinders the biogenesis of mitochondria by decreasing PGC-1α production, and PGC-1α, in turn, controls SIRT3 production.[71]

Exercise

During intense exercise, adrenaline shifts blood flow from the intestines and kidneys to the muscles, heart, eyes, and brain. Lactate is a favorite fuel for our immortal cells, such as the neurons, retinal cells, and cardiomyocytes. Lactic acid is the principal fuel for the heart muscle cells and neurons during exercise, when glucose can be quickly and precipitously exhausted. Lactate easily crosses the blood-brain barrier and is one of, if not the, brain's favorite foods. The retinal pigment epithelial cells also use lactate as fuel.[72] The eyes and brain need more energy during exercise to quickly process and coordinate movement.

Lactate is more than just fuel; it is a signaling molecule. Similar to the response of muscles after intense exercise, in the brain, lactate causes an increase in PGC-1α, and this is associated with an increased expression of mitochondrial DNA.[73] When lactate is used as an energy source, production of hydrogen peroxide (H_2O_2) by mitochondria increases. This induces the expression of hundreds of genes, many involved in energy metabolism and several with mitochondrial reproduction.[74] Thus, exercise not only increases ROS production in non-muscle tissue but also increases the creation of new proteins for mitochondria. The positive effect exercise has on the brain is mediated, in large part, by lactate.

During intense exercise, the muscles become energy-depleted. In the following hours, they recover. Within the first couple of minutes of exercise, glucose is depleted. If available, the muscles will then access glucose stored in the form of glycogen. When glycogen is depleted or unavailable, the muscles burn fat for use as energy.

Exercise increases AMPK activity, which activates the enzymes that convert triglycerides (fats) into glycerol and fatty acids. The muscles also use glycogen or fat during the post-exercise recovery period. If glycogen stores are low, fat is used during recovery. In the unfed state, free fatty acid levels remain elevated for several hours after intense exercise. The fatty acids are converted to energy through the citric acid cycle in the liver, with β-hydroxybutyrate (β-OHB) as a by-product. β-OHB is another fuel for the brain.

A study using one minute, high-intensity "all-out" interval training followed by 75 seconds of low-intensity recovery exercise found a significant increase in SIRT1 and PGC-1α, which was associated with an increase in mitochondrial biogenesis.[75]

P53 is a central regulator for many aspects of organelle and cell survival. The cell makes p53 continuously and breaks it down at about the same rate. AMPK and p38 MAPK are kinase enzymes that phosphorylate p53; this stabilizes it, preventing its destruction, and activating it. P53 promotes the transcription of genes that induce cell component recycling through autophagy and mitophagy in healthy G_0 and G_1 phase cells. After exercise, p53 forms a complex with mitochondrial transcription factor A (Tfam) and mitochondrial DNA (mtDNA).

In mice, after exercise and recovery, there is a marked increase in mRNA for PGC-1α, NRF1, and Tfam. Nuclear respiratory factor 1 (NRF1) is a transcription factor for synapsin, a protein required for neurite extension,[76] as well as for genes involved in heme biosynthesis, mitochondrial DNA replication, and other mitochondrial functions. Mice bred with dysfunctional p53 do not have this response to exercise.[77] If p53 formation is blocked, there is no renewal of mitochondria, and minimal, if any, response to exercise training.

Heat Shock Proteins

The adaptive response to exercise is in part mediated by Heat Shock Response (HSR) from mild heat stress, which leads to the production and activation of heat shock proteins (HSPs). HSPs act as protein chaperones that protect proteins from alterations in their functional structure and aggregation. Mild heat stress during exercise promotes the expression of certain HSPs. Saunas and hot baths can also induce an adaptive heat shock response. Hydrogen sulfide at low, physiologic levels activates the HSR and also promotes autophagy.

Recovery from Aberrant Methylation

DNA methylation alters gene expression; it generally causes clusters of genes on a segment of DNA to be more resistant to expression, however, as the expression of some genes inhibits the expression of other genes; methylation can thus also promote the expression of some genes. DNA methylation has an important control over which genes are expressed and the degree of their expression, and is an important mechanism in health and development. Random methylation is not a good thing, as it keeps the cells from performing their normal tasks. As we age and are exposed to toxins and stressors, aberrant random methylation occurs. Obesity, type 2 diabetes, smoking, exposure to certain environmental toxins, and time increase random methylation. Cellular stress, malnutrition, and aging can cause aberrant methylation of DNA to its histones, which increases or decreases the expression of gene clusters. This epigenetic imprinting can pass from one cell to its daughter cells, and thus pass on the adaptive or maladaptive gene expression. Acetylation of lysine residues in the histone conversely generally facilitates gene expression. There are natural compounds present in foods, however, that help mitigate or even reverse aberrant hypermethylation.

β-Hydroxybutyric acid (β-OHB) is a class 1 histone deacetylase (HDAC) inhibitor that increases p53 expression[78] and improves cognition and memory by promoting the production of BDNF, a neurotrophic growth factor in the hippocampus area of the brain.[79] As a class I HDAC inhibitor, β-OHB can help reprogram maladaptive epigenetic binding of DNA to histones that occurs with aging. β-hydroxybutyrate is synthesized in the liver via the metabolism of fatty acids during the fasting state. It is a ketone that is produced during the catabolism of fat. Several food compounds are Class I HDAC inhibitors that may help reverse hypermethylation.[80]

Sirtuins are a family of proteins, several of which have deacetylase enzyme activity, which facilitates the expression of certain genes. *Dysfunction* of SIRT 1, 2, 3, and 7, all deacetylase enzymes, is associated with neurodegenerative disease.[81] Thus, increased expression or activation of these deacetylase enzymes is thought to help prevent neurodegenerative disease and promote longevity.

Table 19F: Epigenetic Reset Factors [82] [83]

Compound	Impact
N-3 fatty acids: EPA and DHA	Promote reversal of hypermethylation. [84]
EGCG (green tea) Sulforaphane (cruciferous veggies)	HDAC and DNA methyltransferase inhibitors[80]
Butyrate (dietary fiber, cheese, butter. Diallyl sulfide (garlic) Resveratrol (red grapes and berries) Piceatannol (red wine, black grapes) Isoliquiritigenin (licorice root)	Histone deacetylase inhibitors[85, 86] These mostly inhibit Class I HDAC enzymes (HDAC1, HDAC2, HDAC3, and HDAC8). Piceatannol and isoliquiritigenin inhibit multiple HDAC enzymes. Resveratrol also activates SIRT1.
β-hydroxybutyrate (exercise)	HDAC2 and HDAC3 inhibitor
Phenolic compounds: Piceatannol, ferulic acid, catechin, malvidin, pterostilbene, tyrosol.	SIRT 1 activation
Phenolic compounds: Quercetin, luteolin, myricetin, cyanidin, isoliquiritigenin, rutin, apigenin, fisetin, fucoidan. Caffeine.[87]	SIRT 6 activation
Melatonin	Inhibits DNA methyltransferase.[88]

BDNF

Brain-derived neurotrophic factor (BDNF) enhances PGC-1α in the brain, which increases the development of dendritic spines and enhances the differentiation of synapses.[89] BDNF increases neurogenesis (the formation of new neurons) and may be needed for their survival. BDNF improves cognitive function and reduces the risk of neurodegenerative diseases.

Some compounds and factors positively impact BDNF levels: these include theanine, a non-protein amino acid found in tea; high-intensity exercise,[90] walking in new places, foods rich in n-3 fatty acids, adequate restorative sleep, and perhaps, occasional sleep-fasting.

In mice, a (high-fat, high-sugar) Standard American Diet (SAD) has been shown to reduce PGC-1α (and also reduce IGF-1R and SIRT1). The SAD impairs sensorimotor and bladder recovery in mice with spinal cord injuries, reduces axon sprouting, increases the generation of inflammatory microglia in the nervous system, and exacerbates the loss of oligodendrocytes.[91]

DNA Repair

Our bodies contain around 37 trillion cells, and most don't last forever. We replace about 30 billion nucleated cells a day (not counting red blood cells and platelets, which don't have nuclei). Even though the DNA replication mechanism is 99.999999% accurate, there is an error rate of around one base pair per 100 million base pairs copied. Every cell has three billion base pairs to be copied. That comes out to about 30 errors every time a cell gets copied. Ooops!

Fortunately, we have DNA repair mechanisms that find and correct 99 percent of these errors, limiting the number of "typos" to an average of about 3 per cell cycle, but that is still 90 billion errors a day. Most of these don't matter, as they are likely to affect areas of the DNA that are not needed for the function of that particular cell line or may code for a change in an amino acid that does not affect the protein's function significantly. Even when an error does affect a critical function, it becomes likely that the cell does not survive, and thus will be replaced. Thus, we are usually OK. But once in a while, the typo will cause a mutation that causes cancer. If an error occurs in the germ cells (sperm or ova), the mutation may be carried to a child. We want our DNA repair mechanism to work well. The BRCA1 and BRCA2 genes are two of about 130 DNA repair genes; mutations in these genes put people at high risk for breast, ovarian, prostate, and pancreatic cancers. While cancer is of great concern, DNA errors also cause cells to function poorly. Sirtuins, particularly SIRT1 and SIRT6, which are present in the nucleus of the cell, can help activate the transcription and expression of DNA repair genes.

Amyloid plaque in the brain downregulates SIRT6 levels. SIRT1 and SIRT6 have additional functions; SIRT1 protects the brain from ischemic injury, and SIRT6 protects the brain from reperfusion injury and neurotoxicity. SIRT6 downregulates inflammation, promotes metabolic homeostasis, NRF2 expression, and has additional anti-aging effects. SIRT6 levels, however, decline significantly in the brain with age, while SIRT1 levels are maintained.[92] [93] (SIRT2 resides in the cytoplasm of the cell, SIRT3, SIRT4, and SIRT5 are localized in the mitochondria, and SIRT7 is located in the nucleolus where ribosomes are assembled; thus, while these sirtuins are protective, they are not directly involved in DNA repair.)

Various polyphenols activate sirtuins and thus enhance cellular resilience. Cyanidin is the most potent known polyphenolic activator of SIRT6.[94] Cyanidin is an anthocyanin and crosses the blood-brain barrier. It is found in some berries, blackberries, elderberries and aronia berries, raspberries, and in black beans. Other dietary phenols that increase SIRT6 include myricetin, delphinidin, and luteolin. Some polyphenols inhibit SIRT6. These include gallocatechin gallate and catechin. Fucoidan and quercetin can increase or decrease SIRT6 depending on the dose. Nicotinamide riboside acts as a cofactor for several sirtuins.

Elimination of Senescent Cells

Cells age over time, and the polite ones retire and step aside for the greater good, and undergo *apoptosis*, a form of cell death mediated from within the cell. The void is then filled by the growth of adjacent cells, replacing the cell with a healthy new one. Some cells, however, just become sickly but refuse to retire as if they were geriatric members of Congress. Senescence is a state of cellular aging where cells stop dividing but just stay there, being weak and sickly. These worn-out senescent cells release inflammatory cytokines that make the cells around them sick and act as if they were senescent as well. These senescent cells can accumulate and contribute to aging and age-related diseases. As we age, we accumulate more and more poorly functioning, senescent cells.

Our understanding of how to get rid of these old, senile cells is in its infancy. We know of a few "senolytic" agents that will selectively promote apoptosis of senescent cells grown in laboratory culture, and there are some early animal studies, as well as some adventurous biohackers who are experimenting on themselves.

Since proinflammatory cytokines help maintain senescent cells, maintaining an anti-inflammatory environment may help eliminate these cells and may help keep the adjacent cells functioning better. An anti-inflammatory diet and exercise may help reduce the burden of senescent cells.

Advanced Glycation End-products

Advanced Glycation End-products (AGEs) are compounds that can form when proteins or lipids form covalent bonds with sugars. Dietary AGEs (dAGEs) can form in food during its preparation. Endogenous AGEs (eAGEs) form inside the body as a result of elevated blood sugar levels. Some, but not all, AGEs are thought to be causal agents in the development of chronic diseases of aging, including insulin resistance, diabetes, chronic kidney disease, atherosclerosis, and Alzheimer's disease.[95] AGES can cause the cross-linking of collagen, causing stiffening of the arteries, and entrapment and oxidation of LDL cholesterol. Most importantly, AGEs can bind to the RAGE (Receptor for Advanced Glycation End-products) receptors, provoking an inflammatory response. The RAGE receptor's natural ligand is HMGB1, a DNA-binding protein that is released from necrotic cells. RAGE activation elicits an immune response promoting pro-inflammatory gene transcription, which is a good thing when there are necrotic cells that need to be cleaned up, but a bad thing when the only problem is something somebody had for dinner. AGEs are implicated in multiple aspects of aging, including oxidative stress, arterial stiffness, vascular permeability, cataract formation, muscular stiffness, ischemic heart disease, periodontitis, neuropathy, wrinkling of the skin, and other conditions.

For better or worse, it is not as simple as just eliminating dAGES from the diet. Not all dAGEs are associated with risk, and some may have hormetic effects. Unfortunately, testing of the effects of dAGES has focused on representative AGEs that are easy to test for, but this does not help us understand which ones are absorbed or which are toxic. Vegetarians have higher levels of some dAGEs than do carnivores, suggesting that those we have been looking at are likely not dAGEs that cause significant harm.[96] The dAGE (carboxymethyl)lysine (CML) is common in toasted foods during Maillard reactions. However, CML does not cause cross-linking and appears to create little if any health risk. The same appears to be true for other AGEs directly formed from glucose. There is a paucity of data that links dietary AGEs to disease.

Nevertheless, high dietary intake of dAGEs is associated with fatty liver.[97] A large population study found a significant correlation between dAGEs and dementia. DAGE intake was assessed from food frequency questionnaires in over 90,000 British adults over the age of 50, and the presence of dementia was assessed about 12 years later. There was no increase in risk for Alzheimer's disease; however, there was a large (49%) increase in risk of early onset dementia (age <65) and elevated risk for vascular and other non-AD forms of dementia associated with higher dAGE intake.[98] DAGEs in this study may be a proxy for bread consumption, as this is a major source of dAGEs in the diet. The link between dAGEs and early-onset dementia seems unlikely to be causal and may rather reflect an impoverished diet. Glucospane is an AGE associated with collagen cross-linking in the skin of diabetics, and that can be created during the cooking of meat, but there is no epidemiologic data linking dietary glucospane to diseases of aging. This suggests that the high levels of glucosepane found in diabetics are from it being formed in the body as a result of elevated blood sugar, and that these endogenous AGES (eAGES) cause injury.[99] Another large population study failed to find any association of dAGE intake with microvascular function, a target of AGE injury.[100] The effect of dAGEs needs further study.[101] Large effects should be easy to find.

AGEs formed from glyceraldehyde, a metabolic intermediate in fructose metabolism, in contrast, are cytotoxic and dangerous.[102] [103] The AGE that is most clearly linked to disease has been dubbed TAGE: Toxic Advanced Glycation End-product. TAGE forms largely in the liver, from the metabolism of sorbitol and fructose into glyceraldehyde. Sorbitol is converted into fructose, and fructose is metabolized into fructose-1-phosphate and then into pyruvate, which enters the citric acid cycle for the generation of ATP. When there is excess fructose, however, some of the fructose is instead converted into methylglyoxal, and more problematically, glyceraldehyde (GA), which can then accumulate. GA forms TAGE that binds to proteins in the hepatocytes (liver cells), inhibiting protein function and damaging mitochondria, causing the formation of free radicals and killing those cells. This causes the release of TAGE, which poisons other cells. TAGE activates RAGE, causing inflammation.

Glyceraldehyde forms as a result of excessive consumption of sorbitol and fructose. Since table sugar, sucrose, is rapidly split into glucose and fructose, this sugar is a major source of fructose for GA production.

Sweet beverages are quickly digested, providing a heavy dose of fructose. Every cell in the body can use glucose, but the liver is the only organ that can process fructose, so it can become fructose overloaded. Excess glucose can be converted in the body to fructose as a shunt to utilize alternate metabolic pathways, and thus high glucose levels can give rise to GA and TAGE.

TAGE localizes in the soma (the main body) of neurons in Alzheimer's disease. TAGE binds to β-tubulin, which causes it to aggregate into a jumbled mass; this inhibits neurite outgrowth and the ability to make new neuronal connections. TAGE also injures other organs, increasing the risk of cardiovascular disease and heart failure, chronic kidney disease, diabetic retinopathy, female infertility, and fatty liver disease.[104] AGEs accumulate in muscles with age and contribute to muscle wasting and fibrosis.[105]

Methylglyoxal (MGO) forms AGEs with the amino acids: arginine, lysine, and cysteine. Methylglyoxal can modify histones (proteins that help shepherd and protect the DNA strands), and those modifications can increase the risk of cancer.[106] Methylglyoxal appears to play a role in diabetic neuropathic pain.[107] Methylglyoxal is formed during the processing of some foods, and small amounts are also produced by the body during the normal metabolism of glucose, but the body can convert this to lactate.

The major contributor to TAGEs in the body appears to be hyperglycemia, which causes the formation of pathologic levels of MGO and elevated spikes of fructose in the liver, which generate excess glyceraldehyde. The metabolism of alcohol causes the formation of acetaldehyde and other metabolites that can also cause the formation of AGEs.[108] MGO is involved in the development of multiple diseases, including atherosclerosis, hypertension, diabetes, pain, aging, and neurodegeneration.[109] MGO and TAGE disrupt the blood-brain barrier, induce oxidative stress, and cross-link proteins, causing toxic oligomers, resulting in neuroinflammation and apoptosis.[110] GLO1 (lactoylglutathione lyase) is an enzyme that detoxifies MGO. In a study of the brains of adults with Alzheimer's disease, GLO1 levels were 50% higher than normal age-matched controls early during the disease, but decreased with the disease's advancement.[111] This suggests that early in the disease, the cells are trying to adapt to an increased load of MGO and other AGEs, but eventually fail to keep up with the pathologic processes.

With insulin resistance, glucose has more difficulty entering the cell, and there is greater reliance on glycolysis and less on oxidative phosphorylation (OxPhos) by the mitochondria. One of the metabolic intermediates of glycolysis is dihydroxyacetone phosphate (DHAP), which can be converted to methylglyoxal. Hyperglycemia also promotes the formation of other AGEs. Both MGO and hyperglycemia stimulate hypoxia-inducible factor (HIF-1α), which switches metabolism towards glycolysis to help cells survive hypoxia. This is known as the Warburg effect, which allows cancers to survive and spread.[112] Since MGO promotes HIF-1α activation and the transcription of glycolytic proteins, it can form a positive feedback loop. Glycolysis is not as efficient or clean as OxPhos and can generate excess pyruvate, which can overwhelm the mitochondria and lead to the formation of reactive oxygen species (ROS) that injure the cell. Glycolysis can contribute to inflammation. All this contributes to the diseases of aging and neurodegeneration. In a large population study of older adults, higher levels of AGEs were associated with lower muscle mass and strength.[113]

Both MGO and TAGE can be detoxified in the body through the glyoxalase system. The first step is the spontaneous binding of MGO or TAGE to glutathione. The enzyme lactoylglutathione lyase (GLO1) then converts MGO to lactoylglutathione, which is then converted by a second enzyme, hydroxyacylglutathione hydrolase (GLO2), into glutathione and D-lactate. Glutathione can thus be reused, and D-lactate can be converted into pyruvate for use in the citric acid cycle to form ATP. GLO1 is the rate-limiting enzyme.

Several natural compounds present in foods have been found to lower the level of MGO and other AGEs, including a combination of citrus peel and pomegranate extracts,[114] quercetin,[115] cyanidin-3-*O*-galactoside, cyanidin-3-*O*-arabinoside, procyanidin B2,[116] kaempferol,[117] and butyrate formed by commensal bacteria in the colon.[118] Many of these compounds act as hormetic agents, increasing the activation of the transcription factor NRF2 and the production of GLO1 and the recycling of glutathione. Other compounds were found to "trap" MGO, binding to it and neutralizing its toxic effects.

HMOX1

Heme Oxygenase 1 (HMOX1) is an enzyme that degrades heme, which is contained in proteins, such as hemoglobin, myoglobin, and cytochrome P450. During its reaction, iron (Fe2+), biliverdin, and carbon monoxide (CO) are generated. CO in the tiny amount released acts as a gasotransmitter, a signaling molecule. In this situation, CO acts to promote vasodilation, inhibition of platelet aggregation, enhance neurotransmission, modulate inflammation, and cell proliferation, rather than acting as a toxin as when burning fuel in a closed space.

Lower blood levels of HMOX1 are associated with increased risk of dementia. Several dietary factors are associated with higher HMOX1 levels. These include foods high in manganese (whole grains, mollusks [mussels, oysters, clams], legumes, coffee, tea, bananas), phenolic compounds including flavonols and flavonoids, and green tea, as a result of its phenolic compounds.[119] Low-level alcohol intake increases HMOX1 expression.

Notably, high levels of HMOX1 can promote apoptosis. Thus, for most situations, high levels of HMOX1 expression are not beneficial.

[1] Age-related dysregulation of homeostatic control in neuronal microcircuits. Radulescu CI, Doostdar N, Zabouri N, Melgosa-Ecenarro L, Wang X, Sadeh S, Pavlidi P, Airey J, Kopanitsa M, Clopath C, Barnes SJ. Nat Neurosci. 2023 Dec;26(12):2158-2170. doi: 10.1038/s41593-023-01451-z. Epub 2023 Nov 2. PMID: 37919424

[2] Associations of four biological age markers with child development: A multi-omic analysis in the European HELIX cohort. Robinson O, Lau CE, Joo S, Andrusaityte S, Borras E, de Prado-Bert P, Chatzi L, Keun HC, Grazuleviciene R, Gutzkow KB, Maitre L, Martens DS, Sabido E, Siroux V, Urquiza J, Vafeiadi M, Wright J, Nawrot TS, Bustamante M, Vrijheid M. Elife. 2023 Jun 6;12:e85104. doi: 10.7554/eLife.85104. PMID: 37278618

[3] Blood Biochemistry Analysis to Detect Smoking Status and Quantify Accelerated Aging in Smokers. Mamoshina, P., Kochetov, K., Cortese, F. *et al. Sci Rep* 9, 142 (2019). https://doi.org/10.1038/s41598-018-35704-w

[4] The impact of smoking on estimated biological age and body fat composition: A cross-sectional study. Radmilović G, Matijević V, Mikulić D, Rašić Markota D, Čeprnja AR. Tob Induc Dis. 2023 Dec 6;21:161. doi: 10.18332/tid/174663. eCollection 2023. PMID: 38075019

[5] The effects of exercise and diet on oxidative stress and telomere length in breast cancer survivors. Brown JC, Sturgeon K, Sarwer DB, Troxel AB, DeMichele AM, Denlinger CS, Schmitz KH. Breast Cancer Res Treat. 2023 May;199(1):109-117. doi: 10.1007/s10549-023-06868-5. Epub 2023 Mar 18. PMID: 36933050

[6] Effect of comprehensive lifestyle changes on telomerase activity and telomere length in men with biopsy-proven low-risk prostate cancer: 5-year follow-up of a descriptive pilot study. Ornish D, Lin J, Chan JM, Epel E, Kemp C, Weidner G, Marlin R, Frenda SJ, Magbanua MJM, Daubenmier J, Estay I, Hills NK, Chainani-Wu N, Carroll PR, Blackburn EH. Lancet Oncol. 2013 Oct;14(11):1112-1120. doi: 10.1016/S1470-2045(13)70366-8. Epub 2013 Sep 17. PMID: 24051140

[7] Potential reversal of epigenetic age using a diet and lifestyle intervention: a pilot randomized clinical trial. Fitzgerald KN, Hodges R, Hanes D, Stack E, Cheishvili D, Szyf M, Henkel J, Twedt MW, Giannopoulou D, Herdell J, Logan S, Bradley R. Aging (Albany NY). 2021 Apr 12;13(7):9419-9432. doi: 10.18632/aging.202913. Epub 2021 Apr 12. PMID: 33844651

[8] Effect of Modifiable Lifestyle Factors on Biological Aging. Lu WH. JAR Life. 2024 Jun 5;13:88-92. doi: 10.14283/jarlife.2024.13. eCollection 2024. PMID: 38855439

[9] Healthy lifestyle behaviors and transitions in frailty status among independent community-dwelling older adults: The Yabu cohort study. Abe T, Nofuji Y, Seino S, Murayama H, Yoshida Y, Tanigaki T, Yokoyama Y, Narita M, Nishi M, Kitamura A, Shinkai S. Maturitas. 2020 Jun;136:54-59. doi: 10.1016/j.maturitas.2020.04.007. Epub 2020 Apr 18. PMID: 32386667

[10] Hormesis: its impact on medicine and health. Calabrese EJ, Iavicoli I, Calabrese V. Hum Exp Toxicol. 2013 Feb;32(2):120-52. doi: 10.1177/0960327112455069. Epub 2012 Oct 11. PMID: 23060412

[11] Healthy lifestyles and wellbeing reduce neuroinflammation and prevent neurodegenerative and psychiatric disorders. Kip E, Parr-Brownlie LC. Front Neurosci. 2023 Feb 15;17:1092537. doi: 10.3389/fnins.2023.1092537. eCollection 2023. PMID: 36875655

[12] DNA methylation: a cause and consequence of type 2 diabetes. Kim M. Genomics Inform. 2019 Dec;17(4):e38. doi: 10.5808/GI.2019.17.4.e38. Epub 2019 Nov 28. PMID: 31896238

[13] The involvement of NRF2 in the protective effects of diallyl disulfide on carbon tetrachloride-induced hepatic oxidative damage and inflammatory response in rats. Lee IC, Kim SH, Baek HS, et al. Food Chem Toxicol. 2014 Jan;63:174-85PMID:24246655

[14] Biological Functions of Diallyl Disulfide, a Garlic-Derived Natural Organic Sulfur Compound. Song X, Yue Z, Nie L, Zhao P, Zhu K, Wang Q. Evid Based Complement Alternat Med. 2021 Oct 29;2021:5103626. doi: 10.1155/2021/5103626. eCollection 2021. PMID: 34745287

[15] Anthocyanins from purple sweet potato attenuate dimethylnitrosamine-induced liver injury in rats by inducing NRF2-mediated antioxidant enzymes and reducing COX-2 and iNOS expression. Hwang YP, Choi JH, et al. Food Chem Toxicol. 2011 Jan;49(1):93-9. PMID:20934476

[16] Black currant anthocyanins abrogate oxidative stress through NRF2- mediated antioxidant mechanisms in a rat model of hepatocellular carcinoma. Thoppil RJ, Bhatia D, Barnes KF, et al. Curr Cancer Drug Targets. 2012 Nov 1;12(9):1244-57. PMID:22873220

[17] Berry anthocyanins suppress the expression and secretion of proinflammatory mediators in macrophages by inhibiting nuclear translocation of NF-κB independent of NRF2-mediated mechanism. Lee SG, Kim B, Yang Y, et al. J Nutr Biochem. 2014 Apr;25(4):404-11. PMID:24565673

[18] Blackberry extract attenuates oxidative stress through up-regulation of NRF2-dependent antioxidant enzymes in carbon tetrachloride-treated rats. Cho BO, Ryu HW, et al. J Agric Food Chem. 2011 Nov 9;59(21):11442-8. PMID:21888405

[19] Protective effects of ursolic acid in an experimental model of liver fibrosis through NRF2/ARE pathway. Ma JQ, Ding J, Zhang L, Liu CM. Clin Res Hepatol Gastroenterol. 2015 Apr;39(2):188-97. PMID:25459994

[20] Naringenin attenuates CCl4 -induced hepatic inflammation by the activation of an NRF2-mediated pathway in rats. Esmaeili MA, Alilou M.Clin Exp Pharmacol Physiol. 2014 Jun;41(6):416-22. PMID:24684352

[21] Dietary Flavonoid Intake and Cancer Mortality: A Population-Based Cohort Study. Zhou Y, Gu K, Zhou F. Nutrients. 2023 Feb 15;15(4):976. doi: 10.3390/nu15040976. PMID: 36839330

[22] BRCA1 interacts with NRF2 to regulate antioxidant signaling and cell survival. Gorrini C, Baniasadi PS, Harris IS, et al. J Exp Med. 2013 Jul 29;210(8):1529-44. 23857982

[23] Bioactive food components prevent carcinogenic stress via NRF2 activation in BRCA1 deficient breast epithelial cells. Kang HJ, Hong YB, Kim HJ, Wang A, Bae I. Toxicol Lett. 2012 Mar 7;209(2):154-60. PMID:22192953

[24] Antioxidant responses and cellular adjustments to oxidative stress. Espinosa-Diez C, Miguel V, Mennerich D, et al. Redox Biol. 2015 Dec;6:183-97. PMID:26233704

[25] NRF2, a Transcription Factor for Stress Response and Beyond. He F, Ru X, Wen T. Int J Mol Sci. 2020 Jul 6;21(13):4777. doi: 10.3390/ijms21134777. PMID: 32640524

[26] Mitochondrial ALDH2 deficiency as an oxidative stress. Ohta S, Ohsawa I, Kamino K, Ando F, Shimokata H. Ann N Y Acad Sci. 2004 Apr;1011:36-44. doi: 10.1007/978-3-662-41088-2_4. PMID: 15126281

[27] Impact of common ALDH2 inactivating mutation and alcohol consumption on Alzheimer's disease. Seike T, Chen CH, Mochly-Rosen D. Front Aging Neurosci. 2023 Aug 24;15:1223977. doi: 10.3389/fnagi.2023.1223977. PMID: 37693648

[28] Effect of a lifestyle intervention on telomere length: A systematic review and meta-analysis. Buttet M, Bagheri R, Ugbolue UC, Laporte C, Trousselard M, Benson A, Bouillon-Minois JB, Dutheil F. Mech Ageing Dev. 2022 Sep;206:111694. doi: 10.1016/j.mad.2022.111694. Epub 2022 Jun 26. PMID: 35760212

[29] Does Exercise Affect Telomere Length? A Systematic Review and Meta-Analysis of Randomized Controlled Trials. Song S, Lee E, Kim H. Medicina (Kaunas). 2022 Feb 5;58(2):242. doi: 10.3390/medicina58020242. PMID: 35208566

[30] Physical Activity on Telomere Length as a Biomarker for Aging: A Systematic Review. Schellnegger M, Lin AC, Hammer N, Kamolz LP. Sports Med Open. 2022 Sep 4;8(1):111. doi: 10.1186/s40798-022-00503-1. PMID: 36057868

[31] Associations between the New DNA-Methylation-Based Telomere Length Estimator, the Mediterranean Diet and Genetics in a Spanish Population at High Cardiovascular Risk. Coltell O, Asensio EM, Sorlí JV, Ortega-Azorín C, Fernández-Carrión R, Pascual EC, Barragán R, González JI, Estruch R, Alzate JF, Pérez-Fidalgo A, Portolés O, Ordovas JM, Corella D. Antioxidants (Basel). 2023 Nov 15;12(11):2004. doi: 10.3390/antiox12112004. PMID: 38001857 (supplemental data)

[32] The relationship between greenspace exposure and telomere length in the National Health and Nutrition Examination Survey. Ogletree SS, Huang JH, Reif D, Yang L, Dunstan C, Osakwe N, Oh JI, Hipp JA. Sci Total Environ. 2023 Dec 20;905:167452. doi: 10.1016/j.scitotenv.2023.167452. Epub 2023 Sep 28. PMID: 37777139

[33] Green sleep: Immediate residential greenspace and access to larger green areas are associated with better sleep quality, in a longitudinal population-based cohort. Stenfors CUD, Stengård J, Magnusson Hanson LL, Kecklund LG, Westerlund H. Environ Res. 2023 Oct 1;234:116085. doi: 10.1016/j.envres.2023.116085. Epub 2023 May 17. PMID: 37207733

[34] SGLT2 inhibition eliminates senescent cells and alleviates pathological aging. Katsuumi G, Shimizu I, Suda M, Yoshida Y, Furihata T, Joki Y, Hsiao CL, Jiaqi L, Fujiki S, Abe M, Sugimoto M, Soga T, Minamino T. Nat Aging. 2024 Jul;4(7):926-938. doi: 10.1038/s43587-024-00642-y. PMID: 38816549

[35] AMP-activated protein kinase: an energy sensor that regulates all aspects of cell function. Hardie DG. Genes Dev. 2011 Sep 15;25(18):1895-908. doi: 10.1101/gad.17420111. PMID: 21937710

[36] Sensing of energy and nutrients by AMP-activated protein kinase. Hardie DG. Am J Clin Nutr. 2011 Apr;93(4):891S-6. PMID:21325438

[37] Effects of resistance training on cytokines. de Salles BF, Simão R, Fleck SJ, Dias I, Kraemer-Aguiar LG, Bouskela E. Int J Sports Med. 2010 Jul;31(7):441-50. PMID:20432196

[38] Perceived psychological stress and serum leptin concentrations in Japanese men. Otsuka R, Yatsuya H, Tamakoshi K, Matsushita K, Wada K, Toyoshima H. Obesity (Silver Spring). 2006 Oct;14(10):1832-8. PMID:17062814

[39] Comparison of serum adiponectin and tumor necrosis factor-alpha levels between patients with and without obstructive sleep apnea syndrome. Kanbay A, Kokturk O, Ciftci TU, Tavil Y, Bukan N. Respiration. 2008;76(3):324-30. PMID:18487876

[40] Leptin regulates energy metabolism in MCF-7 breast cancer cells. Blanquer-Rosselló Mdel M, Oliver J, Sastre-Serra J, et al. Int J Biochem Cell Biol. 2016 Mar;72:18-26. PMID:26772821

[41] Ghrelin-AMPK Signaling Mediates the Neuroprotective Effects of Calorie Restriction in Parkinson's Disease. Bayliss JA, Lemus MB, Stark R, et al. J Neurosci. 2016 Mar 9;36(10):3049-63. PMID:26961958

[42] New insight into adiponectin role in obesity and obesity-related diseases. Nigro E, Scudiero O, Monaco ML, Palmieri A, Mazzarella G, Costagliola C, Bianco A, Daniele A. Biomed Res Int. 2014;2014:658913. PMID:25110685

[43] The role of adiponectin in cancer: a review of current evidence. Dalamaga M, Diakopoulos KN, Mantzoros CS. Endocr Rev. 2012 Aug;33(4):547-94. PMID:22547160

[44] The important role of sleep in metabolism. Copinschi G, Leproult R, Spiegel K. Front Horm Res. 2014;42:59-72. PMID:24732925

[45] Leptin, obestatin and apelin levels in patients with obstructive sleep apnoea syndrome. Zirlik S, Hauck T, Fuchs FS, Neurath MF, Konturek PC, Harsch IA. Med Sci Monit. 2011 Feb 25;17(3):CR159-64. PMID:21358603

[46] Improved insulin sensitivity and adiponectin level after exercise training in obese Korean youth. Kim ES, Im JA, Kim KC, et al. Obesity (Silver Spring). 2007 Dec;15(12):3023-30. PMID:18198311

47 Pinealectomy increases and exogenous melatonin decreases leptin production in rat anterior pituitary cells: an immunohistochemical study. Kus I, Sarsilmaz M, Colakoglu N, Kukne A, Ozen OA, Yilmaz B, Kelestimur H. Physiol Res. 2004;53(4):403-8. PMID:15311999

48 Intermittent and rhythmic exposure to melatonin in primary cultured adipocytes enhances the insulin and dexamethasone effects on leptin expression. Alonso-Vale MI, Andreotti S, Borges-Silva Cd, et al. J Pineal Res. 2006 Aug;41(1):28-34. PMID:16842538

49 Changes in glucose tolerance and leptin responsiveness of rats offered a choice of lard, sucrose, and chow. Harris RB, Apolzan JW. Am J Physiol Regul Integr Comp Physiol. 2012 Jun;302(11):R1327-39. PMID:22496363

50 Leptin Level and Skipping Breakfast: The National Health and Nutrition Examination Survey III (NHANES III). Asao K, Marekani AS, VanCleave J, Rothberg AE. Nutrients. 2016 Feb 25;8(3). pii: E115. PMID:26927164

51 The effect of myo-inositol supplementation on AMPK/PI3K/AKT pathway and insulin resistance in patients with NAFLD. Aghajani T, Arefhosseini S, Ebrahimi-Mameghani M, Safaralizadeh R. Food Sci Nutr. 2024 Jul 16;12(10):7177-7185. doi: 10.1002/fsn3.4267. eCollection 2024 Oct. PMID: 39479697

52 Gallic acid regulates body weight and glucose homeostasis through AMPK activation. Doan KV, Ko CM, Kinyua AW, et al. Endocrinology. 2015 Jan;156(1):157-68. PMID:25356824

53 The ancient drug salicylate directly activates AMP-activated protein kinase. Hawley SA, Fullerton MD, Ross FA, et al. Science. 2012 May 18;336(6083): PMID:22517326

54 Metformin and salicylate synergistically activate liver AMPK, inhibit lipogenesis and improve insulin sensitivity. Ford RJ, Fullerton MD, Pinkosky SL, et al. Biochem J. 2015 May 15;468(1):125-32. PMID:25742316

55 Salicylate activates AMPK and synergizes with metformin to reduce the survival of prostate and lung cancer cells ex vivo through inhibition of de novo lipogenesis. O'Brien AJ, Villani LA, Broadfield LA, et al. Biochem J. 2015 May 5. PMID:25940306

56 CaMKKβ is involved in AMP-activated protein kinase activation by baicalin in LKB1 deficient cell lines. Ma Y, Yang F, Wang Y, Du Z, Liu D, Guo H, Shen J, Peng H. PLoS One. 2012;7(10):e47900. PMID: 23110126

57 Ca2+/calmodulin-dependent protein kinase kinase is involved in AMP-activated protein kinase activation by alpha-lipoic acid in C2C12 myotubes. Shen QW, Zhu MJ, Tong J, Ren J, Du M. Am J Physiol Cell Physiol. 2007 Oct;293(4):C1395-403. PMID: 17687000

58 S-allyl cysteine attenuates free fatty acid-induced lipogenesis in human HepG2 cells through activation of the AMP-activated protein kinase-dependent pathway. Hwang YP, Kim HG, Choi JH, et al. J Nutr Biochem. 2013 Aug;24(8):1469-78. PMID: 23465592

59 Thyroid hormone activates adenosine 5'-monophosphate-activated protein kinase via intracellular calcium mobilization and activation of calcium/calmodulin-dependent protein kinase kinase-beta. Yamauchi M, Kambe F, Cao X, Lu X, Kozaki Y, Oiso Y, Seo H. Mol Endocrinol. 2008 Apr;22(4):893-903. PMID: 18187603

60 AMPK: a target for drugs and natural products with effects on both diabetes and cancer. Hardie DG. Diabetes. 2013 Jul;62(7):2164-72. PMID: 23801715

61 http://www.brenda-enzymes.info/enzyme.php?ecno=2.7.11.17

62 Genistein, EGCG, and capsaicin inhibit adipocyte differentiation process via activating AMP-activated protein kinase. Hwang JT, Park IJ, Shin JI, et al. Biochem Biophys Res Commun. 2005 Dec 16;338(2):694-9. PMID: 16236247

63 Catechin-induced activation of the LKB1/AMP-activated protein kinase pathway. Murase T, Misawa K, Haramizu S, Hase T. Biochem Pharmacol. 2009 Jul 1;78(1):78-84. PMID:19447226

64 Punicalagin induces apoptotic and autophagic cell death in human U87MG glioma cells. Wang SG, Huang MH, Li JH, Lai FI, Lee HM, Hsu YN. Acta Pharmacol Sin. 2013 Nov;34(11):1411-9. PMID: 24077634

65 Nootkatone, a characteristic constituent of grapefruit, stimulates energy metabolism and prevents diet-induced obesity by activating AMPK. Murase T, Misawa K, Haramizu S, et al. Am J Physiol Endocrinol Metab. 2010 Aug;299(2):E266-75. PMID: 20501876

66 Withdrawal of essential amino acids increases autophagy by a pathway involving Ca2+/calmodulin-dependent kinase kinase-β (CaMKK-β). Ghislat G, Patron M, Rizzuto R, Knecht E. J Biol Chem. 2012 Nov 9;287(46):38625-36. PMID: 23027865

67 Spermidine, a caloric restriction mimetic, provides neuroprotection against normal and D-galactose-induced oxidative stress and apoptosis through activation of autophagy in male rats during aging. Singh S, Kumar R, Garg G, Singh AK, Verma AK, Bissoyi A, Rizvi SI. Biogerontology. 2021 Feb;22(1):35-47. doi: 10.1007/s10522-020-09900-z. Epub 2020 Sep 26. PMID: 32979155

68 Spermidine and spermine delay brain aging by inducing autophagy in SAMP8 mice. Xu TT, Li H, Dai Z, Lau GK, Li BY, Zhu WL, Liu XQ, Liu HF, Cai WW, Huang SQ, Wang Q, Zhang SJ. Aging (Albany NY). 2020 Apr 8;12(7):6401-6414. doi: 10.18632/aging.103035. Epub 2020 Apr 8. PMID: 32268299

69 PGC-1 coactivators: inducible regulators of energy metabolism in health and disease.

Finck BN, Kelly DP. J Clin Invest. 2006 Mar;116(3):615-22. doi: 10.1172/JCI27794. PMID: 16511594

70 Covering the Role of PGC-1α in the Nervous System. Kuczynska Z, Metin E, Liput M, Buzanska L. Cells. 2021 Dec 30;11(1):111. doi: 10.3390/cells11010111. PMID: 35011673

71 Effect of ApoE isoforms on mitochondria in Alzheimer disease. Yin J, Reiman EM, Beach TG, Serrano GE, Sabbagh MN, Nielsen M, Caselli RJ, Shi J. Neurology. 2020 Jun 9;94(23):e2404-e2411. doi:

10.1212/WNL.0000000000009582. Epub 2020 May 26. PMID: 32457210

72 A metabolic switch in brain: glucose and lactate metabolism modulation by ascorbic acid. Castro MA, Beltrán FA, Brauchi S, Concha II. J Neurochem. 2009 Jul;110(2):423-40. PMID:19457103

73 Lactate administration reproduces specific brain and liver exercise-related changes. E L, Lu J, Selfridge JE, Burns JM, et al. J Neurochem. 2013 Oct;127(1):91-100. PMID:23927032

74 Lactate sensitive transcription factor network in L6 cells: activation of MCT1 and mitochondrial biogenesis. Hashimoto T, Hussien R, Oommen S, Gohil K, Brooks GA. FASEB J. 2007 Aug;21(10):2602-12. PMID:17395833

75 A practical model of low-volume high-intensity interval training induces mitochondrial biogenesis in human skeletal muscle: potential mechanisms. Little JP, Safdar A, Wilkin GP, Tarnopolsky MA, Gibala MJ. J Physiol. 2010 Mar 15;588(Pt 6):1011-22. PMID:20100740

76 Human synapsin I mediates the function of nuclear respiratory factor 1 in neurite outgrowth in neuroblastoma IMR-32 cells. Wang JL, Chang WT, Tong CW, Kohno K, Huang AM. J Neurosci Res. 2009 Aug 1;87(10):2255-63. doi: 10.1002/jnr.22059. PMID: 19301426

77 p53 is necessary for the adaptive changes in cellular milieu subsequent to an acute bout of endurance exercise. Saleem A, Carter HN, Hood DA. Am J Physiol Cell Physiol. 2014 Feb 1;306(3):C241-9. PMID:24284795

78 Pathway of programmed cell death and oxidative stress induced by β-hydroxybutyrate in dairy cow abomasum smooth muscle cells and in mouse gastric smooth muscle. Tian W, Wei T, Li B, Wang Z, Zhang N, Xie G. PLoS One. 2014 May 6;9(5):e96775. PMID:24801711

79 Exercise promotes the expression of brain derived neurotrophic factor (BDNF) through the action of the ketone body β-hydroxybutyrate. Sleiman SF, Henry J, Al-Haddad R, et al. Elife. 2016 Jun 2;5. pii: e15092. PMID:27253067

80 Impact of epigenetic dietary compounds on transgenerational prevention of human diseases. Li Y, Saldanha SN, Tollefsbol TO. AAPS J. 2014 Jan;16(1):27-36. PMID:24114450

81 Sirtuin functions and modulation: from chemistry to the clinic. Carafa V, Rotili D, Forgione M, Cuomo F, Serretiello E, Hailu GS, Jarho E, Lahtela-Kakkonen M, Mai A, Altucci L. Clin Epigenetics. 2016 May 25;8:61. doi: 10.1186/s13148-016-0224-3. eCollection 2016. PMID: 27226812

82 Natural polyphenols as sirtuin 6 modulators. Rahnasto-Rilla M, Tyni J, Huovinen M, Jarho E, Kulikowicz T, Ravichandran S, A Bohr V, Ferrucci L, Lahtela-Kakkonen M, Moaddel R. Sci Rep. 2018 Mar 7;8(1):4163. doi: 10.1038/s41598-018-22388-5. PMID: 29515203

83 Role of Sirtuin 1 in the modulation of ER stress-induced apoptosis and autophagy in heart. Da Silva, JP. Thesis. 12-10-2018Universite Paris-Saclay https://theses.hal.science/tel-01894468

84 Fatty acids and epigenetics. Burdge GC, Lillycrop KA. Curr Opin Clin Nutr Metab Care. 2013 Dec 7. PMID:24322369

85 Histone deacetylases as targets for dietary cancer preventive agents: lessons learned with butyrate, diallyl disulfide, and sulforaphane. Myzak MC, Dashwood RH. Curr Drug Targets. 2006 Apr;7(4):443-52. PMID:16611031

86 Identification of HDAC Inhibitors Using a Cell-Based HDAC I/II Assay. Hsu CW, Shou D, Huang R, Khuc T, Dai S, Zheng W, Klumpp-Thomas C, Xia M. J Biomol Screen. 2016 Jul;21(6):643-52. PMID:26858181

87 Caffeine Protects Skin from Oxidative Stress-Induced Senescence through the Activation of Autophagy. Li YF, Ouyang SH, Tu LF, Wang X, Yuan WL, Wang GE, Wu YP, Duan WJ, Yu HM, Fang ZZ, Kurihara H, Zhang Y, He RR. Theranostics. 2018 Nov 10;8(20):5713-5730. doi: 10.7150/thno.28778. eCollection 2018. PMID: 30555576

88 Roles of melatonin in fetal programming in compromised pregnancies. Chen YC, Sheen JM, Tiao MM, Tain YL, Huang LT. Int J Mol Sci. 2013 Mar 6;14(3):5380-401. PMID:23466884

89 Involvement of PGC-1α in the formation and maintenance of neuronal dendritic spines. Cheng A, Wan R, Yang JL, Kamimura N, Son TG, Ouyang X, Luo Y, Okun E, Mattson MP. Nat Commun. 2012;3:1250. doi: 10.1038/ncomms2238. PMID: 23212379

90 Effect of treadmill running on the expression of genes that are involved in neuronal differentiation in the hippocampus of adult male rats. Mojtahedi S, Kordi MR, Hosseini SE, Omran SF, Soleimani M. Cell Biol Int. 2013 Apr;37(4):276-83. doi: 10.1002/cbin.10022. PMID: 23427087

91 A Western diet impairs CNS energy homeostasis and recovery after spinal cord injury: Link to astrocyte metabolism. Kim HN, Langley MR, Simon WL, Yoon H, Kleppe L, Lanza IR, LeBrasseur NK, Matveyenko A, Scarisbrick IA. Neurobiol Dis. 2020 Jul;141:104934. doi: 10.1016/j.nbd.2020.104934. Epub 2020 May 4. PMID: 32376475

92 Is SIRT6 Activity Neuroprotective and How Does It Differ from SIRT1 in This Regard? Tang BL. Front Cell Neurosci. 2017 Jun 8;11:165. doi: 10.3389/fncel.2017.00165. eCollection 2017. PMID: 28642687

93 Emerging Therapeutic Potential of SIRT6 Modulators. Fiorentino F, Mai A, Rotili D. J Med Chem. 2021 Jul 22;64(14):9732-9758. doi: 10.1021/acs.jmedchem.1c00601. Epub 2021 Jul 2. PMID: 34213345

94 Biological and catalytic functions of sirtuin 6 as targets for small-molecule modulators. Klein MA, Denu JM. J Biol Chem. 2020 Aug 7;295(32):11021-11041. doi: 10.1074/jbc.REV120.011438. Epub 2020 Jun 9. PMID: 32518153

95 Advanced glycoxidation and lipoxidation end products (AGEs and ALEs): an overview of their mechanisms of formation. Vistoli G, De Maddis D, Cipak A, Zarkovic N, Carini M, Aldini G. Free Radic Res. 2013 Aug;47 Suppl

1:3-27. doi: 10.3109/10715762.2013.815348. PMID: 23767955

96 Advanced glycation endproducts in food and their effects on health. Poulsen MW, Hedegaard RV, Andersen JM, de Courten B, Bügel S, Nielsen J, Skibsted LH, Dragsted LO. Food Chem Toxicol. 2013 Oct;60:10-37. doi: 10.1016/j.fct.2013.06.052. PMID: 23867544

97 Associations of dietary advanced glycation end products with liver steatosis via vibration controlled transient elastography in the United States: a nationwide cross-sectional study. Xie F, Zhao J, Liu D, Wan Z, Sun K, Wang Y. Eur J Nutr. 2024 Feb;63(1):173-183. doi: 10.1007/s00394-023-03253-2. PMID: 37779113

98 Higher dietary advanced glycation products intake is associated with increased risk of dementia, independent from genetic predisposition. Zhang Y, Jiang F, Liu D, Li X, Ma Z, Zhang Y, Ma A, Qin LQ, Chen GC, Wan Z. Clin Nutr. 2023 Sep;42(9):1788-1797. doi: 10.1016/j.clnu.2023.08.006. PMID: 37586315

99 Glucosepane is a major protein cross-link of the senescent human extracellular matrix. Relationship with diabetes. Sell DR, Biemel KM, Reihl O, Lederer MO, Strauch CM, Monnier VM. J Biol Chem. 2005 Apr 1;280(13):12310-5. doi: 10.1074/jbc.M500733200. PMID: 15677467

100 Habitual intake of dietary advanced glycation end products is not associated with generalized microvascular function-the Maastricht Study. Linkens AMA, Houben AJHM, Kroon AA, Schram MT, Berendschot TTJM, Webers CAB, van Greevenbroek M, Henry RMA, de Galan B, Stehouwer CDA, Eussen SJMP, Schalkwijk CG. Am J Clin Nutr. 2022 Feb 9;115(2):444-455. doi: 10.1093/ajcn/nqab302. PMID: 34581759

101 Evaluation of the effects of dietary advanced glycation end products on inflammation. Demirer B, Fisunoğlu M. Nutr Bull. 2024 Mar;49(1):6-18. doi: 10.1111/nbu.12653. PMID: 38114851

102 Structures of Toxic Advanced Glycation End-Products Derived from Glyceraldehyde, A Sugar Metabolite. Sakai-Sakasai A, Takeda K, Suzuki H, Takeuchi M. Biomolecules. 2024 Feb 8;14(2):202. doi: 10.3390/biom14020202. PMID: 38397439; PMCID: PMC10887030.

103 Effects of Toxic AGEs (TAGE) on Human Health. Takeuchi M, Sakasai-Sakai A, Takata T, Takino JI, Koriyama Y. Cells. 2022 Jul 12;11(14):2178. doi: 10.3390/cells11142178. PMID: 35883620

104 Intracellular Toxic AGEs (TAGE) Triggers Numerous Types of Cell Damage. Takeuchi M, Sakasai-Sakai A, Takata T, Takino JI, Koriyama Y, Kikuchi C, Furukawa A, Nagamine K, Hori T, Matsunaga T. Biomolecules. 2021 Mar 5;11(3):387. doi: 10.3390/biom11030387. PMID: 33808036

105 Advanced Glycation End-Products in Skeletal Muscle Aging. Olson LC, Redden JT, Schwartz Z, Cohen DJ, McClure MJ. Bioengineering (Basel). 2021 Nov 1;8(11):168. doi: 10.3390/bioengineering8110168. PMID: 34821734

106 Reversible histone glycation is associated with disease-related changes in chromatin architecture. Zheng Q, Omans ND, Leicher R, Osunsade A, Agustinus AS, Finkin-Groner E, D'Ambrosio H, Liu B, Chandarlapaty S, Liu S, David Y. Nat Commun. 2019 Mar 20;10(1):1289. doi: 10.1038/s41467-019-09192-z. PMID: 30894531

107 The Type 2 Diabetes Factor Methylglyoxal Mediates Axon Initial Segment Shortening and Alters Neuronal Function at the Cellular and Network Levels. Griggs RB, Nguyen DVM, Yermakov LM, Jaber JM, Shelby JN, Steinbrunner JK, Miller JA, Gonzalez-Islas C, Wenner P, Susuki K. eNeuro. 2021 Oct 6;8(5):ENEURO.0201-21.2021. doi: 10.1523/ENEURO.0201-21.2021. Print 2021 Sep-Oct. PMID: 34531281

108 Advanced glycation end products (AGEs) and other adducts in aging-related diseases and alcohol-mediated tissue injury. Rungratanawanich W, Qu Y, Wang X, Essa MM, Song BJ. Exp Mol Med. 2021 Feb;53(2):168-188. doi: 10.1038/s12276-021-00561-7.. PMID: 33568752

109 Methylglyoxal in the Brain: From Glycolytic Metabolite to Signalling Molecule. Yang Z, Zhang W, Lu H, Cai S. Molecules. 2022 Nov 15;27(22):7905. doi: 10.3390/molecules27227905. PMID: 36432007

110 AGE-RAGE axis culminates into multiple pathogenic processes: a central road to neurodegeneration. Bhattacharya R, Alam MR, Kamal MA, Seo KJ, Singh LR. Front Mol Neurosci. 2023 May 17;16:1155175. doi: 10.3389/fnmol.2023.1155175. PMID: 37266370

111 Age- and stage-dependent glyoxalase I expression and its activity in normal and Alzheimer's disease brains. Kuhla B, Boeck K, Schmidt A, Ogunlade V, Arendt T, Münch G, Lüth HJ. Neurobiol Aging. 2007 Jan;28(1):29-41. doi: 10.1016/j.neurobiolaging.2005.11.007. Epub 2006 Jan 19. PMID: 16427160

112 Normalizing HIF-1α Signaling Improves Cellular Glucose Metabolism and Blocks the Pathological Pathways of Hyperglycemic Damage. Iacobini C, Vitale M, Pugliese G, Menini S. Biomedicines. 2021 Sep 2;9(9):1139. doi: 10.3390/biomedicines9091139. PMID: 34572324

113 Advanced Glycation End Product Accumulation Is Associated With Low Skeletal Muscle Mass, Weak Muscle Strength, and Reduced Bone Density: The Nagahama Study. Tabara Y, Ikezoe T, Yamanaka M, Setoh K, Segawa H, Kawaguchi T, Kosugi S, Nakayama T, Ichihashi N, Tsuboyama T, Matsuda F; Nagahama Study Group. J Gerontol A Biol Sci Med Sci. 2019 Aug 16;74(9):1446-1453. doi: 10.1093/gerona/gly233. PMID: 30329028

114 A Citrus and Pomegranate Complex Reduces Methylglyoxal in Healthy Elderly Subjects: Secondary Analysis of a Double-Blind Randomized Cross-Over Clinical Trial. Bednarska K, Fecka I, Scheijen JLJM, Ahles S, Vangrieken P, Schalkwijk CG. Int J Mol Sci. 2023 Aug 24;24(17):13168. doi: 10.3390/ijms241713168. PMID: 37685975

115 Quercetin, but Not Epicatechin, Decreases Plasma Concentrations of Methylglyoxal in Adults in a Randomized, Double-Blind, Placebo-Controlled, Crossover Trial with Pure Flavonoids. Van den Eynde MDG, Geleijnse JM, Scheijen JLJM, Hanssen NMJ, Dower JI, Afman LA, Stehouwer CDA, Hollman PCH, Schalkwijk CG. J Nutr. 2018 Dec 1;148(12):1911-1916. doi: 10.1093/jn/nxy236. PMID: 30398646

[116] Novel inhibitory effect of black chokeberry (*Aronia melanocarpa*) from selected eight berries extracts on advanced glycation end-products formation and corresponding mechanism study. Tan H, Cui B, Zheng K, Gao N, An X, Zhang Y, Cheng Z, Nie Y, Zhu J, Wang L, Shimizu K, Sun X, Li B. Food Chem X. 2023 Nov 25;21:101032. doi: 10.1016/j.fochx.2023.101032.. PMID: 38235343

[117] The effect of molecular structure of polyphenols on the kinetics of the trapping reactions with methylglyoxal. Zhu H, Poojary MM, Andersen ML, Lund MN. Food Chem. 2020 Jul 30;319:126500. doi: 10.1016/j.foodchem.2020.126500. PMID: 32146288

[118] Butyrate increases methylglyoxal production through regulation of the JAK2/Stat3/NRF2/Glo1 pathway in castration-resistant prostate cancer cells. Hsia YJ, Lin ZM, Zhang T, Chou TC. Oncol Rep. 2024 May;51(5):71. doi: 10.3892/or.2024.8730. PMID: 38577936

[119] Dietary Responses of Dementia-Related Genes Encoding Metabolic Enzymes. Parnell LD, Magadmi R, Zwanger S, Shukitt-Hale B, Lai CQ, Ordovás JM. Nutrients. 2023 Jan 27;15(3):644. doi: 10.3390/nu15030644. PMID: 36771351

20: Broccoli, Garlic, Cacao, and Dates

Essentials

Broccoli and several other cruciferous vegetables; garlic, onions, and other related allium vegetables (leeks, shallots, scallions), chocolate, and certain fruits contain compounds that have hormetic effects that are beneficial to health. They promote the expression of antioxidant and detoxification agents and decrease the risk of cancer and heart disease. They have anti-aging effects. In animal models, the active compound in broccoli decreases cognitive decline and promotes mitochondrial renewal. Frequent consumption of these vegetables is highly recommended.

The active adaptive compounds that provide the hormetic effect in broccoli and related plants are not actually present in the plant, but rather are produced upon damage to the plant's cells. These active compounds, such as sulforaphane, are defense chemicals that are released when insects chew on the plant. Some of these are too toxic to the plant to be kept around, but are produced when the cells are injured. In cruciferous vegetables, injury-causing rupture of intracellular vesicles releases the enzyme myrosinase, which converts glucoraphanin in the cell into the active toxin/hormetic agent sulforaphane. Cooking broccoli at boiling temperatures denatures myrosinase and destroys its activity, and thus prevents the formation of sulforaphane. Furthermore, sulforaphane is unstable and breaks down fairly rapidly as the temperature increases. Garlic contains an analogous compound and enzyme; upon crushing and rupture of the cell walls in the bulb, the enzyme alliinase is released and converts alliin to the active compound allicin.

Thus, broccoli and similar vegetables need to be properly prepared to provide their hormetic effects. Eating a pound of boiled broccoli does not provide an ounce of disease prevention. The salubrious effects of garlic have similar limitations. Cooking prevents the formation and destroys the active compounds that elicit hormetic responses. Stomach acid also inactivates these enzymes.

Cooking, however, does not destroy the fructans and raffinose present in broccoli and onions that cause gastrointestinal gas, bloating, and dysbiosis when consumed in sufficient volume.

Like other hormetic agents, the "dosage" and frequency of consumption of these compounds need to be considered. Men eating cauliflower or broccoli just one time a week had a 45 to 50% lower risk of prostate cancer, and in a study of men diagnosed with prostate cancer, those consuming cruciferous vegetables three times a week had a 59% decrease in cancer progression. A similar three-times-per-week hormetic dosing time frame appears to apply to garlic and other allium vegetables, and for chocolate. There does not appear to be a significant additional hormetic benefit from dosages less than two days apart.

The compounds from cruciferous vegetables and allium prevent cancer and vascular disease as a result of their promotion of antioxidant proteins and compounds. It likely does not require consumption of large "doses" of these compounds to be effective. Both activate Nrf2 and other pathways. Thus, they can be used in place of each other or used in conjunction. Doubling up on their activity overlaps and they share mechanisms of action is unlikely to add to their efficacy. Some pathways are not shared, and thus, there is likely benefit from consuming both.

Heating of cruciferous vegetables, such as broccoli, and allium vegetables, such as garlic, to temperatures over 70°C (158°F), causes rapid breakdown of the activating enzymes and prevents the formation of the beneficial hormetic compounds in these foods. They should not be heated to temperatures of more than 60°C (140°F) and then, only for short periods, to prevent the inactivation of these compounds.

Only a small amount of broccoli is needed if eaten raw and crushed during chewing, or lightly blanched or steamed. About 15 to 20 grams; a medium-sized fleurette. The SANA diet recommends eating a raw or lightly steamed floret of broccoli or a similar amount of raw cauliflower at least once and preferably several times a week.

The most effective way to use garlic is likely to use a garlic press and add the crushed garlic to a salad or other meal just before serving. An appropriate hormetic serving size of garlic for an adult is about 2 grams, about half of a full-sized clove. Dry garlic can also be used, but it is a bit more than two-times as potent by weight. If using dry garlic, the appropriate hormetic serving is about 875 mg, about one slightly rounded quarter teaspoon of garlic powder.

Chocolate also promotes adaptive responses, but the amount of chocolate required to provoke a hormetic response is not trivial. The required dose is made considerably larger if the cocoa is alkalinized, as it is with most cocoa, as this process causes a 60% loss in the total flavonoid content of cocoa, and makes it less bioavailable. Large doses of chocolate have their downsides – it is toxic, and chocolate toxicity does occur in those consuming too much. Additionally, it is often high in sugar, a stimulant that can affect behavior and disturb sleep, especially in children, can trigger migraine, and is an allergen. Natural cocoa powder has a broader hormetic effect, acting on more systems, than does chocolate.

To maximize the hormetic response requires about 13 grams of *natural cocoa*, or about half of a 3.5-ounce 60% chocolate bar for an adult. Alkalized cocoa should not be used when seeking a hormetic effect.

The peak hormetic dose of dates is at about 12 grams. Two dates a day are a healthy hormetic dose, even in T2D.

Stress Response and Cruciferous Vegetables

Sulforaphane (SPH), a compound present in many cruciferous vegetables (CV) such as broccoli, is a direct activator of KEAP1. Sulforaphane thus promotes the release of Nrf2, and in doing so, induces the production of proteins that conjugate and thus aid in the decontamination and elimination of mutagenic heterocyclic amines (HCA) and many other xenobiotics from the cell, and aid in their excretion into the urine. SPH also induces autophagy through the induction of ERK activation.[1] The autophagy and the renewal of cellular components are dependent on oxidative stress signaling induced by SPH.

Cruciferous vegetables (CV) stand out among vegetables for their anti-inflammatory activity and anticarcinogenic potential. These vegetables from the mustard family have a four-petal flower that forms a cross shape and thus are called cruciferous, from the Latin for cross-bearing. Most of the cruciferous vegetables we eat are from the *Brassica* genus, but there are a few closely related vegetables that can also be grouped with them for their anti-carcinogenic potential.

Glucosinolates are compounds found in *Brassica* vegetables. When an insect chews on the plant, it ruptures vesicles within the cell that contain the enzyme myrosinase. The release of myrosinase and its commingling with glucosinolates in the cytosol causes the removal of a glucose molecule from the glucosinolate and converts it into an isothiocyanate (ITC). The ITC has pungent flavors, recognizable in horseradish, mustard, watercress, capers, and other *Brassica* vegetables. Not only do insects eschew the pungent flavor, but ITCs also make them sick. The ITCs are too toxic even for the plants that make them, which is why they keep the enzyme myrosinase in a separate container to avoid activating the toxin. We are interested in the ITC because it activates anti-inflammatory mechanisms.

Glucoraphanin is one of the glucosinolate compounds. It deters insects from feeding on these plants. Myrosinase splits glucoraphanin into glucose plus an ITC, *raphanin*, or *sulforaphane*. Raphanin has antibiotic and antiviral properties, but was judged too toxic for clinical use. Sulforaphane is a natural pesticide, which is the reason that broccoli bothers to make it. Sulforaphane has anti-inflammatory, antioxidant, anti-carcinogenic, and antimicrobial properties.

Another glucosinolate is sinigrin. Sinigrin, present in mustard seed and several other CV, is broken down by myrosinase into glucose and allyl isothiocyanate. Allyl isothiocyanate is antiinflammatory, bactericidal, insecticidal, and nematicidal (worm killing). Most animals don't enjoy its flavor and avoid eating it.

- Glucoraphanin –› glucose + raphanin or sulforaphane (SFN)
- Sinigrin –› glucose + allyl isothiocyanate (AITH)
- Glucotropaeolin –› glucose + benzyl isothiocyanate (BITC)
- Gluconasturtiin –› glucose + phenethyl isothiocyanate (PEITC)
- Glucobrassicin –› glucose + thiocyanate + indole-3-carbinol (I3C)

Table 20A: Glucosinolates in Brassica Vegetables

Glucosinolate	Source
Glucoraphanin: Sulforaphane	Broccoli, cauliflower, Brussels sprouts, cabbage. Lesser amounts in bok choy, kale, collards, Chinese broccoli, broccoli raab, kohlrabi, mustard, turnip, radish, arugula, and watercress.
Sinigrin: Allyl isothiocyanate	Mustard Seed, radish, horseradish, wasabi, and Brussels sprouts
Glucotropaeolin: Benzyl isothiocyanate	Garden nasturtium (*Tropaeolum majus*)
Gluconasturtiin: Phenethyl isothiocyanate	Watercress, horseradish
Glucobrassicin: indole-3-carbinol	Broccoli, cabbage, cauliflower, Brussels sprouts, collard greens, and kale

The glucosinolate, glucobrassicin, is converted to glucose plus an unstable intermediary ITC that spontaneously converts into thiocyanate and indole-3-carbinol. *Indole-3-carbinol* (I3C) is the subject of considerable research for its anti-carcinogenic, anti-atherogenic, and antioxidant effects.

Nevertheless, indole-3-carbinol likely promotes cancer growth. I3C induces P450 CYP1B1 activity and increases the production of 4-hydroxyestrogen, a known carcinogen that promotes breast and prostate cancers. This effect may be amplified in smokers.

When small amounts of I3C, which are likely to be found in food, meet the stomach acid, it is quickly condensed into dimers or trimers, or it can bind with ascorbic acid (vitamin C). Even if stomach acid is not present, most of the I3C from food is quickly condensed, mostly into the I3C dimer (3,3'-diindolylmethane (DIM), and to a lesser amount, the linear trimer (LTR).

In contrast to I3C, DIM suppresses the cytochrome P450 CYP1B1. I3C also induces CYP3A4, while DIM does not. It is most likely that it is DIM, not I3C, that has anti-carcinogenic effects.[2] The I3C *metabolites* shift the production of estrogens to forms that are less favorable for estrogen-responsive tumor growth.[3] They also suppress NF-κB activation;[4] stimulate the cell cycle regulatory proteins p15, p21, and p27; and down-regulate Bcl-2 and Bcl-xL, thereby arresting tumor growth and promoting apoptosis.

DIM appears to act as an androgen receptor antagonist and inhibits the translocation of these receptors to the nucleus of prostate cancer cells, stopping their action. DIM downregulates prostate-specific antigen (PSA). PSA is a glycoprotein that promotes the proliferation, migration, and metastasis of prostate cancer cells.[5] Thus, PSA is more than just a marker of prostate cancer risk; it is a prostate cancer risk factor and growth promoter. Isothiocyanates SFN, BITC, and especially PEITC, found in watercress, suppress the CXCR4 chemokine receptor in prostate cancer cells, and thus, also decrease prostate cancer cell survival and migration.[6]

CV compounds induce the enzyme glutathione S-transferase (GST) via Nrf2. GST conjugates toxic xenobiotic compounds with glutathione so that they can be eliminated from the cell and the body.

Sulforaphane appears to be the isothiocyanate that most actively induces GST activity. Sulforaphane may also act as an anti-carcinogen by inducing the production of pro-apoptotic proteins in the cell[7] and by protecting the mitochondria from oxidative stress through the induction of glutathione peroxidase/reductase enzymes.[8] Sulforaphane is not only an anti-carcinogen; it is cardioprotective,[9] lowers LDL-cholesterol, and has anti-inflammatory effects.[10]

Consumption of broccoli, Brussels sprouts, cabbage, mustard, watercress, rocket, arugula, and other CVs has been associated with decreased risk of many types of cancer. Most studies find about a 20 percent reduction in the rate of various cancers among people consuming higher, rather than lower, amounts of cruciferous vegetables. These results, however, are influenced by genetics. For example, people consuming higher amounts of CVs have a 26% reduction in lung cancer incidence. Individuals with inactive GST enzymes received twice the reduction in risk as those with the active enzyme allele.[11] Similarly, consuming CVs decreased the risk for colorectal neoplasms to a greater extent for individuals with inactive alleles for GST T1.[12]

There are 22 recognized human GST enzymes, and they are expressed in different amounts in different tissues. Their general function is to detoxify xenobiotics as well as some endogenously produced nonpolar (lipid-soluble) toxins. The GST enzymes link a glutathione molecule to a hot spot on the toxin that would otherwise avidly bind to nucleic acids (DNA and RNA) or intracellular proteins, forming adducts. Such adducts can incapacitate proteins and RNA, and may cause mutations when DNA adducts are formed. Conjugation of the xenobiotic with glutathione prevents this, makes the compound water-soluble, and aids in the transport of the conjugate from the cell into the bloodstream and then into the urine.

Eleven percent of European Americans and 23% of African Americans are homozygous for the GST_{P1} variant with reduced glutathione S-transferase activity, and about 20 percent of Americans *have an inactive variant of the* GST_{T1} gene.[13] *About half of Americans of European descent and 28 percent of African Americans have the* GST_{M1} genotype that provides no enzyme activity. Individuals with the impaired GST genotypes are at higher risk of cellular injury and cancer from exposure to potentially genotoxic compounds, such as HCA from meat cooked at high temperatures. It is these individuals, with inactive GST activity, in whom cruciferous vegetables give the greatest reduction in cancer risk.[14]

Sulforaphane acts via the KEAP1 release of Nrf2. By activating the ARE (Table 18-1), it induces various GST enzymes that provide benefits mostly to those with an inactive GST allele, likely by activating other forms of GST, as well as NQO1, UGT, and other ARE enzymes that take over for the crippled GST's role in detoxification. Thus, the detox effects of ITC are especially beneficial for individuals who have impaired

GST alleles and may offer only marginal benefits to those with normal ones.

GSTs are only one family of several cytoprotective proteins that are induced by the ARE. Cruciferous vegetables not only decrease the mutagenicity of HCA and other toxins but also decrease oxidative stress via Nrf2 activation and suppression of NF-κB. These effects are likely shared by everyone.

Not only have the cruciferous vegetables been found to lower cancer risk, but they also lower the risk of heart disease. The mechanism for this is different from that for preventing DNA damage or for improving DNA repair.

When higher doses of SPH are consumed, it increases the induction of the gene for the enzyme PAPOLG (poly(A) polymerase gamma).[15] After PAPOLG has been transcribed, the polymerase enzyme leaves the cytosol and enters the mitochondria. While the mitochondrion has its own DNA, its DNA only has enough space to code for about 31 genes, far fewer than it needs to do its housekeeping and other functions. Most of the proteins that the mitochondria in our bodies use are human proteins encoded in our genes. PAPOLG is one of these; it is the sole polymerase enzyme responsible for DNA synthesis in the mitochondria.[16] Without this enzyme, the mitochondria are kaput. With more of this enzyme available, the mitochondria can renew themselves more efficiently.

For most individuals, consumption of vegetables high in glucoraphanin slows the aging process by promoting mitochondrial renewal and improving the metabolism of lipids. Sulforaphane was found to ameliorate the cognitive dysfunction in an animal model of Alzheimer's disease.[17] Mitochondrial renewal and the anti-free-radical effect from this and ARE protein expression prevent the formation of oxidative products that damage and age the cells.

The GST_{M1} and GST_{P1} enzymes also prevent activation of c-Jun N-terminal kinase 1 (JNK1) and its downstream signaling that results from oxidative stress. GST_{M1} binds ASK1 (apoptosis signal-regulating kinase), and GST_{P1} binds to JNK1, preventing their activation. ASK1 and JNK1 promote chemotherapeutic resistance by preventing the activation of the MAPK → c-Jun.[18] C-Jun can form a dimer with c-Fos to form AP-1. AP-1 is a transcriptional factor that induces gene expression in response to stressors, including cytokines, growth factors, and intracellular infections. C-Jun: c-Fos AP-1 can promote cell growth and differentiation or apoptosis, depending on what else is going on in the cell. When growth is stimulated, AP-1 can promote cancer proliferation; in other circumstances and under other influences, it can promote apoptosis. Under the influence of NF-κB, c-Jun: c-Fos AP-1 promotes growth and proliferation.

Allyl isothiocyanate (AITC) induces G2/M arrest and caspase 9 and caspase 3 activities in glioma and prostate cancer cells, promoting apoptosis; however, it does not do this in normal cells.[19] [20] Sulforaphane (SFN) promotes apoptosis of lung cancer cells, inhibiting histone deacetylase and arresting the cell cycle in the S phase.[21] SFN can also induce G2/M phase arrest; activate caspases 3, 8, and 9 activities; up-regulate BAX, BID, and Fas; and down-regulate the anti-apoptotic protein Bcl-x; thus promoting apoptosis in leukemia cells.[22] SFN promotes the arrest of the cell cycle; increases JNK activity while inhibiting NF-κB, depletes glutathione; and promotes activation of caspase 8 and 9, thus promoting caspase 3 and the activation of apoptotic proteins, all promoting apoptosis.[23] PEITC induces apoptosis via ROS-mediated JNK activation and the upregulation of the Death Receptor proteins, DR4 and DR5, which promote apoptosis. Additionally, PEITC treatment significantly increased TRAIL-induced apoptosis in glioma and oral cancer cells.[24] [25] DIM also sensitizes cancer cells to TRAIL.[26] PEITC has been shown to inhibit the proliferation and promote apoptosis of glioma, lung, ovarian, and leukemia cells.[27]

Even more remarkable than promoting apoptosis in cancer cells, the ITC compounds from cruciferous vegetables do so selectively while protecting normal cells.[28] [29] This may offer normal cells protection from injury from chemotherapy. As a result of ARE expression induced by SFN, there is increased expression of heme oxygenase-1. (HMOX-1) This prevents the creation of ROS during treatment with doxorubicin, which, at least in vitro, protects cardiac stem cells from doxorubicin-induced oxidative stress and cell death.[30] Preconditioning with SFN 24 hours before an ischemic insult has also been demonstrated to protect the blood-brain barrier and decrease neurologic injury from an induced stroke.[31]

Furthermore, the ITCs have been found to sensitize several lines of cancer cells to chemotherapy. ITCs enhance ER+ breast cancer cells to 4-hydroxytamoxifen.[32] PEITC has been shown to reverse cisplatin resistance in biliary tract cancer cells,[33] potentiates the anti-carcinogenic effect of doxorubicin on hepatocarcinoma cells,[34] and enhances Adriamycin-induced apoptosis of osteosarcoma cells.[35]

Thus, the isothiocyanates

- ❖ prevent cancer,
- ❖ selectively promote apoptotic programmed cell death of cancer cells,

- protect normal cells from apoptosis,
- protect non-cancerous cells from chemotherapy, and
- enhance the anticarcinogenic effects of chemotherapy.

Cruciferous vegetables hold great promise for cancer prevention, as well as for the prevention of other diseases of aging.[36] Nevertheless, they can be a bit short on delivery. Several observational dietary intake studies find only weak and often statistically insignificant associations with cruciferous vegetable intake and reduced cancer risk.[37] This is typically the case for European studies, whereas American studies have been considerably stronger.[38] The reason for this difference has been suggested to result from differences in "post-harvest processing." SFN and other ITC are a fragile lot.

Remember that ITCs are not present in these cruciferous vegetables; it is rather their precursors. ITCs are formed when glucosinolates are acted upon by the enzyme myrosinase that is present in vesicles within the cells of the plant. In intact vegetable tissues, these two compounds are separated and only mixed when the cells are crushed, and the vesicles are broken. The purpose of the isothiocyanates is to act as antibiotics and pesticides; so, activation only occurs when the plant cell is damaged, as when munched upon by an insect, rabbit, or human. Enzymatic hydrolysis of glucoraphanin occurs with the cellular disruption that occurs with chewing, cutting, gentle heating, and juicing, wherein the enzyme myrosinase and glucoraphanin can mix.[39] Even then, most of the ITC may be converted to inactive forms, such as sulforaphane nitrile.

Freezing CV greatly diminishes the production of ITCs. Furthermore, heating a cruciferous vegetable to over 70°C (158°F) inactivates myrosinase completely and thereby greatly diminishes the amount of isothiocyanate produced.[40] [41] Sulforaphane and other ITCs are also heat-labile. SFN is stable at 50°C (122°F) but is destroyed at 90°C (194°F).[42] Fully cooked or boiled cruciferous vegetables have insignificant levels of ITCs and have lost their anti-carcinogenic activity. Most of the CV consumed by people is prepared in a way that nullifies their benefits. Light steaming of CVs increases the availability of ITC.

If cruciferous vegetables are briefly heated to 60°C (140°F) and then crushed (chewed) or milled, the amount of sulforaphane produced is greatly increased.[43] A person derives more anti-aging and anticarcinogenic benefits from eating a single sprig of raw broccoli than a pound of boiled broccoli. This may be why cauliflower, which is often eaten raw, has been found in population studies to provide more benefit than broccoli. If myrosinase is inactivated, small amounts of glucosinolates from CV may be converted to ITCs by bacteria in the gut that produce myrosinase, and they can then be absorbed as dithiocarbamates.[44]

Plants that have the myrosinase-glucosinolate defense system include cruciferous vegetables from the mustard family, which include purple cabbage, red cabbage, and broccoli inflorescences. Some closely related plants, including radishes, watercress, garden cress, daikon, and wasabi, are also rich in glucoraphanin.[45] Radishes, radish seed sprouts, and watercress contain glucoraphanin.[46] One advantage of these is that they are usually eaten raw. Radish seedlings and watercress have pleasant spicy flavors.

> The health benefits of cruciferous vegetables can be maximized by eating them raw. They can also be juiced, preferably after heating them to 60°C (140°F). The juice can then be refrigerated (34 – 38° F) for later consumption. If preparing cruciferous vegetables for eating cooked, they should be only very lightly heated to an internal temperature of 60°C (140°F) and eaten while still warm to maximize sulforaphane availability.
>
> Thus, broccoli or other CV can be:
>
> - Blanched in 60°C (140°F) water for 10 minutes
> - Broken into florets and steamed above boiling water for 3 minutes
> - Very briefly microwaved, just until the color darkens slightly
> - Eaten raw.
>
> Garlic also loses its hormetic potency when heated, and likely has its maximal potency when consumed raw, even if in small amounts.

Fresh cruciferous vegetables are recommended over frozen ones. Canning of CV would expose them to sterilizing temperatures, destroying their anticarcinogenic compounds. Snacking on raw cauliflower, broccoli, cabbage (salad or coleslaw), radishes, or CV seed sprouts is a way to ensure that the ITC will be available and not destroyed by heating. Juicing CV can also provide ITC. (Consumption of cabbage and Brussels sprouts is discouraged on the SANA diet.)

Seed sprouts of cruciferous vegetables, for example, from broccoli, radish, and mustard seeds, have very high glucosinolate contents, having 20 to 50 times as much ITC as the mature harvested plants. Only a small amount is required to stimulate Nrf2-induced anti-inflammatory and anti-carcinogenic protection. Additionally, these are usually eaten raw.

Eating one or more servings of cauliflower a week decreases the risk of developing prostate cancer in men by over 50% compared to those men who eat it less than once a month. One or more servings of broccoli a week decreased prostate cancer risk by 45% compared to men who ate it less than once a month[47]. It does not appear to require high doses.

Even more compelling is that the consumption of cruciferous vegetables decreases cancer progression. In a study of men diagnosed with prostate cancer, those in the highest quartile of cruciferous vegetable consumption had a 59% decrease in cancer progression.[48] Those in the highest quartile were consuming broccoli about 3 times a week, or cabbage or cauliflower once a week, compared to the lowest quartile, who reported no CV intake.

Eating two to three servings of properly prepared, fresh CV a week (not boiled broccoli or Brussels sprouts rendered into a paste) is probably sufficient to provide anti-aging and anticancer effects. The most important thing is to make sure that the serving has anti-carcinogenic potential. These studies suggest that large or daily doses of ITC are not required.

Remember, these compounds are seen by the body as toxins and respond through hormesis, rather than as a pharmaceutical type, dose-response effect. There is no evidence of toxicity from eating the small doses of ITC that are encountered when eating CV a few times a week. Moderate doses appear to be safe over the short term,[49]

The recommended hormetic dose of raw, lightly blanched, or steamed broccoli or cauliflower is about 16 grams, just over half of an ounce. This is about the size of a medium fleurette. Consuming a CV every other day or every third day likely provides the maximum benefits.

Garlic and other Allium

Stress Response and Garlic

When garlic is injured by munching insects or otherwise has its cells damaged by crushing, chopping, chewing, and mincing, an enzyme is released from damaged vacuoles in the cell that converts cysteine sulfoxides contained in the cytosol into allicin. Allicin instantly decomposes into diallyl sulfide (DAS) and other compounds. DAS activates Nrf2 and thus, ARE. DAS also activates the Constitutive Androstane Receptor (CAR) that stimulates the transcription of several enzymes involved in endobiotic and xenobiotic metabolism, including several p450 oxidases, sulfotransferases, and glutathione-S-transferases. DAS also inhibits IκBα phosphorylation and translocation of NF-κB to the nucleus.[50] Thus, diallyl sulfide not only increases phase 1 and phase 2 metabolism of endo- and xenobiotics, but it also inhibits the transcription of pro-inflammatory mediators. This effect is likely limited to raw or gently heated garlic.

Garlic, onions, and related *Allium* species, like CV, are rich in sulfur compounds, thiosulfinates in the case of *allium*, which are activated by an enzyme upon injury to their tissues. And like CV, garlic activates Nrf2 and the ARE. Garlic prevents cancer, at least in part, by inhibiting the activation of CYP1A1 and CYP1A2, enzymes that transform HCA to active carcinogens. It is antineoplastic; it promotes apoptosis of cancer cells by arresting the cell cycle at the G2/M checkpoint. Furthermore, it protects the liver from many toxins, including the carcinogen aflatoxin and the chemotherapy drug doxorubicin.[51] [52] Garlic has been called, and may be, the most anticarcinogenic food. Garlic appears to both protect animals from cancer chemotherapy medications[53] and may even enhance the efficacy of some chemotherapy medications.[54]

The principal compound thought to be responsible for garlic's health effects is allium. About one percent of the weight of garlic is composed of allyl-thiosulfinates (ATS), and about 80% of these are the compound alliin. Upon crushing and rupture of the cell walls in the bulb, the enzyme alliinase is released and converts alliin to allicin. Although allicin may be present in the food, it does not reach the bloodstream. Allicin is reactive and is converted into several other compounds, mostly diallyl sulfides (DAS), and lesser amounts of allyl methyl sulfides, diallyl trisulfides (DATS), ajoene, and other compounds. Other ATS in *allium* are converted to S-allyl-cysteine (SAC) and S-allyl-mercaptocysteine (SAMC), other compounds.

Most research points to SAC and SAMC as the important anticancer compounds in garlic.[55] SAC has been shown to bind to estrogen, progesterone, androgen, and glucocorticoid receptors and inhibit their activity.[56] DATS, however, has been demonstrated to inhibit cell cycle progression and decrease mTOR, EGFR, VEGF, and Bcl-2. Ajoene inhibits the proliferation of breast and colon cancer cells and induces apoptosis in human leukemia cells.[57] Consuming the food, rather than isolated garlic extracts, supplies a wide range of anti-carcinogenic substances.

In a study of lung cancer in men, consuming *raw garlic* two or more times a week decreased lung cancer incidence among smokers by nearly one-half. The average amount of raw garlic consumed for this anti-cancer benefit was 30 grams, just over one ounce per week, about half the weight of a medium-sized head of garlic. Even those consuming only around 9 grams per week, about three good-sized cloves of raw garlic a week, had significantly reduced cancer risk.[58]

In a study of the efficacy of garlic on cancer, mice were implanted with sarcoma cells. The mice were then treated with extracts from fresh garlic or garlic leaves, or extracts that had been heated in a microwave oven or boiled. Fresh garlic and its leaves prevented cancer growth, but heating reduced the effects dramatically.[59]

Garlic has anti-thrombotic and anti-hypertensive effects. It inhibits the uptake of LDL-cholesterol by macrophages, which reduces the risk of heart disease. Much of the literature on the effect of cooked vs. raw garlic and other *allium* vegetables has studied their antiplatelet activity (APA), which can easily be tested in the lab (*in vitro).* The APA appears to be related to the presence of allicin, and thus, is likely a helpful indicator of allyl-thiosulfinates activity versus its loss of activity during food preparation.

Steaming raw, quartered onions for one minute raises their internal temperature to 44° C (111° F) and decreases the APA by 18 percent as compared to raw onions. Steaming the onions for 3 minutes raised their internal temperature to 66° C (151° F) and reduced APA by 85%. By six minutes, platelet aggregation *increased* over baseline. Thus, 66° C is sufficient to inactivate alliinase.[60] Garlic has an APA activity about 13 times higher than onions. Boiling or heating intact garlic in an oven set to 200° F for 6 minutes completely inhibits APA activity. Crushing garlic (or onions) before heating allows alliinase to convert alliin into allicin before heating. This extends the APA resistance to heat, but still, APA activity is completely lost in crushed garlic exposed to boiling temperatures in less than 10 minutes.[61] [62] Thus, it is not just that the enzyme alliinase is denatured by heat, but allicin is also destroyed by heating it to a boiling temperature.

At refrigerator temperatures (below 4°C – 39° F), allicin has a half-life of about one year, meaning that it loses half of its activity in that much time. At room temperature (23° C - 73.4° F), the half-life of allicin is nine days. At 37 C° (98.6°F it is 27 hours, and at 42° C (108°F) it is under 17 hours.[63] Extrapolating from this data, the half-life of allicin is estimated to be about 3.5 hours at 50° C (122° F), 43 minutes at 60° C (140° F), less than about 9 minutes at 70° C (158° F), under two minutes at 80°C (176° F), and less than 4 seconds at 90° C (194°F).

Garlic can be sautéed or otherwise cooked to enjoy its flavor and aroma, but it will not provide hormetic health benefits. Garlic can be cooked into food, and more added just before serving to get the hormetic effects.

To obtain the health benefits of garlic, it should be consumed raw or very gently heated. Chopped onions can be added uncooked to salads and other dishes. When garlic is wanted to flavor a cooked food, it can be added, as crushed or finely minced fresh garlic, after the meal is cooked, just before serving, when the food temperature has fallen below 60° C. A temperature of 56° C (133° F) or under is a reasonable serving temperature to prevent thermal injury. Uncooked garlic has a stronger flavor, and thus, the amount needed for flavoring will be lowered. Swallowing garlic whole is not helpful, as alliinase is degraded by stomach acids; the allium must be crushed by chewing.

The best method to obtain the benefits from garlic is likely obtained by putting garlic through a garlic press and using the crushed raw garlic on food. Crushed garlic can be mixed into a salad and stored in the refrigerator until served, preserving the ATS. When properly prepared, less garlic is needed to achieve a peak hormetic dose. This is estimated to be under two grams, every other day.

Dry powdered garlic contains active alliin and alliinase and is stable at room temperature for months. The alliin present in dry garlic powder is converted to allicin within seconds of hydration. Thus, adding garlic powder to a moist dish that is ready to serve is another way to deliver garlic's health benefits. During drying, there is a loss of activity, so even though two-thirds of the weight of fresh garlic has been removed as water, a similar weight of dry powder garlic as fresh garlic is needed to provide the same health benefits.[64] A level ¼-teaspoon of dry garlic powder weighs about 1 gram.

CAUTION: While the low doses of garlic that are likely to be consumed as part of a healthy diet have hormetic effects, high doses can have toxicity. In rats, chronic exposure to a metabolically equivalent daily dose of garlic for humans, approximately 40 mg/kg body weight, increased ARE enzymes. At 50 mg/kg, there was decreased spermatogenesis. Such growth inhibition might be OK for cancer patients, but it is likely problematic for children or pregnant women. At doses equivalent to 80 mg/kg for humans, the rats had a decrease in ARE enzymes and lung and liver damage. Forty mg/kg would be equivalent to two grams of raw garlic or garlic powder a day for a 50 kg (110-pound) woman. Garlic and onions may be toxic to dogs and cats, with some breeds being highly sensitive. Thus, extrapolating garlic toxicity doses from rats may be misleading. Although humans tolerate much higher doses of garlic, the SANA diet recommends a dose of 30 mg/kg of (crushed) raw garlic, a hormetic dose for activating the ARE. This is about 1.9 grams for most adults, somewhere around half of a large clove of garlic. If using dry powdered garlic, the hormetic adult dose is slightly less than half that, about 875 mg.

Water extracts from garlic, such as those in aged garlic extracts, have much lower toxicity than oil extracts, and thus, these would be recommended if higher doses are wanted. Aged garlic extracts are rich in SAC and do not give a garlic breath odor, but they do not provide all of the benefits of fresh garlic in cancer prevention. Garlic oil extracts are not recommended as they may be more toxic and do not contain SAC.

Allergic reactions to garlic are not rare and can be triggered by topical use on the skin, as sometimes used for acne. Garlic capsules generally fail to hydrate and activate the alliinase, and alliinase is inactivated by stomach acid. Thus, garlic capsules are ineffective.

WATERCRESS JUICE

Watercress provides high levels of PEITC, an ITC with anticarcinogenic properties. Here is a distinctive juice with a refreshing bite from the book A Taste of Paradise, made with watercress. (Used with permission.) It is used as a folk remedy in the Caribbean to treat colds and the flu.

Ingredients:

- ½ cup of watercress leaves and stems
- 1 cup orange juice (chilled)
- 1 - 2 tablespoons sugar

PREPARATION: Place the orange juice, watercress, and sugar in a blender and liquefy for one minute at high speed. Serve directly or over ice.

Chocolate

The Latin name for the cacao plant is *Theobroma*; literally, food of the gods. Cocoa and chocolate get DAD scores of 1 to 2. They do not do much for the microbiome. That is not an amazing score for "the food of the gods." The Aztec name from which we get the word chocolate is humbler; xocolatl means 'bitter water'. Nevertheless, cocoa gets a HAR score of 10, depending on its processing.

Cocoa is high in the flavanols (+)-catechin, epicatechin, procyanidin dimers B1 and B2, trimer C1, cinnamotannin A2, and caffeoyl aspartic acid.[65] Some studies show that dark chocolate is additionally high in quercetin and ferulic acid.[66] On the dark side, chocolate contains biogenic amines such as tyramine, which can trigger migraines in some people, especially those with a leaky gut. β-phenylethylamine (βPEA) is found in chocolate, especially when the cocoa beans have been fermented. Chocolate contains the compound theobromine, which is closely related to caffeine.

- Chocolate is widely identified as a trigger for migraine.
- Chocolate provokes behavioral changes, especially in children. Chocolate provides an initial sense of energy and pleasant excitement, but can be followed by depression and moodiness hours to a day later. This effect has often been attributed to βPEA.
- Chocolate contains high levels of the stimulant theobromine, an isomer of caffeine. Theobromine is toxic at high levels.

Chocolate and Sleep

Chocolate can disturb sleep. Chocolate contains caffeine, less than coffee, but depending on the individual and the amount consumed, there may be sufficient caffeine to prevent sleep. Chocolate also contains the alkaloid theobromine, a methylxanthine compound similar to caffeine, but at a level several times higher than its caffeine content. Like caffeine, theobromine binds to adenosine receptors, stimulates wakefulness, and may cause insomnia. Theobromine's effect on wakefulness, however, is milder than that of caffeine. Caffeine is partially metabolized into theobromine. Black and green tea, cola, and guarana also contain caffeine and theobromine.

For most individuals, the half-life of theobromine (TBr) is from five to nine hours.[67] This means that 25% of the TBr is still present in their system 14 hours after the ingestion of chocolate. For someone who metabolizes TBr slowly, the TBr can accumulate from one day to the next. Most people can enjoy small amounts of dark chocolate early in the day to give an energy boost. However, consuming chocolate late in the day may provoke insomnia and irritability. Sleep disturbances from chocolate may be avoided by limiting the amount of chocolate, especially dark chocolate and chocolate desserts, consumed. Even small amounts of chocolate affect behavior and sleep in children.

Death by Chocolate

The toxicity of chocolate to pets from theobromine is well documented. When pets eat chocolate, the effects of TBr toxicity include nausea, vomiting, diarrhea, and increased urination. Poisoning can also cause seizures, cardiac arrhythmia, and death. Less well known is that TBr poisoning from ingestion of chocolate also occurs in humans. Theobromine toxicity is rarely recognized, but it can present in the emergency department, usually in smaller women, presenting with confusion and difficulty walking. It looks like what it is: a drug overdose or poisoning.

Chocolate poisoning, assumed to be caused by excessive TBr, causes hyperventilation, which may trigger panic attack symptoms; confusion, anxiety, agitation, emotional lability, increased urination, hypotension, and tachycardia. Ataxia (difficulty walking) and slurring of the speech have also been reported. Seizures and cardiac dysrhythmias can occur from TBr toxicity.[67].

The usual minimal toxic dose of TBr in humans is about 10 mg per pound (@ 25 mg/kg) of body weight. At this dose, the toxic effects may include sweating, nausea, anorexia, trembling, and severe headache. This may occur in adults consuming 800 to 1500 mg of TBr per day. White chocolate has very low levels of TBr, and a 1½ ounce Hershey milk chocolate bar only has about 75 mg of theobromine. Dark chocolate, however, has much higher levels; an extra dark chocolate bar can have five times the TBr content per ounce as milk chocolate. A three-ounce extra dark 82% cacao bar can have over 700 mg of theobromine (plus over 100 mg of caffeine). Four to five chocolate equivalents (see Table 20B below) are enough to cause toxicity. Spread over several hours, most adults might enjoy a pleasant pharmacologic stimulus without ill effect. Consumption of two dark chocolate bars or their equivalent in brownies, fudge, cake, ice cream, and beverages by a small adult in less than a couple of hours can be sufficient to win a no-expense-paid ambulance ride to the emergency department of one's local hospital. It does not take that much chocolate to land a migraineur in the ER.

Theobromine is metabolized by cytochrome P450 enzymes in the liver. Two different enzymes, CYP2E1 and CYP1A2, appear to be responsible for this process; however, there is genetic variability, and CYP1A2 does not process TBr in some individuals.[68] Further, these enzymes can be inhibited by certain medications, such as cimetidine, ciprofloxacin, contraceptives, and caffeine, or certain foods such as grapefruit and some mushrooms. Enzyme activity is genetically and epigenetically determined and is less active in some people. CYP2E1 and CYP1A2 activity are often lower in the elderly because of slower metabolism and the use of interfering medications. Children may be at risk because of their smaller body mass. Like alcohol, where consumption of two drinks over several hours is unlikely to cause intoxication, but a couple of shots, over a few minutes, can have a potent effect; larger amounts of chocolate over a short time raise blood levels of TBr higher, and induce more risk of toxicity, especially on an empty stomach.

Chocolate and Behavior

Chocolate consumption can trigger hyperactivity, emotional lability, and irritability. This is especially evident in children who are more susceptible, as they are likely to consume more chocolate in relation to their body mass. When my children were small, chocolate was banished from the home, not because of the great highs, with my kids bouncing on the bed, the singing, silliness, and laughter, but because of the terrible tears and fits that followed, lasting longer than the bliss. This response to chocolate is likely the combined effects of caffeine, theobromine, β-phenylethylamine (βPEA), and sugar. Children's frontal lobes are less developed, giving them less control over their emotions and behavior. Thus, children's behavior is more strongly affected by chocolate than is adult behavior.

β-PEA and tyramine are strong agonists for the trace amine receptors TAAR1 and TAAR2. βPEA has been described as the body's endogenous amphetamine.[69] The hyperactivity and pleasure derived from chocolate may result from an amphetamine-like effect of βPEA and the release of NE from nerve terminals. Some chocolate preparations also contain food coloring that may provoke hyperactivity.

Chocolate Headaches

In addition to the toxic effects of TBr, other natural compounds in chocolate can trigger headaches, even at low doses. βPEA from food is usually metabolized quickly by monoamine oxidase (MAO), and thus, has a half-life of only several minutes. MAO-inhibiting medications, however, can cause great increases in the amount of tyramine and βPEA reaching the brain. Diamine oxidase, which breaks down histamine and other bioamines, is inhibited by theobromine, caffeine, βPEA, and TBr, all found in chocolate. Thus, chocolate may trigger migraine in part by inhibiting enzymes that break down histamine and other biogenic amines. When chocolate provokes migraines, it usually occurs 10 or more hours after consuming the chocolate. This suggests a secondary reaction, rather than the direct action of βPEA. βPEA is a preferred ligand for trace amine receptors in the brain, and the delayed onset of migraine suggests an action via the calcitonin gene-related peptide (CGRP). Caffeine withdrawal can also trigger rebound headaches, and this may also occur with theobromine.

Immune Reactions

The delayed adverse reaction to chocolate, which results in migraine, suggests the induction of protein synthesis, as occurs with CGRP and migraine, or may be secondary to delayed (IgG) hypersensitivity reaction requiring the formation of leukotrienes or other secondary responses. Immunologic reactions can also affect sleep and cause irritability and fatigue. Chocolate can also trigger immediate (IgE) allergic reactions. Individuals with immune reactions to chocolate should completely avoid it.

Osteoporosis

Daily chocolate consumption has been found to lower bone density in women[70]. Consumption of high levels of caffeine, more than 3 cups of coffee a day, is also associated with an increased risk of osteoporosis.

Fat

Cocoa butter is not a healthy fat. Chocolate consumption has been associated with an increased risk of developing inflammatory bowel disease (IBD).[71] The SANA program contends that the IBD-associated risk from chocolate is from the cocoa butter rather than from the cocoa, and thus white chocolate would confer risk of IBD, while natural cocoa powder should not.

Benefits of Chocolate

Aside from the pleasure of chocolate, dark chocolate is rich in polyphenols with health benefits.

- It lowers blood pressure in those with hypertension.[72] [73]
- Flavonoid-rich cacao increases blood flow to the coronary arteries.[74] [75]
- In mice with T2D, cacao flavanols were found to improve the mitochondrial structure in their cardiac and skeletal muscles.[76]
- After 3 months of exercise, those consuming dark chocolate had increased pAMPK, PCG1α, and mitochondrial citrate synthase activity in their muscles, and a higher maximal workload, while those doing exercise alone did not.[77]
- Cacao (15 grams) with 55 mg of epicatechin daily increased walking distance in patients with lower extremity peripheral artery disease. It improved blood flow to the lower extremities, activated Nrf2, and protected against oxidative stress and mitochondrial dysfunction.[78] [79]
- It improves insulin sensitivity and beta-cell function in persons with insulin resistance.[80]
- It may prevent LDL cholesterol from becoming oxidized and may increase HDL cholesterol.[81]
- It may improve symptoms in patients with chronic fatigue syndrome.[82]
- Several studies have failed to find any increase in body weight associated with dark chocolate consumption.
- Adults consuming 20 grams of dark chocolate three times a week had lower C-reactive protein levels, showing its anti-inflammatory properties,[83] and it may decrease the formation of TNF-α in response to LPS.
- The French woman, Jeanne Calment, who regularly ate 7 ounces of chocolate a day, died soon after her doctor convinced her to cut back on sweets, at the age of 122.[84]

Cocoa vs. Cacao

Most of the cacao powder used in the U.S. and Europe is sold as cocoa powder. The distinction is the result of a several-century-old spelling mistake. The FDA does not differentiate labeling for cacao and cocoa powders, so it is the vendor's decision on what to call them. Generally, cacao is used by vendors who hope to distinguish themselves from traditional store brands of cocoa, by way of being organically grown and fair-trade products.

Production of Cacao and Chocolate

Raw cacao beans are first fermented for several days and then dried. The next step is to roast them, which develops their flavor and gives them some sweetness. The roasted seeds are then crushed and separated from their hulls, yielding cacao nibs. The nibs are ground to form a thick paste, which, when warmed, is called chocolate liquor, which can be cooled and formed into blocks of raw chocolate. The liquor is about 50% cocoa butter. The cocoa butter can also be separated from the cacao solids. The solids are pressed to separate the cocoa butter, generally leaving 10 – 12% fat, but a higher amount of the fat can be left in the cacao powder. Natural cacao powder is light brown and has an acidic pH (of 5.3 to 5.8). Sugar, lecithin, milk, and other products are added to chocolate to make various types of chocolate.

Cacao is often alkalized to make "Dutch chocolate" to improve the flavor by making the cocoa less acidic, less bitter, smoother, darker, and more soluble in water. Alkalized cacao is used in most commercial cake and brownie mixes, ice cream, and chocolate milk. Alkalization can be done with the nibs or with the cacao solids, and since water is added during the process, the product needs drying, and further roasting is done, giving the cocoa a darker color.[85]

Much of the health benefits of chocolate, including its antioxidant activity, result from chocolate's content of phenolic compounds, which is higher than that of black or green tea or red wine.[86] Dark chocolate, such as bittersweet dark chocolate, is richer in phenolic compounds than milder chocolate. In general, the phenolic content of chocolate is: natural cocoa powder > baking chocolate > dark chocolate or bittersweet baking chips > Dutch chocolate > milk chocolate > chocolate syrup.[87] At appropriate levels, the theobromine and caffeine in chocolate likely help prevent Parkinson's disease through an adenosine-mediated pathway.

Unfortunately, alkalization of cacao results in a 60% loss in total flavonoids and makes the remaining flavonoids less bioavailable.[88] [89] Thus, more alkalized chocolate is required to get a hormetic dose; meanwhile, the amount of theobromine and caffeine remains. Post-harvest processing of cacao can decrease the flavanols to less than one-tenth of their original content.[90] It may not be possible to get an optimal hormetic dose of chocolate flavanols without getting a toxic or near-toxic dose of theobromine. Roasting time and temperature also impact the flavanol and theobromine content of cacao.[91] There is an inverse linear correlation between the degree of alkalization of cocoa to the flavanol content of the end-product. At its natural pH of about 5.5, cacao powder contains an average of around 35 – 40 mg/g of flavonols; with a pH of 7.0, the phenol content is about a third of that, and at a pH of 8.0, the flavanol content is less than 5 mg/gram. Alkalized cocoa powder sold in the U.S. generally contains about 2.0 mg/gram of flavanols, about one-twentieth of the original amount.[92]

Natural cocoa powder is rich in flavonols. I have found no evidence that those labelled natural *cacao* have higher levels than those labelled natural *cocoa* powder.

Baking soda (sodium bicarbonate) is used in baking to generate bubbles to get the baked goods to rise and create the "foam" in cakes, muffins, and soft cookies. Baking soda requires an acid to react with, while baking powder contains its own. Molasses and brown sugar are acidic enough to react with soda to form the carbon dioxide bubbles. Sodium bicarbonate has been used to process cocoa into alkalized cocoa.[93] When natural cocoa is used in baking, it helps produce CO_2 gas from baking soda, thus alkalizing it. Depending on the balance, this may destroy the phenolic activity in baked goods.

The flavanol and procyanidin content in frosting (not recommended) and chocolate milk was unchanged, and that in cookies declined by about 15%. There was a 95% loss of epicatechin in chocolate cakes, and a 100% loss in commercially available cake mixes. If baking powder was used in place of baking soda so that the pH remained acidic (pH around 6.2), the antioxidant and flavanol content was retained.[94] Thus, if baking with natural cacao powder, baking powder, or sufficient acid to neutralize the baking soda should be used to retain flavonol activity.

It appears that there may be a sweet spot for the health effects of dark chocolate. For blood pressure control, 20 grams of dark chocolate daily was found to be equally effective as 40 grams.[95] In another study,[96] a beneficial anti-inflammatory effect was associated with consuming a 20-gram serving of dark chocolate every three days.[97]

Theobromine in chocolate also has an important role. In an analysis of NHANES data, total dietary theobromine from chocolate and coffee was associated with cognitive performance in older adults. In this study, men and women had differential impacts. CERAD (error) scores were lowest for women with a total theobromine intake between 90 and 120 mg/day, with about 35 to 40 percent lower scores than those consuming no theobromine. It might likely be more accurate to say that 700 mg of theobromine per week, in divided doses, was most effective. Women had an L-shaped response curve with no further benefit at higher doses. In men, however, CERAD scores continued to fall by well over 80% among those consuming over 1400 mg of theobromine per week, with an apparently safe dose of up to 350 mg/per day in men. The effect of theobromine-containing foods on CERAD scores was much greater in men, even at the same dose as in women.[98] Additionally, a weak direct correlation between chocolate intake and depression was seen in the NHANES study data in women, but not in men.[99]

Hypothesis: A differential metabolic response to chocolate and theobromine between men and women seems less likely than a differential consumption of chocolate.

Women may be more likely to binge on chocolate, and American women report craving chocolate around their menstrual periods; 24% of American women report perimenstrual chocolate indulgences. Men may be more likely to use chocolate as an energy boost.[100] [101]

The association of chocolate consumption with a higher odds of depression in women but not in men is likely reverse causality; women who are depressed may turn to chocolate as a comfort food and mild psychotropic more commonly than men, who, for example, are more likely to self-medicate with alcohol.

The finding that women have peak benefit from 700 mg of theobromine per week while men may have peak benefit at around 700 mg three times per week might arise from a differential preference in the type of chocolate consumed.

For chocolate to be used for its health benefits, it should be consumed in a healthy format. It may be that when women consume chocolate, it may be more preferentially consumed as alkalinized milk chocolate, chocolate milk, or alkalized cocoa in brownies and cake or other forms that have little hormetic benefit. Occasional high-dose binging of chocolate, especially alkalized chocolate, is also unlikely to provide hormetic benefits.

Theobromine and caffeine neurotoxicity are more commonly seen in women than in men. This likely results from having a lower body mass and perhaps a preference for alkalized chocolate. Women, however, appear to have higher xanthine oxidase activity than men (and Caucasians have higher activity than Blacks); thus, caffeine and theobromine metabolism may be different in women.[102]

The SANA program suggests that a "Hormetic Chocolate Serving Equivalent" based on flavanol activity for chocolate, in which one Serving Equivalent is equivalent to 9 grams of natural cocoa powder, is an appropriate adult hormetic serving size for healthful consumption. Nevertheless, unless the chocolate product is tested and the flavanol content stated, it is hard to create an ideal equivalency table. Even then, we don't know which flavanols, or mix of phenolic compounds in cacao, maximize its health benefits. The hormetic dose range for cacao is fairly wide. For 100% chocolate liquor, the range is from about 11 to 51 grams, with a geometric mean of about 23 grams. Thus, the hormetic range is about half to double the 23-gram dose. For natural cocoa powder, it is about half, with a range of 4.5 to 19.5 grams. Raw cacao has different levels of phenolic compounds and theobromine depending upon the cultivar of the plant, growing conditions, and postharvest processing. The serving equivalent is given to provide a rough comparison of the amount of chocolate in different forms of chocolate.

Chocolate liquor averages 1.22% theobromine and 0.21% caffeine, while cocoa contains 1.89% theobromine and 0.21% caffeine, but there can be a wide variance between samples.[103]

The serving equivalent gives the estimated theobromine level of various natural chocolate preparations, providing a theobromine equivalency and thus some safety against theobromine overdose. It is assumed that it provides a rough polyphenol content equivalency.

Table 20B: Suggested Dark Chocolate Serving Equivalents*

Chocolate	Theobromine @ mg/kg[104]	Serving Equivalent (Approximate Range)	Theobromine per equivalent
Cocoa powder (natural, not alkalinized)	18,900	@ 9 grams (4.5 to 19.5 grams) @ 1.5 level Tbsp.	@ 170 mg
100% Chocolate liquor; Unsweetened Baking Chocolate	12,200	23 grams (11 to 51 grams) (0.39 to 1.8 oz.)	@ 280 mg
70% Dark chocolate	8,540	@ 31 grams (14 to 69 grams) (0.5 to 2.4 oz.)	@ 262 mg
60% Dark Chocolate	7,320	@ 34 g 15.5 to 76 grams (0.55 to 2.7 oz.)	@ 249 mg
Milk Chocolate	1,004	Avoid	

Note that these are approximate doses for promoting a hormetic impact of phenolic compounds in cacao, rather than for theobromine levels present. Note that cocoa powder has a broader hormetic range.

While 9 grams of natural cocoa has a similar *hormetic dose* equivalence to 23 grams of chocolate liquor, the hormetic impact of cocoa and chocolate is not equivalent. A chocolate equivalent of 9 grams of cocoa and 23 grams of 100% chocolate has about the same impact on certain hormetic pathways, but natural cocoa acts on additional hormetic pathways that chocolate does not. Thus, between the two, natural cocoa is the better choice for stimulating broad hormetic effects. The health impact difference between cocoa and chocolate has been attributed to the addition of sugar and fat content,[105] but it is more likely that cocoa butter impedes a broader hormetic effect.

If the health benefits are the excuse to justify eating chocolate, natural cocoa-based products should be selected, and the amount consumed should be limited to about one "dark chocolate serving equivalent", best as one "natural cocoa equivalent" dosed every other day to twice weekly. A tablespoon of cocoa is about the amount that might be used in a cup of mild hot chocolate or a thin slice of chocolate cake.

Natural cocoa powder and products made from it will have less theobromine for the phenolic content than chocolate, and Dutch (alkalized) cocoa has significantly less hormetic impact, but all of the theobromine.

Summary for Chocolate

1. Cacao is a source of phenolic compounds: Cacao is a healthful food high in phenolic compounds. Consuming one chocolate equivalent (9 grams of natural cocoa or 23 grams of 100% chocolate liquor) two to three times a week appears to be sufficient to provide the optimal health benefits from chocolate. Natural cocoa powder has broader hormetic effects than does chocolate, which is thus the preferred ingredient, health-wise, by the SANA program.
2. Cacao can be toxic in high doses, mainly as a result of theobromine. Enjoy it in moderation. The pharmacologic effects of chocolate can cause behavioral effects, especially in children. Keep it away from animals.
3. Cacao is a stimulant and can cause insomnia.
4. Cacao can cause both immune and pseudoallergic reactions.
5. Cacao is a common trigger for migraine headaches.
6. Cacao is fun and can be used as a hormetic agent if used at the proper dose and frequency.
7. Nine grams of natural cocoa powder (about one-third of an ounce) is a healthy hormetic dose.
8. If using cocoa for baking, avoid the use of baking soda to avoid alkalinizing the cocoa, or use enough acidic components (applesauce, molasses) to make sure that the resultant recipe remains slightly acidic.
9. Cocoa butter is an unhealthy fat. White chocolate gets a DAD score of D. For those sensitive, such as those with IBD, milk chocolate scores a C.
10. The SANA program recommends cocoa over chocolate as a hormetic treat.

To substitute cocoa in place of baking chocolate, use 62.5% of the weight of the chocolate being replaced with cocoa, and 37.5% with unsalted butter. Butter is about 80% butterfat, 15% water, and 5% milk solids. To make sweetened chocolate substitutes, the water in the butter helps dissolve the sugar, which is why butter is preferred over coconut oil.

Table 20C: Approximate Grams of Fat and Sugar in 100 Grams of Chocolate, and Percent Weight to Substitute Cocoa, Unsalted Butter, and Sugar in Place of Chocolate.

Chocolate %	Fat (g/100 g)	Sugar (g/100 g)	Cocoa % wt.	Butter % wt.	Sugar % wt.
100% Chocolate (Liquor)	54	0	62	38	0
85% Chocolate Bar	47	13	53	38	15
70% Chocolate Bar	40	27	44	35	30
Bittersweet Chocolate (67%)	39	35	42	31	33
60% Chocolate	33	40	37	29	40
Semisweet Chocolate (57%)	32	46	36	26	43
50% Chocolate	37	50	31	24	50
Cocoa powder	13.7		100	0	0

Using level teaspoons (tsp.) and tablespoons (Tbsp.):

- Table sugar weighs 4.2 grams per level teaspoon (5 ml).
- Butter weighs 4.7 grams per teaspoon, 14.2 grams per tablespoon.
- Cocoa powder weighs 2.6 grams per tsp. and 7.8 grams per Tbsp.

Cocoa to carob: For baking, one oz. (2 Tbsp.) of cocoa powder is equivalent to 3 Tbsp. of carob powder plus 2 Tbsp. of water.

Mud Balls

Messy, potent, delicious:

- 24 grams of natural cocoa
- ½ cup of dense Greek yogurt (can be low-fat)
- Two tablespoons of sugar
- 1/4 cup nut dust (shredded coconut, cashews, pecans, or walnuts, milled into a coarse powder

For this recipe, use extra-dense Greek yogurt, removing much of the whey so that it is thicker than usual. Blend the sugar and cocoa, and then sift them to remove any clumps of cocoa. Mix the cocoa/ sugar blend into the yogurt.

Mill the nuts into a coarse powder and place them in a teacup or custard dish.

Using a teaspoon, drop a one-inch ball of the chocolate yogurt into 1 inch balls into the cup with nut powder and swirl it around to get the ball completely covered in nut powder. Remove the ball and place it on a plate, and repeat the process. Should make about a dozen mud balls. Keep them refrigerated. Thus, each ball should contain about 2 grams of cocoa powder, and thus, 4 to 5 balls make a chocolate equivalent.

Dates

The fruit of date palm trees has an HAR score of around 8. Dates are rich in phenolic and flavonoid compounds, including hydroxybenzoic acids (syringic, protocatechuic, and vanillic acids) and ferulic, p-coumaric, and other hydroxycinnamic acids.[106]

In animal experiments, dates were protective against liver injury, lowering oxidative stress, inflammation, and apoptosis. They suppressed fibrosis, inflammatory cytokines, and DNA fragmentation, and increased adiponectin and the expression of antioxidant enzymes relative to animals that did not receive the dates.[107] [108] In a crossover study of healthy human volunteers, consumption of dates was associated with an increased number of bowel movements and a significant decrease in stool ammonia concentration and fecal water genotoxicity,[109] suggesting that the consumption of dates may lower the risk of colon cancer.

When transgenic mice bred to develop Alzheimer's type dementia (TGAD mice) were fed the standard diet, they showed greater memory deficits, anxiety-type behavior, and impairments in special learning and motor coordination when compared to the same breed of mice that had the diet supplemented with 4% of calories as dates. Plasma Aβ42 was more than 1/3 lower in animals fed dates than in control dementia-prone animals.[110] In a similar study with TGAD mice, a diet with 4% dates lowered markers of oxidative stress and increased NRF2-related antioxidant proteins in the brain.[111]

In a different model, rats were treated with Streptozocin (STZ), a toxin that induces diabetes. STZ rats suffer memory and cognitive injury, and have decreased glutathione in the hippocampus, resulting in oxidative stress. Both control and STZ rats given dates in their diets made fewer mistakes on short and long-term memory tests than either control or STZ rats not given dates. The dates increased the ratio of reduced to oxidized glutathione in the hippocampus.[112]

In another study of transgenic AD mice, the mice had dates, figs, or pomegranate added to their diets. Pomegranate, followed by fig and then dates, lowered levels of inflammatory cytokines in the plasma, lowered levels of Aβ40 and Aβ42 in the cortex and hippocampus, and increased ATP levels in the brain. Brain ATP levels in the TGAD mice were less than 30% of those of normal mice. TDAD mice given pomegranates in the diet had 78% as much brain ATP, those given figs ~60%, and those given dates ~45% as much ATP as normal mice.[113] These fruits appear to lower AD risk in these animals. In a randomized clinical trial, the consumption of three dates a day over the 16-week study was associated with an increased personal assessment of quality of life and improved mental health.[114]

The ideal hormetic dose of dates for adults is around 12 grams, a bit less than half an ounce or two to three dried dates. Consuming dates every other day or every third day likely maximizes the effect.

Blackberries

An easily available source that can be used to get a regular dose of the anthocyanin cyanidin to boost SIRT6 and help protect the brain is a bit of blackberry jam. This is available year-round, when fresh berries and fruits are not available. Elderberry, as jam or tea, is another source of cyanidin. (Please see the caution in Chapter 21.)

Referring to name brands is generally avoided herein, but prepared products may differ significantly from one another. Smucker's Natural Blackberry "fruit spread" (made with sugar) gets a DAD score of 4 and a high HAR score of 10. The minimal effective Hormetic dose is about 6 grams, or one level tsp., and the recommended dose to boost SIRT6 is about 12 grams, or two level tsp.

Hormetic Dose Frequency

Please note that these optimal hormetic dose frequencies are gleaned from the author's reading of epidemiological literature. The only hormetic exposure frequency that has adequate exposure frequency testing data that the author is aware is for exercise training. For exercise, there is data showing that vigorous exercise 3 to 4 times a week is most effective; thus, every other day. Exercise is likely the premier hormetic agent, in part as it acts on multiple systems.

The difference in frequency for the hormetic impact of cacao on men and women that appears in the literature likely results from the differences in type and use of cacao products by men and women rather than inherent physiological differences. Data suggests that the hormetic impact of green tea increases with multiple doses per day above that from once a day.

There are many hormetic agents in the diet. Table 20D, shows some important examples.

There is no reason to think that any particular food has exclusive hormetic properties not available in other hormetic foods. No research suggests piling up on hormetic agents will give better results. Redundant hormetic stimuli would be expected to overload the stress response that causes NRF2 release, and instead stimulate NF-κB or even AP-1, promoting inflammation and even apoptosis. This is seen in exercise; intense exercise 3 to 4 times a week has the most benefit; daily intense exercise, however, has been found *to increase overall mortality* to a level above that of people who never exercise. (Chapter 29).

Different hormetic agents act on different hormetic systems. Thus, it is recommended that a mix of hormetic agents be used. Using a strong hormetic agent, such as broccoli or cocoa, once a week shows strong health benefits in epidemiologic and clinical studies. Consuming them two to three times a week provides further benefits, but does not appear to double the benefits.

High doses of hormetic agents should likely be avoided in pregnant and nursing women and in small children.

Table 20D: Some Suggested Hormetic doses and frequencies.

Food	Approximate Optimal Hormetic Serving	Estimated Optimal Frequency Interval
Broccoli fleurette, raw, well chewed	15 to 30 grams	Every 2nd or 3rd day
Freshly crushed garlic	@ 2 grams	Every 2nd or 3rd day
Natural Cocoa powder or equivalent	See Table 16A	Women: every 3rd or 4th day?
Natural Cocoa powder or equivalent	See Table 16A	Men: every other day
Carob powder	>7 grams	Every other day
Dates	12 grams (@ 2 dates)	Daily
Blackberry jam, 50% fruit	12 grams	Every other day
Wine @12% alcohol	50 ml	Every other day
Guava Paste*	16 grams	Every other day
Coffee	See Chapter 21	One serving daily
Green tea	See Chapter 21	A minimum of 5 - 7 hours
Vigorous Exercise	See Chapter 29	Every other day

Note that Guava paste: 16 grams = 1/25th of a 14-ounce (400 g) pack, may contain @ 40% added sugar. For example, the guava sweet potato sorbet recipe contains about 22 grams of guava paste per 4-oz serving, well within the hormetic dose range.

1 Sulforaphane induces autophagy through ERK activation in neuronal cells. Jo C, Kim S, Cho SJ, Choi KJ, Yun SM, Koh YH, Johnson GV, Park SI. FEBS Lett. 2014 Aug 25;588(17):3081-8. PMID: 24952354

2 Indole-3-carbinol as a chemoprotective agent in breast and prostate cancer. Bradlow HL. In Vivo. 2008 Jul-Aug;22(4):441-5. PMID:18712169

3 Molecular targets and anticancer potential of indole-3-carbinol and its derivatives. Aggarwal BB, Ichikawa H. Cell Cycle. 2005 Sep;4(9):1201-15. PMID:16082211

4 Indole-3-carbinol suppresses NF-kappaB and IkappaBalpha kinase activation, causing inhibition of expression of NF-kappaB-regulated antiapoptotic and metastatic gene products and enhancement of apoptosis in myeloid and leukemia cells. Takada Y, Andreeff M, Aggarwal BB. Blood. 2005 Jul 15;106(2):641-9. PMID:15811958

5 Plant-derived 3,3'-Diindolylmethane is a strong androgen antagonist in human prostate cancer cells. Le HT, Schaldach CM, Firestone GL, Bjeldanes LF. J Biol Chem. 2003 Jun 6;278(23):21136-45. PMID:12665522

6 CXCR4 is a novel target of cancer chemopreventative isothiocyanates in prostate cancer cells. Sakao K, Vyas AR, Chinni SR, Amjad AI, Parikh R, Singh SV. Cancer Prev Res (Phila). 2015 May;8(5):365-74. PMID:25712054

7 D,L-sulforaphane-induced apoptosis in human breast cancer cells is regulated by the adapter protein p66Shc. Sakao K, Singh SV. J Cell Biochem. 2012 Feb;113(2):599-610. PMID:21956685

8 Sulforaphane inhibits mitochondrial permeability transition and oxidative stress.. Greco T, Shafer J, Fiskum G. Free Radic Biol Med. 2011 Sep 21. PMID:21986339

9 Comparison of the protective effects of steamed and cooked broccolis on ischaemia-reperfusion-induced cardiac injury. Mukherjee S, Lekli I, Ray D, Gangopadhyay H, Raychaudhuri U, Das DK. Br J Nutr. 2010 Mar;103(6):815-23. PMID:19857366

10 Sulforophane glucosinolate. Monograph. Altern Med Rev. 2010 Dec;15(4):352-60. PMID:2119425

11 Cruciferous vegetable consumption and lung cancer risk: a systematic review. Lam TK, Gallicchio L, Lindsley K, et al. Cancer Epidemiol Biomarkers Prev. 2009 Jan;18(1):184-95. PMID:19124497

12 Cruciferous vegetables and risk of colorectal neoplasms: a systematic review and meta-analysis. Tse G, Eslick GD. Nutr Cancer. 2014;66(1):128-39. PMID:24341734

13 GST polymorphism and excretion of heterocyclic aromatic amine and isothiocyanate metabolites after Brassica consumption. Steck SE, Hebert JR. Environ Mol Mutagen. 2009 Apr;50(3):238-46. PMID:19197987

14 Cruciferous vegetable consumption and lung cancer risk: a systematic review. Lam TK, Gallicchio L, Lindsley K, et al. Cancer Epidemiol Biomarkers Prev. 2009 Jan;18(1):184-95. PMID:19124497

15 A diet rich in high-glucoraphanin broccoli interacts with genotype to reduce discordance in plasma metabolite profiles by modulating mitochondrial function. Armah CN, Traka MH, Dainty JR, et al. Am J Clin Nutr. 2013 Sep;98(3):712-22. PMID: 23964055

16 A single mutation in human mitochondrial DNA polymerase Pol gammaA affects both polymerization and proofreading activities of only the holoenzyme. Lee YS, Johnson KA, Molineux IJ, Yin YW. J Biol Chem. 2010 Sep 3;285(36):28105-16. PMID: 20513922

17 Amelioration of Alzheimer's disease by neuroprotective effect of sulforaphane in animal model. Kim HV, Kim HY, Ehrlich HY, Choi SY, Kim DJ, Kim Y. Amyloid. 2013 Mar;20(1):7-12. PMID: 23253046

18 Glutathione Transferase (GST)-Activated Prodrugs. Ruzza P, Calderan A. Pharmaceutics. 2013 Apr 2;5(2):220-31. PMID:24300447

19 Allyl isothiocyanate triggers G2/M phase arrest and apoptosis in human brain malignant glioma GBM 8401 cells through a mitochondria-dependent pathway. Chen NG, Chen KT, Lu CC, Lan YH, Lai CH, Chung YT, Yang JS, Lin YC. Oncol Rep. 2010 Aug;24(2):449-55. PMID:20596632

20 Allyl isothiocyanate, a constituent of cruciferous vegetables, inhibits proliferation of human prostate cancer cells by causing G2/M arrest and inducing apoptosis. Xiao D, Srivastava SK, Lew KL, et al. Carcinogenesis. 2003 May;24(5):891-7. PMID:12771033

21 Sulforaphane suppresses in vitro and in vivo lung tumorigenesis through downregulation of HDAC activity. Jiang LL, Zhou SJ, Zhang XM, Chen HQ, Liu W. Biomed Pharmacother. 2016 Mar;78:74-80. PMID:26898427

22 Sulforaphane-induced apoptosis in human leukemia HL-60 cells through extrinsic and intrinsic signal pathways and altering associated genes expression assayed by cDNA microarray. Shang HS, Shih YL, Lee CH, et al. Environ Toxicol. 2016 Feb 2. PMID:26833863

23 Dietary Sulforaphane in Cancer Chemoprevention: The Role of Epigenetic Regulation and HDAC Inhibition. Tortorella SM, Royce SG, Licciardi PV, Karagiannis TC. Antioxid Redox Signal. 2015 Jun 1;22(16):1382-424. PMID:25364882

24 Phenethyl isothiocyanate sensitizes glioma cells to TRAIL-induced apoptosis. Lee DH, Kim DW, Lee HC, etal. Biochem Biophys Res Commun. 2014 Apr 18;446(4):815-21. PMID:24491546

25 Phenethyl isothiocyanate enhances TRAIL-induced apoptosis in oral cancer cells and xenografts. Yeh CC, Ko HH, Hsieh YP, et al. Clin Oral Investig. 2016 Jan 29. PMID:26822174

26 3,3'-diindolylmethane potentiates tumor necrosis factor-related apoptosis-inducing ligand-induced apoptosis of gastric cancer cells. Ye Y, Miao S, Wang Y, Zhou J, Lu R. Oncol Lett. 2015 May;9(5):2393-2397. PMID:26137077

27 In vitro studies of phenethyl isothiocyanate against the growth of LN229 human glioma cells. Su JC, Lin K, Wang Y, Sui SH, Gao ZY, Wang ZG. Int J Clin Exp Pathol. 2015 Apr 1;8(4):4269-76. PMID:26097624

28 ROS Accumulation by PEITC Selectively Kills Ovarian Cancer Cells via UPR-Mediated Apoptosis. Hong YH,

Uddin MH, Jo U, Kim B, Song J, Suh DH, Kim HS, Song YS. Front Oncol. 2015 Jul 28;5:167. PMID:26284193

29 Synergy between sulforaphane and selenium in protection against oxidative damage in colonic CCD841 cells. Wang Y, Dacosta C, Wang W, Zhou Z, Liu M, Bao Y. Nutr Res. 2015 Jul;35(7):610-7. PMID:26094214

30 Sulforaphane prevents doxorubicin-induced oxidative stress and cell death in rat H9c2 cells. Li B, Kim do S, Yadav RK, et al. Int J Mol Med. 2015 Jul;36(1):53-64. PMID:25936432

31 Sulforaphane preconditioning of the Nrf2/HO-1 defense pathway protects the cerebral vasculature against blood-brain barrier disruption and neurological deficits in stroke. Alfieri A, Srivastava S, Siow RC, et al. Free Radic Biol Med. 2013 Dec;65:1012-22. PMID:24017972

32 Sensitization of estrogen receptor-positive breast cancer cell lines to 4-hydroxytamoxifen by isothiocyanates present in cruciferous plants. Pawlik A, Słomińska-Wojewódzka M, Herman-Antosiewicz A. Eur J Nutr. 2016 Apr;55(3):1165-80. PMID:26014809

33 Phenylethyl isothiocyanate reverses cisplatin resistance in biliary tract cancer cells via glutathionylation-dependent degradation of Mcl-1. Li Q, Zhan M, Chen W, Zhao B, et al. Oncotarget. 2016 Mar 1;7(9):10271-82. PMID:26848531

34 Phenethyl isothiocyanate potentiates anti-tumour effect of doxorubicin through Akt-dependent pathway. Eisa NH, ElSherbiny NM, Shebl AM, Eissa LA, El-Shishtawy MM. Cell Biochem Funct. 2015 Dec;33(8):541-51. PMID:26548747

35 Phenethyl isothiocyanate enhances adriamycin-induced apoptosis in osteosarcoma cells. Fan Q, Zhan X, Xiao Z, Liu C. Mol Med Rep. 2015 Oct;12(4):5945-50. PMID:26252906

36 Frugal chemoprevention: targeting Nrf2 with foods rich in sulforaphane. Yang L, Palliyaguru DL, Kensler TW. Semin Oncol. 2016 Feb;43(1):146-53. PMID:26970133

37 Cruciferous vegetables and colo-rectal cancer. Lynn A, Collins A, Fuller Z, Hillman K, Ratcliffe B. Proc Nutr Soc. 2006 Feb;65(1):135-44. PMID:16441953

38 Cruciferous vegetables intake is associated with lower risk of renal cell carcinoma: evidence from a meta-analysis of observational studies. Zhao J, Zhao L. PLoS One. 2013 Oct 28;8(10):e75732. PMID:24204579

39 The activity of myrosinase from broccoli (Brassica oleracea L. cv. Italica): influence of intrinsic and extrinsic factors. Ludikhuyze L, Rodrigo L, Hendrickx M. J Food Prot. 2000 Mar;63(3):400-3. PMID:10716572

40 Effect of meal composition and cooking duration on the fate of sulforaphane following consumption of broccoli by healthy human subjects. Rungapamestry V, Duncan AJ, Fuller Z, Ratcliffe B. Br J Nutr. 2007 Apr;97(4):644-52. PMID:17349076

41 Changes in glucosinolate concentrations, myrosinase activity, and production of metabolites of glucosinolates in cabbage (Brassica oleracea Var. capitata) cooked for different durations. Rungapamestry V, Duncan AJ, Fuller Z, Ratcliffe B. J Agric Food Chem. 2006 Oct 4;54(20):7628-34. PMID:17002432

42 Kinetics of the stability of broccoli (Brassica oleracea Cv. Italica) myrosinase and isothiocyanates in broccoli juice during pressure/temperature treatments. Van Eylen D, Oey I, Hendrickx M, Van Loey A. J Agric Food Chem. 2007 Mar 21;55(6):2163-70. PMID:17305356

43 Heating decreases epithiospecifier protein activity and increases sulforaphane formation in broccoli. Matusheski NV, Juvik JA, Jeffery EH. Phytochemistry. 2004 May;65(9):1273-81. PMID:15184012

44 Chemoprotective glucosinolates and isothiocyanates of broccoli sprouts: metabolism and excretion in humans. Shapiro TA, Fahey JW, Wade KL, et al. Cancer Epidemiol Biomarkers Prev. 2001 May;10(5):501-8. PMID:11352861

45 [Sulforaphane (1-isothiocyanato-4-(methylsulfinyl)-butane) content in cruciferous vegetables]. Campas-Baypoli ON, Bueno-Solano C, Martínez-Ibarra DM, et al. Arch Latinoam Nutr. 2009 Mar;59(1):95-100. PMID:19480351

46 Bioavailability of Sulforaphane from two broccoli sprout beverages: results of a short-term, cross-over clinical trial in Qidong, China.. Egner PA, Chen JG, Wang JB, Wu Yet al. Cancer Prev Res (Phila). 2011 Mar;4(3):384-95. PMID:21372038

47 Prospective study of fruit and vegetable intake and risk of prostate cancer. Kirsh VA, Peters U, Mayne ST, et al; Prostate, Lung, Colorectal and Ovarian Cancer Screening Trial. J Natl Cancer Inst. 2007 Aug 1;99(15):1200-9. PMID:17652276

48 Vegetable and fruit intake after diagnosis and risk of prostate cancer progression.. Richman EL, Carroll PR, Chan JM. Int J Cancer. 2011 Aug 5. PMID:21823116

49 Safety, tolerance, and metabolism of broccoli sprout glucosinolates and isothiocyanates: a clinical phase I study. Shapiro TA, Fahey JW, Dinkova-Kostova AT, et al. Nutr Cancer. 2006;55(1):53-62. PMID:16965241

50 The involvement of Nrf2 in the protective effects of diallyl disulfide on carbon tetrachloride-induced hepatic oxidative damage and inflammatory response in rats. Lee IC, Kim SH, Baek HS, et al. Food Chem Toxicol. 2014 Jan;63:174-85. PMID:24246655

51 Garlic in health and disease. Rana SV, Pal R, Vaiphei K, Sharma SK, Ola RP. Nutr Res Rev. 2011 Jun;24(1):60-71. PMID:24725925

52 Comparison of the chemopreventive efficacies of garlic powders with different alliin contents against aflatoxin B1 carcinogenicity in rats. Bergès R, Siess MH, Arnault I, Auger J, Kahane R, Pinnert MF, Vernevaut MF, le Bon AM. Carcinogenesis. 2004 Oct;25(10):1953-9. PMID:15180943

53 Alleviation by garlic of antitumor drug-induced damage to the intestine. Horie T, Awazu S, Itakura Y, Fuwa T. J Nutr. 2001 Mar;131(3s):1071S-4S. PMID:11238819

54 Evidence of a novel docetaxel sensitizer, garlic-derived S-allylmercaptocysteine, as a treatment option for hormone refractory prostate cancer. Howard EW, Lee DT, Chiu YT, Chua CW, Wang X, Wong YC. Int J Cancer. 2008 May 1;122(9):1941-8. PMID:18183597

[55] Clarifying the real bioactive constituents of garlic. Amagase H. J Nutr. 2006 Mar;136(3 Suppl):716S-725S. PMID:16484550

[56] Garlic Phytocompounds Possess Anticancer Activity by Specifically Targeting Breast Cancer Biomarkers - an in Silico Study. Roy N, Davis S, Narayanankutty A, Nazeem P, Babu T, Abida P, Valsala P, Raghavamenon AC. Asian Pac J Cancer Prev. 2016;17(6):2883-8. PMID:27356707

[57] Garlic: a review of potential therapeutic effects. Bayan L, Koulivand PH, Gorji A. Avicenna J Phytomed. 2014 Jan;4(1):1-14. PMID:25050296

[58] Raw Garlic Consumption and Lung Cancer in a Chinese Population. Myneni AA, Chang SC, Niu R, Liu L, Swanson MK, Li J, Su J, Giovino GA, Yu S, Zhang ZF, Mu L. Cancer Epidemiol Biomarkers Prev. 2016 Apr;25(4):624-33. PMID:26809277

[59] Correlation between antioxidant activity of garlic extracts and WEHI-164 fibrosarcoma tumor growth in BALB/c mice. Shirzad H, Taji F, Rafieian-Kopaei M. J Med Food. 2011 Sep;14(9):969-74. PMID:21812650

[60] Steam-cooking rapidly destroys and reverses onion-induced antiplatelet activity. Hansen EA, Folts JD, Goldman IL. Nutr J. 2012 Sep 20;11:76. PMID:22992282

[61] Effect of raw versus boiled aqueous extract of garlic and onion on platelet aggregation. Ali M, Bordia T, Mustafa T. Prostaglandins Leukot Essent Fatty Acids. 1999 Jan;60(1):43-7. PMID:10319916

[62] Effect of cooking on garlic (Allium sativum L.) antiplatelet activity and thiosulfinates content. Cavagnaro PF, Camargo A, Galmarini CR, Simon PW. J Agric Food Chem. 2007 Feb 21;55(4):1280-8. PMID:17256959

[63] Thermostability of allicin determined by chemical and biological assays. Fujisawa H, Suma K, Origuchi K, Seki T, Ariga T. Biosci Biotechnol Biochem. 2008 Nov;72(11):2877-83. PMID:18997429

[64] Intake of garlic and its bioactive components. Amagase H, Petesch BL, Matsuura H, Kasuga S, Itakura Y. J Nutr. 2001 Mar;131(3s):955S-62S. PMID:11238796

[65] http://phenol-explorer.eu/contents/food/536

[66] http://phenol-explorer.eu/contents/food/439

[67] National Library of Medicine Hazardous Substances Data Bank

[68] Cytochrome P450 isoform selectivity in human hepatic theobromine metabolism. Gates S, Miners JO. Br J Clin Pharmacol. 1999 Mar;47(3):299-305.PMID: 10215755

[69] Trace amines: identification of a family of mammalian G protein-coupled receptors. Borowsky B, Adham N, Jones KA, et al. Proc Natl Acad Sci U S A. 2001 Jul 31;98(16):8966-71. PMID:11459929

[70] Chocolate consumption and bone density in older women. Hodgson JM, Devine A, Burke V, Dick IM, Prince RL. Am J Clin Nutr. 2008 Jan;87(1):175-80.PMID: 18175753

[71] Association of diet and outdoor time with inflammatory bowel disease: a multicenter case-control study using propensity matching analysis in China. Chu X, Chen X, Zhang H, Wang Y, Guo H, Chen Y, Liu X, Zhu Z, He Y, Ding X, Wang Q, Zheng C, Cao X, Yang H, Qian J. Front Public Health. 2024 Jun 17;12:1368401. doi: 10.3389/fpubh.2024.1368401. eCollection 2024. PMID: 38952728

[72] Does chocolate reduce blood pressure? A meta-analysis. Ried K, Sullivan T, Fakler P, Frank OR, Stocks NP. BMC Med. 2010 Jun 28;8:39.PMID: 20584271

[73] Cocoa, Blood Pressure, and Vascular Function. Ludovici V, Barthelmes J, Nägele MP, Enseleit F, Ferri C, Flammer AJ, Ruschitzka F, Sudano I. Front Nutr. 2017 Aug 2;4:36. doi: 10.3389/fnut.2017.00036. eCollection 2017. PMID: 28824916

[74] Acute effect of oral flavonoid-rich dark chocolate intake on coronary circulation, as compared with non-flavonoid white chocolate, by transthoracic Doppler echocardiography in healthy adults. Shiina Y, Funabashi N, Lee K, et al. Int J Cardiol. 2009 Jan 24;131(3):424-9..PMID: 18045712

[75] The Effect of Polyphenol-Rich Interventions on Cardiovascular Risk Factors in Haemodialysis: A Systematic Review and Meta-Analysis. Marx W, Kelly J, Marshall S, Nakos S, Campbell K, Itsiopoulos C. Nutrients. 2017 Dec 11;9(12):1345. doi: 10.3390/nu9121345. PMID: 29232891

[76] Alterations in skeletal muscle indicators of mitochondrial structure and biogenesis in patients with type 2 diabetes and heart failure: effects of epicatechin rich cocoa. Taub PR, Ramirez-Sanchez I, Ciaraldi TP, Perkins G, Murphy AN, Naviaux R, Hogan M, Maisel AS, Henry RR, Ceballos G, Villarreal F. Clin Transl Sci. 2012 Feb;5(1):43-7. doi: 10.1111/j.1752-8062.2011.00357.x. Epub 2011 Nov 7. PMID: 22376256

[77] Beneficial effects of dark chocolate on exercise capacity in sedentary subjects: underlying mechanisms. A double blind, randomized, placebo controlled trial. Taub PR, Ramirez-Sanchez I, Patel M, Higginbotham E, Moreno-Ulloa A, Román-Pintos LM, Phillips P, Perkins G, Ceballos G, Villarreal F. Food Funct. 2016 Sep 14;7(9):3686-93. doi: 10.1039/c6fo00611f. Epub 2016 Aug 5. PMID: 27491778

[78] Cocoa to Improve Walking Performance in Older People With Peripheral Artery Disease: The COCOA-PAD Pilot Randomized Clinical Trial. McDermott MM, Criqui MH, Domanchuk K, Ferrucci L, Guralnik JM, Kibbe MR, Kosmac K, Kramer CM, Leeuwenburgh C, Li L, Lloyd-Jones D, Peterson CA, Polonsky TS, Stein JH, Sufit R, Van Horn L, Villarreal F, Zhang D, Zhao L, Tian L. Circ Res. 2020 Feb 28;126(5):589-599. doi: 10.1161/CIRCRESAHA.119.315600. Epub 2020 Feb 14. PMID: 32078436

[79] Cocoa flavanols, Nrf2 activation, and oxidative stress in peripheral artery disease: mechanistic findings in muscle based on outcomes from a randomized trial. Ismaeel A, McDermott MM, Joshi JK, Sturgis JC, Zhang D, Ho KJ, Sufit R, Ferrucci L, Peterson CA, Kosmac K. Am J Physiol Cell Physiol. 2024 Feb 1;326(2):C589-C605. doi: 10.1152/ajpcell.00573.2023. Epub 2024 Jan 8. PMID: 38189132

[80] Blood pressure is reduced and insulin sensitivity increased in glucose-intolerant, hypertensive subjects after 15 days of consuming high-polyphenol dark chocolate.

Grassi D, Desideri G, Necozione S, et al. J Nutr. 2008 Sep;138(9):1671-6.PMID: 18716168

81 Continuous intake of polyphenolic compounds containing cocoa powder reduces LDL oxidative susceptibility and has beneficial effects on plasma HDL-cholesterol concentrations in humans. Baba S, Osakabe N, Kato Y, et al. Am J Clin Nutr. 2007 Mar;85(3):709-17.PMID: 17344491

82 High cocoa polyphenol rich chocolate may reduce the burden of the symptoms in chronic fatigue syndrome. Sathyapalan T, Beckett S, Rigby AS, Mellor DD, Atkin SL. Nutr J. 2010 Nov 22;9(1):55. PMID: 21092175

83 Regular consumption of dark chocolate is associated with low serum concentrations of C-reactive protein in a healthy Italian population. di Giuseppe R, Di Castelnuovo A, Centritto F, Zito F, De Curtis A, Costanzo S, Vohnout B, Sieri S, Krogh V, Donati MB, de Gaetano G, Iacoviello L. J Nutr. 2008 Oct;138(10):1939-45. doi: 10.1093/jn/138.10.1939. PMID: 18806104

84 Jeanne Calment, World's Elder, Dies at 122. Whitney, CR. New York Times, August 5, 1997

85 Alkalizing Cocoa and Chocolate. Moser A. The Manufacturing Confectioner • June 2015 (31-38). Presented at the PMCA Production Conference. https://www.blommer.com/_documents/Blommer_Alkalizing_Cocoa_and_Chocolate.pdf

86 Cocoa has more phenolic phytochemicals and a higher antioxidant capacity than teas and red wine. Lee KW, Kim YJ, Lee HJ, Lee CY. J Agric Food Chem. 2003 Dec 3;51(25):7292-5. doi: 10.1021/jf0344385. PMID: 14640573

87 Survey of commercially available chocolate- and cocoa-containing products in the United States. 2. Comparison of flavan-3-ol content with nonfat cocoa solids, total polyphenols, and percent cacao. Miller KB, Hurst WJ, Flannigan N, Ou B, Lee CY, Smith N, Stuart DA. J Agric Food Chem. 2009 Oct 14;57(19):9169-80. doi: 10.1021/jf901821x. PMID: 19754118

88 Flavanol and flavonol contents of cocoa powder products: influence of the manufacturing process. Andres-Lacueva C, Monagas M, Khan N, Izquierdo-Pulido M, Urpi-Sarda M, Permanyer J, Lamuela-Raventós RM. J Agric Food Chem. 2008 May 14;56(9):3111-7. doi: 10.1021/jf0728754. Epub 2008 Apr 16. PMID: 18412367

89 Exploring the Nutritional Composition and Bioactive Compounds in Different Cocoa Powders. Razola-Díaz MDC, Aznar-Ramos MJ, Verardo V, Melgar-Locatelli S, Castilla-Ortega E, Rodríguez-Pérez C. Antioxidants (Basel). 2023 Mar 14;12(3):716. doi: 10.3390/antiox12030716. PMID: 36978964

90 Cocoa, Blood Pressure, and Vascular Function. Ludovici V, Barthelmes J, Nägele MP, Enseleit F, Ferri C, Flammer AJ, Ruschitzka F, Sudano I. Front Nutr. 2017 Aug 2;4:36. doi: 10.3389/fnut.2017.00036. eCollection 2017. PMID: 28824916

91 Fate of flavonoids and theobromine in cocoa beans during roasting: Effect of time and temperature. Hermund DB, Larsen LK, Trangbæk SR, Madsen Q-K, Sørensen A-DM, Kaya J, et al. *J Am Oil Chem Soc.* 2024. https://doi.org/10.1002/aocs.12853

92 Impact of alkalization on the antioxidant and flavanol content of commercial cocoa powders. Miller KB, Hurst WJ, Payne MJ, Stuart DA, Apgar J, Sweigart DS, Ou B. J Agric Food Chem. 2008 Sep 24;56(18):8527-33. doi: 10.1021/jf801670p. Epub 2008 Aug 19. PMID: 18710243

93 Alkalizing Cocoa and Chocolate. Moser A. The Manufacturing Confectioner • June 2015 (31-38). Presented at the PMCA Production Conference. https://www.blommer.com/_documents/Blommer_Alkalizing_Cocoa_and_Chocolate.pdf

94 Preservation of cocoa antioxidant activity, total polyphenols, flavan-3-ols, and procyanidin content in foods prepared with cocoa powder. Stahl L, Miller KB, Apgar J, Sweigart DS, Stuart DA, McHale N, Ou B, Kondo M, Hurst WJ. J Food Sci. 2009 Aug;74(6):C456-61. doi: 10.1111/j.1750-3841.2009.01226.x. PMID: 19723182

95 The effect of polyphenol-rich dark chocolate on fasting capillary whole blood glucose, total cholesterol, blood pressure and glucocorticoids in healthy overweight and obese subjects. Almoosawi S, Fyfe L, Ho C, Al-Dujaili E. Br J Nutr. 2010 Mar;103(6):842-50. doi: 10.1017/S0007114509992431. Epub 2009 Oct 13. PMID: 19825207

96 Regular consumption of dark chocolate is associated with low serum concentrations of C-reactive protein in a healthy Italian population. di Giuseppe R, Di Castelnuovo A, Centritto F, Zito F, De Curtis A, Costanzo S, Vohnout B, Sieri S, Krogh V, Donati MB, de Gaetano G, Iacoviello L. J Nutr. 2008 Oct;138(10):1939-45. doi: 10.1093/jn/138.10.1939. PMID: 18806104

97 Regular consumption of dark chocolate is associated with low serum concentrations of C-reactive protein in a healthy Italian population. di Giuseppe R, Di Castelnuovo A, Centritto F, Zito F, De Curtis A, Costanzo S, Vohnout B, Sieri S, Krogh V, Donati MB, de Gaetano G, Iacoviello L. J Nutr. 2008 Oct;138(10):1939-45. doi: 10.1093/jn/138.10.1939. PMID: 18806104

98 Correlation between dietary theobromine intake and low cognitive performance in older adults in the United States: A cross-sectional study based on the National Health and Nutrition Examination Survey. Zhao L, Zhan R, Wang X, Song R, Han M, Shen X. Asia Pac J Clin Nutr. 2023;32(1):120-132. doi: 10.6133/apjcn.202303_32(1).0016. PMID: 36997493

https://apjcn.nhri.org.tw/server/APJCN/32/1/120.pdf

99 Association between dietary theobromine with depression: a population-based study. Li XY, Liu H, Zhang LY, Yang XT. BMC Psychiatry. 2022 Dec 6;22(1):769. doi: 10.1186/s12888-022-04415-y. PMID: 36474233

100 Understanding American premium chocolate consumer perception of craft chocolate and desirable product attributes using focus groups and projective mapping. Brown AL, Bakke AJ, Hopfer H. PLoS One. 2020 Nov 4;15(11):e0240177. doi: 10.1371/journal.pone.0240177. eCollection 2020. PMID: 33147215

101 Chocolate craving and the menstrual cycle. Zellner DA, Garriga-Trillo A, Centeno S, Wadsworth E. Appetite. 2004 Feb;42(1):119-21. doi: 10.1016/j.appet.2003.11.004. PMID: 15036792

[102] Caffeine metabolic ratios for the in vivo evaluation of CYP1A2, N-acetyltransferase 2, xanthine oxidase and CYP2A6 enzymatic activities. Hakooz NM. Curr Drug Metab. 2009 May;10(4):329-38. doi: 10.2174/138920009788499003. PMID: 19519341

[103] Theobromine and caffeine content of chocolate products. Zoumas BL, Kreiser WR, Martin R. Journal of Food Science. August 200645(2):314 – 316. DOI:10.1111/j.1365-2621.1980.tb02603.x

[104] Health benefits and mechanisms of theobromine. Mengjuan Zhang, Haifeng Zhang, Lu Jia, Yi Zhang, Runwen Qin, Shihua Xu, Yingwu Mei, Journal of Functional Foods. 115, 2024, 106126, ISSN 1756-4646, https://doi.org/10.1016/j.jff.2024.106126.

[105] Cocoa, Blood Pressure, and Vascular Function. Ludovici V, Barthelmes J, Nägele MP, Enseleit F, Ferri C, Flammer AJ, Ruschitzka F, Sudano I. Front Nutr. 2017 Aug 2;4:36. doi: 10.3389/fnut.2017.00036. eCollection 2017. PMID: 28824916

[106] http://phenol-explorer.eu/contents/food/913

[107] The Hepatoprotective Effect of Two Date Palm Fruit Cultivars' Extracts: Green Optimization of the Extraction Process. Alqahtani NK, Mohamed HA, Moawad ME, Younis NS, Mohamed ME. Foods. 2023 Mar 13;12(6):1229. doi: 10.3390/foods12061229. PMID: 36981156

[108] Abrogation of carbon tetrachloride-induced hepatotoxicity in Sprague-Dawley rats by Ajwa date fruit extract through ameliorating oxidative stress and apoptosis. Elsadek B, El-Sayed ES, Mansour A, Elazab A. Pak J Pharm Sci. 2017 Nov;30(6):2183-2191. PMID: 29175788

[109] Impact of palm date consumption on microbiota growth and large intestinal health: a randomised, controlled, cross-over, human intervention study. Eid N, Osmanova H, Natchez C, Walton G, Costabile A, Gibson G, Rowland I, Spencer JP. Br J Nutr. 2015 Oct 28;114(8):1226-36. doi: 10.1017/S0007114515002780. PMID: 26428278

[110] Diet rich in date palm fruits improves memory, learning and reduces beta amyloid in transgenic mouse model of Alzheimer's disease. Subash S, Essa MM, Braidy N, Awlad-Thani K, Vaishnav R, Al-Adawi S, Al-Asmi A, Guillemin GJ. J Ayurveda Integr Med. 2015 Apr-Jun;6(2):111-20. doi: 10.4103/0975-9476.159073. PMID: 26167001

[111] Effect of dietary supplementation of dates in Alzheimer's disease APPsw/2576 transgenic mice on oxidative stress and antioxidant status. Subash S, Essa MM, Al-Asmi A, Al-Adawi S, Vaishnav R, Guillemin GJ. Nutr Neurosci. 2015 Aug;18(6):281-8. doi: 10.1179/1476830514Y.0000000134. Epub 2014 Jun 21. PMID: 24954036

[112] Palm Dates Protect Memory Formation in Diabetes Mellitus: Neutralization of Oxidative Stress. Ghaith,IF, Aloubi K, El-Elimat T, et al. August 2023The Open Agriculture Journal 17(1) DOI:10.2174/18743315-v17-230726-2023-29

[113] Long-term dietary supplementation of pomegranates, figs and dates alleviate neuroinflammation in a transgenic mouse model of Alzheimer's disease. Essa MM, Subash S, Akbar M, Al-Adawi S, Guillemin GJ. PLoS One. 2015 Mar 25;10(3):e0120964. doi: 10.1371/journal.pone.0120964. eCollection 2015. PMID: 25807081

[114] Effects of Daily Low-Dose Date Consumption on Glycemic Control, Lipid Profile, and Quality of Life in Adults with Pre- and Type 2 Diabetes: A Randomized Controlled Trial. Alalwan TA, Perna S, Mandeel QA, Abdulhadi A, Alsayyad AS, D'Antona G, Negro M, Riva A, Petrangolini G, Allegrini P, Rondanelli M. Nutrients. 2020 Jan 15;12(1):217. doi: 10.3390/nu12010217. PMID: 31952131

21: Hormetic Beverages

Extracted Overview

Coffee, green tea, and several herbal teas have remarkable hormetic properties that help prevent chronic disease. They are highly recommended as a daily beverage.

For maximum benefit, cold water steeping is recommended for green tea, chamomile, peppermint, and hibiscus tisanes, and even for coffee. This allows a better leaching of the salubrious compounds and avoidance of bitter ones. It also greatly reduced the loss of volatile compounds that quickly evaporate when tea is steeped in hot or boiled water. When properly prepared, these teas are pleasant beverages that don't need sugar to be enjoyed. A cup of the cold-steeped infusions can be warmed (i.e., in a microwave) when a warm beverage is desired. A single tea bag can generally make two servings of iced tea after about 4 hours or more of steeping.

The exception among the teas discussed below is elderberry tea, as if it is not carefully harvested, it may contain toxic compounds; these compounds break down with boiling. Thus, to be extra careful, it is recommended that elderberry tea be boiled.

If in a rush, the teas can be made with hot water; a temperature of 60 to 65°C (140 to 149°F) is the generally recommended temperature for hot steeping, one tea bag for a cup of green tea, steeped 4 minutes.

Individually wrapped foil packs are recommended when tea is purchased unless it is expected that the package will be used within 2 months, so that they remain fresh and potent.

Coffee is recommended for its hormetic effects. For the most part, decaf coffee has similar health benefits to regular coffee. It is recommended that caffeinated beverages not be consumed after about 2:00 in the afternoon to prevent delayed sleep onset. Brewed coffee has a much greater hormetic effect than instant coffee, and medium-dark and dark roasts provide greater health benefits. The suggested daily dose of coffee is 8 to 10 oz. of coffee, but no more than 16 ounces of medium to dark roasted coffee per day. In contrast, up to 6 cups of green tea per day does not interfere with health benefits if spaced across the day. This suggests that the compounds in tea induce hormetic activities with a short turnover time.

For the best hormetic effect, it is recommended that a variety of hormetic beverages be consumed throughout the day.

Drink it black: Adding milk to coffee or tea neutralizes its adaptive benefits.

Parkinson's disease prevention is discussed in this chapter, as caffeine helps prevent this disease.

Fruit juices, dairy, and alcoholic beverages are discussed in other chapters.

Coffee, Teas, and Tisanes

Among the best beverages one can drink for disease prevention, including the prevention of dementia, is the foundation beverage: water. Keep this in mind. When you are thirsty or want something to drink. Water is an essential nutrient. If you want a warm beverage, warm water can be quite satisfying.

Coffee, teas, and herbal tisanes can provide health benefits, and while they may contain some nutrients, the health benefits are mostly derived via a different mechanism. Coffee, tea, and certain tisanes contain hormetic compounds that help the body overcome oxidative stress. They contain phenolic and polyphenolic compounds, several of which trigger activation of the NRF2 pathway. The NRF2 protein, when activated by a stress signal, moves into the nucleus of the cell and promotes the transcription of several other proteins that protect the body from toxins and oxidative stress. This is explained in more detail in Chapter 19. The phenolic compounds in coffee, tea, and certain tisanes can increase the production of antioxidant proteins, and thus protect us from oxidative and other stressors.

There is a range in which this hormetic effect works; too little, of course, does nothing. Excessive amounts fail to provide hormetic benefits, and for some compounds, cause harm. This chapter provides estimates for the Goldilocks, just-right amounts. Fortunately, hormetic doses generally have a fairly wide range, in contrast to pharmacologic dosing, which generally has narrow ranges, and most of the hormetic compounds in these beverages are para-hormetic. This means that although the body reacts to low doses as if they were toxic, they have little actual toxicity in the amounts likely to be consumed in food.

Although these beverages may affect the microbiome, their effect on the microbiome is not their principal mechanism of action. Thus, the DAD scale is not an appropriate metric to describe their impact on health. Their impact on health is better assessed by a Hormetic Adaptation Rating (HAR).

For promoting health, many hormetic agents are best used on an every-other-day basis. Tisanes and coffee, however, work well using a single serving a day for any of these beverages, and tea can be consumed up to several times a day and still provide hormetic benefits. This means that one can have coffee in the morning, decaf green tea at lunch, hibiscus tea in the afternoon, and chamomile tea in the evening. Using a variety of hormetic agents should better stimulate various hormetic and adaptive pathways than using just one. If thirsty after having a serving of one of these beverages, water is a good choice.

Tea and Tisanes

There are lots of things that tea can be made from, and of course, they will have different benefits or health perils. A "tea" is typically a hot water infusion in which dry plant parts are steeped. In more accurate terminology, there is tea made from the leaves of the tea plant (*Camellia sinensis*), and everything else is a tisane, which is often referred to as herbal teas, even when they are not made from herbs.

Tisanes can be made from leaves (yerba mate, peppermint), bark (wild cherry, cinnamon), flowers (chamomile, jasmine, hibiscus), seeds (anise, cardamom, fennel), fruits (lemon, apple, passion fruit), and roots (ginger, peony, liquorice), as some examples.

Brewing temperature and drinking temperature are not the same. Tea can be made with very hot water and made into iced tea, and coffee can be brewed cold and then later heated.

Various temperatures are used to make different brews, as this helps release different compounds from the tea, tisane, or coffee source material. Higher temperatures will cause highly volatile compounds to be released into the air, where their odor may be enjoyed; however, it can diminish the health impact of these volatiles. The process of steeping should be thought of as a differential extraction process, wherein the goal is to coax out the desired compound from the plant material while leaving undesired compounds. This process is controlled by adjusting the steeping temperature and time.

Tea, tisanes, and coffee are generally made with hot, and often boiling water. Drinking beverages at a temperature of 65°C (149°F) or hotter is a risk factor for esophageal cancer.[1] This is common in South America, where mate (pronounced MAH-teh) is consumed hot and sipped through a metal straw. Why they tolerate repeated scalding of their throat and esophagus is beyond strange. It is this repeated injury and healing that gives rise to aberrant cells in the esophagus that lead to cancer, not the compounds present in mate.

It may come as a surprise that when properly prepared, most teas and tisanes, at least the ones covered herein, have a pleasant flavor. They are not bitter or woody, and do not have cardboard overtones. They are pleasant to drink without a sweetener. If they become bitter, unpleasant, or cardboardy flavored, it may be that they are being brewed at too high a temperature or steeped for too long.

While the SANA program does not prohibit the use of a small amount of sugar, honey, or other natural sweeteners in tea and tisanes, when they are properly prepared, they should be pleasant without any need for a sweetener. Thus, the use of sweeteners is discouraged. Properly brewed coffee, however, has bitterness, which is masked by sugar; if sugar is used, the amount is minimized and comes out of the daily sugar budget. (Chapter 8). Properly brewed and cold-brew coffee are considerably less bitter than poorly made coffee.

The reuse of teabags is ill-advised. As a rule of thumb, a first extraction should remove at least 50% and usually closer to 80% of the desirable compounds. Even if only 50% was removed, the second time gives half of that. If 80% of the desirable compounds are removed the first time, the second would be one-fifth as potent, but would likely include more undesirable compounds. It is better to use a greater amount of water in the first extraction, rather than doing sequential extractions.

Tea and tisanes get old and lose their volatile compounds responsible for their aroma. Individually packaged tea bags, especially foil-lined ones, will have a longer shelf life. If you drink tea nearly every day, this should not matter, but if it takes a year to go through a pack, the tea should be better protected. Teas, especially loose teas, should be in a glass or metal container and kept in the dark to prevent oxidation and loss of volatile compounds. When hot steeping, covering the cup with a saucer or pot with a lid while it steeps helps retain those compounds that are more easily lost while the infusion is very hot. Once the tisane has cooled, these flavor compounds are less volatile.

The SANA program recommends cold-brewing for most coffee, tea, and tisanes. Cold-steeping gives better results in terms of flavor and hormetic activity for most infusions. The infusion can be warmed to around 63°C

(145°F) when served. For heating in a microwave, heavy glass (microwave-safe) coffee cups or mugs are recommended, as the mug and handle will not heat up as many ceramic mugs will, and it is easier to see if the tea has been overheated and is steaming. Glass is easy to clean, and safer from contaminants. (Never microwave food in plastic!!!)

For coffee, tea, or tisanes to be effective in lowering the risk of neurodegenerative and other diseases, they need to be consumed regularly, for example, every day or likely at least every other day, to maintain the elevated levels of antioxidant proteins that reduce cell injury. The SANA diet recommends at least one serving of coffee, tea, chamomile, hibiscus, or peppermint tisane daily.

Table 21A: Hormetic Adaptive Response (HAR) Score

Beverage	HAR
Green tea (Cold steeped)	10
Cold-steeped, filtered decaf coffee	10
Cold-steeped, filtered light roast coffee	10
Cold-steeped, filtered dark roast coffee	10
Instant Decaf Coffee	1
Instant coffee	1
Hot brewed decaf, filtered	6
Hot brewed coffee, filtered	6
Hot brewed coffee, unfiltered	5
Chamomile tea (Cold Steeped)	10
Hibiscus (roselle) tea (Cold Steeped)	10
Peppermint tea (Cold Steeped)	10
Elderberry Tea (Cold Steeped)	10
Basil Tea	10

Using hot, near-boiling water kills any bacteria or yeast that may be present in tea or tisane. Using cold-steeping does not. While it is unlikely that any human pathogens will proliferate in cold (38°F, 4°C) steeped, sugar-free infusions, bacteria and yeast are likely to be present on the tea. Most of the risk, however, comes from the water and the equipment used. Use only potable water and make sure the steeping vessel is clean and contamination-free. If there is any concern about possible contamination, the tea or tisane can be pasteurized *after the infusion is made* and the tea or tisane plant materials have been removed. Pasteurization can be done by heating the tea to 170°F (77°C) for 10 to 15 seconds.

Green Tea

Green tea is appreciated for its health benefits. It is particularly rich in the antioxidants epicatechin gallate (ECG), gallocatechin gallate (CGC), and epigallocatechin gallate (EGCG). It may protect those who drink it from metabolic syndrome by helping control weight and increasing insulin sensitivity. It may improve cognitive function, memory, and alertness due to the presence of caffeine, the calming effects of the amino acid L-theanine, and CGC, which may decrease cognitive workload.[2] It may promote dental health by inhibiting plaque formation and inhibiting bacterial growth, preventing gum disease and caries. Green tea appears to lower the risk of several types of cancer. Regular consumption of green tea is associated with a lower risk of heart disease; it reduces blood pressure, may help improve cholesterol levels, and enhances blood vessel function. Finally, and most saliently, EGCG has neuroprotective effects, and green tea may help prevent neurodegenerative diseases such as Alzheimer's and Parkinson's.[3] Tea consumption is associated with a lower risk of ulcerative colitis.[4]

When considering that diabetes, obesity, vascular disease, and periodontal disease are all associated with AD risk, it should not be a surprise that tea that lowers the risk of these conditions lowers the risk of AD. Many hormetic agents are best used no more than once every other day. The minimal time between dosing green to provide additional hormetic effect is about five hours, with a delay of about seven hours giving a fuller hormetic response. This suggests that it acts on specific pathways or proteins that turn over quickly. Green tea can thus be enjoyed and benefits obtained more than once a day, especially if decaffeinated green tea is used, for example, later in the day or evening to avoid interfering with sleep.

If it is properly prepared, green tea (GT) can be considered a health hero. Preparing GT in hot water is like racing to the top of a mountain, only to find a cliff you can crash down if you go too far. *If you use water that is too hot or leave it steep too long, or agitate it enough, it leaches out noxious compounds into the tea that are bitter, astringent, and detrimental to health, making the tea a net negative.* Table 17B shows the degradation of benefits from over-steeped green tea, using a slightly higher temperature than recommended. For 80°C, the best steeping time is 3:00 to 3:30 minutes.

Black tea is black because it is oxidized during the processing of the tea leaves, and thus does not have the antioxidant value that green tea has.

Recommended Preparation using tea bags:

Cold Steep (Recommended): Place two 1.5-gram green tea teabags into a quart container of cold water. Place a lid on it and place the container in the refrigerator. Do not shake or stir. After 4 to 24 hours, remove the tea bags. The tea can be kept for several days.

Hot steep: For green tea, use hot water from a digital water kettle set to a temperature of 75°C (167°F). Place a tea bag in a cup, pour in the hot water, and steep for 4 minutes (for example, using the timer on a smartphone) and then remove the tea bag or otherwise separate the tea leaves from the tea. For decaf green tea (CO_2 extraction), use water heated to 60 - 65°C (140 – 149°F) for four minutes, as its compounds are released more easily; thus, it should be steeped in water at the lower temperature range.

Do not stir or bob the bag in the water. Do not mash it with a spoon. When the alarm goes off in 4 minutes, pull the bag out by its string, let a couple of drops fall into the cup, and discard the bag. The tea should be mild and not bitter or astringent. As soon as the water gets poured into the mug, some heat dissipates into the mug, dropping the temperature several degrees. By the time the 4 minutes have gone by, the temperature of the green tea should be close to drinking temperature. If the tea is too cool, use this method: preheat the cup by pouring hot water into it and dumping out that water just before steeping the tea in it. Covering the cup with a saucer will help retain heat and volatile flavor compounds.

Avoid leaving the tea longer to prevent the leaching of bitter and undesirable compounds into the tea. If it is bitter or astringent, experiment with slightly lower temperatures. If you prefer a stronger tea, use two teabags or bags that are a larger size.

Table 21B: Green Tea (regular) steeped in water with 80°C starting temperature.

Steep Time (min)	HAR	DAD	Flavor
1	10	4	Mild
2	10	4	Mild, pleasant
3	10	4	Good tea flavor
4	10	4	Good tea flavor
5	3	3	Faintly astringent aftertaste
6	3	2	Mildly astringent aftertaste
7	<0	D	Astringent
10	<0	D	Long-lasting astringent aftertaste

Hibiscus Tisane

Hibiscus tisane gets an impressive HAR score. Hibiscus tisane is made from the dried calyces of *Hibiscus sabdariffa* (HS), the tissue at the base of the plant's flowers, not the flower's petals. HS is also known as roselle. Its tea is rich in bioactive phenolic compounds. Hibiscus tisane is another health hero. Among its accolades, it has been shown in clinical trials to have antioxidant properties, and is anti-inflammatory, anti-anemic, and anti-hypertensive. It lowers ApoB and LDL levels and raises HDL cholesterol levels. It helps with weight reduction and protects the kidneys. The use of 2 grams of calyxes per day was typical in many studies of HS tea; some used more, others less. In animal studies, roselle has additionally been found to be neuroprotective and to have sedative, anti-anxiety, and antidepressant effects. It has anti-diabetic, cardioprotective, hepato-protective, anti-ulcer, antiviral, and antibiotic properties.[5] It may be helpful for urinary tract infections,[6] and may have anti-cancer effects for certain tumors (breast, prostate, and others).[7] In a trial, where HS tea was consumed every morning by healthy adults for a month, there was an improvement in balance, grip strength, jump height, and VO_{2MAX}, a measure of maximum workload.[8] In rats on a high-fat diet, roselle reduced cardiac hypertrophy, fibrosis and improved cardiac function.[9]

While hibiscus tea has a sedative effect, consuming it near bedtime may best be avoided as it increases nocturia.

Typically, hibiscus tisane is made by steeping it in 90 – 96°C (195 – 205°F) for 5 – 10 minutes. The five-minute tea is more delicate, and the ten-minute tea is stronger and more acidic.

Preparation:

Cold Steep (*Recommended)*: Place one gram of dry hibiscus sepals per 1 cup (250 ml) serving of cold water into a glass jar. Place a lid on it and place the container in the refrigerator. Do not shake or stir. Allow to steep 4 to 24 hours. Strain out the spent sepals. Keeps well for several days.

Hot steep: Set the kettle to 95°C. If not using a digital kettle, bring water to a boil. Remove from the heat, and allow the water to cool for about 30 to 60 seconds to drop the temperature. The tea can steep in the pot or a cup. Use 1.5 to 2.0 grams of dry sepals in 240 to 300 mL (8 to 10 ounces) of water, serving one person. Add the sepals to the water, cover the container to help keep the water hot and to hold in volatile compounds that add to its flavor, and steep for 8 minutes. Separate the tea from the used calyxes immediately, and then cover again.

Allow the tea to cool to less than 65°C (149°F) before drinking.

While hibiscus calyxes can withstand boiling, they degrade the flavor and rating of the tea. The tea is excellent chilled and served cold, and keeps for several days refrigerated.

Hibiscus calyces are sometimes used in salads, cooked, or in other foods. This should be avoided as they get a D on the DAD scale. This also means that powdered calyxes should not be used.

Peppermint Tea

Peppermint tea has antioxidant properties. As a result of its oils, it helps relax the smooth muscles of the GI tract, increasing transit through the digestive system. Peppermint and its oil can relieve pain related to irritable bowel syndrome (IBS). Peppermint tisane may provide relief for dyspepsia, gastric hypermotility, and nausea. It may help with gastroparesis, as it relaxes the pyloric sphincter, allowing the stomach to empty more quickly. It stimulates bile flow and thus may improve the digestion of fats. On the flip side, it may worsen symptoms of heartburn and gastroesophageal reflux disease (GERD). Thus, those with GERD should avoid drinking this tisane in the evenings before lying down to sleep.

In a trial involving 180 young adults, consumption of peppermint tea improved cognitive performance, increased alertness, memory speed, and memory retention. Peppermint oil was found to improve physical strength, increasing grip strength and jumping distance.[10] Peppermint has antimicrobial properties against some viruses, bacteria, and fungi. The clinical antimicrobial effect is likely small; however, (sugar-free) peppermint tisane consumption may help prevent dental caries, gingivitis, and periodontal disease.[11] Menthol and peppermint oil are not the only active agents in peppermint tea.

Cautious use of peppermint oil can be used and help with abdominal pain in IBS. For use as a medicine, peppermint oil capsules are a more prudent choice. Most clinical trials using peppermint oil used 0.2 ml to 0.4 ml capsules three times a day in adults, and 0.1 to 0.2 ml in children over the age of 8 years.[12] [13] There are about 20 drops in one ml of essential oils; thus, one drop is 0.05 ml and weighs about 20 – 30 mg. An adult medicinal dose of peppermint oil would then be 4 drops. Peppermint oil is about 40% menthol, which is toxic. An overdose can cause coma and death. Medicinal quantities of peppermint oil are not without adverse effects and risks, but these are beyond the scope of this discussion. Peppermint oil should not be given to children under four years old or used by women who are pregnant or breastfeeding. If you are interested in using peppermint oil as a therapeutic agent to treat IBS or abdominal spasm, discuss it with your physician, and with their permission, use capsules that give a premeasured dose.

If peppermint oil is used in beverages for adults, the dose would be two to three drops as a serving.[14] Since the dropper may not stop exactly, aim for two drops. Keep in mind that one drop of peppermint oil is equivalent to about *26 cups* of peppermint tea.[15]

Recommended Preparation:

Cold Steeped peppermint tea: (*Recommended*) Use one gram of dried peppermint leaves per serving. Thus, use two (1.5-gram) peppermint tea bags for 3 servings; so, 24 to 30 ounces of water. Start with chilled water, and let the tisane steep in the refrigerator for about 4 to 24 hours, and then remove the tea bag(s). It should have a spicy peppermint sensation.

Dry peppermint leaf or tea bag: Heat the water in a digital kettle to 70°C (158°F). Pour the hot water over 1 to 1.5 g of dry peppermint leaves in a cup. Cover the tea while it steeps for 4 minutes to trap the essential oils and aroma. If using loose leaves, strain before drinking.

If one tea bag seems too strong, use a larger container and 2 cups of water, and share the tea or save it in the refrigerator for the next day.

Fresh peppermint leaves: Use 5 – 8 fresh leaves. Bruising the leaves will increase the flavor and potency. Heat the water to 82°C (180°F). Place the leaves and hot water in a cup, cover, and steep for 3 – 5 minutes.

Elderberry Tea

Elderberries have an extremely high concentration of cyanidin, about 6 times as much as blackberries and a hundred times that in raspberries, and thus are an excellent source requiring only small quantities.

Note that elderberry leaves, stems, and unripe fruit contain toxic compounds. The elderberry plant contains cyanogenic glycosides, including sambunigrin, which can form cyanide in the body and cause anxiety, dizziness, weakness, mental confusion, headache, nausea, vomiting, abdominal cramps, diarrhea, and such. The risk is greatest from the leaves, stems, and unripe berries. The flowers and dried ripe elderberries contain only very low levels of toxins.[16] Nevertheless, it is still recommended that the berries be boiled for several minutes to reduce toxicity to a safe level. Elderberry is also a low-acid fruit, which makes canning, for example, as a jelly, risky unless it is properly acidified. Even after all this, it is recommended that elderberries be avoided by pregnant and breastfeeding women and small children, as elderberries are an immune stimulant.

Recommended Preparation:

Although boiling the berries is recommended, the tea from boiled berries tastes nasty. Cold brewing elderberry tea is easy and tastes much better. Thus, the recommended preparation is to first cold brew the tea, separate the tea from the berries, and then boil the tea to get rid of any cyanogenic glycosides that might be present. Using high-quality, dried berries and removing any stems before making the tea should make a tea with very low levels of cyanogenic glycosides to begin with.

For cold-steeped elderberry tea, use one gram of dried elderberries per cup of cold water, and refrigerate for 3 to 6 hours. Filter out the seeds, bring the tea to a boil, cover, turn off the heat, and allow the tea to cool for 15 minutes. Those who enjoy larger servings of tea can use one gram of berries per 10 - 12 ounces of water. Some water will be lost during the heating of the tea.

The beneficial hormetic dose of elderberry tisane is small and narrow. One level teaspoon of the dried berries, weighing 2.0 grams, is an appropriate amount to make 2 full servings of tea. Thus, use 2 cups of water to get 2 servings, and limit it to one serving every other day.

Chamomile Tisane

Chamomile (manzanilla) tea is often used for its soothing and sedative properties. It is also traditionally used for stomach complaints. It is a good source of the flavonoids luteolin, apigenin, quercetin, and rutin. It also contains the terpenoids bisoprolol, matricin, and chamazulene. Although used in traditional medicine in many cultures, there is limited clinical research showing any significant efficacy other than being calming. One clinical trial found that it improved glycemic control, insulin levels, and HbA1C in type 2 diabetes and lowered LDL cholesterol when consumed three times a day after meals for 8 weeks.[17] It also decreased serum malondialdehyde levels and increased total antioxidant capacity in the same group of patients.[18] Another study showed that it improved sleep efficiency and reduced depression in postpartum women.[19]

Chamomile tea is typically steeped in near-boiling water for 93°C (200°F) for 5 to 10 minutes. With longer times, it becomes woody and then bitter. Preparing chamomile this way yields a mediocre HAR score and is discouraged.

Recommended Preparation:

Cold Infusion: (*Recommended*) Place a 1-gram chamomile tea bag (or equivalent) per 2 cups (16 ounces) of cold water and allow it to steep in the refrigerator for 4 to 24 hours before removing the tea bag. Use two 1-gram tea bags for one quart of water. The peak hormetic effect is with around 5.3 ounces of the tea, hot or cold (thus three servings per 1-gram tea bag), but 8 ounces (two servings per tea bag) falls within the hormetic range. Alternatively, two 1-gram tea bags can be used to make 24 oz of tea to make 3 8-oz cups of mild chamomile tea. The cold infusion can be kept under refrigeration for one to two days before beginning to lose potency. HAR = 10.

Hot Steep: Pour 70°C (158°F) water into a cup with a (1-gram) chamomile tea bag, and cover. Steep for 3 minutes, remove the tea bag. It should be nearly cool enough to sip. HAR = 10.

Basil Tea

Basil tisane is not a common beverage, but it is pleasant and has a high HAR score. A single fresh (medium to large) leaf is enough for a hormetic serving. Bruise the leaf (i.e., roll it in your palm) and pour 65°C water over it in a cup. Cover, and allow it to steep 3 - 5 minutes; remove the leaf. Fresh leaves can also be used for cold-steeped basil tisane.

Alternatively, dried basil can be used; 1 gram of dried basil for 2 servings. It can be cold-steeped.

Coffee

Coffee is not just permitted on the SANA diet, it is encouraged. Well, at least some coffee for some people.

Coffee gives a mental and energy boost, and coffee drinkers are less likely to be depressed. Taste receptors in the gut respond to the bitter agent in the coffee, stimulating defecation. Coffee contains chlorogenic acid that protects the pancreatic beta cells from endoplasmic reticulum stress, and thus protects against the development of type 2 diabetes.[20] Coffee also suppresses appetite and lowers the risk of obesity.

Perhaps the main reason that people drink coffee is that it contains the stimulant caffeine. Nevertheless, the health benefits from coffee are also derived from phenolic and other compounds in the coffee that activate the transcription of antioxidant and anti-stress proteins. Decaffeinated coffee can also be consumed on the SANA diet.

Coffee and caffeine have risks. High caffeine intake during gestation is associated with fetal loss, low birth weight, and preterm delivery. The general recommendation is that pregnant women limit caffeine intake to less than 200 mg per day, about the amount of caffeine in one large serving (12 ounces) of brewed coffee.[21] However, some studies suggest that this amount may still confer risk to the fetus.[22] The SANA program recommends limiting caffeine to no more than 80 mg a day during pregnancy, about the amount in 6 ounces of American-style coffee or two cups of regular (caffeinated) tea. Caffeine also disturbs sleep.[23] Caffeine has a half-life of about 7 hours in most adults, and thus its consumption should be avoided after about 2 P.M. to avoid delayed sleep onset.

In a study of Americans, the consumption of coffee, caffeinated or decaf, does not increase the odds of having glaucoma; meanwhile, those consuming tea had about one-fourth the risk of glaucoma.[24] In a study of Koreans, drinking tea had no impact on glaucoma, but men who drank coffee had four times the risk of open-angle glaucoma.[25] Caffeine impedes the outflow of aqueous fluid from the front of the eye (the anterior chamber), raising the intraocular pressure (IOP), and thus may promote the onset of glaucoma or its progression.[26] Coffee increases the IOP in the eyes of individuals with ocular hypertension and glaucoma, but does not increase IOP in normal eyes.[27] Caffeinated coffee should be avoided in those with elevated IOP and open-angle glaucoma.

When coffee is (flash) roasted using green coffee beans, the internal temperature in the bean is maintained until the moisture within the seed evaporates off, which takes about six minutes in a 185°C roaster; after which the temperature quickly begins to rise. Under research conditions, the beans had an ideal light roast at 7:00 minutes, medium roast at 7 minutes 24 seconds, dark roast at eight minutes and 3 seconds, and were burned at 9 minutes. Light roasted coffee is slightly less acidic and has higher levels of chlorogenic acids than medium or dark roasts; the levels are about the same for medium and dark roasts. Caffeine levels also fall with roasting; light roast coffee has more caffeine than dark roasts, and medium roasts have an intermediate amount.[28]

Some people suffer gastrointestinal discomfort with coffee consumption, as coffee has several effects on the GI tract. Coffee can stimulate the secretion of the hormone gastrin, which increases acid secretion in the stomach. Ground coffee does this more effectively than instant coffee, and caffeinated coffee increases acid secretion more effectively than decaf. This does not appear to be an effect mediated by caffeine, but by other compounds present in the coffee that are lost during the decaffeination process.[29] Decaf coffee has been found to decrease symptoms of functional dyspepsia as compared to regular coffee.[30] Heartburn symptoms were worse when coffee was taken with a high-fat meal.[31] Dark roasted coffee contains higher levels of compounds that repress stomach acid secretion, such as *N*-methylpyridinium; dark roast coffee may even induce a net decrease in acid secretion.[32] Dark roasted coffee also stimulates less gastric acid than does dark roasted coffee.[33] Thus, if wishing to avoid stomach acidity from coffee, using dark roasted, decaffeinated coffee may help.[34]

Coffee consumption has been suggested to provoke gastroesophageal reflux disorder (GERD). GERD is mediated by relaxation of the lower esophageal sphincter (LES) at the junction of the esophagus and stomach, which can allow stomach contents to seep back up into the esophagus. High doses of caffeinated coffee are associated with GERD, but decaffeinated coffee is not. A meta-analysis study found a non-statistically significant decrease in GERD risk for 1 to 4 cups of coffee per day, and a non-statistically significant increase in risk for 5 or more cups a day.[35] Another meta-analysis study found a near-significant association of coffee drinking and GERD in cross-sectional studies but no effect in case-control studies. This would be consistent with high-coffee intake lifestyle patterns rather than coffee itself promoting GERD.[36]

Several foods provoke GERD symptoms, including high-fat and spicy foods, but also beer, wine, and alcohol, a high-salt diet, carbonated soft drinks or beverages, orange juice, and chocolate.

Health Benefits of Coffee

Coffee drinking lowers the risk of pancreatitis and lowers the risk of gallbladder stone formation, at least in women. The consumption of coffee also lowers the risk of developing and the risk of progression of non-alcoholic fatty liver disease and of chronic liver disease, including that caused by viral hepatitis. Coffee consumption lowers the risk of liver, gallbladder, pancreatic, and endometrial cancers.[37] [38] Coffee also appears to protect women from polycystic ovary syndrome (PCOS), a leading cause of infertility, which is also associated with acne, facial hair, and obesity. Coffee consumption was inversely associated with PCOS risk. One cup of coffee a day was associated with a 72% decreased hazard of anovulatory PCOS.[39] (PCOS is discussed in Chapter 34.)

In one meta-analysis, ulcerative colitis (UC) risk was lower among coffee drinkers, and both UC and Crohn's disease risk were lower among tea drinkers. UC risk was 69% higher, and Crohn's disease risk was 42% higher among those consuming soft drinks.[40] [41] In another meta-analysis, coffee was associated with a lower risk of both UC and Crohn's disease.[42] Coffee helps prevent constipation. Coffee increases the motility of the distal colon in many people, in as little as four but up to 30 minutes, stimulating defecation. Caffeinated coffee is more effective than decaf, but even warm water has some effect on stimulating lower colonic tone.[43] For some people, just smelling coffee works.

Dark roast coffee may help with weight loss more than a light roast. Dark roasted coffee improved weight loss and increased the antioxidant status of red blood cells in subjects over 4 weeks.[44] Dark roast was best at lowering fasting glucose levels in rats, but all coffee reduced insulin levels and insulin resistance, and liver steatosis (fat).[45]

There have been several meta-analyses assessing the impact of coffee on dementia. Some find no benefit while others do. The impact of coffee is hard to study as there is so much variation in the preparation of coffee and in how much is consumed. This variation impacts not only which compounds are present and bioavailable, but also their ratios. Furthermore, coffee has both hormetic and pharmacologic effects, and these may not be optimally balanced; the ideal caffeine level may not come at the same coffee intake level for optimal hormetic effect. Additionally, non-linear relationships are easy to miss, especially when combining various datasets that classify intake differently.

One study that separated intake of caffeinated and decaffeinated coffee found no improvement in cognitive test scores associated with the intake of decaffeinated coffee, but found better cognitive test scores among those who drank regular coffee. The risk of cognitive decline in this study was lowest for those consuming around 160 mg of caffeine per day.[46] Standard American brewed coffee contains about 95 mg in an 8-ounce serving; 160 mg would be about 13 – 14 ounces of American-style coffee. However, we know that caffeine increases cerebral blood flow and improves cognitive test performance even in the young; thus, those taking the cognitive test with coffee in their system would be expected to perform better, whether they had cognitive decline or not.

Coffee lowers the risk of Parkinson's disease (PD) by as much as 37%. A recent study suggests that the risk reduction is associated with the metabolic products of caffeine, theophylline, and paraxanthine; however, this protective effect was not present for women who used postmenopausal hormone treatment. Decaf coffee consumption was not associated with a lower risk of developing PD. This study was performed in Europe. Interestingly, no preventive benefits from coffee were observed in the UK, and the strongest declines in risk were apparent in Germany and Italy.[47] Germans consume considerably higher amounts of coffee (mean: 392 ml/day) than do Italians (mean: 100 ml/day). But the British also consume high amounts of coffee (mean: 475 ml/day). [48] Germans and Italians generally drink dark roasted coffees, while the British prefer a medium roast, and older Brits (those at risk of PD) consume mostly instant coffee. Even though brewed coffee is favored in younger adults, only 24% of in-home coffee in the U.K. is brewed. One in five drinks decaf coffee. More than two-thirds of the coffee consumed in Britain is prepared with milk.[49] [50] The reason that coffee fails to reduce the risk of PD in Britain likely results from its preparation, which counteracts the anti-PD compounds.

Consumption of coffee also lowers the risk of Alzheimer's disease. In a meta-analysis that included 11 follow-up studies, consumption of 1 – 2 cups of coffee per day was associated with a 32% decline in AD risk. Consumption of 3 – 4 cups per day only lowered risk by 21%, and drinking 5 or more cups a day undid any benefits from the first cups.[51] In another meta-analysis that assessed both coffee and tea consumption, the risk of cognitive disorders was 16% lower, and the risk of AD was 26% lower for those consuming 2.5 cups of coffee per day, with a reversal of benefits from intake of higher amounts.

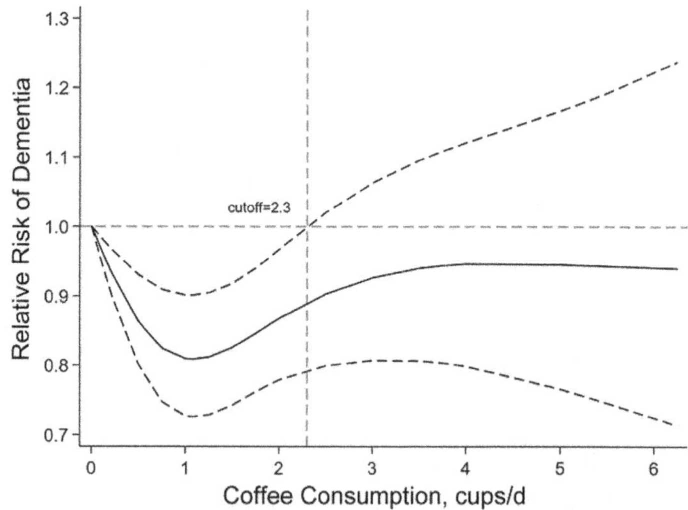

Figure 21A: Hormetic dose-response for dementia risk with coffee, with the lowest risk with one cup per day. (LS Ran, et al.[52]) No statistically significant benefit was apparent beyond 2.3 cups per day. Note that the widening (dashed) confidence estimates give increasingly poor risk estimates at coffee consumption levels over 4 cups a day, and thus, risk estimates above this level are not meaningful. A standard cup of coffee is 6 ounces.

For tea, however, the risk of cognitive disorders declined with the dose of tea up to at least 5.5 cups of tea per day. Green tea has about a quarter as much caffeine per cup (@ 24 – 45 mg) as does coffee (@ 85 – 175 mg). In a dose-response meta-analysis study, the risk of mild cognitive impairment and dementia was lowest among subjects drinking one cup of coffee per day; the benefits diminished with the consumption of higher amounts. This study also found that the risk of dementia and cognitive impairment declines with the dose of up to at least 6 cups of green tea per day, with about a 5% decline in risk for each cup of green tea.[53]

Adaptive Response to Coffee

Rats drinking 2 ml (about half a teaspoon) of coffee daily have 130 percent higher cytosolic NRF2 levels and a 25% increased antioxidant capacity of the liver.[54] A single dose of coffee can raise the level of phase (ARE) enzymes by 20% within an hour.[55] Not only does coffee protect the liver from cancer, but it is also associated with lower rates of depression, type 2 diabetes, and Alzheimer's disease.

When coffee is roasted, sugars in the coffee undergo a Maillard browning reaction, creating pronyl-lysine. Milliard reactants in coffee may have a hormetic effect.[56] [57] Trigonelline, a natural compound in coffee that is also found in peas, oats, and potatoes, decomposes during roasting to form N-methyl pyridinium (NMP). Chlorogenic acids, which are abundant in green coffee, are converted into lactones with light roasting and then converted into phenylindanes with further roasting. Phenylindanes are largely responsible for the lingering bitterness in dark-roasted coffee.[58]

NMP from dark roasted coffee inhibits NF-κB proinflammatory activity by more than 80%.[59] Dark roasted coffee has been found to decrease the number of spontaneous DNA strand breaks (measured in white blood cells) by 27 percent in a group of healthy men.[60] Darker roasts of coffee contain higher amounts of NMP and are more effective in stimulating the release of NRF2 and boosting ARE enzyme transcription than are lighter roasts of coffee. Coffee that has not been toasted does not contain NMP and is not effective in stimulating NRF2.

Coffea arabica has more trigonelline than *Coffea robusta,* and thus *Coffea arabica* can form more NMP. *Coffea robusta* coffee is about 80% higher in caffeine and 25% in phenolic compounds than *Coffea arabica.*

Dark roasts, in comparison to light roasts, appear to be more protective against neurodegeneration. Phenylindanes, which are created during roasting, inhibit the condensation of Aβ and tau proteins that occur during the pathogenesis of AD. Caffeic acid, which is partially destroyed during roasting, inhibits the condensation of α-synuclein fibrillation, a hallmark of PD, at concentrations from 10 to 60 μM,[61] but promotes condensation of α-synuclein fibrillation at concentrations above 100 μM.[62] Thus, dark roasts appear to better protect against neurodegenerative disease unless too much is consumed. This is a hormetic effect; thus, there is a range within which it has its salubrious effects, and beyond that, there is harm.

The transcription of NRF2 appears to respond to positive feedback so that more of the NRF2 protein is made available when the cell is under stress. Coffee not only affects the activation of NRF2, but it also affects the amount of NRF2 transcribed, although this may be secondary to compounds other than NMP in coffee.

The response to NMP in coffee is impacted by genetics. There are several common single-nucleotide promoter-region NRF2 variants relevant to the induction of ARE proteins. For most NRF2 polymorphisms, coffee consumption increases ARE transcription by at least 50 percent. For one of the NRF2 polymorphisms (-653A/G), the response is higher, but for another, found in about 20 percent of the studied population (-651G/A), the ARE response to coffee is significantly muted.[63] Thus, about one in five persons has a limited NRF2 response to the NMP in coffee or to other hormetic agents acting through this pathway.

In a trial, dark roasted coffee rich in NMP was found to lead to a significant weight loss, while light roasted coffee did not. The dark roast was also associated with higher vitamin E levels and higher glutathione levels.[64]

Likely as a result of phenolic compounds, coffee, especially caffeinated coffee, increases the growth of the beneficial *Bifidobacterium* bacteria while inhibiting the proliferation of *Escherichia coli* and *Clostridium* cluster XI bacteria, which are associated with high-fat diets and considered harmful.[65] In obese mice, coffee consumption increased the formation of the SCFAs butyrate and propionate.[66]

Caffeine and Theobromine

Some important health benefits of coffee, tea, and chocolate (Chapters 20, 21) are derived from caffeine in coffee and tea, and likewise, some of the health benefits of chocolate come from a similar compound, theobromine. Theobromine is created during the metabolism of caffeine, and while chocolate contains large amounts of theobromine, it also contains some caffeine. Both agents modulate adenosine receptor activity and have other pharmacologic effects. Caffeine and theobromine are methylxanthines. While they may have some hormetic effects, they principally act as pharmacologic agents interacting with adenosine receptors.

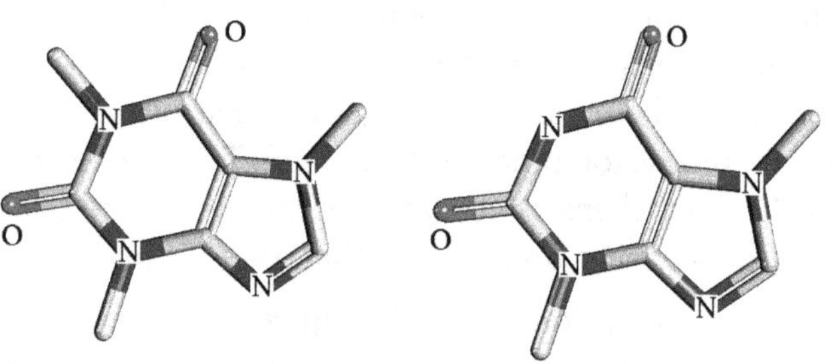

Figure 21A: Structural Similarity of Caffeine and Theobromine

Recent data indicate that caffeine or its metabolites mediate the protective effects of coffee against Parkinson's disease (PD). Mitochondrial dysfunction, causing the generation of reactive oxygen species (ROS) and oxidative stress, is at the core of PD. Caffeine has been found to increase protein levels of Sirtuin 3 (SIRT3) and activation of AMPK, inducing autophagy and mitophagy.[67] Mitophagy is the culling of old and poorly functioning mitochondria. Both caffeine and theobromine induce AMPK phosphorylation; caffeine and theobromine, while not identical, largely act through the same mechanisms, thus the following discussion on caffeine research largely applies to theobromine and vice versa; however, the doses may not be the same.

Caffeine stimulates phosphorylation of AMPK via CaMKII. This activates PGC1α, which promotes mitochondrial biogenesis.[68] [69] Thus, caffeine both helps eliminate old, poorly functioning, ROS-leaking mitochondria and promotes the generation of new, healthier ones. Theobromine has similar activity. Theobromine activates neuronal synaptic transmission while reducing long-term potentiation by activating adenosine-1A receptors and blocking adenosine-2A receptors, respectively. Theobromine was found to protect the hippocampus of mice from loss of neurons when exposed to Aβ42. Additionally, theobromine increases exercise-induced mitochondrial renewal, increasing the beneficial impact of exercise.[70] Caffeine acts similarly.[71] These agents improve cognitive plasticity and memory in TGAD-mice,[72] and may protect against adenosine-2A receptor-mediated stress and glutamate-induced neuronal excitotoxicity.[73]

It should be noted that caffeine and alcohol metabolism significantly slow around the ages of 40 and again around 60, perhaps secondary to lifestyle changes. This is accompanied by a decrease in lipid metabolism.[74] Myosteatosis may influence the decline in metabolic processing of these compounds. The caffeine/theophylline and alcohol "dose" recommendations provided herein are based on research of middle-aged and older adults; thus, although the half-life of these compounds may be longer as we age, adjustments in the amounts are likely not needed other than in extremely older individuals.

Theobromine and caffeine are non-competitive inhibitors of phosphodiesterases (PDEs). Inhibition of PDE4 by theobromine and caffeine in fat cells promotes the utilization of fat for energy and heat production in the metabolically active brown adipocytes, and induces the "browning" of white adipocytes (storage fat) by increasing the mitochondrial mass and activity of these cells. This helps reduce the storage and accumulation of fat in the body. Caffeine also promotes AMPK activation, PGC1α expression, and mitochondrial biogenesis in skeletal muscle.[75] Thus, caffeine and theobromine enhance beta-oxidation, the burning of fat as a fuel, during exercise.

Caffeine and theobromine also inhibit the enzyme PARP-1, thereby decreasing NF-κB and AP-1 activity and their induction of inflammation and apoptosis.[76] Theobromine is further discussed in Chapter 20.

For those with a family history or other elevated risk of Parkinson's, caffeine, as a medicinal supplement (100 mg/ day), is recommended rather than coffee. This avoids vagaries in the caffeine levels in coffee and the risk of excess caffeine exposure. (Please see the section on Parkinson's Prevention, below.)

Brewed Coffee

When brewed coffee is made, using a paper filter has several advantages. First, it helps distribute the hot water more evenly, ensuring a more controlled flow and better flavor extraction. This decreases the amount of coffee grounds that need to be used. The filter prevents small fine particles from entering the brewed coffee, giving a smoother drink. But of course, it is the health impacts of using filters that merit discussion.

Coffee contains the compounds cafestol and kahweol, which are largely unaffected by roasting. They are mostly retained in the coffee grounds when coffee is brewed;[77] however, high amounts are released when coffee is boiled, as with American Cowboy, Norwegian, Scandinavian, Turkish, and Greek coffees, and when using a French press, moka, and espresso coffee makers.[78] Using a paper filter captures most of these compounds, leaving trivial amounts in the coffee. In the Chapter on oil, it was pointed out that some people have high cholesterol levels as a result of a weak feedback mechanism for controlling the level for stopping cholesterol production. Cafestol does something similar; it activates FXR and PXR receptors in the liver, which decreases the feedback loop that limits cholesterol production. This raises serum cholesterol and triglyceride levels. Thus, boiled and French press coffees can raise cholesterol and triglyceride levels. Cafestol also lowers the production of bile acids from cholesterol, which also causes more cholesterol to be retained in the body.[79] Thus, it is recommended that cafestol and kahweol be avoided by filtering coffee through a paper filter. This can be done after the coffee is prepared in a French press, moka pot, or other form of brewing.

There is some lab evidence that coffee may increase HMOX1 expression and NRF2 activation in cell culture, and may play a role in neuroprotection,[80] but there is insufficient evidence of a beneficial effect and more evidence that these compounds are detrimental. HMOX1 is beneficial at moderate levels, but can promote apoptosis at higher levels. It may be that small amounts of cafestol and kahweol, still present in filtered coffee, increase HMOX1 enough to provide benefits, while unfiltered coffee has excessive levels.

Instant Coffee (Not Recommended)

Using instant coffee, the generally recommended instructions are to use 2 grams of coffee granules or powder for 6 oz. of coffee. (Divide the bottles' net weight in grams by the number of servings stated on the label to get the proper concentration.) Standard coffee mugs comfortably hold 9 to 12 ounces of liquid, so it is easy to make dilute instant coffee that does not have a good balance of flavor. When prepared at the correct concentration, the taste is more pleasant, and at least to me, less bitter.

The hormetic range for instant coffee is estimated to be one to six grams of instant coffee per day, thus enough to prepare 3 to 18 oz of coffee, although since different coffees have different amounts of various pro-hormetic compounds, the ideal amounts vary according to the hormetic targets and compounds. Eight ounces (2.5 g of instant coffee) per day is close to ideal, and no more than 16 ounces (5 g of instant coffee should be consumed if drinking it for its health benefits. Instant coffee provides significantly less health benefits than freshly brewed coffee.

Roast Levels

Roast Levels: Cinnamon < Light < Medium < City < Full City < Vienna < French < Italian.

As far as roast levels go, dark roasts have clear health advantages over light roasts, but the difference from a medium-dark "City" to "French" roasts is smaller. Vienna, French, and Italian roasts are considerably darker and have smoky to burnt flavors and higher levels of bitterness. Lightly roasted coffee has lower levels of *N*-methylpyridinium and higher levels of chlorogenic acids than medium and darker roasts, but beyond medium, there is less change in the concentrations of *N*-methylpyridinium and chlorogenic acids.[81]

Recommendation: Coffee has salubrious effects that provide protection from multiple diseases; its consumption is encouraged. The SANA diet suggests drinking 8 but not more than 16 ounces of coffee per day. Brewed coffee is considerably more beneficial (for the prevention of dementia) than instant coffee. Medium-dark or darker roasts are more effective, with light roasts likely to have only minor benefits. Even if not part of the brewing process, it is recommended that the coffee be passed through a paper filter to remove cafestol and kahweol from the coffee. The anti-Parkinson's disease effects of coffee are likely a result of caffeine; Parkinson's disease prevention is discussed below.

Milk and Cream in Coffee and Tea

Cream, creamer, and milk are often added to coffee.

Creamer may contain coloring such as titanium dioxide. Please avoid. Some powdered soy milk would be a better choice.

Coffee with milk or cream and sugar is rich and delicious. Unfortunately, milk and cream neutralize the hormetic benefits of coffee.[82] The common use of milk in coffee may partially explain why coffee consumption in Britain fails to lower the risk of Parkinson's disease.

As with dairy milk, soy milk added to coffee also appears to prevent the adaptive effects of coffee's phenolic compounds.[83]

Adding milk or soy milk to green tea also reduces the bioavailability of some phenolic compounds but increases that of others.[84] In a clinical trial and in lab experiments, adding milk to tea prevented vasorelaxation, and thus prevented tea's beneficial effects on endothelial function and increased blood flow provided.[85] Nevertheless, milk did not impact the absorption of the flavonols quercetin and kaempferol in tea.[86]

There is sufficient evidence that milk can interfere with the health benefits of coffee and tea to recommend that milk not be added to them. I see little reason to add milk to tea other than to mask the bitterness that should not be present if the tea is properly brewed.

But it brings us to a more salient question: Do milk or soy proteins reduce the bioavailability of other hormetic compounds? Are ice cream, frozen yogurt, and smoothies a waste of chocolate, carob, berries, and other hormetic fruits?

The answer to this question appears to be that it depends upon the hormetic compound. Some may bind to milk proteins, delaying their absorption. Other compounds may not be absorbed at all. Some phenolic compounds only become available as a result of microbial fermentation in the colon, and variation in the microbiota population may influence absorption.

In vitro studies suggest enhanced bioavailability of phenolic compounds bound to milk proteins.[87] Anthocyanins from fruit bind mostly to the casein in milk by hydrogen bonding and are easily freed during digestion. Mixing phenolic compounds from black currants into milk was found to protect the phenolic compounds from degradation in the stomach, and thus improve their bioavailable.[88] [89] Thus, while milk may negate some of the benefits of tea and coffee, fruit in yogurt and chocolate froyo seems to be O.K.

Brewing

Coffee can be steamed, boiled, percolated, dripped, cold-brewed, or made with other methods and machines.

The ideal brewing temperature for coffee since the 1950s has been considered to require temperatures from 92–96°C to get "proper extraction", and drip coffee makers are made to maintain water in this temperature range. Hotter water, closer to boiling temperature, extracts acrid, roasty, bitter, and sour attributes into the coffee. Espresso coffee makers can get even higher temperatures, and thus extract more soluble solids from the coffee grounds. Recent research, however, indicates a brewing temperature of 87°C to have flavor indistinguishable from that of 93°C,[90] a temperature with lower scalding risk.

The most important determinant of flavor for freshly ground coffee, when the same beans are used, is the roasting. After that is the extraction. There are three main components to this: grind size, contact time, and temperature. The smaller the grind and the hotter the water, the faster compounds can be transferred from the grounds to the water. To get the freshest and most consistent flavor, the coffee beans should be ground just before brewing. Exposure to air allows the loss of aromatic compounds and degradation of the coffee.

For health benefits, however, the primary goal is to extract compounds that have health benefits and to avoid extracting those that have negative impacts on health. This is most effectively done using ice-water extraction, steeping the coffee grounds under refrigeration for at least 12 and preferably 14 to 24 hours. Cold brewing extracts more caffeine and tends to be less bitter.

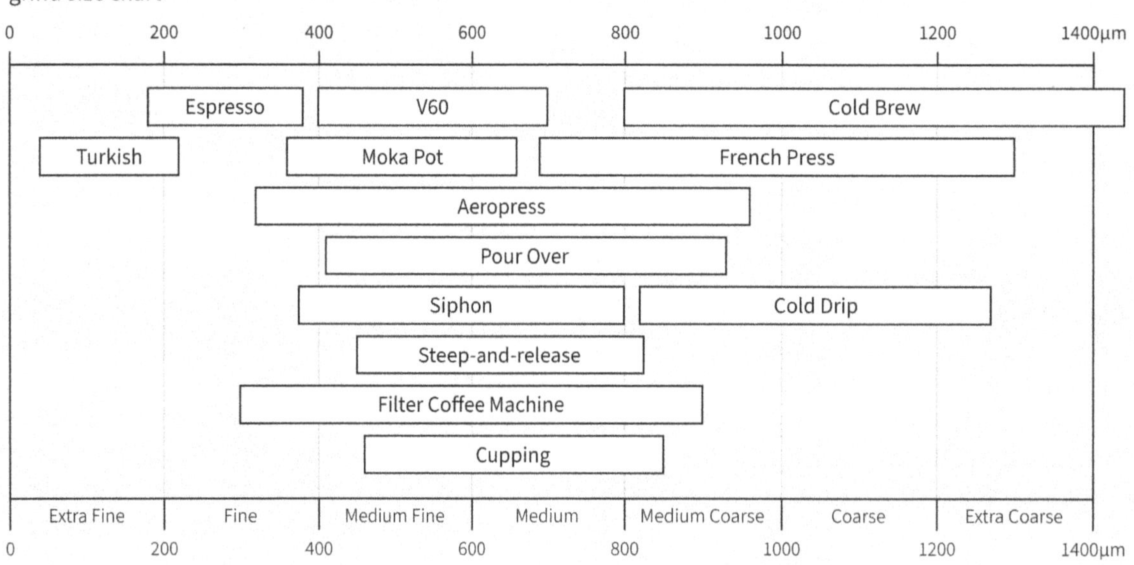

Figure 21B: Grind Size Chart. Courtesy of honestcoffeeguide.com

Table 21D: Coffee Grind Size Impact on Flavor

Under-extraction (Grind is too coarse)	Balanced-Extraction (Appropriate grind)	Over-extraction (Grind is too fine)

Under-extraction (Grind is too coarse)	Balanced-Extraction (Appropriate grind)	Over-extraction (Grind is too fine)
Acidic, sour	Rich, creamy	Bitter
Salty	Complex acidity	Astringent
Lacking sweetness	Sweet	Hollow, dry
Short-lived aftertaste	Great, long-lived aftertaste	Empty

Cold Steeped Coffee: (Recommended) Coffee can be cold-brewed, and this method gives a better HAR score than hot-brewed coffee. Cold brewing extracts a higher amount of caffeine than most other brewing methods and is generally less bitter.

Note: The following recommendation is made not to match any particular style of coffee, or to get the best flavor, but rather to maximize the beneficial effects of coffee on health.

Method: Use coarsely ground coffee beans (about a "French Press" grind). Use chilled water (refrigerator temperature, about 4°C, 38°F), using about 14 ml of water for every gram of coffee grounds. Thus, a 17-gram scoop of coffee for 238 ml, about one cup of water, makes 2 servings. Using a quart glass container, one to 4 cups of cold-steeped coffee can be made. (For 4 servings, use @ 34 grams = @ 1.20 oz of ground coffee) for 2 cups of water to be later diluted 1 to 1. Place the coffee grounds in the jar, followed by a small amount of water. Mix the coffee just enough to make sure it is wet, and then pour in the rest of the water for the amount of coffee grounds (14:1). Place the jar in the refrigerator for 12 to 24 hours. Use a paper filter to separate the coffee from the grounds. Using 2 cups of water and 34 grams of coffee grounds should yield about 300 ml, which can be divided into four (@ 75 ml) servings: Either add hot (near boiling water) or cold water to the 75 ml to dilute it one-to-one, to make 5 oz of coffee, and then heat it if desired. This represents the peak HAR dose. Dividing the 34-gram/300 ml coffee into three 100 ml servings, to be diluted one-to-one, also falls within the hormetic range, and yields about 7 ounces of coffee per serving.

Suggestion: When filtering cold-brewed coffee, first strain the coffee with a fine metal sieve or filter to separate off the grounds, and then filter the coffee with a paper filter as a second step to remove cafestol and kahweol from the coffee. This makes the process quicker and makes clean-up easier.

The dilutions suggested here comply with the Specialty Coffee Association of America standard of 10 grams of ground coffee per 180 ml of water (6 oz.) standard concentration, with this volume as a typical serving size. The volume of water can be adjusted; less water to get a stronger, more to get a milder brew, but the amount of coffee grounds per daily serving should remain the same; about 8.5 grams; no more than 13 grams of coffee grounds should be used per day to stay within the desirable hormetic dose range.

The coffee (concentrate) can be kept refrigerated for several days. It can be warmed to enjoy as a hot beverage or served cold. The coffee should not be returned to the seeping bottle until it has been washed, as some oily residue remains in the jar.

If other brewing methods are used, it is suggested that, if not made using a paper filter, it be passed through one before drinking it. Although they may not get as high a HAR score as cold brew, most brewing methods get a higher score than instant coffee.

Serving Temperature

The "ideal" *serving temperature* for coffee from the barista's point of view is 68 to 70°C (154.5 – 158°F), as this is the temperature at which no one complains that the coffee was served too cold. The preferred sipping temperature for coffee centered around 63°C, perhaps as it stays hot enough not to cool before the cup is finished, and a temperature of about 60°C (140°F) was the preferred drinking temperature by consumers when they controlled the coffee temperature.[91]

Parkinson's Disease Prevention

Like all diseases, but especially irreversible diseases, PD is best prevented. An essential aspect of PD prevention is early detection. Parkinson's disease is a chronic, irreversible disease of the nervous system. It is not limited to the CNS; it also affects the enteric nervous system (ENS). Typically, the first symptom of PD is constipation, with the onset commonly occurring between the ages of 45 to 55; one to two decades before the onset of rigidity, tremor, and cognitive impairment. The next signs of PD develop over about a decade: REM (sleep) Behavior Disorder and excessive daytime sleepiness, often accompanied by depression. The sense of smell becomes dulled (hyposmia), and then orthostatic hypotension often develops, which causes the blood pressure to fall upon standing. About 60% of PD patients have a history of constipation and hyposmia.[92]

PD does not have a single cause, and many people who develop PD have hereditary risks; however, most cases of PD are idiopathic, thus without a known genetic cause. Most PD appears to be caused by one of two pathways, with a small number of patients being affected by both pathways. In one of these causal clusters, there is downregulation of Wnt/β-catenin and thus of neurotrophic factor NEUROD1, which promotes dopaminergic neurogenesis and survival. Wnt/β-catenin also promotes the expression of GRM2. GRM2 encodes the metabotropic glutamate receptor that modulates neurotransmission and synaptic plasticity between the substantia nigra and subthalamic nucleus, and which is essential for the induction of "long-term depression" (LTD). LTD is a dampening mechanism that is important in learning, memory, and motor control, and which may protect the neuronal circuits from excitotoxicity.

The second causal cluster for PD is characterized by enrichment of NF-κB, IL-18, C3AR1, and CASP1 expression, which results in immune activation, inflammation, oxidative stress, and neuronal apoptosis.[93]

In a study of mice with genetic knockdown of Wnt, the animals did not suffer loss of dopaminergic neurons unless they were exposed to a compound that induces mitochondrial damage and oxidative stress.[94] Thus, both impaired Wnt and mitochondrial dysfunction may need to be present to cause neuronal injury in those susceptible to Wnt-associated PD, and avoidance of either may help prevent disease progression.

Caffeine and its metabolite theophylline, but not theobromine, bind to the protein Notum, which interferes with Wnt signaling. Thus, caffeine helps restore Wnt/β-catenin activity.[95] Palmitoleic acid, a fatty acid that is rare in food other than macadamia nuts and sardines, also inhibits Notum-induced degradation of Wnt signaling, and thus, these foods may also help prevent this causal pathway for PD.[96] Caffeine and theobromine promote long-term depression and may also help mitigate excitotoxicity. Thus, those at risk of PD as a result of impaired Wnt/β-catenin activity should receive great benefit from Notum inhibitors. If unsupervised coffee consumption lowers PD risk by 37% (as per the study noted above), and half of those at risk of PD have Wnt/β-catenin susceptibility, it suggests that within this population, caffeine may decrease risk by 74% with even with slipshod dosing. Meanwhile, caffeine would only provide minimal risk reduction from secondary pathways influenced by caffeine, such as AMPK, for those at risk of PD from the inflammatory cluster pathways.

Hormetic factors that reduce inflammatory pathways and oxidative stress should reduce the risk of PD for those susceptible to the second PD causal cluster by down-regulating NF-κB and AP-1-mediated inflammation and apoptosis. "NF-κB-associated" pathways play a role in AD; thus, anti-inflammatory (NRF2) hormetic agents should protect against AD as well, while caffeine would provide only a mild benefit by increasing AMPK activation.

Dysbiosis appears to be a common source of inflammation causing PD. Pathologic dominance of the mucin-digesting species (such as *Akkermansia*) can disrupt the integrity of the mucosal barrier.[97] This can occur when there is insufficient fiber for the production of SCFA for the production of mucin. Some studies implicate a deficit of short-chain fatty acid-producing bacteria in the colon (such as *Bifidobacteria*), which are required for colonocyte health and brain energy during fasting.

Digestion of the mucus liberates cysteine in the colon, which supports the growth of bacteria that produce hydrogen sulfide (H2S) (such as *Clostridia and Desulfovibrio*). H2S is a physiologic gasotransmitter; however, it is neurotoxic in high amounts.[98] Increased mucosal permeability, in part from the degradation of mucin, allows toxins such as LPS to enter the bloodstream from the lumen of the colon, which activates neuroinflammation via TLR4, injuring the brain.[99] [100] It may be the combination of H2S, LPS, and other toxins that promote PD.[101] Metabolic degradation of H2S in the brain requires glutathione; thus, H2S metabolism may also deplete this essential antioxidant.[102, 103] These alterations in the microbiome are well documented in late-stage PD and are almost certainly present in the prodromal stages of the disease. H2S metabolism also needs vitamins B6, B12, and B9 (folate), and iron and zinc as enzymatic cofactors.

Irritable bowel syndrome most frequently manifests with constipation (IBS-C). As with PD, adults with IBS-C commonly have alterations in the sense of smell (and thus taste) and depression.[104] Individuals with IBS are at elevated risk of PD.[105] Those with IBS are also at increased risk of restless leg syndrome, a manifestation of REM Behavior Disorder,[106] a prodromal symptom of PD. Not all patients with IBS develop PD. IBS-C can resolve, perhaps as a result of a change in diet, use of antibiotics, or suppression of other organisms. IBS is much more common in women than in men, while PD is more common in men. Women are thought to be protected from PD by estrogen.

A decline in the sense of smell (hyposmia) can be an early symptom of PD. It does not develop in all PD patients but occurs in most. Hyposmia can begin years or even decades before motor symptoms and can be the first sign of PD. On testing, odor identification (Name this smell) is more sensitive than odor discrimination (Which one of these is chocolate?), followed by odor detection threshold.[107] First, there is a loss in discrimination; the person can tell there is a scent, but confuses it or can't identify it. Later, they lose the perception of smell. Hyposmia is also typical of Alzheimer's disease and is present in many patients by the time mild cognitive impairment (MCI) is diagnosed. Hyposmia in MCI appears to be predictive of AD progression.[108] While some studies suggest that the ability to distinguish certain odors may be lost earlier; banana, licorice, and dill pickle, pineapple, pizza for PD, and banana, cinnamon, clove and garlic for MCI; any loss of smell should be a concern.[109, 110, 111, 112, 113]

The onset of constipation, IBS, or REM Behavior Disorder during middle age should be considered a possible early sign of PD, especially in men. There is some evidence that even after the manifestation of clinical disease, treating the GI microbiome may mitigate PD symptoms.[114] [115] Even late in the disease, fecal material transplant, at least transiently, reduces constipation, leg tremors, anxiety, depression, and improves sleep quality, postural stability, and gait.[116] Normalization of the GI microbiome can improve GI symptoms and decrease the absorption of toxins from the bowel. This should slow PD progression.

The time to treat PD is early in the prodromal phase of the disease before severe damage to the brain has occurred, or earlier. The ENS of the GI tract has considerably more capacity for recovery than does the CNS. Diet and lifestyle modifications should be done as early in the progression of the disease as possible, as there is little recovery of neurons in the brain once they have been lost.

In PD patients with a LRRK2 gene dysfunction, consumption of black tea delayed the age of onset of PD by 5.6 years, but coffee and caffeinated soda did not alter the age of disease onset. In idiopathic-PD patients, coffee consumption was associated with a 2.2-year delay in the age of onset. This lesser amount of protection might be a reflection of only about half of the patients being susceptible to deficits in WNT metabolism. Meanwhile, the consumption of caffeinated soda *lowered* the age of onset by 3.8 years. Green tea did not affect the age of onset of either form of PD.[117] This data suggests that while caffeine helps prevent PD, soda pop and compounds present in coffee other than caffeine may accelerate the disease.

It is my assessment that those with PD, its prodrome, or those at high risk of PD should avoid coffee and other caffeinated beverages and rather take 100 mg to 120 mg of caffeine as a "supplement" daily. Over-the-counter 100 mg caffeine tablets are widely available, and pharmaceutical-quality dosing will ensure receiving a reliable and appropriate dose on a regular daily basis. A four-month supply is about the cost of one cup of coffee at a coffee shop. The amount of caffeine present in coffee is unreliable. Additionally, the frequent failure of coffee to prevent PD suggests that coffee may contain compounds that increase PD risk, or at least inhibit the PD-preventive benefits of caffeine.

Ambroxol is a medication used in Europe to break up phlegm in those with respiratory infections, but has been found to have additional properties. It increases glucocerebrosidase (GCase) expression, which upregulates the Wnt/β-catenin pathway, and thereby promotes neural stem cell differentiation into neurons, and has been shown to decrease infarct size after strokes.[118] Ambroxal promotes the resolution of microglial activation and neuroinflammation, downregulating inflammatory cytokines and enhancing autophagy and lysosomal clearance of misfolded protein, decreasing ER (endoplasmic reticulum) stress.[119]

Ambroxol is a potential PD-preventive agent and therapeutic candidate for those with Wnt/β-catenin-associated PD risk. Since caffeine and Ambroxol upregulate Wnt/β-catenin through different mechanisms; thus, the combination of these agents may provide synergistic effects for the treatment of Wnt/β-catenin cluster type PD. I suggest cell culture synergy studies for Wnt/ β-catenin activity for combinations of caffeine and Ambroxol, followed by an animal model study of PD with Wnt knockdown and oxidative stress.

[1] Loomis D, Guyton KZ, Grosse Y, Lauby-Secretan B, El Ghissassi F, Bouvard V, Benbrahim-Tallaa L, Guha N, Mattock H, Straif K; International Agency for Research on Cancer Monograph Working Group. Carcinogenicity of drinking coffee, mate, and very hot beverages. Lancet Oncol. 2016 Jul;17(7):877-878. doi: 10.1016/S1470-2045(16)30239-X. Epub 2016 Jun 15. PMID: 27318851.

[2] Acute effects of (-)-gallocatechin gallate-rich green tea extract on the cerebral hemodynamic response of the prefrontal cortex in healthy humans. Cha J, Kim HS, Kwon G, Cho SY, Kim JM. Front Neuroergon. 2023 Nov 27;4:1136362. doi: 10.3389/fnrgo.2023.1136362. eCollection 2023. PMID: 38234497

[3] Beneficial effects of green tea: a literature review. Chacko SM, Thambi PT, Kuttan R, Nishigaki I. Chin Med. 2010 Apr 6;5:13. doi: 10.1186/1749-8546-5-13. PMID: 20370896

[4] Diet, Food, and Nutritional Exposures and Inflammatory Bowel Disease or Progression of Disease: an Umbrella Review. Christensen C, Knudsen A, Arnesen EK, Hatlebakk JG, Sletten IS, Fadnes LT. Adv Nutr. 2024 May;15(5):100219. doi: 10.1016/j.advnut.2024.100219. Epub 2024 Apr 8. PMID: 38599319

[5] Physiological Effects and Human Health Benefits of *Hibiscus sabdariffa*: A Review of Clinical Trials. Montalvo-González E, Villagrán Z, González-Torres S, Iñiguez-Muñoz LE, Isiordia-Espinoza MA, Ruvalcaba-Gómez JM, Arteaga-Garibay RI, Acosta JL, González-Silva N, Anaya-Esparza LM. Pharmaceuticals (Basel). 2022 Apr 12;15(4):464. doi: 10.3390/ph15040464. PMID: 35455462

[6] Exploring the Health Benefits and Therapeutic Potential of Roselle (Hibiscus sabdariffa) in Human Studies: A Comprehensive Review. Almajid A, Bazroon A, AlAhmed A, Bakhurji O. Cureus. 2023 Nov 23;15(11):e49309. doi: 10.7759/cureus.49309. eCollection 2023 Nov. PMID: 38024072

[7] Potential Anti-Tumorigenic Properties of Diverse Medicinal Plants against the Majority of Common Types of Cancer. Albahri G, Badran A, Abdel Baki Z, Alame M, Hijazi A, Daou A, Baydoun E. Pharmaceuticals (Basel). 2024 Apr 30;17(5):574. doi: 10.3390/ph17050574. PMID: 38794144

[8] Roselle (Hibiscus sabdariffa L.) calyces tea improves physical fitness of healthy adults. Lubis L, Dewi GT, Supriyan AND, Aprinaldi A, Purba A, Diantini A. Biomed Rep. 2024 Jan 29;20(3):49. doi: 10.3892/br.2024.1737. eCollection 2024 Mar. PMID: 38357241

[9] Roselle is cardioprotective in diet-induced obesity rat model with myocardial infarction. Si LY, Ali SAM, Latip J, Fauzi NM, Budin SB, Zainalabidin S. Life Sci. 2017 Dec 15;191:157-165. doi: 10.1016/j.lfs.2017.10.030. Epub 2017 Oct 21. PMID: 29066253

[10] Phytochemicals for Improving Aspects of Cognitive Function and Psychological State Potentially Relevant to Sports Performance. Kennedy DO. Sports Med. 2019 Feb;49(Suppl 1):39-58. doi: 10.1007/s40279-018-1007-0. PMID: 30671903

[11] Medicinal Plants Used as an Alternative to Treat Gingivitis and Periodontitis. Rani N, Singla RK, Narwal S, Tanushree, Kumar N, Rahman MM. Evid Based Complement Alternat Med. 2022 Sep 6;2022:2327641. doi: 10.1155/2022/2327641. eCollection 2022. PMID: 37941972

[12] https://www.webmd.com/ibs/peppermint-oil-works

[13] Peppermint Oil Am Fam Physician. 2007;75(7):1027-1030. BENJAMIN KLIGLER, M.D., M.P.H., AND SAPNA CHAUDHARY, D.O https://www.aafp.org/pubs/afp/issues/2007/0401/p1027.html

[14] https://www.hollandandbarrett.com/the-health-hub/vitamins-and-supplements/what-is-peppermint-oil/

[15] https://www.dottys-oils.com/doterra-peppermint

[16] Bioactive properties of *Sambucus nigra* L. as a functional ingredient for food and pharmaceutical industry. Młynarczyk K, Walkowiak-Tomczak D, Łysiak GP. J Funct Foods. 2018 Jan;40:377-390. doi: 10.1016/j.jff.2017.11.025. Epub 2017 Dec 22. PMID: 32362939

[17] Effectiveness of chamomile tea on glycemic control and serum lipid profile in patients with type 2 diabetes. Rafraf M, Zemestani M, Asghari-Jafarabadi M. J Endocrinol Invest. 2015 Feb;38(2):163-70. doi: 10.1007/s40618-014-0170-x. Epub 2014 Sep 7. PMID: 25194428

[18] Chamomile tea improves glycemic indices and antioxidants status in patients with type 2 diabetes mellitus. Zemestani M, Rafraf M, Asghari-Jafarabadi M. Nutrition. 2016 Jan;32(1):66-72. doi: 10.1016/j.nut.2015.07.011. Epub 2015 Aug 14. PMID: 26437613

[19] Effects of an intervention with drinking chamomile tea on sleep quality and depression in sleep disturbed postnatal women: a randomized controlled trial.

Chang SM, Chen CH. J Adv Nurs. 2016 Feb;72(2):306-15. doi: 10.1111/jan.12836. Epub 2015 Oct 20. PMID: 26483209

[20] Chlorogenic Acid and Caffeine in Coffee Restore Insulin Signaling in Pancreatic Beta Cells. Ihara Y, Asahara SI, Inoue H, Seike M, Ando M, Kabutoya H, Kimura-Koyanagi M, Kido Y. Kobe J Med Sci. 2023 Mar 2;69(1):E1-E8. PMID: 37088693

[21] How Much Caffeine is Too Much? A Full Guide on Caffeine Overdose | Healthnews https://healthnews.com/nutrition/healthy-eating/caffeine-overdose-what-to-know-before-consuming/

[22] Caffeine intake during pregnancy and adverse outcomes: An integrative review. Rohweder R, de Oliveira Schmalfuss T, Dos Santos Borniger D, Ferreira CZ, Zanardini MK, Lopes GPTF, Barbosa CP, Moreira TD, Schuler-Faccini L, Sanseverino MTV, da Silva AA, Abeche AM, Vianna FSL, Fraga LR. Reprod Toxicol. 2024 Jan;123:108518. doi: 10.1016/j.reprotox.2023.108518. PMID: 38042437

[23] Beverages - a scoping review for Nordic Nutrition Recommendations 2023. Sonestedt E, Lukic M. Food Nutr Res. 2024 Apr 2;68. doi: 10.29219/fnr.v68.10458. eCollection 2024. PMID: 38571923

24 Frequency of a diagnosis of glaucoma in individuals who consume coffee, tea and/or soft drinks. Wu CM, Wu AM, Tseng VL, Yu F, Coleman AL. Br J Ophthalmol. 2018 Aug;102(8):1127-1133. doi: 10.1136/bjophthalmol-2017-310924. Epub 2017 Dec 14. PMID: 29242183

25 Effects of consumption of coffee, tea, or soft drinks on open-angle glaucoma: Korea National Health and Nutrition Examination Survey 2010 to 2011. Bae JH, Kim JM, Lee JM, Song JE, Lee MY, Chung PW, Park KH. PLoS One. 2020 Jul 20;15(7):e0236152. doi: 10.1371/journal.pone.0236152. eCollection 2020. PMID: 32687521

26 Short-term effects of caffeine intake on anterior chamber angle and intraocular pressure in low caffeine consumers. Redondo B, Vera J, Molina R, Jiménez R. Graefes Arch Clin Exp Ophthalmol. 2020 Mar;258(3):613-619. doi: 10.1007/s00417-019-04556-z. Epub 2019 Dec 10. PMID: 31823063

27 The effect of caffeine on intraocular pressure: a systematic review and meta-analysis. Li M, Wang M, Guo W, Wang J, Sun X. Graefes Arch Clin Exp Ophthalmol. 2011 Mar;249(3):435-42. doi: 10.1007/s00417-010-1455-1. Epub 2010 Aug 13. PMID: 20706731

28 Computer vision techniques for modelling the roasting process of coffee (Coffea arabica L.) var. Castillo. Eugenio Ivorra et al. Czech Journal of Food Sciences, 38, 2020 (6): 388–396. https://doi.org/10.17221/346/2019-CJFS

29 Effect of regular and decaffeinated coffee on serum gastrin levels. Acquaviva F, DeFrancesco A, Andriulli A, Piantino P, Arrigoni A, Massarenti P, Balzola F. J Clin Gastroenterol. 1986 Apr;8(2):150-3. doi: 10.1097/00004836-198604000-00009. PMID: 3745848

30 Effects of a non-caffeinated coffee substitute on functional dyspepsia. Correia H, Peneiras S, Levchook N, Peneiras E, Levchook T, Nayyar J. Clin Nutr ESPEN. 2021 Feb;41:412-416. doi: 10.1016/j.clnesp.2020.10.009. Epub 2020 Oct 29. PMID: 33487298

31 Effect of different coffees on esophageal acid contact time and symptoms in coffee-sensitive subjects. Brazer SR, Onken JE, Dalton CB, Smith JW, Schiffman SS. Physiol Behav. 1995 Mar;57(3):563-7. doi: 10.1016/0031-9384(94)00363-a. PMID: 7753895

32 A randomized, double-blind comparison of two different coffee-roasting processes on development of heartburn and dyspepsia in coffee-sensitive individuals. DiBaise JK. Dig Dis Sci. 2003 Apr;48(4):652-6. doi: 10.1023/a:1022860019852. PMID: 12741451

33 A dark brown roast coffee blend is less effective at stimulating gastric acid secretion in healthy volunteers compared to a medium roast market blend. Rubach M, Lang R, Bytof G, Stiebitz H, Lantz I, Hofmann T, Somoza V. Mol Nutr Food Res. 2014 Jun;58(6):1370-3. PMID:24510512

34 Effects of Coffee on the Gastro-Intestinal Tract: A Narrative Review and Literature Update. Nehlig A. Nutrients. 2022 Jan 17;14(2):399. doi: 10.3390/nu14020399. PMID: 35057580

35 Association between coffee intake and gastroesophageal reflux disease: a meta-analysis. Kim J, Oh SW, Myung SK, Kwon H, Lee C, Yun JM, Lee HK; Korean Meta-analysis (KORMA) Study Group. Dis Esophagus. 2014 May-Jun;27(4):311-7. doi: 10.1111/dote.12099. Epub 2013 Jun 24. PMID: 23795898

36 Association between tea consumption and gastroesophageal reflux disease: A meta-analysis. Cao H, Huang X, Zhi X, Han C, Li L, Li Y. Medicine (Baltimore). 2019 Jan;98(4):e14173. doi: 10.1097/MD.0000000000014173. PMID: 30681584

37 Effects of Coffee on the Gastro-Intestinal Tract: A Narrative Review and Literature Update. Nehlig A. Nutrients. 2022 Jan 17;14(2):399. doi: 10.3390/nu14020399. PMID: 35057580

38 Health Effects of Coffee: Mechanism Unraveled? Kolb H, Kempf K, Martin S. Nutrients. 2020 Jun 20;12(6):1842. doi: 10.3390/nu12061842. PMID: 32575704

39 Association between Coffee Consumption and Polycystic Ovary Syndrome: An Exploratory Case-Control Study. Meliani-Rodríguez A, Cutillas-Tolín A, Mendiola J, Sánchez-Ferrer ML, De la Cruz-Sánchez E, Vioque J, Torres-Cantero AM. Nutrients. 2024 Jul 11;16(14):2238. doi: 10.3390/nu16142238. PMID: 39064680

40 Beverage consumption and risk of ulcerative colitis: Systematic review and meta-analysis of epidemiological studies. Nie JY, Zhao Q. Medicine (Baltimore). 2017 Dec;96(49):e9070. doi: 10.1097/MD.0000000000009070. PMID: 29245319

41 Beverage intake and risk of Crohn disease: A meta-analysis of 16 epidemiological studies. Yang Y, Xiang L, He J. Medicine (Baltimore). 2019 May;98(21):e15795. doi: 10.1097/MD.0000000000015795. PMID: 31124976

42 Diet, Food, and Nutritional Exposures and Inflammatory Bowel Disease or Progression of Disease: an Umbrella Review. Christensen C, Knudsen A, Arnesen EK, Hatlebakk JG, Sletten IS, Fadnes LT. Adv Nutr. 2024 May;15(5):100219. doi: 10.1016/j.advnut.2024.100219. Epub 2024 Apr 8. PMID: 38599319

43 Effects of Coffee on the Gastro-Intestinal Tract: A Narrative Review and Literature Update. Nehlig A. Nutrients. 2022 Jan 17;14(2):399. doi: 10.3390/nu14020399. PMID: 35057580

44 Dark roast coffee is more effective than light roast coffee in reducing body weight, and in restoring red blood cell vitamin E and glutathione concentrations in healthy volunteers. Kotyczka C, Boettler U, Lang R, Stiebitz H, Bytof G, Lantz I, Hofmann T, Marko D, Somoza V. Mol Nutr Food Res. 2011 Oct;55(10):1582-6. doi: 10.1002/mnfr.201100248. Epub 2011 Aug 2. PMID: 21809439

45 Effects of coffee with different roasting degrees on obesity and related metabolic disorders. Claudia I. Gamboa-Gómez, et al. Journal of Functional Foods. Vol.111, December 2023, 105889 https://doi.org/10.1016/j.jff.2023.105889

46 Association of Coffee, Decaffeinated Coffee and Caffeine Intake from Coffee with Cognitive Performance in Older Adults: National Health and Nutrition Examination Survey (NHANES) 2011-2014. Dong X, Li S, Sun J, Li Y, Zhang D.

Nutrients. 2020 Mar 20;12(3):840. doi: 10.3390/nu12030840. PMID: 32245123

47 Association of Coffee Consumption and Prediagnostic Caffeine Metabolites With Incident Parkinson Disease in a Population-Based Cohort. Zhao Y, Lai Y, Konijnenberg H, Huerta JM, Vinagre-Aragon A, Sabin JA, Hansen J, Petrova D, Sacerdote C, Zamora-Ros R, Pala V, Heath AK, Panico S, Guevara M, Masala G, Lill CM, Miller GW, Peters S, Vermeulen R. Neurology. 2024 Apr 23;102(8):e209201. doi: 10.1212/WNL.0000000000209201. Epub 2024 Mar 21. PMID: 38513162

48 Association of Coffee Consumption and Prediagnostic Caffeine Metabolites With Incident Parkinson Disease in a Population-Based Cohort. Zhao Y, Lai Y, Konijnenberg H, Huerta JM, Vinagre-Aragon A, Sabin JA, Hansen J, Petrova D, Sacerdote C, Zamora-Ros R, Pala V, Heath AK, Panico S, Guevara M, Masala G, Lill CM, Miller GW, Peters S, Vermeulen R. Neurology. 2024 Apr 23;102(8):e209201. doi: 10.1212/WNL.0000000000209201. PMID: 38513162 SUPPLEMENTARY MATERIALS

49 https://www.bruncher.com/news/10-things-you-didnt-know-about-coffee-in-the-uk/

50 https://learn.bluecoffeebox.com/the-uks-most-popular-coffees/

51 Effect of Daily Coffee Consumption on the Risk of Alzheimer's Disease: A Systematic Review and Meta-Analysis. Nila IS, Villagra Moran VM, Khan ZA, Hong Y. J Lifestyle Med. 2023 Aug 31;13(2):83-89. doi: 10.15280/jlm.2023.13.2.83. PMID: 37970326

52 Alcohol, coffee and tea intake and the risk of cognitive deficits: a dose-response meta-analysis. Ran LS, Liu WH, Fang YY, Xu SB, Li J, Luo X, Pan DJ, Wang MH, Wang W. Epidemiol Psychiatr Sci. 2021 Feb 11;30:e13. doi: 10.1017/S2045796020001183. PMID: 33568254

53 Alcohol, coffee and tea intake and the risk of cognitive deficits: a dose-response meta-analysis. Ran LS, Liu WH, Fang YY, Xu SB, Li J, Luo X, Pan DJ, Wang MH, Wang W. Epidemiol Psychiatr Sci. 2021 Feb 11;30:e13. doi: 10.1017/S2045796020001183. PMID: 33568254

54 Coffee modulates transcription factor NRF2 and highly increases the activity of antioxidant enzymes in rats. Vicente SJ, Ishimoto EY, Torres EA. J Agric Food Chem. 2014 Jan 8;62(1):116-22. PMID:24328189

55 Increase of the activity of phase II antioxidant enzymes in rats after a single dose of coffee. Vicente SJ, Ishimoto EY, Cruz RJ, Pereira CD, Torres EA. J Agric Food Chem. 2011 Oct 26;59(20):10887-92. PMID:21942680

56 Influence of feeding malt, bread crust, and a pronylated protein on the activity of chemopreventive enzymes and antioxidative defense parameters in vivo. Somoza V, Wenzel E, Lindenmeier M, Grothe D, Erbersdobler HF, Hofmann T. J Agric Food Chem. 2005 Oct 19;53(21):8176-82. PMID:16218661

57 Inhibitory effect of bread crust antioxidant pronyl-lysine on two different categories of colonic premalignant lesions induced by 1,2-dimethylhydrazine. Panneerselvam J, Aranganathan S, Nalini N. Eur J Cancer Prev. 2009 Aug;18(4):291-302. PMID:19417676

58 Battling Bitter Coffee: Chemists Identify Roasting As The Main Culprit. Science Daily, Aug. 22, 2007 https://www.sciencedaily.com/releases/2007/08/070821143629.htm

59 Degree of roasting is the main determinant of the effects of coffee on NF-kappaB and EpRE. Paur I, Balstad TR, Blomhoff R. Free Radic Biol Med. 2010 May 1;48(9):1218-27. PMID:20176103

60 Consumption of a dark roast coffee decreases the level of spontaneous DNA strand breaks: a randomized controlled trial. Bakuradze T, Lang R, Hofmann T, Eisenbrand G, Schipp D, Galan J, Richling E. Eur J Nutr. 2015 Feb;54(1):149-56. PMID:24740588

61 Anti-fibrillation potency of caffeic acid against an antidepressant induced fibrillogenesis of human α-synuclein: Implications for Parkinson's disease. Fazili NA, Naeem A. Biochimie. 2015 Jan;108:178-85. doi: 10.1016/j.biochi.2014.11.011. Epub 2014 Nov 22. PMID: 25461276

62 Phenylindanes in Brewed Coffee Inhibit Amyloid-Beta and Tau Aggregation. Mancini RS, Wang Y, Weaver DF. Front Neurosci. 2018 Oct 12;12:735. doi: 10.3389/fnins.2018.00735. eCollection 2018. PMID: 30369868

63 Potential antioxidant response to coffee - A matter of genotype? Hassmann U, Haupt LM, Smith RA, Winkler S, Bytof G, Lantz I, Griffiths LR, Marko D. Meta Gene. 2014 Aug 7;2:525-39. PMID:25606436

64 Dark roast coffee is more effective than light roast coffee in reducing body weight, and in restoring red blood cell vitamin E and glutathione concentrations in healthy volunteers. Kotyczka C, Boettler U, Lang R, Stiebitz H, Bytof G, Lantz I, Hofmann T, Marko D, Somoza V. Mol Nutr Food Res. 2011 Oct;55(10):1582-6. PMID:21809439

65 Chronic coffee consumption in the diet-induced obese rat: impact on gut microbiota and serum metabolomics. Cowan TE, Palmnäs MS, Yang J, Bomhof MR, Ardell KL, Reimer RA, Vogel HJ, Shearer J. J Nutr Biochem. 2014 Apr;25(4):489-95. doi: 10.1016/j.jnutbio.2013.12.009. Epub 2014 Jan 30. PMID: 24629912

66 Effect of coffee or coffee components on gut microbiome and short-chain fatty acids in a mouse model of metabolic syndrome. Nishitsuji K, Watanabe S, Xiao J, Nagatomo R, Ogawa H, Tsunematsu T, Umemoto H, Morimoto Y, Akatsu H, Inoue K, Tsuneyama K. Sci Rep. 2018 Nov 1;8(1):16173. doi: 10.1038/s41598-018-34571-9. PMID: 30385796

67 Caffeine Protects Skin from Oxidative Stress-Induced Senescence through the Activation of Autophagy. Li YF, Ouyang SH, Tu LF, Wang X, Yuan WL, Wang GE, Wu YP, Duan WJ, Yu HM, Fang ZZ, Kurihara H, Zhang Y, He RR. Theranostics. 2018 Nov 10;8(20):5713-5730. doi: 10.7150/thno.28778. eCollection 2018. PMID: 30555576

68 Effect of caffeine on mitochondrial biogenesis in the skeletal muscle - A narrative review. Yamada AK, Pimentel GD, Pickering C, Cordeiro AV, Silva VRR. Clin Nutr ESPEN. 2022 Oct;51:1-6. doi: 10.1016/j.clnesp.2022.09.001. Epub 2022 Sep 13. PMID: 36184193

69 AMPK activation induces mitophagy and promotes mitochondrial fission while activating TBK1 in a PINK1-Parkin independent manner. Seabright AP, Fine NHF, Barlow JP, Lord SO, Musa I, Gray A, Bryant JA, Banzhaf M, Lavery GG, Hardie DG, Hodson DJ, Philp A, Lai YC. FASEB J. 2020 May;34(5):6284-6301. doi: 10.1096/fj.201903051R. Epub 2020 Mar 22. PMID: 32201986

70 Thebromine Targets Adenosine Receptors to Control Hippocampal Neuronal Function and Damage. Valada P, Alçada-Morais S, Cunha RA, Lopes JP. Int J Mol Sci. 2022 Sep 10;23(18):10510. doi: 10.3390/ijms231810510. PMID: 36142422

71 The physiological effects of caffeine on synaptic transmission and plasticity in the mouse hippocampus selectively depend on adenosine A_1 and A_{2A} receptors. Lopes JP, Pliássova A, Cunha RA. Biochem Pharmacol. 2019 Aug;166:313-321. doi: 10.1016/j.bcp.2019.06.008. Epub 2019 Jun 12. PMID: 31199895

72 Blockade of adenosine A_{2A} receptors recovers early deficits of memory and plasticity in the triple transgenic mouse model of Alzheimer's disease. Silva AC, Lemos C, Gonçalves FQ, Pliássova AV, Machado NJ, Silva HB, Canas PM, Cunha RA, Lopes JP, Agostinho P. Neurobiol Dis. 2018 Sep;117:72-81. doi: 10.1016/j.nbd.2018.05.024. Epub 2018 May 31. PMID: 29859867

73 Caffeine acts through neuronal adenosine A2A receptors to prevent mood and memory dysfunction triggered by chronic stress. Kaster MP, Machado NJ, Silva HB, Nunes A, Ardais AP, Santana M, Baqi Y, Müller CE, Rodrigues AL, Porciúncula LO, Chen JF, Tomé ÂR, Agostinho P, Canas PM, Cunha RA. Proc Natl Acad Sci U S A. 2015 Jun 23;112(25):7833-8. doi: 10.1073/pnas.1423088112. Epub 2015 Jun 8. PMID: 26056314

74 Nonlinear dynamics of multi-omics profiles during human aging. Shen X, Wang C, Zhou X, Zhou W, Hornburg D, Wu S, Snyder MP. Nat Aging. 2024 Aug 14. doi: 10.1038/s43587-024-00692-2. Online ahead of print. PMID: 39143318

75 Effect of caffeine on mitochondrial biogenesis in the skeletal muscle - A narrative review. Yamada AK, Pimentel GD, Pickering C, Cordeiro AV, Silva VRR. Clin Nutr ESPEN. 2022 Oct;51:1-6. doi: 10.1016/j.clnesp.2022.09.001. Epub 2022 Sep 13. PMID: 36184193

76 Health benefits and mechanisms of theobromine. Mengjuan Zhang, Haifeng Zhang, Lu Jia, et al. J Funtional Foods. 15, 2024. 2024, 106126, ISSN 1756-4646, https://doi.org/10.1016/j.jff.2024.106126.

77 Is cafestol retained on the paper filter in the preparation of filter coffee? Rendón YM et al. 30 Sep 2017 Food Research International (Food Res Int) 100(1)798-803. https://doi.org/10.1016/j.foodres.2017.08.013

78 Zhang, C.; Linforth, R.; Fisk, I. D. (2012). "Cafestol extraction yield from different coffee brew mechanisms". Food Research International. 49: 27–31. https://doi.org/10.1016/j.foodres.2012.06.032

79 The cholesterol-raising factor from coffee beans, cafestol, as an agonist ligand for the farnesoid and pregnane X receptors. Ricketts ML, Boekschoten MV, Kreeft AJ, Hooiveld GJ, Moen CJ, Müller M, Frants RR, Kasanmoentalib S, Post SM, Princen HM, Porter JG, Katan MB, Hofker MH, Moore DD. Mol Endocrinol. 2007 Jul;21(7):1603-16. doi: 10.1210/me.2007-0133. Epub 2007 Apr 24. PMID: 17456796

80 Neuroprotective Effects of Coffee Bioactive Compounds: A Review. Socała K, Szopa A, Serefko A, Poleszak E, Wlaź P. Int J Mol Sci. 2020 Dec 24;22(1):107. doi: 10.3390/ijms22010107. PMID: 33374338

81 Computer vision techniques for modelling the roasting process of coffee (Coffea arabica L.) var. Castillo. Eugenio Ivorra et al. Czech Journal of Food Sciences, 38, 2020 (6): 388–396. https://doi.org/10.17221/346/2019-CJFS

82 Effect of simultaneous consumption of milk and coffee on chlorogenic acids' bioavailability in humans. Duarte GS, Farah A. J Agric Food Chem. 2011 Jul 27;59(14):7925-31. doi: 10.1021/jf201906p. Epub 2011 Jun 15. PMID: 21627318

83 Effect of simultaneous consumption of soymilk and coffee on the urinary excretion of isoflavones, chlorogenic acids and metabolites in healthy adults. Felberg, I Fara A, Monteiro , et al. Journal of Functional Foods,19A. Dec. 2015 688-699 https://doi.org/10.1016/j.jff.2015.09.059

84 Simultaneous ingestion of dietary proteins reduces the bioavailability of galloylated catechins from green tea in humans. Egert S, Tereszczuk J, Wein S, Müller MJ, Frank J, Rimbach G, Wolffram S. Eur J Nutr. 2013 Feb;52(1):281-8. doi: 10.1007/s00394-012-0330-8. Epub 2012 Feb 25. PMID: 22366739

85 Addition of milk prevents vascular protective effects of tea. Lorenz M, Jochmann N, von Krosigk A, Martus P, Baumann G, Stangl K, Stangl V. Eur Heart J. 2007 Jan;28(2):219-23. doi: 10.1093/eurheartj/ehl442. Epub 2007 Jan 9. PMID: 17213230

86 Effects of infusion time and addition of milk on content and absorption of polyphenols from black tea. Kyle JA, Morrice PC, McNeill G, Duthie GG. J Agric Food Chem. 2007 Jun 13;55(12):4889-94. doi: 10.1021/jf070351y. Epub 2007 May 10. PMID: 17489604

87 Predominance of non-covalent interactions of polyphenols with milk proteins and their health promoting properties. Mao T, Wescombe P, Mohan MS. Crit Rev Food Sci Nutr. 2024 Nov;64(32):11871-11893. doi: 10.1080/10408398.2023.2245037. Epub 2023 Aug 16. PMID: 37584498

88 Preferential Binding of Polyphenols in Blackcurrant Extracts with Milk Proteins and the Effects on the Bioaccessibility and Antioxidant Activity of Polyphenols. Mao T, Akshit F, Matiwalage I, Sasidharan S, Alvarez CM, Wescombe P, Mohan MS. Foods. 2024 Feb 7;13(4):515. doi: 10.3390/foods13040515. PMID: 38397492

89 Structural, Binding and Functional Properties of Milk Protein-Polyphenol Systems: A Review. van de Langerijt TM, O'Mahony JA, Crowley SV. Molecules. 2023 Mar 1;28(5):2288. doi: 10.3390/molecules28052288. PMID: 36903537

90 Batali, M.E., Ristenpart, W.D. & Guinard, JX. Brew temperature, at fixed brew strength and extraction, has

little impact on the sensory profile of drip brew coffee. Sci Rep 10, 16450 (2020). https://doi.org/10.1038/s41598-020-73341-4

91 Impact of beverage temperature on consumer preferences for black coffee. Ristenpart, W.D., Cotter, A.R. & Guinard, JX. Sci Rep 12, 20621 (2022). https://doi.org/10.1038/s41598-022-23904-4

92 Biofluid Markers for Prodromal Parkinson's Disease: Evidence From a Catecholaminergic Perspective. Vermeiren Y, Hirschberg Y, Mertens I, De Deyn PP. Front Neurol. 2020 Jul 15;11:595. doi: 10.3389/fneur.2020.00595. PMID: 32760338

93 A Hybrid Machine Learning and Network Analysis Approach Reveals Two Parkinson's Disease Subtypes from 115 RNA-Seq Post-Mortem Brain Samples. Termine A, Fabrizio C, Strafella C, Caputo V, Petrosini L, Caltagirone C, Cascella R, Giardina E. Int J Mol Sci. 2022 Feb 25;23(5):2557. doi: 10.3390/ijms23052557. PMID: 35269707

94 Conditional Haploinsufficiency of β-Catenin Aggravates Neuronal Damage in a Paraquat-Based Mouse Model of Parkinson Disease. Zhao F, Siedlak SL, Torres SL, Xu Q, Tang B, Zhu X. Mol Neurobiol. 2019 Jul;56(7):5157-5166. doi: 10.1007/s12035-018-1431-z. Epub 2018 Dec 6. PMID: 30519817

95 Caffeine inhibits Notum activity by binding at the catalytic pocket. Zhao Y, Ren J, Hillier J, Lu W, Jones EY. Commun Biol. 2020 Oct 8;3(1):555. doi: 10.1038/s42003-020-01286-5. PMID: 33033363

96 Small-molecule inhibitors of carboxylesterase Notum. Zhao Y, Jolly S, Benvegnu S, Jones EY, Fish PV. Future Med Chem. 2021 Jun;13(11):1001-1015. doi: 10.4155/fmc-2021-0036. Epub 2021 Apr 22. PMID: 33882714

97 Short chain fatty acids-producing and mucin-degrading intestinal bacteria predict the progression of early Parkinson's disease. Nishiwaki H, Ito M, Hamaguchi T, Maeda T, Kashihara K, Tsuboi Y, Ueyama J, Yoshida T, Hanada H, Takeuchi I, Katsuno M, Hirayama M, Ohno K. NPJ Parkinsons Dis. 2022 Jun 1;8(1):65. doi: 10.1038/s41531-022-00328-5. PMID: 35650236

98 Hydrogen Sulfide Produced by Gut Bacteria May Induce Parkinson's Disease. Murros KE. Cells. 2022 Mar 12;11(6):978. doi: 10.3390/cells11060978. PMID: 35326429

99 Altered Gut Microbiome in Parkinson's Disease and the Influence of Lipopolysaccharide in a Human α-Synuclein Over-Expressing Mouse Model. Gorecki AM, Preskey L, Bakeberg MC, Kenna JE, Gildenhuys C, MacDougall G, Dunlop SA, Mastaglia FL, Akkari PA, Koengten F, Anderton RS. Front Neurosci. 2019 Aug 7;13:839. doi: 10.3389/fnins.2019.00839. PMID: 31440136

100 Serum and Fecal Markers of Intestinal Inflammation and Intestinal Barrier Permeability Are Elevated in Parkinson's Disease. Dumitrescu L, Marta D, Dănău A, Lefter A, Tulbă D, Cozma L, Manole E, Gherghiceanu M, Ceafalan LC, Popescu BO. Front Neurosci. 2021 Jun 18;15:689723. doi: 10.3389/fnins.2021.689723. PMID: 34220443

101 *Desulfovibrio* Bacteria Are Associated With Parkinson's Disease. Murros KE, Huynh VA, Takala TM, Saris PEJ. Front Cell Infect Microbiol. 2021 May 3;11:652617. doi: 10.3389/fcimb.2021.652617. eCollection 2021. PMID: 34012926

102 Silica Nanoparticles Promote α-Synuclein Aggregation and Parkinson's Disease Pathology. Yuan X, Yang Y, Xia D, Meng L, He M, Liu C, Zhang Z. Front Neurosci. 2022 Jan 13;15:807988. doi: 10.3389/fnins.2021.807988. PMID: 35095403

103 Acceleration of α-synuclein fibril formation and associated cytotoxicity stimulated by silica nanoparticles as a model of neurodegenerative diseases. Pang C, Zhang N, Falahati M. Int J Biol Macromol. 2021 Feb 1;169:532-540. doi: 10.1016/j.ijbiomac.2020.12.130. PMID: 33352154

104 Subjective Taste and Smell Changes in Conjunction with Anxiety and Depression Are Associated with Symptoms in Patients with Functional Constipation and Irritable Bowel Syndrome. Liu J, Lv C, Wu D, Wang Y, Sun C, Cheng C, Yu Y. Gastroenterol Res Pract. 2021 Sep 18;2021:5491188. doi: 10.1155/2021/5491188. PMID: 34589124

105 Association Between Irritable Bowel Syndrome and Risk of Parkinson's Disease: A Systematic Review and Meta-Analysis. Zhang X, Svn Z, Liv M, Yang Y, Zeng R, Huang Q, Sun Q. Front Neurol. 2021 Sep 22;12:720958. doi: 10.3389/fneur.2021.720958. PMID: 34630293

106 Bidirectional association between irritable bowel syndrome and restless legs syndrome: a systematic review and meta-analysis. Guo J, Pei L, Chen L, Chen H, Gu D, Peng Y, Sun J. Sleep Med. 2021 Jan;77:104-111. doi: 10.1016/j.sleep.2020.12.002. Epub 2020 Dec 4. PMID: 33348297

107 Valid olfactory impairment tests can help identify mild cognitive impairment: an updated meta-analysis. Zhou C, Yang C, Ai Y, Fang X, Zhang A, Wang Y, Hu H. Front Aging Neurosci. 2024 Feb 13;16:1349196. doi: 10.3389/fnagi.2024.1349196. eCollection 2024. PMID: 38419646

108 The role of olfactory dysfunction in mild cognitive impairment and Alzheimer's disease: A meta-analysis. Bouhaben J, Delgado-Lima AH, Delgado-Losada ML. Arch Gerontol Geriatr. 2024 Aug;123:105425. doi: 10.1016/j.archger.2024.105425. Epub 2024 Apr 2. PMID: 38615524

109 Identifying the pattern of olfactory deficits in Parkinson disease using the brief smell identification test. Double KL, Rowe DB, Hayes M, Chan DK, Blackie J, Corbett A, Joffe R, Fung VS, Morris J, Halliday GM. Arch Neurol. 2003 Apr;60(4):545-9. doi: 10.1001/archneur.60.4.545. PMID: 12707068

110 Selective hyposmia and nigrostriatal dopaminergic denervation in Parkinson's disease. Bohnen NI, Gedela S, Kuwabara H, Constantine GM, Mathis CA, Studenski SA, Moore RY. J Neurol. 2007 Jan;254(1):84-90. doi: 10.1007/s00415-006-0284-y. Epub 2007 Feb 14. PMID: 17508142

[111] Olfaction in Parkinson's disease and related disorders. Doty RL. Neurobiol Dis. 2012 Jun;46(3):527-52. doi: 10.1016/j.nbd.2011.10.026. PMID: 22192366

[112] Performance on an Alzheimer-selective odor identification test in patients with Parkinson's disease and its relationship with cerebral dopamine transporter activity. Chou KL, Bohnen NI. Parkinsonism Relat Disord. 2009 Nov;15(9):640-3. doi: 10.1016/j.parkreldis.2009.03.004. PMID: 19329351

[113] Brief Test of Olfactory Dysfunction Based on Diagnostic Features of Specific Odors in Early-Stage Alzheimer Disease. Audronyte E, Sutnikiene V, Pakulaite-Kazliene G, Kaubrys G. Med Sci Monit. 2023 May 27;29:e940363. doi: 10.12659/MSM.940363. PMID: 37243326

[114] Interventional Influence of the Intestinal Microbiome Through Dietary Intervention and Bowel Cleansing Might Improve Motor Symptoms in Parkinson's Disease. Hegelmaier T, Lebbing M, Duscha A, Tomaske L, Tönges L, Holm JB, Bjørn Nielsen H, Gatermann SG, Przuntek H, Haghikia A. Cells. 2020 Feb 6;9(2):376. doi: 10.3390/cells9020376. PMID: 32041265

[115] Fecal microbiota transplantation protects rotenone-induced Parkinson's disease mice via suppressing inflammation mediated by the lipopolysaccharide-TLR4 signaling pathway through the microbiota-gut-brain axis. Zhao Z, Ning J, Bao XQ, Shang M, Ma J, Li G, Zhang D. Microbiome. 2021 Nov 17;9(1):226. doi: 10.1186/s40168-021-01107-9. PMID: 34784980

[116] Neuro-Immunity and Gut Dysbiosis Drive Parkinson's Disease-Induced Pain. Roversi K, Callai-Silva N, Roversi K, Griffith M, Boutopoulos C, Prediger RD, Talbot S. Front Immunol. 2021 Nov 18;12:759679. doi: 10.3389/fimmu.2021.759679. PMID: 34868000

[117] Interaction of Mitochondrial Polygenic Score and Lifestyle Factors in LRRK2 p.Gly2019Ser Parkinsonism. Lüth T, Gabbert C, Koch S, König IR, Caliebe A, Laabs BH, Hentati F, Sassi SB, Amouri R, Spielmann M, Klein C, Grünewald A, Farrer MJ, Trinh J. Mov Disord. 2023 Oct;38(10):1837-1849. doi: 10.1002/mds.29563. Epub 2023 Jul 21. PMID: 37482924

[118] Ambroxol Upregulates Glucocerebrosidase Expression to Promote Neural Stem Cells Differentiation Into Neurons Through Wnt/β-Catenin Pathway After Ischemic Stroke. Ge H, Zhang C, Yang Y, Chen W, Zhong J, Fang X, Jiang X, Tan L, Zou Y, Hu R, Chen Y, Feng H. Front Mol Neurosci. 2021 Jan 20;13:596039. doi: 10.3389/fnmol.2020.596039.. PMID: 33551744

[119] Ambroxol, the cough expectorant with neuroprotective effects. Patzwaldt K, Castaneda-Vega S. Neural Regen Res. 2024 Nov 1;19(11):2345-2346. doi: 10.4103/NRR.NRR-D-23-01664. Epub 2024 Jan 31. PMID: 38526267

22: Alcoholic Beverages

The Distilled Version

First, allow me to apologize to those who enjoy alcoholic beverages, but here is what the data says.

Alcoholic beverages can have a beneficial effect on health, acting as hormetic agents. If used appropriately, the regular consumption of small amounts of alcohol is associated with decreased risk of Alzheimer's disease, type 2 diabetes, several forms of cancer, and heart disease. That being said, alcohol is toxic and a carcinogen. It is the *low dose of a toxic agent* that stimulates a hormetic, adaptive response that lowers disease risk.

The alcoholic beverage that has the best hormetic effect is red wine, as it has a synergistic hormetic effect combining that of alcohol and fermented anthocyanins and tannins from fruit. The grape wine with the best HAR score is (deep red) zinfandel, (not the white stuff!). Blackberry and blueberry wines also have high HAR scores.

The SANA program recommends a dose of 6 ml of absolute alcohol in an alcoholic beverage once, *every-other-day,* as it provides the most effective hormetic effect. This is best consumed in the form of dark wine, which provides hormetic synergy. Six milliliters of absolute alcohol as wine translates to 50 ml (about 1.7 oz.) of red wine at 12% alcohol; about one-third of a standard drink.

For those who enjoy beer, this would mean about 4 ounces of beer every other day. Oh well. Non-alcoholic and very low alcohol beers are available.

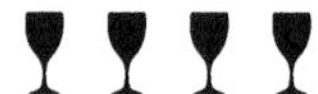

Alcohol

Alcohol is toxic, a neurotoxin, and is classified as a Group 1 carcinogen. The specific alcohol that is present in beverages is ethanol (ETOH). Most other alcohols are far more toxic. As little as 10 ml of methanol (wood alcohol) can cause permanent blindness, and consuming more than 15 ml can cause death. In comparison, there is 17.7 ml of ethanol in a 12-ounce can of beer. For this discussion of alcoholic beverages, alcohol refers exclusively to ethanol.

The simple remedy for alcohol is to avoid it. Nevertheless, many studies show that alcohol can have beneficial effects, including lowering the risk of vascular disease. Teetotalers don't survive as long as those consuming "moderate" amounts of alcohol.

In multiple population studies, moderate alcohol consumption is associated with a lower risk of both vascular dementia and Alzheimer's disease (AD) when compared to persons who never consume alcohol, have less than one drink per week, or drink heavily, typically defined as two or more drinks or "alcohol equivalents" per day. Light consumption of alcohol appears to reduce the incidence of dementia by about 35 to 50% when compared to those who drink no alcohol.[1] [2] [3] In a meta-analysis of 15 studies, risk was lowest for those consuming around 20 grams of alcohol per day, with no difference for men and women.[4] A meta-analysis of wine consumption had similar findings.[5] Another dose-response meta-analysis of alcohol intake and risk of dementia, risk of mild cognitive impairment (MCI), and dementia was associated with the consumption of less than 11 grams of alcohol per day, with a narrow nadir of risk at around 5 grams of absolute alcohol per day.[6]

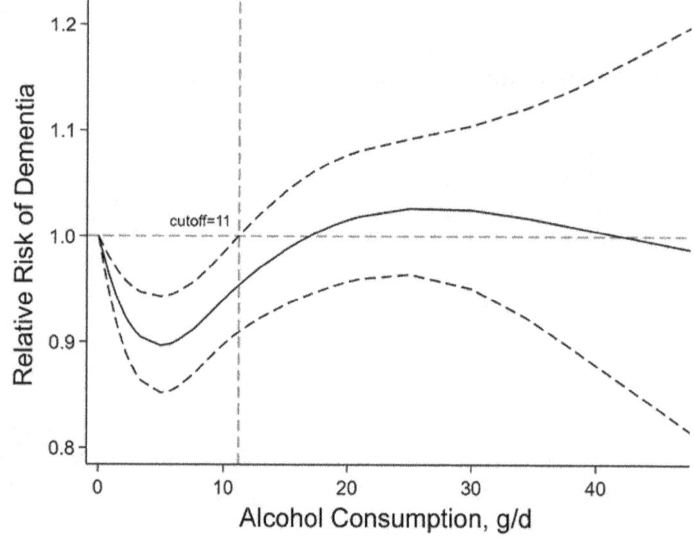

Figure 22A: Hormetic dose-response for alcohol and lower risk of dementia. No statistically significant benefit was seen for those consuming more than 11 grams (13.7 ml absolute alcohol) per day. (LS Ran et al.[7]) The lowest risk was at about 5 grams (@ 6 ml) per day. Note that the decline in slope of the solid line around 40 g/day is not meaningful but rather a function of the widening (dashed) confidence intervals and the lack of meaningful correlation at higher doses where there are few survivors.

In a meta-analysis looking at the relationship between alcohol consumption and diabetes, moderate alcohol consumption was associated with a lower risk of type 2 diabetes than higher or zero intake levels.[8] Data from the UK Biobank shows that dementia risk is lowest when consuming alcohol 3 to 4 times a week.[9]

A meta-analysis for the association between wine consumption and cancer found no association for wine consumption and breast and ovarian cancer, a nonsignificant decrease in risk for colorectal and renal cancers, and a protective effect against skin, pancreatic, lung, and brain cancers.[10] In a meta-analysis, white wine consumption was associated with a 26% increase in risk, while moderate red wine consumption was associated with a 12% decrease in risk of prostate cancer.[11] Heavy wine consumption was found to be associated with as much as a 2.1-fold risk of oral, pharyngeal, and esophageal cancer.[12] Another meta-analysis found a 27% decrease in risk for cardiovascular mortality among wine drinkers, with no difference between men and women.[13] Part of the benefit from alcoholic beverages accrues from the polyphenolic or other compounds present in red wine.[14] It is likely the combination of phenolic compounds and alcohol that reduces disease risk.[15]

Beer consumption has also been associated with a lower risk of cognitive decline, dementia, and cardiovascular disease.[16] Several studies have found that moderate consumption of beer or wine lowers the risk of dementia, but that hard (distilled) liquor does not reduce the risk. Similar to wine, beer contains phenolic compounds. Beer contains antioxidants and the B vitamin folate, which protects against homocysteine accumulation, a risk factor for Alzheimer's disease (AD). Beer also contains readily bioavailable silica, which may serve to reduce the risk from aluminum in drinking water.[17]

(Red) Zinfandel gets a considerably higher Hormetic Adaptive Response (HAR) than does Cabernet Sauvignon, which rates higher than Merlot. White wine gets negative DAD scores. If it is the non-alcohol components of wine and beer that are responsible for their health benefits, then non-alcoholic beer and deep purple grape juice, such as Concord grape juice, may be healthier alternatives than alcoholic beverages. Blackberry and blueberry wines get high HAR scores.

It should not be forgotten that alcohol is a toxic and carcinogenic compound. Nevertheless, with a certain level of exposure, ethyl alcohol can have a hormetic effect.

The SANA program promulgates that the peak beneficial effect of alcohol consumption occurs within a narrow range around 6 ml of absolute alcohol. That is, at a low dose, alcohol can stimulate the expression of proteins that protect the body from other toxins and stressors. This is similar to the effect by which phenolic agents in fruits, and sulfur compounds in broccoli and garlic, mediate their beneficial effects. As a toxin, alcohol stimulates the expression of alcohol detoxifying proteins, including aldehyde dehydrogenases (ALDH), alcohol dehydrogenase, and CYP2E1. Alcohol also increases the expression of HMOX1, which, when expression is moderately increased, protects the brain. HMOX1 dysfunction is seen in AD and Parkinson's disease.[18] Alcohol decreases the expression of PTGS2, the enzyme that produces the inflammatory cytokine PGE2.[19] The impact of alcohol on the expression of various proteins may explain the unusually narrow peak beneficial dose range.

In East Asia, there is a common genetic variant allele of ALDH2, in which this enzyme functions poorly; it affects about 540 million people. This allele is associated with a greater risk of Alzheimer's disease (AD).[20] Lower levels of ALDH1 are found in the substantia nigra in the brains of patients with Parkinson's disease (PD).[21]

ALDH is essential for the prevention of neurodegeneration in animals. Mice bred to have an ALDH2 genetic knockout develop β-amyloid and pTau deposition (markers of AD) in the brain at birth and have cognitive impairment by the age of 3 months. One of the central functions of ALDH in regards to neurodegeneration is that it is responsible for the metabolism of toxic aldehydes, including 4-hydroxynonenal (4-HNE), methylglyoxal, malondialdehyde, acetaldehyde, and formaldehyde, whether they are of endogenous or exogenous origin. (Note: ALDH does not metabolize glyceraldehyde).

4-HNE is a toxic compound produced in the body by lipid peroxidation. While at low levels, 4-HNE can trigger antioxidant defense and compensation mechanisms, at higher levels, it binds to proteins and inhibits their function. It reduces the ability of histones to bind and protect DNA from damage, creating a risk for DNA breaks and mutations. At high levels, 4-HNE causes DNA fragmentation and cell death.

4-HNE is implicated in the causation of neurodegenerative diseases, including AD and PD, as well as that of diabetes, atherosclerosis, cataracts, and cancer.[22] 4-HNE is generated by the oxidation of n-6 polyunsaturated fats such as linoleic and arachidonic acids. 4-HNE is detoxified and removed from the cells by glutathione S-transferases (GST) and aldose reductase in a two-step process. Alternatively, 4-HNE can be metabolized into a non-toxic compound by aldehyde dehydrogenase. However, when excessive levels of 4-HNE are generated by oxidative stress, the cell's detox system gets overloaded, and cell injury or death may occur.

In the brain, 4-HNE leads to dysfunction of glucose and glutamate transporters, promotes synaptic degeneration, increases the risk of DNA oxidation, and impairs energy production. 4-HNE can impair memory by decreasing the activity of choline acetyltransferase and enhancing the production of β-amyloid.[23]

Thus, levels of alcohol consumption that promote the expression of ALDH, both peripherally and in the brain, likely boost 4-HNE metabolism, without increasing other risks. In contrast, upregulation of CYP2E1 enhances the generation of toxic and carcinogenic we are exposed in the environment.[24] CYP2E1 promotes the formation of advanced glycation end products (AGEs), which ALDH helps break down.[25] Finding a balance between increasing ALDH and CYP2E1 expression may explain the unusually narrow hormetic dose range of alcohol.

In the USA, one standard drink is defined as any beverage containing roughly 17.74 ml (0.6 fluid ounces; 14 grams) of pure alcohol. Thus, assuming that 6 ml (4.73 grams) of pure ETOH provides the peak benefit, one standard drink contains 3 times more than the ideal quantity of alcohol appropriate for promoting health. Assuming that a red wine contains 12% alcohol, 50 ml of wine (1.7 oz) would be the ideal dose. For wine that is 13.5% alcohol, a 44 ml dose would be appropriate. For a beer with 5% alcohol, 120 ml (4 oz.) of beer would provide the ideal drink size. For a superlight 2.4% alcohol beer, 250 ml (8.45 oz.) would be the appropriate size,

$$6 \text{ ml} \div \% \text{ ETOH} = \text{volume of beverage}$$
$$6 \text{ ml} \div 0.12 = 50 \text{ ml}$$
$$6 \text{ ml} \div 12 \times 100 = 50 \text{ ml}$$

$$6 \text{ ml} \div 5\% \text{ ABV} \times 100 = 120 \text{ ml}$$
$$6 \text{ ml} \div 2.4\% \text{ ABV} \times 100 = 250 \text{ ml}$$

The SANA program also contends that low-level consumption of alcohol (6 ml) interacts with and creates synergistic potential with phenolic compounds from grapes, which further protect the body from disease. This may also occur for compounds in beer and ale. These phenolic compounds promote the expression of several protective proteins, including glutathione S-transferases, which also act on 4-HNE, as well as on other toxic compounds. Distilled spirits would not be expected to have this synergistic effect.

Studies that show the benefit of alcohol consumption consistently reveal that it is the frequency of consumption that provides benefit. Drinking a six-pack of beer or a bottle of wine on Friday night once a week does not have the same effect as having one beer a day or one glass of wine a day. Binge drinking is far more toxic to the body. For low-dose alcohol to be effective in lowering the risk of neurodegenerative and other diseases, it needs to be consumed regularly.

The SANA program contends that the optimal interval for low-dose alcohol's hormetic effect is around 48 hours, as it is for many other hormetic agents. Thus, dosing to boost and maintain the elevated levels of ALDH and antioxidant proteins that reduce cell injury should be done every other day rather than daily.

Recommendation: Thus, for those who would like to lower their risk of neurodegeneration and other disease through the use of red wine, who do not have problems which preclude or cause risk from low level alcohol consumption, the dose promulgated as being optimal is: 45 to 50 ml of dark red wine (Zinfandel >> Cabernet > Merlot) once every other day or three days a week skipping at least a day between doses. An equivalent amount of concord grape juice or another source of anthocyanins can be consumed on non-wine days. Blackberry wine, which is high in cyanidin, which crosses the blood-brain barrier, has an even better HAR score than dark red zinfandel.

An equivalent dose of beer (usually about 120 ml or 4 ounces) can be used.

Zinfandel, which may be called Primitivo in Europe) It is a sweet, black grape variety that originated in Croatia. Zinfandel is sufficiently superior in terms of health benefits to other red wines tested that it should be considered the grape wine of choice, and other red wines used for health benefits only when zinfandel is unavailable. White zinfandel is not a substitute for zinfandel.

Note: The optimal hormetic interval for grape juice and other sources of anthocyanins is shorter than it is for alcohol. Thus, to maintain a higher hormetic effect, 30 to 100 ml (1 to 3 oz.) of 100% Concord grape juice can be enjoyed on the days between when low-dose wine or beer is taken. Alternatively, to grape juice, other berries can be eaten.

For the 540 million people with poorly functioning ALDH2, the amount of alcohol that enhances ALDH without creating more toxicity may not be the same as for those with more typical ALDH2 function. Certainly, these individuals should avoid doses higher than 6 mL every other day.

For those who are better off without alcohol, 30 ml (about one ounce) of Concord grape juice daily should provide a substantial, healthful hormetic effect. Green tea, chamomile, elderberry, spearmint, and hibiscus tisanes are other beverages with hormetic health benefits. Blackberries and elderberries are high in cyanidins.

Non-alcoholic beer is now widely available. Non-alcoholic beer in the U.S. contains less than 0.5% alcohol by volume. Thus, it would require more than 1.2 liters of non-alcoholic beer to get a 6 ml dose of ethanol. In the UK, low-alcohol (1.2% ABV) beer is available. In the UK, a half-liter can of "non-alcoholic" beer can contain around 6 ml of pure alcohol.

[1] Prospective study of alcohol consumption and risk of dementia in older adults. Mukamal KJ, Kuller LH, Fitzpatrick AL, Longstreth WT Jr, Mittleman MA, Siscovick DS. JAMA. 2003 Mar 19;289(11):1405-13. doi: 10.1001/jama.289.11.1405. PMID: 12636463

[2] Alcohol Consumption and Risk of Dementia and Cognitive Decline Among Older Adults With or Without Mild Cognitive Impairment. Koch M, Fitzpatrick AL, Rapp SR, Nahin RL, Williamson JD, Lopez OL, DeKosky ST, Kuller LH, Mackey RH, Mukamal KJ, Jensen MK, Sink KM. JAMA Netw Open. 2019 Sep 4;2(9):e1910319. doi: 10.1001/jamanetworkopen.2019.10319. PMID: 31560382

[3] Risk of dementia and alcohol and wine consumption: a review of recent results. Letenneur L. Biol Res. 2004;37(2):189-93. doi: 10.4067/s0716-97602004000200003. PMID: 15455646

[4] The relationship between alcohol use and dementia in adults aged more than 60 years: a combined analysis of prospective, individual-participant data from 15 international studies. Mewton L, Visontay R, Hoy N, Lipnicki DM, Sunderland M, Lipton RB, Guerchet M, Ritchie K, Najar J, Scarmeas N, Kim KW, Riedel Heller S, van Boxtel M, Jacobsen E, Brodaty H, Anstey KJ, Haan M, Scazufca M, Lobo E, Sachdev PS; Collaborators from the Cohort Studies of Memory in an International Consortium (COSMIC). Addiction. 2023 Mar;118(3):412-424. doi: 10.1111/add.16035. PMID: 35993434

[5] Association Between Wine Consumption and Cognitive Decline in Older People: A Systematic Review and Meta-Analysis of Longitudinal Studies. Lucerón-Lucas-Torres M, Cavero-Redondo I, Martínez-Vizcaíno V, Saz-Lara A, Pascual-Morena C, Álvarez-Bueno C. Front Nutr. 2022 May 12;9:863059. doi: 10.3389/fnut.2022.863059. eCollection 2022. PMID: 35634389

[6] Alcohol, coffee and tea intake and the risk of cognitive deficits: a dose-response meta-analysis. Ran LS, Liu WH, Fang YY, Xu SB, Li J, Luo X, Pan DJ, Wang MH, Wang W. Epidemiol Psychiatr Sci. 2021 Feb 11;30:e13. doi: 10.1017/S2045796020001183. PMID: 33568254

[7] Alcohol, coffee and tea intake and the risk of cognitive deficits: a dose-response meta-analysis. Ran LS, Liu WH, Fang YY, Xu SB, Li J, Luo X, Pan DJ, Wang MH, Wang W. Epidemiol Psychiatr Sci. 2021 Feb 11;30:e13. doi: 10.1017/S2045796020001183. PMID: 33568254

[8] Moderate alcohol consumption lowers the risk of type 2 diabetes: a meta-analysis of prospective observational studies. Koppes LL, Dekker JM, Hendriks HF, Bouter LM, Heine RJ. Diabetes Care. 2005 Mar;28(3):719-25. doi: 10.2337/diacare.28.3.719. PMID: 15735217

[9] Non-Linear Association of Dietary Polyamines with the Risk of Incident Dementia: Results from Population-Based Cohort of the UK Biobank. Qian M, Zhang N, Zhang R, Liu M, Wu Y, Lu Y, Li F, Zheng L. Nutrients. 2024 Aug 20;16(16):2774. doi: 10.3390/nu16162774. PMID: 39203912

[10] Association between wine consumption and cancer: a systematic review and meta-analysis. Lucerón-Lucas-Torres M, Cavero-Redondo I, Martínez-Vizcaíno V, Bizzozero-Peroni B, Pascual-Morena C, Álvarez-Bueno C. Front Nutr. 2023 Sep 4;10:1197745. doi: 10.3389/fnut.2023.1197745. eCollection 2023. PMID: 37731399

[11] The impact of moderate wine consumption on the risk of developing prostate cancer. Vartolomei MD, Kimura S, Ferro M, Foerster B, Abufaraj M, Briganti A, Karakiewicz PI, Shariat SF. Clin Epidemiol. 2018 Apr 17;10:431-444. doi: 10.2147/CLEP.S163668. eCollection 2018. PMID: 29713200

[12] Ethanol versus Phytochemicals in Wine: Oral Cancer Risk in a Light Drinking Perspective. Varoni EM, Lodi G, Iriti M. Int J Mol Sci. 2015 Jul 27;16(8):17029-47. doi: 10.3390/ijms160817029. PMID: 26225960

[13] Association between Wine Consumption with Cardiovascular Disease and Cardiovascular Mortality: A Systematic Review and Meta-Analysis. Lucerón-Lucas-Torres M, Saz-Lara A, Díez-Fernández A, Martínez-García I, Martínez-Vizcaíno V, Cavero-Redondo I, Álvarez-Bueno C. Nutrients. 2023 Jun 17;15(12):2785. doi: 10.3390/nu15122785. PMID: 37375690

[14] Wine, Polyphenols, and Mediterranean Diets. What Else Is There to Say? Santos-Buelga C, González-Manzano S, González-Paramás AM. Molecules. 2021 Sep 12;26(18):5537. doi: 10.3390/molecules26185537. PMID: 34577008

[15] Red wine induced modulation of vascular function: separating the role of polyphenols, ethanol, and urates. Boban M, Modun D, Music I, Vukovic J, Brizic I, Salamunic I, Obad A, Palada I, Dujic Z. J Cardiovasc Pharmacol. 2006 May;47(5):695-701. doi: 10.1097/01.fjc.0000211762.06271.ce. PMID: 16775510

[16] Effects of moderate beer consumption on health and disease: A consensus document. de Gaetano G, Costanzo S, Di Castelnuovo A, Badimon L, Bejko D, Alkerwi A, Chiva-Blanch G, Estruch R, La Vecchia C, Panico S, Pounis G, Sofi F, Stranges S, Trevisan M, Ursini F, Cerletti C, Donati MB, Iacoviello L. Nutr Metab Cardiovasc Dis. 2016 Jun;26(6):443-67. doi: 10.1016/j.numecd.2016.03.007. Epub 2016 Mar 31. PMID: 27118108

[17] The Nutritional Components of Beer and Its Relationship with Neurodegeneration and Alzheimer's Disease. Sánchez-Muniz FJ, Macho-González A, Garcimartín A, Santos-López JA, Benedí J, Bastida S, González-Muñoz MJ. Nutrients. 2019 Jul 10;11(7):1558. doi: 10.3390/nu11071558. PMID: 31295866

[18] Roles of Heme Oxygenase-1 in Neuroinflammation and Brain Disorders. Wu YH, Hsieh HL. Antioxidants (Basel). 2022 May 8;11(5):923. doi: 10.3390/antiox11050923. PMID: 35624787

[19] Dietary Responses of Dementia-Related Genes Encoding Metabolic Enzymes. Parnell LD, Magadmi R, Zwanger S, Shukitt-Hale B, Lai CQ, Ordovás JM. Nutrients. 2023 Jan 27;15(3):644. doi: 10.3390/nu15030644. PMID: 36771351

[20] Deficiency in mitochondrial aldehyde dehydrogenase increases the risk for late-onset Alzheimer's disease in the Japanese population. Kamino K, Nagasaka K, Imagawa M, Yamamoto H, Yoneda H, Ueki A, Kitamura S, Namekata K, Miki T, Ohta S. Biochem Biophys Res Commun. 2000 Jun 24;273(1):192-6. doi: 10.1006/bbrc.2000.2923. PMID: 10873585

[21] Aldehyde dehydrogenase (ALDH) in Alzheimer's and Parkinson's disease. Grünblatt E, Riederer P. J Neural Transm (Vienna). 2016 Feb;123(2):83-90. doi: 10.1007/s00702-014-1320-1. Epub 2014 Oct 9. PMID: 25298080

[22] Pathological aspects of lipid peroxidation. Negre-Salvayre A, Auge N, Ayala V, Basaga H, Boada J, Brenke R, Chapple S, Cohen G, Feher J, Grune T, Lengyel G, Mann GE, Pamplona R, Poli G, Portero-Otin M, Riahi Y, Salvayre R, Sasson S, Serrano J, Shamni O, Siems W, Siow RC, Wiswedel I, Zarkovic K, Zarkovic N. Free Radic Res. 2010 Oct;44(10):1125-71. doi: 10.3109/10715762.2010.498478. PMID: 20836660

[23] Impact of common ALDH2 inactivating mutation and alcohol consumption on Alzheimer's disease. Seike T, Chen CH, Mochly-Rosen D. Front Aging Neurosci. 2023 Aug 24;15:1223977. doi: 10.3389/fnagi.2023.1223977. eCollection 2023. PMID: 37693648

[24] Structures of human cytochrome P-450 2E1. Insights into the binding of inhibitors and both small molecular weight and fatty acid substrates. Porubsky PR, Meneely KM, Scott EE. J Biol Chem. 2008 Nov 28;283(48):33698-707. doi: 10.1074/jbc.M805999200. Epub 2008 Sep 24. PMID: 18818195

[25] Advanced glycation end products (AGEs) and other adducts in aging-related diseases and alcohol-mediated tissue injury. Rungratanawanich W, Qu Y, Wang X, Essa MM, Song BJ. Exp Mol Med. 2021 Feb;53(2):168-188. doi: 10.1038/s12276-021-00561-7. Epub 2021 Feb 10. PMID: 33568752

23: Condiments

The Essence

Herbs and spices add flavor and spark to food. Many condiments have beneficial antioxidant and hormetic effects. An important concern with herbs and spices is that they are unstable; they are often used infrequently and in small enough amounts that they outlast their shelf lives. Avoid dried herbs and spices that are out of date. Fresh ones are better than dried ones, as long as they are fresh. Whole herbs and spices have longer shelf lives than when in powdered form.

Most herbs and spices are allowed in the SANA diet (if not past their best-by date); however, some herbs and spices should be avoided. These include cloves, black (and white) peppers, and dried red peppers, including paprika, especially for those with active dysbiosis.

Herbs and Spices

First things first. Go to your spice rack and throw all your herbs and spices away! (Joking, but maybe...)

Most herbs and spices have strong aromas, and that is why we use them; they add flavor as a result of their volatile compounds. We can smell them because those aroma molecules are volatile, meaning that they easily escape into the air. Once you open a fresh, sealed spice container, those volatile compounds begin escaping. With time, spices get old and lose their most volatile compounds.

Finely ground herbs and spices age more quickly. Many spices additionally have antioxidant compounds. For some of these compounds, that means that they avidly grab oxygen. When spices are ground into a fine powder, it gives them a greater surface area, which helps increase their flavor but also makes them more exposed to oxygen in the air. Sprinkle-top and flip-top caps that are now common on spice containers often do not make air-tight seals. Thus, the herbs and spices can easily lose their volatile compounds and become oxidized. When this happens, they lose the aromatics that enhance your food and often lose their antioxidant properties; they may instead contain detrimental, oxidized, or even may become toxic compounds. They are not worth putting into your food or your body.

Check the expiration date on your spices; if it is past the "good buy" (AKA the "good bye") date, or if the bottle has been open for more than a year, it is time to get rid of the expired condiment. I suggest replacing your spices with small containers from discount brands, as come next year, it will be easier to throw out a half-used $1 aisle container of sage than a $9 one. Whole spices last longer than ground ones. Using fresh herbs is another great choice for high-quality meal preparation.

Most herb and spice consumption involves the use of small amounts, and unless one is using them heavily, as for pesto or making tea, they most likely don't have a large impact on disease risk. Many have hormetic properties that are beneficial. Thus, the *culinary use* of most herbs and spices (other than expired ones) does not need to be micromanaged. If used as an herbal medicine or tea, more care is needed for proper preparation.

Tables 23A and B: DAD Scores for Herbs and Spices

Herbs	DAD Rating
Basil leaf fresh	4
Spearmint leaf fresh	4
Thyme	4
Cilantro (fresh)	4
Lavender	3
Basil dry leaf	3
Spearmint (dry)	3
Peppermint (dry)	3
Sage, ground powder	3
Rosemary leaf dry	3
Cilantro (dry)	2
Parsley flakes	1
Lemon Grass (fresh)	1
Bay leaf	0
Mexican Oregano (fresh leaf)	0
Oregano, dry	0
Horseradish	
Wasabi	0
Fennel Greens	D

Spices	DAD Rating
Grains of Paradise	4
Ginger root, fresh, skin removed	4
Cardamon seed	4
Fenugreek (seed)	2
Allspice (whole, old)	1
Nutmeg (whole)	1
Coriander	1
Cumin, dry, ground	1
Cinnamon (sticks Mexican)	1
Cinnamon (sticks)	1
Celery Seed	1
Cayenne	0
Turmeric (powder)	A
Fennel seed	A
Ginger (powder)	B
Mustard Seed	0

There are, however, some herbs and spices that should be avoided. At least one is neurotoxic. This should not come as a surprise. Clove oil is used to deaden dental pain, and some dentists report that it kills the nerve in the tooth when there is a caries, causing pain. Some are gastrointestinal irritants, such as red peppers. Some are prone to contamination with fungal toxins.

Turmeric and ginger are underground stems. The skin should be removed before using them. Fresh ginger and turmeric should be used rather than dry powder if being used for their health benefits.

Fenugreek is used in Indian cooking, often in curries, and known as methi. It is a legume with leaves that look like those of the peanut plant. Fenugreek proteins can cross-react with peanut allergens.[1] Thus, it should be avoided by those with severe peanut allergies.

Herbs and Spices to keep out of the SANA diet:

Cloves
Paprika
Smoked Paprika
Black Pepper (*Piper nigrum*)
Dried Red Peppers
Fennel Greens
Parsley

Black Pepper

Black pepper (*Piper nigrum*) is the fruit of a tropical vine. Black peppercorns are harvested green and then cooked and dried. White pepper is the seed of the ripe fruit, with the thin flesh of the outer fruit removed.

Black (and white) peppers are rated D. Black pepper contains well over 50 bioactive compounds, notably several volatile oils (sabinine, caryophyllene, limonene, camphene, and others) that give much of its odor and flavor. Notably, it contains piperine, a compound that interferes with the ability of cells to get rid of many noxious compounds.[2] Black pepper is an irritant and hard on the gut.

In a study of herb and spice contamination with fungal mycotoxins, two-thirds of black pepper and three-fourths of white pepper had ochratoxin A levels above the MTL (maximum tolerable limit) of 15 µg/kg. The average level of ochratoxin A in white pepper was 132 µg/kg, but black pepper at 77 µg/kg was only 5 times above the MTL. The study also notably found that nutmeg was commonly contaminated with ochratoxin A (mean level 68 µg/kg) and also frequently exceeded the MTL of aflatoxin B1. The only herb frequently contaminated with significant amounts of mycotoxins was anise, which was commonly contaminated with ochratoxin (mean levels 5.6 µg/kg).[3] Mycotoxins are further discussed in Chapter 27.

Substitutes: Grains of paradise (*Aframomum melegueta*), a plant in the ginger family, closely related to cardamom. Its seeds have a pungent black pepper-like piquancy and heat, an undertone of cardamom, and a hint of citrus. Virginia pepperweed seed pods have a peppery taste. It grows wild in most of the United States, but does not appear to be commercially exploited for this use. Horse radish can be used as a pepper substitute.

Red Peppers

It is recommended that *dried* red peppers and paprika be avoided. Dried peppers look lovely as a display, but peppers mold easily during the drying process and can have high levels of ochratoxin A (OTA).

For hot red pepper flavor, I suggest using bottled preparations that are made from fresh red peppers that are kept refrigerated after opening, rather than using dried ones.

Individuals with inflammatory bowel disease are especially sensitive to spicy foods and are advised to avoid peppers. Consumption of chili peppers is associated with an increased risk of IBD relapse.[4]

However, Grains of Paradise appears to have beneficial properties.

Several cruciferous plants, relatives of broccoli and cauliflower, are spicy hot. This includes mustard (seed), radish, horseradish, and wasabi (roots), and watercress leaves. None of these gets positive ratings on the DAD scale, and they get negative ratings for those with inflammatory bowel disease. If radishes are peeled, they get a rating of 1, as do their leaves.

Essential Oils

Essential oils are more commonly used as scents, in skin creams, or as medicinal compounds, but are sometimes used as flavorings. For the most part, they should be avoided as a food. Most of those evaluated get a score of D, even when the source plant gets a high score. They are highly concentrated and may be toxic.

Peppermint oil is discussed with peppermint tea.

[1] Characterization of potential allergens in fenugreek (Trigonella foenum-graecum) using patient sera and MS-based proteomic analysis. Faeste CK, Christians U, Egaas E, Jonscher KR. J Proteomics. 2010 May 7;73(7):1321-33. doi: 10.1016/j.jprot.2010.02.011. Epub 2010 Feb 26. PMID: 20219717

[2] Black Pepper, the "King of Spices": Chemical composition to applications. Hammouti B. et al. Arabian Journal of Chemical and Environmental Research.06(1)12-56. 2019. https://www.mocedes.org/ajcer/volume6/AJCER-02-Hammouti-2019.pdf

[3] Public health risk associated with the co-occurrence of aflatoxin B_1 and ochratoxin A in spices, herbs, and nuts in Lebanon. Daou R, Hoteit M, Bookari K, Joubrane K, Khabbaz LR, Ismail A, Maroun RG, El Khoury A. Front Public Health. 2023 Jan 9;10:1072727. doi: 10.3389/fpubh.2022.1072727. eCollection 2022. PMID: 36699892

[4] Dietary risk factors for inflammatory bowel disease in Shanghai: A case-control study. Mi L, Zhang C, Yu XF, Zou J, Yu Y, Bao ZJ. Asia Pac J Clin Nutr. 2022;31(3):405-414. doi: 10.6133/apjcn.202209_31(3).0008. PMID: 36173212

24: Salt and Iodine

Salient Issues

If you have congestive heart failure (CHF), kidney failure or other chronic kidney disease (CKD), or advanced heart disease or severe hypertension, this chapter is not for you. Follow your doctor's or doctors' advice on salt. Even if you don't have these health issues, follow your doctor's advice.

If you don't have a chronic disease such as CHF or CKD, which causes salt retention, and you have a healthy diet, it is inadvisable to consume a low-sodium diet. Low-sodium diets are promulgated by the National Academies of Science, the WHO, the DASH diet, and others. These low-sodium diets are associated with higher, not lower, all-cause mortality risk.

The common electrolyte issue that negatively impacts health is not excess sodium, but rather that people have too little potassium in their diets. If not eating a junk and manufactured food diet, most people should let their palate be their guide to salting their food, and if the diet is not dominated by empty calories (fats and sugars), the diet should be replete with potassium.

Iodine is an essential nutrient. If not using iodized salt or commonly eating dairy and seafood, many people will not get sufficient iodine in their diet. Fast, junk, and manufactured foods are made avoiding the use of iodized salt. If eating all meals at home and using iodized salt, it is likely that people will get an *excessive* amount of iodine in the diet, especially if they consume dairy products such as cheese and yogurt, which are high in iodine. Herein, the recommendation is to use a 50:50 mix of iodized and plain salt if most meals are prepared at home and dairy products are consumed in the diet.

Salt

Salt is the most important condiment; it accentuates the flavor profile of most foods. It also has chemical effects on food; it strengthens the gluten network in bread and slows the growth of yeast, helping the bread to rise more evenly. Salt is 40% sodium and 60% chloride, by weight.

Salt is an essential nutrient. It is needed for maintaining fluid balance, nerve conduction, muscular contraction, and multiple other functions.

How Much Salt?

The World Health Organization (WHO) promulgates a limit of 2,000 mg of sodium in the diet a day. In contrast, the SANA diet does not recommend a low-sodium diet for healthy people. While the Western diet is high in sodium, largely as a result of junk and processed food, sodium overload is not a common health problem in otherwise healthy adults. What is common is a deficit of potassium.

We have been indoctrinated to believe that diets high in sodium raise blood pressure, increase the risk of cardiovascular disease and stroke, and cause kidney disease.

The National Academies of Sciences, Engineering, and Medicine (NAS), the official body that sets Dietary Reference Intakes (RDI) levels in the United States, reduced the RDI for sodium, and therefore for salt and potassium, in 2019. The new RDI for sodium for adults is 1500 mg/day, and the recommended upper limit is 2300 mg of sodium per day.[1]

The RDI is the minimum level that is sufficient for 95% of the population. This means that the NAS considered that five percent of adults would get insufficient sodium in their diets if they had a sodium intake of 1500 mg/day. This should not be considered the minimum requirement to prevent harm for most of the population. The upper limits of 2,000 mg/day by the WHO and 2,300 mg/day by the NAS are recommendations. *There is strong evidence to consider both the upper and lower limits recommended as being wrong and dangerous.*

About 92 percent of the sodium ingested is excreted in the urine, and some is lost in sweat and tears.[2] Thus, the intake of sodium can be closely assessed from urinary sodium. In a national health study, 24-hour urine outputs were collected by 1,103 adults. Only 32 of these had 24-hour urinary sodium excretion less than 2300 mg of sodium; thus, *less than three percent of a random sampling of healthy American adults consume less than the upper recommended intake of salt.*[3] (Since only 92% of the sodium intake shows up in the urine, the actual amount consumed for 2300 mg to be in the urine is 2500 mg; even fewer of these individuals were actually in compliance with this recommendation.)

In a study of over 100,000 adults from around 18 different countries, most people were found to excrete between 3,000 and 6,000 mg of sodium a day, about 20% of people had higher levels, and only 9% had lower amounts of sodium/day in their urine. After a median follow-up of 8.2 years, all-cause mortality was lowest among those excreting 3,500 to 6,000 mg of sodium a day, with the risk being lowest among those with 4,000 to 5,500 mg of sodium in their urine per day. Cardiovascular disease deaths were lowest with levels around 4,000 to 4,500 mg of sodium. The median urinary sodium output was 4.7 g, thus indicating that the median sodium intake of this diverse population from urban and rural communities from rich and poor countries was 5,100 mg per day.[4]

The median potassium excretion level in these populations was about 2,100 mg. All-cause and cardiovascular mortality were lowest among those with urine potassium levels reflecting a dietary intake of *greater than 3000 mg*. Most (93%) of the study population consumed less than 3000 mg of potassium and thus can be assumed to have been at higher disease risk as a result of insufficient potassium consumption. Data from this study suggests that consumption of 4,000 to 4,500 mg of sodium per day with at least 3000 mg of potassium better reflects healthy sodium and potassium intakes for adults. The National Academies also promulgated the consumption of 2,600 mg of potassium for women and 3,400 mg of potassium daily for men as adequate; this recommendation appears sound and coincides with the survival study results.

Even among those with kidney disease, those with 24-hour urinary sodium levels from 2894 to 3649 mg had a lower risk of cardiovascular events, including myocardial infarctions, congestive heart failure, and stroke. Those with daily urinary sodium levels less than 2894 mg had a very similar risk to those with levels 3650 to 4547 mg, and only those in the highest quartile, over 4548 mg of urine sodium, had elevated risk of disease events. The risk of heart disease among those with kidney disease appears to be lowest when the urinary output of sodium is around 3500 mg per day.[5] In the largest controlled trial of dietary sodium restriction in congestive heart failure, a diet with a sodium intake of <1500 mg/day failed to improve survival or reduce cardiovascular-related hospitalization over unrestricted salt intake.[6] In the PURE study, with over 100,000 participants and 3.7 years average follow-up, all-cause mortality was lowest for those with an estimated daily sodium excretion of 4 to 6 g/day, with a nadir of risk at about 5 g/d, and with the median for the population at 4.72 g/day.[7]

Let's assume that the findings from the international study, that a urinary excretion of around 4,500 mg of sodium is optimal for survival in adults. Since 92% of the dietary sodium is excreted in the urine, that would be equivalent to an intake of around 4890 mg of dietary sodium. Table salt is 40% sodium, so if all of the dietary sodium were derived from salt, it would take 12.23 grams of salt to get this much sodium. A teaspoon of salt weighs about 5.7 grams, so the optimal sodium intake for a healthy adult is somewhere around two level teaspoons a day.

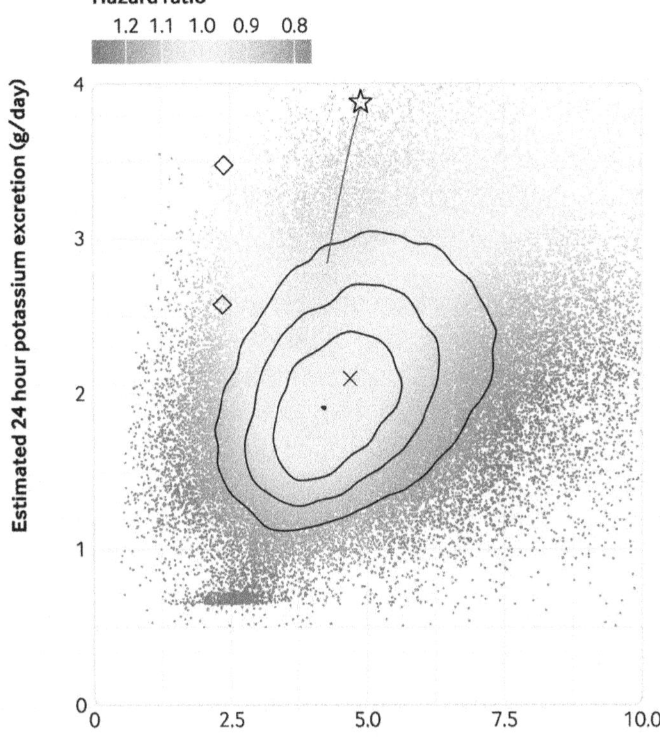

Figure 24A: Plot of urinary sodium and potassium excretion of over 103,000 adults; each dot represents one person; there is confluence in the middle. X marks the median level, and the black dot in the center is the mean. The X thus shows the most typical daily urinary sodium and potassium for adults. The diamonds (upper: men, lower: women) are the "approximate" *upper limit for sodium intake* and recommended potassium *intake* promulgated by the National Academy of Sciences (NAS). It can be seen that it is very rare to find this level of daily *urinary excretion* in the human population. Urinary excretion levels are lower than intake levels; thus, even fewer persons meet the recommended NAS guidelines. The (blue) line shows the lowest-risk Na^+ to K^+ excretion ratio area. This line indicates sodium and potassium excretion levels that are ideal for health. The star is an approximation of the overall data-driven area for the lowest mortality risk for urinary sodium and potassium levels. The outer (orange) dots are in high-risk areas. The contour lines show quartiles of the population; thus, one-fourth of those tested fell within the central contour, and a quarter fell outside of the outer contour line. Almost no one in the world complies with the NAS recommendations, nor should they. Our problem is not excess sodium but rather low potassium intake. From O'Donnell et al. PMCID: PMC6415648

These data suggest that people generally consume an appropriate amount of sodium but insufficient potassium.

Maybe that study got it wrong. Let's explore another.

A study using NHANES data that has comprehensive health and diet information assessed sodium and potassium intake on nearly 14,000 American adults ages 40 to 80, and used a follow-up period averaging over 8 years. The data were controlled for obesity, blood glucose, smoking, age, blood pressure, education, and alcohol intake. Setting the baseline sodium intake to be less than 2300 mg per day, and thus a relative risk (RR) of 1.0, the RR for all-cause mortality was 0.79 for those consuming 2300 – 4600 mg of sodium per day, and 0.69 for those consuming over 4600 mg per day of sodium. Eight years after the diet assessment, all-cause mortality was lowest for those in the high sodium intake group; there was 31% lower mortality for those in the higher than in the lower sodium intake group. When the analysis was limited to middle-aged adults aged 40 – 60, those with the highest intakes of sodium had better survival. For those aged 60 to 80, the lowest all-cause mortality risk for sodium intake was around 4000 mg per day. However, this likely represents bias from the inclusion of older persons with chronic kidney disease (CKD). For those with CKD, the nadir of risk for a sodium intake was between 2500 and 4000 mg of sodium per day; for those without CKD, the risk was lowest for those consuming *over* 4600 mg of sodium per day.

This study also found that all-cause mortality was *higher* for those consuming less than 3500 mg of potassium per day, but the risk was flat above this level. Furthermore, all-cause mortality was lowest when the dietary sodium: potassium intake was at a ratio of 1.20 to one. This was also seen in the data shown (as a blue line) in Figure 24A. A higher or lower ratio was associated with increased risk. Fortunately, healthy diets generally center around this ratio. Dietary potassium intake mostly comes from foods that are naturally low in sodium, such as fruits, vegetables, legumes, and (unsalted) dairy products.[8]

Note in Figure 24A how low the density of the dots is in the recommended sodium/potassium intake areas (diamonds) are especially for men. Not only is it in a high-risk area, but it highlights how impractical the recommendations are; almost no one eats like this. Even the low-risk area has few adherents. Thus, the SANA diet does not suggest trying to manipulate the sodium and potassium intake by those without kidney or heart disease, but rather suggests using salt to taste, as that generally provides appropriate sodium intake for most people not eating fast or manufactured foods that are heavy on salt. Most adults consume sodium by taste and look for salty food when they need more. In health, this usually works appropriately. Low sodium intake can be just as dangerous as excess sodium. Sodium deficits cause weakness and falls in blood pressure. Most adults consume an appropriate amount of sodium.

Where our diets go wrong is that many people don't consume sufficient potassium. Potassium helps maintain healthy blood pressure.[9] Diets that are composed largely of fast, manufactured, refined, and junk foods are likely to be low in potassium. Foods rich in potassium include fruits, vegetables, tubers, legumes, and whole grains. Diets that are high in vegetable oil and sugar are unlikely to have sufficient potassium, as they displace high-potassium foods with empty calories. Adherence to the SANA diet should provide adequate potassium.

Alternatively, a salt substitute that replaces some or most of the salt with potassium can reduce the risk of stroke and other major cardiovascular events in the elderly.[10] Much of this effect may not come from sodium restriction, but rather from increasing potassium intake.

People who chronically add salt to food, even before tasting it, are more likely to have elevated BMIs and greater waist-to-hip ratios, as well as a higher risk of T2D and sleep apnea.[11] [12] This should not be assumed to be a causal relationship. It may rather be associated with a dietary pattern of eating soft, palatable foods that give rise to obesity and insulin resistance.

Fancy pink Himalayan salt comes from an area where goiters and hypothyroidism are endemic, and unless labeled as such, it is not iodized. Pink Himalayan salt gets a bad DAD score and should be avoided.

Iodine

Iodine is an essential mineral that is used by the body to form thyroid hormone. It is critical to brain development during fetal life, and for brain growth during childhood. As an adult, thyroid hormone maintains an appropriate metabolic rate.

During fetal development, maternal thyroid levels have a critical impact on brain development. When children were tested at age 8, both brain volume and IQ levels were associated with the maternal thyroxine (T4) levels during pregnancy. IQs were highest when maternal free T4 was between 15.1 and 15.8 pmol/L. Grey matter and brain cerebral cortex volume were also found to be higher when fT4 levels were in this range. Maternal TSH, which drives thyroid production, was not found to be associated with the child's IQ.[13]

Thus, there is a narrow, optimal maternal free T4 range for thyroid function for neurodevelopment in the fetus.

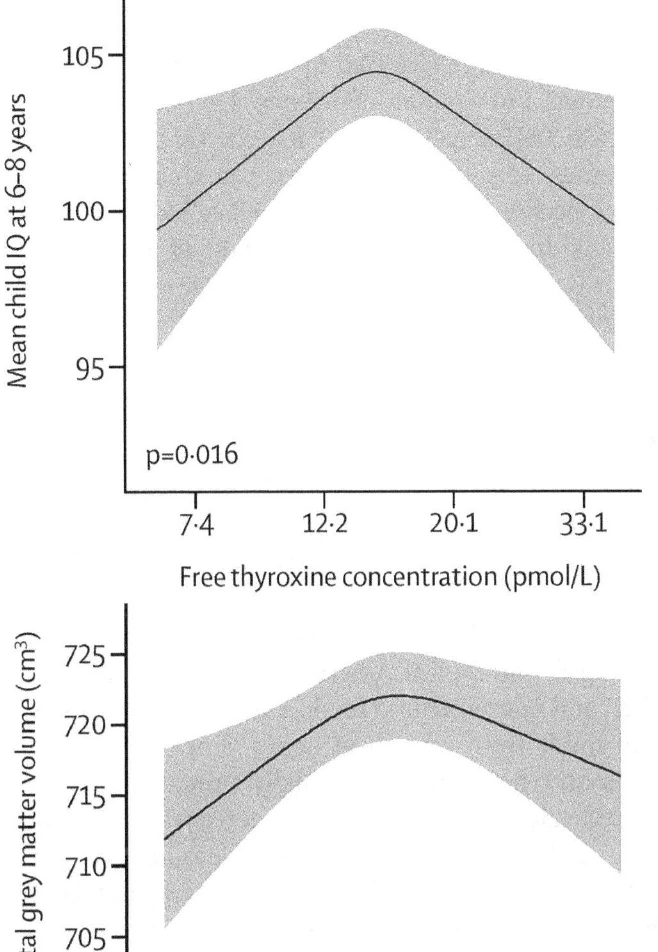

Figure 24B and 24C: Gestational free thyroxine concentration and child's IQ score at age six and grey matter volume from MRI at age eight, excluding women with hypo- or hyperthyroidism. Thus, both hypo- and hyperthyroid states during pregnancy impede neurodevelopment. There is a narrow optimal free T4 range for gestational thyroid status. Note that the scale for fT4 for the graph for grey matter is expanded as compared to the scale for IQ, which might give a false impression that a wider peak optimal range for fT4 for grey matter volume. Permission for use of images graciously granted by H. Tiemeier.[14]

Children born to mothers with gestational hypothyroidism have an increased risk of ADHD, nonverbal cognitive delay, and expressive language delay. The risk for ADHD may be highest when fT4 or iodine is low in the first trimester of pregnancy. Boys whose mothers had subclinical hypothyroidism are more likely to repeat a school grade.[15] Children of women who had even mild gestational iodine deficiency or thyroid insufficiency have an increased risk of ADHD.[16] In a study of nine-year-old children with ADHD, mild iodine deficiency (low urinary iodine levels) was present in 71% of these children.[17] Children with autism spectrum disorder and their mothers have been found to have lower iodine levels than control children and their mothers.[18] Maternal hypothyroidism has also been found to be associated with a 75% increased risk of the offspring developing schizophrenia.

The impact of thyroid hormone on brain development and cognition is not limited to prenatal neurodevelopment. When mildly iodine-deficient children aged 10 – 13 years were treated, their cognition improved.[19] [20] Sufficient dietary iodine and euthyroid function are important for cognitive health throughout the lifespan. In a study of 9,500 adults over 40, both higher and lower fT4 levels were found to be associated with a faster decline in cognitive function over the 8-year follow-up period.[21]

In a meta-analysis including 17 studies and over 340,000 subjects, with an average follow-up of 7.8 years, subclinical *hyperthyroidism* was found to be associated with the risk of dementia, while subclinical *hypothyroidism* was not found to be associated with a higher risk than upper "normal" TSH levels. Nevertheless, TSH (thyroid-stimulating hormone), which stimulates thyroid hormone production, had a U-shaped association with dementia risk. Dementia risk was lowest when the concentration of TSH was 1.55–1.60 mU/L.[22]

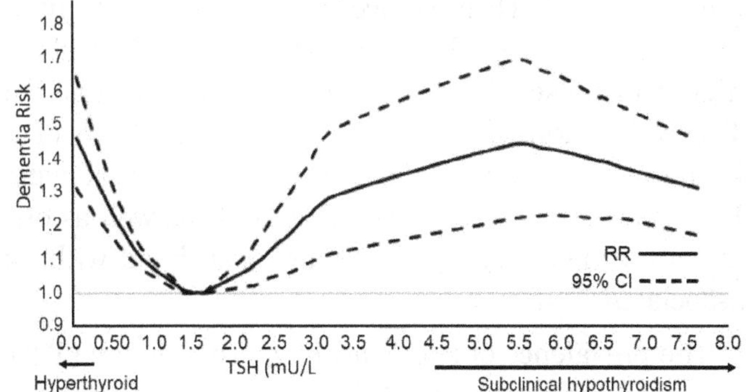

Figure 24D. TSH and dementia risk. [23] This data suggests that the optimal range for thyroid function is narrower than the standard diagnostic range for subclinical hyper- and hypothyroidism. Note that these results would likely have a symmetric U-shape below 5.5 μU/L if plotted on a log scale. In the previous figure, free thyroxine is plotted on a log scale in Figures 24B and 24C.

Hyperthyroidism, defined as a TSH less than 0.2, is associated with a 25% increased hazard of all-cause mortality, and even with subclinical hyperthyroidism, the all-cause mortality risk is 23% higher than for those with normal TSH levels. Most of the increased mortality risk was for cardiovascular events and congestive heart failure.

In contrast, hypothyroidism, defined as a TSH level from 5.0 to 10.0, and even if higher, but asymptomatic in the elderly, appears to be associated with an 8% decline in hazard for all-cause mortality. There is an increased risk (13%) of myocardial infarction for subclinical hypothyroidism, mostly when TSH levels are greater than 10.0, but overall mortality is offset by a lower risk of death from cancer and stroke.[24]

TSH is the standard metric for diagnosing thyroid adequacy. Nevertheless, it has its weaknesses. TSH levels have a circadian cycle. Levels are highest in the early morning hours and lowest during the day. TSH is released in pulses, so levels can vary over several minutes. It responds to temperature, so levels tend to be higher during the winter months. When blood for TSH tests was drawn early in the morning, fasting and again later the same morning, non-fasting, they were on average 26% lower on the second blood draw. TSH levels also increase with age.[25 26]

TSH levels increase during aging, independent of thyroid dysfunction. The body appears to become less sensitive to TSH with age; thus, higher TSH levels may be required to maintain euthyroid function.[27] Thus, making the diagnosis of subclinical hypothyroidism and monitoring treatment based on TSH response may not give a correct assessment of thyroid function in older patients, and subclinical hypothyroidism may be rather the result of "TSH resistance" rather than a reflection of inadequate thyroid hormone activity. TSH levels are higher in those who get low levels of physical activity. The conversion of the mostly inactive T4 form of the hormone to active T3 increases with physical activity.[28] It may be that lack of physical activity, as well as other factors, rather than age itself, are associated with age-associated "TSH resistance".

The prevalence of subclinical hypothyroidism (TSH > 4.5 mU/L) increases from about 2% at age 20 to nearly 14% by age 85, but only 2.3% of the elderly meet the criteria of hypothyroidism with a low thyroxine (T4) level. Low selenium status in the elderly may be a common cause of mild thyroid dysfunction.[29 30] While selenium inadequacy is uncommon in the U.S., eating one Brazil nut each day supplies adequate selenium intake.

Dietary Iodine and Thyroid

Not only is iodine required for the formation of thyroid hormone, but iodine deficiency has been found to increase TSH sensitivity.[31] It may be that excess iodine decreases sensitivity. Aging is commonly associated with a decline in renal function. Since iodine is cleared by the kidneys, the appropriate intake of iodine may be lower in older age as a result of the age-associated decline in renal function.

In some areas, there may be excess iodine in the groundwater. This occurs in some areas of China, Africa (Ethiopia, Kenya, Djibouti, and Algeria), as well as areas of Argentina and Denmark. In contrast, iodine levels are low in the soil of areas that were once covered with glaciers during the last ice age, such as Canada and much of the northern United States.

A majority of the salt (sodium chloride) and other sodium in the typical American diet comes from "fast-food" and manufactured foods, rather than salt added to food made from scratch at home. Since manufactured foods and fast foods are usually prepared with non-iodized salt, many people do not get sufficient iodine in their diets. Additionally, a considerable amount of sodium in prepared foods comes from compounds other than sodium chloride. Cow's milk is the major source of iodine in the American diet; about 60% of the iodine intake comes from dairy products. This means that those who are lactose intolerant or otherwise avoid dairy products often have insufficient iodine in their diet.[32]

Milk is a major source of iodine in the diet, but not always for the best reasons. If the cows drink water high in iodine, it will be found in the milk; however, this is not the usual source.

Cattle grazing or fed feed grown in many northern states, the old goiter belt, and the main dairy states in the U.S. are subject to iodine deficiency. Calves may be born with goiters, may be hairless, and may be weak. Thyroid deficiency in cattle causes low fertility in heifers, low libido, and low sperm count in bulls. (Take that as a hint.)

In addition to low iodine in feed grown in these areas, cattle are often fed goitrogenic compounds. Cyanogenic goitrogens impair iodine uptake by the thyroid gland; some examples are raw soybeans, corn, white clover, beet pulp, and millet. In contrast, progoitrins are compounds that prevent the formation of thyroid hormone; these include onions and *Brassica* plants such as mustard and rapeseed that contain glucosinolates. Rapeseed is used to make canola oil, and the pulp is often included as a source of protein in cattle feed. The effect of *cyanogenic* goitrogens can be overcome with the addition of more iodine in the diet; however, added iodine does not overcome the effects of *progoitrins*, which need to be cut back on to recover thyroid function.[33]

As a result of these factors, cattle feed is usually supplemented with iodine, often using ethylenediamine dihydroiodide (EDDI), to prevent iodine deficiency. The amount used can vary, but levels as high as 5 mg/kg of feed, or about 50,000 µg per animal of iodine, may be given daily.[34] [35] In a 1000 kg animal, that would be equivalent to 50 µg/kg, about 10 times the per-kilogram RDA of iodine for lactating women. Recently, it has been recommended that cattle feed in Europe be limited to 2 mg of iodine per kilo of feed.

Additionally, iodine is commonly used in dairies to disinfect the udder of cows before milking. Under controlled study conditions, milk from control cows (no iodine disinfectant treatment) contained 164 µg of iodine per kg of milk compared to 241 µg/kg using the standard iodine-based cleansing procedure.[36]

In an analysis of 44 samples of non-fat milk, the amount of iodine ranged from 38 to 159 µg/cup.[37] Thus, the issue for iodine in milk is not any inherent risk from the delivery of iodine in milk, but rather that there can easily be a fourfold variation in the amount of iodine present.

A study in a Mexican community revealed that more than one in five children had goiters. Moderate iodine deficiency in these children was associated with a greater than 4-fold risk of low IQ. Iodination of salt has been mandatory in Mexico for more than 60 years, and it was found that 92% of the population used iodized salt. However, when tested, 87% of the salt samples had less iodine than the labeled amount.[38] Loss of iodine from iodized salt can occur in warm and humid conditions, with moisture and air; potassium iodide (KI) easily gets oxidized, forming iodine, which is volatile. The WHO recommends the use of potassium iodate (KIO_3) for salt iodization as it is more stable in warm, humid climates.[39]

One reason that commercial foods usually avoid iodized salt is, in part, a mistaken belief that it alters the flavor of the food. In blinded testing, iodized salt has a discernible impact on the flavor of very few foods. The main reason for not using iodized salt is that iodine can be lost during food preparation and shelf life; thus, labeling the content of iodine would create legal risks, as the content would often be inaccurate. It is safer for the manufacturer to use non-iodized salt, as it provides more reliable labeling of the food.

Age	Male	Female	Pregnancy	Lactation	Tolerable Upper Limit
Birth to 6 months	110	110			Not Established
7–12 Mo	130	130			Not Established
1–3 Yrs	90	90			200
4–8 Yrs	90	90			300
9–13 Yrs	120	120			600
14–18 Yrs	150	150	220/250*	290	900
19+ Yrs	150	150	220/250	290	1100

Table 24D. Recommended Daily Allowances of Iodine: micrograms (µg) per day and upper tolerable limits.

The U.S. Institute of Medicine sets the RDA for iodine as 150 µg (micrograms) per day for those over the age of 13, but 220 µg for pregnant and 290 µg for lactating women. * The WHO and other international bodies recommend higher intakes of iodine during pregnancy than does the American National Academies of Science.

Data from the 2003–2006 NHANES studies revealed that the vast majority of American women of childbearing age, in general, have insufficient iodine intake,[40] and this is exacerbated by the higher demands during pregnancy. Black women were found to have significantly lower iodine intake, as reflected by lower urinary iodine concentrations (UIC), than did White women. Lower UICs in Black women likely result from lower intake of milk and milk products, as Black women are typically lactose intolerant, and dairy is the major source of dietary iodine.[41]

The lowest incidence of subclinical hypothyroidism occurs in pregnant women with urine iodide concentrations (UIC) of 150–249 µg/L, with the nadir around 200 µg/L.[42] Higher UIC levels, above around 600 µg/L, are associated with a higher risk of coronary artery disease, diabetes, obesity, and hypertension.[43] If looking just at cancer mortality and UIC, the lowest risk is at 125 to 170 µg/L.[44] UIC levels over 300 are associated with the odds of clinically relevant depression, with a nadir of risk with UIC at between 150 and 210 µg/L.[45]

A slightly different metric is the urinary iodine to creatinine ratio. In young adults, the optimal urinary iodine to creatinine ratio (UrI/CR ratio) is around 274 µg/g. As renal function declines with age and creatinine levels rise, less iodine may be required in the diet. Less may also be needed with aging as physical activity and the metabolic rate decrease.

Assuming the same dietary distribution of foods would generally be consumed by non-pregnant women and men, it seems rational to set dietary intake of iodine as a ratio to caloric intake, as caloric intake should align with metabolic activity. I suggest that 0.1333 µg of iodine per kcal of dietary intake is the lower limit for adequate intake of iodine, and a target of 0.16 µg of iodine per kcal of food is close to ideal for pregnant women.[46] Thus, for a pregnant woman consuming 2000 calories, the minimal adequate intake would be 266 µg of iodine per day, and an ideal intake would be 350 µg per day. Note that this is two times higher than the RDA, but well below the upper tolerable limits.

Too Much Iodine?

Iodized salt in the US is labeled to contain 45 µg of iodine per gram of salt, but testing has shown it generally contains a bit more, about 47.5 to 50.7 µg/g. One gram of salt contains 388 mg of sodium. If a healthy level of sodium intake is 5,000 grams per day, about 12 grams of salt, and *if all salt in the diet were iodized, the average adult would consume about 540 µg of iodine per day* in addition to that otherwise present in food, such as that in dairy and seafood. That may be too much; perhaps enough to increase the risk of autoimmune thyroid disease,[47] hypothyroidism, or TSH resistance, as well as possibly increasing the risk for depression, coronary artery disease, diabetes, obesity, and hypertension, as cited above.

The iodination level of salt may be set to a standard that is based on an unrealistically low level of salt consumption. This may become more of a problem in older individuals as renal function declines and as retired persons are more likely to have most of their meals at home, if using iodized salt.

Recommendation: If most meals are consumed at home, mixing a container of plain salt and one of iodized salt should provide a level of iodination that is more in line with the dietary needs when consuming salt at a level associated with the lowest all-cause mortality hazard and that is commonly consumed in non-salt-restricted diets.

Some commercially-produced breads (especially bread in the form of hot dog and hamburger buns and lower-cost white bread) use potassium-iodate or calcium-iodate as dough conditioners that allow for quicker leavening and a stronger foam. This type of bread may contain, on average, 200 µg of iodine per slice, while traditionally baked bread contains around 1 µg of iodine per slice. A food nutrition assessment by the US Department of Agriculture found between 469 and 981 µg of iodine per two-ounce hamburger bun made with iodate, as compared to 26 µg of iodine in a 100-gram (4 oz) serving of salmon.[48 49]

A single hamburger bun made with iodate may thus exceed the daily Tolerable Upper Limit of iodine for a teenager, and an average hamburger bun exceeds the upper limit for children under the age of 13. A cheese sandwich made from two slices of iodate-containing bread exceeds the Tolerable Upper Limit of iodine for an eight-year-old. (See table 24A above) Thus, the daily consumption of a typical serving of bread made with iodate has sufficient iodine to provoke hypothyroidism in children! A woman who frequently consumes hamburgers might also get excess iodine from the buns, thus risking subclinical hypothyroidism.

This risk would be expected to rise in the elderly, who are more likely to eat meals at home and who have a decline in renal function, which can curtail the excretion of iodine into the urine. The elderly are generally less physically active, have slower metabolism, and lose less iodine in their sweat.

Unprocessed meat is not high in iodine, but thyrotoxicosis is occasionally caused when an animal's thyroid gland is inadvertently added to hamburger or chorizo, sometimes causing local epidemics of "hamburger thyrotoxicosis".[50]

Some types of seaweed can be very high in iodine. Although seaweed-based iodine supplements may sound like a desirable natural source, they are not recommended as the dose may not be well controlled by the supplement manufacturer. Supplements made from potassium iodide are preferable.[51]

Testing Iodine Intake

For population studies, dietary iodine intake can be assessed by urinary iodine levels (UIC); levels have been periodically assessed in the U.S. population by the NHANES studies since 1971. Urinary iodine levels fell by 50% between 1971 and 1994, but stabilized at a lower level between 2000 and 2014. These lower levels were likely the result of curtailing the use of iodophor sanitizing agents and iodine in feed in dairy cattle, reduced use of iodate in bread, and decreased intake of erythrosine food color in breakfast cereals over this period.[52] Thus, the risk of excess dietary iodine intake has decreased over this period, but the risk of inadequate levels has likely risen.

Unfortunately, while UIC levels are helpful for population studies, they do not tell much more than what an individual had for lunch in terms of iodine intake. A single UIC is a very poor predictor of an individual's iodine intake, as 90% of the iodine consumed is excreted into the urine within 24 hours, and people's diets and water intake change from day to day. To get a reasonably accurate estimate of an individual's general iodine consumption, which is what influences T4 production, it is recommended that ten spot urine samples be done over at least several weeks.[53] Thus, spot urine samples or even 24-hour urine samples only inform about one day's iodine intake, and should not be relied upon for determining iodine sufficiency or excess.

[1] https://www.nap.edu/resource/25353/030519DRISodiumPotassium.pdf (Accessed December 2019)

[2] Percentage of ingested sodium excreted in 24-hour urine collections: A systematic review and meta-analysis. Lucko AM, Doktorchik C, Woodward M, et al.; TRUE Consortium. J Clin Hypertension (Greenwich). 2018 Sep;20(9):1220-1229. doi: 10.1111/jch.13353. PMID:30101426 https://onlinelibrary.wiley.com/doi/full/10.1111/jch.13353

[3] Association Between Urinary Sodium and Potassium Excretion and Blood Pressure Among Adults in the United States: National Health and Nutrition Examination Survey, 2014. Jackson SL, Cogswell ME, Zhao L, , et al. Circulation. 2018 Jan 16;137(3):237-246. doi: 10.1161/CIRCULATIONAHA. 117.029193. PMID:29021321

[4] Joint association of urinary sodium and potassium excretion with cardiovascular events and mortality: prospective cohort study. O'Donnell M, Mente A, Rangarajan S, et al,; PURE Investigators. BMJ. 2019 Mar 13;364:l772. doi: 10.1136/bmj.l772. PMID:30867146

[5] Sodium Excretion and the Risk of Cardiovascular Disease in Patients with Chronic Kidney Disease. Mills KT, Chen J, Yang W, et al.; Chronic Renal Insufficiency Cohort (CRIC) Study Investigators. JAMA. 2016 May 24-31;315(20):2200-10. doi: 10.1001/jama.2016.4447. PMID:27218629

[6] Reduction of dietary sodium to less than 100 mmol in heart failure (SODIUM-HF): an international, open-label, randomised, controlled trial. Ezekowitz JA, Colin-Ramires E, Ros H, et al. The Lancet, Apr. 2, 2022 DOI: https://doi.org/10.1016/S0140-6736(22)00369-5

[7] Urinary sodium and potassium excretion, mortality, and cardiovascular events. O'Donnell M, Mente A, Rangarajan S, McQueen MJ, Wang X, Liu L, Yan H, Lee SF, Mony P, Devanath A, Rosengren A, Lopez-Jaramillo P, Diaz R, Avezum A, Lanas F, Yusoff K, Iqbal R, Ilow R, Mohammadifard N, Gulec S, Yusufali AH, Kruger L, Yusuf R, Chifamba J, Kabali C, Dagenais G, Lear SA, Teo K, Yusuf S; PURE Investigators. N Engl J Med. 2014 Aug 14;371(7):612-23. doi: 10.1056/NEJMoa1311889. PMID: 25119607

[8] Sodium, potassium intake, and all-cause mortality: confusion and new findings. Liu D, Tian Y, Wang R, Zhang T, Shen S, Zeng P, Zou T. BMC Public Health. 2024 Jan 15;24(1):180. doi: 10.1186/s12889-023-17582-8. PMID: 38225648

[9] Association Between Urinary Sodium and Potassium Excretion and Blood Pressure Among Adults in the United States: National Health and Nutrition Examination Survey, 2014. Jackson SL, Cogswell ME, Zhao L, et al. Circulation. 2018 Jan 16;137(3):237-246. doi: 10.1161/CIRCULATIONAHA. 117.029193. PMID:29021321

[10] Effect of Salt Substitution on Cardiovascular Events and Death. Neal B, Wu Y, Feng X, Zhang R, Zhang Y, Shi J, Zhang J, Tian M, Huang L, Li Z, Yu Y, Zhao Y, Zhou B, Sun J, Liu Y, Yin X, Hao Z, Yu J, Li KC, Zhang X, Duan P, Wang F, Ma B, Shi W, Di Tanna GL, Stepien S, Shan S, Pearson SA, Li N, Yan LL, Labarthe D, Elliott P. N Engl J Med. 2021 Sep 16;385(12):1067-1077. doi: 10.1056/NEJMoa2105675. Epub 2021 Aug 29. PMID: 34459569

[11] Dietary Sodium Intake and Risk of Incident Type 2 Diabetes. Wang X, Ma H, Kou M, Tang R, Xue Q, Li X, Harlan TS, Heianza Y, Qi L. Mayo Clin Proc. 2023 Oct 11:S0025-6196(23)00118-0. doi: 10.1016/j.mayocp.2023.02.029. Online ahead of print. PMID: 37921793

[12] Eating habit of adding salt to foods and incident sleep apnea: a prospective cohort study. Li T, Song L, Li G, Li F, Wang X, Chen L, Rong S, Zhang L. Respir Res. 2023 Jan 7;24(1):5. doi: 10.1186/s12931-022-02300-6. PMID: 36611201

[13] Association of maternal thyroid function during early pregnancy with offspring IQ and brain morphology in childhood: a population-based prospective cohort study. Korevaar TI, Muetzel R, Medici M, Chaker L, Jaddoe VW, de Rijke YB, Steegers EA, Visser TJ, White T, Tiemeier H, Peeters RP. Lancet Diabetes Endocrinol. 2016 Jan;4(1):35-43. PMID:26497402

[14] Association of maternal thyroid function during early pregnancy with offspring IQ and brain morphology in childhood: a population-based prospective cohort study. Korevaar TI, Muetzel R, Medici M, et al. Lancet Diabetes Endocrinol. 2016 Jan;4(1):35-43. PMID:26497402

[15] Draft Report: Proposed Approaches to Inform the Derivation of a Maximum Contaminant Level Goal for Perchlorate in Drinking Water (Volume I - Main Report) https://www.regulations.gov/document?D=EPA-HQ-OW-2016-0438-0019

[16] Maternal Mild Thyroid Hormone Insufficiency in Early Pregnancy and Attention-Deficit/Hyperactivity Disorder Symptoms in Children. Modesto T, Tiemeier H, Peeters RP, Jaddoe VW, Hofman A, Verhulst FC, Ghassabian A. JAMA Pediatr. 2015 Sep;169(9):838-45. doi: 10.1001/jamapediatrics.2015.0498. PMID: 26146876

[17] Evaluation of Iodine Deficiency in Children with Attention Deficit/Hyperactivity Disorder. Kanık Yüksek S, Aycan Z, Öner Ö. J Clin Res Pediatr Endocrinol. 2016 Mar 5;8(1):61-6. doi: 10.4274/jcrpe.2406 PMID: 26758811

[18] Analyses of toxic metals and essential minerals in the hair of Arizona children with autism and associated conditions, and their mothers. Adams JB, Holloway CE, George F, Quig D. Biol Trace Elem Res. 2006 Jun;110(3):193-209. doi: 10.1385/BTER:110:3:193. PMID: 16845157

[19] Iodine supplementation improves cognition in mildly iodine-deficient children. Gordon RC, Rose MC, Skeaff SA, Gray AR, Morgan KM, Ruffman T. Am J Clin Nutr. 2009 Nov;90(5):1264-71. doi: 10.3945/ajcn.2009.28145. PMID: 19726593

[20] Iodine supplementation improves cognition in iodine-deficient schoolchildren in Albania: a randomized, controlled, double-blind study. Zimmermann MB, Connolly K, Bozo M, Bridson J, Rohner F, Grimci L. Am J Clin Nutr. 2006 Jan;83(1):108-14. doi: 10.1093/ajcn/83.1.108. PMID: 16400058

[21] Association Between Subclinical Thyroid Dysfunction and Cognitive Decline: Findings From the ELSA-Brasil

Study. Gomes Gonçalves N, Szlejf C, Lotufo PA, Bensenor IM, Suemoto CK. J Gerontol A Biol Sci Med Sci. 2024 Aug 1;79(8):glae169. doi: 10.1093/gerona/glae169. PMID: 38953739

22 Spectrum of thyroid dysfunction and dementia: a dose-response meta-analysis of 344,248 individuals from cohort studies. Tang X, Song ZH, Wang D, Yang J, Augusto Cardoso M, Zhou JB, Simó R. Endocr Connect. 2021 Apr 22;10(4):410-421. doi: 10.1530/EC-21-0047. PMID: 33875615

23 Spectrum of thyroid dysfunction and dementia: a dose-response meta-analysis of 344,248 individuals from cohort studies. Tang X, Song ZH, Wang D, Yang J, Augusto Cardoso M, Zhou JB, Simó R. Endocr Connect. 2021 Apr 22;10(4):410-421. doi: 10.1530/EC-21-0047. PMID: 33875615

24 Subclinical and overt thyroid dysfunction and risk of all-cause mortality and cardiovascular events: a large population study. Selmer C, Olesen JB, Hansen ML, von Kappelgaard LM, Madsen JC, Hansen PR, Pedersen OD, Faber J, Torp-Pedersen C, Gislason GH. J Clin Endocrinol Metab. 2014 Jul;99(7):2372-82. doi: 10.1210/jc.2013-4184. PMID: 24654753

25 Within-Person Variation in Serum Thyrotropin Concentrations: Main Sources, Potential Underlying Biological Mechanisms, and Clinical Implications. van der Spoel E, Roelfsema F, van Heemst D. Front Endocrinol (Lausanne). 2021 Feb 24;12:619568. doi: 10.3389/fendo.2021.619568. eCollection 2021. PMID: 33716972

26 Serum TSH variability in normal individuals: the influence of time of sample collection. Scobbo RR, VonDohlen TW, Hassan M, Islam S. W V Med J. 2004 Jul-Aug;100(4):138-42. PMID: 15471172

27 Iodine deficiency is associated with increased thyroid hormone sensitivity in individuals with elevated TSH. Sun Y, et al. Eur Thyroid J. 2022. PMID: 35324457

28 Association between physical activity and thyroid function in American adults: a survey from the NHANES database. Tian L, Lu C, Teng W. BMC Public Health. 2024 May 10;24(1):1277. doi: 10.1186/s12889-024-18768-4. PMID: 38730302

29 Low selenium status in the elderly influences thyroid hormones. Olivieri O, Girelli D, Azzini M, Stanzial AM, Russo C, Ferroni M, Corrocher R. Clin Sci (Lond). 1995 Dec;89(6):637-42. doi: 10.1042/cs0890637. PMID: 8549083

30 Selenium, zinc, and thyroid hormones in healthy subjects: low T3/T4 ratio in the elderly is related to impaired selenium status. Olivieri O, Girelli D, Stanzial AM, Rossi L, Bassi A, Corrocher R. Biol Trace Elem Res. 1996 Jan;51(1):31-41. doi: 10.1007/BF02790145. PMID: 8834378

31 Iodine deficiency is associated with increased thyroid hormone sensitivity in individuals with elevated TSH. Sun Y, et al. Eur Thyroid J. 2022. PMID: 35324457

32 https://www.theguardian.com/us-news/2019/may/28/bread-additives-chemicals-us-toxic-america

33 Iodine in the feed of cows and in the milk with a view to the consumer's iodine supply. Schöne F, Spörl K, Leiterer M. J Trace Elem Med Biol. 2017 Jan;39:202-209. doi: 10.1016/j.jtemb.2016.10.004. PMID: 27908415

34 Iodine in the feed of cows and in the milk with a view to the consumer's iodine supply. Schöne F, Spörl K, Leiterer M. J Trace Elem Med Biol. 2017 Jan;39:202-209. doi: 10.1016/j.jtemb.2016.10.004. PMID: 27908415

35 https://agriking.com/the-importance-of-micro-minerals-iodin/ (July 2015, Accessed Dec. 2020)

36 Effects of iodine intake and teat-dipping practices on milk iodine concentrations in dairy cows. Castro SI, Berthiaume R, Robichaud A, Lacasse P. J Dairy Sci. 2012 Jan;95(1):213-20. doi: 10.3168/jds.2011-4679. PMID: 22192200

37 National Institutes of Health Office of Dietary Supplements Iodine Fact Sheet for Professionals. https://ods.od.nih.gov/factsheets/Iodine-Health Professional/ (Accessed Dec. 2020)

38 Iodine deficiency and its association with intelligence quotient in schoolchildren from Colima, Mexico. Pineda-Lucatero A, Avila-Jiménez L, Ramos-Hernández RI, Magos C, Martínez H. Public Health Nutr. 2008 Jul;11(7):690-8. doi: 10.1017/S1368980007001243. PMID: 18205986

39 World Health Organization. United Nations Children's Fund & International Council for the Control of Iodine Deficiency Disorders. Assessment of iodine deficiency disorders and monitoring their elimination. 3rd ed. Geneva, Switzerland: WHO, 2007.

40 The CDC's Second National Report on Biochemical Indicators of Diet and Nutrition in the U.S. Population is a valuable tool for researchers and policy makers. Pfeiffer CM, Sternberg MR, Schleicher RL, Haynes BM, Rybak ME, Pirkle JL. J Nutr. 2013 Jun;143(6):938S-47S. PMID:23596164

41 Race-ethnicity is related to biomarkers of iron and iodine status after adjusting for sociodemographic and lifestyle variables in NHANES 2003-2006. Pfeiffer CM, Sternberg MR, Caldwell KL, Pan Y. J Nutr. 2013 Jun;143(6):977S-85S. PMID:23596169

42 Optimal and safe upper limits of iodine intake for early pregnancy in iodine-sufficient regions: a cross-sectional study of 7190 pregnant women in China. Shi X, Han C, Li C, Mao J, Wang W, Xie X, Li C, Xu B, Meng T, Du J, Zhang S, Gao Z, Zhang X, Fan C, Shan Z, Teng W. J Clin Endocrinol Metab. 2015 Apr;100(4):1630-8. doi: 10.1210/jc.2014-3704. Epub 2015 Jan 28. PMID: 25629356

43 Association study of urinary iodine concentrations and coronary artery disease among adults in the USA: National Health and Nutrition Examination Survey 2003-2018. Wu Z, Li M, Liu J, Xie F, Chen Y, Yang S, Li X, Wu Y. Br J Nutr. 2023 Dec 28;130(12):2114-2122. doi: 10.1017/S0007114523001277. Epub 2023 Jul 10. PMID: 37424297

44 Urinary Iodine Concentration and Mortality Among U.S. Adults. Inoue K, Leung AM, Sugiyama T, Tsujimoto T, Makita N, Nangaku M, Ritz BR. Thyroid. 2018

Jul;28(7):913-920. doi: 10.1089/thy.2018.0034. PMID: 29882490

45 Association of Urinary Iodine Concentration with Depressive Symptoms among Adults: NHANES 2007-2018. Chen S, Cui K, Luo J, Zhang D. Nutrients. 2022 Oct 7;14(19):4165. doi: 10.3390/nu14194165. PMID: 36235816

46 Neurodevelopment and Intelligence. Charles Lewis. Chapter 7. Psy Press (February 26, 2022) ISBN-13:978-1938318078
https://books.google.com/books?id=1KhiEAAAQBAJ

47 The protective role of nutritional antioxidants against oxidative stress in thyroid disorders. Macvanin MT, Gluvic Z, Zafirovic S, et al. Front Endocrinol (Lausanne). 2023 Jan 4;13:1092837. doi: 10.3389/fendo.2022.1092837. PMID: 36686463

48 Sources of dietary iodine: bread, cows' milk, and infant formula in the Boston area. Pearce EN, Pino S, He X, Bazrafshan HR, Lee SL, Braverman LE. J Clin Endocrinol Metab. 2004 Jul;89(7):3421-4. doi: 10.1210/jc.2003-032002. PMID: 15240625

49 USDA, FDA, and ODS-NIH Database for the Iodine Content of Common Foods Release 1.0. 2020.

50 Recurrent hamburger thyrotoxicosis. Parmar MS, Sturge C. CMAJ. 2003 Sep 2;169(5):415-7. PMID: 12952802

51 Excess iodine intake: sources, assessment, and effects on thyroid function. Farebrother J, Zimmermann MB, Andersson M. Ann N Y Acad Sci. 2019 Jun;1446(1):44-65. doi: 10.1111/nyas.14041. PMID: 30891786

52 Ibid Ref. 37

53 Ten repeat collections for urinary iodine from spot samples or 24-hour samples are needed to reliably estimate individual iodine status in women. König F, Andersson M, Hotz K, Aeberli I, Zimmermann MB. J Nutr. 2011 Nov;141(11):2049-54. doi: 10.3945/jn.111.144071.. PMID: 21918061

25: Micronutrients

Capsule

For the most part, a healthy diet supplies the micronutrients needed for health; most vitamins and minerals should come from food. Many micronutrient deficits are the result of diets high in refined fats and added sugars that displace the consumption of whole foods.

Supplementation with several vitamins and minerals increases cancer risk and, thus, these supplements should be avoided in middle-aged and older adults. Multivitamin supplements should generally be avoided in older adults.

Vitamins and other supplements should not be expected to reverse most forms of dementia. Nevertheless, preventing deficiencies can help prevent dementia.

Micronutrient supplements should be limited to those needed for specific needs, and the dose should be a physiologic one, not an excessive one, other than when required to treat a specific disorder. Some vitamin and mineral supplements have a place in the treatment of specific diseases, for example, genetic diseases in which an individual does not process the nutrient normally. For most people, the supplement dose should reflect the amount needed to normalize blood levels.

1) When using a micronutrient as a dietary supplement, the dose should be used to fill the gap between the diet and the optimal RDI (recommended daily intake).

2) If using a micronutrient as a medication or to correct a medical condition, the dose needs to be adjusted to the condition, and blood testing should be used to confirm that the dose is working.

❖ Most adults living in temperate and cold climates and those working indoors benefit from vitamin D supplements. A daily dose of 5000 i.u. (25 mcg) of vitamin D3 is appropriate for most older adults living in a temperate climate. Those at risk (of vitamin D deficiency, osteomalacia, infection, diabetes, etc.) should have their blood vitamin D levels checked to confirm that their OH25D3 levels are above 90 nmol/l (36 ng/ml) and ideally around 125 nmol/L (50 ng/ml) regardless of age.

❖ All vegans and most adults over the age of 60 benefit from vitamin B12 supplementation. For adults over the age of 60, 500 to 1000 mcg of cyanocobalamin per day as a chewable tablet is recommended. For young vegan adults, 50 to 100 mcg a day is generally sufficient.

❖ About one in ten people in the U.S. have elevated blood levels of the metabolic intermediate homocysteine (HCY). This occurs most commonly as a result of genetic traits, but can result from nutrient insufficiencies. Elevated HCY levels double the risk of both vascular dementia and Alzheimer's disease. It is also a risk factor for coronary artery disease. Individuals with elevated homocysteine levels (> 8.5 μmol/l) may be able to lower their risk of dementia by supplementing with the 5-MTHF (metafolin) form of vitamin B9 (folate). A dose of 800 mcg a day is generally appropriate. Vitamins B6 and B12 can also help reduce homocysteine levels if there is an inadequacy of these vitamins. Choline can also lower homocysteine levels.

❖ Most people's diets include less choline than the Adequate Intake (AI) level. Vegetarians get about half that of the rest of the population, and vegans typically get even less. Choline may help prevent AD by lowering HCY levels and by helping overcome deficits in lipid metabolism caused by ApeE4. Choline supplements, preferably in the form of αGPC, at a dose of 275 to 300 mg/ day, taken with a meal, is recommended for those at risk of dementia.

❖ Avoid gel caps when possible; if using vitamin gelcaps, bite the capsule to release the contents, and then remove the gel capsule from the mouth. It is my observation that the gelcaps disturb the intestinal mucosa. (Rigid pill capsules are not a problem.)

Micronutrients

Vitamins are essential dietary compounds that our body requires to function. Many vitamins and minerals are required as cofactors for enzymes. Vitamins A and D have hormone-like activity. If we are deficient in any of the various vitamins, our health suffers.

Micronutrients (vitamins and minerals) are like a fan belt on a car. Without the fan belt, the water pump doesn't work, and the engine overheats and gets destroyed. You need one. But putting two or three fan belts on does not make the car work any better. High doses of vitamins are not going to magically improve health. Vitamin requirements are not binary; sufficient or deficient. Rather, there is a range of levels that provide optimal metabolic function of the vitamin. The amount needed in the diet, or as supplements, is different for different individuals as a result of differences in genetics, health status, absorption, etc. The goal is to maintain a level that is optimal for health.

For the most part, nutritional supplements should not be needed, and we should be getting an adequate supply from our diet. We evolved over millions of years to get what we need from food and sunshine. Most people who eat a healthy diet get the vitamins and minerals they need from their diets. However, alcoholics often have nutritional deficiencies. People with intestinal disease or malabsorption often have nutritional deficiencies as a result.

We make hundreds of millions of new cells each day, and some harbor mutations that can become cancer. After the age of 45, caution needs to be used with the use of vitamin supplements, especially those that can increase cancer risk. Vitamins and mineral supplements should be used to overcome deficiencies. For example, iron supplements, along with diet, should be appropriately used to treat iron deficiency-induced anemia, but not until the iron deficiency has been verified and the cause of the deficiency has been determined, and the underlying cause addressed.

While a healthy diet should supply what we need, there are a few nutrients, however, that American adults and especially older adults are commonly deficient in. Some of these deficiencies increase the risk of dementia. Thus, there are some nutritional supplements that most older Americans will benefit from. These will be discussed after providing warnings on some to avoid.

Supplements to Avoid

Before discussing which nutrients merit supplementing, the downside of supplements needs to be addressed. Multiple studies have found that several nutritional supplements increase the risk of cancer and cancer mortality.

Antioxidant vitamins have been the object of multiple studies for the prevention of a wide range of diseases among healthy individuals. For example, a randomized trial for the prevention of prostate cancer among 35,000 men who had been tested for, and found not to have any signs of prostate cancer, were given 400 IU of vitamin E a day for 7 years. The men who received vitamin E during the study had a 17% increase in cancer over those who received the placebo; about 1.6 cases per thousand person-years. Selenium supplements also failed to lower the risk.[1] In another study, 38,000 older women were interviewed about nutritional supplement intake and followed for an average of 22 years. Use of multivitamins was associated with a 2.4 percent *increase* in mortality. Other supplements also increased mortality:

- Zinc by 3.0%
- Magnesium by 3.6%
- Iron by 3.9%
- Vitamin B6 by 4.1%
- Folic acid by 5.9%
- Copper by 18.0%.

Calcium was associated with a decrease in mortality in this population by 3.8%[2]. In a separate study of men and women with an 11-year follow-up of 182,000 patients, multivitamin use did not affect mortality one way or the other.[3]

In a meta-analysis of sixty-seven prevention studies using antioxidants involving over 230,000 patients:[4]

- Vitamin A increased mortality by 16%,
- β-carotene increased mortality by 7%,
- Vitamin E increased mortality by 4%,
- Vitamin C and selenium neither raised nor lowered the risk of mortality.

In 18 blinded clinical trials including 46,000 patients, those taking synthetic vitamin E had no change in mortality rates, but those taking natural vitamin E had a 13 percent increase in mortality.[5] In a placebo-controlled randomized trial for the prevention of prostate cancer, a folic acid supplement or a placebo was given over a ten-year follow-up period. Those who received the folic acid had a 9.7% probability of being diagnosed with prostate cancer during the follow-up period, while only 3.3% of the placebo group were diagnosed with the disease. However, those individuals who had higher serum folate levels but were not vitamin users at baseline were less likely to get prostate cancer.[6] Thus, dietary folate was not a risk, but the use of folic acid as a supplement was.

Why did these supplements cause an increased risk of cancer?

- Vitamin A (and β-carotene, which the body converts to vitamin A), a hormone that promotes cell growth. While it does not cause cells to become cancerous, it helps those aberrant cells proliferate.
- Zinc is a cofactor in vitamin A activity.
- Vitamin E, as α-tocopherol, and Vitamin B9 as folic acid are the wrong forms of the vitamins to supplement with. Taking α-tocopherol actually lowers the levels of other important forms of vitamin E in the body.

- ➢ Copper, iron, and zinc can have pro-oxidative effects and cause an increase in the formation of reactive oxygen species (ROS) that create lipid peroxidation and increase the risk of DNA damage.
- ➢ Gelcaps (typically used with vitamins A, D, and E) are harmful to the intestinal mucosa, getting a DAD rating of D.

There are legitimate reasons to supplement some of these micronutrients. One is to use them to overcome a shortfall in dietary intake or for those with disease conditions that prevent adequate absorption. If using a micronutrient supplement to overcome a dietary shortfall, the nutrient and the dose should reflect that shortfall.

For example, the recommended daily intake of zinc for an adult man is 11 mg per day. If the diet has less than an adequate amount of zinc, for example, containing only half of the recommended amount, the supplement should make up the shortfall. The supplement should be a highly bioavailable form, avoiding ones that are poorly absorbed and that harm the intestine and microbiome. Zinc citrate is highly bioavailable; thus, a reasonable supplemental dose is 6 to 10 mg of zinc, as zinc citrate. Nevertheless, most zinc supplements contain 50 mg or more of poorly utilized forms of zinc. If one looks hard enough, they may find a low-dose zinc citrate tablet that can be cut into an appropriate daily dose. Higher doses of zinc are unlikely to improve health unless there is a specific disease that prevents zinc absorption or its utilization. Higher doses are associated with increased cancer risk.

Supplements that May Be Helpful

The most common micronutrient inadequacies for those consuming the Western diet include magnesium, potassium, vitamin D, vitamin B12, choline, iodine, and iron.

- o Magnesium is present in chlorophyll, in green leafy vegetables, as well as in legumes and whole grains. The SAD (Standard American Diet) is low in magnesium as a result of the consumption of refined foods, sugar, and fat.
- o Potassium is high in fruits, leafy greens, tomatoes, summer and winter squash, legumes, tubers (potatoes, sweet potatoes, carrots, and yogurt. The SAD has inadequate potassium.
- o The reason the western diet often has inadequate amounts of potassium, magnesium, and many other micronutrients is that so much of the nutritional intake is displaced with empty calories from added fats and sugars, and the use of refined grains. Magnesium and potassium inadequacy should be uncommon on the SANA diet.
- o Vitamin D levels are commonly inadequate, as most of us have less exposure to sunlight than our ancestors evolved to have. Vitamin D is discussed in this chapter.
- o Since there is no vitamin B12 (cobalamin)in plants, vegans need to take vitamin B12 supplements. Vitamin B12 deficits are highly prevalent among older adults, including among omnivores. Vitamin B12 absorption is a multistep process. One reason that older adults have a diminished capacity for cobalamin absorption is that they may have dental problems that keep them from chewing their food adequately, or that they have diminished production of saliva. Saliva contains a protein called haptocorrin that protects cobalamin from destruction by stomach acid, and the haptocorrin needs to come into contact with the cobalamin during mastication to protect the vitamin. Another, more common, factor is the accelerated turnover and aging of the parietal cells of the stomach as a result of chronic *Helicobacter pylori* infection. The parietal cells secrete cobalamin-binding intrinsic factor, which is necessary for vitamin B12 absorption. There is often a loss of these cells with aging. Vitamin B12 is discussed below.
- o Most people eating the western diet consume less than the recommended "Adequate Intake" of choline, as established by the National Academy of Medicine. Vegetarians and even more so, vegans, are at a higher risk of having an inadequate choline intake. Choline is essential for brain development, and low intake is associated with the risk of MCI and AD. Thus, choline and its supplementation are discussed in this chapter.
- o Iodine is discussed in Chapter 24.
- o Inadequate iron levels are common, especially among young menstruating women, but are much less common in older adults. Inflammation can make deficiencies worse as it can limit iron uptake from the diet. Iron deficiency during pregnancy limits the brain's development of the fetus and infant. Excess iron, however, is toxic and toxic to the brain. Thus, iron supplementation should be guided by a knowledgeable physician using blood testing. While iron deficiency will not be covered here, for those interested, my book "Neurodevelopment and Intelligence" covers this topic in depth.
- o In addition to vitamin B12, vitamin D, and calcium, a vegan diet can easily have inadequate levels of riboflavin, taurine, carnitine, creatine, β-alanine, and carnosine. These are discussed in Chapter 13 (Protein Requirements).

Vitamin E

There are eight main vitamin E compounds: α, β, δ, and γ tocopherol and α, β, δ, and γ tocotrienol. Vitamin E capsules usually contain only α-tocopherol. The tocotrienol forms of vitamin E have a stronger antioxidant effect and, in rats, inhibit the proliferation of fat cells, and thus may reduce obesity.

Alpha-tocopherol vitamin E supplements increase the risk of hemorrhagic stroke by 22 percent, while decreasing the risk of the more frequently occurring ischemic stroke by 10 percent, which thereby cancels out the overall risk of stroke from vitamin E.[7] Alpha-tocopherol also increases the activity of cytosolic phospholipase A_2, promoting the release of arachidonic acid (AA) and the formation of eicosanoids,[8] including PGE2. Meanwhile, γ-tocopherol, the second most common vitamin E form in the diet, reduces PGE2 synthesis. This results in an increase in prostacyclin, which decreases platelet activity and acts as a vasodilator, thus increasing blood flow and decreasing clotting. γ-Tocopherol would be expected to be beneficial in the prevention of dementia. Bleeding risk is higher in individuals who have vitamin K deficiencies and who supplement with vitamin E but do not replace vitamin K.

PGE_2 also promotes cell proliferation and the development of new blood vessels, which partially explains the increased risk of cancer seen with α-tocopherol supplementation. If the enhanced cytosolic phospholipase A_2 promoted by α-tocopherol activity occurs in animals consuming a balanced n-6 to n-3 fatty acid diet, it should promote the release of eicosatetraenoic acid and EPA and prostacyclin, which would have anti-inflammatory effects and should have anti-carcinogenic effects from reduced fibroblast growth and angiogenesis and increased apoptosis. In individuals eating a Western diet, however, when consuming a high n-6: n-3 fatty acid ratio, α-tocopherol is inflammatory; it increases the proliferation of cancer cells, inflammation, and platelet activation. Walnuts are rich in α-, δ-, and γ-tocopherols.

In cell cultures, tocotrienol, and specifically γ-tocotrienol, induces apoptosis and impairs the growth of breast cancer,[9] prostate cancer,[10] and colon cancer cells.[11] Tocotrienols inhibit cyclooxygenase-2 and prevent PGE_2 formation. These vitaminers are not found in most vitamin E supplements, but are present in whole grain rice and soy.

Table 25A: Impact of Dietary Vitaminers E on Disease

Vitamin E	Impact of Vitaminers E [12 13]
α-tocopherol	Antioxidant, increases phospholipase A2, thus increasing eicosanoid production.
γ-tocopherol	It is better than α-T at trapping NO and other free radicals. Balances Na+ transport. Inhibits the growth of colon cancer cells. Reduces prostaglandin E2 synthesis.
δ-tocopherol	Inhibits the proliferation of prostate cancer cells.
α-tocotrienol	Prevents lipid peroxidation 40 to 60 times more than α-T, and is better at defending cytochrome p-450. Inhibits the proliferation of cancer cells.
γ-tocotrienol	Inhibits cancer cell growth. Antioxidant.
δ-tocotrienol	Anti-thrombotic, most effective vitamin E to prevent and reduce atherosclerotic plaque. Potent antioxidant. Inhibits the growth and proliferation of cancer cells.

Folic Acid

Folic acid, a synthetic form of vitamin B9, is also suspected to cause cancer. In a trial using 1000 micrograms (μg) of folic acid in patients with a history of colonic adenomas, folic acid increased the risk of developing new precancerous lesions by 67%.[14] In lab animals that have had tumor cells implanted, high doses of folic acid, ten times the physiologic requirements, show increased tumor cell growth. In a study of patients with p53-positive colon cancers, both low and high folic acid intake and low vitamin B_6 levels were associated with increased risk. The P53 gene is one of the most commonly mutated genes in cancer. This protein participates in apoptosis, the elimination of cancer cells. When it is mutated, cancer cells resist dying. Excessive intake of folate can promote hypermethylation of the p53 gene, which decreases its expression and ability to promote apoptosis. Hypomethylation, which can occur with folate deficiency, can increase the risk of p53 mutation.

The risk of colon cancer was lowest when total folate intake was between 350 and 600 μg of folate per day.[15] There is no evidence that natural, food-based folates increase cancer risk at higher intake levels.[16] There are several forms of folate; folic acid is the one used for food fortification and in most vitamin tablets, as it is cheap and easy to synthesize. Folic acid is a pre-vitamin B9 that is quite rare in natural foods. The enterocytes and liver only have a limited dihydrofolate reductase (DHFR) capacity for converting folic acid into THF.[17] The amount of folic acid present in fortified foods may not be a problem but consumption of over 200 μg of folic acid a day leads to a build-up of unmetabolized folic acid (UMFA) in the bloodstream, especially in those with allelic variants of the MTHFR gene, present in in about one in ten Americans.[18] UMFA has been associated with a decrease in IL-10 and the number and function of natural killer (NK) immune cells in lab animals and humans.[19] [20] NK cells are essential immune cells that destroy viruses and cancer cells. Excess folic acid and UMFA may increase the losses of active folates from the body, and thus, may cause functional deficiency even with high folate levels. Thus, folic acid should be avoided as a supplement.

Supplements to Lower Dementia Risk

NOTE: The following and any recommendations refer to adults and particularly older adults. Nothing herein should be considered medical advice. Consult your doctor.

Carotenoids: Carotenoids are a class of compounds that have antioxidant effects. A few carotenoids, β-carotene, α-carotene, and β-cryptoxanthin, can be converted into vitamin A in the body, but α-carotene and β-cryptoxanthin only form half as much vitamin A as β-carotene and α-carotene do. In a meta-analysis with 41 studies and over 500,000 subjects, those consuming the highest amounts of carotenoids had a 40% lower mortality rate than those consuming the lowest amounts.[21] In the MIND trial, α-carotene was the carotenoid that was most highly correlated with global cognitive function, as well as episodic memory. Serum lutein, zeaxanthin, and α-carotene were associated with higher semantic memory scores, and lycopene was associated with perceptual speed memory.[22]

The carotenoids lutein, zeaxanthin, and meso-zeaxanthin protect the retina from UV and blue-light injury. They act as antioxidants in the brain and improve sleep and cognitive function. [23] [24] [25] [26] [27] They appear to slow cognitive decline.[28]

The SANA program does not encourage supplementation with carotenoids (unless ordered by a physician for a specific reason, such as using lutein and zeaxanthin for eye health) and discourages supplementation with β-carotene. Rather, the SANA program encourages the consumption of a wide variety of yellow, orange, and red fruits and vegetables. This should provide a better balance of antioxidant carotenoids, including some, such as phytoene and phytofluene, that have received very little study.

Pumpkin, winter squash, carrots, sweet potatoes, mangos, cantaloupes, peaches, and dark green leafy vegetables are great sources of carotenoids. Lycopene is found in tomatoes, watermelon, and red guavas. Consumption of these foods with meals is encouraged as they are much better absorbed in the presence of fat. This is another excuse to make mango, peach, and pumpkin frozen yogurt.

Vitamin D

Recommendation: Vitamin D levels should be assessed and treated when low. Vitamin D should be supplemented as a daily dose sufficient to maintain a serum level of 25-hydroxy-vitamin D (25-OHD3) at around *125 nmol/L.* For most adults, this requires a dose of about 125 μg (5000 IU) of vitamin D3 per day. Vitamin D supplements should be taken with a meal for better absorption. Since vitamin D is made in the skin during the day, the most natural time to take it is with lunch so that it aligns with daylight. Since it is a fat-soluble vitamin, it should be taken with a meal that contains at least some fat.

Not everyone responds to the same dose. Individuals with digestive issues may not absorb it well. Thus, some people will need higher or lower doses to maintain the target level of 25-OHD3. Vitamin D should be taken consistently so that levels can be monitored and then adjusted up or down after testing serum levels.

Vitamin D and Dementia

Vitamin D deficiency is common in the U.S., and especially in northern states during the winter months. Vitamin D is the sunshine vitamin; pre-vitamin D is formed in the skin as a result of UVB light from bright sunshine breaking a chemical bond in cholesterol within the skin. In the winter months, the sun is too low in the sky to effectively make vitamin D. People with darker skin make even less under moderate sunlight conditions. Many dark-skinned women avoid the sun to prevent tanning; thus, vitamin D inadequacy is common in women, even in tropical areas of the world. Many adults, especially in urban areas, work indoors and get little sunshine. Furthermore, as people age, there is a decline in the amount of pre-vitamin D produced in the skin as a result of sun exposure, putting older individuals at higher risk of vitamin D inadequacy.

Thus, most adults need to get vitamin D from food or supplements. Milk is fortified with vitamin D; it contains cholesterol and is irradiated with UV light to form vitamin D. Most adults don't tolerate much milk, and thus miss out on this source. Thus, vitamin D inadequacy and deficiency are common in the US, even in the southern states. I frequently made the diagnosis of osteomalacia in Black female patients when I worked in Tallahassee, Florida. These women are generally lactose intolerant and avoid basking in the sun.

Vitamin D is a hormone with receptors present in every living cell in the body. It participates in the regulation of at least 200 different genes. It plays an important role in regulating inflammation[29] and fighting infection.[30] Vitamin D inhibits TLR4 activation, for example, by bacterial LPS from the gut or the gingiva. Thus, as an example, vitamin D lowers the formation of prostaglandin E2 via PTGS2.[31] Vitamin D intake is associated with better sleep and better cognitive function in the elderly.[32] [33]

The overall prevalence of vitamin D deficiency in U.S. adults, according to a cross-sectional NHANES study, was 41.6%, with deficiency defined as a serum 25-hydroxyvitamin D concentration of less than 50 nmol/L. Deficient levels were present in 82.1 percent of Blacks and 69.2% of Hispanics.[34]

In a meta-analysis of 26 observational and three interventional studies, low vitamin D status was associated with a 26% increase in the risk of dementia. While supplements of 400 IU of vitamin D trended towards lowering dementia risk, it failed to be statistically significant.[35] In another meta-analysis, evaluating five studies, those with vitamin D deficiency (a 25-hydroxy-vitamin D3 (25-OHD3) level of less than 25 - 28 nmol/L) were 54% more likely to develop dementia than those with adequate vitamin D levels (50 to 159 nmol/L).[36]

More recently, a meta-analysis including nine studies found that vitamin D deficiency was associated with a 34% increase in the risk of cognitive impairment, a 42% increase in risk of dementia, and a 57% increase in risk of Alzheimer's Disease (AD). This study identified a deficiency as being a level of less than 40 nmol/L of 25-OHD3. In this study, levels of 77.5 to 100 nmol/L as considered to be optimal for reducing dementia risk.[37]

In a study of people from Great Britain, not only was there an increased risk of AD and all-cause dementia among those with low vitamin D levels, but those taking vitamin D supplements were at lower risk of AD and vascular dementia. Vitamin D insufficiency increased the risk of dementia by 25% for those with ApoE4 and by 19% for those without ApoE4. Serum 25-OHD3 levels over about 70 nmol/L were found to be protective.[38]

Thus, there is considerable evidence that vitamin D sufficiency prevents the development of AD and vascular dementia. Nevertheless, there is a clear lack of evidence that vitamin D supplementation improves cognition among those with dementia.[39] Thus, it should be considered to be preventative, but without the ability to restore lost cognitive function.

The mechanisms by which vitamin D protects the brain have not been established. No correlation between low vitamin D levels in various sections of the brain was found to be associated with any specific pathology. Serum vitamin D levels were, however, found to be associated with fewer chronic microinfarcts.[40] Although vitamin D is needed by the brain, its role in preventing dementia may be the result of it reducing blood platelet cell activation and suppressing platelet-mediated inflammation.[41] Vitamin D may prevent microinfarcts in the brain's vasculature and thus reduce any associated inflammatory impact. Bolstering this mechanistic hypothesis, oral anticoagulants lower the risk of dementia by about 30%.[42]

Optimal Vitamin D Levels

In a young person, one 15-minute-long exposure to the summer sun can cause the equivalent production of vitamin D to a dose of 10,000 IU (250 μg of vitamin D3). In a study of young people from Sao Paulo, Brazil, the summertime average 25-hydroxyvitamin D_3 (25(OH)D) levels for medical students and indoor workers were 103 nmol/L. These were medical students and indoor workers, not outdoor laborers or hunter-gatherers, as were our ancestors, who would have spent most of every day in the sun. Some of the participants, however, went to the beach as many as 5 days a week and spent over 30 minutes in the sun each occasion. A quarter of the participants of this study had levels above 124 nmol/liter, and the top 5 percent had levels over 165 nm/L. The highest 25(OH)D level in this group was 214 nmol/L.[43] Higher 25(OH)D levels were seen in those who frequented the beach.

People who work in the sun generally have high vitamin D levels: a study found that farmers in Puerto Rico had an average 25-OHD3 level of 135 nmol/L, and lifeguards had an average of 148 nmol/L in one study and 166 nmol/L in another.[44]

Non-pregnant women living in two different areas of Africa, who sustain a hunter-gatherer lifestyle, were tested for vitamin D3 levels. The average blood 25(OH)D3 levels were 118.3 nmol/L in one group and 89.0 nmol/L in the other. During pregnancy, the African women's average blood 25(OH)D3 levels were considerably higher, 147.7 and 141.9 nmol/L in the two different communities.[45] This provides an indication of ancestral vitamin D levels during human evolution and suggests that such levels are optimal for human health and that physiologic vitamin D levels are higher in health during pregnancy. Optimal conversion of

25(OH)D3 to the active hormone 1-25(OH)D3 in pregnant women occurs when 25(OH)D3 levels are at least 100 nmol/L.[46]

Another insight into the optimal vitamin D functional levels can be gained by examining the relationship of parathyroid hormone (PTH) with vitamin D. Vitamin D levels are inversely related to PTH levels. PTH raises calcium levels by increasing absorption of calcium from the intestine, increasing reuptake by the kidneys, and by liberating calcium from the bones. When serum calcium levels are low, PTH rises to maintain the narrow physiologic range of calcium required for normal cellular function.

One action of PTH is to induce the enzyme that converts 25-OHD to the active hormone 1,25OHD. 1,25OHD increases the production of the enterocyte calcium pump calbindin-D9k, which transports calcium from the intestinal lumen into the body. The portion of calcium absorbed by the intestine increases with serum 25OHD levels.[47] In an analysis of data from the 2003-2004 NHANES study, including over 8200 Americans, vitamin D levels were inversely associated with PTH levels, with no significance between genders. The average PTH for those with vitamin 25-OHD3 levels less than 40 nmol/L was 53.9 ng/L, for those with vitamin D3 levels 60 – 70, the average PTH level was 42.2 ng/L, and for those with vitamin D3 levels over 100 mmol/L, the average PTH was 31.2 ng/L. PTH levels were found to increase with aging across the lifespan, likely in part from PTH resistance. In a French study of elderly women, it was found that PTH levels fell with higher 25(OH)D3 levels, with a plateau when vitamin D levels were above about 80 nmol/L of 25(OH)D3. Thus, the body scavenges bone stores of calcium to maintain serum calcium if 25(OH)D3 levels are less than 80 nmol/L (32 ng/mL); this suggests that 25(OH)D3 levels less than 80 nmol/L should be considered deficient.[48]

Looking at various studies, the risk of multiple diseases declines as 25(OH)D3 levels rise above 75 nmol/L. Since few urbanites have 25(OH)D3 levels over 100 nmol/L without the use of supplements, there is limited data on a threshold beyond which higher vitamin D levels stop providing additional benefits.

Vitamin D status is also related to bone density. There were fewer fractures and fewer cases of colon cancer risk when vitamin D levels were at 115 nmol/L than at 90 nmol/L. In young Caucasian and Hispanic adults, bone mineral density (BMD) was highest when 25(OH)D3 levels were around 120 nmol/L, although BMD peaks in African Americans with vitamin D levels at about 90 nmol/L.[49] These and other data suggest optimal levels for 25(OH)D3 are around 90 – 120 nmol/l (36 – 48 ng/ml).[50] In a study of white American men aged 30 to 79, bone density was highest in men with 25(OH)D3 levels around 125 nmol/L (50 ng/ml).[51] While bone density was somewhat lower at higher vitamin D levels, this finding might have resulted from the use of vitamin D supplements among those at high risk of bone fracture.

Hypovitaminosis D is associated with insulin resistance. In a study of 126 Californian adults without diabetes, blood glucose levels were inversely related to 25(OH)D3 from low levels to the upper levels present among this population, about 100 nmol/L.[52] The relationship is also seen in children and adolescents.[53] Vitamin D_3 levels are thus associated with improving insulin sensitivity to at least 200 nmol/l. One pathway by which vitamin D prevents diabetes is through its activation of sphingosine kinase.[54] This enzyme lowers ceramide levels and increases S1P. Ceramide increases insulin resistance, decreases the production of insulin, and induces the apoptosis of pancreatic β-cells.[55] S1P inhibits β-cell apoptosis.[56]

Another measure of vitamin D adequacy is to look at muscular activity. Muscular contraction relies on calcium influx into the muscle cells. Several studies have found that vitamin D supplementation decreases falls among the elderly by about 20 percent.[57] In a study of over 4000 Americans over 60 years of age, the time to walk 8 feet was inversely related to 25OHD levels, with a trend to shorter times continuing with 25(OH)D3 levels between 100 and 220 nmol/L.[58] A test of time required to stand up from a sitting position was also performed. In this test, time to stand was also inversely related to 25(OH)D3 levels, but the lowest times were associated with a 25(OH)D3 level around 125 nmol/L, after which times began to increase. The authors pointed out, however, that these higher 25(OH)D3 levels were associated with supplements given to patients with osteoporosis, and thus, the slowing in standing times may have been the result of pre-existing disease rather than from higher vitamin D levels.

In adult men and women, 25(OH)D3 levels below 60 nmol/L were associated with lower blood hemoglobin (Hgb) levels, and peak Hgb levels in men were associated with vitamin D levels between 95 to 125 nmol/L in men. In women, Hgb appeared to continue to rise in association with 25(OH)D3 levels up to 200 nmol/L; however, the number of women with vitamin D levels over 130 nmol/L was small. The RDW% is a measure of the variation in red blood cell volumes and reflects how evenly the red blood cells age and are removed from the bloodstream. A narrower dispersion (a lower score) is favorable. The RDW% increases with aging in adults, and was found to be inversely associated with vitamin D3 levels in the NHANES study, with lower RDW% levels for those with higher 25(OH)D3 levels. Vitamin D3 levels below 75 mmol/L were associated with higher RDW% levels, and even lower values were found for those with vitamin D levels above 100 mmol/L.[59] Thus, vitamin D levels above 95 nmol/L of 25(OH)D3 appear to be consistent with optimal hematopoietic health. This data suggests that optimal 25(OH)D3 levels for health require levels of 100 to 125 nmol/L.

About 100 μg (4000 IU) of vitamin D supplementation daily was needed to maintain vitamin D levels in men living in Omaha, a mid-latitude city in the United States, during the winter months.[60] To maintain a 25(OH)D3 level above 100 nmol/L (≥40 ng/dL), most pregnant women need to supplement with at least 100 μg (4000 IU) of vitamin D per day. Dark-skinned women are at higher risk of vitamin D deficiency, as the melanin in the skin impedes penetration of the UVB light needed to form vitamin D in the skin. Also, dark-skinned women from many cultures avoid the sun to avoid tanning.

There have been several studies that assess the impact of vitamin D supplementation on cognition in the elderly. In some studies, there was improvement seen in some studies but none was found in others. Most of the studies used low doses of vitamin D (600 to 800 IU) rather than optimizing blood levels of vitamin D.[61]

In a study of older persons, those with higher vitamin D levels were 25 to 33% less likely to develop MCI or dementia.[62] In another study of about 2500 older Americans that participated in the NHANES studies from 2011 -2014, both vitamin D intake and serum 25(OH)D3 levels were assessed, and the participants were tested for dementia or brain injury using two cognitive tests: *The Animal Fluency test (AF)* and the *Digit Symbol Substitution Test (DSST)*. In the AF, the subject is asked to name as many animals as possible in 60 seconds. It tests categorical verbal fluency and executive function and is considered to discriminate between normal individuals and those with early dementia. The DSST asks the subject to copy 133 symbol codes for numbers into numbered boxes in 120 seconds. The DSST assesses processing speed and sustained attention.

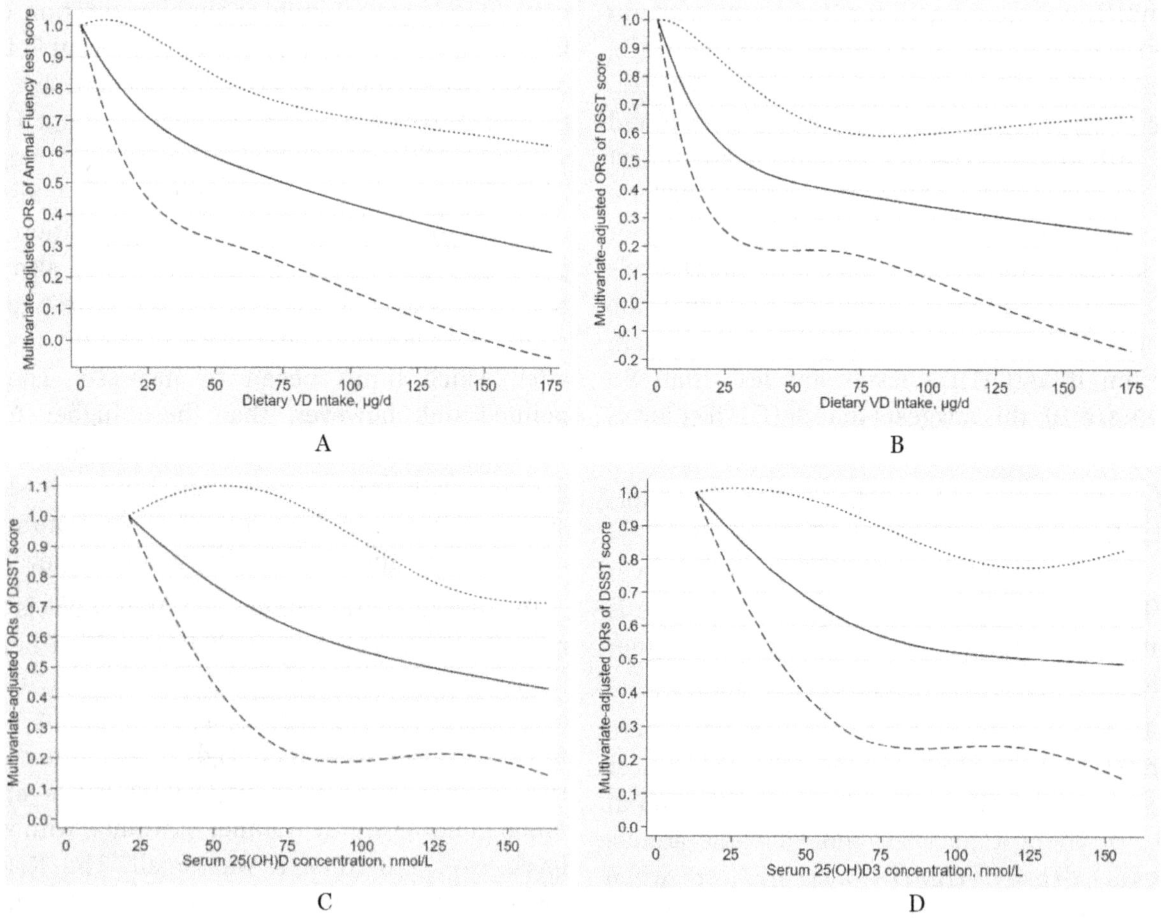

Figure 25A: Vitamin D and dementia risk. A) Animal fluency. B) DSST score for and vitamin D intake. C) Animal fluency D) DSST score for serum 25(OH)D3 level. Image from RuTong Wang et al. PMCID: PMC8467888

In a study that looked at the dose response for both reported vitamin D intake and serum 25(OH)D3 levels, lower cognitive impairment scores were associated with higher vitamin D intake and serum levels. When tested for dementia, higher levels of vitamin D intake and vitamin D blood levels were associated with a lower risk of test scores consistent with brain damage or dementia. Of note, the higher the vitamin D intake and the higher the blood levels, the lower the risk of having a score that was diagnostic of cognitive impairment. While much of the risk reduction was associated with intake of 50 mcg of vitamin D3 a day (2000 IU), further risk reduction was seen for those taking up to 175 mcg (7000 IU) of vitamin D3. Similarly, most of the risk reduction for low scores on the AF and TSST was associated with serum 25(OH)D3 levels above 100 nmol/L (≥40 ng/dL); nonetheless, there may be further risk reduction of low AF scores with 25OHD levels of 150 nmol/L, as shown in Figure 25A.[63] This data suggests that serum vitamin D levels, as measured as 25(OH)D3, should be maintained at a level of at least 100 nmol/L.

While important for maintaining overall health, immune function, bone health, muscle strength, and the prevention of diabetes, it is unlikely that vitamin D can reverse cognitive decline.

Target Dosing for Vitamin D

A reasonable *target* level for serum 25(OH)D3 is 125 nmol/L. It is a level safe from toxicity. Additionally, it gives a large margin for variation within a healthy range. Target levels should be high enough that few in the population have levels associated with risk. Taking sufficient vitamin D supplements to achieve a 25(OH)D3 target level of 125 nmol/L would place most people's 25(OH)D3 level between 100 and 150 nmol/L.

One thousand IU of vitamin D3 (25 mcg) taken daily, on average, raises the 25(OH)D3 level in healthy adults by 17.5 nmol/L (7 ng/mL) at equilibrium.[64] [65] Thus, if an individual's 25(OH)D3 level is 60 nmol/L without supplements, 1000 IU daily would raise the level to 77.5 nmol/L at equilibrium, after about six weeks. Thus, for someone with a background level of 40 nmol/L, it would take 4857 IU a day to achieve a steady state level of 125 nmol/L.

- 25 mcg of vitamin D3 raises 25(OH)D3 levels by 17.5 nmol/L
- (125 nmol/L - Current level in nmol/L) / 17.5 x 1000 IU
- (125 – 40 nmol/L) / 17.5 x 1000 = 4857 or about 5000 IU per day

For an adult not getting sun exposure and getting minimal amounts in the diet, it would take nearly 6000 IU a day (150 mg) to maintain a vitamin D level over 100 nmol/L. Supplementation is especially important for dark-skinned women, and especially for those living further from the equator in the winter months.

Homocysteine

Homocysteine (HCY) is a metabolic intermediary in a metabolic cycle that adds a methyl group to various compounds, an important metabolic function. HCY is recycled into the amino acid methionine, which can then act as a methyl donor again. If the recycling process lags, HCY levels can rise in the body; HCY is a direct and perhaps indirect indicator of vascular and neurodegenerative disease risk. Elevated serum HCY levels are a risk factor for AD and dementia. HCY may cause synaptic dysfunction as an excitotoxin, causing oxidative stress and inflammation, promoting neuronal cell death.[66] HCY also causes endothelial injury, which can initiate atherosclerosis.[67] Elevated HCY causes injury to the small blood vessels of the brain, and this is thought to be the mechanism by which it promotes Alzheimer's disease.[68]

In a study of middle-aged women aged 56 – 67, those with elevated HCY levels already had signs of cognitive decline. HCY over 13 µmol/l was significantly associated with poor verbal and working memory tests.[69] In a 22-year follow-up study, women whose HCY levels were in the upper third of those tested during mid-life were 70% more likely to develop dementia and more than twice as likely to develop AD.[70] These studies reinforce the need to use interventions early, and not wait for a diagnosis of mild cognitive impairment to use preventative interventions.

The principal pathway for recycling HCY requires 5-MTHF (5-methyltetrahydrofolate), the active form of vitamin B9 and vitamin B12. (Figure 25C). A deficiency of either of these vitamins is associated with elevated HCY levels and thus, increased risk of dementia. HCY is also metabolized into cysteine, using pyridoxal L-phosphate, the active form of vitamin B6, as an enzymatic cofactor.

In a study of Hispanics in California, elevated HCY levels were associated with a 2.4 times higher hazard of cognitive impairment or dementia, and those with lower levels of vitamin B12 were at a 61% increased risk.[71] In an Italian population of dementia-free, elderly individuals, those with HCY levels over 15 µmol/l were more than twice as likely to develop AD, and having low folate levels (≤11.8 nmol/L) was associated with a 98% increased hazard of developing AD.[72]

The risk of dementia from elevated HCY may be most clearly illustrated by a study from Japan. As with other studies, HCY levels above 13 – 15 µmol/l are associated with a doubling of risk of both AD and vascular dementia, but the lowest risk is for those with levels between 5 and 8 µmol/l. Note also that levels below 5 µmol/l suggest that very low levels may also convey risk. [73] At least one other study has found that very low HCY levels may increase dementia risk.

Elevated HCY levels can be treated with folate. [74] Elevated HCY may respond to vitamin B12 for those deficient in the vitamin. Vitamin B6 inadequacy can help those with inadequate levels, but this is far less common. Treatment should be based upon blood testing of HCY and retesting of HCY, folate, and vitamin B12 adequacy to assure that proper doses are used.

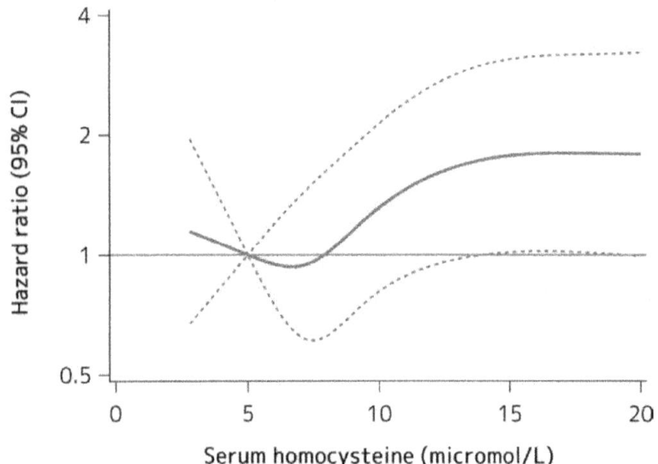

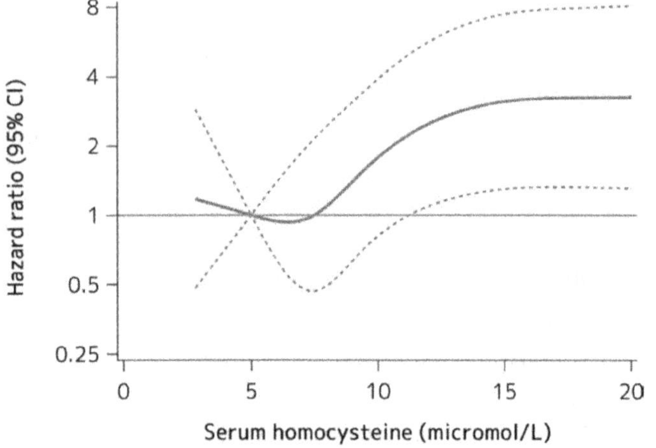

Figure 25A and 25B: Serum Homocysteine and Dementia Risk, 25A: Alzheimer's risk, 25B: Vascular dementia risk. Risk is lowest when serum HCY levels are between 5 and 8 mmol/L. S. Chen et al. PMCID: PMC7231445

Folate

The principal determinant of HCY levels is folate adequacy. Assessment of data from the NHANES study found that those with lower dietary intake of folate had higher odds of scoring poorly on cognitive tests, as compared to those with a higher folate intake. The risk of testing poorly was lowest with a daily folate intake of about 600 mcg of folate per day.[75]

There are several forms of folate; tetrahydrofolate (THF) is the one found in fruits and vegetables. Folic acid is a shelf-stable form that is used to fortify processed foods. Folic acid is a synthetic form of folate that requires enzymatic reduction to form THF. Unfortunately, about 10 percent of the population does not process folate well. L-5-MTHF is the active form of folate and is available as a nutritional supplement, often labelled as metafolin or levomefolic acid.

In meta-analysis, folate supplementation lowers HCY levels in those with mild cognitive impairment (MCI), AD, and vascular dementia (VD), but folate treatment only improved cognition in those with MCI.[76] Another meta-analysis found an improvement in memory but not in cognition or executive function with folate treatment in MCI, but no improvement for those with AD.[77] Another meta-analysis looked specifically at the combination of folate with vitamin B12 supplementation. They found an improvement in Mini-Mental State Examination (MMSE) scores, but no change in the Alzheimer's Disease Assessment Scale-Cognitive Subscale (ADAS-Cog) or measures of daily functioning.[78] A few isolated studies have shown improvement in cognitive testing, especially with the combination of folate with docosahexaenoic acid (DHA).[79]

Nevertheless, currently, the ability of nutritional supplements or medications to reverse dementia is at best minimal. The ability of the brain to form new neurons is limited, and the success is even more curtailed in those who already have dementia and the inflammatory processes that drive it. Folate appears to have the capacity to act as a preventative intervention, but not as a treatment for damage that has already occurred.

Folate Supplementation: Getting adequate folate in the diet is essential for everyone, and most people will get sufficient folate if they consume a whole foods diet rich in fruits and green vegetables. Those with compromised folate metabolism and high HCY levels can benefit from supplementation with the active form of folate, metafolin (5-MTHF). A dose of around 600 - 700 mcg per day of 5-MTHF is recommended for adults with elevated HCY levels. Treatment with vitamin B12, vitamin B6, and choline should also be considered, especially if HCY levels do not respond to folate. Supplementation with the folic acid form of the vitamin as they are associated with an increased risk of cancer. High levels of folate appear to promote cognitive decline in individuals deficient in vitamin B12.[80] Before supplementation with folate, both serum folate and vitamin B12 levels should be tested.

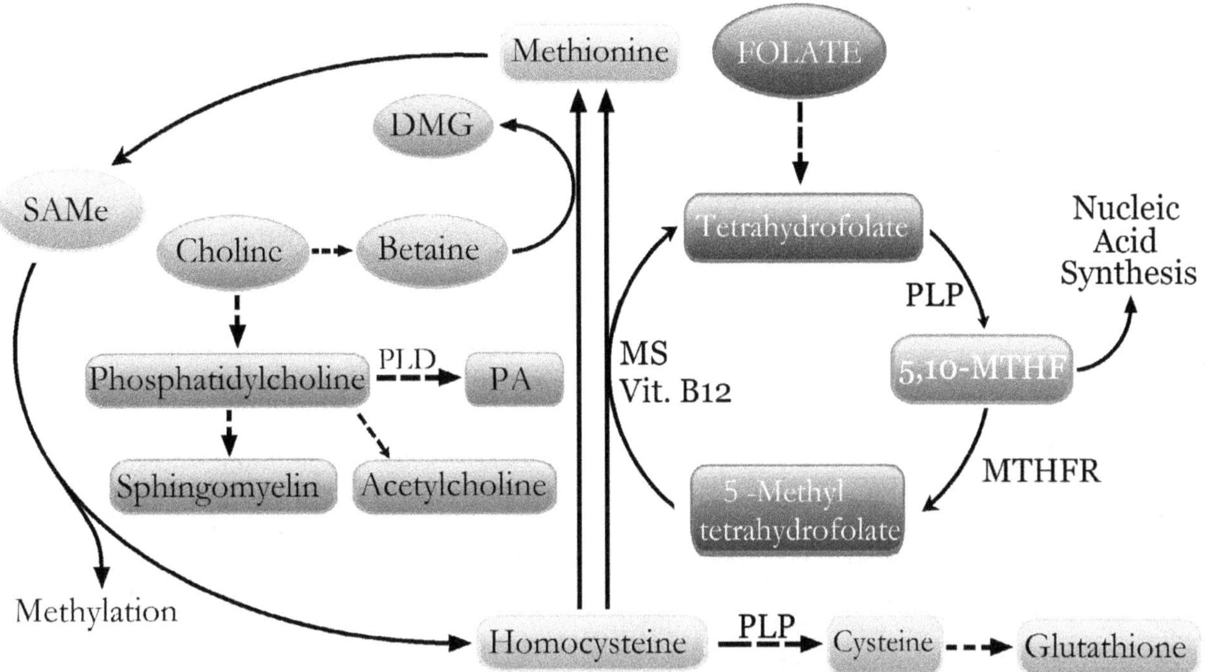

Figure 25C: The methionine cycle. The methionine → SAMe → HCY → methionine cycle principally uses the 5-HTHF form of vitamin B9 and vitamin B12, but can alternatively use betaine (trimethylglycine). PLP: Pyridoxal L-phosphate, vitamin B6. (Right side) In the major pathway, dietary folate is converted to tetrahydrofolate and then 5MTHF, which transfers a methyl group onto HCY to form methionine. Methionine is then converted to S-Adenosylmethionine, which is the methyl donor. HCY can also be recycled into methionine in a more "costly" pathway using choline or betaine (dimethylglycine), donating the methyl group, and converting betaine to dimethylglycine. HCY is also used to form the antioxidant compound glutathione. At least 10% of the population has difficulty converting folic acid into 5-MTHF. Thus, screening for this is important for the prevention of dementia and vascular disease.

Vitamin B6

An extensive meta-analysis assessed the impact of 162 biomarkers in 110 studies for their association with mental disorders. Only a few markers provided convincing evidence of a pathological association with any of the mental diseases studied.[81] Among the few convincing associations, a strong correlation was found for low plasma vitamin B_6 levels among persons with schizophrenia.[82] The study failed to find any association with the most common single-nucleotide variant alteration in vitamin B_6 levels. Thus, the association with low pyridoxal-L-5-phosphate (PLP, P5P, vitamin B_6) levels with schizophrenia is unlikely to have a genetic basis.

Dietary vitamin B6 deficiency is uncommon, as pyridoxine is abundant in a wide variety of foods and is also produced by the enteric bacteria in the large intestine. Nevertheless, 19–27% of the US population has inadequate PLP plasma levels. The reason for this is that PLP becomes sequestered in the tissue during inflammation. PLP is a cofactor in numerous enzymes, including the metabolism of sphingosine 1-phosphate (S1P),[83] kynurenine,[84] and homocysteine, and thus PLP has an important role in inflammation and immunomodulation.[85] Kynurenine dysregulation appears to be common among those with schizophrenia,[86] [87] and its dysregulation is also implicated in AD and other neurodegenerative diseases. PLP is one of the few supplements that appear to help children with autism.

Given its central role in the methionine cycle and in the kynurenine pathway, PLP supplementation seems an obvious low-risk intervention. One cannot assume that a diet with the RDA of PLP will suffice for those with inflammatory conditions. Low PLP levels likely indicate that inflammation is part of the causal pathway, likely as a result of the underlying pathology, but perhaps also contributing to disease progression.

Vitamin B6 Supplementation: Pyridoxal-L-5-phosphate is the active form of vitamin B6. The RDA for vitamin B6 for adults over the age of 51 is 1.7 mg for men and 1.5 mg for women. Large doses can cause sensory neuropathy. A reasonable dose of vitamin B6 as PLP or in one of its other forms may be helpful for those facing AD, PD, schizophrenia, or other neurodegenerative diseases. It is likely to be helpful in other inflammatory diseases, such as IBD, as well. The SANA program recommends 2 to 5 mg of vitamin B6 daily, preferably in the form of PLP, with a limit of no more than 7 mg per day. The underlying cause of inflammation should be addressed. The SAD/Western diet is proinflammatory and should be avoided.

Vitamin B12

With age, vitamin B12 absorption commonly declines, and supplementation is beneficial for most adults by the time they reach retirement age. Although the requirement for vitamin B12 is tiny, a few micrograms per day, vitamin B12 absorption is low, about 1%, thus a dose of 500 to 1000 mcg is usually needed in older adults. Chewable tablets work well for most people; as mentioned previously, saliva contains the protein haptocorrin, which protects the vitamin from degradation by stomach acid. Thus, the tablet needs to be chewed or allowed to dissolve in the mouth to mix it with saliva to be most effective.

Supplementation: While 50 to 100 mcg of vitamin B12 per day (350 to 700 mcg per week) may be sufficient for younger healthy vegans,[88] for older adults, 500 to 1000 micrograms (mcg) per day may be required to maintain sufficient levels; thus, 1000 mcg will cover the need for most older adults.[89] Cyanocobalamin as a chewable tablet is the recommended form for vitamin B12 supplementation.

Vitamin B12 has a wide therapeutic index and is without toxicity when used in reasonable dosages.[90] Thus, there is no appreciable risk of overdose when used at recommended dosages. Pernicious anemia, Sjögren's disease[91] (autoimmune disorders), and other conditions such as small intestinal bacterial overgrowth, celiac disease, and Whipple disease that cause vitamin B12 deficiency should be managed by a medical doctor. Other than in these situations, oral cyanocobalamin is almost always sufficient for age-related decline in vitamin B12 absorption as well as for younger individuals on a low cobalamin diet, such as a vegan diet.

Testing of vitamin B12 levels is recommended for those at risk. (The elderly, those with anemia, family history of dementia, high homocysteine levels, ApoE4, etc.). Testing is not straightforward. Most of the vitamin B12 in the blood is not available to the cells; only that which is bound to the protein transcobalamin. Thus, testing for total vitamin B12 (cobalamin) gives an unreliable picture as to whether levels are adequate or not. The available vitamin B12 can be measured by testing for holotranscobalamin (holoTC). The normal reference value for holoTC is 40 to 200 pmol/l.[92] Functional (surrogate) testing is perhaps better and more inclusive. Testing for homocysteine is not specific for cobalamin inadequacy, but if it is elevated, then the cause can be traced. Methylmalonic acid (MMA) is an intermediary byproduct of metabolism that relies on adenosylcobalamin for its conversion to succinate. If vitamin B12 levels are insufficient, blood levels of MMA rise, and thus indicate vitamin B12 deficiency. Normal methylmalonic acid levels are less than 0.40 µmol/mL. MMA levels can rise due to a decline in renal function even when vitamin B12 levels are adequate; thus, MMA testing may be unreliable in this situation. Fasting urine MMA testing may be more accurate, with urinary methylmalonic acid levels greater than 1.45 µM/mM of creatinine being considered elevated.[93]

Choline

It is stated above that most Americans consume less than the daily Adequate Intake (AI) of choline. This was a bit of an understatement. It is reported that 90% of American adults consume less than the AI for choline (7 mg/kg), including most pregnant and lactating women, which is highly concerning given the crucial role of choline in brain development during fetal life and infancy.

While severe choline deficiency can cause muscle and liver damage, including nonalcoholic fatty liver disease, less severe deficits can cause mood disorders. Adults whose choline levels are inadequate are at elevated risk of suffering from anxiety and depression. In a population study of middle-aged and older adults, only about one in four of the subjects had choline levels associated with a *low risk* of anxiety and depression (>11 μmol/l).[94] In older adults aged 70 to 74, normal blood choline levels were associated with better cognitive function, but poorer function for those with levels below about 10 μmol/l. Cognitive function was also poorer among those with low vitamin B12 status.[95] In a 22-year follow-up study of over 1800 Chinese adults aged 55 to 79, those with a higher intake of choline had less cognitive decline. It is noteworthy that the average dietary choline intake at baseline was only 161 mg/day.[96] The AI for choline for a 70 kg man is 490 mg/day.

Note: Population studies of optimal choline intake can easily be confounded, as the foods highest in choline include red meat, poultry, eggs, and fish. Red meat may, for example, increase the risk of metabolic syndrome, a risk factor for dementia. Fish, being high in n-3 fats, may lower the risk of dementia for other reasons. At the same time, vegans and vegetarians, although having lower intakes of choline, generally have a lower risk of metabolic syndrome and microvascular disease, and thus a lower risk of dementia, despite having inadequate intake of choline. This complicates population studies of the impact of choline in the diet on neurologic health and in determining optimal levels.

Choline is needed for making cell membranes, for sphingomyelin to wrap the nerves, and for the neurotransmitter acetylcholine. As shown in Figure 25C above, choline is also used to recycle HCY into methionine. Individuals with genetic variations in folate metabolism or folate or vitamin B12 inadequacies thus require more choline. Betaine can also spare choline.[97]

Oil and water do not mix. Thus, lipids such as cholesterol and triglycerides are transported in the blood within microscopic packets. Apoproteins (A, B, and E) assist in transporting cholesterol and other lipids throughout the body. They help organize the packet and serve as an address label.

ApoA is associated with HDL-cholesterol and transport of lipids from the periphery, for example, from the arteries to the liver for recycling. ApoB is associated with LDL-cholesterol. It carries dietary lipids from the liver to other organs. If ApoB is not cleared quickly enough, blood levels rise; elevated blood levels of ApoB are associated with an increased risk of atherosclerotic disease, as the particles get stuck in the walls of the blood vessels and cause inflammation and injury. ApoB is discussed in Chapter 15.

ApoE also carries lipids throughout the body, but has a particularly important role in the transport of lipids within and out of the brain. The most common strong genetic risk factor for AD is ApoE4. There are three common genetic variations of ApoE in the population (ApoE2, ApoE3, and ApoE4), and each person gets one copy from each parent. ApoE2 is the least common but the most active. ApoE3 is the most common and is thus considered the reference type. ApoE4 is fairly common, but does not function as well as the other types, and carries a strong risk for AD. Since we get a copy from each parent, the three most common combinations are: ApoE3:ApoE3 medium AD risk, ApoE3:ApoE4 moderate AD risk, or ApoE4:ApoE4 high AD risk.

ApoE4 does not transport lipids as efficiently, and those with this genotype also make less of it. Thus, brain cells of those with the ApoE4 genotype are thought to be at high risk of being overburdened with triglycerides.[98]

I propose that, similar to hepatosteatosis in the liver and myosteatosis in muscles, brain cells can become obese, get overloaded with triglycerides, and develop what I will dub what I will call "neuronosteatosis". This neuronosteatosis causes mitochondrial dysfunction and injury to the cells of the brain, which can lead to ATP starvation, injury, and cell death of neurons. Chubby astrocytes may also impede glymphatic flow during sleep.

Choline can be transformed into phospholipids by the brain. Even though the brain has difficulty getting rid of excess triglycerides because of defective ApoE, it can still convert the fat into phospholipids, which the cells can get rid of using exocytosis, as long as they have access to sufficient choline. Thus, adequate choline may help prevent ApoE4-induced brain injury.

Vegetarians typically consume less than half of the AI for choline, and vegans even smaller amounts. Endogenous choline production is boosted by estrogen; thus, postmenopausal women are at higher risk of choline inadequacy as compared to younger women.[99]

In a study of non-demented adults, those in the top quartile for choline consumption (greater than 382 mg/day) had better verbal and visual immediate and delayed memory scores on testing than those with lower choline intake.[100] In a 12-week double-blinded clinical trial of elderly patients without dementia but with mild memory difficulties, supplementation with 300 mg of choline from egg yolks improved memory and processing speed. Egg yolk contains both choline as phosphatidylcholine (PC), lysophosphatidylcholine (LPC), and α-glycerophosphocholine (α-GPC). PC is converted to LPC by pancreatic phospholipase A2 in the small intestine. LPC and α-GPC are absorbed and transported to the liver. The liver then releases free choline into the bloodstream.[101] α-GPC is water-soluble and easily absorbed.

Choline in foods: Eggs are very high in choline. Two large eggs contain 294 mg of choline. A 100 g serving of salmon has 95 mg. Tofu contains about one mg of choline for every gram, so a 100-gram serving contains 100 mg. An 8-oz. cup of soy milk contains 56 mg of choline. Legumes, potatoes, quinoa, and broccoli contain considerable amounts. Dairy milk contains about 10 – 15 mg of choline per cup, and hard cheese, such as cheddar, contains about 15 – 20 mg per ounce.

Warning: At high dose levels, choline and betaine may be only partially absorbed. The remainder will pass to the colon. Within several days of taking large amounts or in those whose microbiome has already adapted, the choline and betaine will be fermented into TMA, which is absorbed and converted to TMAO in the liver. TMAO is discussed in the chapter on meat (two), as it is a possible risk factor for vascular disease. Thus, large supplemental doses of choline or betaine are discouraged, and forms that have high bioavailability are preferred.

Supplementation: Choline supplementation is recommended for those consuming a diet that does not supply adequate choline. It is especially recommended for those at high risk of AD as a result of having an ApoE4 allele or being at risk of vascular dementias.

α-Glycerophosphocholine (α-GPC) is the form of choline recommended herein, at a dose of 275 to 300 mg daily to supplement that in the diet (equivalent to consuming 2 large eggs). The supplements should be taken with a meal. To have full benefit, especially for those at high risk, adequate folate and vitamin B12 status should be confirmed with blood tests. Optimal free choline levels are likely around 12 μmol/l.

Other Vitamins

Thiamine (Vitamin B1): In a cross-sectional study of over 2400 Americans over the age of 60, higher dietary intake of vitamin B1 (Thiamine) was associated with higher scores on processing speed and executive function tests. Those with daily thiamine intakes in the lowest quartile, less than 0.97 mg/day, scored more poorly. In one set of cognitive tests specifically for Alzheimer's disease, those with dietary thiamine intake levels between 1.34 and 1.82 mg/day had the best scores, while higher intake was not helpful.[102] Another assessment of the same data found an L-shaped curve with lower cognitive scores associated with thiamine levels below about 1.16 mg/day, and little benefit from additional levels.[103] A Chinese study found a more rapid decline in cognitive function over a 5-year follow-up among elderly individuals with *higher* thiamine intake; that is, levels over 1 mg per day, with the slowest decline for those consuming between 0.6 and 1.0 mg/day and a nadir at 0.68 mg per day.[104] A review of the literature concluded that thiamine likely had little direct impact, but that adequate levels were associated with overall good nutrition, and that this overall good nutrition was associated with slower cognitive decline;[105] a sensible assessment. Higher intake may be associated with supplements that provide little benefit. Benfotiamine, a synthetic form of vitamin B1, is discussed below.

Riboflavin (Vitamin B2): In the NHANES data, vitamin B2 (riboflavin) intake less than the recommended daily allowance was associated with poorer scores on the AF, TSST, and the Immediate Recall Test (IRT).[106] I suspect that vitamin B2 in this situation acts as a proxy for an overall poor or restricted diet, alcohol abuse, or disease state, rather than a specific nutrient deficit, as riboflavin deficiency is rare and usually accompanied by other nutrient deficiencies.

Nevertheless, vegans may be deficient in riboflavin intake, as can vegetarians who avoid dairy products, especially when engaging in athletic activities.[107] Adults at risk should supplement with 1.5 to 2 mg of riboflavin a day.

Vitamin C: Vitamin C is an important antioxidant. Deficiency states are associated with depression and cognitive impairment.[108] There is some evidence that vitamin C supplementation may be helpful in subclinical depression.[109] A German study found that patients with mild cognitive impairment (MCI) had lower blood levels of vitamin C and β-carotene than did age matched controls, while no differences were found for blood levels of vitamin E, lycopene or coenzyme Q.[110] There is no reason to expect that supplementation of vitamin C (or β-carotene) can treat or prevent dementia as long as there is not a deficiency of these micronutrients.[111]

Maintaining a healthy and balanced diet is more effective in preventing dementia than supplementing these individual micronutrients. While vitamin C supplementation should not be needed on a healthy diet, Vitamin C may be used as a supplement within the SANA program. Vitamin C supplements may be used, especially during seasons when fruit is less available.

Overall mortality is lowest when daily vitamin C intake is between 100 to 175 mg per day,[112] with higher intake levels decreasing the benefits. Thus, vitamin C appears to have a U-shaped dose-benefit curve. Additionally, only about 60 mg of vitamin C can be absorbed from a meal. Large doses of vitamin C can cause rapid intestinal transit, dysbiosis, cramping, gas, and diarrhea. Thus, there is little, if any, benefit and potential harm from doses over 200 mg.

If vitamin C is used as a supplement, it is recommended that it be at a dose of about 75 mg, be taken with a meal, and preferably be supplemented in the form of ascorbyl palmitate. If the supplement is the only source of vitamin C, this dose can be taken at two different meals during the day.

Vitamin E: It is not that vitamin E does not play a role in the prevention of dementia and other diseases of aging, but rather that α-tocopherol, the most commonly used vitaminer E, is the wrong one and that it lowers the blood levels of other types of vitamin E. In a Finnish 8-year follow-up study of elderly individuals, serum γ-tocopherol, β-tocotrienol, and total tocotrienols were inversely associated with the risk of cognitive impairment.[113] Since these other forms of vitamin E are rarely taken as supplements and are associated with the consumption of whole grains and nuts, and other whole foods, the association with lower risk of cognitive impairment may reflect an overall healthier diet that includes these foods. There is no decrease in all-cause mortality for dietary vitamin E intake beyond 12 mg (18 IU) per day.[114] The use of α-tocopherol as a supplement is discouraged. It is better to get a mix of vitaminers E from a healthy diet.

Vitamin K. An analysis of dietary recall data from the 2011 to 2014 NHANES study found that dietary intake of vitamin K from vegetables (vitamin K1, phylloquinone) was inversely associated with poor cognitive performance in three cognitive domains. Dietary intake of less than around 200 mcg of vitamin K from vegetables was associated with poorer cognitive scores.[115] Vitamin K modulates the metabolism of sphingolipids that myelinate the axons of the nerves and promote neuronal survival.[116] While a plausible protective compound, this analysis fails to separate the impact of vitamin K1 from other compounds in green vegetables. The SANA program does not recommend supplementation with vitamin K1 as a preventive against cognitive decline, but rather encourages a varied plant-based diet.

Other Micronutrients

Taurine, carnitine, and creatine are briefly discussed in Chapter 9 on Protein Requirements, as levels of these compounds may be low in vegans who are not getting sufficient dietary protein. They are mentioned because of the risk of low levels of these important nutrients in the diets of vegans.

Carnitine: Carnitine and creatine are important for energy utilization and the formation of ATP when fatty acids are the fuel source. The neurons' preferred energy source is lactate, which is provided to them by astrocytes in the brain. The astrocyte's preferred fuel is glucose, but they can convert fatty acids into acetate, then to pyruvate, and finally into lactate. This requires adequate carnitine. In theory, carnitine would be especially important for the prevention of AD in those with "neuronosteatosis" and ApoE4, as explained above.

Taurine is a semi-essential amino acid that is critical for the formation of new brain cells and for synapse development.[117] Taurine may protect the brain from excitotoxicity, stress, and ischemic events. It may help downregulate activated microglia and thus help quell their inflammatory activity in the brain. While some studies suggest that higher taurine levels are associated with lower AD hazard and better cognitive scores, other studies do not find differences in brain taurine levels between those with and without AD or dementia.[118] One study found that higher taurine levels in the spinal cerebral fluid were inversely associated with depression and behavioral disturbances, while glutamate was negatively correlated with agitated verbal behavior.[119]

Taurine is an important nutrient for brain health (as well as for metabolic function), and deficiencies should be avoided. Taurine can be synthesized in the body from cysteine, but that can deplete cysteine for its other roles. Vegans need to consume foods high in cysteine, such as legumes, or find other ways to ensure adequate taurine.

Zinc: Zinc is necessary for the expression of the tight junction proteins ZO-1 and occludin.[120] A balanced, healthy diet should provide adequate zinc; however, many low-quality diets do not, and low zinc levels are not uncommon. Zinc supplementation can be helpful in those who have inadequate zinc levels.

Dietary zinc intake has been found to have a narrow, U-shaped correlation with the new onset of diabetes. There was a greater than 50% higher risk for new onset of diabetes among those with total dietary intakes of less than 7.5 mg of zinc per day, and a similar risk for those consuming 13 mg per day, and a doubling of risk for those consuming 17 mg per day. The nadir or risk was for those consuming 10 mg of zinc per day.[121] In a 5.9-year follow-up study of older Chinese adults, those consuming less than 7.9 mg of zinc per day had a more rapid cognitive decline. The inflection point of the L-shaped curve was 8.8 mg per day.[122] Any zinc supplementation should be approached cautiously. If a zinc supplement is used to make up a dietary shortfall, the dose should be about 5 – 7.5 mg per day. Zinc citrate is the recommended supplemental form.

Magnesium: Americans tend not to get sufficient magnesium in their diets. The RDI for magnesium is 400 – 420 mg for younger and older men and 310 – 320 mg for women. The NHANES 2003-2006 nutrition survey found that the average adult consumed 278 mg of Mg per day, and that about half the population was getting insufficient levels in their diets.

Magnesium (Mg) is present in every molecule of chlorophyll, and thus green leafy vegetables such as spinach are good sources of Mg. Dark chocolate is another source of Mg. Nine grams of cocoa, one chocolate equivalent, contains 45 mg of magnesium. Legumes are an excellent source. A 100-gram serving of broccoli contains 21 mg of Mg. A one-cup serving of brown rice contains 86 mg. Nuts, avocados, and bananas are other good sources.

There is a long list of medical conditions that respond to the correction of magnesium deficits. Mg treatment may be helpful for migraine headaches, neuropathic pain, post-operative pain, neonatal neuroprotection, hypertension, endothelial dysfunction, and atherosclerosis. Mg deficits are associated with diabetes, osteoporosis, and sarcopenia.[123]

Mg supplementation is complicated. There are at least a dozen different magnesium salts that are used as supplements. Several of them are poorly absorbed. Only about 4% of the Mg from magnesium oxide is absorbed, and this contributes to its laxative effect. Magnesium carbonate and sulfate also have very low absorption rates. Somewhat better are Mg chloride and citrate. Mg citrate at higher doses is used as a laxative. Mg lactate, Mg gluconate, and Mg malate are considered to have good absorption. Mg glycinate (a.k.a. bisglycinate), orotate, and threonate are considered to have very good absorption. If using a Mg supplement as a nutritional supplement (rather than as a laxative), these are preferred. With higher absorption, smaller doses are required, and gastrointestinal side effects should be minimized.

At the same time, these well-absorbed magnesium salts have larger molecules and thus require a larger mass of the compound to get a dose. Magnesium ions are Mg^{2+}, and thus bind to two anions. Mg oxide has one oxygen (O^{-2}) and has a molecular mass of 40.3, while Mg orotate has two orotate($^{-1}$) molecules and has a molecular mass of 334.4. For a 100 mg supplement of *elemental* magnesium, 166 mg of Mg oxide or 1376 mg of Mg Orotate are needed. Mg threonate would require 1212 mg, Mg citrate 882 mg, and Mg glycinate 709 mg for a 100 mg dose of elemental Mg.

There is a dizzying array of products that claim their Mg supplement is best for the treatment of various conditions. For example, Mg glycinate is often claimed to help with sleep, Mg-L-threonate with dementia prevention, and Mg-orotate to help with cardiac health. When absorbed from the intestinal lumen, the magnesium ion (Mg^{2+}) dissociates from the anionic compound and enters the systemic pool and behaves like magnesium from any other source. The anion is also absorbed and may be used by the body. Malate and citrate can be used for energy in the citric acid cycle. The amino acid glycine can also be used for energy.

Orotate (a.k.a. orotic acid) helps increase the uptake of Mg into cells, particularly those with high energy demand, such as the heart and skeletal muscles. Orotate is an intermediate in the synthesis of cytosine, guanine, and uracil and thus an essential metabolite in DNA and RNA synthesis. Orotic acid was once known as vitamin B13, but was later found to be synthesized in the body from the amino acids glutamine and aspartate. It is present in dairy products, carrots, and beets. Diet is an important contributor to the body's supply of orotate, as orotic acid excretion in the urine falls by about 50% when it is excluded from the diet.[124] Some inborn errors of metabolism can cause elevated urine orotate levels.

L-threonate, which is a naturally occurring product of the oxidative degradation of ascorbic acid (vitamin C), in the body helps transport magnesium across the BBB. Thus, threonate appears to increase magnesium concentration in the brain. Since it is derived from vitamin C, the amount of L-threonate needed to be replete is very likely less than the amount of vitamin C that the body can absorb in a day. This is far less L-threonate than the amount present in a 100 mg dose of elemental Mg.

For both Mg orotate and Mg threonate (MagT), the magnesium content in the supplement may have less impact on well-being (heart and brain health) than the supplement's chelate. MagT is likely a better source of threonate than it is of magnesium, and ideal dosing of threonate is likely 100 mg or less per day. 100 mg of MagT supplies only about 9 mg of elemental magnesium.

There was a warning earlier in this chapter about Mg supplementation being associated with increased mortality risk. This association may have resulted from the underlying reason those people were using magnesium supplements. A common use of magnesium supplements is for constipation, which may result from a diet low in fiber or other GI pathology, including that associated with Parkinson's disease. When used for constipation, poorly absorbed forms of Mg work better. Poorly absorbed Mg may have a negative impact on health.

The best way to get sufficient magnesium is through a healthy diet. If magnesium supplementation is needed, Mg orotate or Mg glycinate is recommended. While Mg can be used to help manage constipation, it is best to find and treat the underlying cause.

Carotenoids: There are several non-vitamin A-forming carotenoids present in food, in contrast to beta-carotene and a few others that do. The carotenoids lutein, xanthin, and mesoxanthin bioconcentrate in the retina and protect it from UV and blue-light injury. These are often used in supplements for the eye. Phytoene and phytofluene are colorless carotenoids that have antioxidant properties. Foods high in phytoene and phytofluene include Cara Caro oranges, tomatoes, carrots, apricots, and watermelon. Tomatoes, guavas, papayas, and apricots are also rich in the carotenoid lycopene. These fruits generally get high DAD scores, in part as a result of the antioxidant impact of these compounds. Several carotenoids have neuroprotective effects. These include fucoxanthin found in brown algae, and crocin and crocetin, which are present in saffron.[125]

Of particular interest for avoiding dementia is the carotenoid **astaxanthin**, as it crosses the blood-brain barrier well and is an effective antioxidant for the brain. Astaxanthin protects the cell membrane from oxidative stress on both the inner and outer surfaces of the cell membrane, reducing oxidative stress. It has anti-inflammatory effects and appears to improve cognition in older adults, especially among those with poorer health. In small clinical trials, it improves working memory and reaction time. In animal models, it protects against AD, and in human studies, it lowers certain markers of AD risk. It has also been found to have positive effects on mental fatigue and to speed up its recovery.[126]

The usually recommended supplemental dose for astaxanthin is 2 to 6 mg/ day, with 18 mg being considered the upper safe limit. Most therapeutic trials use 3 to 4 mg of astaxanthin.

The primary source of most dietary astaxanthin is microalgae, which are fed upon by crustaceans (shrimp, crabs, etc.), which are eaten by fish. Salmon and shellfish are excellent food sources. When used as a supplement, astaxanthin from an algal source is recommended.

Benfotiamine treatment appears to be a safe and potentially efficacious treatment in improving cognitive outcomes in individuals with mild cognitive impairment and mild AD.[127] Benfotiamine is a synthetic prodrug of thiamine (vitamin B1) that has shown promise as a neuroprotective agent, slowing the progression of Alzheimer's disease (AD). Studies indicate that benfotiamine improves cognitive outcomes, prevents loss of body weight and fat mass, improves appetite, lowers advanced glycation end products (AGEs), and decreases apoptotic signaling in the hypothalamus. It appears to mitigate some of the metabolic disturbances associated with AD.[128] [129] [130] It rescues cognitive deficits, reduces amyloid beta burden, and confers neuroprotection against tau phosphorylation and neurofibrillary tangle formation.[131]

One study found that a dose of 300 mg benfotiamine daily over 18 months improved cognitive abilities in patients with mild to moderate AD,[132] while another found benefit using 300 mg twice daily.[133] This is a huge dose, which is highly unlikely to be explained by normal vitamin co-enzymatic function. Considering the studies showing a lack of further reduction in AD risk from a daily dietary intake of thiamine beyond 2 mg a day, it seems unlikely that the benefits of benfotiamine result from it acting as a vitamin. Indeed, one of its effects is providing neuroprotection by the activation of the Nrf2/ARE pathway;[134] something expected with hormetic agents.

One theory holds that benfotiamine, being less well absorbed, remains in the GI tract throughout its course, and that it has an important effect on the GI microbiome, rather the having a direct impact on the brain.[128] Benfotiamine is an anti-inflammatory agent, has been shown to possess protective effects on the gastrointestinal (GI) mucosa.[135] It may act on GI immune and nerve cells in the intestinal wall own regulating inflammation and protecting GI neuronal function. It may be possible to achieve a similar impact using thiamine in enteric capsules or a delayed-release form.

Ergothioneine is discussed at the end of Chapter 29.

[1] Vitamin E and the risk of prostate cancer: the Selenium and Vitamin E Cancer Prevention Trial (SELECT). Klein EA, Thompson IM Jr, Tangen CM, Crowley JJ, Lucia MS, Goodman PJ, et al. JAMA. 2011 Oct 12;306(14):1549-56. PMID:21990298

[2] Dietary supplements and mortality rate in older women: the Iowa Women's Health Study. Mursu J, Robien K, Harnack LJ, Park K, Jacobs DR Jr. Arch Intern Med. 2011 Oct 10;171(18):1625-33. PMID:21987192

[3] Multivitamin use and the risk of mortality and cancer incidence: the multiethnic cohort study. Park SY, Murphy SP, Wilkens LR, et al. Am J Epidemiol. 2011 Apr 15;173(8):906-14. PMID:21343248

[4] Antioxidant supplements for prevention of mortality in healthy participants and patients with various diseases. Bjelakovic G, Nikolova D, Gluud LL, Simonetti RG, Gluud C. Cochrane Database Syst Rev. 2012 Mar 14;2012(3):CD007176. doi: 10.1002/14651858.CD007176.pub2. PMID: 22419320

[5] Unleashing the untold and misunderstood observations on vitamin E. Gee PT. Genes Nutr. 2011 Feb;6(1):5-16. PMID:21437026

[6] Folic acid and risk of prostate cancer: results from a randomized clinical trial. Figueiredo JC, Grau MV, Haile RW, et al. J Natl Cancer Inst. 2009 Mar 18;101(6):432-5. PMID:19276452

[7] Effects of vitamin E on stroke subtypes: meta-analysis of randomised controlled trials. Schürks M, Glynn RJ, Rist PM, Tzourio C, Kurth T. BMJ. 2010 Nov 4;341:c5702. PMID:21051774

[8] Vitamin E increases production of vasodilator prostanoids in human aortic endothelial cells through opposing effects on cyclooxygenase-2 and phospholipase A2. Wu D, Liu L, Meydani M, Meydani SN. J Nutr. 2005 Aug;135(8):1847-53. PMID:16046707

[9] Tocotrienols induce apoptosis in breast cancer cell lines via an endoplasmic reticulum stress-dependent increase in extrinsic death receptor signaling. Park SK, Sanders BG, Kline K. Breast Cancer Res Treat. 2010 Nov;124(2):361-75. PMID:20157774

[10] Gamma-tocotrienol induces apoptosis and autophagy in prostate cancer cells by increasing intracellular dihydrosphingosine and dihydroceramide. Jiang Q, Rao X, Kim CY, et al. Int J Cancer. 2011 Mar 11. PMID:21400505

[11] Inhibition of proliferation and induction of apoptosis by gamma-tocotrienol in human colon carcinoma HT-29 cells. Xu WL, Liu JR, Liu HK, Qi GY, Sun XR, Sun WG, Chen BQ. Nutrition. 2009 May;25(5):555-66. PMID:19121919

[12] Cancer-preventive activities of tocopherols and tocotrienols. Ju J, Picinich SC, Yang Z, Zhao Y, Suh N, Kong AN, Yang CS. Carcinogenesis. 2010 Apr;31(4):533-42. PMID:19748925

[13] Vitamin D supplementation for prevention of mortality in adults. Bjelakovic G, Gluud LL, Nikolova D, et al. Cochrane Database Syst Rev. 2011 Jul 6;(7):CD007470. PMID:21735411

[14] Folic acid for the prevention of colorectal adenomas: a randomized clinical trial. Cole BF, Baron JA, Sandler RS, , etal.; Polyp Prevention Study Group. JAMA. 2007 Jun 6;297(21):2351-9. PMID:17551129

[15] Folate and vitamin B6 intake and risk of colon cancer in relation to p53 expression. Schernhammer ES, Ogino S, Fuchs CS. Gastroenterology. 2008 Sep;135(3):770-80. PMID:18619459

[16] Will mandatory folic acid fortification prevent or promote cancer? Kim YI. Am J Clin Nutr. 2004 Nov;80(5):1123-8. PMID:15531657

[17] Folic acid handling by the human gut: implications for food fortification and supplementation. Patanwala I, King MJ, Barrett DA, et al. Am J Clin Nutr. 2014 Aug;100(2):593-9. PMID:24944062

[18] High concentrations of folate and unmetabolized folic acid in a cohort of pregnant Canadian women and umbilical cord blood. Plumptre L, Masih SP, Ly A, Aufreiter S, Sohn KJ, Croxford R, Lausman AY, Berger H, O'Connor DL, Kim YI. Am J Clin Nutr. 2015 Oct;102(4):848-57. PMID:26269367

[19] High folic acid intake reduces natural killer cell cytotoxicity in aged mice. Sawaengsri H, Wang J, Reginaldo C, Steluti J, Wu D, Meydani SN, Selhub J, Paul L. J Nutr Biochem. 2016 Apr;30:102-7. PMID:27012626

[20] A Daily Dose of 5 mg Folic Acid for 90 Days Is Associated with Increased Serum Unmetabolized Folic Acid and Reduced Natural Killer Cell Cytotoxicity in Healthy Brazilian Adults. Paniz C, Bertinato JF, Lucena MRet al. J Nutr. 2017 Sep;147(9):1677-1685. PMID:28724658

[21] Dietary Antioxidants, Circulating Antioxidant Concentrations, Total Antioxidant Capacity, and Risk of All-Cause Mortality: A Systematic Review and Dose-Response Meta-Analysis of Prospective Observational Studies. Jayedi A, Rashidy-Pour A, Parohan M, Zargar MS, Shab-Bidar S. Adv Nutr. 2018 Nov 1;9(6):701-716. doi: 10.1093/advances/nmy040. PMID: 30239557

[22] Higher circulating α-carotene was associated with better cognitive function: an evaluation among the MIND trial participants. Liu X, Dhana K, Furtado JD, Agarwal P, Aggarwal NT, Tangney C, Laranjo N, Carey V, Barnes LL, Sacks FM. J Nutr Sci. 2021 Aug 16;10:e64. doi: 10.1017/jns.2021.56. PMID: 34527222

[23] Lutein and Zeaxanthin Isomers (L/Zi) Supplementation Improves Visual Function, Performance and Sleep Quality in Individuals using Computer Devices (CDU)–A Double Blind Randomized Placebo Controlled Study Melinda Fernyhough Culver. Biomedical Journal of Scientific & Technical Research

[24] Lutein and Zeaxanthin Isomers Effect on Sleep Quality: A Randomized Placebo-Controlled Trial Melinda Fernyhough Culver, James Bowman and Vijaya Juturu, DOI: 10.26717/BJSTR.2018.09.001775

[25] The Effects of Lutein and Zeaxanthin Supplementation on Cognitive Function in Adults With Self-Reported Mild Cognitive Complaints: A Randomized, Double-Blind, Placebo-Controlled Study. Lopresti AL, Smith SJ, Drummond PD. Front Nutr. 2022 Feb 17;9:843512. doi: 10.3389/fnut.2022.843512. eCollection 2022. PMID: 35252311

[26] Supplemental Retinal Carotenoids Enhance Memory in Healthy Individuals with Low Levels of Macular Pigment in A Randomized, Double-Blind, Placebo-Controlled Clinical Trial.

Power R, Coen RF, Beatty S, Mulcahy R, Moran R, Stack J, Howard AN, Nolan JM. J Alzheimers Dis. 2018;61(3):947-961. doi: 10.3233/JAD-170713. PMID: 29332050

[27] Can Diet Supplements of Macular Pigment of Lutein, Zeaxanthin, and Meso-zeaxanthin Affect Cognition? Wang H, Wang G, Billings R, Li D, Haase SR, Wheeler PF, Vance DE, Li W. J Alzheimers Dis. 2022;87(3):1079-1087. doi: 10.3233/JAD-215736. PMID: 35431251.

[28] Dietary carotenoids and cognitive function among US adults, NHANES 2011-2014. Christensen K, Gleason CE, Mares JA. Nutr Neurosci. 2020 Jul;23(7):554-562. doi: 10.1080/1028415X.2018.1533199. Epub 2018 Oct 16. PMID: 30326796

[29] Calcitriol as a chemopreventive and therapeutic agent in prostate cancer: role of anti-inflammatory activity. Krishnan AV, Moreno J, Nonn L, Swami S, Peehl DM, Feldman D. J Bone Miner Res. 2007 Dec;22 Suppl 2:V74-80. PMID: 18290727

[30] Selective inhibition of the C5a chemotactic cofactor function of the vitamin D binding protein by 1,25(OH)2 vitamin D3. Shah AB, DiMartino SJ, Trujillo G, Kew RR. Mol Immunol. 2006 Mar;43(8):1109-15. PMID: 16115686

[31] Vitamin D attenuates lipopolysaccharide-induced inflammatory response in endothelial cells through inhibition of PI3K/Akt/NF-κB signaling pathway. Zhou W, Yuan G, Wang Q. Pharmazie. 2019 Jul 1;74(7):412-417. doi: 10.1691/ph.2019.9373. PMID: 31288897

[32] Serum Vitamin D_3 Concentration, Sleep, and Cognitive Impairment among Older Adults in China. Xie Y, Bai C, Feng Q, Gu D. Nutrients. 2023 Sep 28;15(19):4192. doi: 10.3390/nu15194192. PMID: 37836477

[33] Association of Dietary Vitamin D Intake, Serum $25(OH)D_3$, $25(OH)D_2$ with Cognitive Performance in the Elderly. Wang R, Wang W, Hu P, Zhang R, Dong X, Zhang D. Nutrients. 2021 Sep 2;13(9):3089. doi: 10.3390/nu13093089. PMID: 34578965

[34] Prevalence and correlates of vitamin D deficiency in US adults. Forrest KY, Stuhldreher WL. Nutr Res. 2011 Jan;31(1):48-54. doi: 10.1016/j.nutres.2010.12.001. PMID: 21310306

[35] A Systematic Review and Meta-Analysis of The Effect of Low Vitamin D on Cognition. Goodwill AM, Szoeke C. J Am Geriatr Soc. 2017 Oct;65(10):2161-2168. doi: 10.1111/jgs.15012. Epub 2017 Jul 31. PMID: 28758188

[36] Vitamin D deficiency as a risk factor for dementia: a systematic review and meta-analysis. Sommer I, Griebler U, Kien C, Auer S, Klerings I, Hammer R, Holzer P, Gartlehner G. BMC Geriatr. 2017 Jan 13;17(1):16. doi: 10.1186/s12877-016-0405-0. PMID: 28086755

[37] Association of Vitamin D Levels with Risk of Cognitive Impairment and Dementia: A Systematic Review and Meta-Analysis of Prospective Studies. Zhang XX, Wang HR, Meng-Wei, Hu YZ, Sun HM, Feng YX, Jia JJ. J Alzheimers Dis. 2024;98(2):373-385. doi: 10.3233/JAD-231381. PMID: 38461506

[38] The associations of serum vitamin D status and vitamin D supplements use with all-cause dementia, Alzheimer's disease, and vascular dementia: a UK Biobank based prospective cohort study. Chen LJ, Sha S, Stocker H, Brenner H, Schöttker B. Am J Clin Nutr. 2024 Apr;119(4):1052-1064. doi: 10.1016/j.ajcnut.2024.01.020. Epub 2024 Jan 29. PMID: 38296029

[39] The Efficacy of Vitamin D Supplementation in Patients With Alzheimer's Disease in Preventing Cognitive Decline: A Systematic Review. Chakkera M, Ravi N, Ramaraju R, Vats A, Nair AR, Bandhu AK, Koirala D, Pallapothu MR, Quintana Mariñez MG, Khan S. Cureus. 2022 Nov 20;14(11):e31710. doi: 10.7759/cureus.31710. eCollection 2022 Nov. PMID: 36569670

[40] Brain vitamin D forms, cognitive decline, and neuropathology in community-dwelling older adults. Shea MK, Barger K, Dawson-Hughes B, Leurgans SE, Fu X, James BD, Holland TM, Agarwal P, Wang J, Matuszek G, Heger NE, Schneider JA, Booth SL. Alzheimers Dement. 2023 Jun;19(6):2389-2396. doi: 10.1002/alz.12836. Epub 2022 Dec 7. PMID: 36479814

[41] Vitamin D Supplementation Modulates Platelet-Mediated Inflammation in Subjects With Type 2 Diabetes: A Randomized, Double-Blind, Placebo-Controlled Trial. Johny E, Jala A, Nath B, Alam MJ, Kuladhipati I, Das R, Borkar RM, Adela R. Front Immunol. 2022 May 26;13:869591. doi: 10.3389/fimmu.2022.869591. eCollection 2022. PMID: 35720377

[42] The effect of oral anticoagulants on the incidence of dementia in patients with atrial fibrillation: A systematic review and meta-analysis. Latif F, Nasir MM, Meer KK, Farhan SH, Cheema HA, Khan AB, Umer M, Rehman WU, Ahmad A, Khan MA, Almas T, Mactaggart S, Nashwan AJ, Ahmed R, Dani SS. Int J Cardiol Cardiovasc Risk Prev. 2024 May 7;21:200282. doi: 10.1016/j.ijcrp.2024.200282. eCollection 2024 Jun. PMID: 38766665

[43] The effect of sun exposure on 25-hydroxyvitamin D concentrations in young healthy subjects living in the city of São Paulo, Brazil. Maeda SS, Kunii IS, Hayashi L, et al J Med Biol Res. 2007 Dec;40(12):1653-9. Epub 2007 Oct 29.PMID: 17713647

[44] Vitamin D supplementation, 25-hydroxyvitamin D concentrations, and safety. Vieth R. Am J Clin Nutr. 1999 May;69(5):842-56. PMID: 10232622

[45] Vitamin D status indicators in indigenous populations in East Africa. Luxwolda MF, Kuipers RS, Kema IP, van der Veer E, Dijck-Brouwer DA, Muskiet FA. Eur J Nutr. 2013 Apr;52(3):1115-25. doi: 10.1007/s00394-012-0421-6. PMID: 22878781

[46] Vitamin D supplementation during pregnancy: double-blind, randomized clinical trial of safety and effectiveness. Hollis BW, Johnson D, Hulsey TC, Ebeling M, Wagner CL. J Bone Miner Res. 2011 Oct;26(10):2341-57. doi: 10.1002/jbmr.463. PMID: 21706518

[47] The Vitamin D requirement in health and disease. Heaney RP. J Steroid Biochem Mol Biol. 2005 Oct;97(1-2):13-9PMID: 16026981

[48] Prevention of rickets and vitamin D deficiency in infants, children, and adolescents. Wagner CL, Greer FR; American

Academy of Pediatrics Section on Breastfeeding; American Academy of Pediatrics Committee on Nutrition. Pediatrics. 2008 Nov;122(5):1142-52. Erratum in: Pediatrics. 2009 Jan;123(1):197. PMID: 18977996

49 Estimation of optimal serum concentrations of 25-hydroxyvitamin D for multiple health outcomes. Bischoff-Ferrari HA, Giovannucci E, Willett WC, Dietrich T, Dawson-Hughes B. Am J Clin Nutr. 2006 Jul;84(1):18-28. Erratum in: Am J Clin Nutr. 2006 Nov;84(5):1253. PMID:16825677

50 Optimal serum 25-hydroxyvitamin D levels for multiple health outcomes. Bischoff-Ferrari HA. Adv Exp Med Biol. 2008;624:55-71. PMID:18348447

51 Serum 25-hydroxyvitamin D and bone mineral density in a racially and ethnically diverse group of men. Hannan MT, Litman HJ, Araujo AB, TC, Holick MF, etal. J Clin Endocrinol Metab. 2008 Jan;93(1):40-6. PMID:17986641

52 Hypovitaminosis D is associated with insulin resistance and beta cell dysfunction. Chiu KC, Chu A, Go VL, Saad MF. Am J Clin Nutr. 2004 May;79(5):820-5. PMID:15113720

53 Hypovitaminosis D in obese children and adolescents: relationship with adiposity, insulin sensitivity, ethnicity, and season. Alemzadeh R, Kichler J, Babar G, Calhoun M. Metabolism. 2008 Feb;57(2):183-91.PMID: 18191047

54 1Alpha,25-dihydroxyvitamin D3 inhibits programmed cell death in HL-60 cells by activation of sphingosine kinase. Kleuser B, Cuvillier O, Spiegel S. Cancer Res. 1998 May 1;58(9):1817-24. PMID:9581819

55 Role of ceramide in diabetes mellitus: evidence and mechanisms. Galadari S, Rahman A, Pallichankandy S, Galadari A, Thayyullathil F. Lipids Health Dis. 2013 Jul 8;12:98. PMID:23835113

56 Sphingosine 1-phosphate is involved in cytoprotective actions of calcitriol in human fibroblasts and enhances the intracellular Bcl-2/Bax rheostat. Sauer B, Gonska H, Manggau M, Kim DS, Schraut C, Schäfer-Korting M, Kleuser B. Pharmazie. 2005 Apr;60(4):298-304. PMID:15881612

57 Fall prevention with supplemental and active forms of vitamin D: a meta-analysis of randomised controlled trials. Bischoff-Ferrari HA, Dawson-Hughes B, et al. BMJ. 2009 Oct 1;339:b3692. PMID: 19797342

58 Higher 25-hydroxyvitamin D concentrations are associated with better lower-extremity function in both active and inactive persons aged > or =60 y. Bischoff-Ferrari HA, Dietrich T, Orav EJ, Hu FB, Zhang Y, Karlson EW, Dawson-Hughes B. Am J Clin Nutr. 2004 Sep;80(3):752-8. PMID:15321818

59 CDC: NHANES Laboratory Data, analyzed by the author. Data Source: 2003-2004 Data. https://wwwn.cdc.gov/nchs/nhanes/search/datapage.aspx?Component=Laboratory

60 Human serum 25-hydroxycholecalciferol response to extended oral dosing with cholecalciferol. Heaney RP, Davies KM, Chen TC, Holick MF, Barger-Lux MJ. Am J Clin Nutr. 2003 Jan;77(1):204-10. doi: 10.1093/ajcn/77.1.204. PMID: 12499343

61 Improving Cognitive Function with Nutritional Supplements in Aging: A Comprehensive Narrative Review of Clinical Studies Investigating the Effects of Vitamins, Minerals, Antioxidants, and Other Dietary Supplements. Fekete M, Lehoczki A, Tarantini S, Fazekas-Pongor V, Csípő T, Csizmadia Z, Varga JT. Nutrients. 2023 Dec 15;15(24):5116. doi: 10.3390/nu15245116. PMID: 38140375

62 Brain vitamin D forms, cognitive decline, and neuropathology in community-dwelling older adults. Shea MK, Barger K, Dawson-Hughes B, Leurgans SE, Fu X, James BD, Holland TM, Agarwal P, Wang J, Matuszek G, Heger NE, Schneider JA, Booth SL. Alzheimers Dement. 2023 Jun;19(6):2389-2396. doi: 10.1002/alz.12836. PMID: 36479814

63 Association of Dietary Vitamin D Intake, Serum $25(OH)D_3$, $25(OH)D_2$ with Cognitive Performance in the Elderly. Wang R, Wang W, Hu P, Zhang R, Dong X, Zhang D. Nutrients. 2021 Sep 2;13(9):3089. doi: 10.3390/nu13093089. PMID: 34578965

64 The Vitamin D requirement in health and disease. Heaney RP. J Steroid Biochem Mol Biol. 2005 Oct;97(1-2):13-9. PMID:16026981

65 An open-label, randomized, 10 weeks prospective study on the efficacy of vitamin D (daily low dose and weekly high dose) in vitamin D deficient patients. Singh V, Misra AK, Singh M, Midha NK, Kumar B, Ambwani S, Bohra GK, Sharma PK. J Family Med Prim Care. 2019 Jun;8(6):1958-1963. doi: 10.4103/jfmpc.jfmpc_272_19. PMID: 31334162

66 The Controversial Role of Homocysteine in Neurology: From Labs to Clinical Practice. Moretti R, Caruso P. Int J Mol Sci. 2019 Jan 8;20(1):231. doi: 10.3390/ijms20010231. PMID: 30626145

67 Mechanism of homocysteine-mediated endothelial injury and its consequences for atherosclerosis. Yuan D, Chu J, Lin H, Zhu G, Qian J, Yu Y, Yao T, Ping F, Chen F, Liu X. Front Cardiovasc Med. 2023 Jan 16;9:1109445. doi: 10.3389/fcvm.2022.1109445. eCollection 2022. PMID: 36727029

68 Cerebral small vessel disease mediates the association between homocysteine and cognitive function. Teng Z, Feng J, Liu R, Ji Y, Xu J, Jiang X, Chen H, Dong Y, Meng N, Xiao Y, Xie X, Lv P. Front Aging Neurosci. 2022 Jul 15;14:868777. doi: 10.3389/fnagi.2022.868777. eCollection 2022. PMID: 35912072

69 Hyperhomocysteinemia is associated with lower performance on memory tasks in post-menopausal women. Clark MS, Guthrie JR, Dennerstein L. Dement Geriatr Cogn Disord. 2005;20(2-3):57-62. doi: 10.1159/000085856. Epub 2005 May 20. PMID: 15908746

70 Midlife homocysteine and late-life dementia in women. A prospective population study. Zylberstein DE, Lissner L, Björkelund C, Mehlig K, Thelle DS, Gustafson D, Ostling S, Waern M, Guo X, Skoog I. Neurobiol Aging. 2011 Mar;32(3):380-6. doi: 10.1016/j.neurobiolaging.2009.02.024.. PMID: 19342123

71 Homocysteine, B vitamins, and the incidence of dementia and cognitive impairment: results from the

Sacramento Area Latino Study on Aging. Haan MN, Miller JW, Aiello AE, Whitmer RA, Jagust WJ, Mungas DM, Allen LH, Green R. Am J Clin Nutr. 2007 Feb;85(2):511-7. doi: 10.1093/ajcn/85.2.511. PMID: 17284751

72 Homocysteine and folate as risk factors for dementia and Alzheimer disease. Ravaglia G, Forti P, Maioli F, Martelli M, Servadei L, Brunetti N, Porcellini E, Licastro F. Am J Clin Nutr. 2005 Sep;82(3):636-43. doi: 10.1093/ajcn.82.3.636. PMID: 16155278

73 Serum homocysteine and risk of dementia in Japan. Chen S, Honda T, Ohara T, Hata J, Hirakawa Y, Yoshida D, Shibata M, Sakata S, Oishi E, Furuta Y, Kitazono T, Ninomiya T. J Neurol Neurosurg Psychiatry. 2020 May;91(5):540-546. doi: 10.1136/jnnp-2019-322366. Epub 2020 Mar 31. PMID: 32234968

74 Blood and CSF Homocysteine Levels in Alzheimer's Disease: A Meta-Analysis and Meta-Regression of Case-Control Studies. Zhang L, Xie X, Sun Y, Zhou F. Neuropsychiatr Dis Treat. 2022 Oct 17;18:2391-2403. doi: 10.2147/NDT.S383654. PMID: 36276430

75 Association between dietary folate intake and cognitive impairment in older US adults: National Health and Nutrition Examination Survey. Zhang K, Li B, Gu Z, Hou Z, Liu T, Zhao J, Ruan M, Zhang T, Yu Q, Yu X, Lv Q. Arch Gerontol Geriatr. 2023 Jun;109:104946. doi: 10.1016/j.archger.2023.104946. Epub 2023 Feb 3. PMID: 36764201

76 Effects of folic acid supplementation on cognitive impairment: A meta-analysis of randomized controlled trials. Xu M, Zhu Y, Chen J, Li J, Qin J, Fan Y, Ren P, Hu H, Wu W. J Evid Based Med. 2024 Mar;17(1):134-144. doi: 10.1111/jebm.12588. PMID: 38465839

77 Efficacy of vitamins B supplementation on mild cognitive impairment and Alzheimer's disease: a systematic review and meta-analysis. Li MM, Yu JT, Wang HF, Jiang T, Wang J, Meng XF, Tan CC, Wang C, Tan L. Curr Alzheimer Res. 2014;11(9):844-52. PMID: 25274113

78 Role of vitamin B12 and folic acid in treatment of Alzheimer's disease: a meta-analysis of randomized control trials. Lee CY, Chan L, Hu CJ, Hong CT, Chen JH. Aging (Albany NY). 2024 May 2;16(9):7856-7869. doi: 10.18632/aging.205788. PMID: 38700503

79 Improving Cognitive Function with Nutritional Supplements in Aging: A Comprehensive Narrative Review of Clinical Studies Investigating the Effects of Vitamins, Minerals, Antioxidants, and Other Dietary Supplements. Fekete M, Lehoczki A, Tarantini S, Fazekas-Pongor V, Csípő T, Csizmadia Z, Varga JT. Nutrients. 2023 Dec 15;15(24):5116. doi: 10.3390/nu15245116. PMID: 38140375

80 High folic acid or folate combined with low vitamin B-12 status: potential but inconsistent association with cognitive function in a nationally representative cross-sectional sample of US older adults participating in the NHANES. Bailey RL, Jun S, Murphy L, Green R, Gahche JJ, Dwyer JT, Potischman N, McCabe GP, Miller JW. Am J Clin Nutr. 2020 Dec 10;112(6):1547-1557. doi: 10.1093/ajcn/nqaa239. PMID: 32860400

81 Evidence-based umbrella review of 162 peripheral biomarkers for major mental disorders. Carvalho AF, Solmi M, Sanches M, Machado MO, Stubbs B, Ajnakina O, Sherman C, Sun YR, Liu CS, Brunoni AR, Pigato G, Fernandes BS, Bortolato B, Husain MI, Dragioti E, Firth J, Cosco TD, Maes M, Berk M, Lanctôt KL, Vieta E, Pizzagalli DA, Smith L, Fusar-Poli P, Kurdyak PA, Fornaro M, Rehm J, Herrmann N. Transl Psychiatry. 2020 May 18;10(1):152. doi: 10.1038/s41398-020-0835-5. PMID: 32424116

82 Decreased serum pyridoxal levels in schizophrenia: meta-analysis and Mendelian randomization analysis. Tomioka Y, Numata S, Kinoshita M, Umehara H, Watanabe SY, Nakataki M, Iwayama Y, Toyota T, Ikeda M, Yamamori H, Shimodera S, Tajima A, Hashimoto R, Iwata N, Yoshikawa T, Ohmori T. J Psychiatry Neurosci. 2018 May;43(3):194-200. doi: 10.1503/jpn.170053. PMID: 29688875

83 Dietary vitamin B6 intake modulates colonic inflammation in the IL10-/- model of inflammatory bowel disease. Selhub J, Byun A, Liu Z, Mason JB, Bronson RT, Crott JW. J Nutr Biochem. 2013 Dec;24(12):2138-43. doi: 10.1016/j.jnutbio.2013.08.005. PMID: 24183308

84 Low plasma vitamin B-6 status affects metabolism through the kynurenine pathway in cardiovascular patients with systemic inflammation. Midttun O, Ulvik A, Ringdal Pedersen E, Ebbing M, Bleie O, Schartum-Hansen H, Nilsen RM, Nygård O, Ueland PM. J Nutr. 2011 Apr 1;141(4):611-7. doi: 10.3945/jn.110.133082. PMID: 21310866

85 Inflammation, vitamin B6 and related pathways. Ueland PM, McCann A, Midttun Ø, Ulvik A. Mol Aspects Med. 2017 Feb;53:10-27. doi: 10.1016/j.mam.2016.08.001. PMID: 27593095

86 Dysregulation of kynurenine pathway and potential dynamic changes of kynurenine in schizophrenia: A systematic review and meta-analysis. Cao B, Chen Y, Ren Z, Pan Z, McIntyre RS, Wang D. Neurosci Biobehav Rev. 2021 Apr;123:203-214. doi: 10.1016/j.neubiorev. 2021.01.018. PMID: 33513412

87 Association of the kynurenine pathway metabolites with clinical, cognitive features and IL-1beta levels in patients with schizophrenia spectrum disorder and their siblings. Noyan H, Erdağ E, Tüzün E, Yaylım İ, Küçükhüseyin Ö, Hakan MT, Gülöksüz S, Rutten BPF, Saka MC, Atbaşoğlu C, Alptekin K, van Os J, Üçok A. Schizophr Res. 2021 Feb 17;229:27-37. doi: 10.1016/j.schres.2021.01.014. PMID: 33609988

88 Exploring Vitamin B12 Supplementation in the Vegan Population: A Scoping Review of the Evidence. Fernandes S, Oliveira L, Pereira A, Costa MDC, Raposo A, Saraiva A, Magalhães B. Nutrients. 2024 May 10;16(10):1442. doi: 10.3390/nu16101442. PMID: 38794680

89 Response of elevated methylmalonic acid to three dose levels of oral cobalamin in older adults. Rajan S, Wallace JI, Brodkin KI, Beresford SA, Allen RH, Stabler SP. J Am Geriatr Soc. 2002 Nov;50(11):1789-95. doi: 10.1046/j.1532-5415.2002.50506.x. PMID: 12410896

90 https://perniciousanemia.org/b12/toxicity/

91 Association of Primary Sjögren's Syndrome and Vitamin B12 Deficiency: A Cross-Sectional Case-Control Study. Urbanski G, Chabrun F, Schaepelynck B, May M, Loiseau M, Schlumberger E, Delattre E, Lavigne C, Lacombe V. J Clin Med. 2020 Dec 16;9(12):4063. doi: 10.3390/jcm9124063. PMID: 33339380

92 Holotranscobalamin, a marker of vitamin B-12 status: analytical aspects and clinical utility. Nexo E, Hoffmann-Lücke E. Am J Clin Nutr. 2011 Jul;94(1):359S-365S. doi: 10.3945/ajcn.111.013458. PMID: 21593496

93 Diagnostic Performances of Urinary Methylmalonic Acid/Creatinine Ratio in Vitamin B12 Deficiency. Supakul S, Chabrun F, Genebrier S, N'Guyen M, Valarche G, Derieppe A, Villoteau A, Lacombe V, Urbanski G. J Clin Med. 2020 Jul 22;9(8):2335. doi: 10.3390/jcm9082335.PMID: 32707915

94 Choline in anxiety and depression: the Hordaland Health Study. Bjelland I, Tell GS, Vollset SE, Konstantinova S, Ueland PM. Am J Clin Nutr. 2009 Oct;90(4):1056-60. doi: 10.3945/ajcn.2009.27493. PMID: 19656836

95 Plasma free choline, betaine and cognitive performance: the Hordaland Health Study. Nurk E, Refsum H, Bjelland I, Drevon CA, Tell GS, Ueland PM, Vollset SE, Engedal K, Nygaard HA, Smith DA. Br J Nutr. 2013 Feb 14;109(3):511-9. doi: 10.1017/S0007114512001249. Epub 2012 May 1. PMID: 22717142

96 Dietary Choline Intake Is Beneficial for Cognitive Function and Delays Cognitive Decline: A 22-Year Large-Scale Prospective Cohort Study from China Health and Nutrition Survey. Huang F, Guan F, Jia X, Zhang J, Su C, Du W, Ouyang Y, Li L, Bai J, Zhang X, Wei Y, Zhang B, He Y, Wang H. Nutrients. 2024 Aug 26;16(17):2845. doi: 10.3390/nu16172845. PMID: 39275163

97 https://ods.od.nih.gov/factsheets/Choline-HealthProfessional/

98 Sienski G., et al. *APOE4* disrupts intracellular lipid homeostasis in human iPSC-derived glia. *Sci Transl Med.* 2021 Mar 3;13(583):eaaz4564. doi: 10.1126/scitranslmed.aaz4564.

99 Choline: The Underconsumed and Underappreciated Essential Nutrient. Wallace TC, Blusztajn JK, Caudill MA, Klatt KC, Natker E, Zeisel SH, Zelman KM. Nutr Today. 2018 Nov-Dec;53(6):240-253. doi: 10.1097/NT.0000000000000302. PMID: 30853718

100 Neuroprotective Actions of Dietary Choline. Blusztajn JK, Slack BE, Mellott TJ. Nutrients. 2017 Jul 28;9(8):815. doi: 10.3390/nu9080815. PMID: 28788094

101 Effects of egg yolk choline intake on cognitive functions and plasma choline levels in healthy middle-aged and older Japanese: a randomized double-blinded placebo-controlled parallel-group study. Yamashita S, Kawada N, Wang W, Susaki K, Takeda Y, Kimura M, Iwama Y, Miura Y, Sugano M, Matsuoka R. Lipids Health Dis. 2023 Jun 20;22(1):75. doi: 10.1186/s12944-023-01844-w. PMID: 37340479

102 Association between dietary vitamin B1 intake and cognitive function among older adults: a cross-sectional study. Jia W, Wang H, Li C, Shi J, Yong F, Jia H. J Transl Med. 2024 Feb 16;22(1):165. doi: 10.1186/s12967-024-04969-3. PMID: 38365743

103 Association of vitamin B1 intake with geriatric cognitive function: An analysis of the National Health and Nutrition Examination Survey (NHANES) from 2011 to 2014. Ji K, Sun M, Hong Y, Li L, Wang X, Li C, Yang S, Du W, Xu K, Zhou H. Heliyon. 2024 Apr 4;10(7):e28119. doi: 10.1016/j.heliyon.2024.e28119. eCollection 2024 Apr 15. PMID: 38601615

104 J-shaped association between dietary thiamine intake and the risk of cognitive decline in cognitively healthy, older Chinese individuals. Liu C, Meng Q, Wei Y, Su X, Zhang Y, He P, Zhou C, Liu M, Ye Z, Qin X. Gen Psychiatr. 2024 Feb 20;37(1):e101311. doi: 10.1136/gpsych-2023-101311. eCollection 2024. PMID: 38390237

105 Role of dietary protein and thiamine intakes on cognitive function in healthy older people: a systematic review. Koh F, Charlton K, Walton K, McMahon AT. Nutrients. 2015 Apr 2;7(4):2415-39. doi: 10.3390/nu7042415. PMID: 25849949

106 Association between vitamin B2 intake and cognitive performance among older adults: a cross-sectional study from NHANES. Ji K, Sun M, Li L, Hong Y, Yang S, Wu Y. Sci Rep. 2024 Sep 20;14(1):21930. doi: 10.1038/s41598-024-72949-0. PMID: 39304710

107 https://ods.od.nih.gov/factsheets/Riboflavin-HealthProfessional/

108 The neuropsychiatric effects of vitamin C deficiency: a systematic review. Plevin D, Galletly C. BMC Psychiatry. 2020 Jun 18;20(1):315. doi: 10.1186/s12888-020-02730-w. PMID: 32552785

109 The effect of vitamin C supplementation on mood status in adults: a systematic review and meta-analysis of randomized controlled clinical trials. Yosaee S, Keshtkaran Z, Abdollahi S, Shidfar F, Sarris J, Soltani S. Gen Hosp Psychiatry. 2021 Jul-Aug;71:36-42. doi: 10.1016/j.genhosppsych.2021.04.006. Epub 2021 Apr 23. PMID: 33932734

110 Dietary antioxidants and dementia in a population-based case-control study among older people in South Germany. von Arnim CA, Herbolsheimer F, Nikolaus T, Peter R, Biesalski HK, Ludolph AC, Riepe M, Nagel G; ActiFE Ulm Study Group. J Alzheimers Dis. 2012;31(4):717-24. doi: 10.3233/JAD-2012-120634. PMID: 22710913

111 A critical review of vitamin C for the prevention of age-related cognitive decline and Alzheimer's disease. Harrison FE. J Alzheimers Dis. 2012;29(4):711-26. doi: 10.3233/JAD-2012-111853. PMID: 22366772

112 Dietary Antioxidants, Circulating Antioxidant Concentrations, Total Antioxidant Capacity, and Risk of All-Cause Mortality: A Systematic Review and Dose-Response Meta-Analysis of Prospective Observational Studies. Jayedi A, Rashidy-Pour A, Parohan M, Zargar MS, Shab-Bidar S. Adv Nutr. 2018 Nov 1;9(6):701-716. doi: 10.1093/advances/nmy040. PMID: 30239557

113 Serum levels of vitamin E forms and risk of cognitive impairment in a Finnish cohort of older adults. Mangialasche F, Solomon A, Kåreholt I, Hooshmand B,

Cecchetti R, Fratiglioni L, Soininen H, Laatikainen T, Mecocci P, Kivipelto M. Exp Gerontol. 2013 Dec;48(12):1428-35. doi: 10.1016/j.exger.2013.09.006. Epub 2013 Oct 7. PMID: 24113154

114 Dietary Antioxidants, Circulating Antioxidant Concentrations, Total Antioxidant Capacity, and Risk of All-Cause Mortality: A Systematic Review and Dose-Response Meta-Analysis of Prospective Observational Studies. Jayedi A, Rashidy-Pour A, Parohan M, Zargar MS, Shab-Bidar S. Adv Nutr. 2018 Nov 1;9(6):701-716. doi: 10.1093/advances/nmy040. PMID: 30239557

115 Association of Dietary Vitamin K Intake With Cognition in the Elderly. Wang A, Zhao M, Luo J, Zhang T, Zhang D. Front Nutr. 2022 Jun 23;9:900887. doi: 10.3389/fnut.2022.900887. eCollection 2022. PMID: 35811956

116 Diet Associated with Inflammation and Alzheimer's Disease. Vasefi M, Hudson M, Ghaboolian-Zare E. J Alzheimers Dis Rep. 2019 Nov 16;3(1):299-309. doi: 10.3233/ADR-190152. PMID: 31867568

117 Taurine Promotes Differentiation and Maturation of Neural Stem/Progenitor Cells from the Subventricular Zone via Activation of $GABA_A$ Receptors. Gutiérrez-Castañeda NE, González-Corona J, Griego E, Galván EJ, Ochoa-de la Paz LD. Neurochem Res. 2023 Jul;48(7):2206-2219. doi: 10.1007/s11064-023-03883-2. PMID: 36862323

118 Taurine Supplementation as a Neuroprotective Strategy upon Brain Dysfunction in Metabolic Syndrome and Diabetes. Rafiee Z, García-Serrano AM, Duarte JMN. Nutrients. 2022 Mar 18;14(6):1292. doi: 10.3390/nu14061292. PMID: 35334949

119 Behavioral correlates of cerebrospinal fluid amino acid and biogenic amine neurotransmitter alterations in dementia. Vermeiren Y, Le Bastard N, Van Hemelrijck A, Drinkenburg WH, Engelborghs S, De Deyn PP. Alzheimers Dement. 2013 Sep;9(5):488-98. doi: 10.1016/j.jalz.2012.06.010. Epub 2012 Nov 14. PMID: 23159046

120 Barrier effects of nutritional factors. Amasheh M, Andres S, Amasheh S, Fromm M, Schulzke JD. Ann N Y Acad Sci. 2009 May;1165:267-73. doi: 10.1111/j.1749-6632.2009.04063.x. PMID: 19538315

121 U-shaped Association Between Dietary Zinc Intake and New-onset Diabetes: A Nationwide Cohort Study in China. He P, Li H, Liu M, Zhang Z, Zhang Y, Zhou C, Li Q, Liu C, Qin X. J Clin Endocrinol Metab. 2022 Jan 18;107(2):e815-e824. doi: 10.1210/clinem/dgab636. PMID: 34448874

122 L-shaped association between dietary zinc intake and cognitive decline in Chinese older people. Meng Q, Liu M, Zu C, Su X, Wei Y, Gan X, Zhang Y, He P, Zhou C, Ye Z, Liu C, Qin X. Age Ageing. 2024 Jan 2;53(1):afae008. doi: 10.1093/ageing/afae008. PMID: 38287702

123 Magnesium. Linus Pauling Institute, Micronutrient Information Center. https://lpi.oregonstate.edu/mic/minerals/magnesium

124 Orotate https://pubchem.ncbi.nlm.nih.gov/compound/1492348

125 Carotenoid Supplementation for Alleviating the Symptoms of Alzheimer's Disease.

Flieger J, Forma A, Flieger W, Flieger M, Gawlik PJ, Dzierżyński E, Maciejewski R, Teresiński G, Baj J. Int J Mol Sci. 2024 Aug 18;25(16):8982. doi: 10.3390/ijms25168982. PMID: 39201668

126 The Effects of Astaxanthin on Cognitive Function and Neurodegeneration in Humans: A Critical Review. Queen CJJ, Sparks SA, Marchant DC, McNaughton LR. Nutrients. 2024 Mar 14;16(6):826. doi: 10.3390/nu16060826. PMID: 38542737

127 Oral benfotiamine reverts cognitive deficit and increase thiamine diphosphate levels in the brain of a rat model of neurodegeneration. Moraes RCM, Singulani MP, Gonçalves AC, Portari GV, Torrão ADS. Exp Gerontol. 2020 Nov;141:111097. doi: 10.1016/j.exger.2020.111097. Epub 2020 Sep 25. PMID: 32987117

128 Synthetic Thioesters of Thiamine: Promising Tools for Slowing Progression of Neurodegenerative Diseases. Bettendorff L. Int J Mol Sci. 2023 Jul 10;24(14):11296. doi: 10.3390/ijms241411296. PMID: 37511056; PMCID: PMC10379298.

129 Benfotiamine protects against hypothalamic dysfunction in a STZ-induced model of neurodegeneration in rats. Moraes RCM, Lima GCA, Cardinali CAEF, Gonçalves AC, Portari GV, Guerra-Shinohara EM, Leboucher A, Donato J Júnior, Kleinridders A, Torrão ADS. Life Sci. 2022 Oct 1;306:120841. doi: 10.1016/j.lfs.2022.120841. PMID: 35907494

130 Benfotiamine and Cognitive Decline in Alzheimer's Disease: Results of a Randomized Placebo-Controlled Phase IIa Clinical Trial. Gibson GE, Luchsinger JA, Cirio R, Chen H, Franchino-Elder J, Hirsch JA, Bettendorff L, Chen Z, Flowers SA, Gerber LM, Grandville T, Schupf N, Xu H, Stern Y, Habeck C, Jordan B, Fonzetti P. J Alzheimers Dis. 2020;78(3):989-1010. doi: 10.3233/JAD-200896. PMID: 33074237

131 Benfotiamine treatment activates the Nrf2/ARE pathway and is neuroprotective in a transgenic mouse model of tauopathy. Tapias V, Jainuddin S, Ahuja M, Stack C, Elipenahli C, Vignisse J, Gerges M, Starkova N, Xu H, Starkov AA, Bettendorff L, Hushpulian DM, Smirnova NA, Gazaryan IG, Kaidery NA, Wakade S, Calingasan NY, Thomas B, Gibson GE, Dumont M, Beal MF. Hum Mol Genet. 2018 Aug 15;27(16):2874-2892. doi: 10.1093/hmg/ddy201. PMID: 29860433

132 Long-Term Cognitive Improvement After Benfotiamine Administration in Patients with Alzheimer's Disease. Pan X, Chen Z, Fei G, Pan S, Bao W, Ren S, Guan Y, Zhong C. Neurosci Bull. 2016 Dec;32(6):591-596. doi: 10.1007/s12264-016-0067-0. PMID: 27696179

133 Benfotiamine and Cognitive Decline in Alzheimer's Disease: Results of a Randomized Placebo-Controlled Phase IIa Clinical Trial. Gibson GE, Luchsinger JA, Cirio R, Chen H, Franchino-Elder J, Hirsch JA, Bettendorff L, Chen Z, Flowers SA, Gerber LM, Grandville T, Schupf N, Xu H, Stern Y, Habeck C, Jordan B, Fonzetti P. J Alzheimers Dis. 2020;78(3):989-1010. doi: 10.3233/JAD-200896. PMID: 33074237

[134] Ibid reference PMID: 29860433

[135] Protective effect of benfotiamine on methotrexate induced gastric damage in rats. Koc S, Erdogan MA, Erdogan E, Yalcin A, Turk A, Erdogan MM. Biotech Histochem. 2021 Nov;96(8):586-593. doi: 10.1080/10520295.2020.1853237. Epub 2020 Dec 16. PMID: 33325753

26: Food Additives

Summary

- The SANA diet promotes proper processing of foods; however, some forms of processing (milling and blending) can increase the speed of eating, stomach emptying, and digestion, which can cause a spike in blood glucose, insulin release, and hunger. Processed food can thus cause overeating.
- Processed foods, grains, for example, may have their germ and bran removed to increase shelf-life and thereby have much of the nutritional benefits removed. Whole grains provide benefits that are not present in refined grains.
- Most of the risk from processed foods, however, comes from food additives.
- The food additives that are most used, and most often overlooked, are refined sugars and oils, and fats. These are empty calories that displace more nutritious foods.
- Read food labels before purchasing food.
- Not all food additives are detrimental. Nevertheless, consider that if the food is "fortified" with vitamins (other than vitamin D in milk), the general reason for doing so is to replace some of the nutrients lost during processing.
- The principal use of food coloring is to fool the consumer's brain into thinking the food is better than it is, making it appear fresher, riper, more natural, and healthier, when it is not. Many food colorants are dangerous. There is no nutritional purpose for food coloring other than to make artificial foods more attractive, especially to children. These additives are best avoided.
- Many and probably most non-digestible emulsifiers and thickening agents disrupt the mucosal layer in the colon and promote dysbiosis and leaky gut.

Processed Foods

Highly processed foods are a risk factor for type 2 diabetes and most likely for type 3 diabetes (Alzheimer's disease). Some of this effect is likely the result of the high glycemic index of many processed foods, as well as the propensity to over-eat highly palatable, refined foods; their lack of fiber; and their high content of fat, sugar, and salt in these foods.

- Grinding, milling, macerating, or blending foods can increase the surface area of the foods, reduce the particle size, and make them quicker to digest. It also often decreases the gastric retention time, so the food can be digested and absorbed more quickly; thus, increasing the glycemic index and raising the blood sugar more than whole food would. Since these foods are milled, they are easy to eat quickly, making overeating likely. Since they spend less time in the mouth, more food may be eaten before satiation is felt.
- Refined foods often have most of their fiber removed. White wheat flour is the basis of many foods. It has had the wheat germ (high in vitamin E and spermidine) removed to improve shelf-life, and the bran has also been removed. White rice has had the bran, which is rich in fiber, lignans, and B vitamins, removed. The lack of soluble fiber (and high glycemic index) increases hunger before the next meal, again promoting high levels of food intake and the deposition of fat.
- The most common and massively used food additives are sugars, including high fructose corn syrup, vegetable oils, and salt. These are empty calories. Most of the added fat is proinflammatory. Sugar, fats, and salt intensify the flavor of the foods. The high glycemic index and the fats are quickly satisfying, making these foods addictive, and this additionally causes overeating and a preference for these foods.
- Highly processed foods are generally less nutritious, obesogenic, proinflammatory, and promote insulin resistance and its associated diseases.
- As discussed in the previous chapter, salt in reasonable amounts is not deleterious, but it can be overused in processed foods.

Food Additives

Food additives are used to enhance the color or flavor of foods to make them more appealing. Additives are also used as preservatives. Often, they are added to processed food to supplement their succulence and savor, but they are also added to foods that are wholesome foods. Not all additives have deleterious effects, and most people can consume them in the amounts found in food with impunity. Others are not that lucky, and they may cause problems.

While much of the health risk of manufactured foods is from caloric food additives, a more insidious issue is non-nutritive food additives. The FDA allows over 2000 food additives to be GRAS.[1] Despite their "Generally Recognized as Safe" status, many have detrimental impacts, while others are innocuous or even have health benefits. Some food additives, such as pectin, may be beneficial to the microbiome. Many food additives alter the balance of the GI microbiome.[2]

Table 26A: Non-Nutritive Food Additive Categories

Additive Category	Common Uses	Typical Usage
Emulsifiers	Maintain or form homogeneous mixtures of non-miscible phases (e.g., water and oil)	Widely used in processed foods, salad dressings, baked goods, and margarine.
Stabilizers	Enhance physical characteristics (e.g., texture, consistency)	Found in ice cream, yogurt, sauces, and processed meats.
Preservatives	Extend shelf life by inhibiting spoilage and microbial growth	Commonly added to canned foods, cured meats, and beverages.
Antioxidants	Prevent oxidation and rancidity in fats and oils	Used in snacks, baked goods, and processed foods.
Sweeteners	Add sweetness without calories (e.g., artificial sweeteners, alcohol sugars)	Found in diet sodas, sugar-free products, and desserts.
Colorants	Enhance visual appeal by adding color.	Widely used in candies, beverages, and processed foods.
Flavor Enhancers	Intensify or modify taste sensations (e.g., monosodium glutamate - MSG)	Commonly found in savory snacks, soups, and restaurant dishes.
Thickeners	Increase viscosity and improve texture	Used in sauces, gravies, and dairy products.
Acidulants	Adjust acidity levels for flavor balance	Present in soft drinks, pickles, and canned fruits.
Anti-Caking Agents	Prevent clumping or sticking of powdered substances	Added to salt, spices, and powdered foods.
Humectants	Retain moisture and prevent drying out: glycerin, glucose, sodium hexametaphosphate.	Found in baked goods, candies, and dried fruits.
Texturizers	Modify texture (e.g., gelling agents, thickeners)	Used in jams, jellies, and dairy products.
Enzymes	Catalyze specific reactions in food processing	Applied in cheese-making, brewing, and baking.
Fiber	May be added for putative health benefits.	Modify bacterial populations, but this may not necessarily be beneficial to health.

Emulsifiers and Thickeners

Emulsifiers bind to both fats and water, and thus help maintain water/fat suspensions. One class of commonly used emulsifiers is phospholipids (lecithin) from soy, eggs, or other natural sources. These are digested and are nutrients.

Non-digestible emulsifiers used in food manufacture include polysorbates (PSB) (20, 40, 60, 80) and carboxymethylcellulose CMC). These agents are used to improve food texture and flavor. They also act as detergents, and since this action is not stopped by digestion, they continue to act as detergents in the small intestine and colon, disrupting the protective mucous lining.

Table 26B: Some Food Additives Ranked by DAD Score

Food Additive	Rating
Hydrolyzed Guar fiber >85% "Sunfiber"	4
Lecithin	3
Polydextrose	2
Oat bran	1
Agar	0
Arrowroot powder	0
Baking Powder, non-aluminum containing	0
Corn or potato starch	0
Baking Soda	0
Gelatin	0
Acacia gum	A
Galactooligosaccharides (GOS) fiber BIOLIGO	A
Inulin	A
Locust bean gum	A
Marshmallow root	A
Sodium Alginate	A
Galactooligosaccharides (GOS) fiber (care4U)	B
Xanthan gum	B
Annatto (powder)	C
Salt, pink Himalayan	C
Psyllium husks	D
Carboxymethyl cellulose	D
Carrageenan CL-220	D
Food Color Blue No. 1	D
Glycerin	D
Xylitol	D
Erythritol	D
Sodium Stearoyl Lactylate	D
Guar gum	D
Baking Powder with aluminum	D

Damage to the mucous layer of the intestine is especially injurious in the colon, as it allows direct contact of the colonocytes with colonic bacteria, thus promoting biofilm formation; bacterial toxin and toxic fermentation product formation and absorption; and microbial transmigration. Detergent emulsifiers such as PSB and CMC should be avoided, especially in infants; individuals with autism; IBD, metabolic syndrome,[3] [4] neuroinflammatory diseases such as migraine, MS, Alzheimer's disease, Parkinson's, schizophrenia; and other diseases that are caused by dysbiosis and leaky gut. PSBs are often used in ice creams, puddings, coconut milk, candies, and in some medications. CMCs are used in baked products, chewing gum, margarine, and peanut butter.

Non-nutritive emulsifiers end up in the colon, where they cause havoc.[5] This may be an inherent result of non-digestible emulsifiers.[6] [7] Carboxymethyl Cellulose (E466) and Polysorbate 80 (E433) have both been shown to increase *Ruminococcus gnavus* and decrease *Bacteroidales* in rats. Polysorbate 80 increased insulin and liver enzyme levels in rats, decreased mucosal thickness, and increased intestinal permeability.[8]

Xanthan gum, a bacterial product, triggers a pro-inflammatory response, which promotes increased cytokine production, especially in adipose tissue. In rats, its consumption increased retroperitoneal IL-6 and TNF.[9]

Carrageenans, maltodextrin, xanthan gum, sorbitan monostearate and glyceryl stearate, Polysorbate-80, and carboxymethylcellulose have been previously discussed in Chapter 15 (Dairy).

Fiber

Fiber is healthy, right? As noted in a previous chapter, carboxymethylcellulose (CMC), a.k.a. cellulose fiber, can be listed on the food ingredient list as fiber. Food manufacturers are highly responsive to market demand for a poorly informed public. How are consumers to know?

Many of the fibers added to manufactured foods have little or no benefit to the commensal bacteria of the gut. Some, such as galactose oligosaccharides (GOS), may be appropriate for infant formula, but not so much for adults.

Inulin is a fiber. It has a DAD score of A, and causes flatulence in healthy persons, and can exacerbate inflammatory bowel disease.[10] Beta-fructans (such as those present in wheat, barley, onions, asparagus, artichokes, Jerusalem artichokes, agave, bananas, chicory, cashews) can have a proinflammatory effect amount those lacking sufficient fermentative microbiota to process this fiber.[11] When there is a dysbiotic microbiome, the same types of fiber that can form short-chain fatty acids that provide benefits in those with a healthy microbiome can instead be fermented into compounds that worsen symptoms with IBS or IBD.[12]

For the most part, my impression is that food manufacturers are trying to give the public what they say they want. Do you want more fiber in your diet? They will manufacture foods with affordable fiber so that you can feel better about your food choices, even if they are good ones, or may cause more problems in a subset of the population. They think that they are being helpful, giving people what they think they want.

If you want fiber that promotes health, eat whole grain rice, beans, oatmeal, fruits, vegetables, and other natural foods that have been properly prepared. Avoid those with low DAD scores.

Sweeteners

Artificial sweeteners, including saccharine, sucralose, and aspartame, induced glucose intolerance in rats, and their intake is associated with an increase in the number of *Bacteroides* spp. and bacteria in the Clostridiales phylum in the intestine. Aspartame impacts the GI microbiome and raises blood glucose levels in animals. Splenda also alters gut microbiota and causes weight gain in animals. Xylitol consumption shifts the rodent intestinal microbial population from gram-negative to gram-positive bacteria. Maltitol and sorbitol likely increase *Lactobacilli and Bifidobacteria.*[13] Both xylitol and, even more, erythritol are suspected to increase the risk of heart disease, as discussed in Chapter 6 (Sugar).

Monk fruit is used as an artificial sweetener and is 200 times sweeter than sugar. While "Generally Recognized as Safe" (GRAS) by the FDA, it is not allowed in food by the European Union.

The history of artificial sweeteners is filled with items that turn out to be worse for health than the sugar they were substituted for. The exception is for type 1 and other insulin-dependent diabetics. A better choice is to avoid excess sugars. For non-diabetics, the SANA diet recommends eating real food and limiting the amount of added sugar in the diet.

Honey, maple syrup, molasses, fruit concentrates, brown sugar, dates, and other natural sugars can be used, but should be considered added sugars.

Advice: Don't try to justify added sugar intake from naturally concentrated sweeteners as being natural or significantly healthier than table sugar. I am not advocating against the use of unrefined sugars, but rather emphasizing that they are still added sugars. Own up to your sweet tooth. Keep the added-sugar intake in the diet to less than 10% of daily caloric intake. Don't use sugar substitutes as a shortcut to eating more sweets, even if they are naturally occurring ones such as xylitol and erythritol (both of which have DAD scores of D). Agave syrup is mostly fructose and should be avoided.

Fructose (generally in the form of high-fructose corn syrup) is used in manufactured food not just as a sweetener, but for other properties. As discussed in Chapter 3 (Fruits), it is used to lower the water activity of certain foods, including baked goods, to deter bacterial and fungal growth. This is a benign and appropriate use, as the amount is fairly low, at least in comparison to soda pop. Fructose, glucose, and honey are used as humectants to soften the texture of some foods.

Allulose, maltitol, and other sweeteners are discussed in Chapter 10.

Food Colorants

Some food colorants are natural; not all natural ones are good for you. Carmine red (E120) is made from beetles that live on cacti in Mexico. Lycopene, which gives tomatoes their red color, is fine. Betanin from beets, anthocyanins from fruits, and beta-carotene from vegetables are beneficial for most people. Annatto causes allergy in some people and is suspected to worsen irritable bowel syndrome (IBS).

The food colorants of most concern to the SANA program are Brilliant Blue FCF (Blue No. 1, E133) and Titanium white. Blue food coloring is not only used to make blue colored foods, but it is also mixed, usually with yellow food coloring, to make green foods; thus, green food coloring is of high concern as well. Titanium white is suspected to damage intestinal mucosal cells and exacerbate inflammatory bowel disease. It is discussed in Chapter 15 (Diary).

There are seven artificial food colorings still in use in the United States. Several others have been removed from the market, usually for their carcinogenic activity. These base colors are mixed to get the desired hue for the food. Beyond the seven, two additional artificial colorings can be legally used. "Citrus Red No. 2" is allowed only for use in coloring the skins of oranges that will not be used in food.[14] Citrus Red No. 2 is a known carcinogen.

Most of the artificial food colorants have been shown to cause tumors or cancers in lab animals. The FDA allows the use of artificial colors primarily because of political pressure, and with the understanding that the amounts consumed in food are quite small. Dyeing the skin of oranges with citrus Red No. 2, a known carcinogen, is allowed as it does not seep into the fruit, but obviously, the peels from these oranges should not be used for marmalade or candies. While the carcinogenic Orange B coloring can still be legally used in hot dogs and sausage casings, manufacturers in the United States voluntarily discontinued making the dye in 1978. Consumption of hot dogs has been associated with the risk of childhood leukemia[15] and brain tumors[16], but that risk is usually attributed to N-nitroso compounds, rather than the food colorant.

Table 26C: Artificial Food Colorings Legal for Use in the United States:

Designation	Name	E number	Cancer or Tumors in Rats or Mice	Color
FD&C Blue No. 1	Brilliant Blue FCF	E133		Dark Blue
FD&C Blue No. 2	Indigotine	E132	Brain	Blue
FD&C Green No. 3	Fast Green	E134	Bladder	Turquoise
FD&C Yellow No. 5	Tartrazine	E102		Yellow
FD&C Yellow No. 6	Sunset Yellow FCF	E110	Kidney Bladder	Orange
FD&C Red No. 3	Erythrosine	E127	Thyroid	Pink
FD&C Red No. 40	Allura Red AC	E129		Red
FD&C Orange B				Orange
FD&C Citrus Red No. 2		E121	Yes	Red

The "E" number is a designation for a food additive used in the European Union.

Allergic reactions have been attributed to Blue No.1, Yellow No.6, and especially to Yellow No. 5, although, as non-proteins, it is more likely that these compounds cause pseudoallergic reactions than true allergic reactions. Tartrazine (Yellow No. 5) has been associated with behavioral problems in children[17] and with pseudoallergic reactions in individuals with leukotriene-associated hypersensitivity (aspirin intolerance). The preservative sodium benzoate can provoke this same reaction. The red dyes are comedogenic when used in cosmetics and thus can provoke acne.[18]

Food additives, especially food colorants, have been suspected of causing behavioral problems, particularly ADD and ADHD, since the 1970s. This remains an area of controversy, as their effect is difficult to study; there are large numbers of variables involved, and different colors and additives are allowed or banned in various countries. Furthermore, these agents only represent a few of the dietary and environmental exposures that affect fluctuating behaviors. The studies that have found that food additives increase hyperactivity have used "cocktails" of food colorings, which included the food preservative sodium benzoate.[19 20] Additionally, studies from other countries included colorants that are not allowed to be added to foods in the United States.

Complicating the study of the effects of food additives, interactions may occur when they are consumed in combination. Brilliant blue, quinoline yellow color (not allowed to be used in the U.S.A.), L-glutamic acid, and the artificial sweetener aspartame all inhibit nerve-fiber growth in cell cultures. Synergistic interactions between these substances can reduce the concentration required to prevent neurite growth by five times or more. When present in combination, these additives result in nerve cell growth inhibition at greatly reduced concentrations[21], as shown in Table 21D. Artificial additives, which may not induce risk at levels consumed in foods when studied individually, may cause injury when combined in a food or when foods are combined in a meal. Note that glutamate is an excitatory neurotransmitter and thus is present in the brain.

Table 26D: Additive Effects of Food Additives on Inhibition of Nerve Growth

Food Additive	Concentration Required to Inhibit Neurite Growth by 50%[21]
Brilliant Blue	51.4 nM
Glutamate	48.7 μM
Brilliant Blue with Glutamate	10 nM with 10 μM
Quinoline Yellow	106 μM
Aspartame	153 μM
Quinoline Yellow with Aspartame	10 μM with 8.06 μM

Some food additives are large, polar (water-soluble) molecules, which are not normally absorbed by the intestines, and thus, have limited potential toxicity. Individuals with an impaired intestinal mucosal barrier, however, may absorb them. The enteric nervous system can also be exposed to artificial food additives that are potential neurotoxins.

Although natural food colorants may sound benign, not all are. Two natural food colorants are of special concern, as they are highly immunogenic. Annatto (also known as bija, bixa, achiote, or roucou) is made from the seed of the *Bixa orellana,* a plant native to South America, where it was used as body paint by native peoples. As a food additive, it can be listed as "natural color," annatto, by the refined chemical names bixin or norbixin, or by the E number E160b.

Table 261E: Some Natural Food Colorings Allowed for Use in the United States:

Name	Source	E Number	Color
Chlorophyll	*Chlorella algae*	E140	Green
Turmeric	*Curcuma longa*	E100	Yellow, orange
Saffron	*Crocus sativus*	E160a	Yellow - Red
Annatto	*Bixa orellana*	E160b	Yellow - Red
Cochineal	*Dactylopius coccus*	E120	Crimson Red
Betanin	Beetroots; *Beta vulgaris*		Deep red
Elderberry juice	*Sambucus* (various species)		Magenta

Immunogenic reaction to annatto is fairly common, and it has been associated with irritable bowel syndrome and behavioral problems. Unfortunately, most labs that test for allergies do not test for immunoreactivity to annatto. It is used as a "lake", a fat-soluble color, for dairy products including cheese, butter, margarine, and ice cream, as well as in some snack foods. Annatto is often hidden in otherwise healthy foods (yellow cheese, butter, vanilla ice cream), not places where allergenic food dyes are expected.

Cochineal (also known as carmine, crimson lake, natural red 4, and E120) is a colorant that gives a crimson red color. FDA regulations require all foods and cosmetics containing cochineal to label their use in the ingredient list. It is made from the pulverized bodies of *Dactylopius coccus,* an insect that lives on prickly pear cactus. During its colonial period, this dye was Mexico's second-most valuable export following silver. As it is an insect product, it is not vegetarian, not kosher, and is Haraam (forbidden) in Islam.

This colorant may be found in candy, beverages, yogurt, or ice cream to impart a red or berry color. Cochineal is immunogenic and can cause mild to severe allergic reactions; however, it is rarely included in panels for immunogenicity testing. Cochineal immunogenicity likely cross-reacts with shrimp, flea, cockroach, and other arthropod immune reactivity.

Caramel, the candy, and caramel coloring can be made by heating sucrose, causing a Maillard reaction. For commercial food coloring, a carbohydrate, usually a sugar such as fructose, sucrose, dextrose, or maltose, is treated with an alkali, acid, or salt. Caramel colors I and II have been determined to have the same toxicological properties as those made by heating sugar. Caramel colors I and II have not been found to pose a significant risk.

Caramel colors III and IV, however, made with ammonia, contain the carcinogen 4-methylimidazole (4-MEI)[22]. A daily intake of 30 µg of MEI-4 has been estimated to impart a 1:100,000 risk of developing cancer. This amount is present in as little as 2.5 ounces of *Coca-Cola* sold in Washington, DC. In California, however, where it is regulated, there is less than 1 µg of MEI-4 in this amount of the beverage.[23] The amounts present in colas vary greatly, and even in California, may exceed levels requiring warning labels for carcinogens.[24]

Caramel color III also contains the compound THI, which inhibits the enzyme S1P lyase, and which thus may affect immune cell activity, especially in the intestine. Caramel color III is used in some beers and confectionery.

The FDA normally restricts food additive carcinogen content to levels below that which imparts a 1:1,000,000 risk of cancer. Use and consumption of Caramel colors III and IV should be abandoned.

Table 26F: Caramel Colorings Allowed for Use in the United States:

Caramel Coloring I	Caramelized Sugar, Malt	E150A	Amber - Brown
Caramel Coloring II	Caustic sulphite caramel	E150B	Amber - Brown
Caramel Coloring III	Ammonia caramel	E150C	Amber - Brown
Caramel Coloring IV	Sulfite ammonia caramel	E150D	Amber - Brown

Food Preservatives

Included among the relatives of cochineal are scale insects and mealybugs. Certain scale bugs are cultivated in Southeast Asia on the branches of plants for the production of sticklac. Lac is a resinous secretion left on the plants by these creatures. This product is used to make shellac, which is used to coat violins. You can also find it in the fruit aisle of your local grocery store, as well, in the candy section.

Lac is a product used to polish and shine grocery store apples. It provides a moisture barrier to help keep the fruit fresh. It is also used on other fruits and in some candies, such as jellybeans, some chocolate treats, some coated chewing gums, and even on some coffee beans. In candies, it may be listed as shellac or as "confectioner's glaze". Yes, this means that apples may not be vegan. Contrary to urban legend, M&M's do not use lac. In candies, it is also used as a moisture barrier, here, to keep moisture out and keep the candy hard. Lac also gives these products a desirable sheen. Lac appears to cause headaches in some individuals. Another reason to avoid or at least peel apples.

Waxes and Oils are also used on many fruits and vegetables to help retain moisture and keep them looking fresh. Cucumbers, for example, often have an oily feel to them. These oils and waxes are mostly petroleum-based products. They are used as moisture barriers to keep the fruits and vegetables from drying out while on display, to improve their shelf life and appearance. The waxes and oils are similar to those used in lip gloss. Chocolate candy often contains paraffin, used to raise the melting temperature to help maintain the candy's shape (for example, chocolate Easter bunnies. Paraffin impedes the absorption of fat-soluble vitamins and, in large quantities, can cause anal leakage.[25]

Sulfites are used as preservatives as they prevent bacterial growth in food. Most wine contains added sulfites, as do many manufactured foods and dried fruits. Sulfites can trigger mast cell degranulation, triggering asthma and other reactions. Most studies report that 3 to 10% of asthmatics are sensitive to dietary exposure to sulfites.[26]

Nitrates and Sodium Benzoate are used as food preservatives to prevent bacterial growth, usually in meat products. These preservatives can cause pseudoallergic reactions by increasing leukotriene production. Sodium Benzoate may provoke ADHD behavior. Nitrates are used to make meat "pink" and appear fresh. When meat preserved with nitrates is cooked, the nitrate can be transformed into carcinogenic nitrosamines.

BHA and BHT: BHA (Butylated hydroxyanisole) and BHT (Butylated hydroxytoluene) are antioxidant food additives. Both are lipid-soluble.

BHA is used to prevent oils and fats from becoming rancid and having objectionable odors. BHA is used in meat products, margarine, cereals, baked goods, snack foods, dehydrated potatoes, chewing gum, beer, animal feed, and cosmetics. BHT is now less frequently used as a food preservative than BHA; however, BHT is still used in food packaging materials and shortening. BHA may thus be contained in foods labeled as containing shortening. BHA and BHT are carcinogenic in some animals. The low levels of BHA and BHT found in food are unlikely to cause significant health risks; probably less health risk than the processed foods in which they are found. By preventing oxidation of fats, they likely decrease the risks associated with eating the processed foods they are contained in.

[1] https://www.fda.gov/food/food-additives-petitions/food-additive-status-list

[2] The Impact of Food Additives on the Abundance and Composition of Gut Microbiota. Zhou X, Qiao K, Wu H, Zhang Y. Molecules. 2023 Jan 7;28(2):631. doi: 10.3390/molecules28020631. PMID: 36677689

[3] Dietary emulsifiers impact the mouse gut microbiota promoting colitis and metabolic syndrome. Chassaing B, Koren O, Goodrich JK, et al. Nature. 2015 Mar 5;519(7541):92-6. PMID:25731162

[4] Translocation of Crohn's disease Escherichia coli across M-cells: contrasting effects of soluble plant fibres and emulsifiers. Roberts CL, Keita AV, et al. Gut. 2010 Oct;59(10):1331-9 PMID:20813719

[5] The Emulsifier Carboxymethylcellulose Induces More Aggressive Colitis in Humanized Mice with Inflammatory Bowel Disease Microbiota Than Polysorbate-80. Rousta E, Oka A, Liu B, Herzog J, Bhatt AP, Wang J, Habibi Najafi MB, Sartor RB. Nutrients. 2021 Oct 12;13(10):3565. doi: 10.3390/nu13103565. PMID: 34684567

[6] Dietary emulsifiers impact the mouse gut microbiota promoting colitis and metabolic yndrome. Chassaing B, Koren O, Goodrich JK, Poole AC, Srinivasan S, Ley RE, Gewirtz AT. Nature. 2015 Mar 5;519(7541):92-6. doi: 10.1038/nature14232. PMID: 25731162

[7] Dietary emulsifiers directly alter human microbiota composition and gene expression ex vivo potentiating intestinal inflammation. Chassaing B, Van de Wiele T, De Bodt J, Marzorati M, Gewirtz AT. Gut. 2017 Aug;66(8):1414-1427. doi: 10.1136/gutjnl-2016-313099. Epub 2017 Mar 21. PMID: 28325746

[8] Food Additive P-80 Impacts Mouse Gut Microbiota Promoting Intestinal Inflammation, Obesity and Liver Dysfunction. Singh RK, Wheildon N, Ishikawa S. SOJ Microbiol Infect Dis. 2016;4(1):10.15226/sojmid/4/1/00148. doi: 10.15226/ sojmid/4/1/00148. PMID: 27430014

[9] A diet including xanthan gum triggers a pro-inflammatory response in Wistar rats inoculated with Walker 256 cells. Silva Rischiteli AB, Neto NIP, Gascho K, Carnier M, de Miranda DA, Silva FP, Boldarine VT, Seelaender M, Ribeiro EB, Oyama LM, Oller do Nascimento CM. PLoS One. 2019 Jun 18;14(6):e0218567. doi: 10.1371/journal.pone.0218567. PMID: 31211796

[10] Supplementation of Low- and High-fat Diets with Fermentable Fiber Exacerbates Severity of DSS-induced Acute Colitis. Miles JP, Zou J, Kumar MV, Pellizzon M, Ulman E, Ricci M, Gewirtz AT, Chassaing B. Inflamm Bowel Dis. 2017 Jul;23(7):1133-1143. doi: 10.1097/MIB.0000000000001155. PMID: 28590342

[11] Unfermented β-fructan Fibers Fuel Inflammation in Select Inflammatory Bowel Disease Patients. Armstrong HK, Bording-Jorgensen M, Santer DM, Zhang Z, Valcheva R, Rieger AM, Sung-Ho Kim J, Dijk SI, Mahmood R, Ogungbola O, Jovel J, Moreau F, Gorman H, Dickner R, Jerasi J, Mander IK, Lafleur D, Cheng C, Petrova A, Jeanson TL, Mason A, Sergi CM, Levine A, Chadee K, Armstrong D, Rauscher S, Bernstein CN, Carroll MW, Huynh HQ, Walter J, Madsen KL, Dieleman LA, Wine E. Gastroenterology. 2023 Feb;164(2):228-240. doi: 10.1053/j.gastro.2022.09.034. PMID: 36183751

[12] Not All Fibers Are Born Equal; Variable Response to Dietary Fiber Subtypes in IBD. Armstrong H, Mander I, Zhang Z, Armstrong D, Wine E. Front Pediatr. 2021 Jan 15;8:620189. doi: 10.3389/fped.2020.620189. eCollection 2020. PMID: 33520902

[13] Food additives and microbiota. Gultekin F, Oner ME, Savas HB, Dogan B. North Clin Istanb. 2019 Jul 17;7(2):192-200. doi: 10.14744/nci.2019.92499. eCollection 2020. PMID: 32259044

[14] Code of Federal Regulations Title 21, Section 74. USFDA revised April 1, 2010

[15] Cured and broiled meat consumption in relation to childhood cancer: Denver, Colorado (United States) Sarasua S, Savitz DA. Cancer Causes Control. 1994 Mar;5(2):141-8. PMID: 8167261

[16] Processed meats and risk of childhood leukemia (California, USA). Peters JM, Preston-Martin S, London SJ, et al. Cancer Causes Control. 1994 Mar;5(2):195-202. PMID: 8167267

[17] Synthetic food coloring and behavior: a dose response effect in a double-blind, placebo-controlled, repeated-measures study. Rowe KS, Rowe KJ. J Pediatr. 1994 Nov;125(5 Pt 1):691-8. PMID: 7965420

[18] Comedogenicity of current therapeutic products, cosmetics, and ingredients in the rabbit ear. Fulton JE Jr, Pay SR, Fulton JE 3rd. J Am Acad Dermatol. 1984 Jan;10(1):96-105. PMID:6229554

[19] Food additives and hyperactive behaviour in 3-year-old and 8/9-year-old children in the community: a randomised, double-blinded, placebo-controlled trial. McCann D, Barrett A, Cooper A, et al. Lancet. 2007 Nov 3;370(9598):1560-7. Erratum in: Lancet. 2007 Nov 3;370(9598):1542. PMID: 17825405

[20] The effects of a double blind, placebo controlled, artificial food colourings and benzoate preservative challenge on hyperactivity in a general population sample of preschool children. Bateman B, Warner JO, Hutchinson E, et al. Arch Dis Child. 2004 Jun;89(6):506-11.

[21] Synergistic interactions between commonly used food additives in a developmental neurotoxicity test. Lau K, McLean WG, Williams DP, Howard CV. Toxicol Sci. 2006 Mar;90(1):178-87. PMID:16352620

[22] http://monographs.iarc.fr/ENG/Monographs/vol101/mono101-015.pdf

[23] Center for Science in the Public Interest, accessed June, 2014 http://www.cspinet.org/new/201206261.html

[24] Consumer Reports: Too many sodas contain potential carcinogen. http://www.cnn.com/2014/01/23/health/consumer-reports-soda-caramel-coloring/ CNN Accessed June 2014.

[25] Laxatives: Types, Purpose, and Side-Effects (patient.info)

[26] Clinical effects of sulphite additives. Vally H, Misso NL, Madan V. Clin Exp Allergy. 2009 Nov;39(11):1643-51. PMID: 19775253

27: Mycotoxins

Simple Summary

There are several hundred mycotoxins, toxic compounds produced by molds and other fungi, that can contaminate food. A few of these are exceptional in that they are both dangerous and widely prevalent. Aflatoxin contamination of food is a major cause of hepatic cancer worldwide. Aflatoxin takes its greatest toll in warmer climates.

Ochratoxin A (OTA) is found in foods contaminated by several species of molds. Ochratoxin A is an acute toxin that damages the kidneys, liver, and the immune system, and is a suspected carcinogen, particularly for the urinary tract. This toxin may be responsible for sporadic epidemic outbreaks of kidney disease. OTA is of particular salience to dementia as it is neurotoxic. Leaky gut increases the absorption of OTA, and it is likely that OTA promotes leaky gut.

Other than cheese that is intentionally inoculated with fungi (i.e., gorgonzola and blue cheese), moldy food should be taken outside of the home and trashed. If black mold spores (the fruiting bodies) are seen on the surface, one can be sure that the mold is growing throughout the food. Similarly, white fuzzy growth on food represents fruiting bodies of mold growing within the food.

Most mycotoxins come from soilborne fungi. Thus, crops in contact with the soil are at high risk of fungal contamination. Peanuts, which grow underground, are often contaminated with mycotoxins.

Moldy food should not be eaten. If mold spores can be seen in one end of a loaf of bread, the rest of the bread should be considered to be contaminated, as the hyphae have most likely grown throughout the loaf. Sweet potatoes, especially if damaged during harvest and not properly stored, can mold. This may appear as black areas or as fuzzy growth on the outside.[1] If the sweet potato flesh is black or turns blackish after cooking, discard it. Dried peppers are so commonly contaminated with mycotoxins that the SANA program advises their avoidance.

Grains are often contaminated by mycotoxins. More than half of the exposure people have to mycotoxins is from the consumption of grains. The preparation process recommended in this book (hydration, pre-soaking with baking soda or vinegar, pressure cooking, and nixtamalization of corn) can decrease the toxicity of mycotoxins by about 85 – 90%.

The FDA does not regulate or monitor the level of OTA in food. I would like to see this change.

Aflatoxin and Other Mycotoxins

Most people are aware that some mushrooms are deadly poisonous. Many people avoid even touching wild mushrooms because of this. While certain mushrooms are famously toxic, not many people die from them. There are, however, other, more insidious, hidden fungal toxins that kill large numbers of people each year. It is estimated that as many as 155,000 people die from liver cancer each year from exposure to just one type of these hidden toxins.[2] Before 1990, aflatoxins were responsible for an estimated 600,000 deaths from hepatocellular cancer each year, but improvements in food quality control in China have greatly reduced the aflatoxin levels there. Still, about one-fourth of the world's food supply has aflatoxin contamination. This exposure to aflatoxin impairs growth in utero and in children and infants. It is an important cause of malnourishment in sub-Saharan Africa and is transferred into breast milk. Aflatoxin is immunosuppressive and thus may increase the risks from infectious disease. It is also a carcinogen.[3]

Ochratoxin A

Ochratoxin A is a nephrotoxic, hepatotoxic, neurotoxic carcinogen that is lightly sprinkled throughout many of the foods we eat. The name does not come from the vegetable okra, but rather from the color ochre, the yellow-brown color of the mold in which the toxin was first isolated. Fungal molds from the genera *Aspergillus*, *Petromyces*, *Neopetromyces*, and *Penicillium* produce ochratoxin A (OTA),[4] and these fungi are common in the environment. Most of the OTA present in foods comes from two species: *Penicillium verruscum*, which is responsible for most OTA contamination in cool and temperate conditions, and *Aspergillus ochraceus*, which is the principal source of ochratoxin in produce in warm and tropical regions. About a quarter of the world's grains are contaminated with mycotoxins, and this contamination is expected to increase with climate warming. For example, in Serbia in 2012, warmer weather was associated with 69% of the corn crop being contaminated with mycotoxins, in an area that had previously been unaffected.[5]

OTA has considerable toxicity to the kidney, perhaps because it is concentrated by the kidney for excretion. OTA exposure is associated with kidney damage and kidney cancer. Nevertheless, the enterocytes lining the intestine likely have the highest exposure to OTA of any cells in the body. OTA inhibits cell growth, inhibits protein synthesis, and impairs sodium-dependent glucose transport in the enterocytes, but increases fructose uptake. OTA lowers transepithelial resistance, an indicator of paracellular permeability. This alteration of the tight junctions between cells then likely allows for an increased absorption of OTA, along with other toxic compounds, into the body.[6] In swine, 66% of a dose of OTA is absorbed, mostly by diffusion. Intestinal absorption is limited (at least in health) by the export of the toxin from the apical surface of the enterocytes back into the lumen. OTA that is absorbed is carried by the portal circulation to the liver, and then into the rest of the body.[7]

OTA adversely impacts the GI microbiome. Some of the alterations to the biome are likely secondary to the toxic effects on the intestinal mucosa, but the OTA also inhibits the growth and metabolism of some bacteria.[8] Feeding OTA to mice causes alterations in the microbiome of the gut. Treated mice had lower levels of *Bacteroides*, *Dorea*, *Escherichia*, *Oribacterium*, *Ruminococcus*, and *Syntrophococcus* and higher levels of *Lactobacillaceae*. In this study, *Lactobacillaceae* was found to absorb and sequester OTA, but did not appear to break it down.[9] This shift in the GI microbiome seen in these mice, when exposed to OTA, is similar to that seen in a meta-analysis of children with autism spectrum disorder (ASD) as compared to peers. [10]

An Italian study, including 172 children with autism and 61 controls, found that blood serum levels of aflatoxin M1, ochratoxin A, and fumonisin B1 were significantly elevated among those with autism. This result is surprising, as siblings of children with ASD served as many of the control subjects, and would thus have been expected to have similar dietary exposure.[11] This suggests that the children with ASD may 1) have leaky gut, and thus absorb higher amounts of these toxins, 2) have differences in OTA sequestration or destruction by the microbiome, or 3) may be less adept at ridding the toxins from their bodies as a result of differences in biotransformation by cytochrome P450 enzymes that detoxify these toxins.

A study including 52 ASD children without genetic syndrome-related autism and 58 healthy controls, including 31 siblings, examined OTA levels in the serum and urine. The *median serum* OTA levels were 0.20 ng/ml in the ASD group, 0.10 ng/ml in the unaffected siblings, and 0.05 ng/ml in the unrelated controls. Median urinary levels were the same in all three groups, suggesting a poorer renal clearance of OTA. *Mean* plasma to urine OTC ratios were 6.67:1 for the ASD group, 4.5:1 for the healthy sib group, and 1.51:1 for the non-related control group. The authors noted that some of the relevant P450 enzymes that act on these mycotoxins are less active in males, under the effect of testosterone, which might explain the increased prevalence of autism in boys.[12] It should be noted that the contemporaneous presence of these toxins may represent host susceptibility, rather than concluding that these toxins caused the neurologic changes leading to autism. The injuries that cause autism most often occur in the early prenatal period. It is plausible that ochratoxin A exposure can promote leaky gut, alter the intestinal biome during pregnancy in the mother, injure or kill neurons, and thus may cause neurodevelopmental injury or delay.

OTA is neurotoxic during the neonatal period in lab animals, causing a reduction in brain weight, particularly in the cerebellar region, where it also causes a deranged cortical structure.[13] Prenatally exposed mice were found to have developmental delays in coordination.[14] At high doses, OTA is teratogenic during critical stages of pregnancy, causing fetal malformations.[15] Prenatal OTA exposure caused microcephaly. There was thinning of the cortex with an increased number of neurons in the somatosensory cortex, but a 28% decrease in the number of synapses per neuron.[16] Normally, axons and dendrites constitute about 60% of cortical volume, so this explains the thinner cortex.[17] OTA is also toxic to the adult brain of mice, causing necrosis of neurons, especially in the midbrain, hippocampus, and striatum.[18] The toxin accumulates in the brain and inhibits protein and DNA synthesis, with neurons being more susceptible to cytotoxicity than are the astrocytes.[19] Much of the neurotoxicity caused by OTA appears to be mediated by oxidative stress.[20]

If OTA promotes leaky gut and ASD in children, it should be assumed to promote leaky gut and neurodegeneration in adults as well.

OTA is also immunotoxic and can cause immunosuppression; it causes a reduction in the size of the spleen, thymus, and lymph nodes, and depression of antibody response and immune modulation. OTA diminishes cytotoxic T lymphocyte activity and reduces the bacteriolytic capability of macrophages.[21] [22] OTA-induced immunosuppression may account for its carcinogenicity.

A study from Europe estimated that the average daily intake of OTA was 33 ng, with 55% of that coming from the consumption of grain.[23] These toxins get into the food supply, and even though the mold may be killed by cooking, the toxin is not destroyed. The toxin is not only found in food but also in water-damaged buildings and heating ducts. When "black mold" is present in a building, it often contains OTA.

Mold loves to grow on food, and has likely evolved the toxin to kill off competitor microbes; OTA is toxic to many bacteria. Rapid drying of grains and other produce greatly limits the growth of molds. For most grains, getting the moisture content below 13–14% halts the growth of the mold and the production of the toxins. Wet harvest conditions can make this impossible.

Mycotoxins in grain fed to animals cause large economic losses; in the U.S., in normal years, mycotoxins cause losses of about $900 million due to lower productivity, susceptibility to disease, and direct toxicity and death of farm animals. Ochratoxin concentrates in the liver and kidneys, so high levels can be found in organ meats and meat products such as salami, which are made from these organs. While many farm animals (swine and fowls) are harmed by OTA toxicity from the grain they are fed, cattle appear not to be affected, as the toxin is degraded, apparently by protozoa in the rumen, greatly limiting bioavailability to these animals.[24]

The typical levels of OTA in the diet might do very little harm to normal individuals, or we would all be in trouble. However, high amounts of OTA from an occasional highly contaminated meal could rise to the level that disrupts the gut microbiome, the mucosal barrier, or causes neurologic injury. If this is the case, then those with difficulty clearing the toxin from their system would be at much greater risk when exposed to a contaminated meal, and especially when food with OTA contamination is consumed repeatedly for several days. The serum half-life of OTA varies among animals; it is about 8 hours in rabbits and 89 hours in pigs, but is generally shorter in smaller animals.[25] Elimination of OTA from the body may be enhanced with xenobiotics that induce certain microsomal P450 enzymes, while other compounds may increase its toxicity.[26]

The fungi that produce OTA in food also produce other mycotoxins, including aflatoxins (AFs), deoxynivalenol (DON), T-2 toxin, zearalenone, and fumonisins. Thus, when food contains one mycotoxin, it likely also contains other toxins. (Think of them as freebies.) Thus, when one toxin is associated with disease in a natural setting, it can be hard to distinguish which toxin, or combination of mycotoxins, actually caused the injury or disease.

AFs are easily absorbed and are an important cause of liver cancer. OTA and fumonisins are not easily absorbed by the enterocytes; thus, they are present throughout the GI tract, and they have more opportunity to affect the GI microbiome. Like OTA, DON affects mucosal immunity, microbiome diversity, and barrier integrity.

OTA and DON in chickens and pigs promote the overgrowth of intestinal *Salmonella,* which may then increase human exposure to *Salmonella* through meat and eggs.[27]

Aflatoxins

Aflatoxins, OTA, and other mycotoxins are produced by several species of Aspergillus, Penicillium, and other molds that live in the soil and help break down decaying vegetable matter. When plants are stressed from drought, water-soaked soils, insect damage, or are poorly adapted to the climate or soil where they are grown, the plant's defenses are weakened. This allows these molds to flourish. These molds can also grow on harvested foods that are stored in warm, humid conditions. In many less-developed areas of the world, grain is often stored in dirt-floored rooms or other less-than-ideal conditions. Improperly stored grain can easily support the growth of molds, and such grain can easily be contaminated with fungal toxins. Mold can also grow in our homes.

Two of the food crops most commonly affected by *Aspergillus* and contaminated with aflatoxin are peanuts, which are affected while still in the ground, and corn that is affected post-harvest. Other crops that may be affected include cereals (wheat, rice, sorghum, and millet), oilseed plants (soybean, sunflower, cotton, and coconut), tree nuts, ginger, peppers (the vegetables, rather than peppercorns), dried figs, vine-dried fruits, and spices.[28] Aflatoxin is so common in peanuts that, despite the use of advanced farming practices to prevent it, aflatoxin is present in trace amounts in almost all peanut butter sold in the United States.

The FDA sets a limit on the aflatoxin content of foods that may be sold.[29] In a study performed in Texas, the foods associated with the highest aflatoxin intake were rice, corn tortillas, and tree nuts; however, not peanut butter or other corn products.[30] The levels encountered in the tortillas tested were high enough to impart risks and be of concern.

Presently, *OTA levels in foods are not regulated in the United States*. Standards should be set.

While aflatoxin toxicity is not thought to be a major carcinogen in the United States, about 70% of the human population is exposed to significant amounts of aflatoxins in their food. This contamination is especially common for those living in warm climates and in areas where food harvest and storage methods do not prevent *Aspergillus* contamination.[31]

Aflatoxins are acute toxins with high case-fatality rates, usually associated with the consumption of corn that has molded. Many outbreaks of acute aflatoxin toxicity have occurred in India and Africa. Acute toxicity can result in liver necrosis. Chronic, lower-level toxin exposure can result in liver cirrhosis. This toxin crosses the placenta and is associated with growth retardation of children in countries where significant amounts of aflatoxin are found in food.[32] These toxins appear more potent and deadly to poorly nourished individuals.

The dangers caused by fungal toxin exposure are growing with global climate change, which supports conditions that favor the robust growth of these molds. *Aspergillus flavus,* a species that produces aflatoxin, prefers drier climates and grows well in the Great Plains of the U.S. In the year 2012, it caused nearly $200 million in losses from *acute toxicity* deaths of farm animals in the U.S.. Aflatoxin contamination also forced a nationwide pet food recall, but not before many companion animals were killed.[33]

Claiming a far greater death toll than it does as an acute poison, aflatoxin is a potent carcinogen. It causes DNA alkylation adducts, resulting in liver cancer. Aflatoxin adducts cause mutations in the p53 gene,[34] a gene that signals for apoptosis, and which helps prevent cells with DNA errors from reproducing. Thus, aflatoxin adducts promote cancer development by preventing p53-induced apoptosis.

Individuals exposed to aflatoxin are 3.4 times more likely to develop hepatocellular carcinoma (HCC). Aflatoxin can cause HCC by itself, but is even more dangerous as a co-carcinogen with hepatitis B (HBV) infection. The presence of hepatitis B surface antigens in the blood, evidence of ongoing HBV disease, increases the risk of HCC by about 7.3 times. Individuals who have HBV surface antigens *and* who are exposed to aflatoxins have nearly 60 times the risk of developing HCC as individuals with neither of these risk factors.[35] HBV infection raises the rate of hepatocyte replacement, and the mycotoxin forms a DNA adduct that causes a loss of p53 function. This creates a perfect storm with more cells dividing, and protection from DNA errors is lost. This interaction amplifies the risk of HCC. In the United States, the HBV infection rate is fairly low, as is the intake of aflatoxin. In China, HBV infection is endemic. In Southeast Asia and parts of Africa, the deadly combination of HVB and aflatoxin exposure is common. Hepatitis C can also cause hepatocellular carcinoma, but it does not appear to interact with aflatoxin. Aflatoxin-induced HCC is common in China,[36] Taiwan,[37] Mexico, and many other regions. It is estimated that nearly a quarter of the 782,000 new cases of HCC each year worldwide are attributable to aflatoxin exposure.[38] [39] Aflatoxin adducts leave molecular traces that can be detected in HCC tumors. Aflatoxin adducts were found in 6 percent of HCC cases in Japan,[40] a country with low levels of exposure to these toxins. In a very small study, about five percent of HCC cases in the U.S. were associated with aflatoxin exposure.[41]

Fumonisins

While aflatoxin is the best studied and most well-known of the fungal carcinogens, it is not the only one common in food. Three hundred to four hundred mycotoxins have been identified, but only about a dozen are recognized as causing a significant burden of animal and human disease. Fungi, including mushrooms, are chemical factories. They make many B vitamins, vitamin D2, ergothioneine, and penicillin. They also produce alcohol, the hallucinogen LSD, and many other toxins. In addition to aflatoxin, two other mycotoxins that appear in the human food supply have been identified as probable carcinogens: OTA and Fumonisins. Fumonisins are common in corn and are associated with esophageal cancer.

There are over fifty species of *Fusarium* fungi that produce toxins, and their toxins, the fumonisins, are not a single chemical class of toxins, but a diverse set of toxins that includes trichothecene and T-2 mycotoxins. Fumonisin B is a neurotoxin that has a large adverse economic impact on agriculture. In a five-year span in the 1990s, during which the weather was wetter than usual, losses to wheat and barley from *Fusarium* fungal contamination totaled more than three billion dollars. *Fusarium* also grows on corn and other grains. This fungus and its toxins are neurotoxic to farm animals that are fed contaminated grain and cause losses of livestock. It is also an acute toxin that can cause abdominal pain, diarrhea, liver damage, and kidney damage. In Russia during the 1930s, *Fusarium*-contaminated grain that was baked into bread led to several outbreaks of acute toxicity. Sixty percent of those affected died, resulting in the deaths of 100,000 persons.

Fumonisin B1, unlike aflatoxin, does not cause DNA adducts and is not genotoxic. Fumonisin B1 acts as a toxin by blocking the enzyme ceramide synthase, which promotes the formation of sphingosine-1-phosphate

(S1P). SIP supports growth and repair, and also supports the growth of tumor cells. Fumonisin B is also a teratogen that causes neural tube defects, such as anencephaly, in humans (in which the fetus forms without a brain).

Fumonisin B is a suspected carcinogen for esophageal cancer in various parts of the world, including within the United States.[42] Mostly, fumonisin B consumption is associated with moldy corn. However, fumonisin B and other *Fusarium* toxins are found on other crops, and also in brine-pickled foods (including fish) where *Fusarium* participate in the fermentation process.

Avoiding Mycotoxins

Ochratoxin A toxin can often be obtained at your local grocer on onions, shallots, and garlic, as well as in cereals, coffee, dried fruit, and red wine. If contaminated foods are eaten, the toxin passes into milk, including human milk.

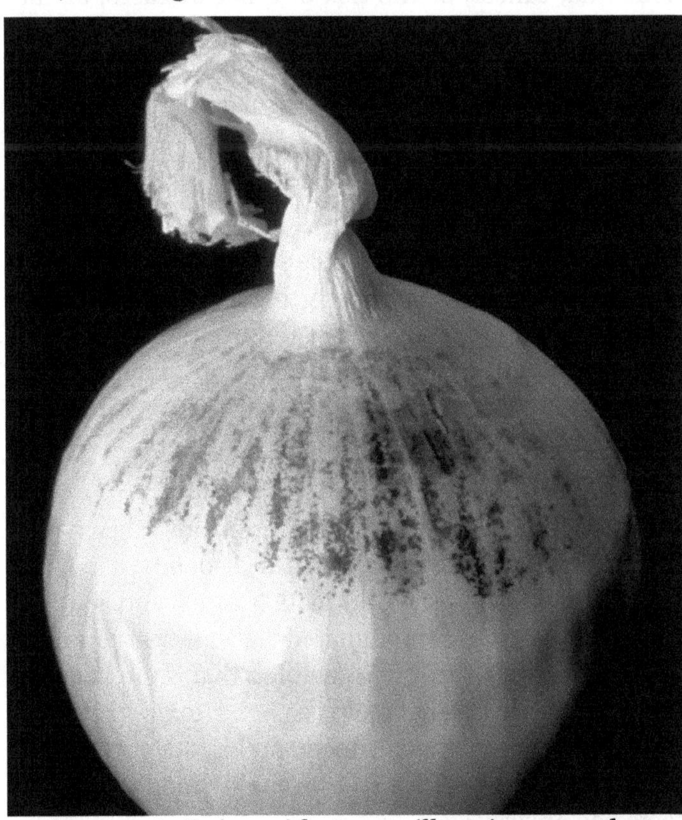

Figure 27A: Onion with *Aspergillus niger* growth.[43]

The black fruiting bodies of *Aspergillus niger* can be seen in the outer layer of the onion in Figure 27A. Note additionally, the softening and depressions around the middle of the onion that was caused by the digestion of pectin in the onion. The mycelium and toxins they produced are most likely spread throughout this onion; the fruiting bodies are visible as a result of their dark color. Some, but not all, strains of *Aspergillus niger* produce the toxin and carcinogen ochratoxin A. Peeling away the black fruiting bodies on the outer layers does not remove the fungus that has invaded the inside layers of the onion. The fruiting bodies are like mushrooms growing out of a log; the fungus is everywhere inside the log; the mushrooms are just the fruiting bodies you can see. The toxin is everywhere the fungus grows.

Rice is commonly contaminated with fungal toxins. In a study of rice grown in the southern United States, 100 samples were tested. All contained aflatoxin.[44] A study from Europe found that imported rice commonly exceeded permissible levels of mycotoxins.[45]

Washing rice can remove some of the fungal spores and may slightly reduce the amount of toxins present. Cooking, and especially pressure cooking rice, lowers the OTA concentration of the rice by 59 to 75%, and pressure cooking further reduces the toxicity of OTA by 20%.[46] Cooking rice also decreases aflatoxin B1 levels in rice and lowers its toxicity.[47] More thorough cooking, longer cooking times, higher temperatures, using more water, and more complete gelation of starches reduce OTA levels and their toxicity. Thus, pre-soaking grains and legumes and increasing the amount of water used reduces OTA levels. Fermentation, as occurs in sourdough bread, lowers OTA levels. Soaking/washing beans in baking soda decreases OTA levels. Washing black pepper with an acetic acid solution lowered OTA levels by about 25%.[48]

Brown Rice: Buy quality brown rice. I purchased American (Louisiana) grown brown rice that, upon close inspection, has numerous partially black grains, and when rinsed after removal of these grains, gave a dirty grey rinse water. Washing rice before cooking it is recommended as it decreases arsenic and mycotoxin levels. The rinse water should not be grey. If this occurs, look for a different brand of brown rice.

The Nixtamalization process used to make masa harina for corn tortillas and hominy reduces the levels of the mycotoxins aflatoxin B1 and fumonisin, generally by 85 to 90 percent.[49] [50] While it is likely that the OTA levels are also minimized by nixtamalization, and several studies found reductions in AFB1 and fumonisin, ochratoxin levels in corn were not addressed.

In yogurt, in an in vitro culture method that may or may not correspond to fermentation in the gut, OTA was completely degraded by *Lactobacillus bulgaricus* and *Streptococcus thermophilus,* and partially degraded by *Bifidobacterium bifidum*.[51] Other enteric genera that have been shown to participate in OTA detoxification are *Acinetobacter, Bacillus,* i.e., *B. subtilis,* and *Eubacterium,* i.e., *E. callanderi*.[52] A healthy GI microbiome may decrease risk from this and similar toxins.

Lessons in Cancer Prevention

Green tea polyphenols have been shown to reduce biomarkers of aflatoxins by over 40%.[53] Black tea polyphenols have also been shown to inhibit DNA adduct formation by lowering the activity of CYP1A1 and CYP1A2.[54]

Lycopene, an antioxidant carotenoid found in tomatoes and certain other fruits (watermelon, guava, papaya, and apricots), also shifts the metabolism of aflatoxin B1, reducing the formation of aflatoxin DNA-adducts to a less toxic metabolite (aflatoxin M1), which is excreted in the urine.[55] However, tomato purée has a more vigorous anti-mutagenic effect in mice exposed to aflatoxin B1 than does pure lycopene.[56] In another study, two other carotenoids, canthaxanthin and astaxanthin, were more effective than lycopene at shifting aflatoxin B1 metabolism to aflatoxin M1 and in preventing DNA adducts and tumor formation. Beta-carotene, the precursor of vitamin A, had no effect.[57] Foods high in astaxanthin include wild-caught salmon, trout, shrimp, and crab.

Dietary chlorophyll, found in green leaves, is highly effective in reducing hepatic DNA adducts in rats exposed to dietary aflatoxin B1 and helps prevent the development of premalignant tumors in the liver and colon. Here, the mechanism is different and preferable to that for tea and tomatoes. Chlorophyll binds to aflatoxin in the diet and prevents it from being absorbed into the body.[58]

Thus, green tea polyphenols (well, perhaps only epigallocatechin-3-gallate), certain carotenoid compounds (but not beta-carotene), and chlorophyll can prevent aflatoxin B1-induced cancers. Since chlorophyll, carotenoids, and green tea polyphenols act through different mechanisms, a diet containing a combination of these would be expected to provide even more comprehensive protection.

But before you run off to your corner NSC (Nutritional Supplement Center) and load up on green tea polyphenols, chlorophyll, and astaxanthin capsules to undo the damage, consider the timing in the mechanisms of these agents. Chlorophyll needs to be in the same meal as the toxin to prevent its absorption. If you have a contaminated corn tortilla for breakfast, a noontime spinach salad will be too late to prevent the absorption of the aflatoxin. And since carotenoids act by inducing the P450 enzymes, they need to be consumed a day or so before exposure to be up and running when the toxin is absorbed to assist in its metabolism. Consuming these compounds after exposure to aflatoxin would be like putting on a Kevlar vest after a gunfight to treat the wounds.

The best bet is to avoid exposure to these and other carcinogens and to have healthy, sustainable eating habits.

Building materials, such as sound-deadening ceiling tiles, easily become sources of black mold, often when there is condensation from air-conditioning ducts. Non-toxic antifungal agents can be added during the manufacture of building materials that are susceptible to molding. Mold-resistant building materials should be mandated for schools and workplaces where there may be children, pregnant women, or other humans of value.

Summary for Fungal Toxins

Obviously, fungal toxins should be avoided. The toxins cannot be seen and are rarely measured. It is hard to assess the impact of these foodborne toxins on dementia, cancer, or the risk of other diseases, as they are hidden in food. Many fungal toxins are inadequately studied and are not tested for. OTA is well known to be toxic, but levels in food are not regulated.

Mold-contaminated foods should be discarded; they are not fit for animals, as they are at just as much risk from these toxins as we are. Just cutting away the fruiting body that makes visible spores does not remove the mold that is typically growing throughout the contaminated food, nor does it remove the toxins. Food with just a little mold on one section should not be salvaged. A handful of mold-contaminated corn kernels contains sufficient toxins to make a truckload of corn illegal to sell into interstate commerce.

Although improperly stored grain is the typical culprit, fruits and vegetables are also hosts to these fungi. Dried figs, prunes, apricots, raisins, and sundried tomatoes can be contaminated. Don't eat or allow children to eat fruit or vegetables that show signs of mold. While this paints molds as being toxic with a very wide brush, even though most molds do not produce carcinogens, why take a risk on moldy food that would taste bad anyway?

The correlation between aflatoxin urinary metabolites and intake of corn tortillas, rice, and tree nuts suggests that the FDA may need to reassess monitoring of aflatoxins for these in foods in the U.S. Aflatoxins are just one of at least several fungal toxins found in food that cause human disease.

Green tea may help prevent aflatoxin-DNA adduct formation.

Not all fungi are toxic or carcinogenic. Some food molds, such as those in blue and gorgonzola cheese, have insignificant toxicity in the amounts typically consumed. Many mushrooms are non-toxic, flavorful, and nutritious, and at least several types of mushrooms have anti-carcinogenic properties. At least 20 different types of mushrooms are currently under study as potential cancer treatments for their antitumor, antioxidant, and immune-stimulating properties. Several of these are culinary mushrooms, including shiitake, white button mushrooms, maitake, and lion's mane mushrooms.[59]

[1] Biomolecular characterization, identification, enzyme activities of molds and physiological changes in sweet potatoes (Ipomea batatas) stored under controlled atmospheric conditions. Oladoye CO, Connerton IF, Kayode RMO, Omojasola PF, Kayode IB. J Zhejiang Univ Sci B. 2016 Apr;17(4):317–32. doi: 10.1631/jzus.B1400328. PMCID: PMC4829637.

[2] Hepatocellular carcinoma: epidemiology and risk factors. Kew MC. J Hepatocell Carcinoma. 2014 Aug 13;1:115-25. PMID:27508181

[3] Aflatoxin Exposure and Associated Human Health Effects, a Review of Epidemiological Studies. Yun Yun Gonga, Sinead Watsona, and Michael N Routledge. 2016 Food Safety Commission, Cabinet Office, Government of Japan http://dx.doi.org/10.14252/foodsafetyfscj.2015026

[4] Biochemical characterization of ochratoxin A-producing strains of the genus Penicillium. Larsen TO, Svendsen A, Smedsgaard J. Appl Environ Microbiol. 2001 Aug;67(8):3630-5. doi: 10.1128/AEM.67.8.3630-3635.2001. PMID: 11472940

[5] Mycotoxin: Its Impact on Gut Health and Microbiota. Liew WP, Mohd-Redzwan S. Front Cell Infect Microbiol. 2018 Feb 26;8:60. doi: 10.3389/fcimb.2018.00060. PMID: 29535978

[6] The mycotoxin ochratoxin A alters intestinal barrier and absorption functions but has no effect on chloride secretion. Maresca M, Mahfoud R, Pfohl-Leszkowicz A, Fantini J. Toxicol Appl Pharmacol. 2001 Oct 1;176(1):54-63. doi: 10.1006/taap.2001.9254. PMID: 11578148

[7] Toxicokinetics and toxicodynamics of ochratoxin A, an update. Ringot D, Chango A, Schneider YJ, Larondelle Y. Chem Biol Interact. 2006 Jan 5;159(1):18-46. doi: 10.1016/j.cbi.2005.10.106. PMID:16293235

[8] Effects of Dietary Mycotoxins on Gut Microbiome. Du K, Wang C, Liu P, Li Y, Ma X. Protein Pept Lett. 2017 May 10;24(5):397-405. doi: 10.2174/0929866524666170223095207. PMID: 28240164

[9] Combination of metagenomics and culture-based methods to study the interaction between ochratoxin a and gut microbiota. Guo M, Huang K, Chen S, Qi X, He X, Cheng WH, Luo Y, Xia K, Xu W. Toxicol Sci. 2014 Sep;141(1):314-23. doi: 10.1093/toxsci/kfu128. PMID: 24973096

[10] Association Between Gut Microbiota and Autism Spectrum Disorder: A Systematic Review and Meta-Analysis. Xu M, Xu X, Li J, Li F. Front Psychiatry. 2019 Jul 17;10:473. doi: 10.3389/fpsyt.2019.00473. PMID: 31404299

[11] Study on the Association among Mycotoxins and other Variables in Children with Autism. De Santis B, Raggi ME, Moretti G, Facchiano F, Mezzelani A, Villa L, Bonfanti A, Campioni A, Rossi S, Camposeo S, Soricelli S, Moracci G, Debegnach F, Gregori E, Ciceri F, Milanesi L, Marabotti A, Brera C. Toxins (Basel). 2017 Jun 29;9(7):203. doi: 10.3390/toxins9070203. PMID: 28661468

[12] Role of mycotoxins in the pathobiology of autism: A first evidence. De Santis B, Brera C, Mezzelani A, Soricelli S, Ciceri F, Moretti G, Debegnach F, Bonaglia MC, Villa L, Molteni M, Raggi ME. Nutr Neurosci. 2019 Feb;22(2):132-144. doi: 10.1080/1028415X.2017.1357793. PMID: 28795659

[13] Developmental abnormalities of mouse cerebellum induced by intracisternal injection of ochratoxin A in neonatal period. Fukui Y, Hoshino K, Kameyama Y. Exp Neurol. 1987 Oct;98(1):54-66. doi: 10.1016/0014-4886(87)90071-9. PMID: 3653334

[14] Postnatal behavioral effects of ochratoxin A in offspring of treated mice. Poppe SM, Stuckhardt JL, Szczech GM. Teratology. 1983 Jun;27(3):293-300. doi: 10.1002/tera.1420270302. PMID: 6879452

[15] Critical period and minimum single oral dose of ochratoxin A for inducing developmental toxicity in pregnant Wistar rats. Patil RD, Dwivedi P, Sharma AK. Reprod Toxicol. 2006 Nov;22(4):679-87. doi: 10.1016/j.reprotox.2006.04.022. PMID: 16781114

[16] Regional difference in the neurotoxicity of ochratoxin A on the developing cerebral cortex in mice. Miki T, Fukui Y, Uemura N, Takeuchi Y. Brain Res Dev Brain Res. 1994 Oct 14;82(1-2):259-64. doi: 10.1016/0165-3806(94)90168-6. PMID: 7842513

[17] Normal development of brain circuits. Tau GZ, Peterson BS. Neuropsychopharmacology. 2010 Jan;35(1):147-68. doi: 10.1038/npp.2009.115. PMID: 19794405

[18] Regional selectivity to ochratoxin A, distribution and cytotoxicity in rat brain. Belmadani A, Tramu G, Betbeder AM, Steyn PS, Creppy EE. Arch Toxicol. 1998 Oct;72(10):656-62. doi: 10.1007/s002040050557. PMID: 9851682

[19] Selective toxicity of ochratoxin A in primary cultures from different brain regions. Belmadani A, Steyn PS, Tramu G, Betbeder AM, Baudrimont I, Creppy EE. Arch Toxicol. 1999 Mar;73(2):108-14. doi: 10.1007/s002040050594. PMID: 10350191

[20] Mechanisms of mycotoxin-induced neurotoxicity through oxidative stress-associated pathways. Doi K, Uetsuka K. Int J Mol Sci. 2011;12(8):5213-37. doi: 10.3390/ijms12085213. PMID: 21954354

[21] Immunotoxic effects of Ochratoxin A in Wistar rats after oral administration. Alvarez L, Gil AG, Ezpeleta O, García-Jalón JA, López de Cerain A. Food Chem Toxicol. 2004 May;42(5):825-34. doi: 10.1016/j.fct.2004.01.005. PMID: 15046829

[22] Immunotoxic activity of ochratoxin A. Al-Anati L, Petzinger E. J Vet Pharmacol Ther. 2006 Apr;29(2):79-90. doi: 10.1111/j.1365-2885.2006.00718.x. PMID: 16515661

[23] Risk Assessment of Ochratoxin a in The Netherlands. Bakker M., Pieters M. 2003. Rijksinstituut voor Volksgezondheid en Milieu RIVM https://rivm.openrepository.com/handle/10029/9185

[24] Effects of ochratoxin a on livestock production. Battacone G, Nudda A, Pulina G. Toxins (Basel). 2010 Jul;2(7):1796-824. doi: 10.3390/toxins2071796. PMID: 22069661

[25] Effects of ochratoxin a on livestock production. Battacone G, Nudda A, Pulina G. Toxins (Basel). 2010 Jul;2(7):1796-824. doi: 10.3390/toxins2071796. PMID: 22069661

26 Effect of cytochrome P450 induction on the metabolism and toxicity of ochratoxin A. Omar RF, Gelboin HV, Rahimtula AD. Biochem Pharmacol. 1996 Feb 9;51(3):207-16. doi: 10.1016/0006-2952(95)02194-9. PMID: 8573185

27 Modulation of intestinal functions following mycotoxin ingestion: meta-analysis of published experiments in animals. Grenier B, Applegate TJ. Toxins (Basel). 2013 Feb 21;5(2):396-430. doi: 10.3390/toxins5020396. PMID: 23430606

28 Mycotoxins in botanicals and dried fruits: a review. Trucksess MW, Scott PM. Food Addit Contam Part A Chem Anal Control Expo Risk Assess. 2008 Feb;25(2):181-92. PMID:18286408

29 Guidance for Industry: Action Levels for Poisonous or Deleterious Substances in Human Food and Animal Feed. August 2000.

30 Aflatoxin and PAH exposure biomarkers in a U.S. population with a high incidence of hepatocellular carcinoma. Johnson NM, Qian G, Xu L, et al. Sci Total Environ. 2010 Nov 1;408(23):6027-31. PMID:20870273

31 Costs and efficacy of public health interventions to reduce aflatoxin-induced human disease. Khlangwiset P, Wu F. Food Addit Contam Part A Chem Anal Control Expo Risk Assess. 2010 Jul;27(7):998-1014. PMID:20419532

32 Mycotoxins and human disease: a largely ignored global health issue. Wild CP, Gong YY. Carcinogenesis. 2010 Jan;31(1):71-82. PMID:19875698

33 Fortified by Global Warming, Deadly Fungus Poisons Corn Crops, Causes Cancer. Mollie Bloudoff-Indelicato Scientific American Jan. 15, 2013

34 Aflatoxin genotoxicity is associated with a defective DNA damage response bypassing p53 activation. Gursoy-Yuzugullu O, Yuzugullu H, Yilmaz M, Ozturk M. Liver Int. 2011 Apr;31(4):561-71. PMID:21382167

35 A follow-up study of urinary markers of aflatoxin exposure and liver cancer risk in Shanghai, People's Republic of China. Qian GS, Ross RK, Yu MC, Yuan JM, Gao YT, Henderson BE, Wogan GN, Groopman JD. Cancer Epidemiol Biomarkers Prev. 1994 Jan-Feb;3(1):3-10. PMID:8118382

36 Hepatitis B, aflatoxin B(1), and p53 codon 249 mutation in hepatocellular carcinomas from Guangxi, People's Republic of China, and a meta-analysis of existing studies. Stern MC, Umbach DM, Yu MC, et al. Cancer Epidemiol Biomarkers Prev. 2001 Jun;10(6):617-25. PMID:11401911

37 p53 mutations, chronic hepatitis B virus infection, and aflatoxin exposure in hepatocellular carcinoma in Taiwan. Lunn RM, Zhang YJ, Wang LY, et al. Cancer Res. 1997 Aug 15;57(16):3471-7. PMID:9270015

38 http://globocan.iarc.fr/Pages/fact_sheets_cancer.aspx Accessed Oct. 2015

39 Population attributable risk of aflatoxin-related liver cancer: systematic review and meta-analysis. Liu Y, Chang CC, Marsh GM, Wu F. Eur J Cancer. 2012 Sep;48(14):2125-36. PMID:22405700

40 Hepatic aflatoxin B1-DNA adducts and TP53 mutations in patients with hepatocellular carcinoma despite low exposure to aflatoxin B1 in southern Japan. Shirabe K, Toshima T, Taketomi A, et al. Liver Int. 2011 Oct;31(9):1366-72. PMID:21745313

41 Does aflatoxin B1 play a role in the etiology of hepatocellular carcinoma in the United States? Hoque A, Patt YZ, Yoffe B, Groopman JD, Greenblatt MS, Zhang YJ, Santella RM. Nutr Cancer. 1999;35(1):27-33. PMID:10624703

42 Mycotoxins. Bennett JW, Klich M. Clin Microbiol Rev. 2003 Jul;16(3):497-516. PMID:12857779

43 Photo by S.K. Mohan, Bugwood.org

44 Mycotoxin Contamination of Rice Grown in the Southern USA. Shier, W.T., Abbas, H.K.. Proceedings of the 8th International Society on Toxinology Asian-Pacific Meeting on Animal Plant and Microbial Toxins, Hanoi, Vietnam, Dec. 2-6, Page 90. 2008

45 Mycotoxins Contamination in Rice: Analytical Methods, Occurrence and Detoxification Strategies. Santos AR, Carreiró F, Freitas A, Barros S, Brites C, Ramos F, Sanches Silva A. Toxins (Basel). 2022 Sep 19;14(9):647. doi: 10.3390/toxins14090647. PMID: 36136585

46 Fate of ochratoxin a during cooking of naturally contaminated polished rice. Park JW, Chung SH, Lee C, Kim YB. J Food Prot. 2005 Oct;68(10):2107-11. doi: 10.4315/0362-028x-68.10.2107. PMID: 16245714

47 Fate of aflatoxin B1 during the cooking of Korean polished rice. Park JW, Lee C, Kim YB. J Food Prot. 2005 Jul;68(7):1431-4. doi: 10.4315/0362-028x-68.7.1431. PMID: 16013381

48 Practical Strategies to Reduce Ochratoxin A in Foods. Lee HJ, Kim HD, Ryu D. Toxins (Basel). 2024 Jan 20;16(1):58. doi: 10.3390/toxins16010058. PMID: 38276534

49 Effect of Nixtamalization on Mycotoxin-Contaminated Corn. José Rodrigo Mendoza and Andréia Bianchini. Nebraska Extension. Jan, 2021 G2329· Index: Food Science & Technology. https://extensionpubs.unl.edu/publication/g2329/na/html/view

50 Mycotoxins during the Processes of Nixtamalization and Tortilla Production. Schaarschmidt S, Fauhl-Hassek C. Toxins (Basel). 2019 Apr 16;11(4):227. doi: 10.3390/toxins11040227. PMID: 30995755

51 Lowering of ochratoxin A level in milk by yoghurt bacteria and bifidobacteria. Skrinjar M, Rasić JL, Stojicić V. Folia Microbiol (Praha). 1996;41(1):26-8. doi: 10.1007/BF02816335. PMID: 9090820

52 Combination of metagenomics and culture-based methods to study the interaction between ochratoxin a and gut microbiota. Guo M, Huang K, Chen S, Qi X, He X, Cheng WH, Luo Y, Xia K, Xu W. Toxicol Sci. 2014 Sep;141(1):314-23. doi: 10.1093/toxsci/kfu128. PMID: 24973096

53 Modulation of aflatoxin biomarkers in human blood and urine by green tea polyphenols intervention. Tang L, Tang M, Xu L, Luo H, Huang T, Yu J, Zhang L, Gao W, Cox SB, Wang JS. Carcinogenesis. 2008 Feb;29(2):411-7. PMID:18192689

54 Inhibitory effect(s) of polymeric black tea polyphenols on the formation of B(a)P-derived DNA adducts in mouse skin. Krishnan R, Maru GB. J Environ Pathol Toxicol Oncol. 2005;24(2):79-90. PMID:15831081

55 Modulation of aflatoxin toxicity and biomarkers by lycopene in F344 rats. Tang L, Guan H, Ding X, Wang JS. Toxicol Appl Pharmacol. 2007 Feb 15;219(1):10-7. PMID:17229449

56 Antimutagenic effects of lycopene and tomato purée. Polívková Z, Šmerák P, Demová H, Houška M. J Med Food. 2010 Dec;13(6):1443-50. PMID:20874227

57 Dietary carotenoids inhibit aflatoxin B1-induced liver preneoplastic foci and DNA damage in the rat: role of the modulation of aflatoxin B1 metabolism. Gradelet S, Le Bon AM, Bergès R, Suschetet M, Astorg P. Carcinogenesis. 1998 Mar;19(3):403-11. PMID:9525273

58 Natural chlorophyll inhibits aflatoxin B1-induced multi-organ carcinogenesis in the rat. Simonich MT, Egner PA, Roebuck BD, et al.Carcinogenesis. 2007 Jun;28(6):1294-302. PMID:17290047

59 Recent developments in mushrooms as anti-cancer therapeutics: a review. Patel S, Goyal A. 3 Biotech. 2012 Mar;2(1):1-15. PMID:22582152

28: Time-Restricted Eating

Diegesis:

Time-restricted eating (TRE) is a popular regimen that is advocated as a means of maintaining and improving health. TRE is a specific form of Intermittent Fasting (which is not otherwise a topic here). In TRE, meals are eaten within an 8 – 12 hour window during the day, and the person fasts for the remaining 12 – 16 hours of each day, including the sleep cycle. Thus, if breakfast is eaten at 7:30 A.M., and supper is completed by 7:30 P.M., with no more food or snacks until the next morning, that would be a 12:12 TRE, which gives 12 hours of fasting and 12 hours during which meals may be consumed. No popcorn while watching Netflix after 7:30 PM, no midnight snacks.

A 16:8 TRE is much more commonly studied, and considerably more restrictive, and would, for example, limit the hours the kitchen and dining hall are open from 7 AM to 3 PM or from 11 AM to 7 PM.

If a 16:8 fasting-to-feeding time ratio does not sound like fun to you, you might be right. Skipping breakfast is associated with a 21% increased risk of type 2 diabetes (T2D).[1] Worse, skipping breakfast is associated with a 27% increased risk of premature death, with a 28% increased risk in cardiovascular disease (CVD) death, and a 34% increase in cancer deaths.[2] Skipping breakfast may promote obesity compared with not eating breakfast. It lowers overall blood sugar and raises GLP-1 levels by about 30%, improving satiety for the entire day.[3] Don't skip breakfast.

The regular skipping of any meals is also not such a great idea. In a large follow-up study of adults over the age of 40, those who regularly skipped meals tended to die sooner. Regular meal skipping was associated with a 30% increase in all-cause mortality and an 83% increased risk of CVD mortality. A 27 to 30% increase in risk of dying is a higher risk than most major risk factors! Skipping breakfast had the strongest adverse risk, followed by skipping dinner (16% increased risk) and skipping lunch (12% increased risk of death). In a 16-year follow-up study of 29,000 American male health professionals, those who skipped breakfast were 21% more likely to develop type 2 diabetes.[4]

Restriction of meal intervals is also not a lovely idea. Among those eating three meals a day, if there was less than 4.5 hours between meals, it increased the risk by 17% as compared to those having 4.6 to 5.5 hours intervals between meals.[5]

Thus, if breakfast is at 8:00 AM and is done in 10 minutes, lunch begins 4.6 hours later at 12:46, taking a leisurely 18 minutes, PM, and supper is served at 5:40 PM, giving half an hour to eat, until 6:00, would be the minimum low-risk time frame for meals. Thus, a 14:10 TRE seems to be the minimum healthy TRE. If a 5.5-hour between-meal span was used and 48 minutes allowed for eating, that would be an 11:48-hour window for eating. If no other food was consumed, that would provide a nearly 12:12 TRE.

Mortality analysis of over 30,000 American adults that participated in NHANES studies, with an average follow-up time of over ten years, found that a night-time fast of less than 10 hours was associated with a 23% increase in overall mortality and a 30% increase of CVD mortality; but if the fast time was greater than 14 hours, all-cause mortality was 36% higher, and the CVD mortality was 37% higher. Eating less than 3 meals a day was associated with a one-third higher risk of all-cause mortality. The safest fasting interval appears to be a nighttime fast from 9 to 11 hours, with the nadir for CVD and overall mortality occurring for those who had a nighttime fast of about 10 hours. Overall mortality was lowest for those eating 5 or more times a day.[6]

Recall from Chapter 19 that biologic age can be estimated from various blood tests to give a biologic age (BA) to chronologic age (BA: CA) score. This was done for 24,000 subjects who participated in the NHANES studies. Using diet history data and blood testing, the BA was calculated using the Klemera–Doubal (KD) and PhenoAge (PA) methods. Compared with eating 3 or fewer times a day, those eating more frequently had lower BA: CA ratios, meaning that they were, on average, physiologically younger than those eating fewer times during the day, with better results from eating up to 8 times a day. The results for optimal nighttime fasting duration were different from the mortality data, however. BA: CA was lowest for those fasting overnight 10 to 14 hours overnight with the lowest BA: CA associated with overnight fasting of about 12.5 hours.[7]

The difference in results from these studies may have arisen from differences in subject age; mortality data is strongly impacted by older persons, many of whom are retired. Thus, older, independently-living, retired adults can eat when they please; their eating schedule is not impacted by work schedules and getting kids off to school in the morning. Mortality data with its 10-hour nadir may be skewed to assess the impact on older individuals, while the biological age nadir of 12.5 hours might be biased, as healthy young and middle-aged people's eating patterns are influenced by their jobs. Those who are not employed may have health habits and issues that impact eating patterns and BA: CA.

A meta-analysis assessing the impact of TRE on type 2 diabetes included 18 small studies with 1169 participants. Each study lasted a minimum of 4 weeks. Most of the studies used 16:8 TRE and a few used 14:10. Overall, TRE failed to have a significant impact on fasting blood glucose, but HbA1c and insulin levels fell significantly, and insulin sensitivity improved, as evidenced by a fall in HOMA-IR, improved. Notably, TRE only showed benefits for glucose metabolism when the eating window began early in the day, with breakfast before 9 AM. The one study with a longer window (13:11) and in which breakfast was early in the day was just as effective as those with short windows and an early breakfast. TRE is not effective as a weight loss method; however, it can have metabolic benefits.

The benefits of TRE are likely the result of synchronizing meals to diurnal rhythms for metabolism, activity, hormonal, and vegetative functions. The gastrointestinal system has its own nervous system and diurnal clock, which needs to be synchronized with daytime activity and nighttime rest of the rest of the body. Meta-analyses that focus specifically on the time of TRE, early or later in the day, have found significant benefits in glycemic metabolism, insulin levels, and blood pressure for those with early eating, but that TRE gives no benefit if eating begins later in the day.[8] [9]

"Eat breakfast like a king, lunch like a prince, and dinner like a pauper."

Controversial nutritionist Adele Davis, 1954

What and When

Various analyses of the NHANES studies, large population studies of Americans over a couple of decades, have revealed that the time at which foods are eaten may impact their effect on health.

Dietary antioxidants appear to have their greatest beneficial impact on health when they are consumed with the evening meal. Much, if not most, of the beneficial effect of antioxidants on lowering all-cause mortality was found to be associated with vegetable consumption at supper time. Consumption of vegetables with dinner or supper was associated with a 31% decreased risk of all-cause mortality, a 23% decrease in CVD mortality, and a 31% decrease in cancer mortality. [10] Individuals who were in the top 20% for the consumption of dietary antioxidants had a 34% lower risk of all-cause mortality. Those in the top quartile for the amount of fruit eaten with dinner were at about 30% decreased mortality risk.[11]

Dietary antioxidants consumed at lunch did not quite reach statistical significance in this study, and those consumed at breakfast did not appear to have any impact on mortality. The consumption of adequate amounts of antioxidant vegetables at suppertime lowered the risk of death sufficiently that the effect was significant for the top 3 quintiles (top 60%) of participants for suppertime antioxidant consumption.

The reason that antioxidants consumed later in the day reduce mortality risk, but not in the morning, may lie in the timing of circadian rhythms for various metabolic processes. The inflammatory response (culling and destruction) is strongest in the afternoons, while more healing, cell repair, and growth take place at night during rest. Nevertheless, the benefit may just as likely be attributed to which vegetables are typically eaten with dinner; tomato sauce, mushrooms, broccoli, cauliflower, garlic, winter squash, and sweet potatoes are usually suppertime vegetables; this may explain why vegetables at this time of day are more beneficial, in contrast to a lettuce salad, cucumbers, tomatoes, or, celery or raw carrots that might be eaten with lunch. The amounts of vegetables consumed with breakfast and lunch are typically smaller than at supper in the Western diet.

In contrast, these analyses found that higher amounts of alcohol-associated antioxidants consumed with dinner were associated with a higher risk of mortality, especially for cancer mortality.[12] Although not specified in the study, alcohol-antioxidants likely refer to wine. Thus, although wine and especially red wine are high in antioxidants, this data suggests that it may usually be consumed in a volume that is harmful (too much wine) or that it is consumed as part of a meal pattern that has an overall negative health impact. For example, wine with supper may reflect a pattern of overeating, the consumption of high-fat meals, or eating charred, red meat, which increases the risk of cancer. Wine consumption with the evening meal may also be associated with considerably later meal times and larger meals. For example, supper time in Italy is commonly from 8:30 to 10:30 p.m., and is somewhat later in Spain.

Another group of researchers analyzed the impact of snacks using the NHANES study data. They found that

- Starchy snacks after breakfast, lunch, or dinner were associated with increased all-cause mortality by 50%.
- Fruit snacks after breakfast were associated with a 22% decrease in the risk of all-cause mortality and a 45% decrease in cancer mortality. Eating fruits with lunch was associated with lower CVD risk.
- A diary snack after supper was associated with a one-third lower risk of CVD death.[13]

These data are intriguing for hypothesis generation, and I love the idea that ice cream, as an after-dinner dairy snack, lowers mortality, but it's wise not to read too much into these studies. It may be that ice cream is not beneficial, but rather that it replaces something worse, such as starchy snacks. Also, the foods categorized as starchy snacks were not specified by the authors; these might include potato and corn chips, popcorn, pretzels, and crackers. Starchy brunch snacks may refer to doughnuts, croissants, and other pastries. The NHANES data does not categorize snack types, so this categorization was done by the study authors.

If one adds the decreases in risk of all-cause mortality associated with dinnertime antioxidant vegetables (34%), dinnertime fruit (33%), fruits for brunch (22%), and evening dairy snack (33%), it adds up to more than 100%. Thus, it sounds as if disciplined mealtime manipulation could make one immortal. Oh well.

Firstly, these overlap and likely measure dietary patterns associated with healthy eating and other healthy lifestyles, so the same risk is being described in different ways in different studies. Secondly, adding multiples does not work mathematically. And thirdly, even if timing meals lowered risk by 50%, that would only, for example, lower the 5-year mortality rate from 300/100,000 to 150/100,000. Death is not something that anyone misses out on.

Trading lower amounts of carbohydrates for higher amounts of protein and, to a lesser degree, for fats at breakfast was found to be associated with a slower rate of cognitive decline in older Chinese adults in a 9-year follow-up study. Overall energy intake at breakfast was not predictive of cognitive decline. In this population, about 76% of the caloric intake of breakfast was carbohydrates, 13% protein, and the remainder was fat. Some common breakfast meals in China include rice porridge, steamed buns, noodles, rice cakes, and fried dough sticks. [14] The increased rate of cognitive decline here is likely explained by an overall impoverished diet excessively dependent on carbohydrates.

The "when" food is eaten may, in large part, be a proxy for "what" is consumed. The hormetic vegetables broccoli, cauliflower, and garlic, which promote antioxidant protein expression, are most commonly consumed with the evening meal. However, if the observation of the impact on the diurnal cycle holds true, suppertime may be a great time for a fruit salad (rich in vitamin C). The evening may also be an advantageous time for a cup of (sugarless) herbal teas that boost antioxidant mechanisms.

BMAL1 is the core circadian clock gene. It helps regulate transcription of various proteins throughout the diurnal cycle so that proteins and enzymes needed for various functions are available when needed. When you think of the protein in a bean burrito or in a slice of cheese, you understand the protein to be stable in your refrigerator over several days. Proteins in our cells are much more ephemeral; many are made and recycled after only a few minutes, others may last a day, and some even longer. But on average, proteins in the cell last less than about 12 hours. There are numerous proteins made only at night, and others only made and used only during the day. BMAL1 helps protect against neurodegeneration by promoting autophagy in the brain, and this can be impaired with poorly functioning BMAL1.[15 16] Autophagy, the recycling of old proteins and cell organelles, is most active in humans at night, while fasting, and during sleep. On the other hand, senescent cells overexpress BMAL1, which impairs apoptosis and promotes inflammation.[17] BMAL1 participates in regulating dopaminergic neuronal survival and may have an important impact on the development of Parkinson's disease.[18] Eating during the day and fasting at night contribute to maintaining the circadian cycle. There is even a circadian cycle to the proliferation of various bacteria in the gut, in response to the secretions regulated by the enteric nervous system.

Late evening meals should be avoided; supper should be completed at least two hours before bedtime. Eating later delays sleep onset and increases waking after sleep onset (WASO) and thus decreases sleep efficiency. Late meals also increase the risk of gastroesophageal reflux. Fried, fatty, and junk foods, as well as spicy foods in the evening, increase acid reflux and heartburn.

Adults who eat less than an hour before bedtime are 2.3 times as likely to wake during the night and sleep about 30 minutes longer, indicating lower sleep efficiency (more time awake during the night) and thus require more time to sleep. The study showed that not eating for two hours before bedtime improved sleep in women; fasting for 3 hours only had small additional benefits. For men, fasting for 3 hours before bedtime was advantageous over a 2-hour evening fast.[19 20] It may be that men are more likely to eat larger supper-time meals, and thus require a longer pre-bed fast time to empty their stomachs. Fat, and perhaps especially unsaturated fats, consumed during the three hours before sleep had the greatest impact on waking after sleep onset (WASO) and poor sleep efficiency.[21]

If a small snack or dessert is eaten in the evening, it should be eaten at least an hour before bedtime and be easily digestible. Such a snack should not be starchy, fatty, or junky foods. The stomach should be nearly empty by bedtime.

A small serving, 3 – 4 oz. serving of ice cream (mostly saturated fat) may not be a problem; research is ongoing. Ice cream made with Greek yogurt should also not be a problem; milk has long been known to help with sleep and has anxiolytic effects.[22] Foods containing lactic acid bacteria (*Lactobacilli*) have also been found to improve sleep quality;[23 24] thus, Greek yogurt-based ice cream (Chapter 16) may be better, while milk and especially low-fat milk consumption is discouraged on the SANA diet.

Alternatively, a small serving of fruit juice or fruit sherbet or sorbet at least an hour before bedtime can be a healthy evening snack, selecting fruit with a high DAD score. Tart cherries, blackberries, and kiwi may help with sleep, so they would be good choices for a sorbet, sherbet, or juice. Ice cream and sorbets melt in the mouth, and the stomach should be empty by bedtime if the ice cream is consumed an hour earlier.

The SANA diet recommends an early breakfast that includes about a quarter to a third of the daily caloric intake; a healthy lunch with fruit 4.5 to 5.5 hours later that includes about quarter of the day's caloric intake; and sitting down to supper between 9 to 11 hours after breakfast, with a meal that contains no more than 40% of the day's calories, but which contains ample soluble fiber, antioxidant vegetables and fruits. At least 20 grams of protein, and at least one-fourth of the day's protein, should be consumed at each of three meals.[25]

Sufficient leucine is required to trigger the building of muscle mass, especially in older adults. (See Chapter 13). Excessive leucine levels, however, drive macrophage mTOR signaling and inflammatory cell signaling and increase cardiovascular risk. Thus, balancing the protein intake across the meals is important, not just to build muscle, but to avoid excess mTOR signaling. For muscle building to occur, amino acid levels need to fall sufficiently between meals to reset the muscle-building signaling. Thus, little protein should be consumed between breakfast and lunch, and between lunch and supper. Also, the meals should be separated by several hours (at least 3) so that leucine and other branched-chain amino acid levels can fall before the next meal. [26 27 28] For older adults, those overweight with fatty muscles, and those with a sedentary lifestyle, dietary protein may need to be concentrated into one or two meals a day in order to get enough leucine to promote muscle synthesis.

Dietary fiber helps fuel the production of short-chain fatty acids, such as butyrate, that help maintain caloric needs and help regulate metabolism through the night. One should wake in the morning with an appetite to enjoy breakfast. This may not occur with overly large, overly late evening meals. If a snack is needed between meals, have a small portion of fruit and a glass of tea or water. To entrain the GI tract and enteric nervous system to the circadian cycle, complete supper 3 hours before bedtime, and avoid snacks or desserts for an hour before bedtime. The body's ability to metabolize sugar is lower at the end of the day, and consumption of sweets is more likely to result in poor sleep and fat accumulation.

The operative aspects of TRE likely boil down to going to bed in the evening with an empty stomach and eating a real breakfast early in the day. This helps align the daytime activity/nighttime rest circadian cycle with the circadian cycle of the gastrointestinal system. If the evening meal is 3 hours before bedtime, and one is in bed for 8 hours, that provides a TRE fasting period of 11 hours. A light, liquid evening snack (ice cream is liquid by the time it enters the stomach) at least an hour before bedtime may not violate the essence of the TRE.

Fasting

Fasting is not recommended by the SANA program. Although it may have benefits, those graces may be more spiritual than physical.

One of the main reasons people fast for health is to induce autophagy, the recycling of old, damaged, and misfolded proteins, as well, to induce mitophagy, the recycling of old, worn-out, and leaky mitochondria. This is a noble goal, but fasting has problems. Fasting is not a way to lose weight; if anything, it may downregulate the metabolic rate and make it easier to gain weight in the future.

Enterocytes lining the small intestine and those in the colon, referred to as colonocytes, require constant energy. Cleansing and fasting rob them of their mainstay of nutrition. Thus, fasting can cause leaky gut. Hospitalized patients on parenteral feeding often develop gram-negative pneumonia as a result of bacteria moving from the bowel into their bloodstream as a result of starving colonocytes and the loss of the mucous barrier that the starvation of colonocytes causes. The bacteria in the blood often get caught as the blood passes through the small blood vessels of the lungs, causing infection.

The upper small intestine relies on glucose as a fuel; glucose is absorbed during digestion, not leaving any for enterocytes downstream. Further along, in the small intestine, the principal source of fuel for the enterocytes is the amino acid glutamic acid. As the chyme (the bolus of digested food remnants) enters and passes through the colon, the cells rely on short-chain fatty acids from bacterial fermentation of fiber for fuel.

The microbiome is constantly eating. Normally, there is a dense, adherent mucous layer that is constantly being produced by the colonocytes that separates them from the contents of the bowel, including the bacteria. As the mucus ages, it becomes less dense, and some bacteria live in this layer and feed on it. As mentioned previously, if the colonocytes don't have food to produce their mucous layer, it still gets consumed until it is gone, and then bacteria can attach directly to the cells. When fasting, the enterocytes have nothing to eat and can't maintain their normal functions, including the production of the mucous layer, IgA to neutralize bacterial adhesion, and other protective mechanisms.

Thus, as appealing as not having to cook, buy groceries, or brush your teeth may be, going hungry for a day or more (fasting) is not recommended on the SANA program. Fasting (for more than 24 hours) is a recipe for a leaky gut.

Autophagic Revival Regime

While fasting is not recommended as part of the SANA program, an occasional autophagic regimen is. This might be in the form of a 36 to 40-hour autophagy diet (starting in the evening, one full day, and until the next morning), which might be done occasionally, or, rarely, a 60 to 64-hour autophagy diet (two days, three nights). This diet promotes autophagy by restricting the diet to foods that promote autophagy.

A modified form of fasting can be done as part of the SANA diet for those interested in promoting autophagy. The cells are constantly making and recycling protein. Recall from Chapter 9 that there is a threshold of leucine in the diet that is needed to trigger the synthesis of new muscle fiber protein. Methionine is another amino acid that plays a role as a metabolic gatekeeper in protein metabolism and autophagy. Methionine, likely as S-adenosylmethionine (SAMe), is a bellwether that acts to indicate if there is a sufficient pool of amino acids in the cell to make proteins, including the regular housekeeping proteins that are constantly being made. Methionine is not just an indicator of amino acid sufficiency. When methionine levels are low, it acts as a signal promoting the recycling of older and less essential proteins. Thus, low levels of methionine promote autophagy. Both methionine and leucine inhibit autophagy,[29] but methionine has a broader impact on various cells, while leucine is more important for muscle protein generation. Both act on mTOR and inhibit autophagy when the supply of amino acids is abundant.[30] Although nutrient sensing and autophagy are primary pathways for metabolic benefits from methionine and leucine restrictions, other pathways are also involved that further promote health and longevity.[31] This includes adaptations in mitochondrial metabolism in response to methionine deficits. Dietary restriction of methionine is associated with better metabolic health and an increased utilization of fat for energy, which may explain its anti-obesity effects. High intakes of methionine are associated with diabetes and obesity.[32]

When there is a scarcity of amino acids, the cell increases the recycling of older proteins so that it can continue making new proteins. This results in new, better-functioning proteins. Methionine is a key amino acid "switch" that helps determine this. If insufficient methionine is available, autophagy gets boosted. By carefully selecting foods that are low in methionine, a short-term methionine-depleting diet can be constructed. Methionine only makes up about two percent of the protein in our bodies.

Methionine restriction (MR) has been found to promote cognitive health in animals, improve learning and memory, decrease anxiety-like behavior, and increase exploratory behavior in mice.[33] MR appears to lower the expression of Aβ and phosphorylated Tau, markers in Alzheimer's disease.[34]

Both continuous MR and intermittent methionine restrictions (IMR) increase longevity by as much as 45% in rodents. [35] IMR improves plasma levels of IGF-1, FGF-21, leptin, and adiponectin.[36] IMR has been found to preserve bone mass better than continuous methionine restriction.[37]

Methionine and cysteine can be interconverted by the body, so their dietary requirements are often stated as the combination of the two. The recommended daily intake for methionine plus cysteine is 19 milligrams per kilogram of body weight, or about 8.6 milligrams per pound.

During methionine restriction, it is important to maintain the recycling of S-adenosyl methionine from homocysteine. This requires sufficient folate (vitamin B9) and vitamin B12. If the methionine restriction is replete with green vegetables, there should be sufficient folate; if not, supplementation with folacin (methyl folate) is recommended.[38] The body stores sufficient vitamin B12 so that a short-term fast for IMR should not deplete B12 levels.

Comparing several food groups, eggs, seafood, meat, and dairy are high in methionine, while legumes, vegetables, cereals, and many nuts are low in methionine. (Macadamia nuts have very little methionine, whereas Brazil nuts have exceptionally high levels.). Dairy is highest in leucine, followed by eggs, beef, pork, and other meats and seafood. Cereals are generally high in glutamic acid. Tomatoes and green peas have exceptionally high levels of glutamic acid, giving them umami flavor and helping nourish the small intestine and colon.[39]

In a study comparing 10 dietary patterns, including the Paleo, Western, DASH, Medi, and others, a plant-based diet was the lowest in leucine and methionine. A plant-based diet is also high in glutamic acid, which is needed for the metabolic activity of the cells lining the distal small intestine. The plant-based diet also supplies an abundance of glycine.[40]

Glycine may help mitigate methionine's anti-autophagic properties by the formation of sarcosine (methylglycine).[41] Thus, a plant-based diet is a naturally low-methionine diet. It can be further tweaked to give a very low methionine diet that promotes autophagy.

Spermidine is a polyamine that plays a different but essential role in autophagy. Spermidine is (indirectly) formed in the body and gut from the amino acid arginine. Spermidine is also present in the diet and can be formed from dietary polyamines, putrescine, and spermine. Dietary citrulline can be converted into arginine, and thus can also help supply spermidine.

Spermidine is enzymatically metabolized by the body into the amino acid hypusine and bound to the proteins EIF5A and EIF5A2, activating them. EIF5A has several functions; one is that it aids in protein translation, and another is that it performs a required step in tagging proteins for autophagy.[42] Spermidine increases the lifespan in animals under experimental conditions by promoting autophagy. Unfortunately, intracellular concentrations of spermidine decline during aging,[43] and this may limit autophagy and other processes that rely on spermidine.

Hypusineated EIF5A appears to be required for neuronal growth and survival,[44] and thus may help prevent the development of dementia. In animal studies, dietary spermidine supplementation helped maintain cerebral mitochondrial and cognitive function.[45]

In a study of over 77 thousand people from the UK over the age of 60, followed for an average of 12 years, those with baseline diets high in natural polyamines (putrescine, spermidine, and spermine) had a lower risk for the development of dementia. The response was U-shaped, with the lowest risk of dementia for those consuming 4.4–5.7 mg of spermine, 10.0–12.3 mg of spermidine, and 13.4–17.8 mg of putrescine per day, with higher and lower levels being less effective. At optimal levels, dietary consumption of these polyamines was associated with a greater than 50% decrease in AD and vascular dementia risk.[46] Thus, at an approximate 1:2:3 ratio of spermine to spermidine to putrescine, at around 32 mg/day, may lower the risk of dementia.

In the UK, the average ratio of polyamines is estimated to be 58 to 98 to 160 µmol of spermine, spermidine, and putrescine, respectively, per day; a ratio quite similar to the 1:2:3 ratio observed to be associated with a lower risk of dementia.[47] Since these polyamines can be converted one to another, there is insufficient evidence to conclude that the ratio of these in the diet has any importance to disease outcome or to determine if 11 mg of spermidine is the ideal amount or if it is 32 mg of total dietary polyamines that is most closely associated with lower dementia risk. What we do learn is that increasing the amounts of polyenes in the diet beyond around 38 mg/day or more than 12.3 mg/day of spermidine was not associated with any further decrease in dementia risk. Rather, there appears to be a loss of risk reduction when these amounts are greatly exceeded.

Cheese, legumes, nuts, seeds, meat, green pepper, chicken liver, and whole grains are high in polyamines. The estimated typical daily dietary intake of polyamines in the diet in Europe is 42 mg. It is 29 mg in the U.S. and 26 mg in Japan. Thus, there does not appear to be any benefit from supplementing polyamines or spermidine when one is consuming a healthy diet. Diets that are likely to be low in polyamines are those filled with empty calories from refined vegetable oils and sugars. Aged cheddar cheese has 200 mg of spermidine and 659 mg of putrescine per kg. Thus, 2 ounces of aged cheddar contains over 11 mg of spermidine and 37 mg of putrescine.

Additionally, the GI microbiota produces polyamines. Supplementing mice with the probiotic *Bifidobacterium animalis (lactis)* increased polyamine levels in the intestine and significantly extended their lifespan; it promoted a downregulation of inflammation-associated genes and improvement of the intestinal barrier function.[48]

The occasion when selecting foods high in spermidine and other polyamines may provide benefits is during a low-methionine, autophagy regimen.

Vegetables that are high in spermidine but low in methionine include: mushrooms, pumpkin and butternut squash, potatoes, arugula (rocket), broccoli, cauliflower, spinach, celeriac, cucumbers, carrots, and okra.

Fruits that are high in spermidine and low in methionine are pears, mangoes, peaches, oranges, tangerines, and melons, including watermelon. Oranges, tangerines, grapefruit, bananas, pumpkin, and plantains are high in putrescine. Oranges, mandarins have around 120 mg per kg of putrescine. Lentils and green peas are high in spermidine.[49] [50]

Soluble fiber is an important component of an autophagic regimen. Fiber feeds the colonocytes and the brain and helps decrease hunger. The food restrictions of this diet, for example, the exclusion of grains, may make it difficult to get sufficient soluble fiber. A daily, several-gram supplement of soluble fiber, such as Sunfiber, beta-glucans, and polydextrose, is recommended during the autophagic regimen.

Rationale

In animals, lifespan can be increased with a 40% restriction in calories, proteins, or methionine. Methionine appears to be the key element to the increase in lifespan. In animals, diets in which methionine intake is restricted by 40 percent, there is a decrease in mitochondrial ROS production and free radical leakage measured in the brain and kidneys,[51] while increasing intake of dietary methionine increases oxidative damage to the liver and heart.[52] In animals, every-other-day (EOD) dietary restriction also decreases mitochondrial oxidative stress by decreasing free radical leak in the complex I mitochondrial respiratory chain proteins and increases longevity[53].

Diets with a 40 percent methionine restriction can achieve mitochondrial ROS reduction. Such a diet may allow the benefits of caloric restriction without fasting or caloric deprivation. The typical mitochondrial life cycle is only seven days; thus, a methionine restriction once a week may promote the culling of weak ones. A 36 to 42-hour methionine-restricted diet should be sufficient to provide such benefits. The 36-hour diet restricts methionine-rich foods for only three meals: from 7 P.M. after supper on one evening, during the next day, and the following morning, returning to a regular lunchtime meal at noon. The 42-hour regimen skips four meals; starting after lunch, a low methionine super, for the next day, and then a normal breakfast the following morning.

The World Health Organization promulgates a daily intake of 0.45 grams of protein per kilogram (0.204 grams per pound) of ideal body weight as the *minimum daily protein intake required for maintaining nitrogen balance.*[54]

Ideal Body Weight

Men: 106 lbs. + (6 lbs. per inch over 60" in height)

48 kg + (1 kg per cm over 150 cm in height)

Women: 100 lbs. + (5 lbs. per inch over 60" in height)

45 kg + (0.85 kg per cm over 150 cm in height)

A 5'8" tall man would have an ideal body weight of 154 pounds (70 kg) and would have a 31.5-gram daily protein requirement. One extra gram of dietary protein is required for individuals doing endurance training.

A 40 percent methionine-restricted diet would supply 60 percent of the dietary methionine requirement, equivalent to 8.37 mg of methionine per kg ideal body weight (3.8 mg per pound). Thus, a 70-kg (154 lb.) ideal body weight individual could consume up to 586 mg of methionine a day on the 40% restricted methionine diet. The methionine requirement is about three percent of the protein requirement. Methionine makes up 3.1% of the protein in chicken eggs, which is considered to be a balanced protein. On average, meals with proteins containing less than 1.86% methionine (60% of 3.1%) would work for this diet.

Assuming a daily dietary intake of 2200 calories for a 70-kg man, a 586 mg methionine restriction would limit meals to an average of less than 0.106% of the calories coming from methionine. Table 28A below shows that there are only a limited number of foods that have methionine at 0.11% or lower. Thus, low-methionine foods, such as fruits, tubers, vegetables, and fats, are needed in this diet. Adding butter or coconut oil to mashed potatoes and squash can be used to add non-protein calories. Clarified butter, ghee, can also be used to lower the protein content. Using the daily allotment of 10 percent of calories as added sugars (honey, molasses, jams), while empty calories, can stave off hunger and avoid methionine.

Note: This diet is not recommended for growing children, adolescents, or pregnant and lactating women.

Table 28A gives the methionine content of a sample of foods, ranked from low to high methionine content. Unless otherwise noted, the portion size is 100 grams of prepared food. Nutrition data for specific foods can be found online at

http://nutritiondata.self.com/tools/nutrient-search

or

https://tools.myfooddata.com/protein-calculator/.

A diet high in fruits and vegetables helps to fill out caloric intake in a methionine-restricted (MR) diet. Use of coconut milk is useful in MR diets, and can be used with breakfast cereal or to make smoothies. Foods in which methionine makes up less than 0.1% of calories (most fruits and vegetables) can be thought of as "low-MR foods" as they lower the methionine ratio in the diet. Some examples of low methionine, high spermidine meals are:

Breakfast: A ripe plantain, baked in its skin in the microwave (cut the ends off, pierce the skin to allow steam to escape, and cover; cook about 120 to 180 seconds, depending on the power of your unit).

Lunch: A salad with cucumbers, tomatoes (with seeds removed), avocado, and bits of cauliflower. Cassava bread or crackers with peach jam. An orange or two tangerines.

Supper: A baked sweet potato with butter, and mung bean cellophane noodles with mushrooms.

Snacks: Macadamia nuts, pears, the usual 16 grams of walnuts or pecans, as the amount of methionine is small. Note that Brazil nuts are extremely high in methionine and should be avoided on the methionine-restricted diet.

Note that pumpkin and butternut squash are listed in Table 28. Sweet potatoes and cooked carrots are better low-methionine choices. Potatoes are shown on the list, but sweet potatoes are the low-methionine choice. Adding butter or ghee, or coconut oil, helps add calories and enriches the flavor. Adding the fat also increases the intestinal absorption of carotenoids from the foods, including lycopene from tomatoes.

Tomatoes are included as the actual amount of methionine is very low, and they are high in glutamic acid, which is needed to nourish the enterocytes. Mushrooms are included as the amount consumed is expected to be small in amounts (one 1.5-inch button mushroom), as they are very high in spermidine (and ergothioneine). Pears, tangerines, peaches, carrots, and pumpkins are high in polyamines. Canned fruit and pumpkin are convenient and available year-round, but not as tasty as fresh pumpkin. While apples and apple sauce are low in methionine, pears are a better choice as they are high in spermidine. Nectarines likely have very similar polyamine content to peaches and are lower in methionine.

Not shown are butter, or the slightly better choice for the methionine restriction, ghee (clarified butter), and coconut oil. Butter has some methionine, but it is allowed, as most of the calories are from fat. Sugars (brown sugar, molasses, etc.) contain no methionine and can be used in small amounts, as with the regular SANA diet.

Cassava is not allowed on the SANA diet (it has a DAD score of D), but tapioca and cassava bread, which use cassava as a raw material, can be used. Similarly, arrowroot flour and cornstarch can be used. Maybe one could make pancakes using banana and arrowroot or tapioca flour.

Coffee, tea, tisanes, and spices are allowed on the autophagy diet.

A 3-gram clove of garlic or ½ tsp. of garlic powder only contains 2 mg of methionine, so they can be used as they are used in small amounts.

Dry onions are allowed (in small amounts), but green onions are too high in methionine. The small buttery "California" (Mexican) avocados are low enough in methionine/ calorie, but the larger green "Florida" ones are not. Cauliflower has considerably less methionine than broccoli. While having more methionine per calorie than ideal, cucumbers and cauliflower have a low density of calories, so the amount of methionine should be small if not eaten in large quantities.

If trying the autophagy regimen, try to eat enough so that you don't go hungry. Ripe plantains (microwaved) and the mung bean noodles really help make the diet filling and easy to comply with. While not specified, cassava bread or crackers are extremely low in methionine, and thus can be used as a platform for fruit spreads, such as blackberry jam, which are allowed, as they are high in calories and low in protein.

Table 28: Low methionine foods

Food Item:	Calories per 100g [kcal]	Grams Protein: Grams/100g	Methionine mg per 100g	Methionine: percent of protein	Protein as a percent of Calories	Methionine as a percent of Calories
Mung bean cellophane noodles dry	956	0.16	2	1.25	0.07	0.00
Tapioca (pearls or flour)	358	0.2	2	1.00	0.22	0.00
Arrowroot flour, corn starch	357	0.3	6	2.00	0.34	0.01
Plantains (yellow, fried)	357	2.5	7	0.28	2.80	0.01
Apples (no skin)	48	0.27	1	0.37	2.25	0.01
Sweet Pickles	122	0.4	3	0.75	1.31	0.01
Pears	63	0.4	2	0.50	2.54	0.01
Tangerines	53	0.8	2	0.25	6.04	0.02
Custard Apple (Annona)	101	1.7	4	0.24	6.73	0.02
Papaya	43	0.5	2	0.40	4.65	0.02
Ketchup	101	1	5	0.50	3.96	0.02
Onions	40	1.1	2	0.18	11.00	0.02
Chayote	19	0.8	1	0.13	16.84	0.02
Plantains (boiled)	121	1.1	7	0.64	3.64	0.02
Cassava	160	1.4	11	0.79	3.50	0.03
Dates	282	2.5	22	0.88	3.55	0.03
Figs	74	0.8	6	0.75	4.32	0.03
Bananas	89	1.1	8	0.73	4.94	0.04
Apricots	48	1.4	6	0.43	11.67	0.05
Mangoes	60	0.8	8	1.00	5.33	0.05
Grapefruit	37	0.5	5	1.00	5.41	0.05
Nectarines	44	1.1	6	0.55	10.00	0.05
Beets (canned)	65	0.8	9	1.13	4.92	0.06
Honeydew Melon	36	0.5	5	1.00	5.56	0.06
Pumpkin	214	3.2	31	0.97	5.98	0.06
Sweet Potato	144	0.9	21	2.33	2.50	0.06
Cherries	63	1.1	10	0.91	6.98	0.06
Ginger root	80	1.8	13	0.72	9.00	0.07
Plums	46	0.7	8	1.14	6.09	0.07
Coconut	354	3.33	62	1.86	3.76	0.07
Kiwi	133	1.1	24	2.18	3.31	0.07
French Fried Potatoes	319	3.8	58	1.53	4.76	0.07
Orange (naval) (not as juice)	49	0.9	9	1.00	7.35	0.07
Pecans	3019	50	568	1.14	6.62	0.08
Coconut milk	197	5	38	0.76	10.15	0.08
Carrots	36	0.8	7	0.88	8.89	0.08
Watermelon	30	0.61	6	0.98	8.13	0.08
Blueberries	57	0.74	12	1.62	5.19	0.08
Grapes (seedless, table)	76	0.5	16	3.20	2.63	0.08
Avocado (California)	167	2	37	1.85	4.79	0.09

Macadamia nuts. dry roasted	1610	33	362	1.10	8.20	0.09
Guava	68	2.6	16	0.62	15.29	0.09
Pineapple	50	0.5	12	2.40	4.00	0.10
Acorn Squash	40	0.8	10	1.25	8.00	0.10
Winter Squash (Acorn)	40	0.8	10	1.25	8.00	0.10
Peaches	39	0.91	10	1.10	9.33	0.10
Snow peas	42	2.8	11	0.39	26.67	0.10
Potatoes	100	2.1	33	1.57	8.40	0.13
Tomatoes	18	0.9	6	0.67	20.00	0.13
Avocado (Florida)	120	2.2	42	1.91	7.33	0.14
Cantaloupe	34	0.8	12	1.50	9.41	0.14
Celery	14	0.7	5	0.71	20.00	0.14
Lettuce, iceberg	14	0.9	5	0.56	25.71	0.14
Walnut, English	654	15.23	236	1.55	9.31	0.14
Rice noodles dry (Chinese)	364	6	144	2.40	6.59	0.16
Dill pickle	12	0.5	5	1.00	16.67	0.17
Shitake mushrooms	56	1.56	25	1.60	11.14	0.18
Garlic	149	6.4	76	1.19	17.18	0.20
Mangoes	146	8.2	91	1.11	22.47	0.25
Cauliflower	25	1.9	20	1.05	30.40	0.32
Green onions	89	7.4	83	1.12	33.26	0.37
Cucumbers (peeled)	32	2.5	32	1.28	31.25	0.40
Broccoli florets	28	3	34	1.13	42.86	0.49
Portabella mushrooms	22	2.11	29	1.37	38.36	0.53
Brazil Nuts	656	14.32	1008	7.04	8.73	0.61

[1] Breakfast skipping and the risk of type 2 diabetes: a meta-analysis of observational studies. Bi H, Gan Y, Yang C, Chen Y, Tong X, Lu Z. Public Health Nutr. 2015 Nov;18(16):3013-9. doi: 10.1017/S1368980015000257. PMID: 25686619

[2] Breakfast skipping and risk of all-cause, cardiovascular and cancer mortality among adults: a systematic review and meta-analysis of prospective cohort studies. Wang Y, Li F, Li X, Wu J, Chen X, Su Y, Qin T, Liu X, Liang L, Ma J, Qin P. Food Funct. 2024 Jun 4;15(11):5703-5713. doi: 10.1039/d3fo05705d. PMID: 38738978

[3] High-energy breakfast with low-energy dinner decreases overall daily hyperglycaemia in type 2 diabetic patients: a randomised clinical trial. Jakubowicz D, Wainstein J, Ahrén B, Bar-Dayan Y, Landau Z, Rabinovitz HR, Froy O. Diabetologia. 2015 May;58(5):912-9. doi: 10.1007/s00125-015-3524-9. Epub 2015 Mar 1. PMID: 25724569

[4] Eating patterns and type 2 diabetes risk in men: breakfast omission, eating frequency, and snacking. Mekary RA, Giovannucci E, Willett WC, van Dam RM, Hu FB. Am J Clin Nutr. 2012 May;95(5):1182-9. doi: 10.3945/ajcn.111.028209. Epub 2012 Mar 28. PMID: 22456660

[5] Meal Skipping and Shorter Meal Intervals Are Associated with Increased Risk of All-Cause and Cardiovascular Disease Mortality among US Adults. Sun Y, Rong S, Liu B, Du Y, Wu Y, Chen L, Xiao Q, Snetselaar L, Wallace R, Bao W. J Acad Nutr Diet. 2023 Mar;123(3):417-426.e3. doi: 10.1016/j.jand.2022.08.119. Epub 2022 Aug 11. PMID: 35964910

[6] Relationship between circadian eating behavior (daily eating frequency and nighttime fasting duration) and cardiovascular mortality. Cheng W, Meng X, Gao J, Jiang W, Sun X, Li Y, Han T, Zhang D, Wei W. Int J Behav Nutr Phys Act. 2024 Feb 26;21(1):22. doi: 10.1186/s12966-023-01556-5. PMID: 38409117

[7] Associations of daily eating frequency and nighttime fasting duration with biological aging in National Health and Nutrition Examination Survey (NHANES) 2003-2010 and 2015-2018. Wang X, Zhang J, Xu X, Pan S, Cheng L, Dang K, Qi X, Li Y. Int J Behav Nutr Phys Act. 2024 Sep 19;21(1):104. doi: 10.1186/s12966-024-01654-y. PMID: 39300516; PMCID: PMC11414321.

[8] The Effect of Early Time-Restricted Eating vs Later Time-Restricted Eating on Weight Loss and Metabolic Health. Liu J, Yi P, Liu F. J Clin Endocrinol Metab. 2023 Jun 16;108(7):1824-1834. doi: 10.1210/clinem/dgad036. PMID: 36702768

[9] Circadian alignment of food intake and glycaemic control by time-restricted eating: A systematic review and meta-analysis. Rovira-Llopis S, Luna-Marco C, Perea-Galera L, Bañuls C, Morillas C, Victor VM. Rev Endocr Metab Disord. 2024 Apr;25(2):325-337. doi: 10.1007/s11154-023-09853-x. Epub 2023 Nov 22. PMID: 37993559

[10] Meal timing of dietary total antioxidant capacity and its association with all-cause, CVD and cancer mortality: the US national health and nutrition examination survey, 1999-2018. Wang P, Jiang X, Tan Q, Du S, Shi D. Int J Behav Nutr Phys Act. 2023 Jul 7;20(1):83. doi: 10.1186/s12966-023-01487-1. PMID: 37420213

[11] Association of dietary total antioxidant capacity and its distribution across three meals with all-cause, cancer, and non-cancer mortality among cancer survivors: the US National Health and Nutrition Examination Survey, 1999-2018. Wang P, Zhao S, Hu X, Tan Q, Tan Y, Shi D. Front Nutr. 2023 Jul 6;10:1141380. doi: 10.3389/fnut.2023.1141380. PMID: 37485382; PMCID: PMC10359731.

[12] Meal timing of dietary total antioxidant capacity and its association with all-cause, CVD and cancer mortality: the US national health and nutrition examination survey, 1999-2018. Wang P, Jiang X, Tan Q, Du S, Shi D. Int J Behav Nutr Phys Act. 2023 Jul 7;20(1):83. doi: 10.1186/s12966-023-01487-1. PMID: 37420213

[13] Association of Meal and Snack Patterns with Mortality of All-Cause, Cardiovascular Disease, and Cancer: The US National Health and Nutrition Examination Survey, 2003 to 2014. Wei W, Jiang W, Huang J, Xu J, Wang X, Jiang X, Wang Y, Li G, Sun C, Li Y, Han T. J Am Heart Assoc. 2021 Jul 6;10(13):e020254. doi: 10.1161/JAHA.120.020254. Epub 2021 Jun 23. PMID: 34157852

[14] Energy and macronutrient intakes at breakfast and cognitive declines in community-dwelling older adults: a 9-year follow-up cohort study. Shang X, Hill E, Li Y, He M. Am J Clin Nutr. 2021 May 8;113(5):1093-1103. doi: 10.1093/ajcn/nqaa403. PMID: 33675345

[15] 0029 The Effect of BMAL1 Expression on Autophagy Activity in Astrocytes. Connor C. Campbell - 30 Apr 2023 - Sleep - Vol. 46, Iss: Supplement_1, pp https://academic.oup.com/sleep/article/46/Supplement_1/A12/7181627

[16] Astrocytes deficient in circadian clock gene Bmal1 show enhanced activation responses to amyloid-beta pathology without changing plaque burden. McKee CA, Lee J, Cai Y, Saito T, Saido T, Musiek ES. Sci Rep. 2022 Feb 2;12(1):1796. doi: 10.1038/s41598-022-05862-z. PMID: 35110643

[17] BMAL1 modulates senescence programming via AP-1. Jachim SK, Zhong J, Ordog T, Lee JH, Bhagwate AV, Nagaraj NK, Westendorf JJ, Passos JF, Matveyenko AV, LeBrasseur NK. Aging (Albany NY). 2023 Oct 10;15(19):9984-10009. doi: 10.18632/aging.205112. Epub 2023 Oct 10. PMID: 37819791

[18] Neuronal deletion of the circadian clock gene Bmal1 induces cell-autonomous dopaminergic neurodegeneration. Kanan MF, Sheehan PW, Haines JN, Gomez PG, Dhuler A, Nadarajah CJ, Wargel ZM, Freeberg BM, Nelvagal HR, Izumo M, Takahashi JS, Cooper JD, Davis AA, Musiek ES. JCI Insight. 2024 Jan 23;9(2):e162771. doi: 10.1172/jci.insight.162771. PMID: 38032732

[19] Associations between bedtime eating or drinking, sleep duration and wake after sleep onset: findings from the American time use survey. Iao SI, Jansen E, Shedden K, O'Brien LM, Chervin RD, Knutson KL, Dunietz GL. Br J Nutr. 2021 Sep 13;127(12):1-10. doi: 10.1017/S0007114521003597. Online ahead of print. PMID: 34511160

[20] Does the Proximity of Meals to Bedtime Influence the Sleep of Young Adults? A Cross-Sectional Survey of University Students. Chung N, Bin YS, Cistulli PA, Chow CM. Int J Environ Res Public Health. 2020 Apr 14;17(8):2677. doi: 10.3390/ijerph17082677. PMID: 32295235

[21] The association between timing of dietary macronutrient and sodium consumption and sleep duration and quality. Baidoo VYA, Alexandria SJ, Zee PC, Knutson KL. Sleep Adv. 2024 Jan 23;5(1):zpae007. doi: 10.1093/sleepadvances/zpae007. eCollection 2024. PMID: 38314117

[22] Milk Collected at Night Induces Sedative and Anxiolytic-Like Effects and Augments Pentobarbital-Induced Sleeping Behavior in Mice. dela Peña IJ, Hong E, de la Peña JB, Kim HJ, Botanas CJ, Hong YS, Hwang YS, Moon BS, Cheong JH. J Med Food. 2015 Nov;18(11):1255-61. doi: 10.1089/jmf.2015.3448. Epub 2015 Jun 4. PMID: 26501383

[23] Effects of lactic acid bacteria-containing foods on the quality of sleep: a placebo-controlled, double-blinded, randomized crossover study. Masafumi Nakagawa et al. Functional Foods in Health and Disease. Vol. 8 No. 12 (2018): December 2018. https://doi.org/10.31989/ffhd.v8i12.572

[24] Daily consumption of Lactobacillus gasseri CP2305 improves quality of sleep in adults - A systematic literature review and meta-analysis. Chu A, Samman S, Galland B, Foster M. Clin Nutr. 2023 Aug;42(8):1314-1321. doi: 10.1016/j.clnu.2023.06.019. Epub 2023 Jun 29. PMID: 37413809.

[25] International Society of Sports Nutrition Position Stand: protein and exercise. Jäger R, Kerksick CM, Campbell BI, Antonio J. J, et al. Int Soc Sports Nutr. 2017 Jun 20;14:20. doi: 10.1186/s12970-017-0177-8. 2017. PMID: 28642676

[26] Defining meal requirements for protein to optimize metabolic roles of amino acids. Layman DK, Anthony TG, Rasmussen BB, Adams SH, Lynch CJ, Brinkworth GD, Davis TA. Am J Clin Nutr. 2015 Jun;101(6):1330S-1338S. doi: 10.3945/ajcn.114.084053. Epub 2015 Apr 29. PMID: 25926513

[27] Identification of a leucine-mediated threshold effect governing macrophage mTOR signalling and cardiovascular risk. Zhang X, Kapoor D, Jeong SJ, Fappi A, Stitham J, Shabrish V, Sergin I, Yousif E, Rodriguez-Velez A, Yeh YS, Park A, Yurdagul A Jr, Rom O, Epelman S, Schilling JD, Sardiello M, Diwan A, Cho J, Stitziel NO, Javaheri A, Lodhi IJ, Mittendorfer B, Razani B. Nat Metab. 2024 Feb;6(2):359-377. doi: 10.1038/s42255-024-00984-2. Epub 2024 Feb 19. PMID: 38409323

[28] A high proportion of leucine is required for optimal stimulation of the rate of muscle protein synthesis by essential amino acids in the elderly. Katsanos CS, Kobayashi H, Sheffield-Moore M, Aarsland A, Wolfe RR. Am J Physiol Endocrinol Metab. 2006 Aug;291(2):E381-7. doi: 10.1152/ajpendo.00488.2005. Epub 2006 Feb 28. PMID: 16507602

[29] Son, S.M., Park, S.J., Stamatakou, E. et al. Leucine regulates autophagy via acetylation of the mTORC1 component raptor. Nat Commun 11, 3148 (2020). https://doi.org/10.1038/s41467-020-16886-2

[30] Methionine is a signal of amino acid sufficiency that inhibits autophagy through the methylation of PP2A. Laxman S, Sutter BM, Tu BP. Autophagy. 2014 Feb;10(2):386-7. doi: 10.4161/auto.27485. Epub 2013 Dec 18. PMID: 24362312

[31] Green, C.L., Lamming, D.W. & Fontana, L. Molecular mechanisms of dietary restriction promoting health and longevity. Nat Rev Mol Cell Biol 23, 56–73 (2022). https://doi.org/10.1038/s41580-021-00411-4

[32] Dai, Z., Zheng, W. & Locasale, J.W. Amino acid variability, tradeoffs and optimality in human diet. Nat Commun 13, 6683 (2022). https://doi.org/10.1038/s41467-022-34486-0

[33] Effects of Dietary Methionine Restriction on Cognition in Mice. Lail H, Mabb AM, Parent MB, Pinheiro F, Wanders D. Nutrients. 2023 Nov 29;15(23):4950. doi: 10.3390/nu15234950. PMID: 38068808

[34] Systems genetics identifies methionine as a high risk factor for Alzheimer's disease. Wang C, Hei Y, Liu Y, Bajpai AK, Li Y, Guan Y, Xu F, Yao C. Front Neurosci. 2024 Jul 16;18:1381889. doi: 10.3389/fnins.2024.1381889. eCollection 2024. PMID: 39081851

[35] Amino acid restriction, aging, and longevity: an update. Austad SN, Smith JR, Hoffman JM. Front Aging. 2024 May 2;5:1393216. doi: 10.3389/fragi.2024.1393216. eCollection 2024. PMID: 38757144

[36] Intermittent methionine restriction reduces IGF-1 levels and produces similar healthspan benefits to continuous methionine restriction. Plummer JD, Johnson JE. Aging Cell. 2022 Jun;21(6):e13629. doi: 10.1111/acel.13629. Epub 2022 May 15. PMID: 35570387

[37] Intermittent Methionine Restriction Reduces Marrow Fat Accumulation and Preserves More Bone Mass than Continuous Methionine Restriction. Plummer JD, Horowitz MC, Johnson JE. Aging Biol. 2024;2:20230019. doi: 10.59368/agingbio.20230019. PMID: 38550776

[38] Wei, F., Liu, S., Liu, J. et al. Separation of reproductive decline from lifespan extension during methionine restriction. Nat Aging 4, 1089–1101 (2024). https://doi.org/10.1038/s43587-024-00674-4

[39] The Roles of Dietary Glutamate in the Intestine. Tomé D. Ann Nutr Metab. 2018;73 Suppl 5:15-20. doi: 10.1159/000494777. Epub 2018 Dec 3. PMID: 30508814.

[40] Dai, Z., Zheng, W. & Locasale, J.W. Amino acid variability, tradeoffs and optimality in human diet. Nat Commun 13, 6683 (2022). https://doi.org/10.1038/s41467-022-34486-0

[41] Glycine and aging: Evidence and mechanisms. Johnson AA, Cuellar TL. Ageing Res Rev. 2023 Jun;87:101922. doi: 10.1016/j.arr.2023.101922. Epub 2023 Mar 31. PMID: 37004845

[42] eIF5A is required for autophagy by mediating ATG3 translation. Lubas M, Harder LM, Kumsta C, Tiessen I, Hansen M, Andersen JS, Lund AH, Frankel LB. EMBO Rep. 2018 Jun;19(6):e46072. doi:

10.15252/embr.201846072. Epub 2018 Apr 30. PMID: 29712776

43 Induction of autophagy by spermidine promotes longevity. Eisenberg T, Knauer H, Schauer A, et al. Nat Cell Biol. 2009 Nov;11(11):1305-14. doi: 10.1038/ncb1975. PMID: 19801973

44 Neuronal growth and survival mediated by eIF5A, a polyamine-modified translation initiation factor. Huang Y, Higginson DS, Hester L, Park MH, Snyder SH. Proc Natl Acad Sci U S A. 2007 Mar 6;104(10):4194-9. doi: 10.1073/pnas.0611609104. PMID: 17360499

45 Spermidine-induced hypusination preserves mitochondrial and cognitive function during aging. Hofer SJ, Liang Y, Zimmermann A, Schroeder S, Dengjel J, Kroemer G, Eisenberg T, Sigrist SJ, Madeo F. Autophagy. 2021 Aug;17(8):2037-2039. doi: 10.1080/15548627.2021.1933299. Epub 2021 Jun 9. PMID: 34105442

46 Non-Linear Association of Dietary Polyamines with the Risk of Incident Dementia: Results from Population-Based Cohort of the UK Biobank. Qian M, Zhang N, Zhang R, Liu M, Wu Y, Lu Y, Li F, Zheng L. Nutrients. 2024 Aug 20;16(16):2774. doi: 10.3390/nu16162774. PMID: 39203912

47 Polyamines in Food. Muñoz-Esparza NC, Latorre-Moratalla ML, Comas-Basté O, Toro-Funes N, Veciana-Nogués MT, Vidal-Carou MC. Front Nutr. 2019 Jul 11;6:108. doi: 10.3389/fnut.2019.00108. eCollection 2019. PMID: 31355206

48 in mice is promoted by probiotic-induced suppression of colonic senescence dependent on upregulation of gut bacterial polyamine production. Matsumoto M, Kurihara S, Kibe R, Ashida H, Benno Y. Longevity PLoS One. 2011;6(8):e23652. doi: 10.1371/journal.pone.0023652. Epub 2011 Aug 16. PMID: 21858192; PMCID: PMC3156754.

49 Occurrence of Polyamines in Foods and the Influence of Cooking Processes. Foods. Muñoz-Esparza NC, Costa-Catala J, Comas-Basté O, Toro-Funes N, Latorre-Moratalla ML, Veciana-Nogués MT, Vidal-Carou MC. 2021 Jul 29;10(8):1752. doi: 10.3390/foods10081752. PMID: 34441529; PMCID: PMC8392025.

50 Polyamines in foods: development of a food database. Atiya Ali M, Poortvliet E, Strömberg R, Yngve A. Food Nutr Res. 2011 Jan 14;55. doi: 10.3402/fnr.v55i0.5572. PMID: 21249159

51 Forty percent methionine restriction decreases mitochondrial oxygen radical production and leak at complex I during forward electron flow and lowers oxidative damage to proteins and mitochondrial DNA in rat kidney and brain mitochondria. Caro P, Gomez J, Sanchez I, Naudi A, Ayala V, López-Torres M, Pamplona R, Barja G. Rejuvenation Res. 2009 Dec;12(6):421-34. doi: 10.1089/rej.2009.0902. PMID: 20041736

52 Effect of methionine dietary supplementation on mitochondrial oxygen radical generation and oxidative DNA damage in rat liver and heart. Gomez J, Caro P, Sanchez I, Naudi A, Jove M, Portero-Otin M, Lopez-Torres M, Pamplona R, Barja G. J Bioenerg Biomembr. 2009 Jun;41(3):309-21. doi: 10.1007/s10863-009-9229-3. Epub 2009 Jul 25. PMID: 19633937

53 Effect of every other day feeding on mitochondrial free radical production and oxidative stress in mouse liver. Caro P, Gómez J, López-Torres M, Sánchez I, Naudi A, Portero-Otín M, Pamplona R, Barja G. Rejuvenation Res. 2008 Jun;11(3):621-9. doi: 10.1089/rej.2008.0704. PMID: 18593280.

54 Protein and amino acid requirements in human nutrition. Joint WHO/FAO/UNU Expert Consultation. World Health Organ Tech Rep Ser. 2007;(935):1-265, back cover. PMID: 18330140

29: Exercise

Summary

It is easy to appreciate the beneficial impact on health. Exercise lowers inflammatory markers, lowers insulin resistance, and improves glycemic control, lowering the risk of diabetes, heart disease, Alzheimer's disease, and cancer. Different types of exercise, however, impact the various disease-causing factors differently; thus, a mix of various exercises helps to reduce the risk of different diseases.

Exercise is associated with a lower risk of breast cancer, lung disease, depression, and the development of dementia.[1] [2] [3] Regular exercise is associated with a 28% decrease in risk of dementia and a 45% decrease in the risk of Alzheimer's disease (AD). Those who don't exercise at all have double the risk of developing AD.[4] Now, consider how much further risk reduction there could be if the exercise were optimized to reduce AD and dementia risk.

Both aerobic and resistance exercise are helpful in reducing the risk of cardiovascular disease and diabetes, with aerobic or the combination of aerobic with resistance training being helpful.[5] [6] Although optimal risk reduction requires a significant amount of exercise, even small amounts of exercise can have great benefits:

- Compared to those who do no exercise, taking an 11-minute walk, at a leisurely 3 miles per hour, 5 days of the week, adds an average of 2 years of life expectancy. That is just a bit more than half a mile, five days a week.[7]
- Five hours (300 minutes) of light activity a day, never breaking a sweat, such as walking and shelving books in a library, lowers all-cause mortality by half (50%) as compared to 200 minutes of very light activity.
- An average of 20 to 25 minutes of vigorous physical activity per day lowers the risk of death by 60%.[8]
- In contrast, being sedentary for eleven hours a day more than doubles the risk of death.
- Even when exercise is begun late in life, it is protective against AD.[9]

Exercise training is typically categorized into four types: Resistance training (RT, i.e., weight lifting), aerobic training (AT, i.e., jogging, dancercise), combination training (RT + AT), and high intensity interval training (HIIT, i.e., repeated high intensity sprints–rest cycles).

Although almost any exercise improves health and lowers the risk of heart disease and diabetes, only exercise that is sufficiently intense to get one short of breath appears to prevent dementia or lower the risk of cancer death. Exercise, especially HIIT, improves mood and sleep.

Exercise provides benefits, especially to the brain, as a hormetic effect by causing brief exposure to oxidative stress and proinflammatory cytokines. Vigorous exercise 3 to 4 days a week appears to be most beneficial, while *vigorous exercise seven days a week increases risk*. We need a day of rest without vigorous exercise.

Excessive vigorous exercise, and especially excessive resistance training (more than an hour a day), begins to reverse the health benefits of exercise. For example, in a study of over 19,000 adults, mortality risk was lowest for those who jogged at an average pace, for 1 to 2.5 hours per week, split between one to three sessions. These light joggers ran at a pace of about 5 MPH (8 K/H). They had a mortality risk of less than one-fourth of that of sedentary non-joggers. Even jogging at this level for less than an hour a week greatly lowered mortality risk, but jogging more than 2.5 hours a week diminished the benefits. In contrast to light jogging, strenuous jogging, more than 7 MPH (11 K/H) and >4 hours/week, or more than a total of 2.5 hours a week with a frequency of >3 times per week, *doubled the all-cause mortality hazard* as compared to sedentary controls.[10] During sustained, intense exercise, there is a fall in perfusion of the intestine, which causes visceral hypoxia and intestinal mucosal injury, and leaky gut.[11]

Thus, a 3-mile (5K) jog, at 5 MPH, taking 36 minutes, twice a week, provides an optimal level of intense exercise for reducing mortality.

The most effective exercise for reducing the risk of dementia is High-Intensity Interval Training (HIIT), in which there are multiple brief bouts of very-high intensity exercise interspaced with recovery periods.

The best exercises, however, are those the individual enjoys and is most willing to perform consistently over time. Thus, the exercise needs to be accessible to the person and enjoyable. Some of the exercises should be ones that can be done at home, so that exercise can be done on rainy days and when schedules are tight. Exercising on a regular basis with a friend helps maintain motivation and consistency in the exercise routine.

Exercise Prescriptions for Those Over 50 for Preventing Dementia

Achieving the optimal exercise level for health and the prevention of dementia and most other chronic diseases is work, but not that much work.

Older adults should consult with their physician and discuss any risk mitigation that should be done before starting a new exercise program that includes vigorous exercise, especially if they are using medications.

A. Start with low, tolerable workloads and work up with time. An exercise program is not a short-term fix, so there is no need to rush to get in shape quickly. Expect to be exercising at the recommended levels for as many years as you want to be healthy. If out of shape, plan on slowly increasing exercise tolerance and fitness over three months.

B. Dementia has multiple causes, and different types of exercise address different risks.

C. By far, the most effective exercises for health maintenance and disease prevention are the ones a person actually does. Choose exercises you enjoy. Make it a habit and exercise with a friend regularly if possible.

D. Music may help make the time more fun, but earbuds can cause hearing loss, especially during intense exercise. Keep the volume low so that you can have a normal conversation when listening to music while exercising.

E. Cognitive function improves only when the exercise intervention includes aerobic or higher intensity levels of exercise.[12] If the exercise does not get the person short of breath, it will have limited efficacy.

F. Stay hydrated and don't get overheated. Either dehydration or overheating defeats the benefits of exercise on the brain and can cause harm.

G. Of the three main categories of exercise, resistance training has the least impact on cognition.

H. Weight-bearing exercise helps preserve and build bone mass, decreasing the risk of osteoporosis and fractures. Fractures are best prevented by preventing falls. Falls are prevented by exercise that maintains muscle strength, coordination, and balance.

I. Avoiding excessive time being sedentary is as important as getting enough exercise.

J. Exercise improves mood, cognition, and sleep quality. Intense exercise may be done in the evening, but should be completed an hour before bedtime.

K. Doing too much exercise can undo the benefits of exercise. Short bursts of intense exercise promote the expression of the body's antioxidant defense system, but sustained levels of intense exercise lead to the generation of more free radicals than the antioxidant system can defend against, resulting in oxidative damage. Excessive exercise may down-regulate the expression of anti-inflammatory cytokines (such as IL-10), putting one at risk of chronic inflammatory disease,[13] and prolonged, intense exercise causes leaky gut.

L. Building and maintaining muscle requires maintaining a positive muscle protein balance. This requires the consumption of sufficient high-quality protein to add muscle, especially on days when heavy exercise is done. The recommended daily protein intake for building and maintaining muscle mass, according to the International Society of Sports Nutrition (ISSN), is 1.4–2.0 g protein/kg body weight/day (g/kg/d), with higher amounts required for resistance training.[14] Protein requirements are discussed in Chapter 13.

M. Note that exercise is not an efficient way to burn fat. Don't bother trying to exercise excess fat mass away. In the long run, it does not work. Compliance with the SANA diet should help lower inflammation and help normalize weight with time. The SANA program encourages people to focus on health, not on body weight.

I. Exercise for Humans

We evolved from hunter-gatherers, who mostly gathered. The gathering involves walking, which is mostly low-intensity exercise. Sometimes they chased prey, and sometimes they ran away from predators and jealous spouses. Sometimes they did some heavy lifting. And sometimes they danced and swam. The Tsimane people, who live in remote Bolivian forests, subsist on hunting, fishing, and some farming. They walk about 15,000 steps a day. Most of them never develop coronary artery calcium deposits. Obesity, hypertension, and diabetes are quite rare in this population. The Ache people of Paraguay cover about 10 km (6 miles) a day, with maybe 1 – 2 km in rapid pursuit. After a hard day, they rest doing more sedentary activities the next day. Their bursts of activity are similar to high-intensity interval (HIIT) exercise, and much of the rest is walking. This is the lifestyle of our development as humans, and we should be able to do it into old age.

Sloth is known as one of the seven deadly sins. Spiritual sloth (acedia) is giving up and not caring about or for one's self or others; nevertheless, in ancient times, the sin of acedia may have been what we now recognize as depression. Physical sloth is a deadly sin in that it can hasten physical corruption and demise. In turn, exercise helps with depression. Exercise is one of the pillars of health, backed by hundreds of studies and clinical trials that document the salubrious effects of physical activity.

Most of these studies have assessed three types of training, plus a combination:

- Resistance Training (RT)
- Aerobic Training (AT)
- High Intensity Interval Training (HIIT)
- A combination of AT and RT (CT)

II. Exercise Recommendations and Guidelines

The health recommendation to do 10,000 steps a day (8 km or 5 miles per day) is not far from what hunter-gatherers do. In contrast, *marathon runners have a higher mass of plaque build-up in their coronary arteries* than do sedentary controls. Jogging a few times a week can give as much as a *6-year increase in life expectancy* as compared to a sedentary lifestyle, but *the benefit is lost with more than 4 hours per week of intense running.* [15]

More than half of adults and children don't get a substantial amount of exercise, and have poorer health as a result. Exercise should not be seen as work, but rather be a pleasurable activity. The best exercises are the ones we evolved to do as part of daily survival and fun. These are ones we can do with our life partners and friends. The best are the ones we enjoy. Pushing the body to its limits is stressful and harmful. Leisure-time activity that lowers stress, or that includes social engagement, can give a double or triple benefit. Two hours of walking in nature each week lowers blood pressure.

Like our ancestors, most of the exercise we should do is walking, with some bursts of activity that are similar to high-intensity interval (HIIT) exercise. As we get older, the two most important exercises for activities of daily living are walking and getting up from a seated position. The most common end of independent living for the elderly occurs when they can no longer get up from the toilet. This is one of the most common disabilities that places the elderly in an assisted living facility or nursing home. Thus, walking and standing from sitting are two exercises that should be included in every exercise regimen. Two hours in nature each week is good for the body and soul.

Physical Activity Recommendations:

Sleep: Eight hours of sleep, at night, in a comfortable, quiet, dark room, in bed (not in a recliner). (At around 8.5 hours in bed, leaves 15.5 hours for activity during the day.)

Occupation: Avoid passing more than half of daytime hours (>7.5 hours) per day in sedentary activities. (Sitting at a desk, sitting in a car or bus, watching TV, sitting in conversation). If your job is mostly sedentary, take breaks as opportunities to briskly walk or climb stairs to get some exercise. Try to get in a brisk walk during the lunch break. Rotate between sitting on a stool, a chair with a backrest, and a standing desk throughout the day. Switching from a chair to a stability ball for half of the workday may help some people retain core strength and improve posture. Even taking 3-minute exercise breaks from watching television in the evening improves sleep and health.[16]

Light Activity: People typically spend about 3 hours a day performing activities of daily living; cooking, cleaning, bathing, laundry, shopping, etc. Many people spend an hour or more on the phone, mostly socializing; spend this time walking or at least standing. Try to find a way to turn your sedentary activity time into light or moderate activity time. Walking 10,000 steps a day while performing light activities provides significant cardiovascular disease risk reduction.

Moderate to vigorous physical activity (MVPA): Do a minimum of 30 minutes of moderate to vigorous activity at least 5 days a week. For example, a brisk, two-mile walk at a pace of 4 miles per hour. Use Table 29B or a similar resource to select activities from 4.1 to 6.9 METS to do for half an hour on most days. Mix it up and do different activities on different days, but get in at least half an hour a day of moderate to vigorous exercise.

The optimal level of MVPA is about 180 total minutes per week. More can be done, but it does not significantly decrease disease risk. This can be done by walking a total of 12 miles per week, at 4 miles per hour. The goal is to exercise at a level of 5 to 7 METs (see chart below). When walking, going to different places rather than the same route each time, promotes great expression of neurotropic agents such as BDNF that stimulate neuronal growth. A treadmill is not effective for promoting BDNF expression in the brain.

Do sustained high-intensity aerobic exercise (*after consulting with one's physician*), preferably high-intensity exercise (more than 7 METs), 2 to 4 times a week. (MVPA is not required on days in which high-intensity exercise is done.) As noted above, a three-mile jog twice a week is enough to get into the Goldilocks zone. This should be aerobic exercise at 70 to 80 percent of the person's predicted maximum heart rate. The workload should be hard enough that the person is getting short of breath, but not so hard that they cannot talk; they should be able to say several words at a time, and their heart rate should not exceed 80% of their age-predicted maximum.

III. HIIT

As an alternative to *sustained* high-intensity exercise, high-intensity interval training (HIIT) exercise is highly recommended (*only after consulting with one's physician*). HIIT is composed of short bursts of near-maximal exercise followed by a brief cool-down, and this is repeated several times. While sustained high-intensity exercise generally has the goal of maintaining the heart rate at 70 to 80% of the person's maximum heart rate, HIIT gets the heart rate over 85% of the maximum heart rate (HRmax), and has a significant anaerobic component. HIIT is likely the most effective exercise for preventing dementia, and may be as well for cancer. HIIT is the quickest and most effective method for building exercise endurance.

HIIT is sometimes called Sprint Interval Training (SIT). An example of HIIT is sprinting (running as fast as possible for 30 to 45 seconds, followed by 4 minutes of walking until the heart rate recovers, before the next sprint/rest cycle, and generally, performing 5 to 6 cycles per session with 2 to 4 sessions a week. HIIT can also be done using a stationary bike to do all-out sprints (which are known as Wingates). For example, doing 30 to 45 seconds of maximum intensity bursts followed by 4 minutes of recovery cycling at 70% of HRmax.

Elite athletes might target HIIT to 75% of VO2max or more, or design their workout to get their rate to 95% their HRmax; for those trying to achieve better health, a more reasonable target is to begin exercising to heart rate that is 70 to 80% of their predicted HRmax (See Table 29C), and then slowly increasing the target heart rate with time towards 85% of the HRmax. The Rate of Perceived Exertion (RPE) is a subjective scale to estimate the VO2 max for targeting exercise level for HIIT. For moderate-intensity HIIT, aim for an RPE of 15, where the effort is hard and one is short of breath enough that one cannot say more than a few words at a time.

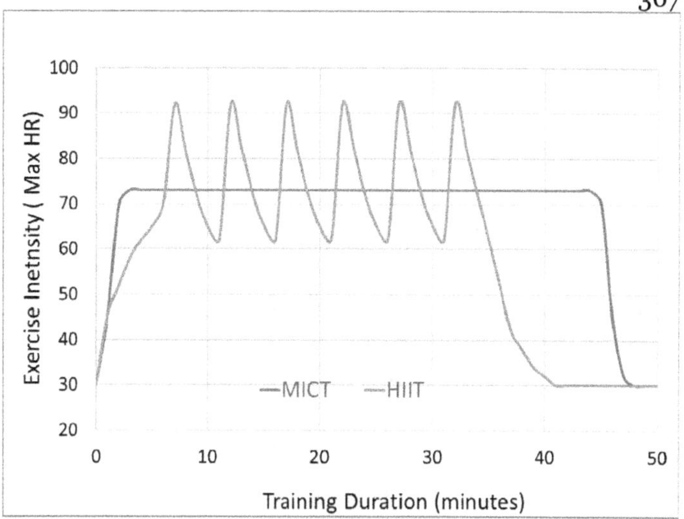

Figure 29A: In a typical moderate-intensity continuous training (MICT) program, the exercise is performed with sufficient intensity to maintain the heart rate at 70 to 80% of the person's HRmax (straight plateau line). In contrast, in high-intensity interval training (HIIT), the goal is to perform multiple bouts of exercise above the lactate threshold (LT), which is associated with achieving a heart rate between 85% to 95% of the HRmax for a short time, followed by a brief recovery period of lower-level exercise.

For HIIT, expect to slowly work up the intensity level over several weeks to months. In young athletes, the goal may be to do only about 10 minutes per week, but it is not as easy as it may sound, as it typically consists, for example, of six 30 to 45-second sprints, three times a week. This is not a treatment for the frail, but should help prevent frailty.

HIIT Elastic Band Training: Especially for senior seniors, adults, elastic band exercise has been demonstrated as an effective exercise for the prevention of dementia. For those in good physical condition, it can be used as an add-on exercise. While generally thought of as a resistance exercise, its true benefits may come from using it as an upper-body HIIT exercise. It does not use sufficient muscle mass to increase the heart rate as much as jogging or an exercise bike, but it can be done at sufficient intensity to induce shortness of breath and increase lactate output from the muscles being used.

Workout: Each elastic band workout session should focus on at least three different muscle groups; i.e., biceps, triceps, pectoral muscles, shoulders, etc. Choose an elastic band thickness that is at least 60 percent of the one-repetition maximum for the given exercise. Perform the exercise quickly, doing as many repetitions as possible for 8 seconds, then rest for 12 seconds, and repeat. Repeat this 20-second cycle 9 – 12 times for a total of 3 to 4 minutes. Rest for a minute and move to the next exercise area.

Note that peak benefits for elastic band exercise occurred at about 250 METs per week. The sweet spot for elastic band exercise is likely around 12 minutes of exercise, three times per week.

IV. Exercise "Snacks"

A study looked at how much break time from sitting was needed to undo the effects of sedentary work. A 5-minute walk break every 30 minutes was needed to lower the area under the curve for blood glucose levels. Nevertheless, even a one-minute break with light intensity walking every hour lowered systolic blood pressure.[17] In a similar study design, a three-minute light intensity walk every thirty minutes lowered fatigue and improved neuroendocrine biomarkers.[18] Five minutes every hour does not seem to be sufficient.[19] Walking up stairs once an hour to break up sedentary time was helpful.[20] When taking bathroom breaks, go to the far one and take the stairs if possible; walking quickly will help. If you get a 15-minute break at work, take a walk, and try to take a brisk walk at lunchtime if possible.[21]

Much of the harm from prolonged sitting can be overcome by high levels of leisure-time activity. To mitigate the impact of prolonged sitting requires the equivalent of about 40 minutes of high-intensity exercise per week, or about 150 minutes of moderate-intensity exercise per week.[22]

V. Dose Response for Exercise and All-Cause Mortality

Several meta-analyses have been done looking at the impact of physical activity on diabetes, cardiovascular disease mortality (CVD), cholesterol levels, risk of stroke, and risk of death. The results are generally similar, with much of the variation coming from the type of exercise engaged in. The following graphs are from a meta-analysis performed by Ekelund et al of over 36,000 adults with a mean age of 62.6 years and almost 6 years of follow-up.[23] The data comes from studies in which the participants were using electronic motion monitors (altigraphs) that measured their activity levels.

Graph 29B shows the impact of being sedentary for more than 7.5 hours a day. This analysis assumes that 7.5 hours of sedentary activity a day is typical in this population. When 12 hours were spent in sedentary activity per day, mortality increased 2.92 times. Graph 29C shows the impact of very light level physical activity (LPA), and uses 200 minutes, just over 3 hours, as a baseline. (The baseline is at 1.0 on the vertical axis.)

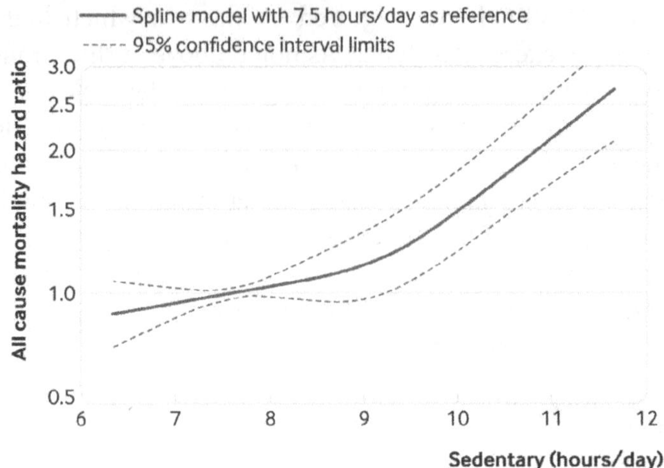

Figure 29B: Risk according to hours of sedentary activity per day

Graph 29C shows that those engaging in fewer minutes of light daily activity had higher mortality, with 1.7 times the risk for those with only 135 minutes of light activity daily. We can also see that an extra 100 minutes of very light physical activity above the typical 200 minutes reduces all-cause mortality by half. It also shows that there is only a trivial additional benefit to very light activity beyond 300 minutes (5 hours) a day. The dotted lines show the confidence intervals, and they get wider at higher exercise levels, indicating that few individuals were exercising at this level; thus, there is less data to make precise estimates from.

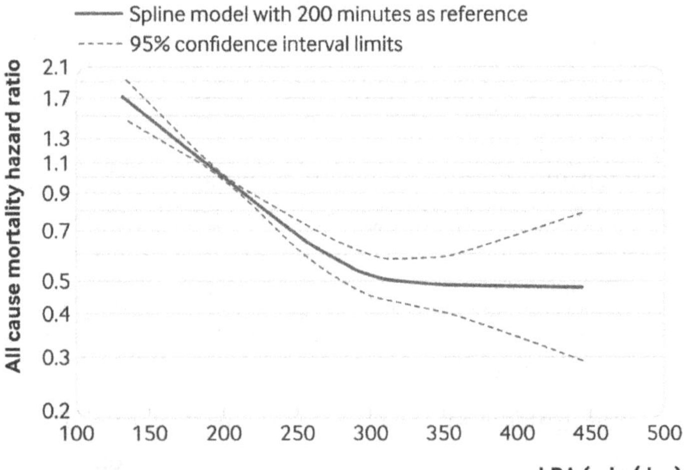

Figure 29C: All-cause mortality risk according to level of very-light physical activity per day

In the next graph (Figure 29D), we see the impact of slightly higher low-level physical activity (HLPA), but activity still considered to be light activity, on mortality. Here, the baseline is at 28 minutes a day. Mortality was lowest for those getting around 75 minutes of "high, light" activity per day, 47 minutes over the baseline. This activity likely included light housework, shopping, and walking, given the populations included in the study.

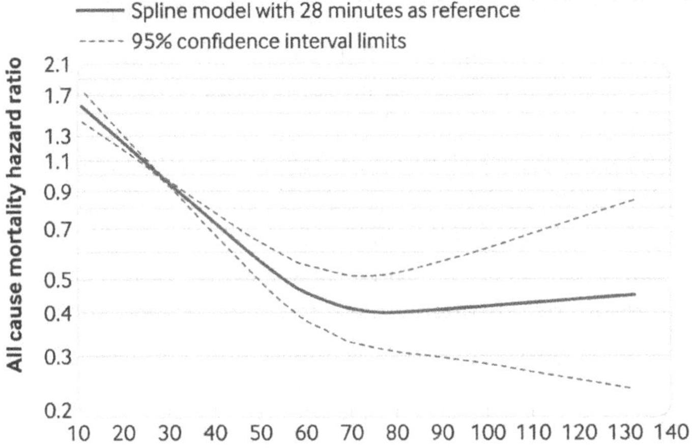

Figure 29D: All-cause mortality risk according to level of light physical activity per day

The final graft (Figure 29E) is for moderate to vigorous exercise, which, for this older population, was equivalent to a brisk walk or more. The nadir of risk was for those doing 20 to 25 minutes of moderately vigorous exercise per day. Note that here, in contrast to lower levels of exercise, the baseline is zero, as many people in this population do none, in comparison to the lower levels, in which the baseline likely represents the average person's activities of daily living. Thus, the benefits of moderate to vigorous exercise in terms of mortality risk reduction should be added to those of lower levels of exercise.

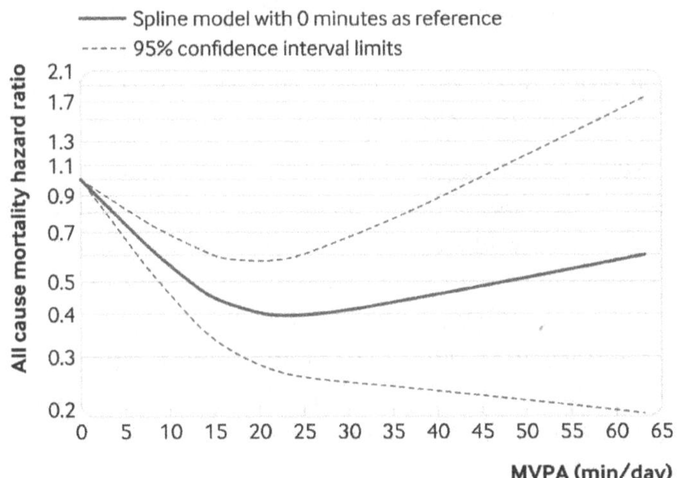

Figure 29E: All-cause mortality risk according to level of moderate to vigorous physical activity per day

What this and similar studies reveal is, firstly, the deleterious impact of sedentary behavior, and, just as importantly, that the amount of exercise needed to lower risk is similar to the activity of our ancestors and current hunter-gatherer people. For this population, near-optimal risk reduction, decreasing risk by half (50%) over being sedentary, required about 300 minutes of very light physical activity or, somewhat better, 75 minutes of higher-level light activity or about 23 minutes of moderate to vigorous activity per day, each reducing risk by about 60%. Please note that higher levels of vigorous activity provide little if any additional risk reduction, and that excess vigorous activity may potentially begin to reverse the benefit.

Let me point out a couple of things. There does not appear to be any downside to long (eight) hours of light activity per day, even in the elderly. We were made for this. Vigorous activity, however, has a hormetic effect. A moderate exposure to vigorous activity improves health and adaptation to stress, and has a subsequent anti-oxidative effect. Excessive vigorous activity is exhausting and damages health.

VI. Detailed Look at Exercise Types

Resistance training (RT) is an exercise that focuses on performing repeated, strong muscle contractions. The archetypal form of RT is weight lifting or the use of weight machines. RT is generally performed by doing repetitions at 70 to 80% of the person's maximum one-time maximal effort. Thus, if one can lift a 100-pound weight once as their maximum, a typical "set" would be to perform 8 to 10 repetitions of lifting 70 to 80 pounds, rest one minute or less, and then repeat with two more sets of that exercise. Typically, in each session, three to five different exercises are performed to work on different body areas. Thus, in a training session, 9 to 15 sets of 8 to 10 "reps" are done. In RT, the principal goal is to build and maintain muscle mass.

Resistance training to build muscle mass increases dietary protein demand, up from the general recommendation of 0.8 grams of dietary protein per kg to greater than 3 grams per kg daily.[24] Failing to provide sufficient protein while building muscle may divert protein from the heart and other vital organs, and thus, may be damaging.

Aerobic Training: In continuous AT, one tries to work at a level that gets the heart and respiratory rate up, but maintains the workload below the lactate threshold (LT).

Exceeding the lactate threshold means that the intensity of the exercise is sufficiently intense that the muscles cannot get enough oxygen to keep up with energy demand using aerobic production of ATP, and anaerobic glycolysis begins to make up the difference. At this point, the muscles begin releasing an increased amount of lactate (lactic acid) into the bloodstream, where it can be measured. Thus, the higher the exercise workload is above the lactate threshold, the greater the proportion of the energy demand is met by anaerobic metabolism.

With aerobic training, the goal is to train at a fairly steady level, generally just below the LT. The heart rate target is at 70 to 80% of the person's maximum heart rate (HRmax). The person's respiratory rate is faster, but they can still say several words at a time. AT includes exercises including brisk walking, jogging, cycling, swimming, aerobics, and many others.

Combined Training is a combination of AT and RT.

High Intensity Interval Training (HIIT), sometimes called Sprint Interval Training (SIT), is a type of exercise with repeated bouts of exercise exceeding the lactate threshold, interspaced with lower intensity for a recovery period. For example, in HIIT, the training may involve a short burst of near-maximal aerobic exercise for 30 to 45 seconds, followed by a few minutes of light aerobic exercise to recover, and then several repeats of this cycle.

The "Norwegian 4x4" HIIT protocol has a warm-up period, followed by 4 minutes of high-intensity exercise above the LT, followed by 4 minutes of exercise at 70% of the HRmax, which is the level at which the muscles can best utilize lactate and thus most efficiently lower blood lactate levels. In the 4 x 4 model, four cycles are done as shown. The goal of 4x4 is to rapidly improve endurance, build aerobic capacity, and raise the lactate threshold for athletes.

Resistance Training

A study that explored the amount of resistance training required to impact cholesterol levels found that 58 minutes per week gave the best results. If more time were devoted to it, the benefits began to decrease. RT even once or twice a week lowered the risk of hypercholesterolemia by about 21%, as compared to no resistance training. Doing more than 60 minutes of RT per week (as the sum of exercise sessions) reverses the benefit.[25] In another study, 60 minutes of RT was found to be associated with the lowest risk of cardiovascular disease (CVD), with risk increasing with more. Doing 130 minutes of RT per week yielded the same level of CVD risk as doing none; more than 130 minutes increased the risk of developing CVD even higher. When considering all-cause mortality, the lowest risk was among those performing 40 minutes of resistance training per week; this lowered CVD risk by about 17%.[26]

Another study found that RT worked best at lowering fasting blood sugar when doing training 2 – 3 times a week, and with doing three sets of 8 – 10 repetitions with less than one minute between sets at a workload of 70 to 80% of the one-repetition weight challenge maximum.[27]

The "one-repetition maximum" (1RM) in weight training is the highest weight that a person can lift for one repetition, and thus represents the maximum contraction force that the person can generate. Using repetitions of the 1RM is a way to maximize muscle mass over 12 to 16 weeks of training. Thus, one resistance training session, exercising 3 body areas, would have 9 sets of 8 to 10 reps. Different exercises can be done on different days. Three to five different exercises can be done in a session, but assume 4 minutes per triplet-set, and thus keep it to 9 to 10 triple-sets per week, divided into two or three sessions. Note that there were diminished benefits beyond 40 to 60 minutes of RT, depending upon the study.

RT helps build and then maintain muscle mass. Having a greater muscle mass helps the uptake of excess glucose from the bloodstream and stores it as glycogen for later use. Thus, it should even out blood sugar and perhaps appetite. Muscle health is a major factor in preventing chronic disease, at least in large part, because of its role in glucose uptake and glycogen storage. Thus, muscle activity and muscle mass help maintain insulin sensitivity.

While there are benefits to RT, it does not appear to be effective in lowering the risk of dementia, and is less effective than other forms of exercise in preventing diabetes, CVD, stroke, cancer, or all-cause mortality. Most studies that combine aerobic training and RT also fail to improve cognitive outcomes. RT causes muscle adaptation and very likely increases HIF1A in the muscle, but not in the brain.

Nevertheless, a particular form of resistance therapy used with older adults, the use of exercise bands, is more effective in improving cognition than regular RT, AT, or CT.[28]

Recommendation: If resistance training is done, optimal levels are for a total of 40 minutes divided into two or three sessions per week. The U-shaped response of RT limits how much should be done.

Aerobic Training

The risk of coronary heart disease (CHD) is high in those who rarely or never exercise. The sweet spot for mild to moderate aerobic exercise is to do it 2 to 6 times a week. CHD risk is about 12% lower among those who do vigorous exercise daily and 20% lower in those who do vigorous exercise once a week. Thus, vigorous exercise once a week is healthier than doing it 7 days a week! In several studies, aerobic exercise performed 4 to 6 days a week provided the highest benefit, with 7 days reversing the benefit. We all deserve a day of rest.

Cardiovascular disease mortality is lowest among those doing 900 to 2400 MET (Metabolic Equivalent of Task) minutes of exercise per week; there is not a lot of difference in health benefit within this range.[29] A brisk walk (4 miles per hour) increases energy consumption to 5 METS; that is, one burns about 5 times as many calories doing a brisk walk as sitting still. Thus, an hour-long brisk walk gives (60 x 5 =) 300 MET minutes. A 30-minute, brisk walk six days a week; 30 x 5 x 6 = 900 MET minutes. Thus, just one mile there-and-back for a total of two miles as a brisk walk 6 days a week, only about 4,000 steps a day, gets one into the lower end of the Goldilocks zone of cardiovascular health benefits. This is in line with other studies that show that 28 minutes a day of moderate-to-vigorous intensity physical activity or 300 minutes of low-level activity is associated with the lowest all-cause mortality.[30] Low-level activity would include shopping (@ 2.3 METs) or indoor work in education, hospitality, and health services (@ 2.5 METs) as examples. One MET hour is roughly equivalent to the expenditure of 1 kcal per kilogram of body weight per hour; therefore, calories burned during an activity can be roughly calculated using the formula. At rest, a 70 kg man needs a caloric intake of about 1680 kcal per day.

Another meta-analysis found that most of the reduction in CVD risk from exercise occurred with the first 2000 MET minutes, with some small additional benefit with further exercise.[31] A Chinese study found that most of the benefits of exercise on all-cause mortality, ischemic heart disease, and stroke occurred at 3600 MET minutes.[32] A study of leisure-time physical activity in American adults found that mortality risk was lowest with about 1350 to 2400 METs per week, although risk did not rise appreciably below 3500 METs.[33] Then again, healthier people are more likely to be physically active. Observational studies may simply be reflecting this. Thus, prospective studies need to be considered.

In a meta-analysis of 26 exercise trials among diabetic patients, moderate to vigorous exercise lowered HbA1c levels, a marker of chronic hyperglycemia, with increased duration of the exercise, but only up to 100 minutes of exercise per week. There was no advantage in terms of HbA1c for times above that. (It should be noted that HbA1c is not a great predictor of disease progression or remission. Fasting glucose, insulin sensitivity (HOMA-IR), and glucose tolerance tests (GTT) are more informative markers of metabolic health.) Studies suggest that moderate-intensity aerobic exercise for at least 150 minutes per week, or vigorous-intensity exercise for 75 minutes, can be very effective in reducing liver fat content and improving non-alcoholic steatohepatitis (NASH).[34] Even low-level activity, such as non-sedentary activity 5 hours (300 minutes) a day, is sufficient to maintain insulin sensitivity and greatly reduce the risk of T2D and CVD. Activity at around 2.5 METs reduces risk if one does a sufficient amount. This is where the 10,000 steps a day recommendation helps.

Aerobic exercise helps lower systolic blood pressure in those with hypertension, but there is no additional advantage to doing more than about 150 minutes of aerobic exercise per week, and little benefit beyond 120 minutes.[35]

Exercise is also good for mental health. In a systematic review and meta-analysis of studies in older adults, exercise decreased depression. Walking and aerobic exercise were the most effective for preventing depression. Yoga was less effective; Qigong and Tai Chi were ineffective. The level of activity that was most effective for preventing depression was aerobic exercise at 800 MET minutes or more per week. One thousand MET minutes (MM) was more effective, but this was the upper limit of data available in the review. For walking, levels greater than 600 MM per week were effective, with stronger effects observed at the review's upper range of around 800 MM. Resistance exercise reduced depression at about 750 MM, but was less effective, and higher levels began to reverse the benefits. [36]

VII. Exercise Intensity

RPE and METS

As exercise intensity increases, so does the heart rate; thus, heart rate is a simple and accessible way to determine exercise workload and oxygen utilization. The Borg Relative Perceived Exertion (RPE) score is another useful and well-validated scale of exercise intensity that correlates well with blood lactate levels during exercise, percent of maximum heart rate (%HRmax), and VO2Max, a measure of oxygen use.[37] [38] [39] Thus, %HRmax and RPE can be used to judge how intensely one is working during exercise. As can be seen in Table 29A, blood lactate levels rise slowly with increasing levels of exercise, but then rise quickly above the lactate threshold. This occurs at a blood lactate level of about 2.5 mmol/L, and at about 45% of the VO2Max, as the body can no longer deliver sufficient oxygen to the muscles to do purely aerobic exercise.

Another measure of the intensity of physical activity is METs (Metabolic Equivalents). One MET is the number of calories (and amount of oxygen) used by the person at rest. Three METs, thus means that a person is working at a level that uses three times as many calories and oxygen as they do when at rest.

HRmax

The predicted maximum heart rate declines with age. There are several methods for calculating the HRmax; this is the HUNT formula is appropriate for people over the age of 30:

Predicted Maximum Heart Rate: 211– (age x 0.64)

Thus, for a 65-year-old, the predicted maximum heart rate would be 169. The targeted sustained, 70 – 80% HRmax for vigorous exercise for a 65-year-old is thus 119 to 136 beats per minute. This is not an exact prediction; only about 67 percent of the population has a maximum heart rate within 11 beats per minute of this prediction.[40] These are estimates and are affected by genetics and the use of certain medications, notably beta blockers. Thus, these should be seen as approximations and not as an exercise prescription.

The Borg scale Rating of Perceived Exertion (RPE) is likely a safer estimate for workload than %HRmax, as it is based on the individual's perception of exertion and shortness of breath.

Table 29A: Levels of Exercise Intensity

Intensity	Borg RPE / METs	Blood Lactate	HRmax %
Rest	6 No exertion at all: doing nothing or resting 1 MET	Blood Lactate @ 1.4	50%
Sedentary	7.5 Extremely light exertion: slightly increased heart rate. 1.5 METs	Can talk fluidly	50-60%
Very light	9 Very light exertion: a gentle walk @ 2.5 METs	Blood Lactate @ 1.5 Can say a sentence at a time.	60 -70%
Light Exercise	11 Light exertion: a person has more than enough energy to continue exercising @ 4 METs	Blood Lactate @ 1.7 Can say a few words at a time.	70 – 80%
Moderate Exercise RPE 12–14	13 Somewhat hard exertion: Exercising is getting more difficult, but is still manageable. @ 5 METs	Blood Lactate @ 2.1	
Vigorous RPE 15–17	15 Hard exertion: Continuing the activity is noticeably more difficult. >6 METs	Blood Lactate @ 3.3 Above the lactate threshold. Can say a word or two at a time.	80 – 90%
	17 Very hard exertion: a person can maintain this level of physical activity if they push themselves; they are very tired. >8 METs	Blood Lactate @ 4.8 Anaerobic Training Hard to say a single word.	90 – 95%
Extremely Hard	19 Very Hard to keep going. >10 METs	Blood Lactate @ 7.4	
Maximal Exertion	20 Maximal Exertion: Complete exhaustion		95 – 100%

Table 29B: Activity Metabolic Equivalents[41]

Physical Activity	METS
Sleep	0.92
Watching television	1
Sitting in church	1.3
Working at a desk	1.5
Cooking	2
Washing dishes	2
Walking 1.7 mph (2.7 km/h) on level ground	2.3
Shopping	2.3
Typical indoor work in education, hospitality, and health services, where a person is active in light activities	2.5
Mowing the lawn with a riding mower	2.5
Walking, level surface 2.5 mph (4 km/h)	3
Vacuuming	3.3
Walking level surface 3.0 mph (4.8 km/h) (20 min/mile)	3.5
Mopping	3.5
Typical construction, logging, and mining work	3.9
Bicycling < 10 mph (16 km/h) leisurely for pleasure	4
Gardening, yard work at moderate effort	4
Walking firm, level surface 3.5 mph (5.6 km/h) (17 min/mile)	4.3
Mowing the lawn, pushing a power mower	4.5
Dancing	4.8
Walking firm, level surface 4 mph (15 min/mile)	5
Golf: walking and pulling clubs	5.3
Stationary bike, 100 watts	5.5
Swimming laps, freestyle, moderate effort	5.8
Playing basketball	6
Jogging 4 mph (15 min/mile) (6.4 km/h)	6
Mowing the lawn, pushing an unpowered mower	6
Hiking, cross-country	6
Tennis	7.3
Walking firm, level surface at 5 mph (12 min/mile)	8.3
Running 5 mph (12 min/mile) (8 km/h)	8.3
Running 6 mph (10 min/mile) (9.7 km/h)	9.8
Playing soccer	10
Running 7 mph (8.6 min/mile) (11.3 km/h)	11
Running 8 mph (7.5 min/mile) (12.9 km/h)	11.8
Running 9 mph (6.7 min/mile) (15.5 km/h)	12.8
Running 10 mph (6 min/mile) (16 km/h)	14.5
Running 12 mph (5 min/mile) (19.3 km/h)	19
Running 14 mph (4.3 min mile) (22.5 km/h)	23

Real METs

METs are sometimes counted in MET minutes and sometimes in MET hours. Let's look at MET Minutes. If one does a brisk walk for four miles over one hour (5 METs for 60 minutes), that is about 300 METs. If instead, they lie on a couch for an hour, they burn 60 METS (1 x 60). Sitting at a desk, looking at YouTube videos, used about 1.5 METs. How much exercise was done by walking? I would argue that the correct way to look at this is that the person did 300 – 60 = 240 *additional METs* or 210 net METs above sedentary (1.5 x 60 = 90). If a person uses zero METs for 5 minutes, they are guaranteed to never use another.

If you assume that the baseline threshold for metabolic benefit of exercise is a doubling of baseline (thus a baseline of 2 METs), then using the Ekelund data shown in the Figures 29 C and D above, 200 minutes at of light activity of 2.3 METS, (690 total METS) would yield 60 METs-2 (METs minus 2) minutes of exercise above the sedentary baseline, and 28 minutes of more active light activity at about 4 METs or 112 total METs) would convert to 56 METs-2 minutes, making 200 minutes of light physical activity burn about the same number of calories as 28 minutes of higher-level light physical activity, after subtracting the threshold.

Cancer: My analysis of cancer prevention trials suggests that exercise at 4 METs or less fails to reduce the risk of cancer. Thus, an hour of brisk walking at 5 METs would be 60 METs-4, and 5 hours of work at 3 METs (walking 3 miles per hour or 15 miles) would be *zero* METs-4.[42]

Aerobic exercise is associated with a 22% decreased risk of death in those diagnosed with breast cancer.[43] The maximum risk reduction was at 3300 MET minutes per week, with no additional benefits for higher levels of physical activity. This is considerably higher than most studies on the dose-response relationship of exercise to health. If 3300 METs is done walking at 4 miles per hour, it would require over 1.5 hours of brisk walking, over 6 miles daily. The very high amounts of exercise required to lower the risk of breast cancer in this study are likely a result of most of the exercise being below the critical threshold for cancer prevention, a level of about 4 METs.

Exercise below 4 METs appears to do little to prevent cancer mortality. Prevention of cancer by exercise has different mechanisms of action than for the prevention of metabolic disease. Exercise for cancer prevention 1) requires short-term induction of inflammatory cytokines, which has a hormetic effect that results in lower levels of sustained inflammation, and 2) gets one short of breath and induces the production of lactate by way of anaerobic respiration, which promotes autophagy and AMPK. Autophagy promotes the recycling of cellular organelles and proteins, and mitophagy causes the elimination of weak, poorly functioning mitochondria that leak free radicals, and stimulates their replacement with new ones. AMPK puts the brakes on the proliferation of new cells.

The benefits of exercise likely have different thresholds below which there is no effect, dependent upon the mechanisms by which the benefit is derived. For T2D, it may be improved insulin sensitivity of the muscles and increased storage of glycogen in the muscles. For cancer, it is likely hormetic induction of antioxidant proteins, replacement of old mitochondria, etc., and the slowing of cancer cell proliferation.

The prevention of dementia likely depends on the prevention of insulin resistance and hyperglycemia, avoidance of vascular disease, vasodilation in the brain, cytokine-induced reduction of inflammation, and the impact of lactate on autophagy in the brain. During exercise, there is a change in the fuel the brain uses; blood glucose levels drop, and lactate levels rise during intense exercise, and the brain is happy to use lactate. During exercise, blood flow to the brain does not increase substantially;[44] nevertheless, exercise promotes the development of small blood vessels in the brain.

Timing of Exercise

In obese adults with microvascular disease, three minutes or more of vigorous exercise in the evening (after 6:00 PM) was the most effective time of the day to exercise, lowering all-cause mortality by 61% as compared to a decrease of 33% for morning and 40% for afternoon exercise.[45] Among middle-aged men, those who exercised in the afternoon and especially evening had reduced insulin resistance as compared to those who exercised in the morning.[46]

The oxidation of fat is about 20% more efficient in the afternoon (4 – 5 PM) than in the morning (7 – 9 AM)[47, 48] although this effect is not seen in all studies.[49] Diabetics who exercise in the afternoon have a considerably greater fall in HbA1c and increased odds of coming off glucose-lowering medications if they exercise in the afternoon as compared to other times of the day.[50]

It appears that for a given amount of physical activity, moderate to vigorous physical activity (MVPA) in the midday (11 AM to 5 PM) lowers all-cause mortality the most; nevertheless, MVPA is better distributed throughout the day. All-cause mortality appears to be the lowest with MVPA distributed to about 50% in the midday, and the rest split evenly between the morning daylight hours (7 – 11 AM) and evening hours (5 – 9 PM).[51] In another study, MVPA exclusively done in the evening (after 5 PM) was not found to lower all-cause or cardiovascular disease risk.[52] High-intensity exercise in the evening appears to improve sleep efficiency and lower wake time after sleep onset (WASO) if done at least half an hour before,[53] and preferably an hour before bedtime.[54] Physical activity at night disturbs the circadian cycle and should be avoided, especially between midnight and 6 A.M.[55] Metabolically, physical activity in the wee hours is risky, and night shift workers pay a toll for it.

VIII. Exercise for Cognitive Function

Various exercises of sufficient intensity are required to activate the different mechanisms that help prevent dementia. Dementia is multicausal. Cerebral insulin resistance, vascular disease, oxidative stress, and inflammation are risk factors for dementia and AD. Most exercise improves insulin sensitivity; moderate to vigorous exercise helps prevent and even reverse insulin resistance and cardiovascular disease. Intense exercise has hormetic effects that promote the expression of antioxidant and anti-inflammatory proteins.

Resistance exercise can build muscle and improve insulin sensitivity; insulin resistance contributes to dementia. Moderate-level aerobic activity lowers the risk of vascular disease; vascular disease is an important cause of dementia and a contributing factor in AD. Intense exercise, enough to get one breathing hard, increases lactate levels. The brain uses lactate as a fuel. Lactate signals for the recycling of old organelles in the cells and the replacement of old, poorly functioning mitochondria with new ones.

Let me preface this section, pointing out that most of the exercise studies done in older adults are done among a population that is not in great shape. The level of exercise that has the best effect on cognitive function is a function of a person's underlying physical condition, and thus their age and comorbidities. The best time to prevent cognitive decline is before it occurs; dementia often subtly begins by the age of 50. Younger persons who would like to prevent cognitive decline may tolerate and require higher levels of exercise intensity to stimulate a hormetic effect. Thus, walking up a gentle slope may cause an increase in heart rate and cause one person to get short of breath (SOB) while it does not for another. Different people thus need different levels of exercise to get to a level that mitigates risk.

A review of 44 studies of individuals over the age of 50 found that a minimum of 724 MET minutes a week was required to observe relevant improvements in cognition, and the levels over 1200 MET minutes provided little additional benefits; however, this was dependent upon the exercise being performed. (The study did not include HIIT training.) Walking was coded as 4.5 METS for moderate and 7.0 METS for vigorous activity. Walking was associated with increased cognitive function, up to at least 1200 METs per week, but very few participants did more than 900 MET minutes per week of walking in these studies.[56]

Cognitive function increased with physical exercise at least up to 1800 METs, but the increase in benefit was not as robust above about 1000 METs. This result may be at least in part an effect of having very few older adult participants doing over 1000 METs per week. In this review, moderate intensity exercise was defined as an average of 4 METs and vigorous activity as an average of 8 METs. The improvements in cognition were similar for lean, overweight, and obese older adults, but the overweight and obese subjects only had cognitive benefits up to 634 METs-min per week. This may have resulted from limitations before which overexercise became unhelpful and even harmful among the overweight. These studies may also not have accounted for the increased burden of obesity (it is harder to climb stairs carrying an extra 50 pounds), and the obese often have diminished respiratory reserve. Being overweight can lead to impaired respiratory function as a result of pressure on the diaphragm, which can increase the work of breathing and reduce lung volume.

A study assessing which form of exercise in the elderly was best for increasing cognition found that it was the use of elastic bands. The optimal exercise for using elastic bands (when used as the sole form of exercise training) was performing 75 minutes of vigorous exercise per week, divided into 3 to 5 sessions, for a total of 376 MET-minutes. This improved cognition more than twice as much as other forms of exercise. The exercise was set to 70 to 80% of the participants' "maximum rate of perceived exertion" (RPE).[57] Using the BORG RPE scale, 70 to 80% RPE for band exercise is equivalent to working very hard, where it is difficult to hard, but not so hard that they have to push themselves or become exhausted.[58 59]

The elastic band exercise studies for improving cognition among the elderly included participants with mild cognitive dementia, and in another study, the elderly who were in wheelchairs.[60]. One program, for example, used elastic band exercises with 15 reps at 65% of the participants' maximal force, 3 times a week.[61] In another trial using elastic bands, high-speed training was more effective for maintaining cognition than low-speed training.[62] The success of elastic band exercise is likely a combination of factors, including the ability of the frail, poorly mobile, or those with poor balance to perform this exercise, but being limited from accomplishing other forms of adequately intense exercise. High-speed elastic band exercise should be considered a method of upper-body HIIT rather than RT.

In another meta-analysis focusing on patients with Alzheimer's disease, the most effective exercise was aerobic exercise at 660 MET Minutes per week, which corresponds to about 150 minutes of moderate intensity exercise or about 75 minutes per week of vigorous exercise. RT was not found to be helpful for those with AD.[63]

HIIT has demonstrated improved cognitive function and brain health in older adults. A 4-week HIIT program was found to significantly enhance cognitive function, physical performance, and electroencephalographic markers in elderly individuals.[64] Between HIIT, *moderate-intensity continuous training (MICT),* and resistance training (RT) in older adults, VO2 max, a measure of exercise capacity, improved the most with HIIT and least with RT. Only HIIT decreased reaction time, thus showing increased processing speed.[65] In a study of college students (no dementia), HIIT improved three tests of cognitive function while MICT improved only one. HIIT also improved subjective vitality, increased positive affect, and decreased negative affect.[66] Thus, HIIT improves mood.

HIIT has been found to improve motor function and neuroplasticity in rats after the induction of an ischemic stroke.[67] In studies of rats with vascular dementia, HIIT was demonstrated to improve cognitive function and increase expression of brain-derived neurotrophic factor (BDNF) in the hippocampus and cerebral cortex; however, this was not observed with MICT.[68] The hippocampus is the area of the brain most affected by AD, and the dentate gyrus of the hippocampus is the area of the brain most susceptible to aging. BDNF plays an important role in memory and learning. AD patients with lower serum BDNF levels have a more rapid deterioration of cognitive function. BDNF helps regulate glucose metabolism and fat oxidation. The HIIT exercise also increases lactate. Lactate promotes the transcription of BDNF (via phosphorylation of CREB). HIIT is also known to stimulate fatty acid oxidation in skeletal muscle more than other forms of exercise. This increases the production of the ketone β-hydroxybutyrate (β-OHB).[69] β-OHB promotes the expression of the protein p53, which promotes autophagy and renewal of cellular organelles. In the brain, this drives a recycling of old, worn-out organelles in the neurons and neuronal support cells. In senescent, aberrant, and cancer cells, β-OHB promotes apoptosis (so long as p53 is not dysfunctional).

A meta-analysis found that among women over the age of 65, participating in regular physical exercise (i.e., three sessions per week for 6 months) improves cognitive scores and increases telomere length (TL).[70] Another meta-analysis found that regular, moderate to vigorous intensity aerobic training for at least 6 months preserves telomere length, while RT and combined AT and RT did not.[71]

IX. Physiological Effects of Exercise

During heavy workload demand, the energy utilization by the muscle can exceed that produced by aerobic oxidative phosphorylation empowered by blood flow delivery of oxygen, and thus, there is an increased production of lactate by the muscles. The reduced levels of oxygen in the skeletal muscles promote the activation of the transcription factor Hypoxia-Inducible Factor-1 (HIF1). HIF1 is a dimer composed of the proteins HIF1A and ARNT. The genes induced by HIF1 include erythropoietin, which increases the generation of red blood cells, vascular endothelial growth factor (VEGF), which induces angiogenesis, vasodilatory agents that increase blood flow, glucose and lactate transporters, and glycolytic enzymes, to increase the metabolism to help adapt the body to the higher workloads.[72]

HIIT is particularly adept at stimulating glycolysis, glycogenesis (for the storage of glycogen in the muscle), and lactate transport proteins in skeletal muscle through its activation of HIF1A. HIF1A is constitutively present in the cytosol of the cell, but is also constantly degraded. During hypoxia, the protein, which degrades HIF1A, is inhibited, allowing for the accumulation of HIF1A and its binding to ARNT for HIF1A activation as a transcription factor. Long-term, regular HIIT increases the basal level of HIF1A.[73]

Under experimental conditions, rats performed equivalent levels of MICT or HIIT 5 days a week for 8 weeks. Their muscles were then analyzed for the levels of monocarboxylate transporter 1 (MCT1) and 4 (MCT4), peroxisome proliferator-activated receptor γ coactivator-1α (PGC-1α), and HIF1A. HIIT increased the level of mRNA for all four proteins, while MICT only increased the level of HIF1A, and even that was at a significantly lower level than that of HIIT.[74] MCT is a lactate transporter, and PGC-1α promotes mitochondrial renewal and improves OXPHOS capacity. Thus, HIIT (anaerobic exercise) has numerous metabolic effects that do not occur with MICT (aerobic exercise).

Among the mechanisms by which exercise helps prevent dementia is the increase in blood flow to the brain. This should not be a surprise, as the brain uses one-fifth of the body's energy and thus oxygen. Exercise helps prevent the shrinkage of the brain during aging. Cardiopulmonary fitness is associated with a greater volume of grey matter in the prefrontal cortex and hippocampus. Exercise increases the production of BDNF (brain-derived neurotrophic factor), which promotes the differentiation and survival of neurons. BDNF is most highly concentrated in the hippocampus and cortex.[75]. Vigorous exercise has hormetic activity, driving autophagy and the recycling of older, worn-out organelles.

Another goal of exercise is to increase growth hormone (GH) and IGF-1 (insulin-like growth factor 1). Short-duration bouts of exercise (6 - 10 min) at intensities that exceed the lactate threshold typically promote substantial GH release in athletes, but have less effect in less fit individuals.

A study tested the impact of a very-rapid cycle-time HIIT exercise program to assess its impact on GH and IGF1. Overweight nurses performed eight-second running sprints, followed by 12 seconds of active recovery cycles (3 cycles per minute) for 6 - 9 minutes at around 90% of the HRmax, 3 times a week. The rapid cycle HIIT effectively raised GH and IGF1 levels and lowered body fat mass, while in comparison, HIIT using 40 40-meter sprints had considerably less effect on GH and IGF1 and body fat mass.[76] The very short HIIT cycles allow the participant to catch their breath between cycles, but do not allow enough time for the heart rate to recover, thus sustaining heart rate at a high level that would be unlikely to be sustainable with other forms of exercise.

In another study, ten 15-second bouts of all-out pedaling against resistance on a cycle ergometer with 1-minute active rest between each interval also increased GH levels.[77] While there is only limited data on the most effective exercises to increase GH, repeated short bursts of exercise that increase the heart rate to 90% of the predicted heart rate for the person's age appear to be effective when the exercise exceeds the lactate threshold. Only a few minutes of exercise at this level is needed, and more can be detrimental.

Another means for assessing the efficacy of exercise is to determine its effects on inflammatory markers. Among adults with type 2 diabetes (T2D), C-reactive protein (CRP), a marker of inflammation, responds best to Combination training (CT), HIIT, and AT. Tumor necrosis factor (TNF) responded best to AT. IL-6 responded best to CT and AT but not to RT or HIIT.[78] HIIT promotes better glycemic control and more visceral weight loss, and lower systolic blood pressure.[79] [80] Unfortunately, these studies failed to assess the impact of each marker on each type of exercise training.

The benefits of exercise are in part a hormetic effect, wherein some stress leads to adaptation and increased muscular efficiency and mass. Too much exercise, however, depletes the body, exhausts it, and can damage the heart and other muscles. Thus, the intensity and duration of the exercise should be targeted. [81]

Exercise, Body Temp, and Intestinal Permeability

Humans are designed to run. Other primates can only run short distances.[82] In a warm climate, humans are the long-distance running champions of the animal world. We can't jump, swim, sprint, or lift heavy weights nearly as well as other animals, but we are the champions at long-distance running.[83] At ambient temperatures with a wet bulb over 28° C (82.4° F), horses are at increased risk for exertional heat illness (EHI), which can cause central nervous system dysfunction, physical collapse, and death.[84] Humans can outdistance horses and other animals in a race,[85] because we are bipedal, have strong gluteal muscles (chimps don't), springy tendons and foot design, we are naked, and we sweat. The lack of fur and the ability to sweat allow us to shed heat, which is our main advantage over other animals. Nevertheless, we can easily overheat, especially in hot weather.

During intense exercise, blood is shunted from the more vegetative organs, the intestine, liver, and kidneys, and flow increases to the muscles, heart, and lungs; organs that are needed for the exercise. Sustained, intense exercise can not only cause visceral hypoxia, but during recovery, there may be reperfusion injury as a result of reactive oxygen species (ROS) generated. These radicals can easily damage the mucosa and increase intestinal permeability, which results in leakage of toxic and inflammatory compounds (such as LPS) from the gut into the body. The inflammatory response to LPS and other endotoxins further weakens the mucosal barrier.[86] [87] The degree of injury is correlated with the core body temperature reached during the exercise. In a review of 16 studies, exercise-induced fever of 39° C was found to increase intestinal permeability in every study.[88] Overheating, such as during heat stroke, appears to increase intestinal permeability on its own, and this is exacerbated by decreased blood flow during exercise and then by reperfusion injury after intense exercise. This intestinal injury promotes systemic inflammation, the very thing we are trying to improve by exercising. Some of the neuropathology observed in horses with EHI may be caused by leaky gut.

Intense exercise should be avoided on hot days. Intense outdoor exercise should not be performed if the heat index is above 90° F (32.2° C). Overheating should be avoided. It is essential to stay hydrated; it has been demonstrated that GI permeability is increased in fluid-restricted runners.[89] The fluid restriction further limits intestinal blood flow, increasing the risk.[90] Hydration during exercise is critical for brain health. Even mild dehydration inhibits the exercise-associated rise in BDNF levels.[91]

The ideal core temperature for exercise is 37.5° C (99.5° F); this is the temperature at which the muscles perform work most effectively. Warm-up exercises literally warm up the muscles.

Stop exercise if the body temperature rises over 38.5° *C (101.3°F). Heat exhaustion is diagnosed with a body temperature of* 100.4*°F (38.3°C)*. There are benefits of getting the temperature up to his level *for a brief time.*

The body acclimates to exercise, heat, and high altitudes (mild hypoxia due to high elevations) through the induction of Hypoxia-Inducible Factor-1 (HIF1) and Heat Shock Proteins (HSP). HIF1 promotes the development of new blood vessels and red blood cells. HSP70 increases the integrity of the intestinal mucosal barrier and reduces the risk of mountain sickness, high-altitude pulmonary edema, and high-altitude cerebral edema. HSP90 increases the plasma volume, decreases sodium in the sweat, and increases blood flow to the organs and skin by inducing endothelial nitric oxide synthase.[92]

Between exercise intensity, exercise duration, and days of exercise, it is the number of days of exercise that best corresponds to acclimation.[93] As we acclimatize, the body adapts so that the same level of exercise causes a smaller rise in body temperature. Thus, accommodation to exercise at higher temperatures or greater altitude should be a gradual process over a week or more. In experimental conditions, the flavonoid quercetin was used in pharmacologic doses during exercise to block heat shock response (2000 mg/day). This treatment caused a failure of heat adaptation to protect the gut from increased permeability and from having endotoxins enter the bloodstream during heat stress.[94]

Two grams of quercetin is many times that normally encountered in the diet; it is about as much quercetin as there is in 200 apples, 500 servings of broccoli, or 16 pounds of onions, some of the foods highest in this compound that is hormetic in low amounts. Quercetin is a hormetic agent that provides benefits at low doses.

Aspirin, NSAID medications, and gluten can increase the risk of impaired intestinal permeability. Pre-exercise treatment with glutamine, arginine, and likely citrulline, amino acids used by the cells lining the intestines, may prevent exercise/heat-induced intestinal permeability.[95] Brief bouts of HIIT training may help prevent intestinal permeability through the induction of HSP70 (heat shock protein 70) and other adaptive mechanisms.

X. Bestowing the Benefits of Exercise on the Infirm, the Incapacitated, or the Indulgent of Indolence:

Feeling lazy? Some of the benefits of heat adaptation can be achieved passively by soaking in a hot bath or sauna. Hot baths have some of the same beneficial metabolic effects as exercise; meanwhile, using a cold clamp (cool baths during experimental conditions, or swimming in cool water) during exercise prevents most of these beneficial effects. The changes that occur with hot baths include increased levels of IL-6, epinephrine and norepinephrine release, growth hormone, cortisol, G-CSF,[96] [97] HSP72,[98] 3-hydroxybutyrate, and lactic acid.[99] Epinephrine release appears to promote lactate utilization.[100] The expected effects of hormones and cytokines resulting from elevated body temperature, elevation from a hot bath, would be to promote mitochondrial reproduction and fission. The net effect of exercise and hot baths, with transient elevation of body temperature, may be the increased turnover rate of mitochondria while protecting the cell from apoptosis. Heat adaptation by HSP72 improves insulin sensitivity, promotes the generation and increased mass of mitochondria, increases glucose uptake by the muscles, decreases the accumulation of fat in the muscles (myosteatosis), lowers inflammation, and fat accumulation in the liver.[101]

Hot baths have some beneficial effects that parallel the effects of intense exercise, but without the work. The core body temperature needs to increase to about 37.5° to 38.5°C.[102] This can be done in a hot bath, hot tub, or sauna. Hot baths also help to improve glucose tolerance[103] and increase insulin sensitivity in type 2 diabetics.[104] Since lactate crosses the blood-brain barrier, hot baths should also benefit mitochondria in the brain.

Taking hot baths with a water temperature of 37.8° – 41.0°C (99.5° – 105.8°F) for 30 minutes a day was found to improve blood sugar levels and cause weight loss in insulin-dependent diabetics.[105] Hot baths are one of the most effective non-pharmacologic treatments for fibromyalgia.[106] Saunas are also helpful,[107] but the time and temperature should be limited to no more than 20 minutes at 80°C (176°F). Higher temperatures or prolonged exposure can cause heat exhaustion and heat stress, nausea, elevated body temperature, as well as depression, anger, fatigue, and confusion, even in healthy young adults.[108] Whether using exercise, baths, or saunas to induce heat adaptation, start with shorter times and lower temperatures, and then gradually increase to the recommended time and intensity.

XI. Ergothioneine

Ergothioneine (EGT) is a non-protein-forming, vitamin-like, amino acid; that is, it is a compound that the human body cannot make but which is needed for full health, and which is exclusively derived from the diet.

EGT appears to be a cofactor for the enzyme 3-mercaptopyruvate sulfurtransferase (MPST), which has several important functions, including coronary vasodilation, mitochondrial activity, and detoxification of cyanide. (The biosynthesis of small amounts of cyanide is a normal physiologic process.) EGT is important enough to the body that it has its own transport protein (SLC22A4) for absorption from the gut and retention in the kidney. Nrf2 is a transcription factor for several antioxidant enzymes. EGT may activate Nrf2 transcription and prevent its degradation.[109] EGT also participates in the recycling of glutathione, the body's major antioxidant.

With exercise training, the amount of EGT in the muscle increases. Exercise induces the transcriptional co-activator PGC-1α; SLC22A4 is among the genes that are upregulated by PGC-1α. Thus, exercise increases how avidly EGT is taken up into the body and the muscles. In the muscles, EGT enhances the ability of the mitochondria to generate ATP in an MPST-dependent process. Increasing dietary EGT in mice increased their spontaneous activity level by ~14%. In mice, the level of muscle EGT nearly doubled with exercise training as compared to sedentary mice. In humans, blood EGT levels increase with both resistance and endurance training.[110]

EGT is solely produced by microbes and fungi. The foods highest in ergothioneine are mushrooms, particularly golden (*Pleurotus citrinopileatus)* and king oyster (*Pleurotus eryngii)* mushrooms. High levels are also present in portobella and button mushrooms (*Agaricus bisporus)*, shitake (*Lentinula edodes*), and porcini mushrooms (*Boletus edulis*). The growth media and growing conditions of the mushrooms appear to have as much impact on the EGT content as does the type of mushroom. Many bacteria produce EGT, and some fermented foods have high levels. Black beans (turtle beans) have been demonstrated to contain moderate levels of EGT; they absorb EGT produced by soil microbes through their roots. Other legumes may also accumulate EGT. Chicken liver has moderate levels as EGT concentrates in the liver. Oat bran also contains some. Most other foods have minimal levels.[111]

EGT was found to protect against brain lipid peroxidation, the accumulation of β-Amyloid in the hippocampus, and neuronal injury in mice.[112] Higher EGT levels are associated with a lower risk of cardiovascular disease and cardiovascular mortality. EGT was also found to provide some protection against liver injury in rats.[113]

Unfortunately, after the age of 60, blood ergothioneine levels decline linearly with age. Still worse, lower EGT levels are associated with more rapid cognitive decline. In a 21-year follow-up study, EGT levels were the metabolite most closely associated with the consumption of a health-conscious food pattern, and EGT was associated with lower cardiovascular and overall mortality.[114] Some small case-control studies have found lower levels of EGT in the blood of older adults with mild cognitive impairment, Parkinson's disease, and dementia, as compared to age-matched healthy controls.[115] Multiple population studies have found preservation of cognitive functioning among older adults who consume mushrooms frequently.

The observation that EGT blood levels fall with age and are associated with chronic disease is unlikely to be the result of dietary changes or mycophobia (avoidance of mushrooms) but rather that the decline in blood level coincides with and results from a decline in physical activity and muscle mass in aging, especially among those with chronic disease. In order to have an optimal supply of EGT for health, sufficient ergothioneine is required in the diet, but the demand side likely comes from physical activity. Young athletes may require a higher dietary intake of EGT to have peak performance than do sedentary elderly individuals. The impact of EGT deficits likely limits performance more in athletes than it does in the sedentary. Nevertheless, EGT should be considered a required nutrient. Mice with higher dietary EGT choose to do more exercise, likely because they have more stamina before feeling like they want to rest.

Consuming several medium-sized button mushrooms each week should provide an adequate supply of EGT. A reasonable supplemental dose is 10 mg, and should not exceed 25 mg per day, even for athletes.

Caution should be used in the use of EGT as a dietary supplement, especially in older adults, as it may protect or enhance the growth of cancer, similar to the effect of vitamin A and some other vitamins.

Table 29C. Heart Rate Target Ranges by Age

Age	HRmax	60% HRmax	70% HRmax	80% HRmax	85% HRmax	90% HRmax
50	179	107	125	143	152	161
51	178	107	125	143	152	161
52	178	107	124	142	151	160
53	177	106	124	142	151	159
54	176	106	124	141	150	159
55	176	105	123	141	149	158
56	175	105	123	140	149	158
57	175	105	122	140	148	157
58	174	104	122	139	148	156
59	173	104	121	139	147	156
60	173	104	121	138	147	155
61	172	103	120	138	146	155
62	171	103	120	137	146	154
63	171	102	119	137	145	154
64	170	102	119	136	145	153
65	169	102	119	136	144	152
66	169	101	118	135	143	152
67	168	101	118	134	143	151
68	167	100	117	134	142	151
69	167	100	117	133	142	150
70	166	100	116	133	141	150
71	166	99	116	132	141	149
72	165	99	115	132	140	148
73	164	99	115	131	140	148
74	164	98	115	131	139	147
75	163	98	114	130	139	147
76	162	97	114	130	138	146
77	162	97	113	129	137	146
78	161	97	113	129	137	145
79	160	96	112	128	136	144
80	160	96	112	128	136	144
81	159	95	111	127	135	143
82	159	95	111	127	135	143
83	158	95	111	126	134	142
84	157	94	110	126	134	142
85	157	94	110	125	133	141
86	156	94	109	125	133	140
87	155	93	109	124	132	140
88	155	93	108	124	131	139
89	154	92	108	123	131	139
90	153	92	107	123	130	138
91	153	92	107	122	130	137
92	152	91	106	122	129	137
93	151	91	106	121	129	136
94	151	91	106	121	128	136
95	150	90	105	120	128	135

[1] High-intensity interval training versus moderate-intensity continuous training on patient quality of life in cardiovascular disease: a systematic review and meta-analysis. Yu H, Zhao X, Wu X, Yang J, Wang J, Hou L. Sci Rep. 2023 Aug 25;13(1):13915. doi: 10.1038/s41598-023-40589-5. PMID: 37626066

[2] Effects of high-intensity interval training on depressive symptoms: A systematic review and meta-analysis. Tao Y, Lu J, Lv J, Zhang L. J Psychosom Res. 2024 May;180:111652. doi: 10.1016/j.jpsychores.2024.111652. Epub 2024 Apr 2. PMID: 38603999

[3] Effect of physical activity on risk of Alzheimer's disease: A systematic review and meta-analysis of twenty-nine prospective cohort studies. Zhang X, Li Q, Cong W, Mu S, Zhan R, Zhong S, Zhao M, Zhao C, Kang K, Zhou Z. Ageing Res Rev. 2023 Dec;92:102127. doi: 10.1016/j.arr.2023.102127. Epub 2023 Nov 17. PMID: 37979700

[4] https://www.alzheimers.org.uk/about-dementia/managing-the-risk-of-dementia/reduce-your-risk-of-dementia/physical-activity

[5] Comparisons of different exercise interventions on glycemic control and insulin resistance in prediabetes: a network meta-analysis. Huang L, Fang Y, Tang L. BMC Endocr Disord. 2021 Sep 6;21(1):181. doi: 10.1186/s12902-021-00846-y. PMID: 34488728

[6] A Meta-Analysis of the Influence on Inflammatory Factors in Type 2 Diabetes among Middle-Aged and Elderly Patients by Various Exercise Modalities. Yang W, Jiao H, Xue Y, Wang L, Zhang Y, Wang B, Teng Z, Li J, Zhao H, Liu C. Int J Environ Res Public Health. 2023 Jan 18;20(3):1783. doi: 10.3390/ijerph20031783. PMID: 36767149

[7] https://www.whyiexercise.com/metabolic-equivalent.html

[8] Dose-response associations between accelerometry measured physical activity and sedentary time and all cause mortality: systematic review and harmonised meta-analysis. Ekelund U, Tarp J, Steene-Johannessen J, Hansen BH, Jefferis B, Fagerland MW, Whincup P, Diaz KM, Hooker SP, Chernofsky A, Larson MG, Spartano N, Vasan RS, Dohrn IM, Hagströmer M, Edwardson C, Yates T, Shiroma E, Anderssen SA, Lee IM. BMJ. 2019 Aug 21;366:l4570. doi: 10.1136/bmj.l4570. PMID: 31434697

[9] Snowdon, David A. (2002). Aging with Grace: What the Nun Study Teaches Us About Leading Longer, Healthier, and More Meaningful Lives. New York, New York: Bantam Books. ISBN 0-553-38092-3.

[10] Dose of jogging and long-term mortality: the Copenhagen City Heart Study. Schnohr P, O'Keefe JH, Marott JL, Lange P, Jensen GB. J Am Coll Cardiol. 2015 Feb 10;65(5):411-9. doi: 10.1016/j.jacc.2014.11.023. PMID: 25660917

[11] Association Between Exercise-Induced Hyperthermia and Intestinal Permeability: A Systematic Review. Pires W, Veneroso CE, Wanner SP, Pacheco DAS, Vaz GC, Amorim FT, Tonoli C, Soares DD, Coimbra CC. Sports Med. 2017 Jul;47(7):1389-1403. doi: 10.1007/s40279-016-0654-2. PMID: 27943148

[12] Physical activity interventions in older adults with a cognitive impairment: A critical review of reviews. de Rondão CA, Mota MP, Esteves D. Aging Med (Milton). 2023 May 24;6(3):290-306. doi: 10.1002/agm2.12256. eCollection 2023 Sep. PMID: 37711255

[13] A Meta-Analysis of the Influence on Inflammatory Factors in Type 2 Diabetes among Middle-Aged and Elderly Patients by Various Exercise Modalities. Yang W, Jiao H, Xue Y, Wang L, Zhang Y, Wang B, Teng Z, Li J, Zhao H, Liu C. Int J Environ Res Public Health. 2023 Jan 18;20(3):1783. doi: 10.3390/ijerph20031783. PMID: 36767149

[14] International Society of Sports Nutrition Position Stand: protein and exercise. Jäger R, Kerksick CM, Campbell BI, Antonio J. J, et al. Int Soc Sports Nutr. 2017 Jun 20;14:20. doi: 10.1186/s12970-017-0177-8. 2017. PMID: 28642676

[15] A Hunter-Gatherer Exercise Prescription to Optimize Health and Well-Being in the Modern World. O'Keefe EL, Lavie CJ. J Sci Sport Exerc. 2021;3(2):147-157. doi: 10.1007/s42978-020-00091-0. Epub 2020 Oct 27. PMID: 38624470

[16] Evening regular activity breaks extend subsequent free-living sleep time in healthy adults: a randomised crossover trial. Gale JT, Haszard JJ, Wei DL, Taylor RW, Peddie MC. BMJ Open Sport Exerc Med. 2024 Jul 16;10(3):e001774. doi: 10.1136/bmjsem-2023-001774. eCollection 2024. PMID: 39027425

[17] Breaking Up Prolonged Sitting to Improve Cardiometabolic Risk: Dose-Response Analysis of a Randomized Crossover Trial. Duran AT, Friel CP, Serafini MA, Ensari I, Cheung YK, Diaz KM. Med Sci Sports Exerc. 2023 May 1;55(5):847-855. doi: 10.1249/MSS.0000000000003109. Epub 2023 Jan 12. PMID: 36728338

[18] Acute effects of breaking up prolonged sitting on fatigue and cognition: a pilot study. Wennberg P, Boraxbekk CJ, Wheeler M, Howard B, Dempsey PC, Lambert G, Eikelis N, Larsen R, Sethi P, Occleston J, Hernestål-Boman J, Ellis KA, Owen N, Dunstan DW. BMJ Open. 2016 Feb 26;6(2):e009630. doi: 10.1136/bmjopen-2015-009630. PMID: 26920441

[19] The Effects Of Interrupting Sedentary Behavior With Hourly Physical Activity On Cardiometabolic Risk Factors In Healthy Adults: 2331Magulas, Melina Meyer; Ekelund, Ulf FACSM; Steene-Johannessen, Jostein.. Medicine & Science in Sports & Exercise 55(9S):p 774, September 2023. | DOI: 10.1249/01.mss.0000987116.56648.29

[20] Metabolic Effect of Breaking Up Prolonged Sitting with Stair Climbing Exercise Snacks. Rafiei H, Omidian K, Myette-Côté É, Little JP. Med Sci Sports Exerc. 2021 Jan;53(1):150-158. doi: 10.1249/MSS.0000000000002431. PMID: 32555024

[21] The Effects of Breaking up Prolonged Sitting Time: A Review of Experimental Studies. Benatti FB, Ried-Larsen M. Med Sci Sports Exerc. 2015 Oct;47(10):2053-61. doi: 10.1249/MSS.0000000000000654. PMID: 26378942

[22] Occupational Sitting Time, Leisure Physical Activity, and All-Cause and Cardiovascular Disease Mortality. Gao W, Sanna M, Chen YH, Tsai MK, Wen CP. JAMA Netw Open.

2024 Jan 2;7(1):e2350680. doi: 10.1001/jamanetworkopen.2023.50680. PMID: 38241049

23 Dose-response associations between accelerometry measured physical activity and sedentary time and all cause mortality: systematic review and harmonised meta-analysis. Ekelund U, Tarp J, Steene-Johannessen J, Hansen BH, Jefferis B, Fagerland MW, Whincup P, Diaz KM, Hooker SP, Chernofsky A, Larson MG, Spartano N, Vasan RS, Dohrn IM, Hagströmer M, Edwardson C, Yates T, Shiroma E, Anderssen SA, Lee IM. BMJ. 2019 Aug 21;366:l4570. doi: 10.1136/bmj.l4570. PMID: 31434697

24 International Society of Sports Nutrition Position Stand: protein and exercise. Jäger R, Kerksick CM, Campbell BI, Antonio J. J, et al. Int Soc Sports Nutr. 2017 Jun 20;14:20. doi: 10.1186/s12970-017-0177-8. 2017. PMID: 28642676

25 Association of Resistance Exercise with the Incidence of Hypercholesterolemia in Men. Bakker EA, Lee DC, Sui X, Eijsvogels TMH, Ortega FB, Lee IM, Lavie CJ, Blair SN. Mayo Clin Proc. 2018 Apr;93(4):419-428. doi: 10.1016/j.mayocp.2017.11.024. Epub 2018 Feb 8. PMID: 29428677

26 Optimum Dose of Resistance Exercise for Cardiovascular Health and Longevity: Is More Better? Lee DC, Lee IM. Curr Cardiol Rep. 2023 Nov;25(11):1573-1580. doi: 10.1007/s11886-023-01976-6. Epub 2023 Oct 14. PMID: 37837559

27 Dose-response relationships of resistance training in Type 2 diabetes mellitus: a meta-analysis of randomized controlled trials. Su W, Tao M, Ma L, Tang K, Xiong F, Dai X, Qin Y. Front Endocrinol (Lausanne). 2023 Sep 25;14:1224161. doi: 10.3389/fendo.2023.1224161. eCollection 2023. PMID: 37818093

28 Optimal dose and type of exercise to improve cognitive function in older adults: A systematic review and bayesian model-based network meta-analysis of RCTs. Gallardo-Gómez D, Del Pozo-Cruz J, Noetel M, Álvarez-Barbosa F, Alfonso-Rosa RM, Del Pozo Cruz B. Ageing Res Rev. 2022 Apr;76:101591. doi: 10.1016/j.arr.2022.101591. Epub 2022 Feb 17. PMID: 35182742

29 Exercise at the Extremes: The Amount of Exercise to Reduce Cardiovascular Events. Eijsvogels TM, Molossi S, Lee DC, Emery MS, Thompson PD. J Am Coll Cardiol. 2016 Jan 26;67(3):316-29. doi: 10.1016/j.jacc.2015.11.034. PMID: 26796398

30 Dose-response associations between accelerometry measured physical activity and sedentary time and all cause mortality: systematic review and harmonised meta-analysis. Ekelund U, Tarp J, Steene-Johannessen J, Hansen BH, Jefferis B, Fagerland MW, Whincup P, Diaz KM, Hooker SP, Chernofsky A, Larson MG, Spartano N, Vasan RS, Dohrn IM, Hagströmer M, Edwardson C, Yates T, Shiroma E, Anderssen SA, Lee IM. BMJ. 2019 Aug 21;366:l4570. doi: 10.1136/bmj.l4570. PMID: 31434697

31 Physical activity policies for cardiovascular health. Ilkka Vuori. UKK Institute for Health Promotion, https://www.google.com/url?sa=t&source=web&rct=j&opi=89978449&url=https://ehnheart.org/wp-content/uploads/2023/05/05737-Physical-activity-report-final-2.pdf

32 Association of regular physical activity with total and cause-specific mortality among middle-aged and older Chinese: a prospective cohort study. Zhou Y, Zhang R, Liu Y, Guo Y, Wang D, He M, Yuan J, Liang Y, Zhang X, Wang Y, Guo H, Wei S, Miao X, Yao P, Wu T, Chen W. Sci Rep. 2017 Jan 4;7:39939. doi: 10.1038/srep39939. PMID: 28051177

33 Leisure time physical activity and mortality: a detailed pooled analysis of the dose-response relationship. Arem H, Moore SC, Patel A, Hartge P, Berrington de Gonzalez A, Visvanathan K, Campbell PT, Freedman M, Weiderpass E, Adami HO, Linet MS, Lee IM, Matthews CE. JAMA Intern Med. 2015 Jun;175(6):959-67. doi: 10.1001/jamainternmed.2015.0533. PMID: 25844730

34 Dose-Dependent Effect of Supervised Aerobic Exercise on HbA_{1c} in Patients with Type 2 Diabetes: A Meta-analysis of Randomized Controlled Trials. Jayedi A, Emadi A, Shab-Bidar S. Sports Med. 2022 Aug;52(8):1919-1938. doi: 10.1007/s40279-022-01673-4. Epub 2022 Apr 1. PMID: 35362859

35 Effects of aerobic exercise on blood pressure in patients with hypertension: a systematic review and dose-response meta-analysis of randomized trials. Jabbarzadeh Ganjeh B, Zeraattalab-Motlagh S, Jayedi A, Daneshvar M, Gohari Z, Norouziasl R, Ghaemi S, Selk-Ghaffari M, Moghadam N, Kordi R, Shab-Bidar S. Hypertens Res. 2024 Feb;47(2):385-398. doi: 10.1038/s41440-023-01467-9. Epub 2023 Oct 23. PMID: 37872373

36 Optimal dose and type of exercise to improve depressive symptoms in older adults: a systematic review and network meta-analysis. Tang L, Zhang L, Liu Y, Li Y, Yang L, Zou M, Yang H, Zhu L, Du R, Shen Y, Li H, Yang Y, Li Z. BMC Geriatr. 2024 Jun 7;24(1):505. doi: 10.1186/s12877-024-05118-7. PMID: 38849780

37 Rating of Perceived Exertion: A Large Cross-Sectional Study Defining Intensity Levels for Individual Physical Activity Recommendations. Grummt M, Hafermann L, Claussen L, Herrmann C, Wolfarth B. Sports Med Open. 2024 Jun 10;10(1):71. doi: 10.1186/s40798-024-00729-1. PMID: 38856875

38 Relationship between the rating of perceived exertion scale and the load intensity of resistance training. Morishita S, Tsubaki A, Takabayashi T, Fu JB. Strength Cond J. 2018 Apr;40(2):94-109. doi: 10.1519/SSC.0000000000000373. PMID: 29674945

39 Associations between Borg's rating of perceived exertion and physiological measures of exercise intensity. Scherr J, Wolfarth B, Christle JW, Pressler A, Wagenpfeil S, Halle M. Eur J Appl Physiol. 2013 Jan;113(1):147-55. doi: 10.1007/s00421-012-2421-x. Epub 2012 May 22. PMID: 22615009

40 Age-predicted maximal heart rate in healthy subjects: The HUNT fitness study. Nes BM, Janszky I, Wisløff U, Støylen A, Karlsen T. Scand J Med Sci Sports. 2013 Dec;23(6):697-704. doi: 10.1111/j.1600-0838.2012.01445.x. Epub 2012 Feb 29. PMID: 22376273.

41 Metabolic equivalents (METS) in exercise testing, exercise prescription, and evaluation of functional capacity. Jetté M, Sidney K, Blümchen G. Clin Cardiol. 1990 Aug;13(8):555-65. PMID:2204507

[42] Unraveling Cancer: Cancer Prevention Even After Diagnosis. Charles Lewis, Psy Press Carrabelle, Fl 2015 Chapter 13.

[43] Dose-response relationship between physical activity and mortality in adults with noncommunicable diseases: a systematic review and meta-analysis of prospective observational studies. Geidl W, Schlesinger S, Mino E, Miranda L, Pfeifer K. Int J Behav Nutr Phys Act. 2020 Aug 26;17(1):109. doi: 10.1186/s12966-020-01007-5. PMID: 32843054

[44] Regulation of increased blood flow (hyperemia) to muscles during exercise: a hierarchy of competing physiological needs. Joyner MJ, Casey DP. Physiol Rev. 2015 Apr;95(2):549-601. doi: 10.1152/physrev.00035.2013. PMID: 25834232

[45] Timing of Moderate to Vigorous Physical Activity, Mortality, Cardiovascular Disease, and Microvascular Disease in Adults With Obesity. Sabag A, Ahmadi MN, Francois ME, Postnova S, Cistulli PA, Fontana L, Stamatakis E. Diabetes Care. 2024 May 1;47(5):890-897. doi: 10.2337/dc23-2448. PMID: 38592034

[46] Timing of physical activity in relation to liver fat content and insulin resistance. van der Velde JHPM, Boone SC, Winters-van Eekelen E, Hesselink MKC, Schrauwen-Hinderling VB, Schrauwen P, Lamb HJ, Rosendaal FR, de Mutsert R. Diabetologia. 2023 Mar;66(3):461-471. doi: 10.1007/s00125-022-05813-3. Epub 2022 Nov 1. PMID: 36316401

[47] Timing matters: diurnal variation of maximal fat oxidation and substrate oxidation rates in metabolic syndrome-a randomized crossover study. Methnani J, Brahim MM, Elhraiech A, Ach T, Latiri I, Zaouali M, Rouatbi S, Bouslama A, Brun JF, Omezzine A, Bouhlel E. Eur J Appl Physiol. 2024 Jun 4. doi: 10.1007/s00421-024-05518-y. Online ahead of print. PMID: 38832982

[48] Timing matters: diurnal variation of maximal fat oxidation and substrate oxidation rates in metabolic syndrome-a randomized crossover study. Methnani J, Brahim MM, Elhraiech A, Ach T, Latiri I, Zaouali M, Rouatbi S, Bouslama A, Brun JF, Omezzine A, Bouhlel E. Eur J Appl Physiol. 2024 Jun 4. doi: 10.1007/s00421-024-05518-y. Online ahead of print. PMID: 38832982

[49] No diurnal variation is present in maximal fat oxidation during exercise in young healthy women: A cross-over study. Robles-González L, Aguilar-Navarro M, López-Samanes Á, Ruiz-Moreno C, Muñoz A, Varillas-Delgado D, Gutiérrez-Hellín J, Helge JW, Ruiz JR, Amaro-Gahete FJ. Eur J Sport Sci. 2023 Jun;23(6):936-942. doi: 10.1080/17461391.2022.2067007. Epub 2022 May 8. PMID: 35437101

[50] Association of Timing of Moderate-to-Vigorous Physical Activity With Changes in Glycemic Control Over 4 Years in Adults With Type 2 Diabetes From the Look AHEAD Trial. Qian J, Xiao Q, Walkup MP, Coday M, Erickson ML, Unick J, Jakicic JM, Hu K, Scheer FAJL, Middelbeek RJW; Look AHEAD Research Group. Diabetes Care. 2023 Jul 1;46(7):1417-1424. doi: 10.2337/dc22-2413. PMID: 37226675

[51] Associations of timing of physical activity with all-cause and cause-specific mortality in a prospective cohort study. Feng H, Yang L, Liang YY, Ai S, Liu Y, Liu Y, Jin X, Lei B, Wang J, Zheng N, Chen X, Chan JWY, Sum RKW, Chan NY, Tan X, Benedict C, Wing YK, Zhang J. Nat Commun. 2023 Feb 18;14(1):930. doi: 10.1038/s41467-023-36546-5. PMID: 36805455

[52] Associations of timing of physical activity with all-cause and cause-specific mortality in a prospective cohort study. Feng H, Yang L, Liang YY, Ai S, Liu Y, Liu Y, Jin X, Lei B, Wang J, Zheng N, Chen X, Chan JWY, Sum RKW, Chan NY, Tan X, Benedict C, Wing YK, Zhang J. Nat Commun. 2023 Feb 18;14(1):930. doi: 10.1038/s41467-023-36546-5. PMID: 36805455

[53] Different Intensities of Evening Exercise on Sleep in Healthy Adults: A Systematic Review and Network Meta-Analysis. Yue T, Liu X, Gao Q, Wang Y. Nat Sci Sleep. 2022 Dec 14;14:2157-2177. doi: 10.2147/NSS.S388863. eCollection 2022. PMID: 36540196

[54] Effects of Evening Exercise on Sleep in Healthy Participants: A Systematic Review and Meta-Analysis. Stutz J, Eiholzer R, Spengler CM. Sports Med. 2019 Feb;49(2):269-287. doi: 10.1007/s40279-018-1015-0. PMID: 30374942

[55] Association between circadian physical activity trajectories and incident type 2 diabetes in the UK Biobank. Bai P, Shao X, Chen L, Zhou S, Lin Y, Liu H, Yu P. Sci Rep. 2024 Mar 18;14(1):6459. doi: 10.1038/s41598-024-57082-2. PMID: 38499679

[56] Optimal dose and type of exercise to improve cognitive function in older adults: A systematic review and bayesian model-based network meta-analysis of RCTs. Gallardo-Gómez D, Del Pozo-Cruz J, Noetel M, Álvarez-Barbosa F, Alfonso-Rosa RM, Del Pozo Cruz B. Ageing Res Rev. 2022 Apr;76:101591. doi: 10.1016/j.arr.2022.101591. Epub 2022 Feb 17. PMID: 35182742

[57] Optimal dose and type of exercise to improve cognitive function in older adults: A systematic review and bayesian model-based network meta-analysis of RCTs. Gallardo-Gómez D, Del Pozo-Cruz J, Noetel M, Álvarez-Barbosa F, Alfonso-Rosa RM, Del Pozo Cruz B. Ageing Res Rev. 2022 Apr;76:101591. doi: 10.1016/j.arr.2022.101591. Epub 2022 Feb 17. PMID: 35182742

[58] Resistance Exercise Program in Cognitively Normal Older Adults: CERT-Based Exercise Protocol of the AGUEDA Randomized Controlled Trial. Fernandez-Gamez B, Solis-Urra P, Olvera-Rojas M, et al. J Nutr Health Aging. 2023;27(10):885-893. doi: 10.1007/s12603-023-1982-1. PMID: 37960912

[59] Rate of perceived exertion (RPE): Scale, what it is, and more (medicalnewstoday.com)

[60] Positive effects of physical training in activity of daily living-dependent older adults. Venturelli M, Lanza M, Muti E, Schena F. Exp Aging Res. 2010 Apr;36(2):190-205. doi: 10.1080/03610731003613771. PMID: 20209421

[61] Effects of 12-Week Resistance Exercise on Electroencephalogram Patterns and Cognitive Function in the Elderly With Mild Cognitive Impairment: A Randomized Controlled Trial. Hong SG, Kim JH, Jun TW. Clin J Sport Med. 2018 Nov;28(6):500-508. doi: 10.1097/JSM.0000000000000476. PMID: 28727639

62 Effect of elastic band-based high-speed power training on cognitive function, physical performance and muscle strength in older women with mild cognitive impairment. Yoon DH, Kang D, Kim HJ, Kim JS, Song HS, Song W. Geriatr Gerontol Int. 2017 May;17(5):765-772. doi: 10.1111/ggi.12784. Epub 2016 Jul 10. PMID: 27396580

63 Effective dosage and mode of exercise for enhancing cognitive function in Alzheimer's disease and dementia: a systematic review and Bayesian Model-Based Network Meta-analysis of RCTs. Yuan Y, Yang Y, Hu X, Zhang L, Xiong Z, Bai Y, Zeng J, Xu F. BMC Geriatr. 2024 Jun 1;24(1):480. doi: 10.1186/s12877-024-05060-8. PMID: 38824515

64 Effects of a High-Intensity Interval Physical Exercise Program on Cognition, Physical Performance, and Electroencephalogram Patterns in Korean Elderly People: A Pilot Study. Lee SM, Choi M, Chun BO, Sun K, Kim KS, Kang SW, Song HS, Moon SY. Dement Neurocogn Disord. 2022 Jul;21(3):93-102. doi: 10.12779/dnd.2022.21.3.93. Epub 2022 Jul 26. PMID: 35949421

65 High-Intensity Interval Training Improves Cognitive Flexibility in Older Adults. Mekari S, Neyedli HF, Fraser S, O'Brien MW, Martins R, Evans K, Earle M, Aucoin R, Chiekwe J, Hollohan Q, Kimmerly DS, Dupuy O. Brain Sci. 2020 Oct 29;10(11):796. doi: 10.3390/brainsci10110796. PMID: 33137993

66 Effect of acute exercise intensity on cognitive inhibition and well-being: Role of lactate and BDNF polymorphism in the dose-response relationship. Ballester-Ferrer JA, Bonete-López B, Roldan A, Cervelló E, Pastor D. Front Psychol. 2022 Dec 9;13:1057475. doi: 10.3389/fpsyg.2022.1057475. PMID: 36570982

67 High-intensity training with short and long intervals regulate cortical neurotrophic factors, apoptosis markers and chloride homeostasis in rats with stroke. Hugues N, Pin-Barre C, Brioche T, Pellegrino C, Berton E, Rivera C, Laurin J. Physiol Behav. 2023 Jul 1;266:114190. doi: 10.1016/j.physbeh.2023.114190. Epub 2023 Apr 11. PMID: 37055005

68 High-intensity interval training improves cognitive impairment of vascular dementia rats by up-regulating expression of brain-derived neurotrophic factor in the hippocampus. Guo C, Yao Y, Ma C, Wang Z. Neuroreport. 2023 May 17;34(8):411-418. doi: 10.1097/WNR.0000000000001903. Epub 2023 Apr 25. PMID: 37104097

69 The Impact of High-Intensity Interval Training on Brain Derived Neurotrophic Factor in Brain: A Mini-Review. Jiménez-Maldonado A, Rentería I, García-Suárez PC, Moncada-Jiménez J, Freire-Royes LF. Front Neurosci. 2018 Nov 14;12:839. doi: 10.3389/fnins.2018.00839. eCollection 2018. PMID: 30487731

70 Physical Activity on Telomere Length as a Biomarker for Aging: A Systematic Review. Schellnegger M, Lin AC, Hammer N, Kamolz LP. Sports Med Open. 2022 Sep 4;8(1):111. doi: 10.1186/s40798-022-00503-1. PMID: 36057868

71 Does Exercise Affect Telomere Length? A Systematic Review and Meta-Analysis of Randomized Controlled Trials. Song S, Lee E, Kim H. Medicina (Kaunas). 2022 Feb 5;58(2):242. doi: 10.3390/medicina58020242. PMID: 35208566

72 Skeletal muscle hypoxia-inducible factor-1 and exercise. Lindholm ME, Rundqvist H. Exp Physiol. 2016 Jan;101(1):28-32. doi: 10.1113/EP085318. Epub 2015 Oct 15. PMID: 26391197

73 High-intensity interval training-induced metabolic adaptation coupled with an increase in Hif-1α and glycolytic protein expression. Abe T, Kitaoka Y, Kikuchi DM, Takeda K, Numata O, Takemasa T. J Appl Physiol (1985). 2015 Dec 1;119(11):1297-302. doi: 10.1152/japplphysiol.00499.2015. Epub 2015 Oct 1. PMID: 26429867

74 The effects of different training modalities on monocarboxylate transporters MCT1 and MCT4, hypoxia inducible factor-1α (HIF-1α), and PGC-1α gene expression in rat skeletal muscles. Ahmadi A, Sheikholeslami-Vatani D, Ghaeeni S, Baazm M. Mol Biol Rep. 2021 Mar;48(3):2153-2161. doi: 10.1007/s11033-021-06224-0. Epub 2021 Feb 24. PMID: 33625690

75 Summary of the effect of an exercise intervention on elderly with mild cognitive impairment: A systematic review and meta-analysis. Xiaotang Liu, Lanjuan Liu, Cheng Liu. Medicine (Baltimore) 2024 Jun 14; 103(24): e38025. Published online 2024 Jun 14. doi: 10.1097/MD.0000000000038025 PMCID: PMC11175880

76 "The Effect of Two Types of High-Intensity Interval Training on Serum Value of GH and IGF-1 in Overweight Nurses." Avazpour, Sahar et al. Asian Journal of Sports Medicine (2020) https://brieflands.com/articles/asjsm-103135

77 High-intensity interval exercise test stimulates growth hormone secretion in children. Dror N, Pantanowitz M, Nemet D, Eliakim A. Growth Horm IGF Res. 2021 Apr-Jun;57-58:101388. doi: 10.1016/j.ghir.2021.101388. Epub 2021 Apr 20. PMID: 33906078

78 A Meta-Analysis of the Influence on Inflammatory Factors in Type 2 Diabetes among Middle-Aged and Elderly Patients by Various Exercise Modalities. Yang W, Jiao H, Xue Y, Wang L, Zhang Y, Wang B, Teng Z, Li J, Zhao H, Liu C. Int J Environ Res Public Health. 2023 Jan 18;20(3):1783. doi: 10.3390/ijerph20031783. PMID: 36767149

79 The effects of high-intensity intermittent exercise training on fat loss and fasting insulin levels of young women. Trapp EG, Chisholm DJ, Freund J, Boutcher SH. Int J Obes (Lond). 2008 Apr;32(4):684-91. doi: 10.1038/sj.ijo.0803781. Epub 2008 Jan 15. PMID: 18197184

80 Effects of aerobic training intensity on resting, exercise and post-exercise blood pressure, heart rate and heart-rate variability. Cornelissen VA, Verheyden B, Aubert AE, Fagard RH. J Hum Hypertens. 2010 Mar;24(3):175-82. doi: 10.1038/jhh.2009.51. Epub 2009 Jun 25. PMID: 19554028

81 Exercise Time and Intensity: How Much Is Too Much? Gottschall JS, Davis JJ, Hastings B, Porter HJ. Int J Sports Physiol Perform. 2020 Feb 28;15(6):808-815. doi:

10.1123/ijspp.2019-0208. Print 2020 Jul 1. PMID: 32365286

[82] Energetic and endurance constraints on great ape quadrupedalism and the benefits of hominin bipedalism. Raichlen DA, Pontzer H. Evol Anthropol. 2021 Jul;30(4):253-261. doi: 10.1002/evan.21911. Epub 2021 Aug 4. PMID: 34347329

[83] Endurance running and the evolution of Homo. Bramble DM, Lieberman DE. Nature. 2004 Nov 18;432(7015):345-52. doi: 10.1038/nature03052. PMID: 15549097

[84] Continuous Monitoring of the Thermoregulatory Response in Endurance Horses and Trotter Horses During Field Exercise: Baselining for Future Hot Weather Studies. Verdegaal, EL, et al. Front. Physiol., 25 August 2021 Sec. Exercise Physiology, 12 - 2021 https://doi.org/10.3389/fphys.2021.708737

[85] https://www.npr.org/sections/health-shots/2015/10/20/450068114/heres-how-you-can-outrun-a-horse

[86] Intestinal epithelial barrier function and tight junction proteins with heat and exercise.

Dokladny K, Zuhl MN, Moseley PL. J Appl Physiol (1985). 2016 Mar 15;120(6):692-701. doi: 10.1152/japplphysiol.00536.2015. Epub 2015 Sep 10. PMID: 26359485

[87] Exercise regulation of intestinal tight junction proteins. Zuhl M, Schneider S, Lanphere K, Conn C, Dokladny K, Moseley P. Br J Sports Med. 2014 Jun;48(12):980-6. doi: 10.1136/bjsports-2012-091585. Epub 2012 Nov 7. PMID: 23134759

[88] Association Between Exercise-Induced Hyperthermia and Intestinal Permeability: A Systematic Review. Pires W, Veneroso CE, Wanner SP, Pacheco DAS, Vaz GC, Amorim FT, Tonoli C, Soares DD, Coimbra CC. Sports Med. 2017 Jul;47(7):1389-1403. doi: 10.1007/s40279-016-0654-2. PMID: 27943148

[89] Fluid restriction during running increases GI permeability. Lambert GP, Lang J, Bull A, Pfeifer PC, Eckerson J, Moore G, Lanspa S, O'Brien J. Int J Sports Med. 2008 Mar;29(3):194-8. doi: 10.1055/s-2007-965163. Epub 2007 Jul 5. PMID: 17614027.

[90] Cardiac output distribution in thermally dehydrated rodents. Horowitz M, Samueloff S. Am J Physiol. 1988 Jan;254(1 Pt 2):R109-16. doi: 10.1152/ajpregu.1988.254.1.R109. PMID: 3276223

[91] Effects of Fluid Ingestion on Brain-Derived Neurotrophic Factor and Cognition During Exercise in the Heat. Roh HT, So WY, Cho SY, Suh SH. J Hum Kinet. 2017 Aug 1;58:73-86. doi: 10.1515/hukin-2017-0074. PMID: 28828079

[92] Heat acclimation and cross tolerance to hypoxia: Bridging the gap between cellular and systemic responses. Ely BR, Lovering AT, Horowitz M, Minson CT. Temperature (Austin). 2014 Jul 8;1(2):107-14. doi: 10.4161/temp.29800. PMID: 27583292

[93] Heat acclimation-induced intracellular HSP70 in humans: a meta-analysis. Nava R, Zuhl MN. Cell Stress Chaperones. 2020 Jan;25(1):35-45. doi: 10.1007/s12192-019-01059-y. Epub 2019 Dec 10. PMID: 31823288

[94] Thermotolerance and heat acclimation may share a common mechanism in humans. Kuennen M, Gillum T, Dokladny K, Bedrick E, Schneider S, Moseley P. Am J Physiol Regul Integr Comp Physiol. 2011 Aug;301(2):R524-33. doi: 10.1152/ajpregu.00039.2011. Epub 2011 May 25. PMID: 21613575

[95] Intestinal epithelial barrier function and tight junction proteins with heat and exercise. Dokladny K, Zuhl MN, Moseley PL. J Appl Physiol (1985). 2016 Mar 15;120(6):692-701. doi: 10.1152/japplphysiol.00536.2015. Epub 2015 Sep 10. PMID: 26359485

[96] Human blood neutrophil responses to prolonged exercise with and without a thermal clamp. Laing SJ, Jackson AR, Walters R, Lloyd-Jones E, Whitham M, Maassen N, Walsh NP. J Appl Physiol. 2008 Jan;104(1):20-6. PMID:17901240

[97] Muscle damage and immune responses to prolonged exercise in environmental extreme conditions. Hassan ES. J Sports Med Phys Fitness. 2016 Oct;56(10):1206-1213. Epub 2015 Sep 1. PMID: 26329839

[98] Elevation of body temperature is an essential factor for exercise-increased extracellular heat shock protein 72 level in rat plasma. Ogura Y, Naito H, Akin S, Ichinoseki-Sekine N, etal. Am J Physiol Regul Integr Comp Physiol. 2008 May;294(5):R1600-7. PMID:18367652

[99] Metabolic and hormonal responses to exogenous hyperthermia in man. Møller N, Beckwith R, Butler PC, Christensen NJ, Orskov H, Alberti KG. Clin Endocrinol (Oxf). 1989 Jun;30(6):651-60. doi: 10.1111/j.1365-2265.1989.tb00271.x. PMID: 2686866

[100] Additive protective effects of the addition of lactic acid and adrenaline on excitability and force in isolated rat skeletal muscle depressed by elevated extracellular K+. de Paoli FV, Overgaard K, Pedersen TH, Nielsen OB. J Physiol. 2007 Jun 1;581(Pt 2):829-39. doi: 10.1113/jphysiol.2007.129049. Epub 2007 Mar 8. PMID: 17347268

[101] Chaperoning to the metabolic party: The emerging therapeutic role of heat-shock proteins in obesity and type 2 diabetes. Henstridge DC, Whitham M, Febbraio MA. Mol Metab. 2014 Aug 30;3(8):781-93. doi: 10.1016/j.molmet.2014.08.003. eCollection 2014 Nov. PMID: 25379403

[102] Human blood neutrophil responses to prolonged exercise with and without a thermal clamp. Laing SJ, Jackson AR, Walters R, Lloyd-Jones E, Whitham M, Maassen N, Walsh NP. J Appl Physiol. 2008 Jan;104(1):20-6. PMID:17901240

[103] HSP72 protects against obesity-induced insulin resistance. Chung J, Nguyen AK, Henstridge DC, Holmes AG, Chan MH, Mesa JL, etal. Proc Natl Acad Sci U S A. 2008 Feb 5;105(5):1739-44. PMID:18223156

[104] Heat treatment improves glucose tolerance and prevents skeletal muscle insulin resistance in rats fed a high-fat diet. Gupte AA, Bomhoff GL, Swerdlow RH, Geiger PC. Diabetes. 2009 Mar;58(3):567-78. Epub 2008 Dec 10. PMID:19073766

[105] Hot-tub therapy for type 2 diabetes mellitus. Hooper PL. N Engl J Med. 1999 Sep 16;341(12):924-5. PMID:10498473

[106] Complementary and alternative medicine in the treatment of pain in fibromyalgia: a systematic review of randomized controlled trials. Terhorst L, Schneider MJ, Kim KH, Goozdich LM, Stilley CS. J Manipulative Physiol Ther. 2011 Sep;34(7):483-96. doi: 10.1016/j.jmpt.2011.05.006. Epub 2011 Jun 24. PMID: 21875523

[107] The multifaceted benefits of passive heat therapies for extending the healthspan: A comprehensive review with a focus on Finnish sauna. Laukkanen JA, Kunutsor SK. Temperature (Austin). 2024 Feb 25;11(1):27-51. doi: 10.1080/23328940.2023.2300623. PMID: 38577299

[108] The influence of extreme thermal stress on the physiological and psychological characteristics of young women who sporadically use the sauna: practical implications for the safe use of the sauna. Podstawski R, Borysławski K, Józefacka NM, Snarska J, Hinca B, Biernat E, Podstawska A. Front Public Health. 2024 Jan 26;11:1303804. doi: 10.3389/fpubh.2023.1303804. eCollection 2023. PMID: 38344040

[109] L-ergothioneine and its combination with metformin attenuates renal dysfunction in type-2 diabetic rat model by activating Nrf2 antioxidant pathway. Dare A, Channa ML, Nadar A. Biomed Pharmacother. 2021 Sep;141:111921. doi: 10.1016/j.biopha.2021.111921. Epub 2021 Jul 30. PMID: 34346315

[110] Ergothioneine boosts mitochondrial respiration and exercise performance via direct activation of MPST. Sprenger HG, Mittenbühler MJ, Sun Y, Van Vranken JG, Schindler S, Jayaraj A, Khetarpal SA, Vargas-Castillo A, Puszynska AM, Spinelli JB, Armani A, Kunchok T, Ryback B, Seo HS, Song K, Sebastian L, O'Young C, Braithwaite C, Dhe-Paganon S, Burger N, Mills EL, Gygi SP, Arthanari H, Chouchani ET, Sabatini DM, Spiegelman BM. bioRxiv. 2024 Apr 10:2024.04.10.588849. doi: 10.1101/2024.04.10.588849. PMID: 38645260

[111] Ergothioneine: an underrecognised dietary micronutrient required for healthy ageing? Tian X, Thorne JL, Moore JB. Br J Nutr. 2023 Jan 14;129(1):104-114. doi: 10.1017/S0007114522003592. PMID: 38018890

[112] Ergothioneine protects against neuronal injury induced by β-amyloid in mice. Yang NC, Lin HC, Wu JH, Ou HC, Chai YC, Tseng CY, Liao JW, Song TY. Food Chem Toxicol. 2012 Nov;50(11):3902-11. doi: 10.1016/j.fct.2012.08.021. Epub 2012 Aug 16. PMID: 22921351

[113] Ergothioneine: an underrecognised dietary micronutrient required for healthy ageing? Tian X, Thorne JL, Moore JB. Br J Nutr. 2023 Jan 14;129(1):104-114. doi: 10.1017/S0007114522003592. PMID: 38018890

[114] Ergothioneine is associated with reduced mortality and decreased risk of cardiovascular disease. Smith E, Ottosson F, Hellstrand S, Ericson U, Orho-Melander M, Fernandez C, Melander O. Heart. 2020 May;106(9):691-697. doi: 10.1136/heartjnl-2019-315485. PMID: 31672783

[115] Ergothioneine: an underrecognised dietary micronutrient required for healthy ageing? Tian X, Thorne JL, Moore JB. Br J Nutr. 2023 Jan 14;129(1):104-114. doi: 10.1017/S0007114522003592. PMID: 38018890

30: Sleep

Summary

Adequate sleep is essential for health.

- Adults are healthiest when getting about 7.7 hours of sleep each night.
- Some people feel fine with fewer hours of sleep; nevertheless, their mental acuity and reaction time suffer just as much as those who feel fatigued with the same amount of sleep deprivation. Some people just feel the effects of sleep deprivation less than others. Give yourself a full 8:15 hours in bed each night. This gives 15 minutes to fall asleep and 15 more to lie awake, relaxing in the morning before starting the day.
- Adequate sleep, preferably sleeping on one's side or prone, increases glymphatic flow and the clearing of metabolic wastes from the brain.
- The pillow should be high enough so that the neck is aligned with the spine during sleep.
- Sleeping on one's side best promotes clearance of metabolic wastes from the brain. *Sleeping in a recliner inhibits this clearance*. Impaired clearance of these toxins is associated with Alzheimer's and Parkinson's diseases.
- Sleep in the dark helps maintain one's circadian clock to the day-night cycle. Going to bed on an empty stomach and avoiding midnight snacks helps align the enteric and central nervous systems to the same phase of the diurnal cycle.
- Late evening meals or midnight snacking, especially with fatty foods, can disrupt the circadian cycle and increase the risk for dysbiosis and leaky gut.
- A healthy enteric microbiota and a diet with sufficient soluble fiber for the production of butyrate during fasting help protect the clearance of metabolic wastes from the brain during sleep, protecting the brain from the development of AD, PD, and other inflammatory brain conditions.
- Sleep deprivation and frequent awakening can impair the consolidation of memory, neuronal health, and the ability for new neuronal development.
- Sleep deprivation, on its own, can cause intestinal dysbiosis and leaky gut.

Sleep Requirements

The optimal amount of sleep for adult humans around the world is about 7 hours and 45 minutes. This is about the length of time that healthy adults will sleep if they have no impediments to sleep: a dark, quiet spot, no appointments, no scheduling imperatives, and no nighttime disturbances. It takes an average of about 15 minutes to fall asleep, and people typically spend about 15 minutes lying awake in the morning before getting out of bed. This is essentially the same 7.7 hours average sleep time and 8.3 hours average time in bed observed in studies of healthy Americans. Thus, healthy adult humans sleep about one-third of their lives away, or at least we are healthiest and perform best when we do.

When sleep times fall below 6 hours, mortality rates rise slightly, as they do for those who sleep more than nine hours. The need for 9 hours of sleep or more is usually caused by poor quality sleep or other sleep disturbances. Infants, children, and adolescents require significantly more sleep time than do adults.

If an adult sleeps for 7.7 hours each night, then they are awake for 16.3 hours a day. Just staying awake for a bit more than an extra two hours greatly degrades performance. By the time that an adult has been awake for 19 hours, their performance in cognitive and motor tasks is equivalent to them having sufficient sleep but a blood alcohol level of 0.05%; this is a blood alcohol level at which it is illegal to drive in most jurisdictions. After being awake for 24 hours, performance is equivalent to having a blood-alcohol level of 0.1%,[1] a level that impairs reaction times, gross motor coordination, and vision.

Table 30A: Typical daily hours in bed needed for sufficient sleep by age

Age	Hours in Bed Needed
Newborn	16.5
3 months	15
9 months	14
2 years	13
3 years	12
5 years	11
9 years	10
14 years	9.6
17	9
22	8.9
30	8.6
40	8.3
50	8.3
60	8.2
70	9

Sleep Deprivation

Many adults make do with much less sleep time without obvious problems. Even when sleep is restricted to only four hours a night, many adults will not complain of feeling fatigued or impaired, even after two weeks of curtailed sleep. People have different thresholds for *feeling* sleep-deprived.[2] Nonetheless, those who feel well when sleep is limited are just as impaired by sleep deprivation; they just don't feel tired. They still suffer just as severe performance deficits as those who do feel tired. Chronic sleep deprivation usually only causes a mild decline in *subjective* functioning. Nonetheless, it can cause a severe decline in attention and reaction times. Surprisingly, people with chronic, severe sleep deprivation often do not feel much worse than those who are only mildly sleep-deprived. Nevertheless, their functioning can be seriously impaired.

Peak functioning, as measured by attention measurements, actually does not depend on sleep, but rather on avoidance of excessive wake time. Being awake too long diminishes focus. The effect of time awake is cumulative. Being awake an additional hour each day for 8 days in a row diminishes the level of focus and attention equivalent to missing one night's sleep; staying awake one extra hour daily for 16 days in a row causes degradation of focus and attention similar to missing two nights' sleep. For adults, performing at full attention and focus is incompatible with being awake for more than about 16 hours per day on average,[3] resulting in our need for about 8 hours of sleep.

Excitatory neurotransmitters, such as glutamate, associated with activity and alertness, can be neurotoxic; with excessive accumulation, they can damage the brain. Sleep provides an opportunity for the brain to detoxify, replenish antioxidants, and repair itself. During sleep, the glymphatic system flushes toxins and metabolic wastes from the cerebrospinal fluid that accumulate during wakefulness.[4]

Sleep deprivation also impairs mitochondrial health. Deprivation of REM sleep can induce the loss of neuronal mitochondria through mitophagy,[5] a process in which the mitochondria, the energy production units of the cell, self-destruct. While an occasional sleep "fast" may help eliminate weak neuronal mitochondria, chronic sleep deprivation diminishes neuronal energy utilization and energy use efficiency.

Several of the genes involved in energy metabolism and encoding Antioxidant Response Element (ARE) proteins have increased transcription during sleep.[6] Melatonin, released from the pineal gland, not only helps induce and maintain the circadian cycle but is also an important antioxidant that helps protect neurons in the central and gastrointestinal nervous systems. During sleep, an accounting of energy utilization and oxidative stress is made, and the degree of stress offers feedback that promotes the appropriate expression of antioxidant proteins. Melatonin is a non-recyclable antioxidant for the nervous system; oxidized melatonin acts as a signaling molecule that promotes the Nrf2 → ARE pathway, which induces the expression of multiple proteins that protect from oxidative stress and endogenous and xenobiotic toxins.

Sleep and the Telomere Length

Reduced telomere length is associated with aging, poorer immune function, and mortality risk. Children with shorter sleep times have shorter telomeres than do children with adequate sleep.[7] Adults who sleep an average of more than 7 hours per night have longer telomeres than those sleeping fewer hours.[8] Men sleeping less than 5 hours had telomeres 6% shorter than those sleeping more than 7 hours.[9] Women with short sleep also have shorter telomeres. Younger women who rotate night shifts, such as nursing staff, have shorter telomeres; however, this was not observed in older women.[10] The difference may be that a younger woman with children in the home may have sleep disturbances or cut sleep short to maintain other activities, while older women with rotating shifts are less likely to be disturbed during their sleep time and are more likely to shortchange their sleep requirements.

Sleep Structure

There are four distinct stages of sleep, and each has a function.

Stage 1 sleep occurs as we first fall asleep. Stage 1 sleep is a transition stage between wakefulness and sleep. If a person is disturbed during this phase, they often deny having been asleep. Sometimes people experience a sensation of falling during this stage. When people are sleep deprived, this stage gets shortened from about 30 minutes to about 10 minutes, thus moving more quickly onto more essential forms of sleep.

After Stage 1, we go into a deeper level of sleep, Stage 2. Sufficient Stage 2 sleep is needed to feel refreshed in the morning. Stage 2 sleep is also the stage of sleep that is most susceptible to curtailment during sleep deprivation; this suggests that Stage 2 sleep is less essential for short-term functioning than are SWS and REM sleep, and thus, Stage 2 can also be sacrificed in favor of SWS and REM when sleep is short-changed.

When getting sufficient sleep, about half of the sleep time is Stage 2 sleep, with most of it occurring during the second half of the night, after the body has gotten sufficient SWS and REM.

The third and deepest stage of sleep is Slow Wave Sleep (SWS). Slow-wave refers to the slow (0.5 to 4 waves per second) “delta brain waves” recorded by an electroencephalogram (EEG) during this phase of sleep. Delta waves are a signal of deep sleep and are considered an indicator of “sleep pressure”. The high amplitude occurs as a result of large areas of the brain activity being synchronized so that the electrical activity adds up to produce these large-amplitude waves.

SWS is a more highly conserved stage of sleep when sleep is deprived. This suggests that SWS is the most essential stage of sleep for health and function. About 75 minutes are spent in SWS during a night’s sleep cycle, even when there is substantial sleep deprivation, as when sleep is limited to only 4 hours. SWS occurs mostly during the first half of the sleep cycle, perhaps to help make sure that we will get enough, even if we are disturbed and can’t get back to sleep. When woken from the deepest part of SWS, the person will often feel groggy and disoriented. Since it takes about 30 minutes to get into SWS, naps that last 30 to 60 minutes will commonly include SWS, and if awoken during this time, one is likely to feel groggy upon awakening.

The fourth type of sleep requires a return from SWS through Stage 2 sleep, back into Stage 1 depth of sleep; however, now there is more active dreaming and rapid eye movement (REM). This stage is called REM sleep, or Stage 1/REM sleep.

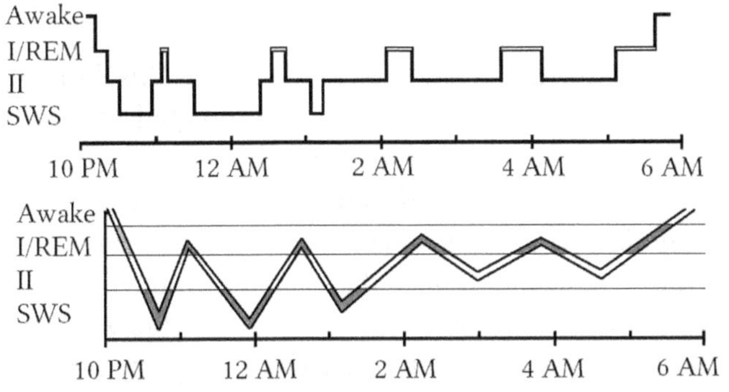

Figures 30A and 30B: These diagrams show a typical night’s sleep stages. Figure A (above) shows the sleep stages as distinct steps, while Figure B illustrates the stages of sleep more as fluctuations in sleep depth. Note that SWS occurs during the first half of the sleep cycle and takes longer to enter than any other phase.

It is typical to have four or five REM cycles during the night’s sleep, with the cycles having longer durations during the latter part of the sleep cycle. During this time, the body is immobilized, which keeps us from acting out our dreams. While we dream during all the sleep stages, it is REM sleep dreams that are most likely to be remembered.

Delta amplitude during sleep decreases with age. Patients with Alzheimer’s disease have very little SWS.[11] Patients with schizophrenia, Parkinson’s syndrome, fibromyalgia, alcoholism, and insulin resistance/type 2 diabetes also have less SWS than healthy individuals.

SWS is the deepest level of sleep and the most important; it is required for survival. This is the phase of sleep during which growth hormone is secreted, and thus it helps with the repair of muscle and other tissues. Glial cells in the brain have their energy levels restored during SWS. BDNF (Brain-derived neurotrophic factor) expression increases during SWS.[12] BDNF promotes neurogenesis and is important for the formation of synapses and the growth of dendrites, and for learning and memory. BDNF is needed for neurodevelopment and for maintaining CNS health. BDNF levels are reduced in several disease conditions, including Alzheimer's disease, schizophrenia, and epilepsy, and low levels are associated with reduced hippocampal volume.[13]

Several hormones are produced and released according to the phase of the diurnal cycle. Cortisol, aldosterone, testosterone, luteinizing hormone, growth hormone, prolactin, thyroid-stimulating hormone, and follicle-stimulating hormone all have diurnal variations and are likely controlled by the effect of light. The autonomic nervous system parasympathetic/sympathetic balance is also influenced by the suprachiasmatic nucleus (SCN) in the brain.[14] Several hormones that impact hunger and the digestive function also have a diurnal cycle, and thus promote hunger during the day rather than during sleep.

Thyroid hormones have a diurnal cycle. Thyroxine (T4) is released in the morning; this helps increase metabolic activity to support physical activity and cell growth. TSH is increased late in the day, near the onset of sleep, and triiodothyronine (T3), which supports nerve growth, is released later in the night. T3 promotes the differentiation of oligodendrocyte precursor cells and the wrapping of nerves with myelin.[15] T3 is thus critical to neurologic development, learning, and healing after injury. Sleep deprivation inhibits thyroid-stimulating hormone release. Some hormones, such as GHRH (growth hormone-releasing hormone) and prolactin, are predominantly released during SWS, while others appear to be impeded during SWS and are rather released during other parts of the sleep cycle.

Melatonin is produced in, and released from, the pineal gland, a tiny neuroendocrine gland about the size of a grain of rice near the center of the brain. Light reception from the retinal ganglion is relayed to the suprachiasmatic nuclei (SCN), activating neurons that stimulate other neurons in the hypothalamus, relaying the signal to the spinal cord, then to the cervical ganglion, and then to the pineal gland. During darkness, the pineal gland makes melatonin, and during light, it does not. *This is also true for nocturnal animals. Melatonin at physiologic levels does not induce sleep, but rather helps entrain the circadian cycle.*[16] While important in the CNS, more than 90% of the body's melatonin is produced by neuroendocrine cells in the gastrointestinal mucosa. Calcification and loss of melatonin production by the pineal gland are common with aging, but appear to have minimal effect on sleep. More salient to the sleep cycle is that the SCN has a high density of melatonin receptors. With aging, the timing of meals thus has an increasing influence over entrainment of the sleep cycle.

Melatonin is also an antioxidant. Administration of melatonin induces fatigue, lowers muscle activity, and helps lower body temperature.[17] Melatonin has been shown to promote the survival of new neurons.[18] Melatonin (high dose, injected) was shown to prevent the cognitive impairment induced by sleep deprivation in rats, reduce oxidative stress, and increase levels of BDNF in the hippocampus.[19] Melatonin helps reset the circadian clock and shorten sleep onset in the evening. Melatonin is used as a sleep aid that can increase deep, short-wave sleep (SWS).

In many animals, one of the most important roles of melatonin is to inhibit LH (luteinizing hormone) and FSH (follicle-stimulating hormone) release. This prevents estrus and fertility during the non-breeding season for the animal. The non-breeding season for different animals depends on the length of gestation, but generally coordinates birth-time to occur in the season when protein-rich foods are most available. For example, green grass in spring promotes milk production in cattle, supplying calves with quality nutrition.

Most sleep medications inhibit short-wave sleep or fail to improve it. GABA agonists, such as benzodiazepines, do not increase SWS in patients with insomnia.[20] Bee balm and some other sedative herbs act as GABAergic agents. Histamine helps us maintain alertness during the day, and thus antihistamines, such as diphenhydramine (sold over-the-counter as Benadryl and Sominex), make people drowsy and promote sleep, but do not help increase SWS. Caution should be used with sedative antihistamines as they can greatly increase the risk of traffic accidents, similar to the risks associated with moderate alcohol intoxication.

Glymphatic Flow (GF)

The exchange of molecules from blood to tissue does not occur across the thick, large arteries and veins, but rather through the tiny, low-pressure, thin-walled capillaries. These capillaries are just large enough for a single red blood cell to pass, in a single file, through the lumens of these capillaries, which have a wall that is only one endothelial cell thick. Water and ions, glucose, lactic acid, uric acid, and other small molecules can pass between the intercellular clefts, and oxygen and carbon dioxide can diffuse through the endothelial cell membranes. The arterial capillary hydrostatic pressure is higher than that of the tissue; this drives water and solutes into the interstitial space (the space in the tissues between the cells). The hydrostatic pressure in the venous capillaries is just low enough, lower than that in the interstitial tissue, that the pressure promotes an equilibrium where water and solutes are reabsorbed into the venous flow, down the concentration gradient. Most lipid-soluble molecules can enter through the lipid membrane of the endothelial cell and then exit on the other side.

The blood-brain barrier is made up of this kind of capillary; however, in addition to endothelial cells, the capillary is surrounded by a thin basal lamina membrane of connective tissue, and within the layers of this membrane are special cells called pericytes that act as the guardians of the blood-brain barrier. Additionally, about 90% of the outer surfaces of the capillaries of the blood-brain barrier (BBB) are covered by astrocyte foot processes. Much of the remaining gap area is covered by neuronal terminals. Thus, other than very small or lipophilic molecules, the BBB is selective. It keeps most water-soluble molecules in or out of the brain.

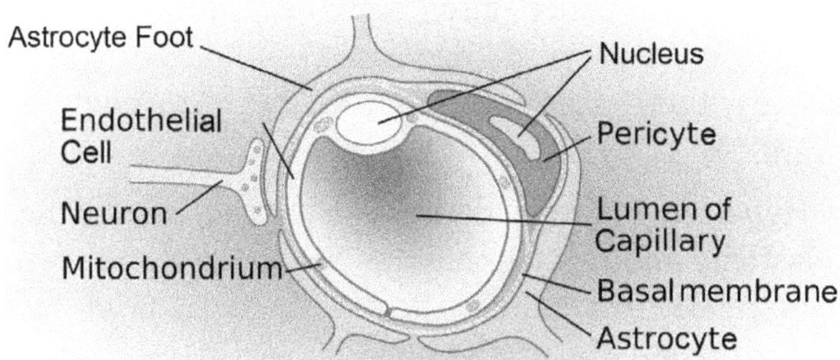

Figure 30C: Cells of the blood-brain barrier.[21]

In peripheral tissues, larger molecules extruded from cells go from the interstitial tissue into the lymphatic drainage. This gives a mechanism for ridding the tissue of waste products, including debris from dead cells and bacteria. The CNS, however, lacks lymphatic drainage.

The central nervous system (CNS), including the spinal cord, is bathed in cerebrospinal fluid (CSF). CSF enters the brain and is carried along the outside of the arteries and their subdivisions as they pass through the brain tissue. CSF is allowed to pass into the interstitium (the space between the cells) of the brain through aquaporin-4 (AQP-4) water channel pores in the foot processes of the astrocytes and into the brain interstitium. A higher pressure on the arterial side creates a convective flow of interstitial fluid through the brain towards the venous capillaries, where the fluid again passes through AQP-4 pores into the venous bloodstream. The absorption of CSF into the venous vasculature also helps propel CSF flow along the outside of the vasculature within the brain.

The convective flow of fluid within the interstitium of the brain, from the arterial to venous capillaries, carries waste products from the neurons and glial cells towards the venous capillaries, which reabsorb the water and electrolytes. Molecular waste products are flushed into the CSF and flow into the CSF of the subarachnoid space, allowing molecules much too large to cross the BBB of the capillaries to be removed from the brain. From the subarachnoid space, these waste products can enter the lymphatic flow of the dura mater that surrounds the CNS. This process of clearing CNS waste products via CSF is referred to as the glymphatic system.[22]

This slow seeping of CSF through the brain tissue, gently washing away spent metabolic wastes and toxins, is called glymphatic flow. Included among the metabolic wastes removed are beta-amyloid (Aβ) protein fragments that are associated with Alzheimer's disease (AD). Accumulation of Aβ40 in the interstitial space slows the flow of CSF into the brain's interstitial space, impeding glymphatic flow.[23] Another protein associated with AD, Tau, also accumulates with decreased glymphatic flow (GF).[24] Diminished GF reduces the clearance of beta-amyloid and Tau from the brain, thus making it more likely for beta-amyloid to form plaques. Alpha-synuclein (α-syn) accumulation in the interstitial space of the brain in Parkinson's disease (PD) also impairs glymphatic flow and is thought to promote PD progression.[25] [26]

While AQP-4 is critical to the formation of CSF, it has to be balanced. Upregulation of AQP-4 in astrocytes, where they attach to capillaries, can result from systemic dehydration, as the brain tries to preserve its hydration. Older people are at increased risk of dehydration encephalopathy as a result of decreased total body water and a diminished sensation of thirst. This can cause a mismatch with excess water entering the astrocytes, causing them to swell or to remain swollen during sleep. During sleep, the astrocytes normally "deflate," allowing more space in the brain interstitium for CSF to flow. Overhydration of the astrocytes results in a decrease in GF and as well, and may also cause protein misfolding in the astrocytes. This process has been reported in AD, PD, multiple sclerosis, traumatic brain injury, epilepsy, and other diseases of the CNS.[27] Brain edema is common in brain injury, and glymphatic flow becomes greatly reduced.

Circadian fluctuation of the hormone vasopressin (AVP) may help to drive CNS glymphatic flow in the brain during sleep. Pharmacologic blockade of the AVP receptor V(1a) can reduce post-traumatic injury brain edema.[28] The thirst regulator in the brain, the subfornical organ, responds to acetylcholine. As we age, we are more susceptible to dehydration as a result of loss of muscle mass and decreased acetylcholine production in the brain. Fluid consumption before bedtime and sleep-time fluid retention induced by AVP (antidiuretic hormone) may maintain a healthy glymphatic flow.

There is a marked increase in glymphatic flow during sleep, and this increase in clearance of toxic metabolites is among the central reasons that sleep is required. During sleep, there is a 60% increase in interstitial volume in the brain, allowing for greater in- and outflow of CSF. The flow rate is higher when the heart rate is slower, and most of the GF occurs during sleep.[29] [30] The rate of GF is highest during

SWS sleep, particularly when delta power is high and other brain wave patterns are low. During slow-wave sleep (0.5 to 4 Hz delta waves), the heart slows considerably as a result of adenosine A1A receptor response, which supports glymphatic flow.[31] During wakefulness, with increased norepinephrine activity, there is very limited GF.[32] Glymphatic clearance is also supported by Theta wave activity during REM sleep.[33] Sleep deprivation disrupts AQP-4 functioning in animal models and thus may degrade sleep quality and glymphatic flow in a feed-forward loop.[34]

In animal testing, sleeping in the lateral recumbent position enhances glymphatic flow as compared to the supine and prone positions. Tracer dye was injected into the brains of rats, and MRI was used to measure the amount of dye retained and the amount cleared. The amount of dye retained by rats sleeping on their right side was less than half of that retained by the animals sleeping on their backs or their bellies. Dye was also cleared from the spinal cord most efficiently in the lateral position, and cleared the least when the animal slept in the prone position.[35] For rats, the prone position is most similar to their waking, upright position.

In humans the most of the venous drainage from the brain flows through the vertebral veins when we are upright and sitting; the internal jugular vein is partially collapsed when we are in the upright position. When lying on our left side (left lateral decubitus position), the left internal jugular vein is collapsed, but the right is widely open, showing venous blood flow. When lying on the right, the left jugular is open. The internal carotid vein is also open when lying in the supine position.[36] Thus, a change in sleeping position from one side to the other during the night may enhance glymphatic flow from one side of the brain to the other.

Other factors that affect glymphatic flow, and thus the clearance of toxic metabolites and waste products from the brain, include arterial and respiratory pulsatility. During inspiration, there is a negative pressure in the chest cavity, and this increases vascular return and lymphatic flow into the venous system. The negative pressure created in the chest by inhalation also likely promotes increased glymphatic flow (GF).[37]

An adequate pulse pressure (the difference between systolic and diastolic pressures) allows a difference between arterial and venous hydrostatic drive, and a higher cardiac diastolic relaxation and cardiac compliance also promote cardiac venous return. With sleep and decreased CNS noradrenergic activity, there is an increase in CSF flow through the brain.

Hypertension can decrease diastolic compliance (elasticity and relaxation of the heart muscle between beats). Heart failure drives higher levels of sympathetic tone (adrenergic activity), which impedes GF. Sleep apnea causes frequent disruption of sleep, impedes deep SWS sleep. Each of these can decrease SWS and thus curtail GF and the removal of toxins from the brain. SWS is accompanied by a lower heart rate and low respiratory rate variability,[38] which facilitates GF.

There is recent evidence that there is a substantial outflow of brain interstitial fluid from the brain through the cribriform plate. This bone lies just below the olfactory bulbs in the brain. Our sense of smell depends upon olfactory nerve fibers in the mucosa of the upper nasal cavity, which pass through the tiny holes in the cribriform plate to carry the signals from the volatile compounds we smell. These tiny perforations also act as one-way valves that allow outflow of glymph as we sleep. With aging and infections, and injury to this area, bone remodeling of the cribriform plate can cause a decline in the number and size of the perforations and cause a decline in the sense of smell and a decrease in GF. In a study of over 560 individuals and 70 post-mortem samples, cribriform plate porosity was found to decrease with age. Cribriform plate porosity was found to be significantly lower among those with AD. It is well established that AD and PD are commonly accompanied by anosmia, a decline or loss of the sense of smell. Long-COVID, which commonly manifests with the loss of the sense of smell, is typically associated with mental fog. This may be caused by interference in GF.[39]

I hypothesize that the cyclic negative nasal airway pressure of breathing during nasal inhalation is essential for gently milking GF through the cribriform plate into the nasal mucosa during sleep. As much as 25 ml of glymph may be slowly drawn through the cribriform plate overnight into the interstitial tissue of the nasal mucosa. This tissue drains into the facial vein and then into the internal carotid vein. Mouth breathing during sleep, which provides less resistance as compared to nasal breathing, may decrease GF into the carotid vein, and would fail to help "milk" the glymph into the nasal mucosal tissue.

In the 19th century, the disparaging terms "adenoidal idiot", "adenoidal moron," and "mouth breather" were used to describe a syndromic facial appearance that was associated with cognitive slowness in children. These children had swollen, inflamed tonsillar adenoids that obstructed the nasal airway and thus were limited to breathing through their mouths, especially during sleep. They suffered from poor concentration, memory problems, attention deficit-hyperactivity, anxiety, language dysfunction, learning disabilities, poor sensorimotor integration and perception, restricted IQ, and poor academic performance.[40] [41] Children with adenoidal airway obstruction can recover with treatment, although it takes several months.[42] The intellectual and behavioral problems are generally assumed to result from sleep deficits; however, perhaps the reduction in GF from loss of nasal breathing contributes to cognitive slowness. As children become adolescents, the tonsils generally shrink, and the nasal respiratory flow improves without treatment, but the cognitive impairment may not completely resolve.

Sleep and the Gut

There is accumulating evidence that inflammation, from the gut or elsewhere, impedes glymphatic flow and promotes AD and PD pathologic processes. LPS and other pathogen-associated molecular patterns (PAMPs) from the gut and gingiva induce CNS inflammation. In contrast, butyrate, produced by healthy commensal bacteria in the colon from dietary fiber, reduces the permeability of the blood-brain barrier (BBB), protecting it from toxins. Butyrate also attenuates the production of proinflammatory cytokines by microglial cells in the brain; thus, butyrate helps reduce inflammatory signaling in the brain that suppresses GF.[43]

Thus, a healthy enteric microbiota and a diet with sufficient soluble fiber for the production of butyrate during fasting help protect GF during sleep and protect the brain from the development of AD, PD, and other inflammatory brain conditions.

Fruit flies are a useful model for studying sleep deprivation, as they can be kept from sleeping with a machine that prevents the fruit flies from landing long enough to sleep, just by vibrating the tubes they are housed in. Keeping fruit flies awake for 15 days kills them. Recent research has identified the cause of death in these sleep-deprived insects; they succumb to oxidative stress injury to their GI tract. If fed antioxidants, these sleep-deprived flies survive a normal lifespan.[44]

After these findings outlining a cause and remedy to sleep depression injury in fruit flies, similar experiments were performed in rats. A 35% reduction of sleep for 10 days caused DNA damage in the liver, lungs, and intestines of rodents. Sleep deprivation caused a 5.3-fold increase in the number of dying cells in the intestinal epithelium.[45] In mice, sleep deprivation appears to be particularly hard on the intestine. The use of antioxidants was shown to protect the rodent intestine from injury,[46] as it did for fruit flies.

Sleep restriction in mice also decreases the transcription of tight junction proteins and increases paracellular permeability across the BBB.[47] Sleep deprivation promotes intestinal dysbiosis and depletes the secondary bile acid deoxycholic acid (DCA), which helps prevent pathobiont overgrowth.[48] In mice, sleep deprivation was found to activate the NLRP3 inflammasome in the colon and the brain and drive Tau pathology as seen in AD.[49] When the sleep-deprived microbiota were transplanted into normal mice, it caused those mice to have similar pathological and behavioral dysfunction as the sleep-deprived mice.[50] Mice with fecal transplants from sleep-deprived mice had neuroinflammation and microglial activity in the hippocampus and medial prefrontal cortex. Sleep deprivation induces gut dysbiosis and inflammatory responses in humans.[51] It weakens immune defenses and can impair the intestinal barriers, allowing toxins such as LPS and even pathogens to enter the bloodstream. This can directly and indirectly cause cognitive impairment as a result of neuroinflammation and microglial activation.[52]

The intestine has a diurnal cycle, with decreased motility at night. Ninety to 95% of the body's melatonin is produced in the gut. Here, it acts to slow motility and guard against oxidative injury. Melatonin is an antioxidant that protects both the CNS and enteric nervous system (ENS) and helps maintain both the CNS and ENS diurnal clocks.

In addition to the need for sleep, our bodies have circadian cycles that tune the metabolism to daytime activity and nighttime quiescence. These cycles do much more than entrain the sleep cycle to help us wake and sleep coincident with dawn and nightfall. The circadian cycles are intimately tied to the release of at least a dozen hormones that control the body's energy use, activity, appetite, digestion, immune function, growth, and healing. Disrupting the circadian cycle can throw these hormonal cycles into disarray.

The intestine has more than 20 types of neuroendocrine cells. These cells comprise the largest endocrine organ of the body.[53]

The diurnal cycle affects the transcription of proteins so that the cells can do the work that needs to be done at the appropriate time. For example, during rest, proteins associated with repair and recycling are made in higher amounts, while during periods of activity, proteins needed for rapid energy use are formed. Nearly one-sixth of all transcribed genes are under diurnal influence. Several core clock-gene transcription factors regulate the diurnal oscillations of protein transcription, including Period (Per), cryptochrome (Cry), Clock, and Bmal (a.k.a. Arntl). These transcription factors activate the expression of numerous genes. For example, the CLOCK and BMAL genes are involved in the growth and repair of muscles.[54]

Different proteins are needed by the brain during the day for activity than during sleep for memory consolidation. Different proteins are also made in the gastrointestinal mucosal cells during the day than at night.

When I think of protein, I usually think of it sitting on my plate staring back at me like two black-eyed peas; just sitting there, not doing much. Most proteins in active metabolism are not static, however, and are quite evanescent. In a study of over 3,750 yeast proteins, most had short-lived regulatory functions; the protein does its job and is retired, that is, recycled. The average half-life of a yeast protein was 43 minutes; 161 proteins had a half-life of under four minutes. [55] [56] The duration of proteins in humans is not so different. In a survey of one hundred human proteins, the half-lives ranged from 45 minutes to 22.5 hours.[57]

After their use, the proteins are broken down and the amino acids recycled. The duration of regulatory proteins in our bodies is similar to this. Thus, there is plenty of time in a 24-hour day to have very different sets of proteins for different functions. Thus, we have many proteins expressed mainly during the active day and others during rest/sleep at night. Similarly, some commensal bacteria in the GI microbiome express different proteins and behave differently during the active/feeding phase of the diurnal cycle than they do during the resting/fasting phase.

The diurnal cycle has a profound influence on metabolism. Of 171 metabolites measured in the plasma, 109 had daily rhythms. In a study of a dozen healthy young men, sleep deprivation attenuated the amplitude of 66 of these metabolites. Being awake for 24 hours was found to cause a significant elevation in tryptophan, serotonin, taurine, and 24 other measured metabolites.[58] In a separate study of a dozen healthy young women, of 130 plasma metabolites measured, 41 were significantly altered, with most rising with sleep deprivation; most notably, phosphatidylcholine. Melatonin also rose in response to the short-term sleep deprivation,[59] likely acting as a signal to nudge these sleep-deprived women to get to bed.

Irritable bowel syndrome and gastrointestinal reflux are associated with sleep disorders and are common among shift workers. Nurses on rotating shifts are twice as likely to have a functional bowel disorder as those working day shifts.[60] Shift work also results in elevated triglyceride levels; increased BMI, waist circumference, and obesity; and a blunted insulin response.[61] Indeed, in addition to the risk of cancer, circadian disruption in shift workers increases the risk of depression, metabolic syndrome, diabetes, cardiovascular disease, cognitive impairment, and premature aging. [62] [63] [64]

When sleep and circadian cycles are normal, there is a surge of glucocorticoid hormones each morning that helps downregulate inflammation.

Since mice are nocturnal, rather than using the light/dark phases, I will describe the diurnal cycle in terms of active/feeding and resting/fasting phases, so studies of mice and other animal study results can be more directly understood in relation to humans.

The mucous layer in the intestine is thicker during the active phase, and bacteria migrate deeper into the mucous layer throughout the active period. In a study of mice, numerous bacteria were adhering to the mucosal cells during the active cycle, but few adherent bacteria by the end of the rest cycle. Messenger RNA and protein expression for the tight junction proteins occludin and claudin-1 are under diurnal control by the clock genes. In mice, claudin-1 and occludin expression are lowest during the early part of the active/feeding phase of the diurnal cycle, and this is associated with increased intestinal permeability. This likely allows for increased uptake of certain nutrients during the feeding phase of the cycle, while increased claudin-1 and occludin expression during the fasting/resting phase decreases intestinal permeability and protects mucosal integrity. Mice with defects in the clock genes that were associated with increased permeability were more susceptible to chemical-induced colitis. [65]

In the intestinal mucosa, an example of diurnal gene expression is REG3G, which encodes for the protein RegIII-gamma, an antibacterial protein produced by Paneth cells in the mucosa of the small intestine. This protein is released during the fasting/resting phase of the cycle. RegIIIγ specifically targets Gram-positive bacteria such as *Clostridia*. Thus, there is a daily cycle where bacteria in the mucous layer are dosed with antibiotic proteins during the fasting period.[66] In mice exposed to constant darkness (since mice are nocturnal, that would be equivalent to a diurnal animal exposed to constant light), there was a dramatic increase in Clostridia in the small intestine.[67]

It is not just intestinal epithelial cells that have diurnal transcriptional oscillations. The circadian rhythm of the commensal microbiome is not limited to a partial die-off from antibacterial proteins followed by recovery. For example, *Enterobacter aerogenes* has swarming activity under the influence of melatonin as a result of melatonin's influence on circadian clock proteins within the bacteria.[68] Other bacteria in the microbiome respond to the diurnal difference in body temperatures that occurs between day and night.[69]

Testing a sample of the genes expressed by the intestinal microbiome of mice revealed that 404 of 1552 of the bacterial genes tested had distinct oscillations in their expression across the diurnal cycle. Many of these genes are for proteins that are involved in the degradation of mucus, and others are for flagellar proteins involved with bacterial motility. Thus, the commensal bacteria are doing different things during different parts of the day.

Nfil3 is a transcriptional regulator that represses the transcriptional activity of the Clock genes Per1 and Per2.[70] Nfil3 expression is selectively activated in the enterocytes by Gram-negative, motile bacteria that produce the immune-activating PAMPS (pathogen-associated molecular patterns), flagellin, and LPS, such as *Salmonella typhimurium* and *E. coli*. Dendritic immune cells of the lamina propria in contact with these bacteria secrete IL-23, which stimulates innate lymphoid cells (ILC3) that secrete IL-22, which promotes Nfil3 expression by the enterocytes. This causes alterations in circadian lipid metabolism that result in increased uptake of lipids from the lumen during the resting phase. This resulted in obesity in an animal model that could be prevented by inhibiting any of the various steps in this pathway.[71] Thus, dysbiosis can affect the circadian clock in the intestinal epithelial cells, increase weight gain, and promote metabolic syndrome. Moreover, a high-fat diet was found to decrease diurnal oscillatory variance in the microbiota population and phenotype.[72]

About 20% of the GI microbiome species in humans undergo diurnal fluctuations.[73] The relative abundance of *Firmicutes*, such as *Clostridia*, within the lumen of the cecum, proliferates and dominates the microbiome during the activity/feeding phase, but their populations greatly decline during the fasting/resting period, while the relative abundances of *Bacteroidetes* and *Verrucomicrobia* peaked during fasting/resting and bottomed out during feeding and activity. *Lactobacillaceae* in the cecal lumen increased during the fasting/resting phase and rapidly declined with feeding and activity. A high-fat diet dampens the circadian oscillations in the microbiome population in mice, similar to that of having the mice under constant exposure to light, even when food is restricted to feeding during times of activity.[74]

Different microbiome communities can perform different functions at different times in the circadian cycle. During feeding/activity, the cecal microbiome metabolizes food remnants, bile, and enzymes that remain in the food bolus after having passed through the small intestine. The microbiota has different symbiotic effects in different locations in the intestine and during different phases of the diurnal cycle. Disturbances in the circadian rhythms in the intestine cause dysbiosis, which can promote metabolic disease that favors weight gain, obesity, and diabetes. Sleep deprivation increases the appetite for starchy and sweet foods. Jet lag and shift work are associated with leaky gut and a decreased GI microbiome diversity. Shift work is associated with an increased risk of breast and other cancers. Shift workers are prone to obesity, metabolic syndrome, and type 2 diabetes.[75] Dysbiosis can promote intestinal inflammation that causes obesity in mice.[76] The inflammatory signaling is exacerbated by a high-fat diet.[77]

In animal models of jet lag, dysbiosis results from irregular feeding times and induces glucose intolerance and obesity in the animals. The resulting alterations in the microbiota can then be transferred to another animal via fecal transplant, causing the transfer of dysbiosis, even when the host animal has normal feeding times.[78] This suggests that a temporary disruption in diurnal wake times and feeding cycles can cause long-term sustained dysbiosis in an individual.

Microbiome diversity is correlated with increased sleep efficiency and total sleep time and inversely correlated with wake time during the sleep period. Recall that sleep efficiency is the percent of time spent sleeping from the time one lies down to sleep until they wake up in the morning before getting out of bed. The populations of both *Bacteroidetes* and *Firmicutes,* which are generally major populations of the commensal microbiome, are associated with sleep efficiency, IL-6, and abstract thinking ability. Meanwhile, a study found that *Lachnospiraceae*,

Corynebacterium, and *Blautia,* which are common in dysbiosis, were associated with adverse sleep factors.[79]

A study that examined sleep restrictions in mice and humans, however, only found mild alterations in the microbiome, with no loss in biodiversity. In one study, the men were restricted to 4 hours of sleep per night for five consecutive nights.[80] In another study, the subjects were allowed 4¼ hours of sleep for two nights in a row; there were changes in the makeup of the microbiome, but no loss in beta diversity.[81] Short-term sleep restriction thus does not appear to be sufficient to cause dysbiosis in healthy adults. Occasional short-term sleep loss is not harmful and may even provide benefits, as discussed below. Longer-term sleep deprivation, however, has different effects.

Taken as a whole, these data suggest that the type and timing of meals likely have more impact on the circadian cycle of the gut than does sleep. Jet lag eating can cause dysbiosis. Shift work can cause dysbiosis and an increased appetite for fatty foods. [82] Fatty foods have a considerable impact on the GI microbiome, as a result of their slower digestion and the increased requirements for lipase and bile, which impact the microbiota. Additionally, melatonin, an important antioxidant for the gut, is produced while the gut is at rest, and production falls in favor of serotonin during activity.

Severe sleep deprivation causes oxidative injury in the intestine and leaky gut. Although dysbiosis can cause leaky gut, leaky gut can also cause dysbiosis. Not only does leaky gut allow toxins and pathogens to get into the body, but it also allows fluids and proteins to leak out into the intestinal lumen. Thus, leaky gut can cause alterations in the biome and promote pathogenic overgrowth. More importantly, oxidative injury to the mucosa decreases its ability to form a protective mucus layer and produce anti-microbial enzymes that modulate the microbiome. Thus, injury to the mucosa can cause dysbiosis, which sustains mucosal dysfunction and dysbiosis.

Sleep deprivation causes loss of dendritic spines in the CA1 neurons, preventing memory consolidation. Growth hormone (GH) increases the density of mushroom-shaped dendritic spines in large pyramidal cells in the CA1 region of the hippocampus and increases the length of the dendritic trees in the prefrontal cortex.[83] GH participates not only in brain development but also in neuroplasticity, and thus, in learning throughout life. It is during SWS that GH-releasing hormone (GHRH) is released. The hippocampus is the area of the brain that has the most neurogenesis in adults. Neurogenesis in the adult hippocampus is required for mood regulation and certain types of memory processes.[84] This neurogenesis continues into old age in health but fails in Alzheimer's disease,[85] where new neurons arise but do not survive.

Sleep deprivation impairs the protein synthesis in the brain that supports the structural changes in neuronal connectivity needed for synaptic efficiency, learning, and encoding memory.[86] This plasticity is surprisingly fast. In rats, pyramidal neuron spines in the medial prefrontal cortex grow and retract within the 24-hour diurnal cycle. During the active phase of their diurnal cycle, there is an increase in basilar dendrite length and complexity of basilar spines on the dendrites, which retract during the sleep cycle. This suggests that sleep may be essential for consolidating relevant memory and pruning the irrelevant information from the memory. Psychosocial stress has been found to reduce or eliminate these diurnal changes, and thus impair plasticity.[87]

Synaptic plasticity is needed for learning and memory. In common parlance, this is often referred to as "rewiring of the brain". Synaptic plasticity also affects the regulation of emotions and mood. Impaired synaptic plasticity causes cognitive impairment, mood disturbances, and disrupted emotional regulation. Sleep fragmentation, which is similar to what occurs in people who awaken or are disturbed frequently during the night, also causes a marked decrease in the proliferation and survival of cells in the hippocampus of rodents. Selective REM sleep deprivation decreases neurogenesis, the proliferation, and survival of new neurons, in the hippocampal area of the brain in adult animals, while it enhances the survival of older neurons. Thus, the loss of REM sleep prevents learning and adaptation.

Sleep deprivation-induced loss of neurogenesis is associated with depressive symptoms and can lead to major depressive disorder. About 90% of depressed individuals report sleep disturbances. Poor sleep is also associated with suicide and relapse into depression. Since the body prioritizes SWS, it is a deficit of REM sleep that is most common in depressed individuals. Most antidepressant medications improve sleep and help restore hippocampal neurogenesis.[88] While both REM and SWS appear to be required for the development of fully developed neurons, inhibition of REM sleep is sufficient to reduce the neurogenesis in the hippocampus by more than half.[89] A deficit of REM sleep results in fewer and weaker new neurons. [90]

REM sleep also appears to be central to autophagy in the neurons, which is required to keep neurons healthy.

Autophagy is a process in which the cell tags organelles and proteins for recycling (ubiquitination), which allows the removal of older proteins and organelles. Although neurons are post-mitotic and thus can last a lifetime, autophagy keeps these cells fresh and vital. It is as if you had a 1957 Ford pickup truck, but changed out each part with time as needed, except for the VIN number plate. New fenders, new engine block, carburetor, doors, new seats and mirrors, et cetera. It would be a new, old model car. A pickup of Theseus. This is how the neurons can live for many decades without degradation; they are constantly replacing parts. A critical step in this process appears to require REM sleep.

Without REM and autophagy, the neurons build up waste, and the mitochondria become inefficient. This creates an increase in oxidative stress and oxidative injury. Eventually, it can lead to neuronal death. This is thought to contribute to neurodegenerative disorders such as Parkinson's disease and Alzheimer's disease.[91] A study has reported that the impairments of hippocampal neurogenesis caused by sleep deprivation could be prevented by blocking the rise in both corticosterone and IL-1β formation, which occur as a result of wakefulness.[92] It is thus not the lack of sleep but rather the excess of wakefulness and elevations in IL-1β and corticosterone that inhibit neuronal proliferation.

Although the development of new neurons in the CNS greatly diminishes by the age of three, there are some areas of the brain in which adult neurogenesis continues, albeit at a much lower rate. Notably, there is continued neurogenesis in the dentate gyrus (DG) of the hippocampus, an area involved in distinguishing similar memories (for example, visiting the same place on multiple occasions). Neural stem and progenitor cells (NSCs) in the subgranular zone generate new neurons throughout life. There is also evidence of adult neurogenesis in other parts of the brain, including the hypothalamus, subventricular zone, amygdala, striatum, and neocortex. NSC daughter cells from the hippocampus can even migrate to other areas of the brain and form various types of neurons or glial cells in response to injury; however, the generation of new neurons in adults is limited.

The NSCs in the dentate gyrus are thought to help adapt the emotional response to the environment. Post-mortem studies of patients with major depressive disorder have fewer NSCs in the DG than those without depression, and antidepressant medications are associated with an increased number of NSCs in the DG in some studies. New neurons in the anterior (ventral) DG appear to aid in emotional response, while those in the posterior (dorsal) DG are more involved in cognitive function. Deficits in adult neurogenesis in the DG have been found in post-traumatic stress disorder (PTSD), schizophrenia, and Alzheimer's disease.

These new neurons may be needed for pattern recognition, encoding temporal information, and promoting cognitive flexibility. Logically, we associate the results of an action sequentially; if something in the environment causes injury, we learn to avoid it. If we cannot distinguish ordinal timing (what came before what), we cannot integrate causation and discern where the danger arises in the environment. Difficulties with this may occur in PTSD and anxiety, where innocuous stimuli may trigger a danger response.[93]

Insufficient or fractured sleep can disrupt the formation of hippocampal BDNF, and thus prevent the survival and maturation of newborn neurons and glial support cells in adults.

When a person fails to get sufficient sleep over several days, the sleep deficit accumulates. Recovery can take more than three full nights of sleep to recover normal cognitive and neurobehavioral performance. Repeated short sleep on weekdays is thus not recovered over a weekend. The person, however, may subjectively feel well. Adolescents appear to be more susceptible than adults to sleep deficits and take longer to recover.

Short-term sleep loss impairs neural plasticity but also impairs the development of new neurons. Long-term sleep deprivation (excess wake time) has far worse effects. It is not just the loss of new neurons from neural stem and progenitor cells (NSCs) but also the loss of astrocytes and oligodendrocytes that are also derived from NSC/progenitor cells that are essential for supporting the neurons and their functions. Additionally, excess wake time increases the production of pro-inflammatory cytokines TNF-α, IL-1β, and IL-6 by the microglia, immune cells in the brain, causing a neuroinflammatory response.

Neural stem cells in the brain can differentiate into neurons, astrocytes, or oligodendrocytes, and in health, more than half of NSCs differentiate into neurons. About 10 – 15% of the cells in the brain are microglia; these cells are plastic in nature and can act similarly to dendritic immune cells, monitoring for antigens, or as tissue macrophages. Most of the time, the microglia are quiescent, but they can become reactive when there is immune activation or if they sense injury. When this occurs, they become phagocytic and start gobbling up debris from dead or injured cells.

When the microglia are activated, they cause a shift in the differentiation of NSCs, from the predominant formation of new neurons to the predominant formation of oligodendrocytes and astrocytes. Brain trauma, infection, or other injury or cause of neuroinflammation (such as LPS from bacteria) triggers activation of the microglia, leading to the release of TNF, IL-6, and IL-1β. These cytokines both downregulate NSC proliferation and shift cell differentiation away from neurogenesis in favor of the formation of oligodendrocytes and astrocytes.

Even peripheral LPS can inhibit neurogenesis; injection of LPS into the abdominal cavity in mice was found to do this. In other experiments, TNF or IL-6 overexpression in the brain of mice has been demonstrated to induce neuronal death, while IL-1β reduced NSC proliferation.

In contrast, microglia in the alternate activation (repair) state produce anti-inflammatory cytokines IL-4 and IL-10, which restore the pro-neuronal differentiation balance to NSC proliferation and help promote the survival of these cells.[94]

Sleep Fasting?

A single night of short sleep *increases* the expression of antioxidant enzymes in the locus coeruleus (LC) neurons in the brain stem and areas of the brain that help maintain alertness. Thus, an occasional night of poor sleep or a loss of sleep due to nighttime activity is not harmful (as long as it does not include eating).

After a few days of excess wakefulness, however, there is no longer an increase of antioxidant enzymes, but rather an increase in reactive oxidative species (ROS) and the formation of a toxic waste product called lipofuscin, not only indicating mitochondrial injury but also irreversible aging of the neuron. Lipofuscin is created during lipid and protein peroxidation by free radicals generated by poorly functioning mitochondria. Unfortunately, most cells have very limited, if any, capacity for getting rid of lipofuscin, so it accumulates in the cell. Lipofuscin is both a sign of ROS damage and aging and a cause of cell senescence and cell death. Thus, ROS damage and lipofuscin accumulation impair cell rejuvenation in post-mitotic cells such as neurons. Lipofuscin accumulation in the retina is associated with, and considered a causal factor in, age-related macular degeneration. In the brain, it appears that the microglia participate in the removal of lipofuscin from the neurons, but accumulate the pigment themselves, and thus, injure themselves in the process to a point where they can no longer protect the neurons.[95]

The neurons only have very limited mechanisms for the removal of lipofuscin, and when sufficiently excessive amounts accumulate, the cell dies. In mice, four weeks of chronic short sleep caused a 40% loss of both LC neurons and orexinergic neurons, which did not recover even after a month of recovery sleep.[96] Orexins are hypothalamic hormones that regulate appetite and sleep.

There have been a few studies on "therapeutic sleep deprivation" as a treatment for major depressive disorder and as a means of promoting brain health. Some studies have found that occasional shorting of REM sleep, by getting up out of bed 3 to 4 hours earlier than usual, while preserving SWS, may be helpful against depression. The effect size appears to be small, and the benefit fleeting. Thus, while occasional early rising may have some beneficial effects on depression, this therapy does currently have sufficient benefit even under controlled conditions to merit its use.[97] [98]

[1] Fatigue, alcohol and performance impairment. Dawson D, Reid K. Nature. 1997 Jul 17;388(6639):235. PMID:9230429

[2] Systematic interindividual differences in neurobehavioral impairment from sleep loss: evidence of trait-like differential vulnerability. Van Dongen HP, Baynard MD, Maislin G, Dinges DF. Sleep. 2004 May 1;27(3):423-33. PMID: 15164894

[3] The cumulative cost of additional wakefulness: dose-response effects on neurobehavioral functions and sleep physiology from chronic sleep restriction and total sleep deprivation. Van Dongen HP, Maislin G, et al. Sleep. 2003 Mar 15;26(2):117-26. PMID: 12683469

[4] Sleep drives metabolite clearance from the adult brain. Xie L, Kang H, Xu Q, et al. Science. 2013 Oct 18;342(6156):373-7. PMID:24136970

[5] Paradoxical sleep deprivation impairs spatial learning and affects membrane excitability and mitochondrial protein in the hippocampus. Yang RH, Hu SJ, Wang Y, Zhang WB, Luo WJ, Chen JY. Brain Res. 2008 Sep 16;1230:224-32. 18674519

[6] Why we sleep: the temporal organization of recovery. Mignot E. PLoS Biol. 2008 Apr 29;6(4):e106. PMID:18447584

[7] Sleep Duration and Telomere Length in Children. James S, McLanahan S, Brooks-Gunn J, Mitchell C, Schneper L, Wagner B, Notterman DA. J Pediatr. 2017 Aug;187:247-252.e1. PMID:28602380

[8] Telomere length is associated with sleep duration but not sleep quality in adults with human immunodeficiency virus. Lee KA, Gay C, Humphreys J, Portillo CJ, Pullinger CR, Aouizerat BE. Sleep. 2014 Jan 1;37(1):157-66. PMID:24470704

[9] Short sleep duration is associated with shorter telomere length in healthy men: findings from the Whitehall II cohort study. Jackowska M, Hamer M, Carvalho LA, Erusalimsky JD, Butcher L, Steptoe A. PLoS One. 2012;7(10):e47292. PMID:23144701

[10] Associations between rotating night shifts, sleep duration, and telomere length in women. Liang G, Schernhammer E, Qi L, Gao X, De Vivo I, Han J. PLoS One. 2011;6(8):e23462. PMID:21853136

[11] Sleep evoked delta frequency responses show a linear decline in amplitude across the adult lifespan. Colrain IM, Crowley KE, Nicholas CL, Afifi L, Baker FC, Padilla M, Turlington SR, Trinder J. Neurobiol Aging. 2010 May;31(5):874-83. doi: 10.1016/j.neurobiolaging.2008.06.003. PMID:18657881

[12] Oroxylin A Induces BDNF Expression on Cortical Neurons through Adenosine A2A Receptor Stimulation: A Possible Role in Neuroprotection. Jeon SJ, Bak H, Seo J, Han SM, Lee SH, Han SH, Kwon KJ, Ryu JH, Cheong JH, Ko KH, Yang SI, Choi JW, Park SH, Shin CY. Biomol Ther (Seoul). 2012 Jan;20(1):27-35. doi: 10.4062/biomolther.2012.20.1.027. PMID:24116271

[13] Brain-derived neurotrophic factor is associated with age-related decline in hippocampal volume. Erickson KI, Prakash RS, Voss MW, Chaddock L, Heo S, McLaren M, Pence BD, Martin SA, Vieira VJ, Woods JA, McAuley E, Kramer AF. J Neurosci. 2010 Apr 14;30(15):5368-75. doi: 10.1523/JNEUROSCI.6251-09.2010. PMID:20392958

[14] Coordinated regulation of circadian rhythms and homeostasis by the suprachiasmatic nucleus. Nakagawa H, Okumura N. Proc Jpn Acad Ser B Phys Biol Sci. 2010;86(4):391-409. PMID:20431263

[15] Micropillar arrays as a high-throughput screening platform for therapeutics in multiple sclerosis. Mei F, Fancy SP, Shen YA, et al. Nat Med. 2014 Aug;20(8):954-60. PMID:24997607

[16] The Effects of Light and the Circadian System on Rhythmic Brain Function. von Gall C. Int J Mol Sci. 2022 Mar 3;23(5):2778. doi: 10.3390/ijms23052778. PMID: 35269920

[17] The Pineal Gland and Melatonin. Richard Bowen, VIVO Pathophysiology Colorado State Univ. http://www.vivo.colostate.edu/hbooks/pathphys/endocrine/otherendo/pineal.html

[18] Inhibition of hippocampal neurogenesis by sleep deprivation is independent of circadian disruption and melatonin suppression. Mueller AD, Mear RJ, Mistlberger RE. Neuroscience. 2011 Oct 13;193:170-81. doi: 10.1016/j.neuroscience.2011.07.019. PMID:21771640

[19] Melatonin ameliorates cognitive impairment induced by sleep deprivation in rats: role of oxidative stress, BDNF and CaMKII. Zhang L, Zhang HQ, Liang XY, Zhang HF, Zhang T, Liu FE. Behav Brain Res. 2013 Nov 1;256:72-81. doi: 10.1016/j.bbr.2013.07.051. PMID:23933144

[20] Sleep EEG power spectra, insomnia, and chronic use of benzodiazepines. Bastien CH, LeBlanc M, Carrier J, Morin CM. Sleep. 2003 May 1;26(3):313-7. PMID:12749551

[21] Schematic sketch showing the blood-brain barrier. https://commons.wikimedia.org/wiki/File:Blood-brain_barrier_02.png Image by Armin Kübelbeck

[22] The Glymphatic System in Central Nervous System Health and Disease: Past, Present, and Future. Plog BA, Nedergaard M. Annu Rev Pathol. 2018 Jan 24;13:379-394. doi: 10.1146/annurev-pathol-051217-111018. PMID:29195051

[23] Suppression of glymphatic fluid transport in a mouse model of Alzheimer's disease. Peng W, Achariyar TM, Li B, Liao Y, Mestre H, Hitomi E, Regan S, Kasper T, Peng S, Ding F, Benveniste H, Nedergaard M, Deane R. Neurobiol Dis. 2016 Sep;93:215-25. doi: 10.1016/j.nbd.2016.05.015. Epub 2016 May 24. PMID: 27234656

[24] Impaired glymphatic function and clearance of tau in an Alzheimer's disease model. Harrison IF, Ismail O, Machhada A, Colgan N, Ohene Y, Nahavandi P, Ahmed Z, Fisher A, Meftah S, Murray TK, Ottersen OP, Nagelhus EA, O'Neill MJ, Wells JA, Lythgoe MF. Brain. 2020 Aug 1;143(8):2576-2593. doi: 10.1093/brain/awaa179. PMID: 32705145

[25] Decreased AQP4 Expression Aggravates α-Synuclein Pathology in Parkinson's Disease Mice, Possibly via Impaired Glymphatic Clearance. Cui H, Wang W, Zheng X, Xia D, Liu H, Qin C, Tian H, Teng J. J Mol Neurosci. 2021 Dec;71(12):2500-2513. doi: 10.1007/s12031-021-01836-4. Epub 2021 Mar 26. PMID: 33772424

[26] Interaction Between the Glymphatic System and α-Synuclein in Parkinson's Disease. Zhang Y, Zhang C, He XZ, Li ZH, Meng JC, Mao RT, Li X, Xue R, Gui Q, Zhang GX, Wang LH. Mol Neurobiol. 2023 Apr;60(4):2209-2222. doi: 10.1007/s12035-023-03212-2. Epub 2023 Jan 13. PMID: 36637746

[27] Dehydration and Cognition in Geriatrics: A Hydromolecular Hypothesis Adonis Sfera, Michael Cummings, Carolina Osorio Front Mol Biosci. 2016; 3: 18. doi: 10.3389/fmolb.2016.00018 PMCID: PMC4860410

[28] Arginine-vasopressin V1a receptor inhibition improves neurologic outcomes following an intracerebral hemorrhagic brain injury. Manaenko A, Fathali N, Khatibi NH, Lekic T, Hasegawa Y, Martin R, Tang J, Zhang JH. Neurochem Int. 2011 Mar;58(4):542-8. doi: 10.1016/j.neuint.2011.01.018. PMID:21256175

[29] Theoretical analysis of wake/sleep changes in brain solute transport suggests a flow of interstitial fluid. Thomas JH. Fluids Barriers CNS. 2022 Apr 13;19(1):30. doi: 10.1186/s12987-022-00325-z. PMID: 35418142

[30] Glymphatic System Dysfunction and Sleep Disturbance May Contribute to the Pathogenesis and Progression of Parkinson's Disease. Scott-Massey A, Boag MK, Magnier A, Bispo DPCF, Khoo TK, Pountney DL. Int J Mol Sci. 2022 Oct 26;23(21):12928. doi: 10.3390/ijms232112928. PMID: 36361716

[31] Increased glymphatic influx is correlated with high EEG delta power and low heart rate in mice under anesthesia. Hablitz LM, Vinitsky HS, Sun Q, Stæger FF, Sigurdsson B, Mortensen KN, Lilius TO, Nedergaard M. Sci Adv. 2019 Feb 27;5(2):eaav5447. doi: 10.1126/sciadv.aav5447. PMID:30820460

[32] During wakefulness, with norepinephrine stimulation, there is very limited GF. Hauglund NL, Pavan C, Nedergaard M. Current Opinion in Physiology 2020, 15:1–6 https://doi.org/10.1016/j.cophys.2019.10.020

[33] Continuous theta burst stimulation facilitates the clearance efficiency of the glymphatic pathway in a mouse model of sleep deprivation. Liu DX, He X, Wu D, Zhang Q, Yang C, Liang FY, He XF, Dai GY, Pei Z, Lan Y, Xu GQ. Neurosci Lett. 2017 Jul 13;653:189-194. doi: 10.1016/j.neulet.2017.05.064. PMID: 28576566

[34] Aquaporin-4 Water Channel in the Brain and Its Implication for Health and Disease. Mader S, Brimberg L. Cells. 2019 Jan 27;8(2). pii: E90. doi: 10.3390/cells8020090. PMID:30691235

[35] The Effect of Body Posture on Brain Glymphatic Transport. Lee H, Xie L, Yu M, Kang H, Feng T, Deane R, Logan J, Nedergaard M, Benveniste H. J Neurosci. 2015 Aug 5;35(31):11034-44. doi: 10.1523/JNEUROSCI.1625-15.2015. PMID: 26245965

[36] Collapsibility of the internal jugular veins in the lateral decubitus body position: A potential protective role of the cerebral venous outflow against neurodegeneration. Simka M, Czaja J, Kowalczyk D. Med Hypotheses. 2019 Dec;133:109397. doi: 10.1016/j.mehy.2019.109397. Epub 2019 Sep 11. PMID: 31526984

[37] Collapsibility of the internal jugular veins in the lateral decubitus body position: A potential protective role of the cerebral venous outflow against neurodegeneration. Simka M, Czaja J, Kowalczyk D. Med Hypotheses. 2019 Dec;133:109397. doi: 10.1016/j.mehy.2019.109397. Epub 2019 Sep 11. PMID: 31526984

[38] Respiratory rate variability in sleeping adults without obstructive sleep apnea. Gutierrez G, Williams J, Alrehaili GA, McLean A, Pirouz R, Amdur R, Jain V, Ahari J, Bawa A, Kimbro S. Physiol Rep. 2016 Sep;4(17). pii: e12949. doi: 10.14814/phy2.12949. PMID:27597768

[39] Impairment of CSF Egress through the Cribriform Plate plays an Apical role in Alzheimer's disease Etiology. Ricardo Zaragoza, Daniel Miulli, Samir Kashyap, Tyler A Carson, Andre Obenaus, Javed Siddiqi, Douglas W Ethell. medRxiv 2021.10.04.21264049; doi: https://doi.org/10.1101/2021.10.04.21264049

[40] Neurocognitive abilities in children with adenotonsillar hypertrophy. Kurnatowski P, Putyński L, Lapienis M, Kowalska B. Int J Pediatr Otorhinolaryngol. 2006 Mar;70(3):419-24. doi: 10.1016/j.ijporl.2005.07.006. Epub 2005 Oct 10. PMID: 16216342

[41] Psychiatric disorders and symptoms severity in patients with adenotonsillar hypertrophy before and after adenotonsillectomy. Soylu E, Soylu N, Yıldırım YS, Sakallıoğlu Ö, Polat C, Orhan I. Int J Pediatr Otorhinolaryngol. 2013 Oct;77(10):1775-81. doi: 10.1016/j.ijporl.2013.08.020. Epub 2013 Aug 28. PMID: 24011939

[42] Gomaa M A, Mamdouh H, khalaf Z, Abd El-hakeem WH, Zaky EA. (2021) Cognitive Impairment in Children with Adenotonsillar Hypertrophy. J. Neuroscience and Neurological Surgery. 8(1); DOI:10.31579/2578-8868/147

[43] Glymphatic System Pathology and Neuroinflammation as Two Risk Factors of Neurodegeneration. Szlufik S, Kopeć K, Szleszkowski S, Koziorowski D. Cells. 2024 Feb 5;13(3):286. doi: 10.3390/cells13030286. PMID: 38334678

[44] https://www.quantamagazine.org/why-sleep-deprivation-kills-20200604/

[45] Cell injury and repair resulting from sleep loss and sleep recovery in laboratory rats. Everson CA, Henchen CJ, Szabo A, Hogg N. Sleep. 2014 Dec 1;37(12):1929-40. doi: 10.5665/sleep.4244. PMID: 25325492

[46] Sleep Loss Can Cause Death through Accumulation of Reactive Oxygen Species in the Gut. Vaccaro A, Kaplan Dor Y, Nambara K, Pollina EA, Lin C, Greenberg ME, Rogulja D. Cell. 2020 Jun 11;181(6):1307-1328.e15. doi: 10.1016/j.cell.2020.04.049. PMID: 32502393

[47] Sleep restriction impairs blood-brain barrier function. He J, Hsuchou H, He Y, Kastin AJ, Wang Y, Pan W. J Neurosci. 2014 Oct 29;34(44):14697-706. doi: 10.1523/JNEUROSCI.2111-14.2014. PMID: 25355222

[48] Nicotinamide Mononucleotide Ameliorates Sleep Deprivation-Induced Gut Microbiota Dysbiosis and Restores Colonization Resistance against Intestinal Infections. Fang D, Xu T, Sun J, Shi J, Li F, Yin Y, Wang Z, Liu Y. Adv Sci (Weinh). 2023 Mar;10(9):e2207170. doi: 10.1002/advs.202207170. Epub 2023 Jan 25. PMID: 36698264

49 NLRP3-mediated autophagy dysfunction links gut microbiota dysbiosis to tau pathology in chronic sleep deprivation. Zhao N, Chen X, Chen QG, Liu XT, Geng F, Zhu MM, Yan FL, Zhang ZJ, Ren QG. Zool Res. 2024 Jul 18;45(4):857-874. doi: 10.24272/j.issn.2095-8137.2024.085. PMID: 39004863

50 Intestinal dysbiosis mediates cognitive impairment via the intestine and brain NLRP3 inflammasome activation in chronic sleep deprivation. Zhao N, Chen QG, Chen X, Liu XT, Geng F, Zhu MM, Yan FL, Zhang ZJ, Ren QG. Brain Behav Immun. 2023 Feb;108:98-117. doi: 10.1016/j.bbi.2022.11.013. Epub 2022 Nov 24. PMID: 36427810

51 Gut microbiota modulates the inflammatory response and cognitive impairment induced by sleep deprivation. Wang Z, Chen WH, Li SX, He ZM, Zhu WL, Ji YB, Wang Z, Zhu XM, Yuan K, Bao YP, Shi L, Meng SQ, Xue YX, Xie W, Shi J, Yan W, Wei H, Lu L, Han Y. Mol Psychiatry. 2021 Nov;26(11):6277-6292. doi: 10.1038/s41380-021-01113-1. Epub 2021 May 7. PMID: 33963281

52 Sleep Deprivation and Gut Microbiota Dysbiosis: Current Understandings and Implications. Sun J, Fang D, Wang Z, Liu Y. Int J Mol Sci. 2023 May 31;24(11):9603. doi: 10.3390/ijms24119603. PMID: 37298553

53 The Role of Microbiome in Insomnia, Circadian Disturbance and Depression. Li Y, Hao Y, Fan F, Zhang B. Front Psychiatry. 2018 Dec 5;9:669. doi: 10.3389/fpsyt.2018.00669. PMID: 30568608

54 CLOCK and BMAL1 regulate MyoD and are necessary for maintenance of skeletal muscle phenotype and function.Andrews JL, Zhang X, McCarthy JJ, et al. Proc Natl Acad Sci U S A. 2010 Nov 2;107(44):19090-5. PMID: 20956306

55 In vivo half-life of a protein is a function of its amino-terminal residue. Bachmair A, Finley D, Varshavsky A. Science. 1986 Oct 10;234(4773):179-86. PMID:3018930

56 Quantification of protein half-lives in the budding yeast proteome. Belle A, Tanay A, Bitincka L, Shamir R, O'Shea EK. Version 2. Proc Natl Acad Sci U S A. 2006 Aug 29;103(35):13004-9. doi: 10.1073/pnas.0605420103. PMID: 16916930

57 Proteome half-life dynamics in living human cells. Eden E, Geva-Zatorsky N, Issaeva I, et al. Science. 2011 Feb 11;331(6018):764-8. PMID:21233346

58 Effect of sleep deprivation on the human metabolome. Davies SK, Ang JE, Revell VL, et al. Proc Natl Acad Sci U S A. 2014 Jul 22;111(29):10761-6. doi: 10.1073/pnas.1402663111. PMID: 25002497

59 Effect of acute total sleep deprivation on plasma melatonin, cortisol and metabolite rhythms in females. Honma A, Revell VL, Gunn PJ, Davies SK, Middleton B, Raynaud FI, Skene DJ. Eur J Neurosci. 2020 Jan;51(1):366-378. doi: 10.1111/ejn.14411. PMID: 30929284

60 Functional bowel disorders in rotating shift nurses may be related to sleep disturbances.. Zhen Lu W, Ann Gwee K, Yu Ho K. Eur J Gastroenterol Hepatol. 2006 Jun;18(6):623-7. PMID:16702851

61 Appetite-regulating hormones from the upper gut: disrupted control of xenin and ghrelin in night workers. Schiavo-Cardozo D, Lima MM, Pareja JC, Geloneze B. Clin Endocrinol (Oxf). 2012 Dec 1. PMID:23199168

62 Total and cause-specific mortality of U.S. nurses working rotating night shifts. Gu F, Han J, Laden F, Pan A, et al. Am J Prev Med. 2015 Mar;48(3):241-52. PMID:25576495

63 Shifting eating to the circadian rest phase misaligns the peripheral clocks with the master SCN clock and leads to a metabolic syndrome. Mukherji A, Kobiita A, Damara M, et al. Proc Natl Acad Sci U S A. 2015 Dec 1;112(48):E6691-8. PMID:26627260

64 The impact of the circadian timing system on cardiovascular and metabolic function. Morris CJ, Yang JN, Scheer FA. Prog Brain Res. 2012;199:337-58. PMID:22877674

65 Expressions of tight junction proteins Occludin and Claudin-1 are under the circadian control in the mouse large intestine: implications in intestinal permeability and susceptibility to colitis. Kyoko OO, Kono H, Ishimaru K, Miyake K, Kubota T, Ogawa H, Okumura K, Shibata S, Nakao A. PLoS One. 2014 May 20;9(5):e98016. doi: 10.1371/journal.pone.0098016. PMID: 24845399

66 Microbiota Diurnal Rhythmicity Programs Host Transcriptome Oscillations. Thaiss CA, Levy M, Korem T, Dohnalová L et al. Cell. 2016 Dec 1;167(6):1495-1510.e12. doi: 10.1016/j.cell. 2016.11.003. PMID: 27912059

67 Light exposure influences the diurnal oscillation of gut microbiota in mice. Wu G, Tang W, He Y, Hu J, Gong S, He Z, Wei G, Lv L, Jiang Y, Zhou H, Chen P. Biochem Biophys Res Commun. 2018 Jun 18;501(1):16-23. doi: 10.1016/j.bbrc.2018.04.095. PMID: 29730287

68 Human Gut Bacteria Are Sensitive to Melatonin and Express Endogenous Circadian Rhythmicity. Paulose JK, Wright JM, Patel AG, Cassone VM. PLoS One. 2016 Jan 11;11(1):e0146643. doi: 10.1371/journal.pone.0146643. PMID: 26751389

69 Entrainment of the Circadian Clock of the Enteric Bacterium Klebsiella aerogenes by Temperature Cycles. Paulose JK, Cassone CV, Graniczkowska KB, Cassone VM. iScience. 2019 Sep 27;19:1202-1213. doi: 10.1016/j.isci.2019.09.007. PMID: 31551197

70 https://www.genecards.org/cgi-bin/carddisp.pl?gene=NFIL3

71 The intestinal microbiota regulates body composition through NFIL3 and the circadian clock. Wang Y, Kuang Z, Yu X, Ruhn KA, Kubo M, Hooper LV. Science. 2017 Sep 1;357(6354):912-916. doi: 10.1126/science.aan0677. PMID: 28860383

72 Effects of diurnal variation of gut microbes and high-fat feeding on host circadian clock function and metabolism. Leone V, Gibbons SM, Martinez K, et al. Cell Host Microbe. 2015 May 13;17(5):681-9. doi: 10.1016/j.chom.2015.03.006. PMID: 25891358

73 Microbiome diurnal rhythmicity and its impact on host physiology and disease risk. Nobs SP, Tuganbaev T, Elinav E. EMBO Rep. 2019 Apr;20(4):e47129. doi: 10.15252/embr.201847129. PMID: 30877136

[74] Diet and feeding pattern affect the diurnal dynamics of the gut microbiome. Zarrinpar A, Chaix A, Yooseph S, Panda S. Cell Metab. 2014 Dec 2;20(6):1006-17. doi: 10.1016/j.cmet.2014.11.008. PMID: 25470548

[75] The Role of Microbiome in Insomnia, Circadian Disturbance and Depression. Li Y, Hao Y, Fan F, Zhang B. Front Psychiatry. 2018 Dec 5;9:669. doi: 10.3389/fpsyt.2018.00669. PMID: 30568608

[76] Replication of obesity and associated signaling pathways through transfer of microbiota from obese-prone rats. Duca FA, Sakar Y, Lepage P, et al. Diabetes. 2014 May;63(5):1624-36. PMID:24430437

[77] High fat diet-induced gut microbiota exacerbates inflammation and obesity in mice via the TLR4 signaling pathway. Kim KA, Gu W, Lee IA, et al. PLoS One. 2012;7(10):e47713. PMID:23091640

[78] Transkingdom control of microbiota diurnal oscillations promotes metabolic homeostasis. Thaiss CA, Zeevi D, Levy M, Zilberman-Schapira G, Suez J, Tengeler AC, Abramson L, Katz MN, Korem T, Zmora N, Kuperman Y, Biton I, Gilad S, Harmelin A, Shapiro H, Halpern Z, Segal E, Elinav E. Cell. 2014 Oct 23;159(3):514-29. doi: 10.1016/j.cell.2014.09.048. PMID: 25417104

[79] Gut microbiome diversity is associated with sleep physiology in humans. Smith RP, Easson C, Lyle SM, Kapoor R, Donnelly CP, Davidson EJ, Parikh E, Lopez JV, Tartar JL. PLoS One. 2019 Oct 7;14(10):e0222394. doi: 10.1371/journal.pone.0222394. PMID: 31589627

[80] Human and rat gut microbiome composition is maintained following sleep restriction. Zhang SL, Bai L, Goel N, Bailey A, Jang CJ, Bushman FD, Meerlo P, Dinges DF, Sehgal A. Proc Natl Acad Sci U S A. 2017 Feb 21;114(8):E1564-E1571. doi: 10.1073/pnas.1620673114. PMID: 28179566

[81] Gut microbiota and glucometabolic alterations in response to recurrent partial sleep deprivation in normal-weight young individuals. Benedict C, Vogel H, Jonas W, Woting A, Blaut M, Schürmann A, Cedernaes J. Mol Metab. 2016 Oct 24;5(12):1175-1186. doi: 10.1016/j.molmet.2016.10.003. PMID: 27900260

[82] Dietary inflammatory index scores differ by shift work status: NHANES 2005 to 2010. Wirth MD, Burch J, Shivappa N, Steck SE, Hurley TG, Vena JE, Hébert JR. J Occup Environ Med. 2014 Feb;56(2):145-8. PMID:24451608

[83] Intracerebroventricular administration of growth hormone induces morphological changes in pyramidal neurons of the hippocampus and prefrontal cortex in adult rats. Olivares-Hernández JD, García-García F, Camacho-Abrego I, Flores G, Juárez-Aguilar E. Synapse. 2018 Jul;72(7):e22030. doi: 10.1002/syn.22030. PMID:29405381

[84] Born this way: Hippocampal neurogenesis across the lifespan. Kozareva DA, Cryan JF, Nolan YM. Aging Cell. 2019 Oct;18(5):e13007. doi: 10.1111/acel.13007. PMID: 31298475

[85] Adult hippocampal neurogenesis is abundant in neurologically healthy subjects and drops sharply in patients with Alzheimer's disease. Moreno-Jiménez EP, Flor-García M, Terreros-Roncal J, et al. Nat Med. 2019 Apr;25(4):554-560. doi: 10.1038/s41591-019-0375-9. PMID: 30911133

[86] The tired hippocampus: the molecular impact of sleep deprivation on hippocampal function. Havekes R, Abel T. Curr Opin Neurobiol. 2017 Jun;44:13-19. doi: 10.1016/j.conb.2017.02.005. PMID:28242433

[87] Diurnal rhythm and stress regulate dendritic architecture and spine density of pyramidal neurons in the rat infralimbic cortex. Perez-Cruz C, Simon M, Flügge G, Fuchs E, Czéh B. Behav Brain Res. 2009 Dec 28;205(2):406-13. doi: 10.1016/j.bbr.2009.07.021. PMID:19643147

[88] Modulation of Adult Hippocampal Neurogenesis by Sleep: Impact on Mental Health. Navarro-Sanchis C, Brock O, Winsky-Sommerer R, Thuret S. Front Neural Circuits. 2017 Oct 12;11:74. doi: 10.3389/fncir.2017.00074. PMID:29075182

[89] Rapid eye movement sleep deprivation contributes to reduction of neurogenesis in the hippocampal dentate gyrus of the adult rat. Guzman-Marin R, Suntsova N, Bashir T, Nienhuis R, Szymusiak R, McGinty D. Sleep. 2008 Feb;31(2):167-75. PMID:18274263

[90] New neurons in the adult brain: the role of sleep and consequences of sleep loss. Meerlo P, Mistlberger RE, Jacobs BL, Heller HC, McGinty D. Sleep Med Rev. 2009 Jun;13(3):187-94. doi: 10.1016/j.smrv.2008.07.004. PMID:18848476

[91] Association between autophagy and rapid eye movement sleep loss-associated neurodegenerative and patho-physio-behavioral changes. Chauhan AK, Mallick BN. Sleep Med. 2019 Nov;63:29-37. doi: 10.1016/j.sleep.2019.04.019. PMID:31605901

[92] Sleep and adult neurogenesis: implications for cognition and mood. Mueller AD, Meerlo P, McGinty D, Mistlberger RE. Curr Top Behav Neurosci. 2015;25:151-81. doi: 10.1007/7854_2013_251. PMID:24218292

[93] Concise Review: Regulatory Influence of Sleep and Epigenetics on Adult Hippocampal Neurogenesis and Cognitive and Emotional Function. Akers KG, Chérasse Y, Fujita Y, Srinivasan S, Sakurai T, Sakaguchi M. Stem Cells. 2018 Jul;36(7):969-976. doi: 10.1002/stem.2815. PMID:29484772

[94] Factors that influence adult neurogenesis as potential therapy. Shohayeb B, Diab M, Ahmed M, Ng DCH. Transl Neurodegener. 2018 Feb 21;7:4. doi: 10.1186/s40035-018-0109-9. PMID: 29484176

[95] A Sequential Study of Age-Related Lipofuscin Accumulation in Hippocampus and Striate Cortex of Rats. Singh KS, Patro N, Kumar P. Ann Neurosci. 2018 Dec;25(4):223-233. doi: 10.1159/000490908. PMID:31000961

[96] Neural Consequences of Chronic Short Sleep: Reversible or Lasting? Zhao Z, Zhao X, Veasey SC. Front Neurol. 2017 May 31;8:235. doi: 10.3389/fneur. 2017.00235. PMID:28620347

[97] Antidepressant effects of acute sleep deprivation are reduced in highly controlled environments. Goldschmied JR, Boland E, Palermo E, Barilla H, Dinges DF, Detre JA,

Basner M, Sheline YI, Rao H, Gehrman P. J Affect Disord. 2023 Nov 1;340:412-419. doi: 10.1016/j.jad.2023.07.116. Epub 2023 Aug 6. PMID: 37553017

[98] Therapeutic sleep deprivation for major depressive disorder: A randomized controlled trial. Xu YH, Wu F, Yu S, Guo YN, Zhao RR, Zhang RL. J Affect Disord. 2024 Sep 15;361:10-16. doi: 10.1016/j.jad.2024.06.005. Epub 2024 Jun 4. PMID: 38844163

31: Periodontal Disease and Its Prevention

Bite-Sized Sum-up

There is mounting evidence that periodontal disease contributes to the development of Alzheimer's disease (AD). Similar to intestinal dysbiosis, the bacteria that thrive in periodontitis produce LPS that can cross the blood-brain barrier and promote inflammatory injury. The journey from the oral cavity to the brain is not a long stretch.

The human oral microbiome houses about 770 different microorganisms. The microbiota forms the dental biofilm (dental plaque) on the surface of the teeth. In healthy conditions, the microbiome is dominated by gram-positive bacteria, which live in a commensal relationship and don't cause harm.[1] Upsetting the balance can cause disease.

- Periodontitis is likely a causal contributor in the development of about 40% of AD cases.
- A healthy diet, such as the SANA diet, is associated with a lower risk of periodontal disease.
- Diets rich in dairy products are associated with a lower risk of periodontal disease.
- Individuals with low serum vitamin D are at elevated risk of developing periodontal disease (PDD).
- Insulin resistance may be a risk factor for dental disease.
- Adequate dental hygiene greatly lowers the risk and can help in the recovery from PDD.
    - Use fluoridated toothpaste without glycerin. Stannous fluoride is likely more effective than sodium fluoride for treating established periodontal disease, but it can cause the teeth to become rough. Sodium fluoride is sufficient to help prevent periodontitis and dental caries.
    - Floss at least once daily. Glide waxed floss is a recommended brand.
    - Use a water-flosser using warm water daily.
    - Use an essential oil mouthwash twice daily to complete the dental hygiene regimen.

Periodontal Disease

Periodontal Disease is highly prevalent; *about one in three American adults over the age of 30 has periodontal disease*. In young women, PDD is a common cause of preterm birth and low birthweight; PDD can cause fetal death. PDD is a risk factor for Alzheimer's dementia and a suspected risk factor for cardiovascular and other chronic diseases.

Some common signs of periodontitis include:

- Red, swollen, or tender gums
- Gums bleed with brushing or flossing
- Persistent metallic or foul-smelling breath
- Receding gums and gaps between teeth
- Loose or sensitive teeth

Dental Caries: The oral mucosa is an ideal environment for both commensal and pathogenic bacteria. Dental caries is the most common chronic disease in the human population. The bacteria *Streptococcus mutans* have a unique ability to adhere to the surface of the teeth as a result of their ability to convert sucrose from the diet into a sticky polysaccharide that forms plaque. The fermentation of sucrose and other sugars produces acids that demineralize the teeth, causing caries. The yeast, *Candida albicans,* has a symbiotic relationship with *S. mutans,* which increases plaque formation. *S. mutans* then ferments sucrose and other sugars into lactic acid, which dissolves the tooth enamel.[2]

PPD: Periodontal disease is a common, chronic oral infection that is common among older adults, and which puts people at risk of cognitive decline. A meta-analysis including 47 studies found that poor periodontal health was associated with a 23% increased risk of cognitive decline and a 21% increased risk of dementia. Loss of one or more teeth had a similar impact on risk. Extensive loss of teeth from PDD was associated with a 50% increased risk of cognitive decline.[3] There appears to be a linear relationship between the number of teeth lost and the risk of cognitive impairment and dementia.[4]

In recent years, it has been recognized that periodontal disease is a strong risk factor for Alzheimer's disease (AD) in the general population, but especially for those with other risk factors, such as those with the APOε4/4 genotype. Tooth loss and inconsistent tooth brushing are risk factors for the development of AD. Women who brushed three times a day were only 38 percent as likely to develop AD as those brushing once daily. Clinical periodontitis is associated with lower cognitive function among non-demented persons. AD patients with active *Porphyromonas gingivalis (P. gingivalis)* periodontitis have a more rapid decline in function when compared to those not affected.[5] Additionally, alterations in the intestinal flora have been associated with risk for AD.[6]

Diet and oral hygiene are important risk determinants for PDD. The Western diet, high in sugar and fats, increases the risk of PDD. Diets deficient in beta carotene, vitamin C, and vitamin D increase risk. Diets high in polyphenols are associated with a lower risk.[7]

Analysis of data on 9,820 American adults over the age of 30 who participated in the National Health and Nutrition Examination Surveys (NHANES) from 2009-2014 found that 36% of the participants had PDD. The odds for PDD were 1.99 times higher for men as compared to women, 3.2 times higher for those with less than a high school education, more than 2-fold higher for non-Caucasians, 2.4 times higher for those living in poverty, 3 times higher for current smokers, 39% higher for the morbidly obese (BMI ≥30), 63% higher for diabetics, and 44% higher for single adults. Subjects who did not use dental floss were twice as likely to have PDD as those who did.[8] Currently, the impact of flossing on PDD is controversial; it may be that it effectively prevents the disease, or it may be that those who floss are more fastidious about their overall dental hygiene, dental care, and overall health.

In a study of older adults, those brushing three times daily were one-third as likely to have dementia as those brushing 1 – 2 times, and were 5.5 times as likely to have dementia as those who never brushed. After adjusting for other variables, of several metrics of PDD severity, only bleeding on probing was significantly more common among dementia patients.[9] In a case-control study of elderly patients in Spain, those with more severe dementia were 11 times more likely to have fewer natural teeth.[10]

Poor dental health, however, may be the result of cognitive decline and dementia. Studies of the elderly have found an inverse association between cognition and daily oral hygiene, and a direct association was found for the accumulation of bacterial plaque and gingival bleeding with cognitive impairment and dementia.[11] [12] In a study of 60 community-dwelling subjects with mild to moderate AD, cognitive scores declined six times more quickly over six months for those with periodontal disease than for those without.[13]

It may not be only that individuals with cognitive impairment forget to brush and floss. Frailty in the elderly is commonly associated with oral hypofunction (OHF). OHF includes oral dryness and decreased muscular function of the lips, tongue, masseter, and pharyngeal muscles involved in chewing and swallowing.[14] OHF is surprisingly common in people over the age of 65; in one investigation, over 30% of those over the age of 65 met the diagnostic criteria for OHF.[15] In another study, at least one criterion of OHF was present in 19% of those aged 32 – 64, 45% in those 65 – 74, 75% among those 74 – 84, and in 90% of those over the age of 85.[16] Oral-muscular function likely reflects overall muscular loss with aging, but can be improved with diet and exercise.[17]

Oral dryness can be the result of autoimmune disease (Sjögren's syndrome), but more commonly is the result of medications, especially those with anticholinergic effects.[18] About one in three persons over the age of 65 has either dry mouth (xerostomia) or reduced salivary flow.[19] Lack of salivary flow increases the risk of PDD and tooth decay. Older adults are more likely to mouth breathe during sleep, further impeding the antibiotic effects of saliva in the mouth. Obstructive sleep apnea (OSA) severity is correlated with the severity of PDD. A meta-analysis found a 65% increased risk of PDD among those with OSA.[20] Mouth breathing associated with OSA exacerbates xerostomia and dental caries. Both conditions are associated with systemic inflammation.[21]

The question remains: does PDD cause cognitive decline and AD, or is it a case of reverse causality? It has been demonstrated that the induction of periodontal disease exacerbates cognitive decline and AD pathology in mice bred to be genetically susceptible to AD. The pathology was found to be associated with the up-regulation of interleukin 1-beta (IL-1β) and tumor necrosis factor-alpha (TNF-α), which induce systemic and cerebral inflammatory responses.[22]

Porphyromonas gingivalis (*P. gingivalis* or *Pg*) is a Gram-negative, non-motile bacterium that plays a central role in periodontal disease. Interestingly, it does not cause PDD on its own, but only in combination with other bacteria. Pg has been linked to AD and rheumatoid arthritis, and is theorized to promote atherosclerosis.

The outer membrane vesicles of *Pg* encase several key virulence factors (LPS, gingipains, and fimbriae). Pg gingipains are protease enzymes that can act on tau protein in the brain, transforming it into a neurotoxic product that contributes to the progression of AD. *Pg* LPS promotes the TLR4 inflammatory cascade; the bacteria's s fimbriae induce the TLR2 inflammatory pathway. These cause cerebral inflammatory response and increase BBB permeability.[23]

Gingivitis and periodontitis are polymicrobial infections with *Pg*, commonly in association with spirochetes and other bacteria. Other bacteria commonly present in PDD are *Aggregatibacter actinomycetemcomitans* (*Aa*), *Actinomyces naeslundii (An)*, *Campylobacter rectus* (*Cr*), *Fusobacterium nucleatum* (*Fn*), *Prevotella intermedia* (*Pi*), *Tannerella forsythensis (Tf)*, and *Treponema denticola* (*Td*), all of which release inflammatory mediators and toxins.

Pg increases the production of hydrogen sulfide in the mouth. Although the bacterium *P. gingivalis* cannot cause periodontal disease on its own, it induces a shift in the microbial population of the mouth and increases the virulence of otherwise commensal oral bacteria that, in the absence of *P. gingivalis,* will not act as pathogens.[24 25]

P. gingivalis produces some hydrogen sulfide (H_2S), but it greatly increases the growth and invasiveness of other species that are highly efficient at converting cysteine, homocysteine, and glutathione to H_2S, including *Treponema denticola* and various *Fusobacterium* species.[26] In these bacteria, the enzyme L-cysteine desulfidase converts cysteine into H2S, ammonia, and water.[27] While H_2S is often present in bad breath, halitosis results from the stench of methanethiol, dimethyl sulfide, and other sulfides emanating from the mouth as a result of bacterial fermentation. H_2S is not a major factor in halitosis, as humans cannot smell H_2S nearly as well as we can detect methanethiol.

P. gingivalis may cause AD by gaining entry into the CNS. Persons colonized with this bacterium can have transient bacteremia with minimal injuries to the gums, and this can cause the bacteria to translocate to the liver, coronary arteries, placenta, or other tissues. The history of vascular exposure to P. gingivalis appears universal in patients with coronary artery disease. In mice, brain exposure to P. gingivalis allows the production of toxic gingipains.

In a post-mortem tissue study of ten AD cases and ten age-matched controls, LPS from *P. gingivalis* was present in four of the AD patient brains, but not found in the brains of any of the control patients.[28] Brain infection with *Pg* or other periodontal pathogens is likely not required to cause an inflammatory response in the brain. These bacteria release membrane vesicles containing proinflammatory and toxic compounds that can make their way into the brain.[29]

Several treponemal bacteria are found in periodontal disease. It is well known that *Treponema pallidum*, the causative agent of syphilis, can cause neurosyphilis, a form of chronic brain infection that can cause mania, psychosis, depression, and dementia. In a study of the post-mortem frontal lobes of the brains of AD, assessing six different Treponema species found in periodontal disease, 14 of 16 AD patients were found to have the presence of at least one Treponema, while only 4 of 18 control brains did; an odds ratio of 3.5.[30]

In mice, oral infection with *Treponema denticola* causes resorption of the alveolar bone around the teeth. *T. denticola* colonization of brain tissue causes neuroinflammation in the hippocampus, a main area of brain injury in AD, and promotes hyperphosphorylation of the tau protein.[31]

As discussed in the chapter on sleep, glymphatic flow (GF) through the tiny holes in the cribriform plate of the skull, from the base of the brain into the olfactory nasal mucosa, is essential for brain health. Loss of GF occurs in AD. Also discussed was the loss of the sense of smell is common in both AD and Parkinson's Disease (PD) patients. Periodontitis is also accompanied by a loss of the sense of smell, with over half of patients reporting it.

With aging and inflammation, there is a loss of the perforations in the cribriform plate. [32] This loss is associated with a loss in the sense of smell, as these perforations allow olfactory nerve fibers to communicate between the nasal mucosa and the brain. The loss of these perforations also impedes the cleansing activity of the GF, which causes a buildup of Aβ and other toxic compounds in the brain, causing AD and promoting Parkinson's disease.

Let me suggest that the loss of perforations in the cribriform plate is not a normal aspect of aging, but rather the result of pathologic bone remodeling (PBR). PBR occurs in PDD as a result of the chronic tissue inflammation and immune mediators, including TNF, IL-1, IL-6, and RANKL.[33] *Treponema denticola* expresses proinflammatory compounds that activate TLR4 and express chymotrypsin-like proteinase.[34] It is one of the bacteria that causes PBR of the alveolar bone. It is likely that *Treponema denticola* and other bacteria associated with PDD promote chronic inflammation and bone remodeling of the cribriform plate, and that promote the loss of perforations in the cribriform plate over time, degrading the sense of smell.

Treatment and preventive care for PPD are likely critical to the prevention of dementia. Antibiotic treatment with an antibiotic that makes its way into the glymphatic flow may be a necessary aspect of treatment to get clearance of these pathogens from the cribriform/olfactory mucosa.

Is it possible for pathological bone remodeling to be replaced by healthy bone remodeling, and thus restoration of cribriform plate patency? Perhaps. There is a constant turnover of bone, and healthy remodeling can theoretically replace dysfunctional remodeling.[35] As long as there are viable nerve fibers through the perforation, there is hope for recovery. Surgical intervention may be possible to restore glymphatic flow through an obstructed cribriform plate.

Antibodies to *Borrelia burgdorferi*, another spirochete and the causative agent of Lyme disease, were found in about 8% of AD patients but not in any of the 51 control subjects, and in a study of both cerebral spinal fluid and blood, about four times as many AD patients showed antibodies to this spirochete. In a separate study, about one in four AD patients had *B. burgdorferi* detected in the brain.[36]

Diet and Periodontal Disease

Periodontitis is a chronic and progressive disease in which damage accumulates with age. The Western diet, which is high in fat and refined sugars, increases PDD risk. In a meta-analysis of three studies, people consuming a Mediterranean diet had about 23% lower risk of PDD; however, the study narrowly missed statistical significance.[37] In the NHANES data, PDD risk has been found to correlate with the energy-adjusted dietary inflammatory index (E-DII), a metric of dietary factors that have been associated with inflammatory blood markers such as cytokines. Those in the highest tertile for E-DII were 53% more likely to have periodontitis than those in the lowest tertile.[38] [39] The DII is also linearly associated with tooth loss.[40] A meta-analysis including 19 studies found that diets high in inflammation-promoting foods increased PDD risk by 39%, while plant-based diets were associated with an 8% lower PDD risk, and in dairy-rich diets, PDD risk was 24% lower.[41] The SANA (Symbiotic Anti-inflammatory Nutritional Agendum) diet is designed to be anti-inflammatory and thus should lower the risk of PDD.

Diets rich in polyphenols appear to be protective against PDD. Thus, green tea and other sugarless tisanes may be protective.[42] Several hormetic beverages, which are rich in phenolic compounds, have activity against periodontal organisms.[43] These include green tea and cocoa.[44] The SANA program also encourages the consumption of (sugarless) ginger root, hibiscus, and yerba maté teas for the prevention and quelling of PDD. Phenolic compounds present in some fruits, such as cranberries, tart cherries, and certain other berries, have preventative effects against PDD pathogens.[45] [46] [47]

The consumption of sweet beverages is associated with tooth loss, but does not appear to be an important risk factor for PDD. Alcohol consumption is associated with both tooth loss and PDD. Milk and coffee consumption in those aged over 60 was associated with a lower risk of PDD. [48] Consumption of high-sugar beverages is associated with an increase in acid-producing bacteria in the mouth, and commensal species are less common.[49]

In a study of young non-obese young adults, the number of dental caries was found to be correlated with insulin resistance; this correlation might be due to the effect of sugar in the diet. In vitro, doses of myoinositol sufficient to increase insulin sensitivity exerted a regenerative action on endothelial cells and fibroblasts, which were used as surrogates for dental alveolar cells, and in mice, myoinositol stimulated bone calcium uptake and the growth of mandibular chondrocytes, osteoblasts, and osteoprogenitors.[50] Thus, insulin resistance is likely to be a risk factor for PDD, and myoinositol, which helps improve insulin sensitivity, may help prevent and improve the condition. Proper preparation of grains (Chapter 9) increases myoinositol availability.

Vitamins

An analysis of NHANES data found that people whose diets were lower in vitamins were more likely to have PDD. The researchers divided the population into those with dietary intakes above or below the median for each vitamin, rather than by adequate or inadequate intake. For each vitamin, those with a diet higher in the upper half of vitamin intake had a lower risk of PDD. The odds ratios for the various vitamins were similar, suggesting that the lower risk was associated with a healthier overall diet. Certain vitamins, however, had greater statistical significance, suggesting that diets rich in these vitamins may be mechanistically protective against PDD. These were vitamins E, D, and B6. Additionally, the carotenoids α- and β-carotene and lutein+zeaxanthin (measured together) were protective, while lycopene and β-cryptoxanthin were not.[51] The study did not assess folate.

The median vitamin E intake of 7.48 mg/day for this study was well below the recommended daily intake (RDA) of 15 mg, indicating that most of the U.S. population is not getting sufficient vitamin E. Nevertheless, the median vitamin B6 intake was 2.455 mg, which was well above the 1.5 and 1.7 mg RDA for older women and men, respectively. This begs the question: Is the RDA for vitamin B6 set below the level that provides optimal health?

Vitamin E is found in many foods, but whole grains are an important source. Vitamin B6 is widely distributed in whole foods. The carotenoids are found in high amounts in yellow and orange fruits and vegetables, and these are also high in vitamin B6. Other foods high in both vitamin B6 and carotenoids include green leafy vegetables such as spinach and avocados, which are high in vitamin E.

Vitamin C: A few studies have found that vitamin C intake is inversely related to periodontitis. Plasma ascorbic acid levels are lower in those with the disease.[52] [53] This does not indicate that vitamin C supplements will or will not help prevent periodontitis, but rather that those consuming a diet rich in fruits were at lower risk of this condition.

Vitamin D: Vitamin D appears to be protective from periodontal disease, with an inverse linear association between gingival inflammation and vitamin D level. Vitamin D protects against bone loss, inhibits activation of TLR4, and promotes immune function.[54] In a clinical trial, a modest dose of vitamin D (1000 IU) improved bleeding on probing, probing depth, the furcation index, and other metrics in patients with periodontitis as compared to the control patients.[55] In the NHANES study, those with serum vitamin D levels less than 50 nmol/l were twice as likely to have PDD as those with higher levels.[56]

Environmental Factors and Toxins

Other risk factors for periodontal disease, beyond diet and personal oral hygiene, include environmental pollutants, including blood lead level, phthalates, and polychlorinated biphenyls (PCBs). Data from the National Health and Nutrition Examination Study (NHANES), including 8,884 Americans, found that elevated blood levels of several PCBs were associated with a doubling in the odds of having periodontal disease.

The odds of having PDD are also associated with blood lead and cadmium levels, and urine antimony levels. Other pollutants, including phenanthrene, fluorine, benzene, styrene, dioxins, naphthol, and toluene, were found to be commonly elevated in persons with PDD.[57] Self-administered air pollution from smoking is another risk factor for periodontal disease.

Oral Hygiene

As mentioned above, dental flossing among adults was associated with a halving of the risk of PDD. Brushing the teeth, especially if brushing multiple times a day, also decreases the risk.

Using mouthwash is recommended. Some evidence may come from studies of pregnant women; periodontal disease is a strong risk factor for poor outcomes of pregnancy. In a meta-analysis assessing women with periodontal disease, dental scaling and root planing plus mouthwash reduced the risk of preterm birth by 63% and low birth weight by 46%, while scaling and root planing alone did not improve these metrics.[58]

Clinical trials indicate that the following regimen effectively reduced supragingival plaque:

- Brushing for one minute, twice daily with soft soft-bristle toothbrush and fluoride toothpaste, plus
- Flossing, at least once a day, plus
- Using a water flosser (such as a Waterpik)
- Rinsing for 30 seconds twice daily with an (preferably non-alcoholic) essential oil mouthwash.

This regimen has a short-term bactericidal effect on the plaque without killing all the bacteria in the mouth. This allows repopulation of the plaque with commensal species that mitigate plaque above and below the gingival margin.[59] This regimen reduces the abundance of *P. gingivalis* and *F. nucleatum* more effectively than brushing and flossing or brushing and mouthwash alone, and also reduces gingivitis, halitosis, and acid-forming bacteria in the plaque.[60]

Using a water-flosser reduced inflammation, reduced probing depth, and improved clinical attachment levels, in comparison to brushing or brushing and flossing. Water-flossing has been shown to reduce the colonization of spirochetes and *Prevotella intermedia* below the gumline.[61]

Essential oil (EO) mouthwashes are as effective as chlorhexidine,[62] the standard that other mouthwashes that others are generally compared to. Alcohol-free 0.05% cetylpyridinium chloride mouthwash appears to be as effective as 0.12% chlorhexidine gluconate mouthwash, but has less staining of the teeth.[63] Essential oils in the EO mouthwashes penetrate the plaque biofilm and destroy the microorganisms. The alcohol in mouthwash is used to carry the antibiotic compounds, but the alcohol is not at a high enough concentration to effectively kill bacteria. Alcohol consumption increases the risk of PDD and is toxic to the mucosa. When compared in a short-term cross-over study, the plaque reduction from EO mouthwash with or without alcohol was not statistically different, while those without alcohol were rated as being more acceptable to the users.[64]

Recommendations:

- Toothpaste: Fluoridated toothpaste containing stannous fluoride is likely more effective than sodium fluoride for established periodontal disease, but it can cause the teeth to become rough. Sodium fluoride is sufficient to help prevent caries and periodontitis. Zinc citrate in toothpaste helps remineralize the teeth. Having sufficient amounts of zinc in the diet, or using a low-dose zinc supplement (6 – 10 mg of zinc as zinc citrate daily), is likely more effective as the zinc gets secreted in the saliva.
- Use a quality, soft-bristle toothbrush. Bush at least twice daily.
- Floss: Glide, waxed. Use at least once daily and additionally when the need is felt.
- Use a water-flosser using warm water daily.
- Mouthwash: Use a non-alcoholic mouthwash with eucalyptus, menthol, and thymol essential oils. (i.e., Listerine Zero). Vigorously swish 15 ml of EO mouthwash around in the mouth for 30 seconds twice daily at the final step in the dental hygiene regimen, before spitting it out.

[1] Analysis the Link between Periodontal Diseases and Alzheimer's Disease: A Systematic Review. Borsa L, Dubois M, Sacco G, Lupi L. Int J Environ Res Public Health. 2021 Sep 3;18(17):9312. doi: 10.3390/ijerph18179312. PMID: 34501899

[2] https://en.wikipedia.org/wiki/Streptococcus_mutans

[3] Periodontal health, cognitive decline, and dementia: A systematic review and meta-analysis of longitudinal studies. Asher S, Stephen R, Mäntylä P, Suominen AL, Solomon A. J Am Geriatr Soc. 2022 Sep;70(9):2695-2709. doi: 10.1111/jgs.17978. Epub 2022 Sep 8. PMID: 36073186; PMCID: PMC9826143.

[4] Dose-Response Meta-Analysis on Tooth Loss with the Risk of Cognitive Impairment and Dementia. Qi X, Zhu Z, Plassman BL, Wu B. J Am Med Dir Assoc. 2021 Oct;22(10):2039-2045. doi: 10.1016/j.jamda.2021.05.009. PMID: 34579934

[5] Periodontitis and Cognitive Decline in Alzheimer's Disease. Ide M, Harris M, Stevens A, Sussams R, Hopkins V, Culliford D, Fuller J, Ibbett P, Raybould R, Thomas R, Puenter U, Teeling J, Perry VH, Holmes C. PLoS One. 2016 Mar 10;11(3):e0151081. doi: 10.1371/journal.pone.0151081. PMID:26963387

[6] The gut microbiome in human neurological disease: A review. Tremlett H, Bauer KC, Appel-Cresswell S, Finlay BB, Waubant E. Ann Neurol. 2017 Mar;81(3):369-382. doi: 10.1002/ana.24901. PMID:28220542

[7] Nutrition as a Key Modifiable Factor for Periodontitis and Main Chronic Diseases. Martinon P, Fraticelli L, Giboreau A, Dussart C, Bourgeois D, Carrouel F. J Clin Med. 2021 Jan 7;10(2):197. doi: 10.3390/jcm10020197. PMID: 33430519

[8] Associations between single and multiple dietary vitamins and the risk of periodontitis: results from NHANES 2009-2014. Liang F, Lu M, Zhou Y. Front Nutr. 2024 Apr 8;11:1347712. doi: 10.3389/fnut.2024.1347712. PMID: 38650639 (Supplemental Materials)

[9] Oral Health Status in Older People with Dementia: A Case-Control Study. Lopez-Jornet P, Zamora Lavella C, Pons-Fuster Lopez E, Tvarijonaviciute A. J Clin Med. 2021 Jan 27;10(3):477. doi: 10.3390/jcm10030477. PMID: 33514062

[10] Oral Health Status in Older People with Dementia: A Case-Control Study. Lopez-Jornet P, Zamora Lavella C, Pons-Fuster Lopez E, Tvarijonaviciute A. J Clin Med. 2021 Jan 27;10(3):477. doi: 10.3390/jcm10030477. PMID: 33514062

[11] Oral Hygiene in the Elderly with Different Degrees of Cognitive Impairment and Dementia. Gil-Montoya JA, Sánchez-Lara I, Carnero-Pardo C, Fornieles-Rubio F, Montes J, Barrios R, Gonzalez-Moles MA, Bravo M. J Am Geriatr Soc. 2017 Mar;65(3):642-647. doi: 10.1111/jgs.14697. PMID: 28024093

[12] Oral Health Status in Older People with Dementia: A Case-Control Study. Lopez-Jornet P, Zamora Lavella C, Pons-Fuster Lopez E, Tvarijonaviciute A. J Clin Med. 2021 Jan 27;10(3):477. doi: 10.3390/jcm10030477. PMID: 33514062

[13] Periodontitis and Cognitive Decline in Alzheimer's Disease. Ide M, Harris M, Stevens A, Sussams R, Hopkins V, Culliford D, Fuller J, Ibbett P, Raybould R, Thomas R, Puenter U, Teeling J, Perry VH, Holmes C. PLoS One. 2016 Mar 10;11(3):e0151081. doi: 10.1371/journal.pone.0151081. PMID: 26963387

[14] Association between intrinsic capacity and oral health in older patients in a frailty clinic. Miyahara S, Maeda K, Kawamura K, Matsui Y, Satake S, Arai H, Umegaki H. Eur Geriatr Med. 2024 Aug;15(4):1119-1127. doi: 10.1007/s41999-024-00956-5. Epub 2024 Mar 5. PMID: 38438830

[15] Evaluating the effect of management on patients with oral hypofunction: A longitudinal study. Onuki W, Magara J, Ito K, Ita R, Kawada S, Tsutsui Y, Nakajima Y, Sakai H, Tsujimura T, Inoue M. Gerodontology. 2023 Sep;40(3):308-316. doi: 10.1111/ger.12655. Epub 2022 Sep 6. PMID: 36065761

[16] Associations between Oral Hypofunction Tests, Age, and Sex. Hatanaka Y, Furuya J, Sato Y, Uchida Y, Shichita T, Kitagawa N, Osawa T. Int J Environ Res Public Health. 2021 Sep 29;18(19):10256. doi: 10.3390/ijerph181910256. PMID: 34639564

[17] Impact of oral health guidance on the tongue-lip motor function of outpatients at a dental hospital. Hatanaka Y, Furuya J, Sato Y, Uchida Y, Osawa T, Shichita T, Suzuki H, Minakuchi S. Gerodontology. 2022 Mar;39(1):83-89. doi: 10.1111/ger.12599. Epub 2021 Oct 24. PMID: 34689371

[18] The Challenge of Medication-Induced Dry Mouth in Residential Aged Care. Thomson WM, Smith MB, Ferguson CA, Moses G. Pharmacy (Basel). 2021 Oct 1;9(4):162. doi: 10.3390/pharmacy9040162. PMID: 34698291

[19] The occurrence of xerostomia and salivary gland hypofunction in a population-based sample of older South Australians. Thomson WM, Chalmers JM, Spencer AJ, Ketabi M. Spec Care Dentist. 1999 Jan-Feb;19(1):20-3. doi: 10.1111/j.1754-4505.1999.tb01363.x. PMID: 10483456

[20] Periodontitis and obstructive sleep apnea's bidirectional relationship: a systematic review and meta-analysis. Al-Jewair TS, Al-Jasser R, Almas K. Sleep Breath. 2015 Dec;19(4):1111-20. doi: 10.1007/s11325-015-1160-8. Epub 2015 Mar 24. PMID: 25801281

[21] Oral Health Implications of Obstructive Sleep Apnea: A Literature Review. Maniaci A, Lavalle S, Anzalone R, Lo Giudice A, Cocuzza S, Parisi FM, Torrisi F, Iannella G, Sireci F, Fadda G, Lentini M, Masiello E, La Via L. Biomedicines. 2024 Jun 21;12(7):1382. doi: 10.3390/biomedicines12071382. PMID: 39061956

[22] L-1β and TNF-α play an important role in modulating the risk of periodontitis and Alzheimer's disease. Wang RP, Huang J, Chan KWY, Leung WK, Goto T, Ho YS, Chang RC. J Neuroinflammation. 2023 Mar 13;20(1):71. doi: 10.1186/s12974-023-02747-4. PMID: 36915108

[23] Analysis the Link between Periodontal Diseases and Alzheimer's Disease: A Systematic Review. Borsa L, Dubois M, Sacco G, Lupi L. Int J Environ Res Public Health. 2021 Sep 3;18(17):9312. doi: 10.3390/ijerph18179312. PMID: 34501899

24 Low-abundance biofilm species orchestrates inflammatory periodontal disease through the commensal microbiota and complement. Hajishengallis G, Liang S, Payne MA, Hashim A, Jotwani R, Eskan MA, McIntosh ML, Alsam A, Kirkwood KL, Lambris JD, Darveau RP, Curtis MA. Cell Host Microbe. 2011 Nov 17;10(5):497-506. doi: 10.1016/j.chom.2011.10.006. PMID:22036469

25 Mouse model of experimental periodontitis induced by Porphyromonas gingivalis/ Fusobacterium nucleatum infection: bone loss and host response. Polak D, Wilensky A, Shapira L, Halabi A, Goldstein D, Weiss EI, Houri-Haddad Y. J Clin Periodontol. 2009 May;36(5):406-10. doi: 10.1111/j.1600-051X.2009.01393.x. PMID:19419440

26 Estimation of bacterial hydrogen sulfide production in vitro. Basic A, Blomqvist S, Carlén A, Dahlén G. J Oral Microbiol. 2015 Jun 29;7:28166. doi: 10.3402/jom.v7.28166. eCollection 2015. PMID:26130377

27 BRENDA https://brenda-enzymes.org/enzyme.php?ecno=4.4.1.28

28 Determining the presence of periodontopathic virulence factors in short-term postmortem Alzheimer's disease brain tissue. Poole S, Singhrao SK, Kesavalu L, Curtis MA, Crean S. J Alzheimers Dis. 2013;36(4):665-77. doi: 10.3233/JAD-121918. PMID: 23666172

29 Bacterial Membrane Vesicles: The Missing Link Between Bacterial Infection and Alzheimer Disease. Butler CA, Ciccotosto GD, Rygh N, Bijlsma E, Dashper SG, Brown AC. J Infect Dis. 2024 Sep 10;230(Supplement_2):S87-S94. doi: 10.1093/infdis/jiae228. PMID: 39255395

30 Molecular and immunological evidence of oral Treponema in the human brain and their association with Alzheimer's disease. Riviere GR, Riviere KH, Smith KS. Oral Microbiol Immunol. 2002 Apr;17(2):113-8. doi: 10.1046/j.0902-0055.2001.00100.x. PMID: 11929559

31 *Treponema denticola* Induces Alzheimer-Like Tau Hyperphosphorylation by Activating Hippocampal Neuroinflammation in Mice. Tang Z, Cheng X, Su X, Wu L, Cai Q, Wu H. J Dent Res. 2022 Jul;101(8):992-1001. doi: 10.1177/00220345221076772. Epub 2022 Feb 22. PMID: 35193423

32 Impairment of CSF Egress through the Cribriform Plate plays an Apical role in Alzheimer's disease Etiology. Ricardo Zaragoza, Daniel Miulli, Samir Kashyap, Tyler A Carson, Andre Obenaus, Javed Siddiqi, Douglas W Ethell. medRxiv 2021.10.04.21264049; doi: https://doi.org/10.1101/2021.10.04.21264049

33 Role of periodontal ligament fibroblasts in periodontitis: pathological mechanisms and therapeutic potential. Huang Y, Tang Y, Zhang R, Wu X, Yan L, Chen X, Wu Q, Chen Y, Lv Y, Su Y. J Transl Med. 2024 Dec 21;22(1):1136. doi: 10.1186/s12967-024-05944-8. PMID: 39709490

34 Infection and apoptosis associated with inflammation in periodontitis: An immunohistologic study. Listyarifah D, Al-Samadi A, Salem A, Syaify A, Salo T, Tervahartiala T, Grenier D, Nordström DC, Sorsa T, Ainola M. Oral Dis. 2017 Nov;23(8):1144-1154. doi: 10.1111/odi.12711. Epub 2017 Aug 7. PMID: 28686335

35 Molecular Signaling Pathways and MicroRNAs in Bone Remodeling: A Narrative Review. Singh M, Singh P, Singh B, Sharma K, Kumar N, Singh D, Mastana S. Diseases. 2024 Oct 12;12(10):252. doi: 10.3390/diseases12100252. PMID: 39452495

36 Alzheimer's disease - a neurospirochetosis. Analysis of the evidence following Koch's and Hill's criteria. Miklossy J. J Neuroinflammation. 2011 Aug 4;8:90. doi: 10.1186/1742-2094-8-90. PMID: 21816039

37 The Mediterranean diet and periodontitis: A systematic review and meta-analysis. Aalizadeh Y, Khamisi N, Asghari P, Safari A, Mottaghi M, Taherkhani MH, Alemi A, Ghaderi M, Rahmanian M. Heliyon. 2024 Aug 5;10(15):e35633. doi: 10.1016/j.heliyon.2024.e35633. eCollection 2024 Aug 15. PMID: 39170303

38 Dietary inflammatory potential is associated with poor periodontal health: A population-based study. Li A, Chen Y, Schuller AA, van der Sluis LWM, Tjakkes GE. J Clin Periodontol. 2021 Jul;48(7):907-918. doi: 10.1111/jcpe.13472.. PMID: 33899265

39 Association between Dietary Inflammatory Index and Periodontitis: A Cross-Sectional and Mediation Analysis. Machado V, Botelho J, Viana J, Pereira P, Lopes LB, Proença L, Delgado AS, Mendes JJ. Nutrients. 2021 Apr 5;13(4):1194. doi: 10.3390/nu13041194. PMID: 33916342

40 Diet-borne systemic inflammation is associated with prevalent tooth loss. Kotsakis GA, Chrepa V, Shivappa N, Wirth M, Hébert J, Koyanagi A, Tyrovolas S. Clin Nutr. 2018 Aug;37(4):1306-1312. doi: 10.1016/j.clnu.2017.06.001. Epub 2017 Jun 9. PMID: 28633943

41 Assessing periodontitis risk from specific dietary patterns: a systematic review and meta-analysis. Fan RY, Chen JX, Chen LL, Sun WL. Clin Oral Investig. 2025 Jan 3;29(1):43. doi: 10.1007/s00784-024-06125-z. PMID: 39751926

42 Nutrition as a Key Modifiable Factor for Periodontitis and Main Chronic Diseases. Martinon P, Fraticelli L, Giboreau A, Dussart C, Bourgeois D, Carrouel F. J Clin Med. 2021 Jan 7;10(2):197. doi: 10.3390/jcm10020197. PMID: 33430519

43 Propolis, Aloe Vera, Green Tea, Cranberry, Calendula, Myrrha and Salvia Properties against Periodontal Microorganisms. Figueiredo LC, Freitas Figueiredo N, da Cruz DF, Baccelli GT, Sarachini GE, Bueno MR, Feres M, Bueno-Silva B. Microorganisms. 2022 Oct 31;10(11):2172. doi: 10.3390/microorganisms10112172. PMID: 36363764

44 Anti-cariogenic effects of polyphenols from plant stimulant beverages (cocoa, coffee, tea). Ferrazzano GF, Amato I, Ingenito A, De Natale A, Pollio A. Fitoterapia. 2009 Jul;80(5):255-62. doi: 10.1016/j.fitote.2009.04.006. PMID: 19397954

45 Cranberry proanthocyanidins: natural weapons against periodontal diseases. Feghali K, Feldman M, La VD, Santos J, Grenier D. J Agric Food Chem. 2012 Jun 13;60(23):5728-35. doi: 10.1021/jf203304v. Epub 2011 Nov 29. PMID: 22082264

46 Effects of a tart cherry (Prunus cerasus L.) phenolic extract on Porphyromonas gingivalis and its ability to impair the oral epithelial barrier. Ben Lagha A, Pellerin G, Vaillancourt K, Grenier D. PLoS One. 2021 Jan

26;16(1):e0246194. doi: 10.1371/journal.pone.0246194. eCollection 2021. PMID: 33497417

47 Effects of a Berry Polyphenolic Fraction on the Pathogenic Properties of *Porphyromonas gingivalis.* Vaillancourt K, Ben Lagha A, Grenier D. Front Oral Health. 2022 Jun 16;3:923663. doi: 10.3389/froh.2022.923663. eCollection 2022. PMID: 35784661

48 Beverages Consumption and Oral Health in the Aging Population: A Systematic Review. Zupo R, Castellana F, De Nucci S, Dibello V, Lozupone M, Giannelli G, De Pergola G, Panza F, Sardone R, Boeing H. Front Nutr. 2021 Oct 27;8:762383. doi: 10.3389/fnut.2021.762383. eCollection 2021. PMID: 34778347

49 Altered salivary microbiota associated with high-sugar beverage consumption. Fan X, Monson KR, Peters BA, Whittington JM, Um CY, Oberstein PE, McCullough ML, Freedman ND, Huang WY, Ahn J, Hayes RB. Sci Rep. 2024 Jun 11;14(1):13386. doi: 10.1038/s41598-024-64324-w. PMID: 38862651

50 Correlation between tooth decay and insulin resistance in normal weight males prompts a role for myo-inositol as a regenerative factor in dentistry and oral surgery: a feasibility study. Barbaro F, Conza GD, Quartulli FP, Quarantini E, Quarantini M, Zini N, Fabbri C, Mosca S, Caravelli S, Mosca M, Vescovi P, Sprio S, Tampieri A, Toni R. Front Bioeng Biotechnol. 2024 Jul 31;12:1374135. doi: 10.3389/fbioe.2024.1374135. eCollection 2024. PMID: 39144484

51 Associations between single and multiple dietary vitamins and the risk of periodontitis: results from NHANES 2009-2014. Liang F, Lu M, Zhou Y. Front Nutr. 2024 Apr 8;11:1347712. doi: 10.3389/fnut.2024.1347712. eCollection 2024. PMID: 38650639

52 Grapefruit consumption improves vitamin C status in periodontitis patients. Staudte H, Sigusch BW, Glockmann E. Br Dent J. 2005 Aug 27;199(4):213-7, discussion 210. doi: 10.1038/sj.bdj.4812613. PMID: 16127404

53 The prevalence of inflammatory periodontitis is negatively associated with serum antioxidant concentrations. Chapple IL, Milward MR, Dietrich T. J Nutr. 2007 Mar;137(3):657-64. doi: 10.1093/jn/137.3.657. PMID: 17311956

54 Vitamin D and Periodontal Health: A Systematic Review. Shah M, Poojari M, Nadig P, Kakkad D, Dutta SB, Sinha S, Chowdhury K, Dagli N, Haque M, Kumar S. Cureus. 2023 Oct 26;15(10):e47773. doi: 10.7759/cureus.47773. eCollection 2023 Oct. PMID: 37899906

55 One-year effects of vitamin D and calcium supplementation on chronic periodontitis. Garcia MN, Hildebolt CF, Miley DD, Dixon DA, Couture RA, Spearie CL, Langenwalter EM, Shannon WD, Deych E, Mueller C, Civitelli R. J Periodontol. 2011 Jan;82(1):25-32. doi: 10.1902/jop.2010.100207. Epub 2010 Sep 1. PMID: 20809866

56 Associations between single and multiple dietary vitamins and the risk of periodontitis: results from NHANES 2009-2014. Liang F, Lu M, Zhou Y. Front Nutr. 2024 Apr 8;11:1347712. doi: 10.3389/fnut.2024.1347712. eCollection 2024. PMID: 38650639

57 Epidemiologic evaluation of NHANES for environmental Factors and periodontal disease. Emecen-Huja P, Li HF, Ebersole JL, Lambert J, Bush H. Sci Rep. 2019 Jun 3;9(1):8227. doi: 10.1038/s41598-019-44445-3. PMID: 31160648

58 DIFFERENTIAL IMPACT OF PERIODONTAL TREATMENT STRATEGIES DURING PREGNANCY ON PERINATAL OUTCOMES: A SYSTEMATIC REVIEW AND META-ANALYSIS. Le QA, Eslick GD, Coulton KM, Akhter R, Lain S, Nassar N, Yaacoub A, Condous G, Leonardi M, Eberhard J, Nanan R. J Evid Based Dent Pract. 2022 Mar;22(1):101666. doi: 10.1016/j.jebdp.2021.101666. Epub 2021 Nov 12. PMID: 35219458

59 Quantitative analysis of the effects of brushing, flossing, and mouthrinsing on supragingival and subgingival plaque microbiota: 12-week clinical trial. Min K, Bosma ML, John G, McGuire JA, DelSasso A, Milleman J, Milleman KR. BMC Oral Health. 2024 May 17;24(1):575. doi: 10.1186/s12903-024-04362-y. PMID: 38760758

60 Quantitative analysis of the effects of brushing, flossing, and mouthrinsing on supragingival and subgingival plaque microbiota: 12-week clinical trial. Min K, Bosma ML, John G, McGuire JA, DelSasso A, Milleman J, Milleman KR. BMC Oral Health. 2024 May 17;24(1):575. doi: 10.1186/s12903-024-04362-y. PMID: 38760758

61 Evaluation of the Safety of a Water Flosser on Gingival and Epithelial Tissue at Different Pressure Settings. C. Ram Goyal, BDS; Jimmy G. Qaqish, BSc; Reinhard Schuller, MSc; and Deborah M. Lyle. Compendium of Continuing Education in Dentistry. June 2018 39(2).

62 Can Chemical Mouthwash Agents Achieve Plaque/Gingivitis Control? Van der Weijden FA, Van der Sluijs E, Ciancio SG, Slot DE. Dent Clin North Am. 2015 Oct;59(4):799-829. doi: 10.1016/j.cden.2015.06.002. PMID: 26427569

63 Efficacy of 0.05% cetylpyridinium chloride mouthwash as an adjunct to toothbrushing compared with 0.12% chlorhexidine gluconate mouthwash in reducing dental plaque and gingival inflammation: A randomized control trial. Oo MMT, Oo PH, Saddki N. Int J Dent Hyg. 2023 Feb;21(1):195-202. doi: 10.1111/idh.12614. Epub 2022 Aug 17. PMID: 35946123

64 Alcohol-free essential oils containing mouthrinse efficacy on three-day supragingival plaque regrowth: a randomized crossover clinical trial. Marchetti E, Tecco S, Caterini E, Casalena F, Quinzi V, Mattei A, Marzo G. Trials. 2017 Mar 31;18(1):154. doi: 10.1186/s13063-017-1901-z. PMID: 28359280

32: Indoor Air Quality

Filtered Content

- ❖ Air pollution is a common contributing cause of vascular disease, dementia, and death.
- ❖ Indoor air pollution has a greater impact on health than outside air; we spend much more time indoors, and indoor air quality is generally worse than outside air. Unless one lives in a highly polluted area or close to a highway or busy intersection, the outside air is usually cleaner than the air in your home. Open the windows when the weather allows it.
- ❖ Particulate Matter (PM) air pollution, including industrial and roadway pollution, pollen, dander, and mold spores, can be greatly reduced in the home with the use of MERV 13 and HEPA filters. If you live in an area with moderate to high levels of PM 0.1 exposure, use a dedicated HEPA filter in your bedroom
- ❖ Activated charcoal air filters are an effective means for removing volatile organic compounds, odors, and certain noxious gases from indoor air in the home.
- ❖ Damp mopping and damp-cloth dusting also help reduce PM in the air of the home. Declutter your home from dust-collecting knick-knacks.
- ❖ Never allow anyone to smoke in your home.
- ❖ Pets create significant amounts of allergens and lower air quality. Cat dander stays in the home for months to years even after the cat is gone.
- ❖ Mold can be mitigated by keeping the humidity inside the building between 30 and 50%.
- ❖ Do not bring shoes worn outdoors into the house. They can carry particulate matter, including lead, cadmium, and other toxic wastes, into the home
- ❖ Most of the risk from microplastics likely comes from airborne exposure. They can be filtered out using MERV 13 or higher and HEPA filters.
- ❖ Use a vacuum cleaner with a HEPA filter. Otherwise, the vacuum just resuspends and creates more small, dangerous PM into the air to be breathed.
- ❖ Make sure your dryer vent is cleaned and functioning properly regularly. Clean the radiator vents on your refrigerator regularly.
- ❖ The roadway can be an area with extremely high PM pollution. Have a HEPA/Charcoal cabin filter put into your vehicle and change it every 12,000 miles
- ❖ If you have the choice, use electric rather than gas appliances in your home. Gas appliances create air quality risks from NOx, carbon monoxide, and carbon dioxide.
- ❖ If you have gas appliances in the home, and especially if there are at-risk individuals in the home (pregnant women, small children, individuals with heart or lung disease, or impaired cognition, get a high-sensitivity carbon monoxide sensor to monitor levels
- ❖ Make sure that the flame and air entrainment of gas appliances are properly adjusted and maintained.
- ❖ If you have a gas range or oven:
  - o Make sure your hood vent actually vents to the outside of the building.
  - o Always use the vent fan while cooking. Preferably, use the back burners to better capture and vent fumes. Use the low fan setting for low gas usage, but use high fan speeds if frying or if using higher fuel levels, such as when using multiple burners and baking.
  - o To ensure the hood works properly, replacement air needs to enter the house at a rate equivalent to that being removed. Depressurization by the vent fan can cause backdraft of combustion gases from other gas appliances, which vent passively; the fan can pull exhaust gas from the gas water heater or furnace into the home. Always open a window enough so that there is sufficient inflow of fresh air to balance the outflow of exhaust from the vent.
  - o At a typical low-speed vent fan setting of 150 cubic feet per minute, an opening of about 20 square inches of window opening is needed to balance the pressure. Thus, opening a 30-inch wide window, one inch should be sufficient. A range hood vent at high speed may vent 600 cubic feet per minute and would require an 80 square inch opening. Thus, a 30-inch wide window would need to be opened just less than three inches.
- ❖ Carbon Dioxide can easily build up in energy-efficient modern homes and buildings to a level that impairs thinking and judgment, even when there are no gas appliances. An air quality monitor that measures CO2 and guides the need for air exchange in the home.Radon gas is an invisible threat. Every home in EPA radon level 1 and 3 zones should be tested for radon, especially those with a basement. Modern, energy-efficient buildings leak little air, and thus are more likely to retain radon, elevating the risk of exposure to dangerous levels of radon gas. If there is variation in terrain, even within a county, there can be large differences in radon risk between homes in the same area.

Air Pollution

Air pollution is deadly. The World Health Organization (WHO) estimates that 3.7 million people die prematurely each year as a result of outdoor air pollution. Many of those reside in highly polluted, densely populated urban areas of Asia. If the deaths from indoor air pollution, including indoor air pollution from cooking over coal and wood and other solid fuel, are considered, the WHO estimates that air pollution causes 7 million premature deaths each year, about *one in eight of all deaths* worldwide. Most of these deaths are from stroke, ischemic heart disease, COPD, and lung cancer, but over 650,000 respiratory infection deaths among children less than five years old are attributed to air pollution.[1 2]

Air pollution is a major cause of vascular disease. A 2016 study found that 19% of all cardiovascular disease (CVD) deaths worldwide were caused by air pollution; a greater number of CVD deaths than those caused by tobacco, obesity, or diabetes.[3] Official European Union estimates attributed 420,000 premature deaths to air pollution in 2016, and calculated that air pollution reduced the average life expectancy in Europe by 2.2 years. Eastern Europe, northern Italy, and Turkey had even higher reductions in life expectancy from air pollution.[4 5]

In India, there are a million premature deaths from outdoor air pollution each year, and another million deaths from indoor air pollution, largely from cooking over solid fuel.[6] A study published in 2019 estimated that seven million people were dying each year from air pollution. That is *one in eight of all deaths* worldwide, with most of these deaths resulting from coronary artery and cerebrovascular disease, but also secondary to heart failure, cardiac arrhythmias, hypertension, and diabetes caused by pollution.[7] A will be discussed below, air pollution is also a cause of dementia.

The death toll from air pollution is much lower in the United States and Canada, where the population density is lower and there are better pollution controls; here, there are *only* about 85,000 deaths per year from PM, mostly from outdoor air pollution. The Los Angeles basin in California has annual average $PM_{2.5}$ (particulate matter smaller than 2.5 microns) levels that exceed the EPA 12.5 μg/m³ limit for long-term exposure.

There are many sources of air pollution, including that from volcanoes, forest fires, dust from the deserts, and dust from the plowing of agricultural lands. The principal type of air pollution that will be discussed herein are those resulting from combustion, and mostly pollution from the combustion of fossil fuels used in the production of energy; coal for electrical power generation and the production of steel, cement, and other industrial products; natural gas and propane for heating and cooking; and gasoline, kerosene, diesel, and bunker fuel for moving cars, jets, trucks, and ships. Organic materials, such as wood used for fuel and cooking, or from forest fires and the burning of trash, plastic, and burning buildings, are significant sources of air pollution from the combustion of hydrocarbons.

This discussion is focused on indoor air quality; as individuals, we can control our indoor air quality, but we have very little power to control outdoor air quality. Also, unless one lives in a particularly polluted area, such as heavy traffic areas or a busy intersection, the air in the home is generally more polluted than the outside air. This is especially true if there is a smoker in the home or if cooking with gas. On average, Americans spend about 90% of their time indoors, and most of that is at home. Thus, indoor air quality is both an important determinant of health and one we have agency over.

Air pollution can be better understood if segregated into two parts: particulate matter and gases. The discussion on gases will be limited to gases produced in the home.

Particulate Matter

In the U.S., about 20% of the population lives in high-traffic areas. Particulate Matter (PM) pollution in the U.S. is nothing to brag about, but exposure to dangerous levels of PM is much less prevalent in the U.S. than in most developed countries, where urban populations are exposed to high levels of PM pollution.[8] Spatial mapping of PM shows that 24 percent of the population of Toronto, Canada, 41% of the population in New Delhi, India, 66% of the population of Beijing, 67% of the population of Paris, and 96% of the population of Barcelona live in areas of high levels of traffic-related air pollution. Beijing and Mexico City had the highest concentrations of PM, but it was localized, so lower percentages of the populations were exposed.[9]

Particulate matter (PM) larger than about 10 microns is mostly filtered or trapped by the upper airways during breathing. The particles above 10 microns usually have a sufficient mass that they collide with mucosal membranes as they move through the nose, and get caught in the moist mucous film that covers the turbinates in the nose.

The mucosa is well supplied with blood and stays moist and warm. The mucous membranes in the respiratory tract act to warm and humidify the air we breathe, so that when we are at rest and inhaling through the nose, by the time the air reaches the lungs, the air has been warmed to near body temperature and humidified to nearly 100 percent relative humidity. As air is drawn into the nose during inhalation, the nasal turbinates create turbulence in the airflow so that there is a high level of contact of air with the mucosa as it is drawn in towards the lungs. The angular momentum of larger dust particles in the air, those particles larger than about 10 microns, makes it highly likely that they collide with the mucosa as the air careens around the turbinates. Thus, PM10 can enter the lower airway, while larger dust particles are mostly excluded. We end up swallowing those dust particles. For the most part, they are poorly absorbed by the intestinal tract.

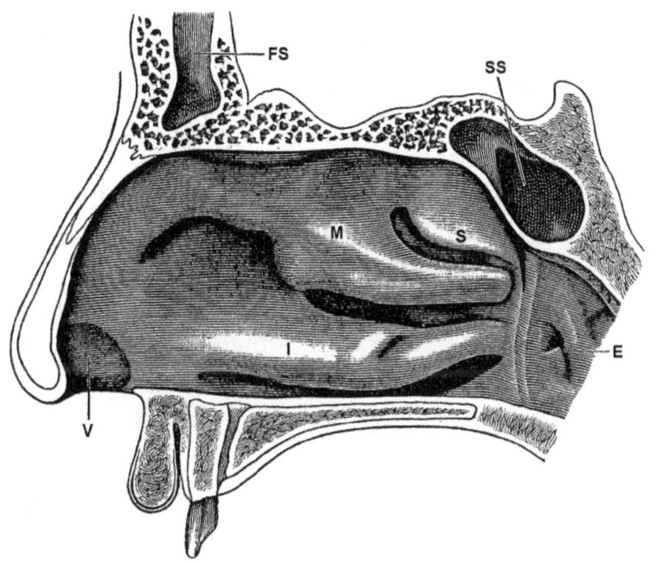

Figure 21-1: A cutaway diagram of the nasal turbinates. S, M, I: superior, middle, and inferior turbinates, FS: frontal sinus, SS: sphenoid sinus, E: Opening of the Eustachian tube, V: nasal vestibule.

Particulate matter (PM) between 2.5 and 10 microns is largely carried in and out of the lungs, exiting in the exhaled breath. PM smaller than about 2.5 microns ($PM_{2.5}$) is much more likely to get deep in the lungs and get deposited there.

Ultrafine particulate (UFP) pollution is PM pollution smaller than 0.1 micron (<100 nm) in diameter. Ultrafine PM can deposit into the alveoli, the tiny gas exchange units of the lung, and can cross into the bloodstream. These ultra-fine airborne particles can also cross the olfactory epithelium in the nose, gaining access to the central nervous system through the olfactory and trigeminal nerves. Thus, it is the fine, and very likely ultra-fine, particulate matter pollution that carries the greatest toxic potential.

For example, UFP exposure is associated with increased blood pressure in children, while $PM_{2.5}$ greater than 0.1 microns is not.[10] In an in vitro study, exposure of the rat brain to PM from environmental pollution, it was only the UFP that caused the neuronal loss. These and other data suggest that the toxicity of PM is inversely proportional to the size of the particles.[11] In a study of children and young adults who had been killed in accidents, ultrafine PM was observed in olfactory bulb neurons, and its presence was associated with the accumulation of Aβ42 and alpha-synuclein; thus, an indication of risk for Alzheimer's and Parkinson's diseases.12 Unfortunately, there are relatively few studies of UFP and its impacts.

The composition of the PM pollution also varies by size; large PM10 is predominantly made up of metals, inorganic compounds, and ions, while ultrafine $PM_{0.1}$ is predominantly composed of organic compounds, including polyaromatic hydrocarbons (PAH).[13] [14] [15]

Air pollution impairs the sense of smell. Autopsies of young people killed in trauma from areas with high levels of air pollution had higher levels of COX-2 (an inflammatory intermediate), Aβ, and α-synuclein in the olfactory nerves, while these were not present in the autopsies of people of the same age killed in areas with low air pollution.[16] Manganese and vanadium are examples of metals particularly toxic to the olfactory bulb.[17] [18] NO2, a product of high-temperature combustion, is also associated with olfactory dysfunction.[19] It should be kept in mind, however, that isolating causal agents of injury from air pollution is difficult, as air pollution is almost always a soup of toxins rather than single compounds.

Particle size has a significant impact on the bioactivity of air pollutants. Water-soluble chemicals are much more likely to be bioavailable. They are much more easily absorbed into the body, and also more easily enter the food chain. For example, aluminum, titanium, iron, and chromium are poorly water-soluble even as particles smaller than 2.5 microns, while sodium is highly water-soluble, irrespective of particle size. Cadmium particles greater than 2.5 microns have minimal water solubility but are easily soluble when smaller. Zinc, copper, nickel, cobalt, and lead have much greater solubility when the particle size is below 2.5 microns. Manganese (Mn) with a PM 2.5–10 microns has about 50% solubility, but is 100% soluble when less than 0.25 microns. Thus, ultrafine particles are not only more likely to enter the body, but they are also more likely to be absorbed and have toxic effects. Vanadium and nickel PM0.25, which are produced from the combustion of vehicle fuels, are particularly active among metal particles in creating reactive oxygen species (ROS) and thus are likely to cause injury.[20] Mn exposure to the nasal mucosa is a risk for Parkinson's disease. This risk can come from welding, the use of street drugs processed with manganese compounds, or even showering in water with high Mn levels, which creates aerosols containing Mn.

Roadway pollution is responsible for a large amount of particulate matter. The sources of the PM from roadways and vehicular traffic come from brake pads, tire wear, the roadway surfaces themselves, and dust and dirt on the roadway, in addition to tailpipe emissions. Small amounts come from rust and the deterioration of vehicles. Contributions from the roadway itself include silica dust from cement and bitumen dust from asphalt.

The greatest single contributor to roadway $PM_{2.5}$ is diesel exhaust. Nevertheless, the combined contribution of brake, tire, and road surface wear is greater than that from diesel exhaust. Even though there are far more cars than diesel vehicles on the road, the actual contribution to $PM_{2.5}$ from car exhaust is tiny compared to that from tires and brakes. It is projected that as cars and trucks modernize, their emissions will fall; however, brake, tire, and road wear emissions are expected to rise. Electric vehicles using regenerative braking create much less brake-pad wear and PM pollution, but weigh more as a result of their batteries and thus have greater tire wear.

Urban areas often become pollution canyons, in which the particulate matter is dispersed into the air and then resettles in the street. It is disturbed by the traffic and then settles back down, accumulating with time. Since these areas have stop-and-go traffic, they have more brake material than freeways. As a result of frequent starts and stops, vehicles have about 50 percent more tire wear per mile in urban areas than highway driving, and about seven to eight times more brake-wear-induced particulate matter production. A heavy vehicle, such as a bus, creates about five times the tire, brake, and road abrasion PM as does a standard car.[21] However, if they carry more passengers who would otherwise be in cars, the total contribution to air pollution can be reduced, especially since mass transit can reduce traffic congestion. Trucks carrying very heavy loads can deform, spall, and crack roadways, leading to rapid degradation and thus greatly contributing to the formation of PM as smaller pieces of road detritus are created. Ice and freezing also damage roadways. Asphalt and cement surfaces wear and release particles. Stop-and-go traffic also creates much more exhaust, as acceleration from a stop takes more energy and vehicles spend more time idling at a standstill.

Additionally, road paint may contain lead, cadmium, chromium, and zinc. As the paint weathers and wears, it becomes part of the PM of the road. Although lead is banned for house paint, it is still allowed to be used in paint for industrial uses. It may be found in car paint, and in most areas, in road and parking lot paint. Road and industrial paint can also contain the toxic heavy metals cadmium and chromium.[22] [23]

Tires are a large contributor to PM roadway pollution. In 2001, the annual volume of dust from tire emissions in Japan was calculated to be 2.1 kg (about 3 lbs.) per person (463 million pounds).[8] The U.S. has 0.797 vehicles per person compared to Japan's 0.591; average Japanese cars are smaller and lighter than those used in the U.S., and the average annual distance driven in Japan is about a quarter of that driven by American drivers.[24] [25] The U.S. is also a much larger country, and goods need to be transported greater distances. Thus, the per capita contribution of PM from tires is much greater in the U.S. than in Japan. In Germany, annual tire emissions have been measured to be as high as 657 kg per kilometer (2331 pounds) of PM per mile) on busy roadways. Tire emissions are higher in cold climates where snow tires are used, as these tires are manufactured to have higher coefficients of friction and wear more quickly. Tire wear is higher on cement than on asphalt, as cement is more abrasive.[26]

Tires are made of and release natural and synthetic rubber particles. PM from tires contains soot, cadmium, copper, lead, zinc, and organotin compounds. Many organotin (carbon-tin) compounds are neurotoxic.

> More than half of the mature coho salmon returning from the sea to spawn in rivers in the Pacific Northwest of the United States die of cardiorespiratory distress once reaching the rivers and streams, before they can spawn. The cause has been recognized as a result of exposure to urban stormwater runoff into the streams.[27] The toxin was identified in 2020 as 6PPD-quinone, which has an LD_{50} of 0.8μg/L of stream water for the fish. 6PPD is added to vehicle tires to prevent ozone-induced damage to the tires. With tire wear, 6PPD is released in the tire dust, and with oxidation is converted to 6PPD-quinone, which washes into the streams with the rain. The salmon are likely not the only animals susceptible to this highly toxic compound.[28]

When horses pulled wagons, leather was used as a friction material for brakes; however, it wears out quickly and does not work well when wet. Later, in early cars, camel hair or cotton fiber pads impregnated with asphalt and rubber resin were used, but would catch fire at a temperature of about 300°F, a temperature easily reached by breaking. In the 1920s, asbestos was introduced and worked well, but it has the downside of causing the otherwise rare lung cancer, mesothelioma.

Better resins were developed over the years, and by the 1980s, asbestos was replaced by fiberglass.

Modern brake pads are composed of a surprising array of materials; cashew shell dust helps with compression, improves braking at cold temperatures, and reduces noise. Barium sulfate improves wear resistance and is stable at high temperatures. Lead, tin, copper sulfide, molybdenum disulfide, and antimony trisulfide are used as lubricants. Lead oxide is used as a friction modifier. Chromium dioxide raises the coefficient of friction. Aluminum oxide adds wear resistance. Molybdenum trioxide helps prevent thermal fade if brakes overheat. Asbestos is still found in aftermarket replacement brake pads. Brake pads may contain phenolic or other resins and may contain mica, copper, zinc, titanium, iron, paper, graphite, rubber, ceramic spheres, aramid fiber, vermiculite, zirconium silicate, Kevlar, brass chips, and other materials.[29] [30] All these can end up as PM air pollution from brake wear.

Driving down a dirt road on a dry summer day stirs up a cloud of dust: the faster one drives and the less aerodynamic the vehicle is, the larger the dust cloud is. If there is not much wind, most of the dust will settle back down on the dirt road or nearby. Particulate matter acts in the same way. The suspension time in the air depends on the shape and density of the PM.

Non-fibrous, roughly spherical particles larger than 200 microns don't stay airborne long or move far, as they are just too heavy. As the diameter of a particle increases, its volume, and thus mass, increase by the cube of its diameter. Thus, spherical particles with a diameter of 100 μm have a volume of 1000 times that of 10 μm particles, and a billion million times greater than 0.1 μm particles; thus, particles composed of the same compound have much greater mass as their diameter increases. While larger, traffic-created particulate pollution can contaminate the soil near the roadway and get into the water runoff that pollutes streams and lakes, it does not travel far in the air. Roadway PM larger than 20 μm do not stay suspended in the air long, and particles greater than 10 μm generally have sufficient mass to be caught by the upper airway mucosa. These particles then get swallowed rather than entering the lower airway. Thus, it is mostly PM_{10} (particles smaller than 10 μm) that are considered a health concern.

Not all PM is from traffic and combustion. Another human-caused type of particulate matter air pollution is dust from desertification. Deforestation and desertification in Central Asia give rise to intermittent dust storms that increase particulate matter in the air in Eastern China, South Korea, and Taiwan. In a study from South Korea, the increased levels of dust in the air during these storms were associated with a 13% increase in the risk of suicide on the days when the storm dust levels were high, and there was a 20% increase in suicides when the storms were of long duration.[31] Desert dust also increases the risk of cardiovascular disease mortality, with risk increasing by 2% for every 10 μg of dust per cubic meter of air.[32]

This risk is not limited to East Asia. Desert dust exposure was found to be associated with increased hospital ER visits and mortality in Southern Europe[33] and the Middle East.[34] Airborne desert PM has a significant impact on health in Mali, Mauritania, Niger, and northern Nigeria, countries on the western edge of the Sahara, where extremely high levels of desert dust are present. [35]

Small particulate pollution exposure decreases rapidly with distance from the source. At 100 meters (328 feet) from the roadway, the concentration of $PM_{0.25}$ drops by about 80%, and after 150 meters, the ultrafine PM pollution is dispersed into the background level for the local area. Thus, those within 100 meters of a busy street or roadway are those most highly exposed.[36]

Generally, about 40% of the *mass* of aerodynamically available PM is $PM_{0.25}$, thus smaller than 0.25 μm. About 20 percent of the PM mass is between 0.25 and 2.5 μm, and another 40 percent of the PM_{10} is larger, from 2.5 to 10 μm. Thus, even though the total mass of the larger particles is similar to small particles, there are hugely more very small $PM_{0.25}$ particles than there are large ones.[37]

Since the dust usually settles on or near the roadway, it is repeatedly launched and recycled into the air with traffic. During this cycle, some of the particulate matter can be further broken into smaller particles, while new material is added to the roadway. Thus, the PM in pollution canyons undergoes repeated wearing as it falls back to the ground and is cycled through engines, breaking it into smaller, more dangerous PM particles. Time spent in these areas gives high exposure to these particles.

Data on the health effects of PM and other forms of pollution are dependent upon the data that can be collected. Many, especially older studies, investigated the associations between PM_{10} and health, as that was the data available. Most studies on the health effects of air pollution in recent years assess $PM_{2.5}$, as daily $PM_{2.5}$ estimates are now available in the U.S. with a resolution of one-fourth square kilometer from satellite data. Satellites using the Moderate Resolution Imaging Spectroradiometer (MODIS) can measure various wavelengths of visible and infrared light and capture data that accurately correlates with aerosols near ground level. Using samples of ground data, neural networks can use satellite data to create daily or weekly maps of $PM_{2.5}$ specific to areas about one-third of a mile across. This allows estimates of exposure specific to the address of study subjects by date, allowing for accurate exposure data over time. For example, PM exposure can be assessed at different phases of pregnancy to estimate exposure for a woman's residential address.[38]

PM and the Brain

PM is not a single thing. It is more like a dirty snowball that collects various pollutants. One of the common components of PM in some areas is ammonium nitrate. It forms in the air from two gases, NO and ammonia.[39] Ammonium nitrate (NH_4NO_3) is the same chemical compound that is used as fertilizer and in explosive devices. Ammonium nitrate, under the right pollution and atmospheric conditions, may make up a significant portion of the mass of PM. At normal atmospheric temperatures, ammonium nitrate forms crystals that are hygroscopic and hold on to moisture and other compounds from the air.[40] Thus, it can form particles with numerous other pollutants.

The $PM_{2.5}$ read by the MODIS satellite is composed mostly of peroxynitrite, compounds that later break down into ozone and NO_2, as well as other nitrates, sulfates, ammonia, carbon, dust, and sea salt aerosols. [41] When tissue is exposed to peroxynitrite (NO_3^-), it causes chemical modification of proteins that cause them to be recognized as damage-associated molecular patterns (DAMPs) that are recognized by TLR4 receptors as part of the innate immune system. These peroxynitrite-modified proteins cause proinflammatory signaling and activate the production of α-synuclein, heat shock protein 60 (HSP60), and high-mobility group box 1 protein (HMGB1) as part of the immune response. Inhalation of peroxynitrite into the lungs amplifies lung inflammation.[42] Absorption of peroxynitrite by the olfactory mucosa may allow uptake of these DAMPs into the brain.

Ambient air pollution is rarely a single chemical compound. Thus, most studies of the health impact of air pollution can't identify the compounds or the mechanism of action causing the disease. When a study looks at particulate matter, it may explain a mode of exposure, but typically does not tell what the dirty little snowballs are composed of. If a study looks at NOx in the air, it does not preclude the presence of other pollutants. Some studies will look at blood levels to determine the exposure to certain chemical pollutants that can be measured in the blood, but that still does not rule out exposure to other pollutants. Furthermore, the toxic effect of pollution on the brain may not be from a single compound, but rather from additive or interactive effects of the exposures. Having stated those cautions, let's look at some of the evidence.

When cell cultures of neuronal tissue were exposed in a lab to ultra-fine particulate pollution collected from the air near the Interstate 10 freeway in Los Angeles, California, it inhibited neuronal growth, reduced neuronal viability, and increased inflammatory markers. When mice were exposed to the same or similar ultrafine PM, it increased the level of inflammatory cytokines and the amount of APP (amyloid precursor protein) formed by the brain, the source protein for Aβ, which forms plaques in the brain typical of Alzheimer's disease (AD). When otherwise healthy dogs from a polluted area of Mexico City were compared to dogs from Tlaxcala, an area of low pollution, the brains from dogs from Mexico City had higher levels of inflammatory markers, higher levels of APP and Aβ plaques, and had white matter lesions in the brain.[43] The annual average $PM_{2.5}$ levels were as high as 70 micrograms per cubic meter of air (μg/m³) in the southwestern parts of Mexico City in the year 2000. Fortunately, with the adoption of better pollution controls, levels have fallen are generally to the low 20 μg/m³ in recent years.[44]

Several population studies have compared the risk of Alzheimer's disease among those living in areas of high air pollution levels to populations who live in less air-polluted areas. One of these studies examined the records of 9.8 million Medicare enrollees living in 50 cities near the northeast coast, from Maryland to Maine. Those living in cities with higher particulate pollution were more likely to have a hospital admission with the diagnosis of AD, Parkinson's disease (PD), and dementia. For each microgram/m³ of $PM_{2.5}$ in the air of these cities, the diagnosis rate of PD and dementia both increased by 7 percent, and the diagnosis rate of AD increased by 15 percent. An exposure differential of 5 μg/m³ of $PM_{2.5}$ doubled the rate of AD diagnosis.[45] Another large population study included all 2.1 million native-born residents of the province of Ontario, Canada, between the ages of 55 to 85 who were free of dementia in April of 2001. Over 12 years, 257,816 persons from this population, about one in eight, developed dementia. For every quartile increase in $PM_{2.5}$, the hazard of dementia increased by four percent.[46] In a study from Taiwan, however, an increase in $PM_{2.5}$ of 4.34 μg/m3 increased AD risk by 38 percent.[47]

In yet another study of 3647 women aged 65 to 79 without dementia from 48 different states were followed for up to 15 years and assessed for changes in cognitive function. Data on $PM_{2.5}$ exposure were taken from the Environmental Protection Agency (EPA) based on the city of their residences during the study period. Women living in areas where $PM_{2.5}$ exceeded the 3-year US National Ambient Air Quality Standard average of 12 µg/m³ were 92 percent more likely to develop dementia than those exposed to lower levels. Exposure to high levels of $PM_{2.5}$ was especially hazardous to women who carried the high-risk Apo ε4/4 genetic variant. Their risk of dementia increased by 264%.[48] The 18.7 million residents of the Los Angeles basin are thus exposed to air pollution levels associated with a near doubling of the risk of AD, with some residents (those with APO ε4/ε4) having more than three times the risk of AD as they would have if they lived in an area with cleaner air.

Long-term $PM_{2.5}$ exposure is associated with an increased risk of respiratory, cardiac, and cancer mortality. Living in areas with a 10 µg/m3 or higher level of $PM_{2.5}$ for five years had increased all-cause mortality risk by 45%, increased the risk of lung cancer by about a third, more than doubled the risk of cardiovascular disease, and more than tripled the risk of death from pneumonia, as compared to those exposed to lower levels of $PM_{2.5}$.[49] In adults, exposure to particulate matter smaller than 2.5 microns was also found to be associated with increased prevalence of major depressive disorders and to have deleterious effects on memory.

It does not require lifetime exposure to air pollution to cause brain injury. In autopsies of the brains of children 11 to 17 years of age from highly polluted areas of Mexico City that had been killed in accidents, there was already an accumulation of PM material in the brain and the presence of Aβ42, amyloid plaques, and α-synuclein, thus early evidence of risk for Alzheimer's disease and Parkinson's disease. These changes were evident even among those with the low-risk APOε3/ε3 genotype. These accumulations of toxic proteins were not found in the autopsies of children from areas of Mexico with low air pollution.[50]

In a separate study by the same researchers, the highest hazards from air pollution appeared among girls with the APOε4/ε4 genotype who are in the top quartile for body mass index (BMI). The girls exposed to high levels of $PM_{2.5}$, who are in the top quartile of BMI and carry the APOε4/ε4 allele, had a 1.5 to 2 standard deviation decrement in full-scale IQ, *equivalent to a loss of 22 to 30 IQ points,* as compared to APOε3/ε3 boys and girls. These girls were found to have elevated fasting glucose and low vitamin D levels. Children from high $PM_{2.5}$ areas show high leptin levels and food-reward dysregulation as compared to clean air areas.

Several studies have linked the risk of autism spectrum disorder (ASD) to prenatal exposure to PM. In a study including 14,400 births, women exposed to more than 10 µg/m₃ of PM_{10} during the third trimester of pregnancy were 38% more likely to bear a child who would be later diagnosed with ASD than women with lower exposure levels.[51] Another study found a doubling of the risk of autism among children in the highest quartile of prenatal exposure to traffic pollution, and a tripling of risk for those in the top quartile of exposure during the first year of life. This study could not discern the risk contributed by PM_{10}, $PM_{2.5}$, and NO_2 gas.[52]

In the Nurses' Health Study II, which included over 115,000 American female nurses, children of women exposed to $PM_{2.5}$ pollution (>12.4 µg/m³) were at a 65% to 106% increased risk of ASD, when compared to those in the lowest quartile of exposure (<12.4 µg/m³). Thus, 75% of the women in the study were exposed to PM levels that increased the risk of ASD in their child by an average of 85%. Those exposed to higher levels of $PM_{2.5}$ in the first and second trimesters only were about 25% more likely to be diagnosed with ASD, while those exposed only in the third trimester were 49% more likely to be diagnosed with ASD. Larger PM ($PM_{2.5}$ to PM_{10}) did not contribute to risk.[53]

Microplastics and Microfibers

Microplastics generated from the wear and tear of plastics and microfibers are another form of PM pollution. Solid plastics create microparticles as they wear, age, and degrade.

A large amount of microplastics end up in the water, where they are consumed by zooplankton; the microplastics can block their intestines, killing them. Microplastics are also filtered by mollusks and other aquatic filter feeders. The particles can then move up the food chain fish, and into other animals such as humans. While not discounting the environmental concerns caused by microplastics, the focus of this book is human health, especially as it relates to longevity and prevention of dementia. The impacts of micro- and nanoplastics on human health have only recently begun to be studied.

MNPs have been demonstrated to alter immune function (increasing inflammation and impeding healing), and cause DNA damage, promoting mutations and the risk of cancers. In a study published in 2025, patients with higher concentrations of MNPs in their airways were found to have more lung lesions on CT scans. Smokers were found to have higher levels of MNPs in their lungs.[54] This may be the result of smoking causing injury to the cilia in the airways that help clear foreign matter that settles on the mucous membranes.

A study published in the New England Journal of Medicine in 2024 assessed the consequences of micro- and nanoplastics (MNPs) in the carotid arteries of 257 adults with an average age of 72. Participants were divided into two groups based on whether MNPs were present in the intimal layer of the carotid artery or not. The two groups did not differ by the level of carotid stenosis, hypertension, blood lipid levels, the presence of diabetes, smoking, or medication use. They were followed for about 3 years (33.7 months on average). Those with MNPs present in the carotid intima were 4.5 times more likely to suffer a non-fatal MI or stroke, or die within 3 years, than those without carotid MNPs after adjusting for other cardiovascular risk factors.

Interestingly, of the nine plastics evaluated, only polyethylene and a smaller amount of polyvinyl chloride (PVC) were present in the intimal lining of the carotid arteries. Some of it was present within macrophages. Those with MNPs had considerably less collagen in the intima and had higher levels of inflammatory cytokines, including IL-1, IL-6. TNF and CD68. This study found that nanoplastics smaller than 200 nm (0.2 μM), rather than larger microplastics, were deposited into the intima. Other studies have found MNPs up to 10 μm in the placenta, up to 15 μm in breast milk and urine, up to 30 μm have been found in the liver, and up to 88 μm in the lung samples. MNPs up to 700 nm have been found in whole blood.[55]

For particulate matter from combustion, it is mainly $PM_{0.25}$ (particles 250 nm or smaller) that confer risk, as it is these particles that are most likely to lodge in the lung and to be absorbed. From here, they can make their way into the circulation and across the blood-brain barrier. Airborne PM is also absorbed into the nasal mucosa and then into the trigeminal and olfactory nerves, and then carried directly into the brain.

A recent study found a 50% increase in the amount of MNPs in the brain when comparing samples collected in 2014 and 2024. Surprisingly, MNPs levels were seven to 30 times higher in the brain than in the kidneys or liver, organs that usually help with the elimination of foreign materials. As in the carotid artery intima, a smaller size indicated a higher risk. In this study, polyethylene (PE) was the dominant plastic found. Polypropylene (PP), PVC, and lesser amounts of other MNPs were also present in the brain. The study also found that decedents diagnosed with dementia had a significantly higher average mass of MNPs (@10x higher) than did the brains of normal control brains. The MNPs were located primarily within inflammatory cells and along the walls of the brain's vasculature. While it appears likely that microplastics have a deleterious impact on the brain, it is possible that defects in the BBB of those with dementia facilitate the transfer of MNPs into the brain. Thus, the increased presence of MNPs does not establish a causal role of MNPs in dementia. Most of the MNPs particles in the brain were in the 100 to 200 nm size (PM0.1 to PM0.2).[56] This is consistent with the size of PM airborne particles that are easily deposited in the lungs.

MNP may also create dementia risk as a result of its impact on the gut. There is growing evidence that microplastics disrupt the gastrointestinal microbiome and increase translocation of LPS into the bloodstream by damaging the intestinal epithelial barrier. MNPs also promote immune activation and inflammation in the intestines. Small MNPs can cross the BBB, where they provoke inflammation and microglial activation, resulting in neurotoxicity and neurodegeneration.[57] Additionally, MNP promotes cellular senescence by causing mitochondrial dysfunction, which promotes ROS production, impairs autophagy, and activates the DNA damage response.[58]

Why is polyethylene (PE) the dominant MNP in the body? A likely reason is simply that PE is the most highly produced plastic resin in the world, and that it is the one we are most exposed to. Polyethylene (33.5%), polypropylene (19.5%), and polyester (18%) comprise over 70% of all plastics produced. PE is particularly easy to work with, considered to be non-toxic, and is long-lived. PE is used in plastic bags, plastic cups, and bottles, which are used in our homes, as well as in the water pipes in our homes.[59] Polypropylene (PP) is commonly used in molded plastics, carpets and rugs, non-woven clothing, air filters, including face masks, and diapers. Polyester (PET) is used in fabrics, including those used in clothing and car tires, and as a wood finish, including musical instruments.

The high load of PE MNPs in the body may be influenced by the ease with which it produces MNPs or how easily it produces MNPs of a size that easily enters the body, either through ingestion or respiration. While we may bioaccumulate PE more than other plastics, higher exposure to PE MNPs is the most likely reason for its dominance in the tissues.

It should also not be assumed that just because PE is the most common MNP in the lung and brain, it is associated with the highest disease risk. Risk may not just be caused by the presence of MNPs, but may be caused by phthalates, bisphenols, toxic metals, and other compounds present in the plastics.

Some plastics are considerably more toxic than others. Two of the most noxious and ubiquitous plastics are PVC and polystyrene. Before its use in toys was banned in 2009, some toys made of polyvinylchloride (PVC) contained as much as 40% of their mass as phthalates, endocrine disruptors that cause birth defects, infertility, and behavioral problems. PVC is commonly made with organotin added to it to prevent its degradation. Many organotin compounds are neurotoxic, and others interfere with immune function. PVC was previously made with cadmium as a stabilizer, a metal well known for its renal toxicity. PVC has been known to be a carcinogen since 1974.[60] The Biden administration initiated a risk assessment of vinyl chloride under the Toxic Substances Control Act, in a move to possibly ban it from commerce in the U.S.,[61] and PVC bans are also being considered in the European Union. Polystyrene (Styrofoam) is another widely used toxic plastic that easily enters the environment and forms MNPs. It's toxic to the lungs, liver, and kidneys.[62 63 64]

If MNPs act similarly to PM from combustion, the most damaging MNPs are those that are airborne and small; $PM_{0.25}$ MNPs that are captured in the lung and nasal mucosa and then move into the blood vessels and brain.

Microplastics in the Home

In the home and office, MNPs are mostly from clothing and fabrics, including carpets. While cotton and paper form microfibers, they are easily biodegradable and are not thought to cause significant harm to humans or the environment. One of the greatest contributors of microfibers and MNPs in the home is the wear and tear of fabrics. Synthetic microfiber is of much greater risk than organic ones, such as those from cotton, as the synthetics are not easily biodegraded and last in the environment a long time, thus creating a cumulative exposure risk.

Washing and drying clothing is a major source of MNPs in the environment. An average of about 0.3% of the mass of a new garment was recovered as MNPs from the filtered wash water from washing machines. Top-loading machines produced on average seven times more microfiber than front-loading machines, as front-loading machines use less water and are gentler on clothes.[65] Synthetic microfibers from laundry, which end up in the Great Lakes, appear to be a major source of MNPs in tap water and beer made in that region. Using a front-load washer, shorter washing times, and cold water can reduce wear on clothing and MNP pollution.[66]

Driers are an even greater source of MNPs, producing 1.4 to 40 times as many MNPs as washing clothes. A fifteen-minute dryer cycle was found to release half a million polyester MNPs into the dryer exhaust (not including the lint that is trapped in the lint filter). With larger loads of polyester laundry, the MNPs count was higher.[67] The abrasive action of the tumbling and the heat cause wear that produces more MNPs.

Although laundry is the major source of MNPs from the home into the environment, it is likely not the greatest hazard within the home. Carpets, clothing, bedding, plastic containers, shoes, cords, toys, or any other plastic items can create MNPs, especially with wear and aging. Some MNPs come into the home from the outside. Both MNPs and PM from combustion can come on clothing and shoes.

Children, and especially infants, are more highly exposed to indoor PM pollution as they are closer to and spend more time on the floor. The heaviest concentration of PM is in the first 10 inches above the floor. Children also have a higher metabolic demand for O2 for their body mass, and thus breathe in more air (and air pollutants) for their body mass, causing a higher exposure risk.

Microplastic Consumption

Although ingestion of MNP is likely less harmful than inhalation exposure, eating MNP should be avoided. Avoid storing food in plastic containers, and never microwave food in plastic containers. Heat-resistant glass or ceramic containers are far safer and, being reusable, create less environmental waste. Avoid washing plastic containers in the dishwasher. Use a wooden cutting board rather than a plastic one. In general, avoid plastic when it comes to food. Styrofoam cups, plates, and take-out boxes should be avoided and should never be used for reheating food or beverages in a microwave.

Bisphenol A (BPA) is an endocrine disruptor present in plastics. Because the public is aware of this, many products labelled as no-BPA now instead contain BPS or BPF, which may be just as harmful., Thermoprinting paper, used in cash register receipts, is made with a plastic coating that contains bisphenol A (BPA) or its substitutes, and it easily rubs off. These receipts are often bagged with one's groceries. The health risks from MPN ingestion may be dominated by the toxic compounds found in the plastics, rather than plastics in general.

PM Mitigation for the Home

Air Filters

Air filters can remove particulate matter, including MNPs, those from desert sand and destructive farming practices, combustion, and pollen and mold spores.

The PM that most easily escapes filtration turns out to be particles around 0.3 microns in diameter. They have sufficient mass and momentum to be carried through, yet are small enough to be difficult to capture. They are also in a size range considered to carry risk. Most heavy metals, for example, are easily soluble when they have a diameter of less than 0.25 microns, and thus can be absorbed via the olfactory mucosa directly into the brain.

The Minimum Efficiency Reporting Value (MERV) rating of air filters is designed to indicate how well an air filter removes larger particles, 3.0 to 10.0 µm. Filters with higher MERV scores remove particles more efficiently. A MERV 8 filter removes about 85% of these larger particles. To remove fine PM, as well as bacteria, viruses, and spores, a HEPA filter is needed. A filter with an MERV rating of 13 or higher complies with the HEPA standard.

HEPA (High-Efficiency Particulate Absorbing) filters are designed to capture ultrafine particles, but do not remove smoke, fumes, or gases. Particles around 0.3 microns are the most difficult to filter. Larger particles are blocked from passing through the filter in the way that a screen prevents mosquitoes from passing through; they are just bigger than the mesh, and can't get through. Particles less than about 0.1 are captured by diffusion interception and impaction. The matting of the filter acts like an obstacle course for these fine particles, and they collide with the fibers of the filter, preventing their passage. Thus, HEPA filters capture very fine particles, including viruses (0.02 to 0.3 µm). The standard for HEPA filters is to capture 99.97% of particles at 0.3 µm. Thus, they capture other particles at even greater efficiency. HEPA filters have been demonstrated not only to capture COVID-19 viruses from the air but also to decrease the viral load from surfaces in the room. ULPA (Ultra-Low Penetration Air) filters clear a minimum of 99.999% of particles as small as 0.12 microns from the air. They are designed for use in cleanrooms and other critical environments such as microchip manufacturing.

If a HEPA filter is being used to lower viral load, it is recommended that the blower speed be sufficient to filter the volume of air in the room every ten minutes. This requires a clean air delivery rate (CADR; in cubic feet per minute) of about 65 for every 100 square feet of floor space in a room with eight-foot ceilings. Thus, the recommended airflow to clean room air for airborne viral control is a CADR of about 2/3rds of the floor space for most homes and office buildings.[68]

A filter, obviously, only cleans the air while the blower is running. Thus, a HEPA filter on a ventilation and air conditioning (HVAC) unit does not clean the air when it is not heating or cooling unless non-heat/cooling cycle air circulation is done. Some thermostats allow the HVAC blower to be turned independently of the heat and cooling. Running an HVAC blower continuously, however, causes condensation that has collected on the coils during cooling to re-evaporate into the room, rather than to condensate and drain. This thus defeats the dehumidification process and can promote the growth of mold, worsening air quality in the building. Thus, continuous running of the HVAC blower is not ideal. Thermostats that allow the blowers to be used intermittently, for example, for 10 minutes every half hour, are recommended to improve indoor air quality. In contrast, free-standing HEPA air filters, which do not act as dehumidifiers, can be left running and used in a single room, such as a bedroom, to purify the air in that space.

HEPA filters in HVAC units can use prefilters for larger particles to extend the life of the more expensive HEPA filter. HEPA filters need to be replaced, generally every 6 to 12 months, depending on the usage situation and air quality. Dirty air filters do not work well.

HEPA filters are a very reasonable choice for homes, schools, office buildings, buses, and public buildings to improve air quality and decrease disease transmission. They were installed in most airliners to decrease the spread of disease during the COVID-19 pandemic, and hopefully, this move to protect passengers will be sustained.

Central Air Conditioning:

Use a MERV 13 or higher air conditioning filter in your home as a whole-house filter, and change it regularly. The unusual recommendation is to replace it every 3 months or less.

Deeper filters, for example, a 4" deep filter, will have deeper pleats and thus more surface area for particle removal. This provides a slower air flow across the filter media and is effective in removing small particles. While more expensive, the deeper filter should not need to be replaced as frequently, and thus may cost less over time. Using a deep filter requires that a deep filter housing be installed in the HVAC air handler.

Free-standing HEPA Air Purifiers:

Freestanding HEPA air filters, typically with an activated charcoal air filter, can be used in bedrooms and other areas where people spend several hours each day.

The HEPA filter should ideally be capable of four to six complete air changes per hour (ACH) in a room. A 12 by 14 foot bedroom with 8-foot ceilings has a volume of 1334 cubic feet minus furnishings. To get five ACH per hour would require an air purifier that can do an air exchange every 12 minutes. Thus, an air purifier for a room this size should be rated to provide an air flow of about 111 cubic feet per minute.

Since the free-standing HEPA/charcoal filters are intended to be used during sleep, the air filter should be quiet. Pre-cleaning the air by running the filter at a higher speed setting in the evening, and then reducing the speed setting during sleep hours, can allow clean room air with very little fan noise using a quality filter.

On their own, HEPA filters only remove particles, but do not remove gases from the air. Many free-standing air purifiers include a charcoal (activated carbon) filter, which can capture odors and certain other gases. These charcoal filters can reduce the levels of many volatile organic compounds, odors, and some gases, including sulfur dioxide, ammonia, NO2, and hydrogen sulfide.

Cleaning

Vacuuming: Vacuum cleaners without HEPA filters can worsen indoor air quality by both resuspending PM and by shearing it into smaller, and thus more dangerous, particles. Because vacuuming can increase PM levels, it should not be done with small children or other susceptible persons in the room. While carpets create MNPs, they also trap dust, lowering the amount of PM that is recirculated into the air with foot traffic and movement. Carpets are dirty dirt magnets.

Noisy vacuum cleaners should be avoided as they can contribute to hearing damage. If purchasing a new vacuum, look not only for one that is HEPA rated, but also for one that has a low noise level.

Damp Mopping is an effective method for removing dirt, including PM that has settled on the floor.

Dusting: Use a damp dusting or a microfiber cloth to capture dust more effectively. Dust evenly to capture rather than to disperse the dust. "Feather dusting" just resuspends PM and allergens back into the air. Microfiber cloths carry a positive charge that the PM is attracted to. Rinse the dust cloth frequently. Consider wearing a particle mask during dusting. Vacuum after dusting rather than before, as a vacuum (with a HEPA filter) will help eliminate some of the dust that has been disturbed. Don't leave out the dusting of ceiling fans, blinds, and light fixtures.

Dust Mites and Mold: While not generally considered to be PM, dust mites and mold create allergens that can easily impact health.

- High humidity encourages the growth of dust mites and mold. Dust mites and mold can be controlled by keeping the humidity between 30% and 50%.
- Wash bedding regularly. Although it will create more outdoor MNPs, if allergies are a problem, clean bedding can decrease exposure to allergens.
- Avoid purely decorative pillows and shams, as well as knick-knacks and schlocky items that collect dust, especially in the bedroom. Get rid of unnecessary clutter.
- Pillows and stuffed animals can be frozen in the freezer for 24 – 48 hours to kill dust mites.
- Avoid having a furry pet. If you have a furry pet, groom them frequently, ideally outdoors, to minimize the amount of dander in your home.

The dominant protein that triggers human allergies to cats is known as Fel d 1. Fel d 1 is very difficult to remove from the home, and can remain for months after a cat has vacated the home. When cats groom, the saliva gets on their fur and then into the environment. Cat food made with LiveClear contains a protein from chicken eggs that neutralizes Fel d 1 in the cat's saliva. After 6 weeks on the LiveClear, the production of Fel d 1 by cats has been found to decrease by nearly half. This may be enough to eventually lower the severity of allergy symptoms of those affected, if the home is thoroughly cleaned and the cat is washed. This chow is about five times as expensive as cat chow without it from the same brand.[69]

Shoes: Shoes should be removed upon entering the home to prevent tracking in dirt that will end up in the air in your home. Have a shoe bench in your mudroom or at the entrance to your home. If you park your vehicle in your garage, have a shoe bench there. Have a dedicated pair of sandals or slippers for use in the house. Inside and outside door mats can greatly decrease the amount of PM and dirt brought into the home on shoes. They need to be cleaned regularly.

Smoking and vaping: Obviously, tobacco smoke creates both carbon monoxide, PM, and other indoor pollutants, and that increases disease risk for everyone in the home.

Your Vehicle: Cars and trucks are spaces that have extremely high exposures to PM, including both roadway and MNP pollution, as well as toxic gases from fuel combustion and off-gassing of plastic if the vehicle is new. Since people are frequently getting in and out of the vehicle, they are bringing in road and other dirt on their shoes. It is not uncommon for vehicles to get wet and have mold growth.

HEPA filters in vehicles have been demonstrated to lower cabin $PM_{2.5}$ from over 800 μg/m3 in outside air in a testing chamber to well below 12 μg/m3 (to below the test instrument's level of detection) within a few minutes.[70]

Aftermarket HEPA/Carbon cabin air filters are available for most vehicles and can provide much cleaner air for the driver and passengers.

Keep your vehicle clean and free of trash. Clean the floor mats regularly.

Gases

To understand air pollution, it is helpful to understand the normal composition of gases in the air. Other than water vapor, air is composed principally of nitrogen in the form of N_2. Nitrogen gas comprises about 78% of all the gases in the air. Nitrogen gas is formed by pairs of nitrogen atoms bound by a triple covalent bond (N:N). About 21 percent of the gas in the air is oxygen in the form of O_2, which is bound by a divalent bond (O:O). Argon comprises most of the remaining one percent of gases in the air. Argon is inert, meaning that it is extremely resistant to forming compounds with other elements, and thus, does not form toxic compounds except under extraordinary conditions. After accounting for N2, O2, and Ar, other gases make up about 0.045 percent of the atmosphere.

Outdoor air has low levels of carbon dioxide (CO_2). For most of the last 2 million years, the atmosphere contained between 0.0213 and 0.0283 percent CO_2. This began to slowly increase in the industrial era, with an increase in world population and the great increase in the use of fossil fuels. By the time I was born, atmospheric CO_2 levels were around 0.0310 percent (310 ppm). The CO2 content in the atmosphere in February 2025 was 0.0427 percent (427 ppm), and will almost surely be higher when you read this.[71]

Exhaled breath contains around one hundred times this amount, as metabolic oxidation converts fuel and O_2 into energy and CO_2. The exhaled breath contains up to around four percent CO_2 (40,000 ppm) and as little as 17 percent oxygen.

The remaining 0.004 percent of gases naturally occurring in the atmosphere are mostly neon, helium, methane, krypton, and hydrogen (in descending order of concentration). Note that several of the gases that are naturally present in the atmosphere in low amounts, helium, neon, argon, and krypton, are noble gases. Noble gases under standard conditions have extremely low reactivity, which is why they don't combine with other materials and thus stay free in the air. They are considered to be inert as they don't form compounds in the atmosphere or our bodies. This also means that they are not toxic.

Science tidbit: Earth's gravity is insufficient to prevent small amounts of hydrogen and helium from escaping into space. These are the lightest and most kinetic (fast-moving) gases, and they float towards the upper atmosphere where they can be blown away by solar wind and other forces. The Earth loses about 3 kg of hydrogen each second, the amount of hydrogen in about 27 liters of water; thus, the Earth's atmosphere loses the amount of hydrogen in 2.3 million liters of water each day, about the amount needed to fill an Olympic-sized pool. In about a billion years, when the sun will be around 10 percent brighter than it is now, the increased energy will accelerate the escape of hydrogen gas from the atmosphere sufficiently that all of the hydrogen from every bit of water on the planet will billow off into space.

Under ambient atmospheric conditions, the water vapor content of the atmosphere varies widely, largely dependent on temperature. On average, water vapor makes up about 0.4 percent of the gas in the atmosphere. However, in dry arctic conditions, it may be as low as 0.01%. In steamy, wet, tropical environments, water vapor can comprise over 4% of the gas in the air. This is enough to create a noticeable increase in the difficulty in breathing during exercise.

Gaseous Air Pollutants

The most prominent gaseous atmospheric pollutants created during the combustion of fossil fuels are nitrogen oxides (NO_x), carbon dioxide (CO_2), carbon monoxide (CO), ozone (O_3), sulfur dioxide (SO2), and particulate matter (PM). Hydrogen cyanide (H·C:N) is also produced from the burning of natural and synthetic materials that contain C:N bonds, such as cotton, wool, silk, polyurethane, and nylon. Cyanide gas formed during a house fire can kill. Industry also produces many other volatile gases. Among these are endocrine disruptors known to promote cancer. For example, women who work in the automotive industry with the plastics used in a car's interiors are five times more likely to develop breast cancer than other workers.[72] The "new car smell" comes from the off-gassing of the same volatile compounds that cause breast cancer in workers.

In atmospheric chemistry, NO_x is a term of art that refers to the sum of two gases: nitric oxide (NO) and nitrogen dioxide (NO_2). During the high-temperature combustion of fuels, Atmospheric nitrogen gas (N:N) is oxidized by oxygen (O:O), forming two molecules of NO. NO is a free radical that can then react with O2 in the air, forming nitrogen dioxide: $2\ NO + O_2 \rightarrow 2\ NO_2$. NO_2 is a brown, toxic gas that may be visible in air pollution. Nitric oxide should not be confused with the anesthetic gas nitrous oxide (N_2O).

The cleanest burning and purest fossil fuel in common use is probably natural gas, making it the simplest to describe. With the name "natural gas", one might think that it would be benign, but it is only natural in the way that swamp gas, farts, and sewer gas are natural. A more accurate name than natural gas would be "petrochemical gas". When petrochemical gas is mined and leaves the wellhead, it typically contains about 90% alkane gases (methane, ethane, propane, butane, and pentane) and may contain up to 8% CO2, 5% nitrogen, and 5% hydrogen sulfide (H_2S). For domestic and most commercial use, petrochemical gas is processed so that the "natural gas" delivered for use is almost pure methane.[73]

Petrochemical gas also contains small amounts of other gases, including helium; petrochemical gas mines are the source of the helium that fills lighter-than-air balloons that provide levity at celebratory events.

Helium originates from the alpha decay of the radioactive metals uranium and thorium deep within the Earth. U238 → Th234 + α; U235 → Th231 + α; and Th232 → Ra228 + α. The free alpha particles pick up an electron from their environment and become the stable gaseous element helium. Enough helium gets captured in natural gas pockets underground that natural gas can contain up to 2.7% helium. Since helium is lighter than air and is a non-reactive noble gas that does not form compounds, once free from its early bonds, it floats towards the upper atmosphere. Sixteen hundred metric tons of helium are produced by radioactive decay each year and are carried away from Earth by the solar wind, mostly from near the poles.[74] That is a lot of helium being lost, but if it did not escape and had been retained in the atmosphere, as would occur if the planet had a greater mass and stronger gravity, we would all sound like Donald Duck when we spoke.

After the refinement of petrochemical gas, a small amount of methanethiol (mercaptan) (CH_3SH) is added to the methane. Methanethiol and hydrogen sulfide (H_2S) are both products of putrefaction (anaerobic fermentation of amino acids), are flammable, and have putrid, repulsive odors. H_2S is quite toxic. H2S smells of rotten eggs, while mercaptan smells more of rotten cabbage and garlic. Methanethiol is one of the principal gases responsible for halitosis and the smell of flatus (bad breath and farts), and causes the odor in the urine that occurs after eating asparagus. Methanethiol has similar toxicity as hydrogen sulfide but has a mean detection odor threshold of 0.0000002 ppm, many times higher than H_2S (0.001 ppm), and thus can be smelled at much lower concentrations.[75] Methanethiol is added to natural gas so that gas leaks can be detected, as methane is odorless.

Hydrocarbon Fuels

It can be understood that fuel use is most efficient when it is completely oxidized; this occurs at the correct oxygen–fuel ratio for that fuel. For methane, it is one molecule of CH4 and two of O2. This also gives the peak temperature for that fuel. For methane and other alkane fuels, combustion at the ideal stoichiometric ratio results in the highest energy production, the most CO2, and the highest combustion temperature, which also causes the highest amount of NOx to be produced. With less ideal air–fuel ratios, the fuel is less completely burned, resulting in high production of CO, VOC, and other hydrocarbons, and poor fuel efficiency.

Pure methane (CH_4) burns most efficiently at an oxygen–fuel ratio of 2-to-1. The principal products of the full combustion of hydrocarbon fuels such as methane (CH_4) are CO_2 and water vapor.

$$CH4 + 2\ O2 \rightarrow CO2 + 2\ H2O$$

An air–fuel ratio of about 2-to-1 for methane gives a 9.53:1 ratio by volume and a 17.2:1 ratio by weight. This gives the best conversion to heat and the most complete utilization of fuel. Processed natural gas is at least 90% methane, but may contain other gases, so the actual stoichiometric air to natural gas ratio averages about 9.61 to one by volume.

With the correct fuel-to-air mixture, natural gas burns at around 1960°C (3560°F) and has a compact blue flame with perhaps a hint of yellow at the tip of the hotter inner cone in the center of the flame. In contrast, propane burns most efficiently with a fuel-to-air ratio of 23.9:1, with a flame temperature of 1967° C (3573° F).

If there is too little air for complete combustion (a rich fuel-air mixture) on a gas stove, oven, water heater, or furnace, it produces less heat, gives a larger, yellow flame, and greater production of carbon monoxide and soot from the partial combustion of fuel. More unburned natural gas may be released into the home.

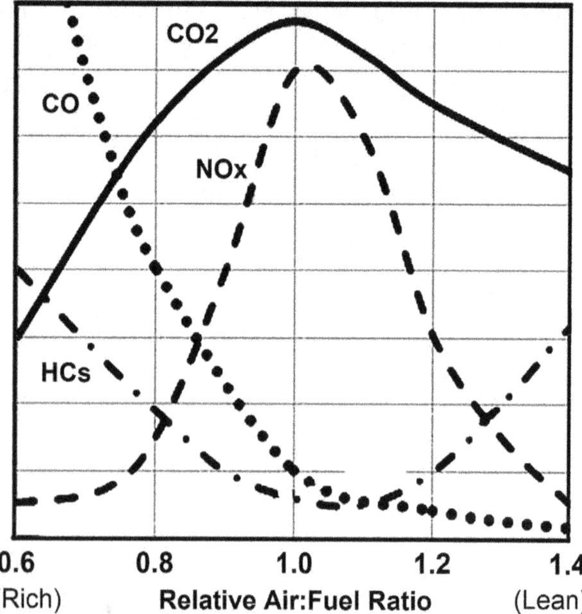

Figure 32A: Air–fuel ratio and Emissions. The most complete combustion gives the highest temperature, and thus the most NOx; meanwhile, high levels of CO are caused by burning with insufficient O2 (fuel-rich) combustion. Both rich and lean mixes leave some fuel unburned and emitted into the environment.

Entrainment of too much air (a lean fuel-air mixture) can also cause inefficient burning of fuel and thus increase the amount of volatile organic compounds released into the atmosphere or home.

> Internal combustion (gasoline) engines in cars shoot for a 14.7-to-1 air-to-fuel ratio (by weight) or 14.1:1 for E10 gasoline containing 10% ethanol. Power output (torque) for gasoline peaks with an air–fuel ratio of about 13:1, and has lower NO_X production, but this creates considerably more CO, volatile organic compounds (VOC), and particulate matter pollution. A lean mixture gives better fuel economy and the highest NO production, and also creates the risks of high-temperature pre-ignition detonation (knocking) that can damage the engine. A 14.7 air: fuel mix provides a balance of near-optimal power output with much lower CO and hydrocarbon output, but has a high NO production. The catalytic converter on cars reduces NO_X to N2 and oxidizes much of the CO to CO_2 and hydrocarbons to CO_2 and H_2O.

Carbon Monoxide (CO)

Carbon dioxide is usually considered non-toxic except in high levels, and water vapor is water. The body is designed to get rid of CO_2. The OSHA (Occupational Safety and Health Administration) Permissible Exposure Level (PEL) for CO2 is 9000 ppm, and the lethal level is around 90,000 ppm. This is equivalent to a CO_2 concentration in the air of 9 percent, and a displacement of O_2 concentration in the air from 21 percent down to 19 percent. At these levels, the body can't get rid of CO2, and the body is suffocated. We will come back to CO2 later.

Carbon monoxide, on the other hand, is highly toxic. The OSHA time-weighted average PEL for CO for workers is 50 ppm for 8 hours, with a short-term recommended exposure maximum of 200 ppm.[76] The National Institute for Occupational Safety and Health (NIOSH) recommends limiting CO exposure to less than an eight-hour time-weighted average of 35 ppm.

Carbon monoxide levels of 600 to 1000 ppm cause headaches. At 1000 ppm, CO causes confusion, drowsiness, and nausea. At 2000 ppm, it causes unconsciousness within 10 minutes, and at 4000 ppm, death in five minutes. CO poisoning is mostly associated with exposure to indoor air pollution, where levels can accumulate.

Hemoglobin in the red blood cells carries oxygen to the tissues. Hemoglobin in the red blood cells (RBCs) does this by quickly and gently binding to oxygen in the blood as it passes through the lungs, where O_2 easily diffuses across the thin membranes of the alveoli. Then, when the blood circulates to the tissues, where the oxygen content is lower, hemoglobin generously releases most of the O2.

The first way in which CO acts as a toxin is that it binds to the hemoglobin in the red blood cells and prevents the blood from carrying and delivering oxygen to the tissues. In other words, it causes hypoxia. CO_2 is mostly dissolved in the blood plasma and easily exchanges from the blood in the lungs into the exhaled breath. In contrast, CO directly binds hemoglobin at the same sites as oxygen does. Worse, CO binds to hemoglobin (Hgb) 218 times more avidly than does oxygen, forming carboxyhemoglobin (COHb), and in doing so, effectively outcompetes oxygen, preventing Hgb from carrying oxygen. Additionally, CO shifts the oxygen dissociation of the remaining oxyhemoglobin so that it does not release oxygen to the tissues as readily. Since CO binds more strongly than does O_2, COHb tends to accumulate with exposure time until an equilibrium of CO in the blood and tissues is reached.[77]

Cigarette smokers generally have COHb levels below two percent; however, those smoking more than two packs per day can have levels of COHb over 10 percent. Several hours of exposure to CO at 12 ppm would be expected to increase COHb to two percent; it would take a CO of about 73 ppm to raise it to 10 percent. Although these heavy smokers are not without symptoms of hypoxia and exercise intolerance, and have some decline in mental acuity, they can appear to function fairly normally with COHb levels that would make most persons ill. Their bodies have adapted to CO poisoning; some have increased red blood cell mass (polycythemia) as part of this adaptation.

At CO levels below 30 ppm, or a COHb level of around five percent, healthy adults have no obvious symptoms of toxicity. Non-smoking coronary artery disease patients, however, were found to have an increase in angina and dysrhythmia during exercise with a COHb of 2.4 percent on experimental short-term exposure to CO.[78] Thus, some individuals are at considerably increased risk from CO exposure.

In addition to its hypoxic effects, carbon monoxide poisons the body in other ways. Just as CO binds to the heme molecules in hemoglobin, it binds to heme molecules in many other heme-containing proteins. These include myoglobin in muscles, neuroglobin in the brain, and thus inhibit the delivery of O2 to the muscles and brain.

CO binds to heme in myoglobin in the muscles and heart even more strongly than it does to hemoglobin in the blood. It can cause dysrhythmia, hypotension, and decreased cardiac output. Even at fairly low levels, CO decreases exercise capacity and at high levels causes severe weakness. CO adherence binding to neuroglobin can put the brain at additional risk from hypoxic insults by depleting oxygen in the brain. Inhibition of cytochrome by CO in the mitochondria inhibits cellular respiration, decreases energy production, and increases the formation of free radicals and oxidative damage. CO inhibition of catalases, which break down hydrogen peroxide in the cell, further promotes free radical injury. During recovery from CO intoxication, re-oxygenation injury creates further free radical-induced oxidative injury that can trigger apoptosis of brain cells. CO causes more severe injury to areas of the brain where the blood supply is less robust or the oxygen demand is higher. Another protein inhibited by CO is NPAS2, a transcription factor that promotes the production of proteins that control circadian rhythms.[79]

CO also inhibits ATP production in the mitochondria by inactivating cytochrome, causing the creation of free radicals that injure the cell.CO poisons the enzyme sulfite oxidase that is required for the regeneration of reduced cytochrome C and a major pathway for H2S and cyanide elimination. CO inhibits NADPH oxidases (NOX), which are essential for multiple functions. It inhibits nitric oxide synthase, which forms NO, and guanylate cyclase, which forms cGMP. CO inhibits catalase, which breaks down H2O2. These are just a sampling of the enzymes and pathways that CO can poison.

While exposure to CO in the environment has a fairly good correlation with the COHb level, COHb levels are poorly correlated with the degree of toxic manifestations in patients. People exposed to CO at toxic levels in a room may have widely varying reactions, with some having a mild headache, others having severe signs of poisoning, and others collapsing into a coma. Some of this has to do with physical and metabolic activity, with children being at higher risk. Individuals with compromised cardiovascular function, heart or lung disease, or anemia are also at higher risk.

Background levels of CO in the air are around 0.05 to 0.12 ppm. In urban environments with traffic, the levels may range from 17 to 53 ppm; restaurants where people smoke may have similar levels. CO levels may be as high as 100 ppm in underground parking lots or road tunnels. As noted above, the 8-hour OSHA limit for workers is 50 ppm.[80]

Common symptoms of moderate acute CO toxicity include headache, dizziness, nausea and vomiting, drowsiness, weakness, confusion, disorientation, and irritability. Some individuals have an increased heart or respiratory rate; others do not. Intoxication can cause visual disturbances. More severe toxicity can cause flaccidity or spasticity of the muscles. Heart problems occur especially in those with pre-existing heart disease. Seizures, coma, and death can occur.

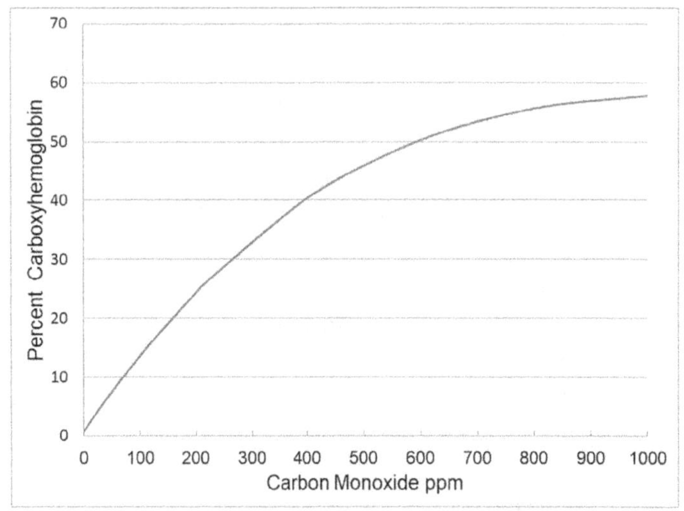

Figure 32B: Carboxyhemoglobin levels associated with carbon monoxide exposure

In healthy individuals, symptoms from COHb levels below 5% are generally mild; however, those with heart disease may have an increase in arrhythmias and angina even with 2.5% COHb. At 5%, there is decreased exercise tolerance, and above this level, there is decreased cognitive functioning, attention, driving performance, and fine sensorimotor control. At a COHb of 20%, there is shortness of breath on moderate exertion, and some individuals have headaches. With a

COHb of 30%, there is impaired judgment, fatigue, and headache. At COHb levels from 40 to 50, most individuals have headache, dizziness, drowsiness, disorientation, confusion, irritability, and nausea. Some will have convulsions, collapse, and become comatose. At higher levels, these effects will occur more quickly.

Acute, moderately severe carbon dioxide poisoning is very often misdiagnosed, as its symptoms can be confused with flu, food poisoning, or gastroenteritis, especially when the victim and family are not aware of the CO exposure. Infants may be diagnosed as having colic. CO poisoning is most common in the winter months when windows are closed and the home is heated, a time when flu and gastroenteritis are common. Doctors should consider CO poisoning in the differential diagnosis of flu-like symptoms that present without a fever.

Acute, high-level CO exposure sufficient to raise COHb levels about 40% can also cause delayed injury to the brain. CO levels sufficient to increase COHb to above 40% can result in white matter and basal ganglia lesions, memory deficits, personality changes, difficulty with learning, and attention. CO toxicity can cause Parkinson's disease-like manifestations with movement disorders and mask-like facial expression, as well as urinary incontinence, peripheral neuropathy, psychosis, and dementia.

The basal ganglia are areas of the brain most sensitive to CO, but CO injury is also common in the cerebral white matter, hippocampus, and cerebellum. Carbon monoxide injury to the brain can often be seen as demyelination injury, evident on an MRI.[81] A delayed neuropsychiatric syndrome occurs in about one in five patients after acute CO injury. Manifestations of this syndrome include memory deficits, personality changes, difficulties with learning and attention, a mask-like facial expression, urinary incontinence, peripheral neuropathy, psychosis, dementia, and movement disorders.

Carbon Monoxide Sources

Considerably more CO is produced when hydrocarbons are burned in an atmosphere with lower levels of O2 and higher levels of CO_2. Thus, as air is recycled into the combustion process in a closed space and O2 is consumed, CO2 is produced, and dangerous levels of CO can be produced. This is why turning on a gas oven and opening the oven door to heat a room can be deadly. Wood fires produce high levels of CO as the fuel: air mixture is rarely ideal; thus, proper venting of a fireplace is essential. Improperly functioning fireplace flues are not uncommon. While there are several indoor air pollutants, other than tobacco smoke, carbon monoxide is the most common acute lethal toxin. At least 430 Americans die from CO poisoning each year, and about 50,000 are diagnosed and treated in emergency departments. Likely, far more are never diagnosed. Other common causes of acute CO toxicity arise from the use of charcoal grills, camp stoves, or lanterns indoors or in tents, and from the use of gasoline-powered engines, such as generators in or near an enclosed space, even a garage, for example, with the large door open.[82] Fumes from the garage can vent into the home, poisoning people inside. People are sometimes poisoned by fumes from a motor running near an open window.

When a gas stove is correctly adjusted to have a small blue flame, almost all the carbon in the gas is converted to CO2, with only negligible amounts of carbon monoxide produced. However, as soon as a pot is placed on the burner, CO production rises. The levels of CO produced decline as the pot heats up, but the temperature never rises enough (without melting the pot) to prevent CO formation. Using a higher flame to quickly heat a pot greatly increases CO production, without increasing the heat proportionately. A single gas burner can raise the CO level in a closed kitchen to 20 to 100 ppm. About half of kitchen ranges raise CO levels above the EPA standard of 9 ppm, and five percent raise levels above 200 ppm.[83]

The design of gas ovens ensures that CO is produced, generally from 100 to 800 ppm of CO. Thus, venting of the kitchen is essential, especially when long baking times are used, for example, baking a large turkey with stuffing for over three hours, as compared to a tray of cookies baked for 12 minutes. Exposure to CO and NO_2 from a gas stove can be mitigated with the use of a stove vent/fan that vents to the outdoors. Even if there is a vent with a blower, a window needs to be opened enough to allow an equal volume of fresh air inflow into the room as is vented to the outdoors.[84]

Electric ranges only produce CO when food is burned. This includes the burning that occurs during the cleaning cycle of electric ovens. When food is burned or a cleaning cycle is done, the room should be vented.

Nitrogen Dioxide

When air is heated sufficiently, as it is during the combustion of many fuels, it causes the decomposition of nitrogen gas in the air. The nitrogen ions are reactive and attack O2 in the air, forming nitric oxide in an endothermic reaction, consuming much more energy than is released:

$$O_2 + N_2 \rightarrow 2\,NO$$

When nitric oxide is exposed to oxygen in the air, it is further oxidized to nitrogen dioxide:

$$2\,NO + O_2 \rightarrow 2\,NO_2.$$

Any form of high-temperature combustion over 1500° C in air can create NO, with the amount rising with the combustion temperature. Natural gas burning at 1960° C is easily hot enough to produce considerable amounts of NOx.

High amounts of NO_2 are produced in automobile exhaust and from nuclear explosions. Both of these are responsible for the significant depletion of the ozone layer.[85] Most of the health consequences of NO_2, however, come from indoor air exposure, as this is where we spend the majority of our lives, and because significant NO_2 levels can accumulate in closed spaces.

The most commonly recognized health risk from NO_2 is to the lungs. NO_2 is a respiratory irritant that can cause or exacerbate asthma, especially in children. I speculate that it may act to cause injury as a result of the formation of acids. Some of the NO_2, on contact with the moist respiratory epithelium, is converted to nitrous acid (HNO_2) and nitric acid (HNO_3).

$$4\,NO + O_2 + 2\,H_2O \rightarrow 4\,HNO_2$$

and

$$2\,NO_2\,(N_2O_4) + H_2O \rightarrow HNO_2 + HNO_3$$

Nitrous acid may irritate the lungs; however, nitric acid is a considerably stronger acid than nitrous acid. Nitric acid is a strong oxidizing acid that readily reacts with organic molecules. HNO_3 reacts with proteins, causing a xanthoproteic reaction in which aromatic amino acids become nitrated, and thus injure the cells of the respiratory tract.

A Canadian study found a dose-response association for small for gestational age births with exposure to NO_2 and found that the association was stronger for NO_2 than it was for fine particulate matter ($PM_{2.5}$) air pollution.[86] This indicates that NO_2 causes SGA births and fetal loss. In a study of about 69,000 pregnancies in Boston, every increase in exposure of 10 ppb NO_2 lowered the live birth rate by 13%. The risk was highest for exposure occurring during the 15th week of pregnancy. In a study of 95,000 live births in Israel, for every 10-ppb exposure to NO_2, there was an 18% decrease in live births; the peak risk was at the 16th week of pregnancy.[87]

NOx and the Brain

Exposure to NO_2 has also been found to increase the risk of dementia. NO_2 and nitric oxide (NO) exposure are associated with an increased risk of Parkinson's disease.[88]

In the study of older adults from Ontario previously cited, for every quartile of NO_2 exposure, the hazard for dementia increased by 10 percent. While ozone exposure was not associated with an increase in dementia in this study, [89] the study cited from Taiwan found that an increase of 10.91 ppb in ozone (O_3) increases AD risk by 211%.[90] A study of older adults in Sweden showed a 38% increase in AD and a 47% increase in vascular dementia for those in the highest versus the lowest quartile of NO_x exposure.

In a study of older adults, environmental NO_2 exposure was found to be associated with a 2-fold risk for depression for each 10μg/m^3 of exposure, and the odds of the subjects being on antidepressant medication were also higher among those with higher NO_2 exposure.[91]

There is considerable evidence that NO_2 causes adverse effects on the neurodevelopment of infants and children.

A principal target of nitric oxide is the activation of the enzyme guanylate cyclase. NO in the air, NO formed from nitroglycerin, or other decomposition of NO2 into NO may activate guanylate cyclase C, an enzyme present on the surface of neurons. The increased activation of this enzyme can promote excitotoxicity to the neurons, deregulate attention and neurodevelopment,[92] and may downregulate nerve cell proliferation.[93]

In a study performed in Spain, children aged 11 to 22 months were assessed using the Bayley Scales of Infant Development.[1] Fourteen-month-old children living in homes with a gas cooker had three-point lower Bayley developmental scores than did children in homes with electric ranges. In homes where the gas cooker was used less frequently or used with an exhaust fan, the association was weaker.[94] In another study, exposure to NO_2 from gas cookers was found to be associated with inattention and inversely associated with cognitive function in 4-year-old children.[95]

A study examining birth cohorts from six European countries and the timing of air pollution levels over twenty years found that air pollution exposure during pregnancy was associated with reduced psychomotor

---

[1] The Bayley Scale of Infant and Toddler Development is used to assess cognitive, motor and communicative development in infants and babies that are too young for IQ testing. As with IQ scoring, the Bayley Scale has a mean of 100 and a standard deviation of 15 points. It has a range of 40 to 160.

development in the intrauterine exposed child, with NO2 having the highest correlation to impaired development.[96]

Mitigation of Indoor CO and NOx

Most of the NO_2 exposure in the home comes from gas cooktops and ovens. Gas heaters, water heaters, and clothes dryers require venting to the outdoors to prevent the gases from accumulating in the home, with the principal concern being the avoidance of carbon monoxide accumulation in the room. Water heaters, boilers, and dryers are also usually placed in unoccupied areas of the home, and thus should pose less risk of NO2 exposure as long as they function properly.

While much lower amounts of CO are produced when a stove or oven has a properly adjusted air–fuel ratio, a correctly burning gas flame produces significant amounts of NO and NO_2. It should thus be understood that the efficient production of high levels of NOx during the use of gas appliances is the best-case scenario when burning fuels.

The nichrome heating elements used in most electric stoves have a melting point of 1400° C, below the 1500° C temperature at which nitrogen gas begins to decompose. The peak temperature of electric stove elements runs at temperatures much lower than this. Thus, electric ovens and stoves do not produce NOx.

Home Carbon Monoxide Detectors

As an odorless, tasteless, and colorless gas, the only way to detect CO in the home is with a CO detector. Thus, it is surprising that the standard for home CO detectors is laxer than it is for the workplace. The UL 2034 standard is set for the alarm *not to sound* until CO levels are high enough to cause a blood COHb of 10%, a dangerous level. This level is sufficiently dangerous that if the CO detector alarm sounds, the occupants are advised to call 9-1-1, evacuate, and not re-enter the premises until emergency services have determined that the building is safe to reoccupy.[97] The detectors are not designed to prevent CO intoxication, but rather to report it.

CO alarms use time-weighted averages, so they will sound more quickly at higher levels. While the OSHA eight-hour recommended ceiling for CO exposure is 35 ppm for 8 hours and the Permissible Exposure Limit (PEL) is 50 ppm for 8 hours, a home alarm is *prohibited* from sounding unless the CO level has been between 30 and 69 ppm for 30 days! The UL 2034 standard mandates that if the CO detector has a digital display, as long as the CO level is less than 30, *it must display a default level of zero* unless a button is pressed to show the actual reading. For CO levels of 70–149 ppm, the alarms will not sound for at least one hour, but must sound before 4 hours, and levels must be between 150 and 399 ppm for ten to 50 minutes for the alarm to sound.

The Kiddie™ ultra-sensitive monitor does not comply with UL standards, as it will beep at lower CO levels, as low as 20 ppm for 20 minutes.[98] Ultra-sensitive CO detectors (such as the Kidde KN-COU-B) can display the CO level down to 10 ppm and will alarm if the air is over 20 ppm for 20 to 115 minutes or over 70 ppm for 20 to 70 minutes, about half the time that regular detectors wait for 150 and 400 ppm levels. The ultra-sensitive detectors cost more but can be recommended for people with lung disease, heart conditions, or other medical conditions that make the individual more susceptible to CO. Pregnant women should consider themselves in the susceptible category if they live in a home with gas appliances or one heated with wood. Infants should also be considered susceptible individuals.

A 2015 analysis put the annual cost of accidental acute CO poisoning (resulting in hospitalization or death) in the U.S. at $1.3 billion.[99] This estimate does not include the cost of exacerbations of heart and lung disease that are caused by lower-level CO exposures. Having operational *smoke alarms* in homes has been found to reduce the risk of injury or death from a home fire by 88 percent. CO monitors should reduce risk.

Mitigating CO Production

Carbon monoxide formation can be curtailed by proper adjustment of the flame height and regular, proper maintenance of the burners so that they have the correct air-fuel ratio, as well as proper venting.

Gas burners on stoves have an air intake adjustment that allows for the control of the air-fuel mix. If the flame is yellow-orange, the mix is too rich, and more air intake is needed to avoid excess production of carbon monoxide and soot. Soot on the bottom of pots indicates an excessively rich fuel-to-air mix. Avoiding the use of an excessively high flame in an attempt to accelerate cooking will help prevent CO overproduction. Cooking in water does not get faster with more vigorous boiling.

If the flame is very tall and wispy blue, it can indicate a lean fuel-air mix, which is less hazardous, but can reduce efficiency and increase NOx production. While injurious, NOx is not nearly as dangerous as CO.

The vent should be used whenever cooking is done on a gas stove. The back burners should preferentially be used, as the stove vent hood more efficiently captures and vents combustion gases produced from the back burners as compared to the front burners.

The speed of the hood vent should be appropriate for the amount of fuel used and the amount of NOx, CO, and CO2 being produced. For one burner, a low fan speed is appropriate, while higher speeds are needed when more fuel is burned. The amount of air vented by the hood must be balanced with fresh air inflow into the room. If not, there can be a backflow of combustion gases being passively vented from the water heater, furnace, or other gas appliance back into the home.

A slow setting on a hood vent is typically about 100 to 200 cubic feet per minute (CFM). To balance a 150 CFM vent, a window opening of about 20 square inches is needed; thus, opening a 24-inch-wide window by one inch is sufficient. For a 600 CFM vent flow, 80 square inches of window opening are needed; thus, a 24" wide window would need to be opened about 3.4 inches.

Unfortunately, some kitchens are not designed with the gas stove up against an outside wall so that the stove can be vented to the outdoors. I rented an apartment for a while with a gas stove and oven in which the hood vented through a grease filter back into the room rather than to the outdoors. A grease filter with a fan may help remove oil vapors from the air, but it just recirculates CO2, CO, and NOx. There is no building code requirement for gas stoves in the home to have venting to the outdoors.

The creation of NOx can be avoided in the home with the use of electrical appliances (oven, stove, furnace, water heater, fireplace), rather than using natural gas, propane, or other fuel. Any cooking range on a kitchen island creates risks, especially to children. They are hard to vent properly, and thus, gas ranges on an island should be avoided.

Carbon Dioxide in the Home

The buildup of indoor carbon dioxide has not been much of a concern in the home, school, or most non-industrial workplaces. CO2 is considered to have extremely low toxicity. The principal concern has been limited to the displacement of oxygen to the point that it causes hypoxia.

Even in an all-electric home, carbon dioxide (CO2) levels can build up, as we produce it as a primary metabolic byproduct. Even at rest during sleep, when metabolic activity is at its lowest, CO2 can build up in a room. For example, if two average adults were to sleep in an airtight 12 x 12-foot bedroom with an 8-foot high ceiling, the CO2 level would rise from about 425 ppm to over 10,000 ppm. Fortunately, doors leak, there are vents, and air conditioning fans that circulate air throughout the house. In the past, most houses were leaky. Modern, energy-efficient houses, however, are much tighter. Nowadays, CO2 levels can easily rise to 2000 - 4000 ppm in a bedroom at night, or even higher in a poorly ventilated room.

The American Society of Heating, Refrigerating, and Air-Conditioning Engineers (ASHRAE) recommends that indoor CO2 levels be kept below 1000 ppm.

When CO2 levels rise above 1000 ppm, cognitive performance and sleep quality decline. At a room CO2 level of 1400 ppm, basic cognitive function scores drop by 25%, and scores for complex problem solving drop by 50%![100] Another reason that I could not concentrate in a classroom with 50 other kids and a nun. It was enough to addle the brain.

There are two people (no pets) in my home, with all-electric appliances (no gas-burning appliances) and central air conditioning circulating the air, and we sleep with the bedroom door open. The CO2 level in my home easily rises by 700 ppm to over 1100 ppm if the windows are closed overnight. Opening the windows to get cross ventilation (with the HVAC fan on) to better mix the air can drop the level to below 425, that of the outside. The first time I tried the monitor, the levels were stupidly high; around 1400 ppm.

While not directly deadly, poor decision-making and poor sleep quality lead to real-life consequences, even if they don't directly cause permanent disability.

Indoor CO2 Mitigation

The simplest and most cost-effective remedy is to open windows to get cross-ventilation in the home. Even opening a couple of windows one inch to get cross-ventilation can drastically lower CO2 accumulation.

Doors can be left open during the night to avoid a buildup in bedrooms. Having larger spaces under the door allows for greater ventilation and airflow return to the central air handler. Larger space under the door, however, allows more noise transmission.

Setting the HVAC to have the fan run intermittently, even when not heating or cooling, to circulate air throughout the home will help mix air throughout the house. The levels in the home will rise, but levels in the bedrooms will not get as high, allowing for better sleep.

In hot or cold climates where the windows need to be closed for energy efficiency, an energy recovery ventilator (ERV) or heat recovery ventilator (HRV) can be used to exchange indoor air with outdoor air.

Since it is such a common issue, air quality monitoring for CO2 may be as important as CO monitoring. If a CO2 monitor is used, set the alarm to 1000 to 1200 ppm, and adjust the home's ventilation until the alerts become rare events.

Radon

Radon is an invisible, odorless, radioactive gas that is emitted from rock, and that is the second most common cause of lung cancer, second only to smoking.

Homes with a basement are at considerably higher risk of having higher radon levels, and exposure risk is higher in the basement. Having a basement can promote the accumulation of high levels of radon in the home, even in areas without high radon levels. Cracks in the basement floor or wall, gaps around pipes, and sump pits are areas where radon gas can leak in. As with other gases, risk increases with a tighter, more energy-efficient, modern home.

The World Health Organization recommends building mitigation if radon levels are 2.7 pCi/L or higher, while the EPA recommends mitigation in homes and other buildings if radon levels are 4.0 pCi/L or higher. The EPA data and recommendations were developed in 1993, when the median home age was 27 years (thus, on average, built in 1966). This was before energy-efficient homes and HVAC were common. Because homes are much tighter than in the past, the risk of radon accumulation in a house is much greater today. Even if the home is older, the risk has likely increased, as most homes have been upgraded to improve energy efficiency.

The U.S. Environmental Protection Agency (EPA) map https://www.epa.gov/radon/epa-map-radon-zones provides county-level radon levels scored one to three. Homes in areas 1 and 2 should be tested for radon, especially if the home has a basement.

It is important to understand that there can be a great variation in radon emission within the same county, depending on the geological terrain and the building. My sister lives in a zip code area where the average radon level in homes is 1.7 PCi/L, but the levels in her basement were as high as 11.4 before mitigation. Testing was only done after her stage 4 lung cancer diagnosis. More detailed radon data can be found by searching for radon levels by zip code.

Mitigation is straightforward and involves the repair of cracks and providing ventilation of the basement.

Other Indoor Gases and Pollutants

Homes, especially new homes, manufactured homes, and recently upgraded homes (recently repaired or painted, new carpets, new furniture, etc.), can have off-gassing of a variety of noxious chemicals.

Formaldehyde and other Volatile Organic Compounds: Formaldehyde in the air can irritate the eyes, nose, and throat, and cause wheezing, coughing, and trigger allergic reactions. Prolonged exposure can increase the risk of cancer. Formaldehyde can off-gas from plywood, particleboard, paints, glues, adhesives, and certain cleaning products. Home air quality monitors are available that measure formaldehyde (HCHO) and usually also measure total volatile organic compounds (TVOC), which includes the measurement of HCHO and other volatile organic compounds (VOCs), such as benzene, toluene, and xylene. These monitors typically also monitor PM and CO2.

The most practical methods for mitigation of volatile organic compounds, such as formaldehyde from a building, are primary prevention (not bringing them into the home as building materials, for example), and secondly, ensuring sufficient fresh air exchange, as well as the need for CO2 removal from the home. To avoid health risks from and other noxious gases in the home, avoid their use during building.

While particulate filters, such as MERV or HEPA filters, do not remove O3, CO, NO, NO2, SO2, radon, or other gases from the air, charcoal air filters can reduce the levels of many noxious gases, including benzene, formaldehyde, and most other VOCs. They also remove most odors from the air. Charcoal filters can reduce the levels of certain gases, including NO2, sulfur dioxide, and reduce the levels of ozone levels by as much as 70%. While charcoal filters can absorb small amounts of carbon monoxide and radon, they are not an effective means of removing either of these gases.

Frying: Cooking in oil, which is highly discouraged by the SANA program, can produce large amounts of VOCs, including formaldehyde, acetaldehyde, furans, PAHs, benzene, acrolein, crotonaldehyde, and other toxic, volatile gases. It can additionally be a large source of PM that can contribute to lung and CVD risk.[101] Frying meat or fish creates large amounts of these compounds as well. Thus, it is not only eating these foods that is damaging to health, but it is also detrimental to breathe the air pollution created during their preparation. Cooking using a wok produces high amounts of lung carcinogens as a result of the high cooking temperature used.[102]

Range hood vents can help lower household exposure to volatile compounds created during frying, and the use of range hoods has been found to lower the risk of cooking-related lung cancer among those exposed by 50%.[103] Range hood ventilation should be used at high speed when frying, as there is a higher production of toxic fumes than just those from burning fuel. Fumes from frying are created even when cooking on an electric range. Air frying also creates VOCs and PM. If using an air fryer, it should be done in an area that can be easily vented.

Use of the range hood also vents steam and heat created during cooking to the outdoors, helping keep the house cooler and less humid during the summer.

Fireplaces: Having a crackling fire in a hearth may conjure up nostalgia for a cozy Christmas or curling up in a blanket with hot chocolate on a winter evening, but burning wood to heat a home, or worse, as a decorative flourish, is inappropriate in today's climate. We don't need any additional smoke, particulate pollution, carbon dioxide, or other gases added to our atmosphere, neighborhoods, or the air in our homes. Fireplaces are inefficient and waste energy even when not being used. They increase the risk of both house fires and wildfires. Relegate that bit of nostalgia to the past.

Atmospheric Mercury

Mercury (Hg) is neurotoxic. Since 1997, the annual release of Hg into the atmosphere, which was mostly from coal-fired power plants, has decreased in the U.S. by about 75%, mostly as a result of flue gas desulfurization, but also as a result of shifting to the use of natural gas for power generation. Nevertheless, the global atmospheric Hg releases increased by 9% between 1990 and 2010 as a result of the increased coal-powered electricity production in China and India.[104] Nevertheless, atmospheric mercury only accounts for about one percent of the mercury in the biosphere, with most of the mercury being stored in the soil, ocean, and surface water. Thus, the Hg remains in our environment.[105] A considerable amount of the mercury that enters the atmosphere from the burning of coal, production of cement, and gold processing in Asia comes down in the rain on the West Coast of the United States, and ends up in rivers, lakes, and fish. Florida has a substantial amount is its rain from power plants in Texas.

If people are exposed to gaseous mercury downwind of power plants, cement factories, steel mills, waste incinerators, gold mining operations, some of that mercury will show up in their hair, and some will be in their brains, where it is unlikely to be measured. Five years after the exposure ends, the mercury will still be present in the brain, but it will not be present in the blood, urine, feces, or hair.

Elemental mercury is a liquid at body temperature. In its liquid form, Hg is poorly absorbed from the GI tract (less than 0.1 percent), and thus it has comparatively low toxicity. However, metallic mercury is volatile at room temperature, and gaseous elemental mercury (GEM) is lipid-soluble and easily diffuses across the alveoli of the lungs and is carried in the blood. GEM can enter the red blood cells, where it can be oxidized by the enzyme catalase and then converted into insoluble divalent inorganic mercury in the RBCs.

It is mercury in the brain that is of greatest toxicity. GEM can also cross the blood-brain barrier and the placenta. In the brain, GEM becomes ionized. In its ionized form, it is no longer lipid-soluble and thus gets trapped in the brain, where it causes neurotoxicity, especially in the fetus and young children. Mercury appears to be less toxic to mature than to developing neurons and other brain cells. Methylmercury is lipid-soluble and is also well absorbed and can cross the blood-brain barrier (BBB) and placenta. In the brain, it causes focal necrosis of neurons and destruction of glial cells.

The half-life of mercury in the blood is about 60 to 65 days, which corresponds to the average remaining survival time of the red blood cells. Absorbed mercury undergoes enterohepatic circulation, being repeatedly excreted into the bile and reabsorbed from the intestine. Thus, it is only slowly eliminated from the body into the feces. Methylmercury that enters the cells that are desquamated (GI mucosa cells, skin cells, and hair) also allows the disposal of organic mercury from the body. Negligible amounts pass into the urine.[106, 107]

Some of the inhaled mercury vapor can make it to the CNS. Once inside the brain, mercury becomes ionized and trapped, giving mercury in the brain an extremely long half-life. Here, it can cause significant injury. Inorganic mercury has a long half-life in primates, perhaps around one year. The half-life for organic mercury in the human brain is much longer; modeling from autopsies gives a half-life of 27.4 years.[108]

The most common exposure to a significant amount of Hg is from organic mercury ingested from the consumption of fish. Mercury has varying toxicity depending on host factors. In a study of mice, oral ingestion of 16 mg/kg of methyl mercuric chloride killed two-thirds of male mice, but the minimum lethal dose in the same breed of female mice was 40 mg/kg. Toxicity also varies by the strain of mice. As different mice respond so differently to the same dose, it should be assumed that the mouse dose-response may not model the human dose-response accurately. Neonatal monkeys given 0.5 mg Hg/kg/day as methyl mercuric chloride in infant formula for 4 weeks had stumbling and falling by the end of the exposure. Following the cessation of exposure, neurologic injury progressed; the animals developed abnormal reflexes, shrieking, crying, and tantrums, blindness, and coma. Monkeys fed 0.05 mg Hg/kg/day from birth to age 3–4 showed impaired spatial vision, and with continued dosing to age 6.5–7 had decreased fine motor performance, clumsiness. By age 14, there was decreased sensitivity to touch and hearing loss.

Mercury in the Home

Some potential sources of elemental mercury contamination in the home are fluorescent lights, mercury thermometers, and some older light switches and thermostats. When it is contained in glass, there is no risk, but if a thermometer or fluorescent lamps are broken, the mercury and its vapors are released. Even a few beads of mercury can raise air mercury levels to harmful levels, and the longer the exposure, the greater the risk. Mercury vapor and tiny droplets are hard to remove from clothing, furniture, carpet, and floors, and may slowly evaporate for months or years, continuing to expose those in the home to mercury.[109]

If fluorescent lights or other mercury-containing items break in the home, the mercury will slowly evaporate and be inhaled.

Mitigation

Mercury cleanup is not a simple task, and depending on local regulations, it may require calling in a Hazmat team. Cleaning tiny liquid beads of mercury is not easy, and those captured in carpet and cracks end up evaporating into the air in the home over time. Vacuuming mercury can increase its evaporation into GEM. Even the trash from the cleanup is considered hazardous waste that should not be included with regular garbage.

Clean-up methods for a small mercury release can be Googled. Here is a link to a document that describes how to clean up a *small* mercury spill in the home. (www.health.ny.gov/environmental/chemicals/mercury/docs/cleaning_up_a_small_mercury_spill.pdf).

Thus, mercury thermometers should also be used in the home or schools. Fluorescent tubes contain more mercury than compact fluorescent lights. Imported fluorescent bulbs typically have higher mercury content than do name-brand bulbs. Compact fluorescent bulbs are being phased out in favor of LED lights. When a compact fluorescent bulb breaks, the level of mercury vapor in the immediate area may be several times the maximum OSHA 8-hour exposure limit for mercury.[110]

I encourage those who still have any fluorescent lights, thermometers, or other mercury-containing items in their home to remove them and take them to a hazardous waste collection site. The hazard of breakage is too high to keep them in the home.

If living downwind from an industrial source of mercury pollution, activated charcoal filters are an efficient means of capturing GEM. Note that these filters should be considered hazardous waste when they are ready to be disposed of. If there is a small release of mercury into the home, for example, from a broken compact fluorescent bulb, an air purifier with activated charcoal can help further remove GEM from the room after it has been cleaned and aired out.

Fish can be a large source of dietary mercury. Chapter 14 lists fish that should be avoided. Rice, which was noted to bioconcentrate arsenic and cadmium in Chapter 13, appears to do the same trick with methyl mercury (MeHg). Generally, the levels of MeHg in rice are low enough not to exceed the reference intake for mercury. Nevertheless, in areas of high mercury contamination, where rice constitutes a large portion of calories for young children, such as in Bangladesh, the exposure is considered sufficient to cause intellectual losses.[111] Fun fact: When tested, baby cereals and teething biscuits made from rice had 61 and 92 times more MeHg, and 9.4 and 4.7 times more arsenic in them, respectively, than those made from wheat or oats.[112]

Children and adults may also be exposed to mercury as a result of dental amalgams used in the treatment of dental caries.[113] Vaccines for older children and adults may contain thiomersal, which is degraded into MeHg. Thiomersal is still used in childhood vaccines in some countries as a preservative, as it is less expensive than alternatives. (A quite odd justification.) Skin whitening creams and anti-acne treatments (mostly from Asia) may contain Hg^{2+}. The use of these products has been associated with the development of nephrotic syndrome in adults.[114] Imported discount and counterfeit cosmetics, toothpaste, and other personal care products of questionable origin should be avoided.

1 https://www.who.int/mediacentre/news/releases/2014/air-pollution/en/ (Accessed Feb. 2019)

2 Air pollution estimates. WHO 2104, https://www.who.int/phe/health_topics/outdoorair/databases /FINAL _HAP_AAP_BoD_24March2014.pdf?ua=1

3 Developing a Clinical Approach to Air Pollution and Cardiovascular Health. Hadley MB, Baumgartner J, Vedanthan R. Circulation. 2018 Feb 13;137(7):725-742. doi: 10.1161/CIRCULATIONAHA.117.030377. PMID: 29440198

4 https://www.eea.europa.eu//publications/air-quality-in-europe-2018 and Air-quality-in-europe 2019-final 21102019.pdf

5 Health effects of particulate matter: Policy implications for countries in eastern Europe,

Caucasus and central Asia. World Health Organization 2013 ISBN 978 92 890 0001 7

6 Air pollution in India and related adverse respiratory health effects: past, present, and future directions. Khilnani GC, Tiwari P. Curr Opin Pulm Med. 2018 Mar;24(2):108-116. doi: 10.1097/MCP.0000000000000463. PMID: 29300211

7 Novel evidence for a greater burden of ambient air pollution on cardiovascular disease. Mannucci PM, Harari S, Franchini M. Haematologica. 2019 Dec;104(12):2349-2357. doi: 10.3324/haematol.2019.225086. PMID: 31672903

8 Half the world's population are exposed to increasing air pollution. Shaddick G, Thomas ML, Mudu P, Ruggeri G, Gumy S. npj Clim Atmos Sci 3, 23 (2020). https://doi.org/10.1038/s41612-020-0124-2 https://www.nature.com/articles/s41612-020-0124-2

9 Populations potentially exposed to traffic-related air pollution in seven world cities. Su JG, Apte JS, Lipsitt J, Garcia-Gonzales DA, Beckerman BS, de Nazelle A, Texcalac-Sangrador JL, Jerrett M. Environ Int. 2015 May;78:82-89. doi: 10.1016/j.envint.2014.12.007. PMID: 25770919

10 Blood Pressure and Same-Day Exposure to Air Pollution at School: Associations with Nano-Sized to Coarse PM in Children. Pieters N, Koppen G, Van Poppel M, De Prins S, Cox B, Dons E, Nelen V, Panis LI, Plusquin M, Schoeters G, Nawrot TS. Environ Health Perspect. 2015 Jul;123(7):737-42. doi: 10.1289/ehp.1408121. PMID:25756964

11 Particulate matter neurotoxicity in culture is size-dependent. Gillespie P, Tajuba J, Lippmann M, Chen LC, Veronesi B. Neurotoxicology. 2013 May;36:112-7. doi: 10.1016/j.neuro.2011.10.006. PMID:22057156

12 Long-term air pollution exposure is associated with neuroinflammation, an altered innate immune response, disruption of the blood-brain barrier, ultrafine particulate deposition, and accumulation of amyloid beta-42 and alpha-synuclein in children and young adults. Calderón-Garcidueñas L, Solt AC, Henríquez-Roldán C, Torres-Jardón R, Nuse B, Herritt L, Villarreal-Calderón R, Osnaya N, Stone I, García R, Brooks DM, González-Maciel A, Reynoso-Robles R, Delgado-Chávez R, Reed W. Toxicol Pathol. 2008 Feb;36(2):289-310. doi: 10.1177/0192623307313011. PMID:18349428

13 The emerging risk of exposure to air pollution on cognitive decline and Alzheimer's disease - Evidence from epidemiological and animal studies. Kilian J, Kitazawa M. Biomed J. 2018 Jun;41(3):141-162. doi: 10.1016/j.bj.2018.06.001. PMID:30080655

14 Chemical composition of size-resolved particulate matter at near-freeway and urban background sites in the greater Beirut area. Daher N, Sabila NA, Shihadeh A, Jaafar M, et al Atmospheric Environment 80:96-106 · December 2013 DOI: 10.1016/j.atmosenv.2013.08.004

15 Size-segregated composition of particulate matter (PM) in major roadways and surface streets. Kam w, Liacos JW, Schauer JJ, Delfino RJ, Sioutas C. Atmospheric Environment 55(12)90-97 Aug. 2012. https://doi.org/10.1016/j.atmosenv.2012.03.028

16 Effects of Ambient Air Pollution Exposure on Olfaction: A Review. Ajmani GS, Suh HH, Pinto JM. Environ Health Perspect. 2016 Nov;124(11):1683-1693. doi: 10.1289/EHP136. PMID: 27285588

17 Functional and morphological olfactory bulb modifications in mice after vanadium inhalation. Colín-Barenque L, Pedraza-Chaverri J, Medina-Campos O, Jimenez-Martínez R, Bizarro-Nevares P, González-Villalva A, Rojas-Lemus M, Fortoul TI. Toxicol Pathol. 2015 Feb;43(2):282-91. doi: 10.1177/0192623314548668. PMID: 25492423

18 Vanadium exposure induces olfactory dysfunction in an animal model of metal neurotoxicity. Ngwa HA, Kanthasamy A, Jin H, Anantharam V, Kanthasamy AG. Neurotoxicology. 2014 Jul;43:73-81. doi: 10.1016/j.neuro.2013.12.004. PMID: 24362016

19 Nitrogen dioxide pollution exposure is associated with olfactory dysfunction in older U.S. adults. Adams DR, Ajmani GS, Pun VC, Wroblewski KE, Kern DW, Schumm LP, McClintock MK, Suh HH, Pinto JM. Int Forum Allergy Rhinol. 2016 Dec;6(12):1245-1252. doi: 10.1002/alr.21829. PMID: 27620703

20 Size-resolved particulate matter (PM) in urban areas: toxico-chemical characteristics, sources, trends and health implications. Nancy Daher. Doctoral Dissertation, University of Southern California, December 2013 Chapter 5; pp 105 – 130.

21 Call for evidence on brake, tyre and road surface wear July 2018 UK Department for Transportation, Dept. for Environment, Food & Rural Affairs

22 Time to ban lead in industrial paints and coatings. Gottesfeld P. Front Public Health. 2015 May 18;3:144. doi: 10.3389/fpubh.2015.00144. 2015. PMID:26042214

23 Lead and Other Metals in Traffic Paint in Washington State. Hazardous Waste and Toxics Reduction Program. May 2015 Publication 15-04-018

24 https://www.nationmaster.com/country-info/stats/Transport/Road/Motor-vehicles-per-1000-people (Accessed Feb. 2019)

25 https://tradingeconomics.com/japan/passenger-cars-per-1-000-people-wb-data.html (Accessed Feb. 2019)

26 Particulate Matter from the Road Surface Abrasion as a Problem of Non-Exhaust Emission Control. Penkala M, Oprondnik P, Rogula-Kozłowska W, et al. Environments 5(9) · January 2018 DOI: 10.3390/environments5010009

27 An urban stormwater runoff mortality syndrome in juvenile coho salmon. Chow MI, Lundin JI, Mitchell CJ, Davis JW, Young G, Scholz NL, McIntyre JK. Aquat Toxicol. 2019 Sep;214:105231. doi: 10.1016/j.aquatox. 2019.105231. PMID: 31295703

28 A ubiquitous tire rubber-derived chemical induces acute mortality in coho salmon. Tian Z, Zhao H, Peter KT, Gonzalez M, et al. Science. 2021 Jan 8;371(6525):185-189. doi: 10.1126/science.abd6951. PMID: 33273063

29 Compositions, Functions, and Testing of Friction Brake Materials and Their Additives. Oak Ridge National Laboratory ORNL/TM-2001/64, Sept. 2001

30 Chemical fractionation and mobility of traffic-related elements in road environments. Adamiec E. Environ Geochem Health. 2017 Dec;39(6):1457-1468. doi: 10.1007/s10653-017-9983-9. PMID:28551883

31 Association between dust storm occurrence and risk of suicide: Case-crossover analysis of the Korean national death database. Lee H, Jung J, Myung W, Baek JH, Kang JM, Kim DK, Kim H. Environ Int. 2019 Dec;133(Pt A):105146. doi: 10.1016/j.envint.2019.105146. PMID: 31630066

32 Impact of Desert Dust Events on Cardiovascular Disease: A Systematic Review and Meta-Analysis. Domínguez-Rodríguez A, Báez-Ferrer N, Abreu-González P, Rodríguez S, Díaz R, Avanzas P, Hernández-Vaquero D. J Clin Med. 2021 Feb 12;10(4):727. doi: 10.3390/jcm10040727. PMID: 33673156

33 Desert Dust Outbreaks in Southern Europe: Contribution to Daily PM10 Concentrations and Short-Term Associations with Mortality and Hospital Admissions. Stafoggia M, Zauli-Sajani S, Pey J, Samoli E, et al.. PMID: 26219103

34 Short-term effects of particulate matter during desert and non-desert dust days on mortality in Iran. Shahsavani A, Tobías A, Querol X, Stafoggia M, Abdolshahnejad M, Mayvaneh F, Guo Y, Hadei M, Saeed Hashemi S, Khosravi A, Namvar Z, Yarahmadi M, Emam B. Environ Int. 2020 Jan;134:105299. doi: 10.1016/j.envint.2019.105299. PMID: 31751828

35 Half the world's population are exposed to increasing air pollution. Shaddick G, Thomas ML, Mudu P, Ruggeri G, Gumy S. npj Clim Atmos Sci 3, 23 (2020). https://doi.org/10.1038/s41612-020-0124-2 https://www.nature.com/articles/s41612-020-0124-2

36 Study of ultrafine particles near a major highway with heavy-duty diesel traffic. ZAhu Y, Hinds WC, Kim S, Shen S, Sioutas C. Atmospheric Environment 36 (2002) 4323–4335

37 Chemical composition of size-resolved particulate matter at near-freeway and urban background sites in the greater Beirut area. Daher n, Saliba N, Shihadeh AL, Jaafa M, et al. Atmospheric Environment, 80(12)96-106. Dec. 2013. https://doi.org/10.1016/j.atmosenv.2013.08.004

38 Assessing PM2.5 Exposures with High Spatiotemporal Resolution across the Continental United States. Di Q, Kloog I, Koutrakis P, Lyapustin A, Wang Y, Schwartz J. Environ Sci Technol. 2016 May 3;50(9):4712-21. doi: 10.1021/acs.est.5b06121. PMID:27023334 See also supplemental materials

39 Formation of urban fine particulate matter. Zhang R, Wang G, Guo S, Zamora ML, Ying Q, Lin Y, Wang W, Hu M, Wang Y. Chem Rev. 2015 May 27;115(10):3803-55. doi: 10.1021/acs.chemrev.5b00067. PMID:25942499

40 Size-resolved particulate matter (PM) in urban areas: toxico-chemical characteristics, sources, trends and health implications. Nancy Daher. Doctoral Dissertation, University of Southern California, December 2013.

41 Assessing PM2.5 Exposures with High Spatiotemporal Resolution across the Continental United States. Di Q, Kloog I, Koutrakis P, Lyapustin A, Wang Y, Schwartz J. Environ Sci Technol. 2016 May 3;50(9):4712-21. doi: 10.1021/acs.est.5b06121. PMID:27023334 See also supplemental materials

42 Chemical modification of pro-inflammatory proteins by peroxynitrite increases activation of TLR4 and NF-κB: Implications for the health effects of air pollution and oxidative stress. Ziegler K, Kunert AT, Reinmuth-Selzle K, Leifke AL, Widera D, Weller MG, Schuppan D, Fröhlich-Nowoisky J, Lucas K, Pöschl U. Redox Biol. 2020 Oct;37:101581. doi: 10.1016/j.redox.2020.101581. PMID: 32739154

43 The emerging risk of exposure to air pollution on cognitive decline and Alzheimer's disease - Evidence from epidemiological and animal studies. Kilian J, Kitazawa M. Biomed J. 2018 Jun;41(3):141-162. doi: 10.1016/j.bj.2018.06.001. PMID:30080655

44 Particulate air pollutants, APOE alleles and their contributions to cognitive impairment in older women and to amyloidogenesis in experimental models. Cacciottolo M, Wang X, Driscoll I, Woodward N, Saffari A, Reyes J, Serre ML, Vizuete W, Sioutas C, Morgan TE, Gatz M, Chui HC, Shumaker SA, Resnick SM, Espeland MA, Finch CE, Chen JC. Transl Psychiatry. 2017 Jan 31;7(1):e1022. doi: 10.1038/tp.2016.280. PMID:28140404

45 Long-term PM2.5 Exposure and Neurological Hospital Admissions in the Northeastern United States. Kioumourtzoglou MA, Schwartz JD, Weisskopf MG, Melly SJ, Wang Y, Dominici F, Zanobetti A. Environ Health Perspect. 2016 Jan;124(1):23-9. doi: 10.1289/ehp.1408973. PMID:25978701

46 Exposure to ambient air pollution and the incidence of dementia: A population-based cohort study. Chen H, Kwong JC, Copes R, Hystad P, van Donkelaar A, Tu K, Brook JR, Goldberg MS, Martin RV, Murray BJ, Wilton AS, Kopp A, Burnett RT. Environ Int. 2017 Nov;108:271-277. doi: 10.1016/j.envint.2017.08.020. PMID:28917207

47 Ozone, particulate matter, and newly diagnosed Alzheimer's disease: a population-based cohort study in Taiwan. Jung CR, Lin YT, Hwang BF. J Alzheimers Dis. 2015;44(2):573-84. doi: 10.3233/JAD-140855. PMID:25310992

48 Ibid Reference 44: PMID:28140404

49 Long-Term PM2.5 Exposure and Respiratory, Cancer, and Cardiovascular Mortality in Older US Adults. Pun VC, Kazemiparkouhi F, Manjourides J, Suh HH. Am J Epidemiol. 2017 Oct 15;186(8):961-969. doi: 10.1093/aje/kwx166. PMID: 28541385

50 Ibid Ref. 12. PMID:18349428

51 Particulate matter exposure, prenatal and postnatal windows of susceptibility, and autism spectrum disorders. Kalkbrenner AE, Windham GC, Serre ML, Akita Y, Wang X, Hoffman K, Thayer BP, Daniels JL. Epidemiology. 2015 Jan;26(1):30-42. doi: 10.1097/EDE.0000000000000173. PMID:25286049

52 Traffic-related air pollution, particulate matter, and autism. Volk HE, Lurmann F, Penfold B, Hertz-Picciotto I, McConnell R. JAMA Psychiatry. 2013 Jan;70(1):71-7. doi: 10.1001/jamapsychiatry.2013.266. PMID:23404082

53 Autism spectrum disorder and particulate matter air pollution before, during, and after pregnancy: a nested case-control analysis within the Nurses' Health Study II Cohort. Raz R, Roberts AL, Lyall K, Hart JE, Just AC, Laden F, Weisskopf MG. Environ Health Perspect. 2015 Mar;123(3):264-70. doi: 10.1289/ehp.1408133. PMID:25522338

54 The Hidden Impact of Microplastics on Respiratory Health. Callari, M. Pulmonology News (from Medscape) March 2025 1(1)1, 3-4.

55 Microplastics and Nanoplastics in Atheromas and Cardiovascular Events. Marfella R, Prattichizzo F, Sardu C, et al. N Engl J Med. 2024 Mar 7;390(10): 900-910. doi: 10.1056/NEJMoa2309822. PMID: 38446676

56 Bioaccumulation of microplastics in decedent human brains. Nihart AJ, Garcia MA, El Hayek et al. Nat Med. 2025 Apr;31(4):1114-1119. doi: 10.1038/s41591-024-03453-1. PMID: 39901044

57 Mind over Microplastics: Exploring Microplastic-Induced Gut Disruption and Gut-Brain-Axis Consequences. Sofield CE, Anderton RS, Gorecki AM. Curr Issues Mol Biol. 2024 Apr 30;46(5):4186-4202. doi: 10.3390/cimb46050256. PMID: 38785524

58 Molecular and Cellular Effects of Microplastics and Nanoplastics: Focus on Inflammation and Senescence. Mahmud F, Sarker DB, Jocelyn JA, Sang QA. Cells. 2024 Oct 29;13(21):1788. doi: 10.3390/cells13211788. PMID: 39513895

59 https://en.wikipedia.org/wiki/Polyethylene

60 Chemical Agents and Related Occupations: Vinyl Chloride. https://www.ncbi.nlm.nih.gov/books/NBK304420/

61 EPA Begins Process to Prioritize Five Chemicals for Risk Evaluation Under Toxic Substances Control Act https://www.epa.gov/newsreleases/epa-begins-process-prioritize-five-chemicals-risk-evaluation-under-toxic-substances

62 As the world swims in plastic, some offer an answer: Ban the toxic two. Wicker A. MONGABAY. Jan3, 2024. https://news.mongabay.com/2024/01/as-the-world-swims-in-plastic-some-offer-an-answer-ban-the-toxic-two/

63 Exposure of Human Lung Cells to Polystyrene Microplastics Significantly Retards Cell Proliferation and Triggers Morphological Changes. Goodman KE, Hare JT, Khamis ZI, Hua T, Sang QA. Chem Res Toxicol. 2021 Apr 19;34(4):1069-1081. doi: 10.1021/acs.chemrestox.0c00486. PMID: 33720697

64 Effects of Polystyrene Microplastics on Human Kidney and Liver Cell Morphology, Cellular Proliferation, and Metabolism. Goodman KE, Hua T, Sang QA. ACS Omega. 2022 Sep 19;7(38):34136-34153. doi: 10.1021/acsomega.2c03453. PMID: 36188270

65 Microfiber Masses Recovered from Conventional Machine Washing of New or Aged Garments. Hartline NL et al. Environ. Sci. Technol. 2016, 50, 21, 11532–11538. https://doi.org/10.1021/acs.est.6b03045

66 The Most Hidden Source of Microfibers in the Great Lakes is Our Laundry. March 3 2020. Flow. https://forloveofwater.org/the-most-hidden-source-of-microfibers-in-the-great-lakes-is-our-laundry/

67 Microfibers Released into the Air from a Household Tumble Dryer. Danyang Tao, Kai Zhang, Shaopeng Xu, Huiju Lin, Yuan Liu, Jingliang Kang, Tszewai Yim, John P. Giesy, and Kenneth M. Y. Leung Environmental Science & Technology Letters 2022 9 (2), 120-126 https://doi.org/10.1021/acs.estlett.1c00911

68 https://www.webmd.com/lung/news/20201103/can-portable-air-cleaner-protect-you-from-covid (Accessed April 2021)

69 Hypoallergenic Pet Food: Myth or Magic Solution? https://www.aaoallergy.org/hypoallergenic-pet-food-myth-or-magic-solution/

70 https://www.tesla.com/blog/putting-tesla-hepa-filter-and-bioweapon-defense-mode-to-the-test (Accessed April 2021)

71 https://www.co2.earth/

72 Breast cancer risk in relation to occupations with exposure to carcinogens and endocrine disruptors: a Canadian case-control study. Brophy JT, Keith MM, Watterson A, et al. Environ Health. 2012 Nov 19;11:87. PMID:23164221

73 http://naturalgas.org/overview/background/ (Accessed January 2019)

74 Helium sources and uses. University of Pittsburg. http://researchservices.pitt.edu/helium/sourcesanduses

75 Hydrogen sulfide: https://haz-map.com/Agents/22 Methanethiol: https://haz-map.com/Agents/192

76 NIOSH Pocket Guide to Chemical Hazards #0105". National Institute for Occupational Safety and Health *(NIOSH)*.

77 Oxygen and carbon monoxide equilibria of human adult hemoglobin at atmospheric and elevated pressure. Rodkey FL, O'Neal JD, Collison HA. Blood. 1969 Jan;33(1):57-65. PMID:5763633

78 Carbon Monoxide Poisoning (CO). Centers for Disease Control and Prevention. https://www.cdc.gov/dotw/carbonmonoxide/index.html (Accessed January 2019)

79 Toxicological Profile for Carbon Monoxide. Wilbur S, Williams M, Williams R, et al. Atlanta (GA): Agency for Toxic Substances and Disease Registry (US); 2012 Jun

80 Causes and clinical significance of increased carboxyhemoglobin. Higgins C.2005. https://acutecaretesting.org/en/articles/causes-and-clinical-significance-of-increased-carboxyhemoglobin (Accessed June 2021)

81 Carbon monoxide poisoning. Blumenthal I. J R Soc Med. 2001 Jun;94(6):270-2. PMID:11387414

82 Carbon Monoxide Poisening (CO). Centers for Disease Control and Prevention. https://www.cdc.gov/dotw/carbonmonoxide/index.html (Accessed January 2019)

83 Carbon Monoxide Poisoning: Gas-fired Kitchen Ranges (AEN-205). Iowa State University Dept. of Agriculture and Biosystems Engineering. (Accessed January 2019)

84 Carbon Monoxide Myths. https://carbonmonoxide myths.com/f-a-q/ (Accessed January 2019)

85 Effects of Nuclear Explosions. Nuclearweapon archive.org.

86 A national study of the association between traffic-related air pollution and adverse pregnancy outcomes in Canada, 1999-2008. Stieb DM, Chen L, Hystad P, et al. Environ Res. 2016 Jul;148:513-526. doi: 10.1016/j.envres.2016.04.025. PMID:27155984

87 Traffic-related Air Pollution and Pregnancy Loss. Kioumourtzoglou MA, Raz R, Wilson A, Fluss R, Nirel R, Broday DM, Yuval, Hacker MR, McElrath TF, Grotto I, Koutrakis P, Weisskopf MG. Epidemiology. 2019 Jan;30(1):4-10. doi: 10.1097/EDE.0000000000000918. PMID:30199416

88 The impact of air pollution to central nervous system in children and adults. Sram RJ, Veleminsky M Jr, Veleminsky M Sr, Stejskalová J. Neuro Endocrinol Lett. 2017 Dec;38(6):389-396. PMID:29298278

89 Ibid Ref. 46. PMID:28917207

90 Ozone, particulate matter, and newly diagnosed Alzheimer's disease: a population-based cohort study in Taiwan. Jung CR, Lin YT, Hwang BF. J Alzheimers Dis. 2015;44(2):573-84. doi: 10.3233/JAD-140855. PMID:25310992

91 Effect of long-term exposure to air pollution on anxiety and depression in adults: A cross-sectional study. Vert C, Sánchez-Benavides G, Martínez D, Gotsens X, Gramunt N, Cirach M, Molinuevo JL, Sunyer J, Nieuwenhuijsen MJ, Crous-Bou M, Gascon M. Int J Hyg Environ Health. 2017 Aug;220(6):1074-1080. doi: 10.1016/j.ijheh.2017.06.009. PMID: 28705430

92 Role for the membrane receptor guanylyl cyclase-C in attention deficiency and hyperactive behavior. Gong R, Ding C, Hu J, Lu Y, Liu F, Mann E, Xu F, Cohen MB, Luo M. Science. 2011 Sep 16;333(6049):1642-6. doi: 10.1126/science.1207675. PMID:21835979

93 Intestinal cell proliferation and senescence are regulated by receptor guanylyl cyclase C and p21. Basu N, Saha S, Khan I, Ramachandra SG, Visweswariah SS. J Biol Chem. 2014 Jan 3;289(1):581-93. doi: 10.1074/jbc.M113.511311. PMID:24217248

94 Indoor air pollution from gas cooking and infant neurodevelopment. Vrijheid M, Martinez D, Aguilera I, et al; INMA Project. Epidemiology. 2012 Jan;23(1):23-32. doi: 10.1097/EDE.0b013e31823a4023. PMID:22082993

95 Association of early-life exposure to household gas appliances and indoor nitrogen dioxide with cognition and attention behavior in preschoolers. Morales E, Julvez J, Torrent M, de Cid R, Guxens M, Bustamante M, Künzli N, Sunyer J. Am J Epidemiol. 2009 Jun 1;169(11):1327-36. doi: 10.1093/aje/kwp067. PMID:19395695

96 Air pollution during pregnancy and childhood cognitive and psychomotor development: six European birth cohorts. Guxens M, Garcia-Esteban R, Giorgis-Allemand L, et al. Epidemiology. 2014 Sep;25(5):636-47. doi: 10.1097/EDE.0000000000000133. PMID: 25036432

97 Carbon Monoxide Alarm Considerations for Code Authorities. Underwriters Laboratories.

98 https://www.kidde.com/home-safety/en/us/ products/fire-safety/co-alarms/kn-cou-b/ Carbon Monoxide Monitor User Guide. (Accessed February 2019)

99 Cost of accidental carbon monoxide poisoning: A preventable expense. Hampson NB. Prev Med Rep. 2015 Dec 3;3:21-4. doi: 10.1016/j.pmedr.2015.11.010. eCollection 2016 Jun. PMID:26844181

100 Fossil Fuel Combustion Is Driving Indoor CO_2 Toward Levels Harmful to Human Cognition. Karnauskas KB, Miller SL, Schapiro AC. Geohealth. 2020 May 16;4(5):e2019GH000237. doi: 10.1029/2019GH000237. PMID: 32426622

101 Assessing Impacts of Additives on Particulate Matter and Volatile Organic Compounds Produced from the Grilling of Meat. Liu X, Xing W, Xu Z, Zhang X, Zhou H, Cai K, Xu B, Chen C. Foods. 2022 Mar 14;11(6):833. doi: 10.3390/foods11060833. PMID: 35327256

102 Elevated levels of volatile organic carcinogen and toxicant biomarkers in Chinese women who regularly cook at home. Hecht SS, Seow A, Wang et al. Cancer Epidemiol Biomarkers Prev. 2010 May;19(5):1185-92. doi: 10.1158/1055-9965.EPI-09-1291. PMID: 20406956

103 Impact of cooking oil fume exposure and fume extractor use on lung cancer risk in non-smoking Han Chinese women. Chen TY, Fang YH, Chen HL, et al. Sci Rep. 2020 Apr 21;10(1):6774. doi: 10.1038/s41598-020-63656-7. PMID: 32317677

104 Observed decrease in atmospheric mercury explained by global decline in anthropogenic emissions. Zhang Y, Jacob DJ, Horowitz HM, Chen L, Amos HM, Krabbenhoft DP, Slemr F, St Louis VL, Sunderland EM. Proc Natl Acad Sci U S A. 2016 Jan 19;113(3):526-31. doi: 10.1073/pnas.1516312113. PMID: 26729866

105 A review of global environmental mercury processes in response to human and natural perturbations: Changes of emissions, climate, and land use. Obrist D, Kirk JL, Zhang L, Sunderland EM, Jiskra M, Selin NE. Ambio. 2018 Mar;47(2):116-140. doi: 10.1007/s13280-017-1004-9. PMID: 29388126

[106] A toxicokinetic model for predicting the tissue distribution and elimination of organic and inorganic mercury following exposure to methyl mercury in animals and humans. II. Application and validation of the model in humans. Carrier G, Bouchard M, Brunet RC, Caza M. Toxicol Appl Pharmacol. 2001 Feb 15;171(1):50-60. PMID:11181111

[107] The toxicity of mercury. Broussared LA, Hammett-Stabler CA, Winecker RE, Ropero-Miller JD. Laboratory Medicine Aug. 2002 33(8)614 – 25. https://academic.oup.com/labmed/article-abstract/33/8/614/2657245

[108] The retention time of inorganic mercury in the brain--a systematic review of the evidence. Rooney JP. Toxicol Appl Pharmacol. 2014 Feb 1;274(3):425-35. doi: 10.1016/j.taap.2013.12.011. PMID:24368178

[109] Toxicological profile for mercury. U.S. Dept. of Health and Human Services Agency for Toxic Substances and Disease Registry. https://www.atsdr.cdc.gov/ToxProfiles/tp.asp?id=115&tid=24 March 1999.

[110] Mercury vapor release from broken compact fluorescent lamps and in situ capture by new nanomaterial sorbents. Johnson NC, Manchester S, Sarin L, Gao Y, Kulaots I, Hurt RH. Environ Sci Technol. 2008 Aug 1;42(15):5772-8. doi: 10.1021/es8004392. PMID: 18754507

[111] Total mercury and methylmercury in rice: Exposure and health implications in Bangladesh. Wang Y, Habibullah-Al-Mamun M, Han J, Wang L, Zhu Y, Xu X, Li N, Qiu G. Environ Pollut. 2020 Oct;265(Pt A):114991. doi: 10.1016/j.envpol.2020.114991. PMID: 32574891

[112] Co-exposure to methylmercury and inorganic arsenic in baby rice cereals and rice-containing teething biscuits. Rothenberg SE, Jackson BP, Carly McCalla G, Donohue A, Emmons AM. Environ Res. 2017 Nov;159:639-647. doi: 10.1016/j.envres.2017.08.046. PMID: 28938205

[113] A significant dose-dependent relationship between mercury exposure from dental amalgams and kidney integrity biomarkers: a further assessment of the Casa Pia children's dental amalgam trial. Geier DA, Carmody T, Kern JK, King PG, Geier MR. Hum Exp Toxicol. 2013 Apr;32(4):434-40. doi: 10.1177/0960327112455671. PMID: 22893351

[114] Nephrotic syndrome caused by exposures to skin-lightening cosmetic products containing inorganic mercury. Chan TYK, Chan APL, Tang HL. Clin Toxicol (Phila). 2020 Jan;58(1):9-15. doi: 10.1080/15563650.2019.1639724. PMID: 31314603

33: Meat Two: Noxious Compounds

Genesis 1:29: God said, "See, I give you every seed-bearing plant that is upon all the earth and every tree that has seed-bearing fruit; they shall be yours for food".

While being a rich source of protein and a source of easily absorbed iron, the consumption of red meat, and especially processed meat, is strongly discouraged on the SANA Diet. This chapter is included to explain some reasons for avoiding meat, especially red meat.

This chapter has in part been adapted from the author's book "Neurodevelopment and Intelligence," thus explaining its focus on the impact of nutrition on the developing brain.

N-Nitrosyl Compounds

Consumption of meat increases the risk of cancer. Some of this risk is not inherent to the meat, but rather from the mode of the meat's preparation. The meat that carries the highest cancer risk is processed meat, with much of this risk coming from N-nitrosyl compounds (NNC) that are formed during the preparation and digestion of meats that have been processed with nitrates and nitrites.

Nitrates and nitrites are added to meat to give it a pink color, making it appear fresh, but they also deter bacterial growth. Lunch meats, baloney, salami, deli meats, and canned hams are examples of processed meats that are treated with nitrates or nitrites. Cooking processed meat at high temperatures (above about 300° F (150°C) promotes NNC formation (i.e., fried bologna). Stomach acid can also induce NNC formation from preserved meats. The nitrosation of amino acids in food can cause the formation of nitrosamines, many or most of which are indirect mutagens and carcinogens. Nitrosamines get metabolized into alkylating agents that can modify nucleobases in the DNA, causing random mutations, some of which cause cell dysfunction or cell death, and some of which cause cancer.

Curing, drying, and smoking meats can also promote the formation of NNCs when the meats are cooked or exposed to stomach acid. Salted fish and nicotine in tobacco are additional sources of NNC exposure. Of the 120 NNCs tested, about 80% are carcinogens; some are extremely potent carcinogens. The carcinogenic ones cause DNA adducts that result in mutations. Consumption of processed meats is also strongly associated with diabetes risk, as some NNCs are toxic to the β-cells of the pancreas and are pro-inflammatory.

Interestingly, the cancer risk imposed by NNCs appears to be largely confined to cancers of the mucosa that is directly exposed to NNCs, and of the brain. Thus, NNCs cause esophageal, stomach, colon, and rectal cancers, as well as brain cancers. The liver, an organ highly exposed to dietary NNCs, contains high levels of the DNA repair protein MGMT, which can thus undo most of the DNA damage caused by these compounds when they reach the liver via the portal circulation during digestion.

About 12 percent of adults do not express MCMT in the brain, and these individuals are 4.5 times more likely to develop brain tumors than are those who do. MGMT develops in the fetal brain during development. At six to eight weeks of development, 75% of fetuses do not express MGMT in the brain. By 19 weeks, 88% of fetuses have the same percentage as adults. Thus, there is an increased risk from NNC exposure during the first half of fetal life. Notably, prenatal exposure to processed meats increases the risk of brain cancer in children by 50%. Meanwhile, the gestational consumption of fresh fish lowers the risk of brain cancer in the child by 30%. Prenatal consumption of yellow-orange vegetables by the mother lowers the risk of brain cancer in the child by 20%, and a higher versus lower intake of grains lowers the risk by 10%.[1]

The GI mucosa is injured by NNCs, and thus, these compounds can affect the microbiome and mucosal barrier.

Dietary NNCs, in addition to their carcinogenic effect on the brain, may cause neurological or developmental injury. NNCs are neurotoxic, and the nitroso compound, N-ethyl-N-nitrosourea (ENU), has been found to disrupt developmental neurogenesis and alter memory formation in lab animals. Prenatal exposure to ENU is used to create brain tumors in animals for the study of potential anti-cancer treatments.[2] Prenatal exposure to ENU in mice disrupts developmental neurogenesis, is toxic to the neural stem cells, and alters memory formation. Additionally, ENU exposure in adult mice impairs spatial memory, alters behavior, and disrupts the generation of new neurons in the subventricular zone and dentate gyrus of the brain.[3]

Thus, NNCs from processed meats and other foods should be considered probable developmental neurotoxins, especially from exposure during the first half of pregnancy. NNCs likely act as neurotoxins throughout life. The one-in-eight individuals who do not express MGMT in the brain should be expected to be highly susceptible to neurologic injury from NNCs.

Heterocyclic Amines

Another set of compounds formed during the preparation of meat is the heterocyclic amines (HCA). About 15 to 20 HCA are suspected human carcinogens, and at least 17 HCA can be produced during the cooking of meat, particularly when it is cooked at higher temperatures. Stewing and simmering meat does not cause the formation of HCA; boiling or pressure cooking produces trivial amounts, and even microwave cooking of meat does not produce HCA as long as the meat does not dry out. Baking and roasting meats produce low levels of HCA as long as the meat does not dry out. Frying meat produces more; high-temperature frying still more; and grilling, especially flame grilling, where there is searing or charring, creates very high amounts of HCA. As long as the water content of the meat keeps the temperature at the boiling point or below (212° F), very little HCA is created. Once the surface of the meat dries or gets crispy, high amounts of HCA are produced.

Disrupting the cells of the meat allows sugars and amino acids in the cells to leak out, and this aids in the formation of HCA and glucosepane.

> Glucosepane is the principal cross-linked advanced glycation end-product (AGE) in the human body. It promotes arteriosclerosis, stiffening of the joints, wrinkling of the skin, and aging of the eyes.[4] AGEs bind to the receptor for AGE (RAGE), which promotes an increase in Aβ42 and the phosphorylation of Tau protein, key steps in the development of Alzheimer's disease.[5]

The recipe for glucosepane is one part lysine and one part arginine, heated in the presence of the reducing sugar glucose, with a small amount of water. The ingredients for HCA are creatine plus another amino acid and a simple sugar (glucose, fructose, galactose), heated to a temperature of 123 – 300° C (275 – 572° F). These conditions are easily met during the cooking of meat, especially if the muscle cells have been disrupted. The longer the cooking time and the higher the temperature, the more HCA is formed. At the upper range of cooking temperatures, HCA is very rapidly formed. Pressure cooking meat at 121° C is hot enough to cause HCA formation.

The freeze-thaw cycling, grinding (hamburger), and mechanical tenderization of meat disrupt the muscle cells and allow leakage of amino acids, glucose, and water from the intracellular space, greatly enhancing the formation of glucosepane during cooking. Pressing down on a hamburger patty to press out the fluid and have it sizzle on the grill is an excellent method for creating high amounts of HCA and glucosepane. The pan drippings (often used to make gravy) from cooking meat or fish have high amounts of HCA.

Various HCAs absorbed from the diet are further metabolized in the body into aminoimidazoarenes (AIA), which are pre-carcinogens that are further metabolized in the body to aryl nitrenium ions that form DNA adducts, causing mutations, and thus cancer.[6] Most mutagens are also teratogenic, and thus can cause birth defects and increase the risk of cancer in the child.

Carcinogenic HCA compounds can be found in the breast milk of rats fed meat cooked at high temperatures, and DNA adducts of these carcinogens are found in the organs of their pups.[7] Carcinogenic HCA are also found in human breast milk.[8] More dangerously, carcinogenic HCA crosses the placenta, and aryl nitrenium DNA adducts can be found in the organs of fetal primates that have been exposed to HCA from food in their mother's diet.[9]

The time of highest risk for mutations that can cause genetic disease and cancer is during cell division. Risk is especially elevated during the S phase, during which the DNA replicates and is highly exposed. In this phase, it is more likely that breaks in the DNA strand undergo an aberrant repair and thus result in a mutation. Fetal life and infancy are times of high risk for mutation due to the high rate of cell division during growth. Mice exposed to carcinogenic HCA in the first days of life formed liver cancers at middle age from doses that were a minuscule fraction of the chronic exposure dose required to cause cancer in adult mice.[10]

Almost all of the ova in a woman's ovaries are formed during her fetal life, before she was born. Thus, exposure to DNA adducts during pregnancy, resulting in female offspring, can potentially cause mutations that do not appear until the following generation. For males, sperm stem cells develop during early adolescence; thus, this is a time at which epigenetic imprinting or germ cell mutations can readily occur and create risk for the progeny. Exposure to mutagens at these times has the potential for germline mutations that can be passed down to later generations.

Pregnancy, infancy, and adolescence are periods when mutagens and carcinogens should be vigilantly avoided. And not just by women. It takes around 77 days for sperm to form from stem cells. Those who plan to be fathers should be especially careful to avoid exposure to mutagens and carcinogens during the three months before conception.

Breast development mainly occurs during early adolescence, and thus is a time when exposure to carcinogens can greatly increase the risk for the development of breast cancer later in adult life.

Are HCA neurotoxic?

2-Amino-1-methyl-6-phenylimidazo[4,5-b] pyridine (PhIP) is one of the most abundant HCA present in red meat that has been cooked at high temperatures. It is a human carcinogen. Mice exposed to dietary PhIP have been found to have oxidative damage of hippocampal synaptic proteins and higher levels of Beta-secretase 1 (BACE1) and the generation of Aβ, Aβ aggregations, tau protein phosphorylation, and damage to cholinergic neurons; all consistent with Alzheimer's disease processes.[11]

Harmane is another HCA that is produced during the cooking of meat, with levels more than twice as high in chicken as in beef. Harmane is a neurotoxin associated with tremors, movement disorders, and the development of Parkinson's disease (PD) in humans.[12] In a study that investigated the relative neurotoxicity of three subclasses of HCA compounds that are formed as a result of consuming cooked meat, five AIA, two β-carbolines (harmane and norharman), and an α-carboline were tested in rat midbrain cultures. All of the HCAs tested were selectively toxic to dopaminergic neurons, and thus are possible risk factors for PD. Among these eight HCAs, there was a 50-fold differential in neurotoxicity. Notably, neurotoxicity was not correlated with the carcinogenic potency of the HCA.[13] A recent study found that AIA binds to neuromelanin, which is then taken up by dopaminergic neurons in the brain, with subsequent oxidative toxicity specifically affecting these neurons.[14]

While HCA is toxic in cell culture, it cannot simply be assumed that there is a neurotoxic effect at the dose levels likely to be present in food.

The β-carbolines harmane and norharman, which are two of the most potent HCA neurotoxins in vitro, are not only present in cooked meats but are also found in coffee, tobacco smoke, and toasted bread.[15] Harmane is formed by burning tryptophan. Harmane and norharman are also present in cocoa and several herbs. Harmane, a lipophilic compound, concentrates in the brain at levels 55 times higher than in the blood plasma. Nevertheless, these two compounds do not appear to be neurotoxic in the context of commonly consumed food. Harmane and norharman have pharmacologic activity, acting as monoamine oxidase (MAO) inhibitors that may protect the brain from oxidative damage. While the effect may be from compounds other than β-carbolines, coffee and tobacco, two of the largest exposure sources of these compounds, are both associated with a lower risk of Parkinson's disease. This may be a hormetic effect, where low doses of these or other compounds in these foods provide a protective mechanism.

In a study that screened over a thousand medicinal compounds for agents that would increase the expression of EAAT2 (a.k.a. glutamate transporter 1, GLT-1) in human fetal astrocytes, harmane was among the most potent compounds.[16] EAAT2 is a transporter protein that takes glutamate up from the synaptic cleft, and thus terminates excitatory activity. EAAT2 is essential to prevent excitotoxicity.

Harmane is also a potent inhibitor of DYRK1, which participates in the development of brain morphology. In Down Syndrome, trisomy of chromosome 21 increases the expression of DYRK1; mice with one copy of this gene have reduced viability, a smaller brain, alterations in pyramidal cell structure, and cognitive impairment.[17] Thus, either insufficient or excess DYRK1A activity harms neurodevelopment. The inhibition of DYRK1 by harmane also promotes the activation of a transcription factor that increases the proliferation of pancreatic beta cells.[18] The seeds of Syrian rue contain high levels of harmane and are an abortifacient and hallucinogen. Harmane should thus be considered a developmental toxin.

β-carbolines can be converted in the brain to N-methyl-β-carboline cations, which are neurotoxic. It may be that β-carbolines have an insignificant carcinogenic or neurotoxic effect on their own, but they easily react with other compounds to form carcinogens and toxins.[19] While β-carbolines in food seem unlikely to promote adult neurotoxicity, HCA, such as AIA, are unlikely to be benign.[20]

Meat cooked at high temperatures produces carcinogenic HCA, some of which may have neurotoxic effects. Processed meat, especially when cooked at high temperatures, is also mutagenic, carcinogenic, and neurotoxic. These should be avoided by pregnant and lactating women, children, and those seeking to preserve their health and intelligence.

The SANA diet proscribes all mammalian meat, and advises avoidance of most other animal flesh other than oily fish, which it advises should be steamed or poached to keep cooking temperatures low, to prevent the formation of toxic compounds. The SANA diet allows occasional consumption of poultry, but advises that that be limited to white meat, cooked at or preferably below the boiling temperature; in part to prevent the formation of toxic compounds, but also to improve digestibility.

Sialic Acids

Humans are somewhat unique among mammals; we cannot make the sialic acid N-glycolylneuraminic acid (Neu5Gc) as do most other mammals, including most other primates, because of a mutation in the CMAH gene that all humans have. Sialic acids are among the sugars that adorn glycoproteins on the outer surface of cells. They have multiple functions, including self-recognition by the immune system.

Many viruses and other pathogens gain entry into the cell by adhering to specific sialic acid configurations on glycoproteins residing on the cell's outer membrane. Some time in our distant past, one of these diseases came close to driving humans to extinction. According to this theory, the disease, perhaps an ancient malaria parasite, strongly preferred binding to Neu5Gc rather than N-acetylneuraminic acid (Neu5Ac) on glycoproteins on the red blood cells, allowing the parasite to infect cells bearing Neu5Gc. The sole survivors of the plague were those early hominids that had a genetic mutation that prevented them from forming Neu5Gc. The hominids whose red blood cells bore Neu5Gc did not survive the disease, leaving no descendants.[21] The disease caused a genetic bottleneck; we are the descendants of those ancestors who could make Neu5Ac, the precursor of Neu5Gc, but not the final product.

Perhaps that species of malaria died out with those humans, but don't feel bad, there are over 200 other Plasmodium species, five of which can cause human malaria infections by binding to Neu5Ac-containing glycoproteins. These parasites are quite adaptable. They have been around for at least 15 million years, and quickly mutate to survive the medications we use in attempts to control them. Also, it is only a small number of malaria parasites that infect primates; 150 species of malaria infect birds, and 90 species infect lizards.

Evolution has an uncanny intelligence. The malaria parasite causes an infected individual to be a more attractive meal for uninfected mosquitoes,[22] but once infected, the mosquitoes are more attracted to non-infected hosts.[23] Thus, the parasite manipulates the metabolism of the host and the disease insect vector to increase the efficiency of their transmission.

Malaria, mostly as a result of *Plasmodium falciparum,* remains a major cause of death and disability in the world today.

Both intrinsic and extrinsic sialic acids may be involved in immunity and inflammation. The intrinsic sialic acid Neu5Ac is part of the glycoprotein of cells lining the blood vessels, and elevated serum levels are present in cardiovascular disease, likely reflecting the degree of vascular injury.[24] [25] Neu5Ac is also a component of neuronal cell membranes.

Humans can also have elevated levels of *extrinsic* Neu5Gc in the blood serum; elevated Neu5Gc levels are associated with vascular disease,[26] atherosclerosis, and coronary artery disease. Higher Neu5Gc blood levels are also associated with cancer risk.

While our bodies cannot make Neu5Gc, it can be present in the diet, as it is found in mammalian meat and milk whey, and it is absorbed from the diet. Beef has higher Neu5Gc levels than pork or lamb, while rabbit meat has considerably lower levels. Liver and sausage have much higher amounts of Neu5Gc than does muscle tissue. Consumption of sheep or goat milk or cheese promotes very high levels of Neu5Gc antibody reactivity as compared to cow's milk or even beef, with Roquefort cheese, made of sheep's milk, causing 30 times the impact of Gouda or Swiss cheese prepared from cow's milk. Yogurt has lower levels than milk, and hard cheese has lower levels than soft cheese. Rabbit meat has very low levels compared to other mammals. Buffalo cheese has even lower levels than bovine cheese. Poultry, eggs, and fish, not being mammalian, do not contain Neu5Gc.[27]

Although we lost the ability to make this sialic acid, we retain the enzymes that incorporate Neu5Gc into our cell surface glycoproteins. Exogenous Neu5Gc that is absorbed from the diet is absorbed into the cells and can be incorporated onto tissue glycoproteins during their formation. Cooking does not break Neu5Gc down. While humans no longer make Neu5Gc, the proteins that preferentially attach Neu5Ac or Neu5Gc onto glycoproteins remain. Thus, Neu5Gc that shows up in the diet can be placed on cells, with some cell types giving a preferential placement of Neu5Ac or Neu5Gc over the other. The immune system may then recognize cells bearing these sialic acids as foreign and respond to them as foreign or infected cells.

Neu5Gc consumption is associated with the risk of vascular disease. It is possible that Neu5Gc is an innocent bystander and just a marker of meat consumption; the elevated risk of vascular disease, metabolic syndrome, cancer, and inflammation associated with higher Neu5Gc levels in the body may be secondary to other factors present in or associated with meat consumption. Whether dietary Neu5Gc causes vascular disease or cancer or is simply a marker of its consumption remains a matter of ongoing investigation and controversy.[28]

What is of principal interest herein is whether Neu5Gc promotes inflammation and specifically neuroinflammation. Theoretically, consuming mammalian meat and whey may increase the risk of inflammation and autoimmune disease.[29] Since Neu5Gc is non-human, there is a concern that Neu5Gc glycoproteins may be recognized as foreign antigens. In a small study, most patients with multiple sclerosis (MS) were found to have antibodies to Neu5Ac and Neu5Gc, and antibody levels to sialic acid were considerably higher in MS patients than in patients with non-inflammatory neurologic disease or infectious neurological diseases.[30]

Meat during Pregnancy

A diet very high in meat consumption before pregnancy is associated with a 4-fold risk of having a child with autism spectrum disorder (ASD). Nevertheless, an unbalanced diet composed mostly of vegetables was also associated with increased risk (2.2-fold risk of ASD). The same study also found that taking calcium supplements during pregnancy was associated with a 50% reduction in the risk of a child developing ASD.[31] Women with autoimmune conditions are 34% more likely to have a child with ASD. Maternal immune thyroid disease increases the risk of ASD by 30%.[32] This creates a concern that dietary Neu5Gc from the consumption of mammalian meat may directly or indirectly increase ASD risk.

Several of the 14 human Sialic acid-binding immunoglobulin-type lectins (Siglecs) preferentially bind to Neu5Gc over Neu5Ac. Lectins are carbohydrate-binding proteins, and Siglecs are cell surface proteins, primarily found on immune cells, that bind to sialic acids. In addition to being expressed on immune cells, Siglec-5 and Siglec-14 are expressed on the amniotic epithelium, Siglec-6 is expressed by the placenta, and Siglec-11 is expressed by microglial cells in the CNS.[33] Expression of Siglet-11 in microglia is unique to humans and is neuroprotective, while Siglet-16 is inflammatory.[34] Modulators of Siglec-11 are being studied as potential treatments for neurodegenerative diseases such as AD and PD.[35] Thus, alterations in the type of sialic acids on cell surface glycoproteins can alter the immune response.

One of the genes that was most differentially expressed in the placentas of women with preeclampsia as compared to women with normal pregnancies was Siglec-6. Notably, the placental expression of Siglec-6 and the disease preeclampsia are both uniquely human and do not occur in other primates.[36] In a study of vegan women, only one of 775 (0.13%) vegan mothers had symptoms of preeclampsia.[37] This is remarkably (35 times) lower than the 4.6% incidence of preeclampsia in the general population of pregnant women.[38]

Meat consumption is associated with vascular inflammation; the placenta is a vascular organ. Inflammation of the placenta is injurious to the fetus, even if Neu5Gc does not directly affect neuro-development. Thus, consumption of mammalian meat and whey proteins may contribute to the pathology of preeclampsia.

Dietary intake of Neu5Gc may be a significant risk for gestational immunoreactivity from the consumption of meat and dairy. In contrast, eggs, fish, and poultry meat (chicken, turkey, and duck) would not be expected to confer this risk. Bovine dairy products do contain significant amounts of Neu5Gc, but far less than those from sheep and goats. Yogurt has less Neu5Gc than milk,[39] and hard cheeses have lower levels than soft cheeses.

Similar to the loss of the CMAH gene activity, which prevents the formation of Neu5Gc, humans and, in this case, Old World monkeys, lack a functioning gene for another immune-recognition glycoprotein carbohydrate that almost all other mammals have: GGTA1. GGTA1 codes for glycoprotein alpha-galactosyl-transferase-1, which links galactose molecules to form galactose-α-1,3-galactose, a.k.a. alpha-gal (α-gal). α-gal is a foreign antigen present in mammalian meat and dairy products; it is normal to form IgG antibodies to it. However, it is also possible to form IgE antibodies to it. This generally occurs after being bitten by a lone star tick (that presumably previously feasted on another mammal during an earlier stage of its development). IgE to α-gal can cause α-gal syndrome (AGS), a potentially life-threatening allergic reaction, usually 4 – 6 hours after eating meat or dairy products. Reactions range from hives to anaphylaxis. The treatment for AGS is the avoidance of mammal meat and dairy for two years.[40]

TMAO

Ideally, when food is eaten, the proteins are completely broken down during digestion, and the amino acids and small peptides are absorbed in the small intestine. When this occurs, there should not be any formation of TMAO.[41]

Meat, however, is typically incompletely digested; some of the meat becomes "fiber" that is fermented by bacteria in the gut. When this occurs, the nutrient L-carnitine is converted by gut bacteria into γ-butyrobetaine (γBB) or crotonobetaine. γBB is then converted into trimethylamine (TMA) by *Emergencia timonensis* or other gut bacteria.[42] Some of the other bacteria that can generate TMA include *Acinetobacter, Citrobacter, Escherichia, Klebsiella,* and *Proteus* species.[43] Crotonobetaine accelerates atherosclerosis in mice and may interact with γBB in causing vascular disease.[44] Choline, lecithin, and betaine that reach the colon can also be fermented by microbiota in the gut, inducing the formation of TMA.

TMA has the unpleasant odor of rotting fish.

Trimethylaminuria is an autosomal recessive genetic disorder in which there is an alteration in the FMO3 gene; this defect slows TMA metabolism, raising TMA levels in the body. People with this disorder have a fishy odor in their urine, sweat, and breath after the consumption of foods high in choline. TMA can also cause halitosis from infections and give rise to the fishy odor from bacterial vaginosis.

TMA is absorbed from the colon into the portal circulation and metabolized in the liver to trimethylamine N-oxide (TMAO), which smells like fresh fish. While this may seem like an improvement, individuals with elevated TMAO blood levels are at elevated risk of cardiovascular disease, myocardial infarctions, heart failure, diabetes, strokes, and perhaps cancer. TMAO causes vascular inflammation, oxidative stress, DNA damage, and platelet reactivity.[45] [46] [47] [48] [49]

TMAO crosses the blood-brain barrier and can be measured in the cerebrospinal fluid.[50] In vitro, TMA appears to compromise BBB function, while TMAO may enhance tight junction function.[51] [52]

If the nutrients carnitine, choline, or betaine are not absorbed by the small intestine, they can be fermented in the colon into γBB and then into TMA. Since meat contains phosphatidylcholine as part of the cell membrane, undigested meat that enters the colon thus provides both choline and carnitine for the creation of TMA and, later, TMAO. Thus, L-carnitine in meat and betaine, choline, lecithin, and phosphatidylcholine from various foods can be converted into TMAO by colonic bacteria.

L-carnitine is an important nutrient as it carries acetyl groups from the metabolism of fatty acids across the mitochondrial membrane for beta-oxidation for the utilization of fat in ATP production. L-carnitine is an essential nutrient for premature infants; however, by full-term, we can make carnitine from dietary amino acids.

How does undigested meat or other sources of TMA enter the colon? Moving through the GI tract sequentially:

A. Eating very large quantities of these nutrients might prevent them from being fully digested if the consumption exceeds the system's capacity or needs.

B. Meat needs to be chewed sufficiently so that the pieces are small enough to be fully digested. Swallowing large pieces of meat may prevent full digestion. People who are missing teeth or eating hurriedly may swallow large pieces of meat that evade complete digestion.

C. Lack of stomach acid. Stomach acid helps break down the meat and denatures proteins, making them more easily accessible to digestive enzymes. Medications that block stomach acid, or loss of acid production from chronic infection with *H. pylori,* can thus prevent the full digestion of meat.

D. Pancreatic or other digestive enzyme insufficiencies. If lipase, proteases, or peptidases are insufficient to digest the meat, it will end up in the colon, where it is fermented.

E. Dumping syndrome and other causes of rapid emptying of the stomach and/or rapid small intestinal transit. If the bolus does not have sufficient time to be digested, it can enter the colon undigested. Thus, lactose intolerance, as an example, lactose ingestion with a meal may cause rapid transit of chyme containing partially undigested meat to enter the colon. Other causes of accelerated small intestinal transit include small intestinal bacterial overgrowth (SIBO), excess sorbitol, spicy foods, some artificial sweeteners, and certain medications such as erythromycin, which increases small bowel motility.

F. Any conditions that cause steatorrhea (fatty stools) may increase the transport of phosphatidylcholine and other lipids to enter the colon, where they can be fermented into γBB and thus TMA. This can occur in pancreatic insufficiency, liver damage, celiac disease, diseases of the small intestine, and parasitic infections such as *Giardia.*

It may be that only high levels of TMAO cause damage; there is likely a threshold below which there is no injury from TMAO. Thus, chronic low-level production may not cause any injury, while peak levels, even of short duration, may induce harm. For example, eating a large steak may cause short-term, but very high levels, which might induce injury. Nevertheless, individuals who frequently eat red meat are more likely to harbor a population of bacteria that are adept at converting creatine and choline into γBB and TMA and crotonobetaine.

In a trial of healthy American adults consuming a diet with 25% of calories as protein from red meat, white meat, or non-meat in cross-over diets, TMAO levels were only elevated with the consumption of red meat. In some subjects, red meat raised TMAO levels ten times more than did white meat. TMAO levels were not associated with dietary choline in any of the three diet groups. In this study, dairy and eggs were included in the diet for all three diets. Red meat consumption was associated with a lower renal clearance rate of TMAO.[53] Thus, red meat (mammalian meat) can cause an increase in TMAO, even in healthy subjects without digestive disorders. In a review of several studies, fish consumption was also associated with increased TMAO levels. Low-dose aspirin (81 mg/day) appears to lower TMAO production and blood levels.[54]

Marine fish and crustaceans have high levels of TMAO, as it protects their proteins from distortion from the pressure of the water column on them; thus, fish living deeper in the water have higher TMAO levels. TMA is the result of bacterial decomposition of TMAO in the flesh of dead fish and contributes to the unpleasant smell of fish that is going bad.[55]

Eggs and TMAO

Eggs are a rich source of choline, in the form of phosphatidylcholine, and thus, there has been concern that consumption of eggs may cause detrimental amounts of TMA formation. In a dose-response study in which subjects consumed zero to six hard-boiled eggs in a single meal, there was a clear increase in TMAO levels several hours after the consumption of multiple eggs. However, the amount of TMAO elevation in response to the number of eggs varied greatly among different participants, with some having very little response to one or two eggs, while others had a much more pronounced elevation in the production of TMAO as measured in the blood and urine.[56] This likely reflects the availability of bacteria that process TMA. Overcooked eggs and long-boiled eggs are difficult to digest; thus, the mode of cooking the egg may also influence TMA production. It is the yolk of the egg that contains the choline that can be fermented into TMA. Thus, the SANA diet specifies the time and temperature for cooking eggs in the shell to maximize digestibility.

In a randomized study, overweight postmenopausal women were given either two eggs or a yolk-free substitute every day for four weeks. Women consuming two eggs with yolks had higher plasma levels of the nutrients choline and betaine, but TMAO was not increased in comparison to the women not consuming egg yolks.[57] In another randomized crossover study, young healthy men and women were given either oatmeal or 2 eggs for breakfast daily for 4 weeks, and then, after a three-week wash-out, switched to the other breakfast for another 4 weeks. There were no changes in plasma TMAO.[58]

In another study wherein participants consumed three eggs per day for four weeks, there was no increase in TMAO, but choline levels did increase.[59] In another 14-week crossover study, after a two-week egg-free washout, young healthy participants were assigned to consume 1, 2, and 3 eggs per day, each for 4 weeks. Eating one to three eggs per day was associated with an increase in HDL cholesterol (which is associated with lower atherosclerosis risk). Neither LDL nor TMAO levels increased with the consumption of two to three eggs per day.[60]

TMAO levels were also recorded in a study in which nutritionally at-risk, Amerindian infants in Ecuador aged 6–9 months were randomized to consume one egg a day for 6 months. At follow-up, those consuming eggs had significantly increased TMAO levels. (Mean of egg-eaters: 4.1 μmol/L as compared to 2.6 μmol/L in control children.) While higher than the control infants, these TMAO levels are not high, if using vegetarian adults as a norm,[61] and considerably lower than levels associated with cardiovascular disease,[62] [63] although caution should be used in comparing levels between studies, as different methods may have been used. Additionally, one egg a day for an infant would be about equal to an adult consuming 4 eggs per day, if adjusting for metabolic and caloric intake.

Other than the top study, in which hard-boiled eggs were consumed, the method of preparation was not discussed in these studies. Over-cooked (boiled) eggs are poorly digested, as are overcooked fried eggs. Preparation likely affects the absorption, and thus the amount of choline that reaches the colon, where it can be fermented.

Another issue complicating the interpretation of TMAO risk is that plasma TMAO levels are inversely related to renal function. Thus, while TMAO may injure the kidneys, TMAO levels rise with a decline in renal function. In a study assessing TMAO risk, after adjusting for renal clearance rates in a high-risk population, TMAO was no longer a risk factor for stroke or heart failure.[64] Thus, studies evaluating TMAO risk need to adjust for renal clearance.[65] Children and other young and healthy individuals may be at low risk from TMAO as a result of high renal function, maintaining low serum levels, even when there are moderate levels of TMAO production. To better understand the body's production of TMAO from different diets, 24-hour urinary collection may be required, or at least correction for renal clearance. Animal studies do suggest risk, so the risk is not limited to those with renal decline.

The facility to produce TMAO appears to be associated with the commensal community of the colon. Those eating a plant-based diet are less likely to harbor bacteria that readily form TMA, while those eating a Western diet have an abundance of these bacteria. Thus, occasional consumption of moderate portions of fish or other flesh is unlikely to maintain a sufficient population of *E. timonensis* or other bacteria required to ferment carnitine into γBB.[66]

The SANA recommendation on egg consumption is to prepare them properly so that they are easily digested. Healthy individuals with normal renal function appear unlikely to be harmed by eating up to three eggs a day, but this may not be the case if the eggs are poorly digested or the person has a decline in renal function. Avoid overcooking eggs.

Consumption of red meat increases TMAO even in healthy individuals. White meat does not have this effect. Fish, especially deep-water fish, contain significant levels of TMAO. It appears to be the metabolites of carnitine, crotonobetaine, and γ-butyrobetaine, from red meat, rather than choline, that increase TMA and TMAO production in human studies.[67]

As long as digestion is normal, the risk from normal amounts of dietary choline should not pose a risk. The risk is even lower among those who consume a diet rich in various plant fibers, whose enteric microbiome is dominated by *Bacteroidetes*.

While choline that enters the colon can be metabolized by enteric bacteria to TMA and then converted into atherogenic TMAO in the liver, phosphatidylcholine appears to escape or at least be considerably less susceptible to this fate, perhaps as over 90% of the phosphatidylcholine in the diet is absorbed. Phosphatidylcholine supplements to the diet, not exceeding the AI (Adequate Intake level), are unlikely to cause injury in those with normal digestion and absorption.

Consumption of red meat is associated with inflammation and increased BMI. NNC from nitrates or nitrites in processed or cured meats consumed during pregnancy can increase the risk of brain cancer in the child, and some NNC may be metabolized into compounds toxic to neuronal stem cells. The HCA PhIP, which forms during high-temperature cooking of red meat, is neurotoxic, enters the placenta, and is present in breast milk. Neu5Gc from meat, especially from organ meat and from milk, and especially sheep and goat whey, is easily absorbed from the diet and integrated into glycoproteins. Neu5Gc-adorned glycol-proteins can promote autoimmune activity. Incorporation of Neu5Gc into these cell membrane proteins may increase the risk of preeclampsia, neurodegenerative diseases, and autoimmune diseases. TMAO from the consumption of red meat, at least in theory, may injure the vasculature.

Phenylacetylglutamine: Another byproduct of fermentation, created when microbes in the lower gut break down dietary protein that has not been adequately digested and absorbed, such as meat, is phenylacetylglutamine (PAG). When the amino acid phenylalanine gets fermented in the colon, it can become acetylated to form phenylacetic acid (PAA), which is absorbed back into the body where it becomes conjugated with glutamine and glycine in the liver or kidney, forming PAG.[68] PAG enhances platelet activation and thrombosis, and is a risk factor for heart attack, heart failure, stroke, and death.[69] [70]

Meat and the Kidney

As outlined in Chapter 3 (Table 3A), the fermentation of various amino acids in the gut can produce toxic metabolites. Among these is p-cresyl sulfate (PCS). PCS is produced from the fermentation of aromatic amino acids (phenylalanine, tryptophan, and tyrosine. PCS is a uremic toxin that causes oxidative stress, increases inflammatory cytokines and TGF-β1 expression, promotes insulin resistance, damages renal tubular cells, and causes kidney dysfunction. The fermentation of tryptophan in the colon results in the formation of indoxyl sulfate (IS), which is toxic to the kidneys, heart, bones, and brain. IS is a potent uremic toxin and also causes altered mental status in those with chronic kidney disease, resulting in apathetic behavior, reduced motor activity, and impairment of motor coordination and memory.[71] The consumption of red meat is associated with increased levels of PCS, IS, and TMAO.[72] In a follow-up study examining dietary patterns, those in the top 25% for the consumption of red meat were 73% more likely to develop chronic kidney disease (CKD) as compared to those in the lowest quartile.[73] The risk of CKD was linearly associated with processed meat consumption. The risk of CKD, however, has a U-shaped curve when it comes to overall protein consumption, with the lowest level for those consuming around 75 mg of protein per day. [74] It is not protein, but red meat, that imparts CKD risk.

Nutrients from Meat

Fatty Acids

Meat is an important source of fat in the diet. This is not just the visible fat that is seen in marbled ribeye steak, chicken skin, or just when fatty tissues are added to hamburger to make it "juicier".

Hamburger meat is generally 30% fat, although it may be as high as 40% fat. Fat provides nine calories of energy per gram, while protein provides four calories of energy. After cooking, a three-ounce, 70% lean (30% fat) hamburger contains 61% of its calories as fat. Even a 90% lean hamburger (10% fat) has 49% of its calories as fat, and a 97% super lean hamburger (3% fat) has 26% of its calories as fat.

The reason that there is so much fat in even healthy lean muscle tissue is that the external and internal cell membranes, including those of organelles such as mitochondria, are a bilipid membrane that is in large part composed of fatty acids. These fatty acids are mostly in the form of phospholipids or sphingolipids, each molecule of which contains two fatty acid groups. A high-fat diet causes myosteatosis, with storage of fat within the muscle cells. Feeding cattle with a corn-based diet also causes myosteatosis.

The presence of fat in meat is not inherently unhealthy; we require certain fats in our diet. The fatty acids linoleic acid (18:2, n-6) and linolenic acid (18:3, n-3) are essential polyunsaturated fatty acids that, like amino acids and vitamins, cannot be synthesized by our bodies, or for that matter, by the bodies of chickens, cows, crows, goats, or fish. And this is where the problems arise.

Most animals, including humans, who eat a natural diet and food in the natural food chain, will consume foods with a roughly 1:1 to 1:2 ratio of n-6 to n-3 fats. Cattle, grazing on grass, have an n-6 to n-3 fats ratio of about 1.5 to 1 in their flesh, reflective of the ratio of these fats in the grass they eat. A problem arises when animals for meat production are fed on corn or other products that have a high n-6 to n-3 ratio. Corn, which makes up about 90% of the diet of cattle raised in feedlots, has an n-6 to n-3 ratio of *45 to 1*, and this becomes reflected in the meat of these animals. The calves are kept in the feedlots for about 140 days before being butchered. The reason for such a short time is that harvest around the end of the adolescent growth spurt gives the highest feed-to-meat ratio, and thus the best return on investment. Furthermore, if these animals are kept in a feedlot for even a few more weeks, they often sicken and die. Even during the 20-week feedlot experience, these are not healthy animals; most of the antibiotics used in the United States are administered to animals in feedlots to keep the animals from getting sick. Corn is also a major component of feed for chickens, which are generally slaughtered at 42 days of age in the E.U. and at around 47 days in the U.S. If you have noticed that your fried chicken legs are smaller than when you were a kid, it is because chickens take about 12 weeks to mature, and it used to be typical to harvest them at 10 to 12 weeks of age, rather than the current 6 to 7 weeks of age. A chicken used to be large enough to feed a family, but is now more like a personal pizza. Corn is also a major component of feed for laying hens, and thus a source of fatty acids contained in eggs.

It is estimated that 70% of the calories consumed by Americans come directly or indirectly from corn. Only a tiny amount is from sweet corn (corn on the cob) or popcorn. Most of the corn is large-kernelled, starchy field corn. Some corn is used to make corn flakes, cornbread, tortillas, corn chips, and cornstarch. Many more calories from corn are present in the diet as corn oil and corn syrup, and hidden in the diet as the corn-fed animals whose products we eat.

Soybeans, which are also used as animal feed, have a 7:1 n-6 to n-3 ratio, which is less extreme than corn, but still proinflammatory. Rapeseed cake has a 2 to 1 ratio. Many vegetable oils, including sunflower, safflower, peanut, and sesame seed oils, have significant amounts of n-6 fats but are devoid of n-3 fats; their n-6 to n-3 ratio is thus roughly one to zero.

Most meat sold in the United States has a fat content with a very high n-6 to n-3 ratio. Diets with high n-6 to n-3 ratios are proinflammatory and associated with chronic diseases, such as coronary artery disease, acne, asthma, pulmonary disease, arthritis, obesity, and cancer.[75 76 77 78] Grass-fed beef and mutton, which is generally range-fed, should have lower n-6 to n-3 ratios.

An inflammatory milieu is hard on the brain; high levels of n-6 fatty acids are associated with neuro-oxidative stress. High n-6 to n-3 ratios are associated with an increased risk of diseases of dementia, seizure disorders, chronic headaches, and sleep disorders.[79 80] High n-6 to n-3 ratio diets and blood levels are associated with mood disorders, self-harm and suicidal behavior, psychosis, impulsivity and aggression, bipolar syndrome, and major depression.[81 82 83 84] Children with high cellular n-6 to n-3 ratios are at higher odds of having ASD, ADHD, learning disorders, depression, and a high n-6 to n-3 ratio is associated with a lower IQ and poorer neurodevelopment.[85 86 87 88 89] For example, in a study of 6-month-old infants, those whose mothers were in the lowest quartile of dietary n-6 to n-3 ratio during pregnancy had higher mental development and psychomotor development on the Bayley Scales of Infant Development than those in the higher three quartiles of n-6 to n-3 fat intake.[90]

Numerous trials using fish oil supplements have been performed and, at best, show mild benefits. The results reflect the weak approach. The underlying issue is a diet packed with high levels of n-6 fats; adding a relatively small amount of n-3 fats is an inefficient means for correcting the excess n-6 fats in the cellular membranes resulting from the extreme imbalance of polyunsaturated fats in the diet, as well as overall fatty diets. A more effective approach is to limit the amount of n-6 and other fats in the diet. This is difficult to do on the standard American diet.

The SANA diet recommends against the consumption of mammalian meat, and ranks chicken as an A (avoid). Nevertheless, if one chooses to eat chicken, it is suggested that free-range chicken and free-range chicken eggs be chosen. Coldwater fatty fish are high in the fatty acids EPA and DHA; very-long-chain n-3 fats, as a result of a food chain based on cold water algae. Farm-raised catfish and tilapia have the n-6 to n-3 ratio given by their diets. Farm-raised catfish are fed pellets made of soybeans, corn, and wheat, and thus have an n-6 to n-3 ratio more similar to chicken than to wild-caught fish.

Choline and Betaine

Choline is a nutrient that is essential for brain development and health, and is also a nutrient that is commonly consumed in quantities below the Recommended Daily Allowance. Choline is structurally and functionally similar to a non-protein-forming amino acid. While our metabolism can synthesize small amounts of choline, they are insufficient. When placed on low choline diets, adults develop fatty liver disease and liver and muscle damage.

Choline is used in the formation of the neurotransmitter and neuromodulator acetylcholine. Acetylcholine activity is not limited to synapses in the CNS, where it is important for learning and memory; it is also the major neurotransmitter for the autonomic nervous system. Acetylcholine activates muscular activity, affects glandular function, gastrointestinal activity, vascular tone, and sweating. In addition to being a precursor for the neurotransmitter acetylcholine, choline is needed for the formation of sphingomyelin for the formation of the myelin sheath in the white matter of the brain and nerves.

Most of the choline in the diet, and almost all of that from animal sources, comes in the form of phosphatidylcholine (PC). Foods high in PC include lean meat (especially liver), fish, egg yolks, shrimp, dairy, and legumes such as soy. Most seeds contain some PC, but not in high levels. Some vegetables, such as broccoli and cauliflower, provide a significant amount of choline, while most vegetables have lower amounts. The meat of grazing animals is high in PC; they form it from choline present in the leaves of plants they graze on. Nevertheless, it is difficult for humans to get sufficient choline from a vegan diet without legumes.

Phosphatidylcholine is the predominant phospholipid in the diet and the body. PC and other phospholipids have two long-chain fatty acids. During digestion, one of the fatty acids is removed by pancreatic phospholipase A2, resulting in lysoPC and a free fatty acid. Both of these are readily absorbed by enterocytes in the small intestine. PC is then reconstructed in the enterocyte by adding a fatty acid back to lysoPC.[91] PC is fat-soluble and transported into triglyceride-rich chylomicrons. In contrast, choline is water-soluble, and dietary choline is absorbed by enterocytes of the small intestine via specific choline transport proteins. Choline is then transported into the interstitial space and enters the portal circulation. It is carried to the liver, and there, converted to PC. About 95% of the choline in the body is in the form of phosphatidylcholine.[92]

PC is a major component of the lipid membrane of the cells, and a major component of the surfactant of the lungs that keeps the alveoli from collapsing. Choline is in part converted into the vitamin-like compound betaine (trimethylglycine) in the body. Betaine is a nutrient that is found in high concentrations in quinoa, spinach, beets, wheat, and saltwater fish. Betaine acts as an osmolyte in the cell. Under osmotic stress (dehydration), cells pull in electrolytes and other organic osmolytes such as sorbitol to maintain osmotic pressure and keep sufficient water in the cell. Excessive electrolytes, however, can interfere with protein conformation and function. Betaine also holds water in the cells, but unlike sorbitol, it does not interfere with protein configuration or function.

Betaine helps recycle homocysteine to methionine in a secondary pathway to that using 5-MTHF in the methylation cycle; the enzyme betaine homocysteine methyltransferase (BHMT) uses betaine to convert homocysteine (HCY) to methionine. This enzyme requires zinc as a cofactor.[93] Here, betaine acts as a methyl donor, and trimethylglycine is converted to dimethylglycine. The use of betaine in the remethylation of HCY into methionine is a minor pathway; it can help, but not overcome defects in the folate pathway.[94] Nevertheless, this pathway is considerably more active and perhaps essential during pregnancy and fetal life.

Choline levels in the cord blood of infants are three times higher than those in the maternal blood,[95] and choline levels in the amniotic fluid are ten times higher than those in the maternal blood. This is indicative of the increased demand for choline during development. The fetus drinks the choline-laden amniotic fluid,[96] which activates fetal α7-nicotinic acetylcholine receptors, which facilitate the maturation of GABA inhibitory synapses and the development of cerebral inhibition.

Choline insufficiency can cause muscle and liver damage. Choline deficiency in adults causes non-alcoholic fatty liver disease (NAFLD), thus contributing to a disease that affects one in four American adults and half of all obese adults. Choline deficiency is one of the very few single-nutrient deficiencies that increases spontaneous carcinogenesis; this risk results from chronic fatty liver injury. Choline is protective against fatty liver disease; this effect may be mediated in part by betaine.[97] Low vitamin D status may also increase the risk of NAFLD.[98] [99] [100]

(The role of choline in Alzheimer's disease and its supplementation is discussed in Chapter 25)

Choline and the Developing Brain

In women, lower gestational plasma choline levels were associated with lower infant gestational age at birth, poorer behavioral development at 3 months of age, and poorer development of inhibitory neurons. Among women with low plasma choline levels, those given choline supplements bore infants at a higher gestational age, with higher neurodevelopment and less social withdrawal and attention problems at the age of 40 months.[101]

In a non-interventional, cross-sectional follow-up study, children of women in the top quartile of choline consumption measured during the second trimester of pregnancy (mean 404 mg/day as compared to those in the lowest quartile, consuming 266 mg of choline per day), had higher visuospatial memory and verbal and nonverbal intelligence scores at age seven.[102] The effect size, however, was not particularly large; perhaps equivalent to one to three IQ points. First-trimester choline intake was found to have a smaller association that did not reach statistical significance. Note, however, that the mean intake of choline for women in the top quartile of choline intake was 404 mg of choline per day; less than the RDA for choline in pregnant women of 450 mg/day. This indicates that fewer than one in eight pregnant women in the study population consumed adequate choline.

In a study of 154 mother-infant dyads, maternal blood was collected at 16 and 36 weeks of gestation and assayed for choline, betaine, dimethylglycine, methionine, homocysteine, cysteine, folate, total B12, and holotranscobalamin (a marker of B12 status); all factors that participate in the methionine cycle. The estimated mean choline intake was 383 g/day. The infants were tested with the Bayley Scales of Infant Development at age 18 months. Plasma choline and plasma betaine levels at 16 weeks of gestation were both associated with infant cognitive scores.[103]

In a Canadian study of toddlers, the dietary intake of choline and betaine was assessed using three-day food records at age one and again one year later. The mean intake of total choline (choline plus betaine) was 174 mg/day at age one and 205 mg/day at age two. Only 28.1% of one-year-olds and 44.2% of two-year-olds met the RDA for choline intake. Children with higher plasma betaine levels at age two had better visual-motor development.[104] In a study of 5-year-old children from Seychelles, plasma betaine levels, but not choline levels, were positively associated with language scores on the Preschool Language Scale.[105]

As seen in the rat studies, the effect of choline supplementation during gestation may protect the developing brain from injury. Supplementation with 2,000 mg of choline per day during pregnancy in women who drank alcohol had infants with closer to normal processing speeds, more catch-up growth in weight and head circumference in the first year of life, as compared to those not getting the supplement.[106]

In a study of women with gestational infections, 41% had elevated CRP levels. Infants from these pregnancies had decreased self-regulation at one year of age. Among these women, children of mothers who had higher choline levels had better inhibition of auditory cerebral response, and at one year of age had similar self-regulation to infants of healthy pregnancies.[107]

In another study, maternal serum choline and C-reactive protein (CRP), a marker of inflammation, were measured. Women with choline levels below 7.06 μM had more stress and depression than did women with higher choline levels. Infants of mothers with higher choline levels had larger head circumferences, and the children had higher processing speeds. Higher maternal CRP levels were associated with slower processing speed in the infants, but this effect was mitigated by higher choline levels, at least in males;[108] the brain of male infants appears to be more sensitive to CRP-associated inflammation.[109] At age four, the children of mothers with lower choline levels in this population had more attention problems and social withdrawal.[110]

An observational study found that plasma choline levels at 16 weeks of gestation were associated with Bayley Scales of Infant Development scores at 18 months of age. Choline supplemented as phosphatidylcholine is now generally recommended during pregnancy, and is even more important for women whose children are at increased risk of behavioral problems or schizophrenia. A daily dose of PC from 3000 to 5000 mg, equivalent to 450 to 750 mg of choline, appears to be appropriate as a supplement during pregnancy.[111] Adding such a supplement to typical dietary PC intake would give a total daily intake of about 750 to 1150 mg of choline per day.

Phosphatidylcholine supplementation during pregnancy is associated with a lower incidence of attention problems and less social withdrawal in the offspring at 40 months, as compared to children in the placebo group.[112] Early evidence suggests that prenatal PC supplementation (but not choline supplements) may significantly diminish the risk of the development of schizophrenia among those with a genetic proclivity to it.[113]

In a double-blinded RCT of maternal choline supplementation, infants were assessed at 4, 7, 10, and 13 months of age. The women in the low choline (LC) groups took 480 mg of PC per day, and those in the high choline (HC) groups took 930 mg of PC per day. Children of mothers from the HC group were found to have significantly faster reaction times. Among the women in the LC group, those who took the choline supplement on more days had children with faster reaction times than those who took it fewer days during the third trimester.[114]

There are four main phosphatidates in the lipid membranes of the cell: Phosphatidylcholine (PC), phosphatidylethanolamine (PE), phosphatidylserine (PS), and phosphatidylinositol (PI). PC is the most abundant of these in the body. For example, in the rat liver, PC comprises 70% of the phospholipids; PE 27%, and PS 3%. In the rat brain, however, PS is much more abundant, making up about 17% of the phosphatidates, with PE composing 46%, and PC only 37% PC. The ratios are similar in humans. Phosphatidylserine levels are greatly increased in the brain, especially in the gray matter, while phosphatidylethanolamine dominates in the white matter.

Multiple studies have demonstrated that the use of oral phosphatidylserine supplementation can help slow age-related decline in neurologic function, such as the loss of dendrites in the hippocampus with age, and improve cognitive function.[115] [116] PS supplements have also been found to improve exercise tolerance and recovery, and lower cortisol response to stress.[117] These studies have focused on resilience to injury and aging rather than neurodevelopment; nevertheless, phosphatidylserine is essential for brain development and function.

Phosphatidylserine is especially abundant in the inner leaf of the cell membrane in neural tissues, where it is metabolically active, participating in signaling that stimulates neuronal growth and survival. PS in the brain is primarily formed from PC via the enzyme phosphatidylserine synthase 1 (PSS1) in a reaction in which serine is added to, and choline is removed from PC.

PC + serine <—> PS + choline

The favored substrate for PSS1 in the brain is PC 18:0, 22:6; this is phosphatidylcholine in which one fatty acid is stearic acid (18:0), and the other docosahexaenoic acid (DHA, C22:6, n-3). To a lesser extent, oleic acid (18:1, 9) can be used in place of stearic acid in PS, and this occurs slightly more often in the white matter of the brain. Similarly, DHA and oleic acid (18:1, n-9) are the dominant fatty acid components of PE in the white matter of the brain, with the PE in the gray matter slightly more likely to contain stearic acid than oleic acid.

Stearic acid can be formed in the body; in contrast to DHA is an n-3 fatty acid. Although DHA can be synthesized from the essential fatty acid α-linolenic acid (ALA; 18:3 n-3), the efficiency of this conversion is low. Thus, the diet must contain sufficient ALA, and it is advantageous for the diet to contain significant amounts of DHA.[118] The most abundant source of dietary DHA is oily fish, and the incorporation of DHA into PS in the brain explains the better neurodevelopment of children whose mothers consumed oily fish during pregnancy. PC with oleic acid (18:1) may also be incorporated in place of stearic acid, especially in the white matter of the brain. PE in the brain also has DHA and 18:0 or 18:1 as the dominant fatty acids.[119] Serine is a non-essential amino acid, and thus can be manufactured in the body from other amino acids.

The food highest in phosphatidylserine is brain, but consumption of neurologic tissue should be avoided because of the risk of prion diseases such as Mad Cow Disease. Other foods high in PS are the fish mackerel, herring, tuna, chicken heart and liver, and white beans. Lower levels of PS are present in chicken breast, beef, and pork.[120] The body can interconvert the phosphatidates, and most of the PS in the brain is derived from PC; thus, dietary PS does not appear to be required for health when there is adequate PC in the diet.

With aging, however, the enzyme PSS1 and PEMT (phosphatidylethanolamine methyltransferase), which form PC, may not function as well and thus limit the formation of PS in the brain. Thus, PS supplements and foods such as mackerel may be helpful for the prevention of cognitive decline. Some supplements that have helped improve neurologic functions in previous studies include naturally derived mixtures of phospholipids. Thus, unless head-to-head studies comparing PS to PE or PC for cognitive function show otherwise, it may be that any of them can help. Dietary n-3 fatty acids, and especially DHA or EPA, which can be converted to DHA, may also act as limiting factors for neuronal health and brain development.

The Upper Tolerable Limit of choline intake is 3,500 mg per day. High levels cause fishy body odor and gastrointestinal side effects from the fermentation of the choline into TMA. Choline, bound to phospholipids in the form of PC from egg yolk, is absorbed four times more efficiently than choline salts as supplements.[121] This should be taken to indicate that more choline is absorbed as PC, and that *several times less choline remains unabsorbed,* and thus, is liable to fermentation into TMA. If supplements are used, they should be in the form of PC or preferably as L-α-glycerophosphorylcholine, rather than as choline salts.

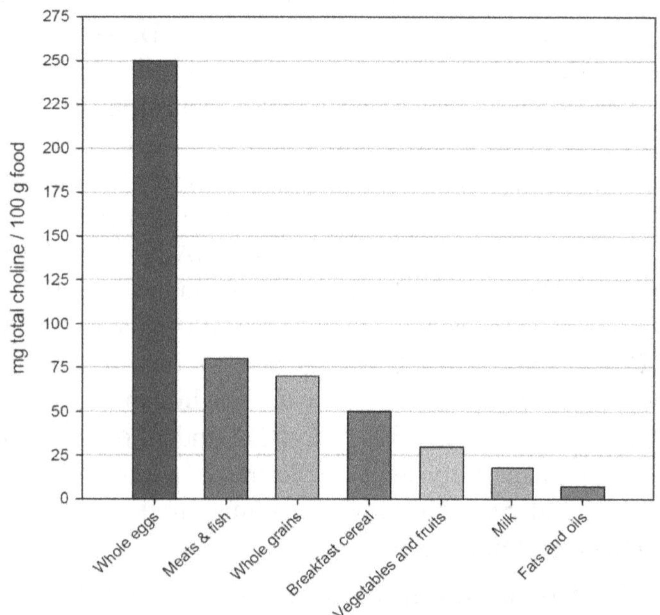

Figure 33A: Choline content in various food groups.[122]

It is common among the American population to have a dietary intake of choline below the recommended daily allowance (RDA). Part of this may arise from a misplaced cholesterol phobia. As demonstrated by the studies on the consumption of one to three eggs, HDL was raised with egg consumption, while LDL levels were unchanged; thus, presumably lowering cardiovascular disease risk. PC in the meal decreases cholesterol absorption; soluble fiber and many plant phytosterols also lower cholesterol absorption.[123]

Eggs are an excellent source of PC. One large egg contains 147 mg of easily absorbed choline, and thus, two large eggs would supply 65% of the daily adequate intake level for a pregnant woman. Since choline from eggs in the form of PC is well absorbed, the risk of TMA formation is low as long as the intestinal function is normal. In the studies cited above, consumption of one to three eggs a day raised choline and HDL levels without increasing TMAO levels.

BMAA

An uncommon but interesting dietary cause of neurodegeneration results from the consumption of cycad seed. It is not the cycad plant but a soil bacterium, a cyanobacterium, that produces the toxic non-protein-forming amino acid, β-methylamino-L-alanine (BMAA). BMAA is taken up by the plant and concentrates in the fleshy covering of the cycad seed. When vervet monkeys with ApoE4 were given BMAA orally, they developed brain lesions identical to Alzheimer's disease. BMAA crosses the BBB into the brain, but seems to get trapped there, where it acts as an excitotoxin that induces oxidative stress.

Nevertheless, eating cycad seed flour alone does not explain the high incidence of amyotrophic lateral sclerosis/ parkinsonism–dementia complex (ALS/PDC) among the Chamorro people of Guan who consume cycad flour. Large bats called flying foxes feed on the cycad seed coat and bioconcentrate BMAA. These flying foxes are considered a delicacy. Pigs and other animals that eat the cycad seed can also bioaccumulate BMAA. It is eating animals that bioconcentrate BMAA that appears to cause ALS/PDC in the Chamorro.[124] If you are visiting the island of Guam and are offered fried flying fox, I will remind you that it is considered a "D" for please, politely Decline to Dine on this delicacy.

Guam is not the only place where BMAA accumulates in the brain and is associated with AD and amyotrophic lateral sclerosis (ALS). Brain tissue from deceased ALS patients in North America has been found to have higher levels of BMAA than did the brains of people of the same age dying of other causes.[125] One food that is very high in BMAA is shark fin.[126] Sharks, as top predators, bioaccumulate BMAA in their muscles and fins. Sharks get a rating of D for this, as well as for being predators. Lobsters are also predators and bioaccumulate BMAA.[127] Lobsters, especially older ones, become cannibalistic and eat smaller ones. This occurs more when the environment is stressed, and there is less other food available for them to eat. Lobsters served in restaurants are generally 5 to 7 years old, but can live well past 100 years, all that time, accumulating BMAA.

Studies from China and Egypt have shown that some leafy vegetables[128] and some grains (corn and sorghum, but not wheat)[129] will contain high BMAA levels if irrigated with water contaminated with BMAA-producing cyanobacteria. While not normally used in protein, BMAA can sneak in and be used in place of the amino acid serine in proteins. While this is a possible direct risk for human consumption, the far greater risk would be from the consumption of meat from animals that were fed plant matter high in BMAA, as with the case of cycad seed. The highest levels of BMAA are in the brain. Consumption of the brain of any animal is banned on the SANA diet, for this and other reasons, including mad cow and similar diseases.

Cycad also contains β-sitosterol β-d-glucoside (BSSG), another neurotoxic compound that enhances the aggregation and cytotoxicity of alpha-synuclein.[130]

[1] Unraveling Cancer: Cancer prevention even after diagnosis. Chapter 18, pp 173-179. Charles A Lewis. Psy Press Carrabelle, FL. July 2016. ISBN: 1535593725, 9781535593724

[2] Immunotherapeutic effects of T11TS/S-LFA3 against nitrosocompound mediated neural genotoxicity. Mukherjee J, Sarkar S, Ghosh A, Duttagupta AK, Chaudhuri S, Chaudhuri S. Toxicol Lett. 2004 May 2;150(3):239-57. doi: 10.1016/j.toxlet.2004.01.016. PMID: 15110076

[3] Exposure to N-ethyl-N-nitrosourea in adult mice alters structural and functional integrity of neurogenic sites. Capilla-Gonzalez V, Gil-Perotin S, Ferragud A, Bonet-Ponce L, Canales JJ, Garcia-Verdugo JM. PLoS One. 2012;7(1):e29891. doi: 10.1371/journal.pone.0029891. PMID: 22238669

[4] Characteristics, formation, and pathophysiology of glucosepane: a major protein cross-link. Sjöberg JS, Bulterijs S. Rejuvenation Res. 2009 Apr;12(2):137-48. doi: 10.1089/rej.2009.0846. PMID: 19415980

[5] Advanced Glycation End Products Modulate Amyloidogenic APP Processing and Tau Phosphorylation: A Mechanistic Link between Glycation and the Development of Alzheimer's Disease. Batkulwar K, Godbole R, Banarjee R, Kassaar O, Williams RJ, Kulkarni MJ. ACS Chem Neurosci. 2018 May 16;9(5):988-1000. doi: 10.1021/acschemneuro.7b00410. PMID: 29384651

[6] Unraveling Cancer: Cancer prevention even after diagnosis. Chapter 17, pp 159-172. Charles A Lewis. Psy Press Carrabelle, FL. July 2016. ISBN: 1535593725, 9781535593724

[7] Metabolism of the food-derived carcinogen 2-amino-1-methyl-6-phenylimidazo[4,5-b]pyridine by lactating Fischer 344 rats and their nursing pups. Davis CD, Ghoshal A, Schut HA, Snyderwine EG. J Natl Cancer Inst. 1994 Jul 20;86(14):1065-70. PMID:8021955

[8] Evidence for the presence of mutagenic arylamines in human breast milk and DNA adducts in exfoliated breast ductal epithelial cells. Thompson PA, DeMarini DM, Kadlubar FF, et al. Environ Mol Mutagen. 2002;39(2-3):134-42. PMID:11921181

[9] DNA adducts of 2-amino-3-methylimidazo[4,5-f]quinoline (IQ) in fetal tissues of patas monkeys after transplacental exposure. Josyula S, Lu LJ, Salazar JJ, et al. Toxicol Appl Pharmacol. 2000 Aug 1;166(3):151-60. PMID:10906279

[10] Comparative carcinogenicity of 4-aminobiphenyl and the food pyrolysates, Glu-P-1, IQ, PhIP, and MeIQx in the neonatal B6C3F1 male mouse. Dooley KL, Von Tungeln LS, Bucci T, Fu PP, Kadlubar FF. Cancer Lett. 1992 Mar 15;62(3):205-9. PMID:1596864

[11] PhIP exposure in rodents produces neuropathology potentially relevant to Alzheimer's disease. Syeda T, Foguth RM, Llewellyn E, Cannon JR. Toxicology. 2020 May 15;437:152436. doi: 10.1016/j.tox.2020.152436. PMID: 32169473

[12] Quantification of the neurotoxic beta-carboline harmane in barbecued/grilled meat samples and correlation with level of doneness. Louis ED, Zheng W, Jiang W, Bogen KT, Keating GA. J Toxicol Environ Health A. 2007 Jun;70(12):1014-9. doi: 10.1080/15287390601172015. PMID: 17497412

[13] Selective dopaminergic neurotoxicity of three heterocyclic amine subclasses in primary rat midbrain neurons. Cruz-Hernandez A, Agim ZS, Montenegro PC, McCabe GP, Rochet JC, Cannon JR. Neurotoxicology. 2018 Mar;65:68-84. doi: 10.1016/j.neuro.2018.01.009. PMID: 29408373

[14] Neuromelanin Modulates Heterocyclic Aromatic Amine-Induced Dopaminergic Neurotoxicity. Lawana V, Um SY, Rochet JC, Turesky RJ, Shannahan JH, Cannon JR. Toxicol Sci. 2020 Jan 1;173(1):171-188. doi: 10.1093/toxsci/kfz210. PMID: 31562763

[15] Relative exposure to beta-carbolines norharman and harman from foods and tobacco smoke. Herraiz T. Food Addit Contam. 2004 Nov;21(11):1041-50. doi: 10.1080/02652030400019844. PMID: 15764332

[16] Harmine, a natural beta-carboline alkaloid, upregulates astroglial glutamate transporter expression. Li Y, Sattler R, Yang EJ, Nunes A, Ayukawa Y, Akhtar S, Ji G, Zhang PW, Rothstein JD. Neuropharmacology. 2011 Jun;60(7-8):1168-75. doi: 10.1016/j.neuropharm.2010.10.016. PMID: 21034752

[17] Development of a novel selective inhibitor of the Down syndrome-related kinase Dyrk1A. Ogawa Y, Nonaka Y, Goto T, Ohnishi E, Hiramatsu T, Kii I, Yoshida M, Ikura T, Onogi H, Shibuya H, Hosoya T, Ito N, Hagiwara M. Nat Commun. 2010 Oct 5;1:86. doi: 10.1038/ncomms1090. PMID: 20981014

[18] A high-throughput chemical screen reveals that harmine-mediated inhibition of DYRK1A increases human pancreatic beta cell replication. Wang P, Alvarez-Perez JC, Felsenfeld DP, Liu H, Sivendran S, Bender A, Kumar A, Sanchez R, Scott DK, Garcia-Ocaña A, Stewart AF. Nat Med. 2015 Apr;21(4):383-8. doi: 10.1038/nm.3820. PMID: 25751815

[19] Biological significance of aminophenyl-β-carboline derivatives formed from co-mutagenic action of β-carbolines and aniline and o-toluidine and its effect on tumorigenesis in humans: A review. Totsuka Y, Wakabayashi K. Mutat Res. 2020 Feb-Mar;850-851:503148. doi: 10.1016/j.mrgentox.2020.503148. PMID: 32247557

[20] Bioactive β-Carbolines in Food: A Review. Piechowska P, Zawirska-Wojtasiak R, Mildner-Szkudlarz S. Nutrients. 2019 Apr 11;11(4):814. doi: 10.3390/nu11040814. PMID: 30978920

[21] Colloquium paper: uniquely human evolution of sialic acid genetics and biology. Varki A. Proc Natl Acad Sci U S A. 2010 May 11;107 Suppl 2(Suppl 2):8939-46. doi: 10.1073/pnas.0914634107. PMID: 20445087

[22] Malaria infection increases bird attractiveness to uninfected mosquitoes. Cornet S, Nicot A, Rivero A, Gandon S. Ecol Lett. 2013 Mar;16(3):323-9. doi: 10.1111/ele.12041. PMID: 23205903

[23] Mechanisms of Plasmodium-Enhanced Attraction of Mosquito Vectors. Busula AO, Verhulst NO, Bousema

T, Takken W, de Boer JG. Trends Parasitol. 2017 Dec;33(12):961-973. doi: 10.1016/j.pt.2017.08.010. PMID: 28942108

24 Correlation of serum N-Acetylneuraminic acid with the risk and prognosis of acute coronary syndrome: a prospective cohort study. Li MN, Qian SH, Yao ZY, Ming SP, Shi XJ, Kang PF, Zhang NR, Wang XJ, Gao DS, Gao Q, Zhang H, Wang HJ. BMC Cardiovasc Disord. 2020 Sep 10;20(1):404. doi: 10.1186/s12872-020-01690-z. PMID: 32912159

25 Sialic acid metabolism as a potential therapeutic target of atherosclerosis. Zhang C, Chen J, Liu Y, Xu D. Lipids Health Dis. 2019 Sep 14;18(1):173. doi: 10.1186/s12944-019-1113-5. PMID: 31521172

26 Human species-specific loss of CMP-*N*-acetylneuraminic acid hydroxylase enhances atherosclerosis via intrinsic and extrinsic mechanisms. Kawanishi K, Dhar C, Do R, Varki N, Gordts PLSM, Varki A. Proc Natl Acad Sci U S A. 2019 Aug 6;116(32):16036-16045. doi: 10.1073/pnas.1902902116. PMID: 31332008

27 Association between Neu5Gc carbohydrate and serum antibodies against it provides the molecular link to cancer: French NutriNet-Santé study. Bashir S, Fezeu LK, Leviatan Ben-Arye S, Yehuda S, Reuven EM, Szabo de Edelenyi F, Fellah-Hebia I, Le Tourneau T, Imbert-Marcille BM, Drouet EB, Touvier M, Roussel JC, Yu H, Chen X, Hercberg S, Cozzi E, Soulillou JP, Galan P, Padler-Karavani V. BMC Med. 2020 Sep 23;18(1):262. doi: 10.1186/s12916-020-01721-8. PMID: 32962714 Supplementary Materials 1 and 2

28 Challenging the Role of Diet-Induced Anti-Neu5Gc Antibodies in Human Pathologies. Soulillou JP, Cozzi E, Bach JM. Front Immunol. 2020 Jun 9;11:834. doi: 10.3389/fimmu.2020.00834. PMID: 32655538

29 Are humans prone to autoimmunity? Implications from evolutionary changes in hominin sialic acid biology. Varki A. J Autoimmun. 2017 Sep;83:134-142. doi: 10.1016/j.jaut.2017.07.011. PMID: 28755952

30 Xenogeneic Neu5Gc and self-glycan Neu5Ac epitopes are potential immune targets in MS. Boligan KF, Oechtering J, Keller CW, Peschke B, Rieben R, Bovin N, Kappos L, Cummings RD, Kuhle J, von Gunten S, Lünemann JD. Neurol Neuroimmunol Neuroinflamm. 2020 Feb 3;7(2):e676. doi: 10.1212/NXI.0000000000000676. PMID: 32014849

31 Maternal dietary patterns, supplements intake and autism spectrum disorders: A preliminary case-control study. Li YM, Shen YD, Li YJ, Xun GL, Liu H, Wu RR, Xia K, Zhao JP, Ou JJ. Medicine (Baltimore). 2018 Dec;97(52):e13902. doi: 10.1097/MD.0000000000013902. PMID: 30593205

32 Maternal autoimmune diseases and the risk of autism spectrum disorders in offspring: A systematic review and meta-analysis. Chen SW, Zhong XS, Jiang LN, Zheng XY, Xiong YQ, Ma SJ, Qiu M, Huo ST, Ge J, Chen Q. Behav Brain Res. 2016 Jan 1;296:61-69. doi: 10.1016/j.bbr.2015.08.035. PMID: 26327239

33 Possible Influences of Endogenous and Exogenous Ligands on the Evolution of Human Siglecs. Angata T. Front Immunol. 2018 Dec 4;9:2885. doi: 10.3389/fimmu.2018.02885. PMID: 30564250

34 Human-specific microglial Siglec-11 transcript variant has the potential to affect polysialic acid-mediated brain functions at a distance. Hane M, Chen DY, Varki A. Glycobiology. 2021 Apr 1;31(3):231-242. doi: 10.1093/glycob/cwaa082. PMID: 32845322

35 What are SIGLEC11 modulators and how do they work? June 2024. https://synapse.patsnap.com/article/what-are-siglec11-modulators-and-how-do-they-work

36 Colloquium paper: uniquely human evolution of sialic acid genetics and biology. Varki A. Proc Natl Acad Sci U S A. 2010 May 11;107 Suppl 2(Suppl 2):8939-46. doi: 10.1073/pnas.0914634107. PMID: 20445087

37 Preeclampsia and reproductive performance in a community of vegans. Carter JP, Furman T, Hutcheson HR. South Med J. 1987 Jun;80(6):692-7. doi: 10.1097/00007611-198706000-00007. PMID: 589760

38 Preeclampsia: Clinical features and diagnosis. Phyllis August, Baha M Sibai UPtoDate https://www.uptodate.com/contents/preeclampsia-clinical-features-and-diagnosis (accessed May 2021.

39 [Study on the correlation between dietary N-glycolylneuraminic acid intake and chronic inflammation state of body]. Zhuang YY, Zheng HY, Lan H, Li HW. Zhonghua Yu Fang Yi Xue Za Zhi. 2020 Jun 6;54(6):668-672. doi: 10.3760/cma.j.cn112150-20191021-00802. PMID: 32842284

40 https://www.cdc.gov/ticks/alpha-gal/index.html

41 In older women, a high-protein diet including animal-sourced foods did not impact serum levels and urinary excretion of trimethylamine-N-oxide. Dahl WJ, Hung WL, Ford AL, Suh JH, Auger J, Nagulesapillai V, Wang Y. Nutr Res. 2020 Jun;78:72-81. doi: 10.1016/j.nutres.2020.05.004. PMID: 32544852

42 l-Carnitine in omnivorous diets induces an atherogenic gut microbial pathway in humans. Koeth RA, Lam-Galvez BR, Kirsop J, Wang Z, Levison BS, Gu X, Copeland MF, Bartlett D, Cody DB, Dai HJ, Culley MK, Li XS, Fu X, Wu Y, Li L, DiDonato JA, Tang WHW, Garcia-Garcia JC, Hazen SL. J Clin Invest. 2019 Jan 2;129(1):373-387. doi: 10.1172/JCI94601. PMID: 30530985

43 Trimethylamine and Trimethylamine N-Oxide, a Flavin-Containing Monooxygenase 3 (FMO3)-Mediated Host-Microbiome Metabolic Axis Implicated in Health and Disease. Fennema D, Phillips IR, Shephard EA. Drug Metab Dispos. 2016 Nov;44(11):1839-1850. doi: 10.1124/dmd.116.070615. PMID: 27190056

44 Crotonobetaine is a proatherogenic but microbiota metabolite of L-Carnitine. Koeth R, Culley M, Wang Z, et al. J Am Coll Cardiol. 2019 Mar, 73 (9_Supplement_1) 14

45 Trimethylamine N-Oxide Generated by the Gut Microbiota Is Associated with Vascular Inflammation:

New Insights into Atherosclerosis. Liu Y, Dai M. Mediators Inflamm. 2020 Feb 17;2020:4634172. doi: 10.1155/2020/4634172. PMID: 32148438

46 Gut microbe-generated metabolite trimethylamine N-oxide and the risk of diabetes: A systematic review and dose-response meta-analysis. Zhuang R, Ge X, Han L, Yu P, Gong X, Meng Q, Zhang Y, Fan H, Zheng L, Liu Z, Zhou X. Obes Rev. 2019 Jun;20(6):883-894. doi: 10.1111/obr.12843. PMID: 30868721

47 Trimethylamine-N-oxide as One Hypothetical Link for the Relationship between Intestinal Microbiota and Cancer - Where We Are and Where Shall We Go? Chan CWH, Law BMH, Waye MMY, Chan JYW, So WKW, Chow KM. J Cancer. 2019 Oct 8;10(23):5874-5882. doi: 10.7150/jca.31737. PMID: 31737123

48 Association of L-α Glycerylphosphorylcholine With Subsequent Stroke Risk After 10 Years. Lee G, Choi S, Chang J, Choi D, Son JS, Kim K, Kim SM, Jeong S, Park SM. JAMA Netw Open. 2021 Nov 1;4(11):e2136008. doi: 10.1001/jamanetworkopen.2021.36008. PMID: 3481758

49 Microbiota-dependent metabolite trimethylamine-N-oxide is associated with disease severity and survival of patients with chronic heart failure. Trøseid M, Ueland T, Hov JR, Svardal A, Gregersen I, Dahl CP, Aakhus S, Gude E, Bjørndal B, Halvorsen B, Karlsen TH, Aukrust P, Gullestad L, Berge RK, Yndestad A. J Intern Med. 2015 Jun;277(6):717-26. doi: 10.1111/joim.12328. PMID: 25382824

50 The Gut Microbial Metabolite Trimethylamine-N-Oxide Is Present in Human Cerebrospinal Fluid. Del Rio D, Zimetti F, Caffarra P, Tassotti M, Bernini F, Brighenti F, Zini A, Zanotti I. Nutrients. 2017 Sep 22;9(10):1053. doi: 10.3390/nu9101053. PMID: 28937600

51 Effects of gut-derived trimethylamines on the blood-brain barrier. McArthur S, Fonseca S, Carvalho AL, Snelling T, et al. March 2018 ARUK - Alzheimer's Research UK Conference 2018 https://www.researchgate.net/publication/326849311_Effects_of_gut-derived_trimethylamines_on_the_blood-brain_barrier

52 Gut microbes and metabolites as modulators of blood-brain barrier integrity and brain health. Parker A, Fonseca S, Carding SR. Gut Microbes. 2020;11(2):135-157. doi: 10.1080/19490976.2019.1638722. PMID: 31368397

53 Impact of chronic dietary red meat, white meat, or non-meat protein on trimethylamine N-oxide metabolism and renal excretion in healthy men and women. Wang Z, Bergeron N, Levison BS, Li XS, Chiu S, Jia X, Koeth RA, Li L, Wu Y, Tang WHW, Krauss RM, Hazen SL. Eur Heart J. 2019 Feb 14;40(7):583-594. doi: 10.1093/eurheartj/ ehy799. PMID: 30535398

54 Gut Microbe-Generated Trimethylamine *N*-Oxide From Dietary Choline Is Prothrombotic in Subjects. Zhu W, Wang Z, Tang WHW, Hazen SL. Circulation. 2017 Apr 25;135(17):1671-1673. doi: 10.1161/CIRCULATIONAHA. 116.025338. PMID: 28438808

55 Utility of Plasma Concentration of Trimethylamine N-Oxide in Predicting Cardiovascular and Renal Complications in Individuals With Type 1 Diabetes. Winther SA, Øllgaard JC, Tofte N, Tarnow L, Wang Z, Ahluwalia TS, Jorsal A, Theilade S, Parving HH, Hansen TW, Hazen SL, Pedersen O, Rossing P. Diabetes Care. 2019 Aug;42(8):1512-1520. doi: 10.2337/dc19-0048. PMID: 31123156

56 Effect of egg ingestion on trimethylamine-N-oxide production in humans: a randomized, controlled, dose-response study. Miller CA, Corbin KD, da Costa KA, Zhang S, Zhao X, Galanko JA, Blevins T, Bennett BJ, O'Connor A, Zeisel SH. Am J Clin Nutr. 2014 Sep;100(3):778-86. doi: 10.3945/ajcn.114.087692. PMID: 24944063

57 Whole egg consumption increases plasma choline and betaine without affecting TMAO levels or gut microbiome in overweight postmenopausal women. Zhu C, Sawrey-Kubicek L, Bardagjy AS, Houts H, Tang X, Sacchi R, Randolph JM, Steinberg FM, Zivkovic AM. Nutr Res. 2020 Jun;78:36-41. doi: 10.1016/j.nutres.2020.04.002. PMID: 32464420

58 Compared to an Oatmeal Breakfast, Two Eggs/Day Increased Plasma Carotenoids and Choline without Increasing Trimethyl Amine N-Oxide Concentrations. Missimer A, Fernandez ML, DiMarco DM, Norris GH, Blesso CN, Murillo AG, Vergara-Jimenez M, Lemos BS, Medina-Vera I, Malysheva OV, Caudill MA. J Am Coll Nutr. 2018 Feb;37(2):140-148. doi: 10.1080/07315724.2017.1365026. PMID: 29313753

59 Effects of Egg Consumption and Choline Supplementation on Plasma Choline and Trimethylamine-N-Oxide in a Young Population. Lemos BS, Medina-Vera I, Malysheva OV, Caudill MA, Fernandez ML. J Am Coll Nutr. 2018 Nov-Dec;37(8):716-723. doi: 10.1080/07315724.2018.1466213. PMID: 29764315

60 Intake of up to 3 Eggs/Day Increases HDL Cholesterol and Plasma Choline While Plasma Trimethylamine-N-oxide is Unchanged in a Healthy Population. DiMarco DM, Missimer A, Murillo AG, Lemos BS, Malysheva OV, Caudill MA, Blesso CN, Fernandez ML. Lipids. 2017 Mar;52(3):255-263. doi: 10.1007/s11745-017-4230-9. PMID: 28091798

61 Intestinal microbiota metabolism of L-carnitine, a nutrient in red meat, promotes atherosclerosis. Koeth RA, Wang Z, Levison BS, Buffa JA, Org E, Sheehy BT, Britt EB, Fu X, Wu Y, Li L, Smith JD, DiDonato JA, Chen J, Li H, Wu GD, Lewis JD, Warrier M, Brown JM, Krauss RM, Tang WH, Bushman FD, Lusis AJ, Hazen SL. Nat Med. 2013 May;19(5):576-85. doi: 10.1038/nm.3145. PMID: 23563705

62 Associations among serum trimethylamine-N-oxide (TMAO) levels, kidney function and infarcted coronary artery number in patients undergoing cardiovascular surgery: a cross-sectional study. Mafune A, Iwamoto T, Tsutsumi Y, Nakashima A, Yamamoto I, Yokoyama K, Yokoo T, Urashima M. Clin Exp Nephrol. 2016

Oct;20(5):731-739. doi: 10.1007/s10157-015-1207-y. PMID: 26676906

63 Plasma Trimethylamine N-Oxide, a Gut Microbe-Generated Phosphatidylcholine Metabolite, Is Associated With Atherosclerotic Burden. Senthong V, Li XS, Hudec T, Coughlin J, Wu Y, Levison B, Wang Z, Hazen SL, Tang WH. J Am Coll Cardiol. 2016 Jun 7;67(22):2620-8. doi: 10.1016/j.jacc.2016.03.546. PMID: 27256833

64 Plasma trimethylamine n-oxide is associated with renal function in patients with heart failure with preserved ejection fraction. Guo F, Qiu X, Tan Z, Li Z, Ouyang D. BMC Cardiovasc Disord. 2020 Aug 28;20(1):394. doi: 10.1186/s12872-020-01669-w. PMID: 32859154

65 Utility of Plasma Concentration of Trimethylamine N-Oxide in Predicting Cardiovascular and Renal Complications in Individuals With Type 1 Diabetes. Winther SA, Øllgaard JC, Tofte N, Tarnow L, Wang Z, Ahluwalia TS, Jorsal A, Theilade S, Parving HH, Hansen TW, Hazen SL, Pedersen O, Rossing P. Diabetes Care. 2019 Aug;42(8):1512-1520. doi: 10.2337/dc19-0048. PMID: 31123156

66 Potential TMA-Producing Bacteria Are Ubiquitously Found in Mammalia. Rath S, Rud T, Pieper DH, Vital M. Front Microbiol. 2020 Jan 9;10:2966. doi: 10.3389/fmicb.2019.02966. PMID: 31998260

67 Impact of chronic dietary red meat, white meat, or non-meat protein on trimethylamine N-oxide metabolism and renal excretion in healthy men and women. Wang Z, Bergeron N, Levison BS, Li XS, Chiu S, Jia X, Koeth RA, Li L, Wu Y, Tang WHW, Krauss RM, Hazen SL. Eur Heart J. 2019 Feb 14;40(7):583-594. doi: 10.1093/eurheartj/ehy799. PMID: 30535398

68 Role of the Gut Bacteria-Derived Metabolite Phenylacetylglutamine in Health and Diseases. Krishnamoorthy NK, Kalyan M, Hediyal, et al. ACS Omega. 2024 Jan 8;9(3):3164-3172. doi: 10.1021/acsomega.3c08184. eCollection 2024 Jan 23. PMID: 38284070

69 Gut Microbiota-Generated Phenylacetylglutamine and Heart Failure. Romano KA, Nemet I, Prasad Saha P, Haghikia A, Li XS, et al. Circ Heart Fail. 2023 Jan;16(1):e009972. doi: 10.1161/CIRCHEARTFAILURE. 122.009972. PMID: 36524472

70 A Cardiovascular Disease-Linked Gut Microbial Metabolite Acts via Adrenergic Receptors. Nemet I, Saha PP, Gupta N, et al. 2020 Mar 5;180(5):862-877.e22. doi: 10.1016/j.cell.2020.02.016. PMID: 32142679

71 Neurobehavioral effects of uremic toxin-indoxyl sulfate in the rat model. Karbowska M, Hermanowicz JM, Tankiewicz-Kwedlo A, Kalaska B, Kaminski TW, Nosek K, Wisniewska RJ, Pawlak D. Sci Rep. 2020 Jun 11;10(1):9483. doi: 10.1038/s41598-020-66421-y. PMID: 32528183

72 Red meat intake in chronic kidney disease patients: Two sides of the coin. Mafra D, Borges NA, Cardozo LFMF, Anjos JS, Black AP, Moraes C, Bergman P, Lindholm B, Stenvinkel P. Nutrition. 2018 Feb;46:26-32. doi: 10.1016/j.nut.2017.08.015. Epub 2017 Sep 19. PMID: 29290351

73 A Prospective Study of Dietary Meat Intake and Risk of Incident Chronic Kidney Disease. Mirmiran P, Yuzbashian E, Aghayan M, Mahdavi M, Asghari G, Azizi F. J Ren Nutr. 2020 Mar;30(2):111-118. doi: 10.1053/j.jrn.2019.06.008. Epub 2019 Aug 14. PMID: 31422013

74 Dietary Protein Sources and Risk for Incident Chronic Kidney Disease: Results From the Atherosclerosis Risk in Communities (ARIC) Study. Haring B, Selvin E, Liang M, Coresh J, Grams ME, Petruski-Ivleva N, Steffen LM, Rebholz CM. J Ren Nutr. 2017 Jul;27(4):233-242. doi: 10.1053/j.jrn.2016.11.004. Epub 2017 Jan 5. PMID: 28065493

75 The relationship of diet and acne: A review. Pappas A. Dermatoendocrinol. 2009 Sep;1(5):262-7. PMID:20808513

76 Omega-3 polyunsaturated fatty acids modify the inverse association between systemic inflammation and cardiovascular fitness. Farley G, Riggs DW, Bhatnagar A, Hellmann J. Clin Nutr. 2021 Jun;40(6):4097-4105. doi: 10.1016/j.clnu.2021.02.006. PMID: 33618966

77 Fatty Acid Profile of Mature Red Blood Cell Membranes and Dietary Intake as a New Approach to Characterize Children with Overweight and Obesity. Jauregibeitia I, Portune K, Rica I, Tueros I, Velasco O, Grau G, Trebolazabala N, Castaño L, Larocca AV, Ferreri C, Arranz S. Nutrients. 2020 Nov 10;12(11):3446. doi: 10.3390/nu12113446. PMID: 33182783

78 The association of dietary intake and supplementation of specific polyunsaturated fatty acids with inflammation and functional capacity in chronic obstructive pulmonary disease: a systematic review. Atlantis E, Cochrane B. Int J Evid Based Healthc. 2016 Jun;14(2):53-63. doi: 10.1097/XEB.0000000000000056. PMID: 26134547

79 Omega-3 fatty acids: potential role in the management of early Alzheimer's disease. Jicha GA, Markesbery WR. Clin Interv Aging. 2010 Apr 7;5:45-61. PMID:20396634

80 Low omega-6 vs. low omega-6 plus high omega-3 dietary intervention for chronic daily headache: protocol for a randomized clinical trial. Ramsden CE, Mann JD, Faurot KR, et al. Trials. 2011 Apr 15;12:97. PMID:21496264

81 Fats and factors: lipid profiles associate with personality factors and suicidal history in bipolar subjects. Evans SJ, Prossin AR, Harrington GJ, Kamali M, Ellingrod VL, Burant CF, McInnis MG. PLoS One. 2012;7(1):e29297. doi: 10.1371/journal.pone.0029297. PMID: 22253709

82 Omega-3 and Omega-6 Polyunsaturated Fatty Acids in Bipolar Disorder: A Review of Biomarker and Treatment Studies. Saunders EF, Ramsden CE, Sherazy MS, Gelenberg AJ, Davis JM, Rapoport SI. J Clin

Psychiatry. 2016 Oct;77(10):e1301-e1308. doi: 10.4088/JCP. 15r09925. PMID: 27631140

83 Effects of Omega 3 Fatty Acids on Main Dimensions of Psychopathology. Bozzatello P, De Rosa ML, Rocca P, Bellino S. Int J Mol Sci. 2020 Aug 21;21(17):6042. doi: 10.3390/ijms21176042. PMID: 32839416

84 Essential fatty acids and their role in conditions characterised by impulsivity. Garland MR, Hallahan B. Int Rev Psychiatry. 2006 Apr;18(2):99-105. PMID: 16777664

85 Protective effects of dietary supplementation with natural ω-3 polyunsaturated fatty acids on the visual acuity of school-age children with lower IQ or attention-deficit hyperactivity disorder. Wu Q, Zhou T, Ma L, Yuan D, Peng Y. Nutrition. 2015 Jul-Aug;31(7-8):935-40. doi: 10.1016/j.nut.2014.12.026. PMID: 26015389

86 Omega-3 and Omega-6 Polyunsaturated Fatty Acid Levels and Correlations with Symptoms in Children with Attention Deficit Hyperactivity Disorder, Autistic Spectrum Disorder and Typically Developing Controls. Parletta N, Niyonsenga T, Duff J. PLoS One. 2016 May 27;11(5):e0156432. doi: 10.1371/journal.pone.0156432. PMID: 27232999

87 The Role of Omega-3 Fatty Acids in Developmental Psychopathology: A Systematic Review on Early Psychosis, Autism, and ADHD. Agostoni C, Nobile M, Ciappolino V, Delvecchio G, Tesei A, Turolo S, Crippa A, Mazzocchi A, Altamura CA, Brambilla P. Int J Mol Sci. 2017 Dec 4;18(12):2608. doi: 10.3390/ijms18122608. PMID: 29207548

88 Omega-3 polyunsaturated essential fatty acids are associated with depression in adolescents with eating disorders and weight loss. Swenne I, Rosling A, Tengblad S, Vessby B. Acta Paediatr. 2011 Jul 6. PMID:21732977

89 Higher maternal plasma docosahexaenoic acid during pregnancy is associated with more mature neonatal sleep-state patterning. Cheruku SR, Montgomery-Downs HE, Farkas SL, et al. Am J Clin Nutr. 2002 Sep;76(3):608-13. PMID:12198007

90 Association between maternal intake of n-6 to n-3 fatty acid ratio during pregnancy and infant neurodevelopment at 6 months of age: results of the MOCEH cohort study. Kim H, Kim H, Lee E, Kim Y, Ha EH, Chang N. Nutr J. 2017 Apr 18;16(1):23. doi: 10.1186/s12937-017-0242-9. PMID: 28420388

91 Dietary phospholipids and intestinal cholesterol absorption. Cohn JS, Kamili A, Wat E, Chung RW, Tandy S. Nutrients. 2010 Feb;2(2):116-27. doi: 10.3390/nu2020116. PMID: 22254012

92 Choline and betaine in health and disease. Ueland PM. J Inherit Metab Dis. 2011 Feb;34(1):3-15. doi: 10.1007/s10545-010-9088-4. PMID: 20446114

93 https://brenda-enzymes.org/enzyme.php?ecno=2.1.1.5#

94 Cerebrospinal fluid and plasma total homocysteine and related metabolites in children with cystathionine beta-synthase deficiency: the effect of treatment. Surtees R, Bowron A, Leonard J. Pediatr Res. 1997 Nov;42(5):577-82. doi: 10.1203/00006450-199711000-00004. PMID: 9357926

95 Choline and homocysteine interrelations in umbilical cord and maternal plasma at delivery. Molloy AM, Mills JL, Cox C, Daly SF, Conley M, Brody LC, Kirke PN, Scott JM, Ueland PM. Am J Clin Nutr. 2005 Oct;82(4):836-42. doi: 10.1093/ajcn/82.4.836. PMID: 16210714

96 Dietary Reference Intakes for Thiamin, Riboflavin, Niacin, Vitamin B6, Folate, Vitamin B12, Pantothenic Acid, Biotin, and Choline (1998) Chapter: 12 Choline , page 405 National Academies Press, 1998 https://www.nap.edu/read/6015/chapter/14#405

97 Alleviatiin of dietary cirrhosis with betaine and other lipotropic agents. Best CH, Ridout JH, Lucas CC. Can J Physiol Pharmacol. 1969 Jan;47(1):73-9. doi: 10.1139/y69-012. PMID: 4178227

98 Phospholipase D and Choline Metabolism. Onono FO, Morris AJ. Handb Exp Pharmacol. 2020;259:205-218. doi: 10.1007/164_2019_320. PMID: 32086667

99 Racial and Ethnic Disparities in Nonalcoholic Fatty Liver Disease Prevalence, Severity, and Outcomes in the United States: A Systematic Review and Meta-analysis. Rich NE, Oji S, Mufti AR, Browning JD, Parikh ND, Odewole M, Mayo H, Singal AG. Clin Gastroenterol Hepatol. 2018 Feb;16(2):198-210.e2. doi: 10.1016/ j.cgh.2017.09.041. PMID: 28970148

100 Serum 25-hydroxyvitamin-D and nonalcoholic fatty liver disease: Does race/ethnicity matter? Findings from the MESA cohort. El Khoudary SR, Samargandy S, Zeb I, Foster T, de Boer IH, Li D, Budoff MJ. Nutr Metab Cardiovasc Dis. 2020 Jan 3;30(1):114-122. doi: 10.1016/j.numecd.2019.09.004. PMID: 31761548

101 Black American Maternal Prenatal Choline, Offspring Gestational Age at Birth, and Developmental Predisposition to Mental Illness. Hunter SK, Hoffman MC, McCarthy L, D'Alessandro A, Wyrwa A, Noonan K, Christians U, Nakimuli-Mpungu E, Zeisel SH, Law AJ, Freedman R. Schizophr Bull. 2021 Jul 8;47(4):896-905. doi: 10.1093/schbul/sbaa171. PMID: 33184653

102 Choline intake during pregnancy and child cognition at age 7 years. Boeke CE, Gillman MW, Hughes MD, Rifas-Shiman SL, Villamor E, Oken E. Am J Epidemiol. 2013 Jun 15;177(12):1338-47. doi: 10.1093/aje/kws395. PMID: 23425631

103 Early second trimester maternal plasma choline and betaine are related to measures of early cognitive development in term infants. Wu BT, Dyer RA, King DJ, Richardson KJ, Innis SM. PLoS One. 2012;7(8):e43448. doi: 10.1371/journal.pone.0043448. PMID: 22916264

104 Plasma Betaine Is Positively Associated with Developmental Outcomes in Healthy Toddlers at Age 2 Years Who Are Not Meeting the Recommended Adequate Intake for Dietary Choline. Wiedeman AM, Chau CMY, Grunau RE, McCarthy D, Yurko-Mauro K, Dyer RA, Innis SM, Devlin AM. J Nutr. 2018 Aug

1;148(8):1309-1314. doi: 10.1093/jn/nxy108. PMID: 29986040

105 Choline status and neurodevelopmental outcomes at 5 years of age in the Seychelles Child Development Nutrition Study. Strain JJ, McSorley EM, van Wijngaarden E, Kobrosly RW, Bonham MP, Mulhern MS, McAfee AJ, Davidson PW, Shamlaye CF, Henderson J, Watson GE, Thurston SW, Wallace JM, Ueland PM, Myers GJ. Br J Nutr. 2013 Jul 28;110(2):330-6. doi: 10.1017/ S0007114512005077. PMID: 23298754

106 Efficacy of Maternal Choline Supplementation During Pregnancy in Mitigating Adverse Effects of Prenatal Alcohol Exposure on Growth and Cognitive Function: A Randomized, Double-Blind, Placebo-Controlled Clinical Trial. Jacobson SW, Carter RC, Molteno CD, Stanton ME, Herbert JS, Lindinger NM, Lewis CE, Dodge NC, Hoyme HE, Zeisel SH, Meintjes EM, Duggan CP, Jacobson JL. Alcohol Clin Exp Res. 2018 Jul;42(7):1327-1341. doi: 10.1111/acer.13769. PMID: 29750367

107 Higher Gestational Choline Levels in Maternal Infection Are Protective for Infant Brain Development. Freedman R, Hunter SK, Law AJ, Wagner BD, D'Alessandro A, Christians U, Noonan K, Wyrwa A, Hoffman MC. J Pediatr. 2019 May;208:198-206.e2. doi: 10.1016/j.jpeds.2018.12.010. PMID: 30879727

108 Maternal prenatal choline and inflammation effects on 4-year-olds' performance on the Wechsler Preschool and Primary Scale of Intelligence-IV. Hunter SK, Hoffman MC, D'Alessandro A, Walker VK, Balser M, Noonan K, Law AJ, Freedman R. J Psychiatr Res. 2021 Sep;141:50-56. doi: 10.1016/j.jpsychires.2021.06.037. PMID: 34174557

109 Male fetus susceptibility to maternal inflammation: C-reactive protein and brain development. Hunter SK, Hoffman MC, D'Alessandro A, Noonan K, Wyrwa A, Freedman R, Law AJ. Psychol Med. 2021 Feb;51(3):450-459. doi: 10.1017/S0033291719003313. PMID: 31787129

110 Prenatal choline, cannabis, and infection, and their association with offspring development of attention and social problems through 4 years of age. Hunter SK, Hoffman MC, D'Alessandro A, Wyrwa A, Noonan K, Zeisel SH, Law AJ, Freedman R. Psychol Med. 2021 Jan 25:1-10. doi: 10.1017/S0033291720005061. PMID: 33491615

111 Prenatal Primary Prevention of Mental Illness by Micronutrient Supplements in Pregnancy. Freedman R, Hunter SK, Hoffman MC. Am J Psychiatry. 2018 Jul 1;175(7):607-619. doi: 10.1176/appi.ajp.2018.17070836. PMID: 29558816

112 Perinatal Phosphatidylcholine Supplementation and Early Childhood Behavior Problems: Evidence for CHRNA7 Moderation. Ross RG, Hunter SK, Hoffman MC, McCarthy L, Chambers BM, Law AJ, Leonard S, Zerbe GO, Freedman R. Am J Psychiatry. 2016 May 1;173(5):509-16. doi: 10.1176/appi.ajp.2015.15091188. PMID: 26651393

113 Perinatal choline effects on neonatal pathophysiology related to later schizophrenia risk. Ross RG, Hunter SK, McCarthy L, Beuler J, Hutchison AK, Wagner BD, Leonard S, Stevens KE, Freedman R. Am J Psychiatry. 2013 Mar;170(3):290-8. doi: 10.1176/appi.ajp.2012. 12070940. PMID: 23318559

114 Maternal choline supplementation during the third trimester of pregnancy improves infant information processing speed: a randomized, double-blind, controlled feeding study. Caudill MA, Strupp BJ, Muscalu L, Nevins JEH, Canfield RL. FASEB J. 2018 Apr;32(4):2172-2180. doi: 10.1096/fj.201700692RR. PMID: 29217669

115 Dendritic spine loss in hippocampus of aged rats. Effect of brain phosphatidylserine administration. Nunzi MG, Milan F, Guidolin D, Toffano G. Neurobiol Aging. 1987 Nov-Dec;8(6):501-10. doi: 10.1016/0197-4580(87)90124-2. PMID: 3431625

116 Effects of Dietary Food Components on Cognitive Functions in Older Adults. Ozawa H, Miyazawa T, Miyazawa T. Nutrients. 2021 Aug 16;13(8):2804. doi: 10.3390/nu13082804. PMID: 34444965

117 Phospholipids and sports performance. Jäger R, Purpura M, Kingsley M. J Int Soc Sports Nutr. 2007 Jul 25;4:5. doi: 10.1186/1550-2783-4-5. PMID: 17908342

118 Essential Fatty Acids https://lpi.oregonstate.edu/mic/ other-nutrients/essential-fatty-acids (Accessed Sept 2021)

119 Phosphatidylserine inl the brain: metabolism and function. Kim HY, Huang BX, Spector AA. Prog Lipid Res. 2014 Oct;56:1-18. doi: 10.1016/j.plipres.2014.06.002. PMID: 24992464

120 https://en.wikipedia.org/wiki/Phosphatidylserine (Accessed Sept. 2021)

121 Natural Choline from Egg Yolk Phospholipids Is More Efficiently Absorbed Compared with Choline Bitartrate; Outcomes of A Randomized Trial in Healthy Adults. Smolders L, de Wit NJW, Balvers MGJ, Obeid R, Vissers MMM, Esser D. Nutrients. 2019 Nov 13;11(11):2758. doi: 10.3390/nu11112758. PMID: 31766273

122 USDA Database fo the Choline Content of Common Foods, Releases Two. Patterson KY, Bhagwat SA, Williams JR et al. USDA Nutriuent Data Laboratory Jan, 2008.

123 Food Ingredients That Inhibit Cholesterol Absorption. Jesch ED, Carr TP. Prev Nutr Food Sci. 2017 Jun;22(2):67-80. doi: 10.3746/pnf.2017.22.2.67. PMID: 28702423; PMCID: PMC5503415.

124 https://en.wikipedia.org/wiki/%CE%92-Methylamino-L-alanine

125 Beyond Guam: the cyanobacteria/BMAA hypothesis of the cause of ALS and other neurodegenerative diseases. Bradley WG, Mash DC. Amyotroph Lateral Scler. 2009;10 Suppl 2:7-20. doi: 10.3109/17482960903286009. PMID: 19929726

126 Cyanobacterial neurotoxin β-N-methylamino-L-alanine (BMAA) in shark fins. Mondo K, Hammerschlag N, Basile M, Pablo J, Banack SA, Mash

DC. Mar Drugs. 2012 Feb;10(2):509-520. doi: 10.3390/md10020509. PMID: 22412816

127 Detection of cyanobacterial neurotoxin β-N-methylamino-l-alanine within shellfish in the diet of an ALS patient in Florida. Banack SA, Metcalf JS, Bradley WG, Cox PA. Toxicon. 2014 Nov;90:167-73. doi: 10.1016/j.toxicon.2014.07.018. PMID: 25123936

128 Transfer of a cyanobacterial neurotoxin, β-methylamino-l-alanine from soil to crop and its bioaccumulation in Chinese cabbage. Li B, Yu S, Li G, Chen X, Huang M, Liao X, Li H, Hu F, Wu J. Chemosphere. 2019 Mar;219:997-1001. doi: 10.1016/j.chemosphere.2018.12.104. PMID: 30682765

129 Presence of the neurotoxin β-N-methylamino-L-alanine in irrigation water and accumulation in cereal grains with human exposure risk. Mohamed ZA, Elnour RO, Alamri S, Hashem M, Campos A, Vasconcelos V, Badawye H. Environ Sci Pollut Res Int. 2024 May;31(21):31479-31491. doi: 10.1007/s11356-024-33188-y. PMID: 38635096

130 Chronic exposure to dietary sterol glucosides is neurotoxic to motor neurons and induces an ALS-PDC phenotype. Tabata RC, Wilson JM, Ly P, Zwiegers P, Kwok D, Van Kampen JM, Cashman N, Shaw CA. Neuromolecular Med. 2008;10(1):24-39. doi: 10.1007/s12017-007-8020-z. PMID: 1819647

34: Other Diseases

The SANA program and diet present a healthy lifestyle that is designed to promote the prevention and recovery of most chronic diseases. Nevertheless, various conditions have particularities that require some additional dietary recommendations or restrictions that merit discussion. A few of those situations will be briefly summarized here.

Inflammatory Bowel Disease (IBD)

Those with IBD should greatly benefit from compliance with the SANA diets as compared to eating a standard American Western diet.[1] There are a few foods, however, that are more problematic in IBD than for the general population and that additionally need to be avoided by those with IBD. These include: Hot peppers,[2] mustard, wasabi, annatto (Bixa), sesame seeds, sunflower seeds, celery, raw carrots, and raw onions. Additionally, for those with IBD and IBS, adding fiber may increase inflammation when there is active dysbiosis. Thus, fiber should be added slowly. The DAD scores of high fiber foods generally reflect this; those with letter grades are more likely to incite inflammation.

While it is a general recommendation, those with IBD appear to be especially sensitive to cocoa butter and should thus avoid chocolate, especially white and milk chocolates.[3] Confections made with natural cocoa powder, without added cocoa butter, are likely O.K. Processed foods containing non-nutritive emulsifiers and gums need to be cautiously avoided for those with IBD. (Chapters 16 and 26)

Beer, ale, may be a problem for those with IBD. Wine consumption should be kept to 6 ml of absolute ethanol every other day, as described in Chapter 22.

Those with IBD should completely avoid foods with DAD scores of B or lower when healthy, and should stay away from any foods ranked A or lower during exacerbations of IBD to heal.

In mice, sweet beverages, when combined with a high-fat diet (HFD), provoked intestinal mucosal inflammation and submucosal edema. As compared to an HFD alone, adding sugar sugar-sweetened beverage increased the proliferation of IBD-related pathogenic bacteria, and exacerbated HFD-induced colitis by promoting a shift from a commensal microbiome into a pathogenic one.[4]

Soda pop is deadly for those with IBD. Among patients with IBD, consuming more than one can (250 ml) of sugar-sweetened beverages a day increased all-cause mortality by 97%. Consumption of more than one serving of artificially sweetened beverages increased cardiovascular mortality by 78% in IBD patients.[5] Such beverages are prohibited on the SANA program.

Parkinson's Disease (PD)

The only deviation in the SANA diet for those with or at high risk of PD found in this research was for decaffeinated coffee. Decaf coffee should be strongly avoided by this population as it rates a decidedly negative DAD score. Decaf green tea and chocolate are not a problem. Since caffeine consumption strongly protects against the development of PD, it is recommended that coffee and caffeinated beverages be avoided in this population and that they instead take a daily dose of 100 to 120 mg of caffeine in the morning each day as a supplement. Taking the pharmaceutical preparation of caffeine should avoid the vagaries of caffeine content in different coffees and other compounds, which are potentially detrimental.

One-hundred-milligram caffeine tablets are available over the counter.

Type 2 Diabetes (T2D)

Adherence to the SANA program should greatly improve the health of those with T2D who are consuming a Western diet. If switching from a Western diet to the SANA diet, diabetics should monitor their blood sugars; they may need a reduction in their medications.

The SANA diet does require some adaptations for those with diabetes. Diabetics need to greatly restrict sugars and sweets and items and avoid such as sweetened breakfast cereals.

Diabetics should be very cautious with consuming fruit juices and limit the amounts. For orange juice, the maximum serving size is 2.5 fluid ounces (@75 ml). An average orange makes about 2 oz. of juice. It is better to eat an orange, which contains fiber and gives a slower release of sugars. (The exception is when using orange juice in an emergency to raise blood sugar.) Diabetics should also avoid smoothies, as they also speed up the digestion of the blended foods.

There are a few dietary DAD score idiosyncrasies for those with T2D. Bananas have a DAD score of zero, but get an A in diabetics. They have too much carbs and sugar in relation to overall nutritional value; thus, they should be avoided by those with T2D.

Attention Deficit Hyperactivity Disorder (ADHD)

ADHD is largely a lifestyle disease; it is at least exacerbated if not mostly caused by poor diet and sleep habits. A diet that protects against leaky gut, such as the SANA diet, is imperative to restoring health in those with ADHD, but disordered sleep, physical activity, and screen time also need to be addressed. Sleep disturbances contribute to disrupted intestinal membrane integrity.

For recovery from ADHD, regular sleep and rise times need to be maintained; the enteric nervous system of the gut needs to be entrained to the diurnal cycle. This requires regular meal times and avoiding late evening meals or snacks. (as discussed in Chapter 21, Time Restricted Eating)

Although serotonin is generally thought of as a calming neurotransmitter of the central nervous system, 90% of the serotonin made by the body is produced by enterochromaffin cells in the intestine. Most of the body's melatonin is also produced by the intestines. The production of these compounds has a strong diurnal cycle, which is impacted by eating time. Those with ADHD should not eat for two hours before their regular bedtime.

Stimulants such as caffeine should be avoided during the second half of the day, especially for those with ADHD and others who have difficulty maintaining a regular sleep cycle. Chocolate should be avoided as it contains theobromine, a stimulant, as well as other compounds that affect mood.

Adequate exercise is strongly encouraged for those with ADHD; although busy, most people with ADHD do not get sufficient exercise.

The impact of artificial lighting on sleep onset delay should not be underestimated. Fluorescent light, daylight LEDs, and screens (TV, computer, phones) have high levels of blue light that act as a signal to the brain that it is still daytime. This suppresses melatonin and disrupts the sleep cycle. Sleep cycles are commonly disrupted in ADHD, and sleep deprivation is common.

Lowering light levels in the home in the evening, using lights with less blue light (warmer rather than cooler colors, and lower K values, i.e., 3,000K rather than 5,000K), and avoiding looking at screens for at least an hour before bedtime should help avoid delayed sleep onset. Blue-blocking glasses and settings that lower blue light on monitors may help. Exciting activities in the evening should also be avoided for those with ADHD, including exciting (scary, emotionally charged, violent, and ugly) shows.

A regular daily routine, with meals at the same time each day, and regular rise and sleep times, is important for resolving ADHD. Adequate sleep time is a must. Table 30A shows sleep time requirements by age. Many parents underestimate the sleep needs of children and adolescents, as well as their own. Lowering the lights and maintaining a calm home atmosphere an hour before bedtime helps prepare for sleep. Not feeling sleepy is not a guarantee that one is getting sufficient sleep.

Autism Spectrum Disorder (ASD) is not the result of the child having a leaky gut.[6] Autism is a syndrome with multiple causes; some genetic, some environmental, but with most cases being a combination of both. The pathological events that cause autism usually occur early in gestation, between the 8th to 12th week of pregnancy. Maternal leaky gut during this part of pregnancy is a likely contributing factor in the causation of ASD; however, this has not been confirmed.

Gastrointestinal issues, including leaky gut, are highly prevalent among children with ASD. In children with autism, leaky gut may increase the severity of behavioral issues, may make the child feel worse, and may prevent adaptation. Thus, a healthy diet that prevents leaky gut is very likely to be helpful to a child with ASD.

Pregnancy

While not a disease, pregnancy is a special time that has profound consequences on the life of the offspring and can also be a time of great health risk for its mother.

The SANA diet is very appropriate *before and during* pregnancy, as well as when breastfeeding. The SANA diet is geared to reduce the risk of diabetes, and thus should help prevent gestational diabetes. Being low in empty calories, it is a very nutritious diet. A meta-analysis of ten studies, including 54,000 pregnancies, found that women consuming a diet with a high Dietary Inflammatory Index were about 25 to 33% more likely to develop gestational diabetes.[7] The SANA diet was designed to be an anti-inflammatory diet.

Diet before the onset of pregnancy impacts the outcome. Women eating a low-quality diet before pregnancy are at higher risk of preterm birth, small for gestational age, low birthweight infants, and neonatal intensive care unit admission.[8] In another study, starchy diets and those high in caffeine before the onset of pregnancy were associated with an increased risk of poor outcomes of pregnancy.[9] [10] The SANA program recommends that caffeine be limited to no more than about 80 mg per day during pregnancy, about the amount in 6 ounces of standard American-style brewed coffee or two cups of green tea.

The SANA program does not recommend veganism during pregnancy or breastfeeding because of the difficulty in getting several micronutrients, as explained in the section on veganism in Chapter 13. Nevertheless, the SANA program does recommend the avoidance of red meat, especially during pregnancy.

Pregnant women need more vitamin D than non-pregnant people. The target serum 25OHD3 level during pregnancy is 140 to 150 mmol/l. This is the level women have living in a natural human environment during pregnancy.[11] Vitamin D raises erythropoietin (EPO) levels. EPO is the hormone that controls the production of red blood cells, and more blood and iron stores are needed for pregnancy. Parathyroid hormone, which increases when vitamin D levels are insufficient, inhibits the production of erythropoietin, inhibits erythropoiesis, promotes erythropoietin resistance, and causes fibrosis of the bone marrow.[12] [13] In a study of twin births, women with 25-hydroxyvitamin D levels over 70 nmol/L (28 ng/dL) were 60% less likely to have preterm delivery than women with lower vitamin D levels.[14] Adequate levels of vitamin D decrease the risk of giving birth to an infant that is small for gestational age.[15] Vitamin D supplementation at 6,000 – 7,000 IU (150 – 175 mcg) per day is recommended during pregnancy.

Anemia is a major risk for the fetus and the pregnant woman. The most critical time for brain development is during fetal life and infancy, and it is dependent upon the mother's red blood cell count and oxygen-carrying capacity, as well as the woman's iron stores needed for the baby's growth and development. Thus, women should be replete with iron before the onset of pregnancy. The red blood cell mass is the safest way to store iron in the body.

In addition to iron, being replete in vitamin A and D, zinc, and selenium, all help to optimize the red blood cell mass; these nutrients help maintain a high hemoglobin level.

The best way to get vitamin A is a diet rich in yellow-orange vegetables and fruits, such as winter squash and pumpkin, sweet potatoes, tomatoes, mangoes, peaches, mandarins, and papayas. These not only supply carotenoids that are converted into vitamin A but also supply other carotenoids such as lutein, zeaxanthin, meso-zeaxanthin, and phytoene that cross the placental and blood-brain barriers and act as antioxidants. Yellow-orange vegetable consumption during pregnancy decreases the risk of the child developing brain cancer.

Sufficient zinc and selenium are also needed for optimal production of red blood cells. Adequate selenium is associated with a lower risk of having a small for gestational age infant. Eating one Brazil nut on most days supplies the RDA for selenium. (Two Brazil nuts contain too much selenium.) Of course, adequate iron is needed, especially during the second trimester. Chicken liver (DAD score 0) is an excellent source of readily available iron.

Short sleep is associated with anemia.[16] [17] Short sleep promotes inflammation, and inflammation promotes the anemia of chronic disease, during which iron absorption falls. Anemia is also associated with and provokes insomnia.[18] Iron deficiency can cause insomnia and sleep disturbances. Sleep deficits during pregnancy are associated with increased risk of cesarean section.

Calcium and folate supplementation should ideally be started before the onset of pregnancy, and at the onset if not done before. Calcium supplements during pregnancy decrease the risk of autism. The likely mechanism for this is that taking supplements sidesteps the resorption of calcium from the mother's bones. When calcium is resorbed from the bones during pregnancy, any lead, cadmium, manganese, or other toxic metals sequestered in the bone are also released, exposing the fetus to these toxins. Ensuring adequate calcium intake and absorption, supported by sufficient vitamin D, is crucial during pregnancy to minimize maternal bone resorption.

Folate in the form of 5-MTHF (see Chapter 25 Micronutrients) supplementation has also been found to greatly decrease the risk of the child having autism. It should be supplemented from the onset of pregnancy or before. The most critical risk period for the development of autism is likely between 8 and 12 weeks, thus in the first trimester of pregnancy.

I recommend that women avoid red meat (meat from mammals) during pregnancy, as I suspect that preeclampsia risk is associated with exposure to Neu5Gc (See Chapter 32 Meat Two). While cow's milk contains some Neu5Gc, levels are lower. Sheep and goat's milk have higher Neu5Gc levels than cow's milk does. Thus, unless dairy from cows cannot be used, goat and sheep milk and cheese are not recommended during pregnancy.

The recommendation for the consumption of dairy is slightly modified for pregnancy. The branched-chain amino acids in whey are helpful for fetal growth. Thus, regular yogurt is recommended rather than Greek yogurt during pregnancy and breastfeeding. Whole milk can be used if the woman is not lactose intolerant, but fermented milk (kefir and yogurt) is still recommended over liquid milk. Low-fat milk should be avoided. Full-fat cow's milk cheeses can be eaten.

Preterm delivery (PTD) and low birth weight (LBW) are grave dangers for infants. Risk can be greatly reduced by avoiding infections. The chapter on periodontal disease is highly relevant for pregnant women. Preferably, when planning pregnancy or at the onset of pregnancy, women should be seen by a dentist and assessed for periodontal disease, as it is a major risk factor for PTD and LBW. Good oral hygiene with the use of mouthwash (preferably a non-alcoholic, essential oil-based mouthwash) can reduce the risk of PTD by 63% and LBW by 46%. Avoiding gestational diabetes also reduces risk.

Bacterial vaginosis is another risk factor for PTD and LBW. Lactobacilli in fermented foods such as yogurt may decrease the risk of vaginal infections; however, the most helpful Lactobacilli species for this are not present in yogurt; specific vaginal probiotics may be appropriate for women at risk.[19]

While this chapter briefly addresses the topic of infant neurodevelopment, readers seeking more comprehensive information on fetal/maternal health and child development, including the topics of ADHD and autism, will find further details and discussion in my two-volume book, "Neurodevelopment and Intelligence," accessible on Google Books at:
https://www.google.com/books/edition/_/1KhiEAAAQBAJ

Morning Sickness and Hyperemesis Gravidarum (HG)

Hyperemesis gravidarum is a severe form of morning sickness that can pose a danger to the mother and fetus. HG, severe nausea and vomiting in pregnancy can have lifetime consequences for the child; increasing the lifetime risk of anxiety disorder (OR 1.74), sleep disorders (OR 2.94), hospitalization for neurologic problems (OR 1.5), developmental disorders (OR 1.51), increased risk of attention deficit hyperactivity disorder, autism, and testicular cancer (OR 1.6). HG-exposed children were found to have smaller brain cortices and cognitive and motor problems.[20 21]

It is not surprising that the diet has a significant causative role in this disease. HG is more common in women who are overweight or obese before they become pregnant.

When women were ranked by their dietary inflammatory index score, those in the top third were 65% more likely to develop HG than those in the lower third.[22] The SANA diet should substantially lower this risk.

In a study that looked at dietary patterns, women whose diet were characterized by high consumption of sugar-free colas, sugary drinks, and coffee drinks were at greatest risk of HG, while those characterized by the consumption of dairy products, eggs, water, and yogurt were at the lowest risk followed by those whose diets were high in fish, shrimp, unprocessed poultry and meat.[23] In another study, women whose diets were high in carbohydrates and added sugars, primarily from soft drinks, were at higher risk of nausea and vomiting in pregnancy.[24]

The SANA diet is an anti-inflammatory diet that warns against the consumption of sugary beverages, and thus should greatly lower the risk of hyperemesis gravidarum and morning sickness. A diet rich in digestible protein is recommended to avert HG; thus, the consumption of dairy, eggs, seafood, and fatty fish is recommended. Poultry can be eaten as advised in Chapter 13, but red meat should be avoided.

Polycystic Ovary Syndrome (PCOS)

PCOS is a syndrome, meaning it has a cluster of disease conditions. These include insulin resistance, a tendency to obesity, hirsutism (e.g., increased facial hair), severe acne, depression, infertility, and all the diseases associated with metabolic syndrome (heart disease, T2D, stroke), and the risk of endometrial cancer. Since the SANA diet reduces insulin resistance, it should help lower the risk of developing many of these diseases.

As many as 15% of women of reproductive age have PCOS. Many women with PCOS were thin throughout adolescence, but become overweight or obese by the age of thirty; their menstrual irregularities typically predate the weight gain. Thus, PCOS in these women is not caused by insulin resistance but rather secondary to it. Thus, while the insulin resistance needs to be addressed, the underlying disorder also needs to be treated.

Both environmental and genetic factors are involved in the development of PCOS. Most women cluster into one of two groups: the "metabolic type" and the "reproductive type" of PCOS, although there is overlap, and some women have both types. The reproductive type is primarily caused by alterations in sex hormone feedback mechanisms, while the metabolic type is primarily the result of glucose metabolism and insulin resistance.[25] The underlying cause needs to be addressed. For the metabolic type, the SANA diet should be of significant benefit as it addresses metabolic syndrome.

For women with the reproductive type of PCOS, the underlying cause, hyperandrogenism, needs to be addressed. Steroid hormones are interconverted, including testosterone into estrogen by the enzyme aromatase; thus, hypofunction of the enzyme aromatase, and likely hyperfunction of the enzyme 21-hydroxylase, which converts progesterone into corticosteroids, may occur in PCOS. Other steroid-modifying enzymes and pituitary feedback loops are also involved. These mechanisms result in an increase in testosterone and a decrease in estrogen synthesis, causing acne, hirsutism, and ovarian dysfunction, and elevation of corticosteroids, which promotes weight gain, which then promotes insulin resistance, as a simplified explanation.

A contributing cause for some cases of PCOS is fetal exposure to androgens. Women with PCOS have high androgen levels, imparting risk to their daughters, creating a transgenerational risk for the disease. This is a result of epigenetic imprinting rather than being a typical hereditary condition.[26] Thus, metabolic PCOS in the mother may promote reproductive PCOS in the daughter. Hypothetically, this impacts the setpoint for what the woman's body deems a normal testosterone to estrogen ratio, altering the expression of aromatase and other enzymes that control steroid metabolism.

Melatonin inhibits aromatase expression,[27] and thus, this supplement is best avoided in women with PCOS. Certain antioxidants have been found to help with PCOS.[28] The SANA diet goes further by being an anti-inflammatory diet.

Coffee consumption has been found to have a strong inverse association with the risk of PCOS and its associated infertility. One cup of coffee per day was found to be associated with a 72% lower risk of anovulatory PCOS.[29] A serving of coffee (8 oz.) typically contains between 70 and 140 mg of caffeine. I suggest that the total daily dose of caffeine not exceed one cup of coffee in PCOS, as higher doses may inhibit this effect. Green tea, which has 30 – 50 mg of caffeine, or matcha with 60 – 70 mg per serving, can also be used as a source of caffeine.

Other nutrients that have beneficial effects on PCOS include myoinositol, genistein, and L-carnitine. Niacinamide and vitamin C may be helpful.[30] Consumption of citrus fruit (tangerines and oranges) is encouraged for those with PCOS.

A small to medium morning dose of caffeine and a citrus fruit (whole rather than as juice) are recommended as a daily regimen for those with PCOS.

Metformin is commonly used in the treatment of PCOS. Both metformin and myoinositol increase insulin sensitivity by activating AMPK and by increasing the expression of GLUT4, which increases glucose uptake by the cells.[31] In meta-analyses, myoinositol has been found to have similar efficacy in the treatment of PCOS with fewer side effects, and myoinositol lowers triglyceride (fat) levels in the blood.[32] [33] [34] Myoinositol lowers the risk of metabolic syndrome and is important for thyroid hormone synthesis, insulin signaling, nerve guidance, and fat metabolism. It also helps in the treatment of depression and anxiety.[35] For treating PCOS, 2,000 to 2,500 mg of myoinositol per day is recommended. As discussed in Chapter 9, soaking rice helps convert phytic acid into myoinositol. Consumption of brown rice is recommended for PCOS over that of white rice.

The hormone 17 beta-estradiol 17-dehydrogenase-2 (HSD17B2) promotes the synthesis of estrogen and decreases the signs of PCOS. Genistein enhances the expression of HSD17B2[36] and has significant estrogenic effects on multiple tissues.[37] Tofu and other soy-based products are high in genistein and are recommended to be frequently consumed by women with PCOS. Sesame seeds (tahini) appear to negatively impact steroid hormone feedback regulation in women with PCOS and thus should be avoided in PCOS. This is likely due to the effect of enterolactone generated during the digestion of sesame seeds.[38]

Supplementation with carnitine is helpful in treating infertility in women with polycystic ovary disease (PCOS).[39] As discussed in Chapter 13, there are only trivial amounts of carnitine in foods from plants, other than tempeh, a fermented food. Carnitine helps with the metabolism of fats and helps in the treatment of PCOS. Red meat, while high in carnitine, is not part of the SANA diet. Dairy (yogurt, cheese, etc.) contains substantial amounts of carnitine. Tofu is not only high in genistein, but it is also rich in lysine and methionine, the amino acids the body uses to form carnitine. If L-carnitine is used as a supplement to help in the treatment of PCOS, it is recommended that it be taken with and split between meals for best absorption. A healthier approach is to maintain a low-fat diet, greatly curtailing the need for high amounts of carnitine in the diet. Acetyl carnitine is generally considered to be better absorbed than L-carnitine and is thus the preferred form for supplementation.

Exposure to environmental toxins such as PFAS increases the risk of PCOS[40] and thus needs to be avoided.

Cancer

Cancer is not a disease, but rather a class of diseases. Every cancer is unique, so making generalizations about what diet is most appropriate for those with cancer can be problematic.

Cancer patients should heed the warnings in Chapter 25 and avoid vitamin A and several other vitamins and mineral supplements, as several of these increase cancer proliferation and mortality among those with cancer. It is far better just to eat a healthy diet. Vitamin D is the greatest exception. Vitamin B12 will also be needed by most older cancer patients.

Many people advocate a vegan diet for those diagnosed with cancer. In a meta-analysis, a vegan diet was found to be associated with a lower risk of the incidence of cancer, but there was no difference in the risk of cancer mortality.[41] Vegans were about 15% less likely to develop cancer, but just as likely to die from cancer, suggesting that they may be at a slightly higher risk of dying from cancer if it develops. I was unable to find any data demonstrating that adopting a vegan diet after the diagnosis of cancer improved survival or cure rates.

In a meta-analysis of 15 follow-up studies assessing the impact of total fat intake, there was no difference in breast cancer or overall mortality between high and low-fat diets. Diets high in saturated fats were associated with an increase in breast cancer deaths.[42] Nevertheless, another meta-analysis found no difference in breast cancer mortality when comparing women with the highest and lowest categories of animal fat intake,[43] and another meta-analysis that looked at serum levels of SFA, MUFA, PUFA, n-3 PUFA, and n-6 PUFA, found that only monounsaturated fats appeared to be associated with breast cancer risk.[44]

Studies that examine cancer incidence associated with diet may not elucidate which dietary components improve survival after a diagnosis of cancer has been made.

The SANA diet is a low-fat diet, as it is a healthier and more nutritious diet than one high in added fat and added sugar, with empty calories. As discussed in Chapter 13, a diet with sufficient protein improves cancer survival. This is hard to do on a vegan diet. Most animal-based foods, including fish, eggs, and dairy, contain substantial amounts of fat.

As with healthy persons, the SANA diet recommends that those with cancer keep total fat calories below their protein caloric intake. Carnitine (discussed in Chapter 13), which is produced from amino acids in protein, is needed to utilize fat for energy. Carnitine and palmitic acids interact in at least some cancers to kill cancer cells, while diets high in palmitic acid (C16:0) alone may promote cancer cell proliferation.[45] [46] Beet tallow and butter contain 26% of their calories as palmitic acid. Chicken flesh is 23% palmitic acid. Palm oil is 45% C16:0, while coconut oil, in contrast, contains 8%. The lack of carnitine in relation to palmitic acid may be a risk for cancer growth.

Consuming a diet with high amounts of protein increases survival in those with cancer. Protein intake should be around 1.2–1.5 g protein/kg of body mass per day. One way to do this is to use lower-fat dairy products such as low-fat Greek yogurt and low-fat cheeses, as mozzarella, and fro-yo, so that more of the caloric intake is as protein, assuming that caloric intake remains the same. It is easier to get a nourishing, high-protein diet when avoiding empty calories, such as sugar-sweetened foods and vegetables, and those made with vegetable oils.

As mentioned in Chapter 13, black beans and chickpeas, which are high in isoflavones, a diet high in fiber, sufficient vitamin D, and recreational exercise, lower the mortality risk among women with breast cancer. Soy products (Tofu, tempeh, soy milk) likely improve survival for women with estrogen receptor-positive breast cancer. Fiber may act by binding bile acids and preventing the formation of secondary bile acids and by binding steroid hormone conjugates that are excreted in the bile, thus decreasing reabsorption of steroid hormones. Thus, the high fiber diet may be more effective in hormone-sensitive cancers than in those that are not.

[1] Diet, Food, and Nutritional Exposures and Inflammatory Bowel Disease or Progression of Disease: an Umbrella Review. Christensen C, Knudsen A, Arnesen EK, Hatlebakk JG, Sletten IS, Fadnes LT. Adv Nutr. 2024 May;15(5):100219. doi: 10.1016/j.advnut.2024.100219. Epub 2024 Apr 8. PMID: 38599319

[2] Dietary risk factors for inflammatory bowel disease in Shanghai: A case-control study. Mi L, Zhang C, Yu XF, Zou J, Yu Y, Bao ZJ. Asia Pac J Clin Nutr. 2022;31(3):405-414. doi: 10.6133/apjcn.202209_31(3).0008. PMID: 36173212

[3] Association of diet and outdoor time with inflammatory bowel disease: a multicenter case-control study using propensity matching analysis in China. Chu X, Chen X, Zhang H, Wang Y, Guo H, Chen Y, Liu X, Zhu Z, He Y, Ding X, Wang Q, Zheng C, Cao X, Yang H, Qian J. Front Public Health. 2024 Jun 17;12:1368401. doi: 10.3389/fpubh.2024.1368401. eCollection 2024. PMID: 38952728

[4] Sugar-sweetened beverages exacerbate high-fat diet-induced inflammatory bowel disease by altering the gut microbiome.Shon WJ, Jung MH, Kim Y, Kang GH, Choi EY, Shin DM. J Nutr Biochem. 2023 Mar;113:109254. doi: 10.1016/j.jnutbio.2022.109254. PMID: 36572070.

[5] Associations of sugar-sweetened beverages, artificially sweetened beverages, and natural juices with cardiovascular disease and all-cause mortality in individuals with inflammatory bowel disease in a prospective cohort study. Dan L, Fu T, Sun Y, Ruan X, Lu S, Chen J, Wang X. Therap Adv Gastroenterol. 2023 Nov 8;16:17562848231207305. doi: 10.1177/17562848231207305. PMID: 37954536; PMCID: PMC10637157.

[6] The search for gastrointestinal inflammation in autism: a systematic review and meta-analysis of non-invasive gastrointestinal markers. Mathew NE, McCaffrey D, Walker AK, Mallitt KA, Masi A, Morris MJ, Ooi CY. Mol Autism. 2024 Jan 17;15(1):4. doi: 10.1186/s13229-023-00575-0. PMID: 38233886

[7] Impact of dietary inflammatory index on gestational diabetes mellitus in normal and overweight women: a systematic review and meta-analysis of observational studiesLiu RL, Chen XQ, Zheng QX, Li JN, Zhu Y, Huang L, Pan YQ, Jiang XM.. Asia Pac J Clin Nutr. 2024 Sep;33(3):298-312. doi: 10.6133/apjcn.202409_33(3).0002. PMID: 38965719; PMCID: PMC11389818.

[8] Quality of periconceptional dietary intake and maternal and neonatal outcomes. Yee LM, Silver RM, Haas DM, Parry S, Mercer BM, Iams J, Wing D, Parker CB, Reddy UM, Wapner RJ, Grobman WA. Am J Obstet Gynecol. 2020 Jul;223(1):121.e1-121.e8. doi: 10.1016/j.ajog.2020.01.042. Epub 2020 Jan 23. PMID: 31981510

[9] High starchy food intake may increase the risk of adverse pregnancy outcomes: a nested case-control study in the Shaanxi province of Northwestern China. Huang L, Shang L, Yang W, Li D, Qi C, Xin J, Wang S, Yang L, Zeng L, Chung MC. BMC Pregnancy Childbirth. 2019 Oct 21;19(1):362. doi: 10.1186/s12884-019-2524-z. PMID: 31638947

[10] Caffeine intake during pregnancy and adverse outcomes: An integrative review. Rohweder R, de Oliveira Schmalfuss T, Dos Santos Borniger D, Ferreira CZ, Zanardini MK, Lopes GPTF, Barbosa CP, Moreira TD, Schuler-Faccini L, Sanseverino MTV, da Silva AA, Abeche AM, Vianna FSL, Fraga LR. Reprod Toxicol. 2024 Jan;123:108518. doi: 10.1016/j.reprotox.2023.108518. PMID: 38042437

[11] Vitamin D status indicators in indigenous populations in East Africa. Luxwolda MF, Kuipers RS, Kema IP, van der Veer E, Dijck-Brouwer DA, Muskiet FA. Eur J Nutr. 2013 Apr;52(3):1115-25. doi: 10.1007/s00394-012-0421-6. PMID: 22878781

[12] Vitamin D Level and Its Correlation With Hemoglobin In Pediatric Sickle Cell Disease Patients. Busse JA, Seelaboyina KN, Malonga G, Setty MJ. Blood (2013) 122 (21): 4677. https://doi.org/10.1182/blood.V122.21.4677.4677

[13] Vitamin D and anemia: insights into an emerging association. Smith EM, Tangpricha V. Curr Opin Endocrinol Diabetes Obes. 2015 Dec;22(6):432-8. doi: 10.1097/MED.0000000000000199. PMID: 26414080

[14] Maternal 25-hydroxyvitamin D and preterm birth in twin gestations. Bodnar LM, Rouse DJ, Momirova V, et al; Eunice Kennedy Shriver (NICHD) Maternal-Fetal Medicine Units (MFMU) Network. Obstet Gynecol. 2013 Jul;122(1):91-98. doi: 10.1097/AOG.0b013e3182941d9a. PMID: 23743453.

[15] Maternal dietary consumption of legumes, vegetables and fruit during pregnancy, does it protect against small for gestational age? Martínez-Galiano JM, Amezcua-Prieto C, Salcedo-Bellido I, González-Mata G, et al. BMC Pregnancy Childbirth. 2018 Dec 11;18(1):486. doi: 10.1186/s12884-018-2123-4. PMID: 30537936

[16] Relationship between Self-Reported Sleep Duration and Risk of Anemia: Data from the Korea National Health and Nutrition Examination Survey 2016-2017. Chun MY, Kim JH, Kang JS. Int J Environ Res Public Health. 2021 Apr 28;18(9):4721. doi: 10.3390/ijerph18094721. PMID: 33925225

[17] Night Sleep Duration and Risk of Incident Anemia in a Chinese Population: A Prospective Cohort Study. Liu X, Song Q, Hu W, Han X, Gan J, Zheng X, Wang X, Wu S. Sci Rep. 2018 Mar 5;8(1):3975. doi: 10.1038/s41598-018-22407-5. PMID: 29507334

[18] Anemia and insomnia: a cross-sectional study and meta-analysis. Neumann SN, Li JJ, Yuan XD, Chen SH, Ma CR, Murray-Kolb LE, Shen Y, Wu SL, Gao X. Chin Med J (Engl). 2020 Dec 21;134(6):675-681. doi: 10.1097/CM9.0000000000001306. PMID: 33725707

[19] Neurodevelopment and Intelligence: Impacts of Nutrition, Environmental Toxins, and Stress. (Volumes 1 and 2. Charles A Lewis. Psy Press, Carrabelle FL. 2022 ISBN-13: 978-1938318078 and 978-1938318085

[20] Long-term health outcomes of children born to mothers with hyperemesis gravidarum: a systematic review and meta-analysis. Nijsten K, Jansen LAW, Limpens J, Finken MJJ, Koot MH, Grooten IJ, Roseboom TJ, Painter RC. Am J Obstet Gynecol. 2022 Sep;227(3):414-429.e17. doi: 10.1016/j.ajog.2022.03.052. PMID: 35367190

[21] Hyperemesis gravidarum and the risk of offspring morbidity: a longitudinal cohort study. Auger N, Padda B, Bégin P, Brousseau É, Côté-Corriveau G. Eur J Pediatr. 2024 Sep;183(9):3843-3851. doi: 10.1007/s00431-024-05647-8. Epub 2024 Jun 17. PMID: 38884821

[22] Association between Dietary Inflammatory Index and Hyperemesis Gravidarum. Nutrients.Zhi S, Zhang L, Cheng W, Jin Y, Long Z, Gu W, Ma L, Zhang S, Lin J. 2024 Aug 8;16(16):2618. doi: 10.3390/nu16162618. PMID: 39203755; PMCID: PMC11357208.

[23] Association between Dietary Patterns and the Risk of Hyperemesis Gravidarum. Cheng W, Li L, Long Z, Ma X, Chen F, Ma L, Zhang S, Lin J. Nutrients. 2023 Jul 25;15(15):3300. doi: 10.3390/nu15153300. PMID: 37571237

[24] Nausea and vomiting in pregnancy: associations with maternal gestational diet and lifestyle factors in the Norwegian Mother and Child Cohort Study. Chortatos A, Haugen M, Iversen PO, Vikanes Å, Magnus P, Veierød MB. BJOG. 2013 Dec;120(13):1642-53. doi: 10.1111/1471-0528.12406. PMID: 23962347

[25] Distinct subtypes of polycystic ovary syndrome with novel genetic associations: An unsupervised, phenotypic clustering analysis. Dapas M, Lin FTJ, Nadkarni GN, Sisk R, Legro RS, Urbanek M, Hayes MG, Dunaif A. PLoS Med. 2020 Jun 23;17(6):e1003132. doi: 10.1371/journal.pmed.1003132. PMID: 32574161

[26] Animal Models to Understand the Etiology and Pathophysiology of Polycystic Ovary Syndrome. Stener-Victorin E, Padmanabhan V, Walters KA, Campbell RE, Benrick A, Giacobini P, Dumesic DA, Abbott DH. Endocr Rev. 2020 Jul 1;41(4):bnaa010. doi: 10.1210/endrev/bnaa010. PMID: 32310267

[27] Melatonin as an Oncostatic Molecule Based on Its Anti-Aromatase Role in Breast Cancer. Jin Y, Choi YJ, Heo K, Park SJ. Int J Mol Sci. 2021 Jan 4;22(1):438. doi: 10.3390/ijms22010438. PMID: 33406787

[28] Distinct subtypes of polycystic ovary syndrome with novel genetic associations: An unsupervised, phenotypic clustering analysis. Dapas M, Lin FTJ, Nadkarni GN, Sisk R, Legro RS, Urbanek M, Hayes MG, Dunaif A. PLoS Med. 2020 Jun 23;17(6):e1003132. doi: 10.1371/journal.pmed.1003132. eCollection 2020 Jun. PMID: 32574161

[29] Association between Coffee Consumption and Polycystic Ovary Syndrome: An Exploratory Case-Control Study. Meliani-Rodríguez A, Cutillas-Tolín A, Mendiola J, Sánchez-Ferrer ML, De la Cruz-Sánchez E, Vioque J, Torres-Cantero AM. Nutrients. 2024 Jul 11;16(14):2238. doi: 10.3390/nu16142238. PMID: 39064680

[30] A Properly Balanced Reduction Diet and/or Supplementation Solve the Problem with the Deficiency of These Vitamins Soluble in Water in Patients with PCOS.

Szczuko M, Szydłowska I, Nawrocka-Rutkowska J. Nutrients. 2021 Feb 26;13(3):746. doi: 10.3390/nu13030746. PMID: 33652684

[31] The insulin-sensitizing mechanism of myo-inositol is associated with AMPK activation and GLUT-4 expression in human endometrial cells exposed to a PCOS environment. Cabrera-Cruz H, Oróstica L, Plaza-Parrochia F, Torres-Pinto I, Romero C, Vega M. Am J Physiol Endocrinol Metab. 2020 Feb 1;318(2):E237-E248. doi: 10.1152/ajpendo.00162.2019. Epub 2019 Dec 24. PMID: 31874063

[32] Comparative efficacy of oral insulin sensitizers metformin, thiazolidinediones, inositol, and berberine in improving endocrine and metabolic profiles in women with PCOS: a network meta-analysis. Zhao H, Xing C, Zhang J, He B. Reprod Health. 2021 Aug 18;18(1):171. doi: 10.1186/s12978-021-01207-7. PMID: 34407851

[33] The effects of inositol supplementation on lipid profiles among patients with metabolic diseases: a systematic review and meta-analysis of randomized controlled trials. Tabrizi R, Ostadmohammadi V, Lankarani KB, Peymani P, Akbari M, Kolahdooz F, Asemi Z. Lipids Health Dis. 2018 May 24;17(1):123. doi: 10.1186/s12944-018-0779-4. PMID: 29793496

[34] Inositol is an effective and safe treatment in polycystic ovary syndrome: a systematic review and meta-analysis of randomized controlled trials. Greff D, Juhász AE, Váncsa S, Váradi A, Sipos Z, Szinte J, Park S, Hegyi P, Nyirády P, Ács N, Várbíró S, Horváth EM. Reprod Biol Endocrinol. 2023 Jan 26;21(1):10. doi: 10.1186/s12958-023-01055-z. PMID: 36703143

[35] https://en.wikipedia.org/wiki/Inositol

[36] Uterine Patterning, Endometrial Gland Development, and Implantation Failure in Mice Exposed Neonatally to Genistein. Jefferson WN, Padilla-Banks E, Suen AA, Royer LJ, Zeldin SM, Arora R, Williams CJ. Environ Health Perspect. 2020 Mar;128(3):37001. doi: 10.1289/EHP6336. PMID: 32186404

[37] Effects of chronic genistein treatment in mammary gland, uterus, and vagina. Rimoldi G, Christoffel J, Seidlova-Wuttke D, Jarry H, Wuttke W. Environ Health Perspect. 2007 Dec;115 Suppl 1(Suppl 1):62-8. doi: 10.1289/ehp.9367. PMID: 18174952

[38] Mammalian lignans and genistein decrease the activities of aromatase and 17beta-hydroxysteroid dehydrogenase in MCF-7 cells. Brooks JD, Thompson LU. J Steroid Biochem Mol Biol. 2005 Apr;94(5):461-7. doi: 10.1016/j.jsbmb.2005.02.002. Epub 2005 Mar 16. PMID: 15876411

[39] Effects of L-carnitine supplementation for women with polycystic ovary syndrome: a systematic review and meta-analysis. Mohd Shukri MF, Norhayati MN, Badrin S, Abdul Kadir A. PeerJ. 2022 Sep 16;10:e13992. doi: 10.7717/peerj.13992. eCollection 2022. PMID: 36132218

[40] Environmental Exposure to Emerging Alternatives of Per- and Polyfluoroalkyl Substances and Polycystic Ovarian Syndrome in Women Diagnosed with Infertility: A Mixture Analysis. Zhan W, Qiu W, Ao Y, Zhou W, Sun Y, Zhao H, Zhang J. Environ Health Perspect. 2023 May;131(5):57001. doi: 10.1289/EHP11814. Epub 2023 May 3. PMID: 37134253

[41] Vegetarian, vegan diets and multiple health outcomes: A systematic review with meta-analysis of observational studies. Dinu M, Abbate R, Gensini GF, Casini A, Sofi F.

Crit Rev Food Sci Nutr. 2017 Nov 22;57(17):3640-3649. doi: 10.1080/10408398.2016.1138447. PMID: 26853923

42 Dietary fat and breast cancer mortality: A systematic review and meta-analysis. Brennan SF, Woodside JV, Lunny PM, Cardwell CR, Cantwell MM. Crit Rev Food Sci Nutr. 2017 Jul 3;57(10):1999-2008. doi: 10.1080/10408398.2012.724481. PMID: 25692500

43 Summary and meta-analysis of prospective studies of animal fat intake and breast cancer. Alexander DD, Morimoto LM, Mink PJ, Lowe KA. Nutr Res Rev. 2010 Jun;23(1):169-79. doi: 10.1017/S095442241000003X. Epub 2010 Feb 25. PMID: 20181297

44 Dietary total fat and fatty acids intake, serum fatty acids and risk of breast cancer: A meta-analysis of prospective cohort studies. Cao Y, Hou L, Wang W. Int J Cancer. 2016 Apr 15;138(8):1894-904. doi: 10.1002/ijc.29938. Epub 2015 Dec 9. PMID: 26595162

45 A HIF-1α inhibitor combined with palmitic acid and L-carnitine treatment can prevent the fat metabolic reprogramming under hypoxia and induce apoptosis in hepatocellular carcinoma cells. Matsufuji S, Kitajima Y, Higure K, Kimura N, Maeda S, Yamada K, Ito K, Tanaka T, Kai K, Noshiro H. Cancer Metab. 2023 Dec 8;11(1):25. doi: 10.1186/s40170-023-00328-w. PMID: 38066600

46 PA suppresses antitumor immunity of T cells by disturbing mitochondrial activity through Akt/mTOR-mediated Ca^{2+} flux. Sun S, Xu H, Zhao W, Li Q, Yuan Y, Zhang G, Li S, Wang B, Zhang W, Gao X, Zheng J, Zhang Q. Cancer Lett. 2024 Jan 28;581:216511. doi: 10.1016/j.canlet.2023.216511. PMID: 38013049

Appendix A: Glossary

4-hydroxy-2-nonenal (4-HNE): A product of lipid peroxidation and used as a biomarker of oxidative stress in the body.

Aberrant DNA Methylation: Carbon methyl groups tend to randomly stick to the DNA with time, sort of like dust particles. These make it harder for the RNA copies of the gene to be made during transcription, and thus inhibit the cell from making proteins. This occurs with aging and is accelerated by smoking and environmental stressors. By silencing tumor suppressor genes or inhibiting the repression of oncogenes, aberrant DNA methylation can promote cancer.

Activator Protein-1 (AP-1): A transcription factor composed of Jun and Fos that can promote cell growth, differentiation, and apoptosis, often in response to cytokines or growth factors.

AD: Alzheimer's Disease, the most common form of dementia, accounts for 60 to 80% of dementia. The occurrence increases with age. The pathologic findings in AD typically include amyloid plaques, neurofibrillary tangles, and loss of synapses in the brain.

Adaptive mechanism: Any mechanism by which the body compensates to protect itself from noxious stimuli, helping it adapt to stress and injury. Examples include the production of antioxidant enzymes.

Advanced glycation end-products (AGEs): A class of natural compounds that form through non-enzymatic binding of sugars to proteins, nucleic acids, or lipids. Excessive endogenous formation of these compounds can occur with hyperglycemia. Accumulation of AGEs is associated with the risk of diabetes, atherosclerosis, cardiovascular disease, and ageing.

Agency: An individual's sense of being able to control their actions and direct their actions to achieve their goals.

All-cause mortality: The sum of mortality from various injuries and diseases. It is a good indicator of the overall impact of various exposures on health.

Allicin, A.K.A. diallyl thiosulfinate, is a compound produced from allin (S-allylcysteine sulfoxide) in garlic when there is tissue injury. It is noxious to insects and many microbes, and acts as a defense compound for garlic. In humans, it has protective hormetic effects. Allicin gives garlic its distinct odor. It is thought to have cardioprotective properties and to lower lung cancer risk.

Alleles: Slight variations in genes that may be normal variation (such as eye color or blood type) or may place the person at risk for disease. ApoE4 is one such allele of ApoE.

Alpha-synuclein: A protein that collects in the brain and is a marker of certain forms of Parkinson's Disease (PD). In PD, alpha-synuclein can polymerize to form Lewy Bodies, a pathological marker of the disease.

ALS (Amyotrophic Lateral Sclerosis): A neurodegenerative disease. Formerly called Lou Gehrig's disease, after a famous baseball player who suffered from it. In ALS, there is degeneration of motor neurons, leading to muscle weakness and atrophy.

Amyloid plaques: A conglomeration of Aβ protein fragments that is commonly present in the brain of patients with Alzheimer's disease.

Amyloid precursor protein (APP): A protein formed in the brain that likely serves to protect the brain from infection. Depending on the activity of various enzymes, cleavage products of APP can form beta-amyloid, which participates in the causation of Alzheimer's disease.

Angiogenesis: The formation of new blood vessels. Angiogenesis occurs in the healing of wounds, but also in the development of cancer.

Anthocyanins: A class of flavonoid compounds found in flowers and fruits.

Antinutrients: Compounds in some plants that can interfere with the absorption of nutrients. Some examples include phytates, tannins, and saponins. Many anti-nutrients in food can be mitigated by proper preparation and cooking methods (described in this book).

Antioxidant enzymes: Enzymes that help protect cells from damage caused by free radicals. Among these are the enzymes of the Antioxidant-Response Element, including superoxide dismutase, catalase, and glutathione peroxidase.

Antioxidant-Response Element (ARE): A large set of adaptive enzymes and other proteins that are often expressed as a group in response to noxious stimuli. ARE transcription can be induced by activation of Nrf2.

Antioxidant: A substance that helps protect cells from damage caused by free radicals. Free radicals are unstable molecules that can damage cells and contribute to the development of chronic diseases.

Apoε: Apoprotein E is a lipid transport molecule. There are three common alleles (variants) in the human population: Apoε2, Apoε3, and Apoε4. Everyone gets one Apoε gene from each parent; thus, each of us has two. Those with Apoε4/4 are at high risk of developing AD in their 70s; those with Apoε3/4 (having one high and one average risk gene are at high risk, but lower risk than those with two Apoε4 genes. The Apoε2 allele carries a lower risk than does the Apoε3 allele.

Apoptosis: A form of cell death mediated from within the cell. It can be thought of as cell self-sacrifice. Apoptosis plays a crucial and likely daily role in preventing cancer through the elimination of aberrant cells. The failure of apoptotic pathways is typical in cancer cells.

Autophagy: Autophagy is a process where the cell breaks down old or damaged parts and recycles the materials. In autophagy, older and often worn-out or poorly functioning proteins or organelles are marked for removal and then recycled into their component amino acids. Think of autophagy as a cell's recycling and renewal system. Autophagy becomes less vigorous with aging. Dysfunctional autophagy is linked to neurodegenerative diseases.

Aβeta: Amyloid beta is a protein fragment of APP suspected of having an immune function, but when cut into certain fragments increases the risk of AD.

Aβ42: A specific amyloid precursor protein fragment that is highly associated with the development of AD and amyloid plaques. Aβ42 has a higher propensity for aggregation than other amyloid beta fragments and is associated with a higher risk of forming plaques.

Biological age: An estimate of a person's aging in contrast to their calendar age, based on the average biological age of persons of a given calendar age. Thus, for example, a person may have the frailty of an average 85-year-old while only being 72. Lifestyle has a major impact on the difference between a person's biological age from their calendar age.

Bipolar disorder: A mental disorder characterized by episodes of both manic behavior and severe depression.

Brain-Derived Neurotrophic Factor (BDNF): A neuronal growth factor protein essential for the growth, differentiation, and survival of neurons in the brain. BDNF has a crucial role in learning, memory, and mental health. Walking in new places and having new experiences enhances the production of BDNF.

BRCA1 and BRCA2: These are two very different genes, but both are involved in DNA repair. Some people have genetic alleles of these genes that do not function well, putting them at high risk of hereditary breast, ovarian, and other solid cancers.

Caries: One or more dental cavities. The word caries is both singular and plural. Caries result from the chronic demineralization of tooth enamel by acids produced principally by the bacteria *Streptococcus mutans*.

Catalase (CAT): One of several antioxidant proteins produced by the body. It catalyzes the decomposition of hydrogen peroxide into oxygen and water, thus protecting the cell from oxidative damage that can result from hydrogen peroxide produced in the cell.

Catechin: A flavonoid compound present in green tea and cacao. Catechin provides antioxidant benefits.

Cell proliferation: Growth in the number of cells as a result of cellular division. Also called cell growth.

Chronological age: A person's calendar age.

CNS: The Central Nervous System, including the brain and spinal cord

Commensal: A long-term symbiotic interaction in which members of one species gain benefits while those of the other species either benefit or are unharmed.

Cytokine: Cytokines are a class of signaling proteins produced by cells that influence the behavior primarily of nearby cells by way of cell surface receptors. Many promote inflammation, while others suppress inflammation. Some cytokines include the interleukins, TGF (tissue growth factors), interferons, and tumor necrosis factor.

Cytoprotective proteins: Proteins, including antioxidant enzymes, that protect the cell from stress and injury. Examples include heat shock proteins and enzymes such as glutathione peroxidase.

Cytosol: The main inside area of a cell, excluding the nucleus.

DAD Rating: The Defense Against Dysbiosis score is a metric used in this book to describe how beneficial or detrimental a food is to the microbiome and general health. The best rating is 4, while a rating of zero is neutral. Letter scores of A to D are detrimental, with foods ranked D being the most damaging.

DAMPs (Danger-associated molecular patterns): Molecules that signal danger to the immune system. LPS and flagellin are examples of DAMPs. DAMPs act by activation of cell surface toll-like receptors (TLRs).

Dementia: A gradual loss of mental abilities, including reasoning ability, judgment, and memory loss, severe enough to interfere with the activities of daily living. There are multiple forms of dementia, the most common being Alzheimer's disease.

DNA adducts: Chemicals, either formed within the body or from the environment, that covalently bind to the DNA. These can impact the DNA function and cause mutations during DNA replication. DNA adducts can induce cancer or cause cellular dysfunction. Tobacco smoke, industrial and transportation pollutants, and diet can be environmental sources of DNA adducts. Polycyclic aromatic hydrocarbons (PAHs) from burnt matter, including meat, fungal toxins, and alcohol, can cause the formation of DNA adducts.

DNA methylation: The addition of methyl groups (single carbon atoms with three hydrogen atoms) to specific DNA sequences. The addition of these methyl groups causes the DNA to be more adherent to histone proteins, which makes the DNA more resistant to transcription. Methylation of a gene decreases its expression. DNA methylation is a key component of epigenetic programming and epigenetic effects.

DNA methylation age: A metric of biological age based on tests of the methylation, usually of white blood cells.

DNA Repair: Multiple mechanisms are present in the cell to reconnect broken strands of DNA or to repair certain errors. When these mechanisms fail, there is an increased risk of cancer and age-related diseases.

Dysbiosis: An imbalance in the microbiome, where the community of microorganisms promotes inflammation or disease. This can occur, for example, in the mouth, colon, or vagina. Dysbiosis is associated with inflammation, obesity, and many other disease conditions.

Enteric Dysbiosis: An imbalance in the gut microbiome, the community of microorganisms living in the intestines, in which harmful bacteria dominate beneficial ones.

Enterocytes: Cells lining the small intestine that absorb nutrients. These cells maintain the intestinal barrier.

Expression: See gene expression.

Ferroptosis: A type of programmed cell death distinct from apoptosis. It is dependent upon iron ions and is characterized by lipid oxidation. It may play a role in the elimination of aberrant cells at risk of developing into cancer.

Fibrolytic bacteria: Bacteria that can digest complex carbohydrates that humans cannot. They are essential for health. One of their roles is to convert soluble fiber into short-chain fatty acids.

Flagellin: A protein found in some bacteria that can also trigger an inflammatory response by activating toll-like receptor 5 (TLR5).

Flavones: A specific class of phenolic compounds that is common in many foods, including herbs.

Flavonoid compounds: A group of over 5000 naturally occurring phytochemicals found in plants with the same basic structure. The subgroups include: Flavonols, Flavones, Anthocyanidins, Isoflavonoids, and Neoflavonoids. Many have health benefits, typically through hormetic activity, stimulating the ARE, and thus offering benefits as antioxidants.

Frailty: Loss of physiologic reserves, strength, and capacity to rebound from injury with aging. The diagnosis of frailty is based on the presence of at least three of the following: unintentional weight loss, slow walking speed, weakness (low grip strength), low physical activity, and exhaustion. Frailty increases the risk of falling, fractures, hospitalization, and mortality in older adults.

Gene expression: The process by which genetic information stored in DNA is transformed into functional proteins and peptides. It involves several steps: Transcription: The DNA sequence is copied into RNA. Translation: The RNA is used as a blueprint to build a protein. The level of expression of a gene determines how much of that protein is produced.

Genetic mutation: The change of one or more nucleic acids in the DNA structure that causes an alteration in a codon, and thus a change in the transcribed RNA. Mutations may be point mutations with the substitution of a single nucleotide, or may involve larger areas of a gene, as a result of insertions, deletions, or frameshift mutations.

GI microbiome: The microbiome of the gastrointestinal tract, which plays a crucial role in digestion, nutrient absorption, and immune function.

Glutathione: The body's main antioxidant compound. It is a small peptide composed of three amino acids. It is recycled by glutathione reductase. Glutathione is also used by the body to help eliminate many toxins from the body.

Glutathione reductase (GR): An enzyme that recycles oxidized glutathione into reduced glutathione, allowing it to act as an antioxidant again. GR helps maintain the cellular redox balance and thus helps prevent oxidative injury.

Glutathione S-transferases (GST): An enzyme that binds glutathione to electrophilic compounds, which lowers the toxicity of the compound and makes it easier for the compound to be excreted from the cell and the body. It is essential for protecting the body from environmental toxins.

Glycemic index: A system for ranking carbohydrates based on how quickly they raise blood sugar levels. High-GI foods cause blood sugar to spike quickly, while low-GI foods cause a more gradual rise in blood sugar. Sugar-sweetened beverages have a high glycemic index.

Greenspace: Open space and natural areas set aside from development. In urban areas, these may represent parks with public access or be buffers between areas of development. Urban green spaces reduce stress and improve mental health in urban populations that have access to them.

HAR: See Hormetic Adaptive Response

Healthspan: In contrast to the total years of life (the lifespan), healthspan refers to years of health.

Heme oxygenase (HMOX1): HMOX1 is an enzyme that breaks heme from red blood cells and other sources down into biliverdin, iron, and carbon monoxide. HMOX1, thus, protects against the toxic and oxidative impacts of heme from senescent RBCs. The carbon monoxide produced acts as a vasodilator, and biliverdin is converted into bilirubin, which has antioxidant properties.

Homeostatic dysregulation: Disruption of the body's ability to compensate for stressors or maintain its normal internal environment and metabolic balance.

Hormesis: An adaptive response, usually to a chemical compound, that at low dose exposure strengthens the body's resilience to stressors and toxins.

Hormetic adaptive response (HAR): The HAR is a score used in this book to rate the strength of dietary agents at stimulating an adaptive response on a scale of 1 to 10. Rating: It is a proprietary rating of hormetic reaction to foods and other stimuli to help describe the relative adaptive impact of various foods. Scores are zero to 10, with 10 being foods with very strong adaptive responses.

Hormetic agent: Any compound or stimulus that promotes a hormetic adaptive response. Examples of hormetic agents include exercise, sulforaphane from broccoli, and catechin in cocoa.

Horvath DNAmAge clock: A metric of biological age that measures DNA methylation. It is considered to be one of the most accurate metrics of biological age. It is used to study the impact of various interventions on aging.

Hyperglycemia: Elevated blood sugar levels. Hyperglycemia is a hallmark of diabetes and closely linked to its adverse outcomes, including diabetic retinopathy and neuropathy.

IBD: Inflammatory Bowel Disease, such as Crohn's disease and ulcerative colitis.

Inflammaging: Inflamm-aging – biological aging which occurs as a result of chronic or repetitive low-grade sterile inflammatory response. Strategies for avoiding inflammaging include exercise and an anti-inflammatory diet, such as the SANA diet.

Innate Immunity: In contrast to adaptive immunity with the formation of antibodies, innate immunity recognizes DAMPs and PAMPs (such as LPS and lipoteichoic acid. Innate immunity provides a non-specific but rapid response to pathogens. This is especially important for responding to pathogens the immune system has not encountered before.

Insulin Resistance: A highly common metabolic condition in which the body has decreased sensitivity to insulin. Thus, higher levels of insulin are required to control blood glucose levels. Insulin resistance underlies metabolic syndrome, is present in most cases of PCOS, and is near universal in type 2 diabetes.

Klemera-Doubal Method: A metric of biological age that uses common blood tests. It has limited predictive utility in individuals, but can be useful for population studies. Phenotype age (eyeball assessment of age by an average person) is likely a stronger predictive assessment of biological age than the Klemera-Doubal method.

Leaky gut: A condition in which there is increased intestinal permeability. In this theoretical condition, the intestinal barrier weakens, allowing the passage of harmful substances like toxins and bacteria into the bloodstream. (Note: The existence and significance of leaky gut is a matter of ongoing scientific debate.) Leaky gut appears to be associated with many highly prevalent chronic diseases, including AD.

Life expectancy: The remaining expected years of life for a person. The life expectancy of a newborn in the U.S.A. is about 77.5 years; the life expectancy of a 70-year-old man in the U.S. is 84.4, as they have survived many earlier risks. Life expectancy is influenced by lifestyle habits, genetics, educational level, and access to medical care.

Lifespan: The total time between birth and death of an individual.

Lipolytic bacteria: Bacteria that break down fat. Lipolytic bacteria can over-proliferate in the gut if there is fat malabsorption or if the diet is very high in fat.

Lipopolysaccharides (LPS): Molecules found in the outer cell wall of gram-negative bacteria. LPS triggers an inflammatory response in the body as a result of the innate immune response to it.

Lipoteichoic acid: A component of the cell wall of gram-positive bacteria to which there is an innate immune inflammatory response.

Longitudinal study: A research design that follows participants over time to observe how a factor (e.g., diet) might influence the development of a condition (e.g., AD). Longitudinal studies are useful for finding causal relationships to environmental influences.

LPS: See Lipopolysaccharides

Meta-analysis: A statistical method that combines data from multiple studies to assess the overall effect of a particular intervention or exposure (e.g., fruit consumption) on a specific outcome (e.g., Alzheimer's Disease). Meta-analyses help resolve conflicting results between individual studies.

Metabolic age: This is a metric of biological age that compares one's basal metabolic rate (BMR) and compares typical BMRs at various ages. It measures how much energy the body uses at rest. The BMR falls with age as the body's muscle-to-adipose ratio declines in aging. The SANA program, including diet, exercise, and sleep hygiene, can increase the BMR and thus help reduce the metabolic age in those in whom it is higher than their calendar age.

Methyl group: A carbon atom bonded to three hydrogen atoms. Methyl groups are a basic building block of organic compounds. Methyl group deposition impacts epigenetic regulation.

Methylglyoxal (MGO): A highly reactive, endogenous byproduct of the glycolytic pathway. MGO can accumulate and have toxic effects when there is impaired metabolism of glucose, hyperglycemia, or oxidative stress. Endogenous AGEs such as MGO are linked to accelerated biological aging.

Microbiome: The entire community of microorganisms (bacteria, fungi, viruses) inhabiting a particular environment, such as the human gut.

Micronutrients: Vitamins and minerals that the body needs in small amounts to function properly. They are essential for many bodily processes, including growth, development, and metabolism.

Mitochondria: The cellular organelle that is mostly responsible for converting energy from sugars and fat into ATP as an energy supply for metabolic processes. They are key players in apoptosis.

Mitophagy is a special type of autophagy that specifically targets mitochondria, the cell's powerhouses. It's like taking your old, broken-down car to thc junkyard to be recycled for parts. By removing damaged mitochondria, the cell can improve its overall health and function.

Multiple sclerosis (MS): An autoimmune disease of the CNS characterized by injury to the myelin sheath surrounding nerve fibers. Because of the disruption of communication, different areas of the CNS, including the spinal cord, may be affected. Some patients with MS have remissions and relapses, while others have steadily progressive disease.

Mutualism: A long-term symbiotic interaction in which members of two different species gain benefits from coexisting with each other.

Neurodegeneration: The degeneration of neurons and neuronal pathways of the central nervous system. It is generally progressive and irreversible.

Neuroinflammation: Inflammation of the CNS. It may result from infection, traumatic injury, or other disease processes.

NF-κB: A Protein complex that acts as a transcription factor for inflammatory mechanisms, including the production of inflammatory cytokines. NF-κB is involved in immune responses and cell survival.

Nixtamalization: A process used to treat corn, which improves its nutritional value and makes it more digestible. It also improves the flavor and gives the corn cohesiveness, allowing it to be used to make dough for tamales.

NO2: Nitrogen dioxide, an air pollutant gas. A tailpipe emission from internal combustion engine cars.

NOAEL: No-observed-adverse-effect level.

NOx: Nitrogen oxidative products, which result from the high-temperature oxidation of nitrogen (air used for combustion). Although oxygen is needed to burn fuel, nitrogen gas, which makes up nearly 80% of air, is also taken into the combustion chamber and exposed to high-temperature oxidation.

Nrf2: A transcription factor that promotes the expression of the Antioxidant-Response Element proteins.

Polyphenolic compounds: A class of compounds present in many plants that are part of the plant's defense mechanism against predation by insects and against microbes. These include flavonoids, tannins, and lignans. Many have hormetic effects in the diet. Others act as fiber. Some foods high in polyphenolic compounds include fruits such as berries, teas, and cacao.

Pro-inflammatory diet: The Standard American Diet (SAD), which is high in polyunsaturated fats, sugars, and red meat, promotes inflammation. Diets that promote obesity are generally pro-inflammatory.

Protein misfolding: After RNA is read by the ribosome, the primary protein is like a string of beads, with each amino acid representing a bead. To become functional, most proteins need to be folded in the endoplasmic reticulum. Errors in the folding can occur; some errors can be corrected, others cannot. Environmental stress and mutations can cause misfolding. Misfolded proteins can trigger the unfolded protein response (UPR), which attempts to restore normal folding, but can also initiate apoptosis if the damage is irreparable. Aggregates of misfolded proteins can thus cause cell death and contribute to diseases such as AD, PD, prion (i.e., mad cow disease), and other neurodegenerative diseases.

Proteolytic bacteria: These bacteria are adapted to the fermentation of protein. They produce protease enzymes and often live in anaerobic environments. Tissue infection with proteolytic bacteria is quite dangerous.

RBC: Red Blood Cell.

Reactive nitrogen species (RNS): Highly reactive nitrogen molecules. These act as signaling molecules, vasodilators, and immune response against pathogens; however, overproduction can induce oxidative damage. RNS include nitric oxide (NO), nitrogen dioxide (NO_2), nitrite (NO_2), nitrate (NO_3^-), peroxynitrite ($ONOO^-$), and S-nitrosothiols (RS-NO)

Reactive oxygen species (ROS): Unstable, highly reactive oxygen-containing molecules that can cause oxidative injury to the cell. The production of energy by the mitochondria is a major source of ROS, which can cause damage to the DNA, RNA, and other components of the cell.

SANA Diet: Symbiotic Antiinflammatory Nutrition Agendum. A diet and overall health program designed to promote health and the prevention of chronic disease. Sana means to heal in Spanish.

Schizophrenia: A severe thought disorder that causes disorganized thinking and can cause delusional thinking and hallucinations. Its onset is generally in the late teen years to the early twenties. It may be caused by excitotoxicity. Early treatment decreases disease severity. Between 0.3 and 0.7% of U.S. adults are affected, and about 40% of those affected are untreated at any given time. Environmental factors, including cannabis and other recreational drug use, and air pollution, are contributing causes of this disease.

Seed coat: The outer covering of a seed, which plays a role in dormancy and the regulation of germination. It also contains compounds that protect the seed from microbial and insect attack.

Sepsis: A bacterial infection in which bacteria multiply in the blood. The symptoms of sepsis result from an extreme immune response, leading to overwhelming inflammation and organ failure. It is commonly fatal.

Short-chain fatty acids (SCFAs): Fatty acids produced by the fermentation of dietary fiber in the colon. SCFAs, such as butyrate, propionate, and acetate, play a vital role in gut health and provide energy for colonic cells.

Sirtuins: A family of endogenous enzymes that act in metabolism and stress response, and which impact aging. Some influence gene expression, and others promote mitochondrial renewal, gene expression, apoptosis, and cell proliferation.

Skin (in the context of food): The outer layer of fruits, vegetables, tubers, and seeds.

Sleep Deprivation: A state of impaired mental, emotional, and physical functioning and health caused by insufficient sleep duration or sleep depth. Chronic sleep deprivation is associated with increased risk of cardiovascular disease, diabetes, which increases the risk of dementia. Sleep deprivation is also linked to mental health disorders.

Social isolation: A state where an individual has insufficient social engagement, support, and connections, such that they suffer distress from loneliness and a negative impact on mental and physical health. Social isolation is associated with increased mortality and cognitive decline.

SOD1 (Superoxide dismutase): SOD1 is an enzyme that catalyzes the conversion of superoxide radicals into hydrogen peroxide and oxygen. This enzyme is crucial in protecting mitochondria from oxidative stress. SOD1 helps mitigate oxidative stress that can promote neurodegenerative diseases such as ALS and PD.

Sofrito: A traditional seasoning for food in Spain and Latin America that includes sautéed garlic, onions, tomatoes, and other spices such as cilantro. The recipes vary by location.

Soluble fiber: A type of fiber that dissolves in water and can be fermented by gut bacteria, producing beneficial short-chain fatty acids. Some well-known sources of soluble fiber include oats and legumes.

Sulforaphane (SFN): A sulfur-containing compound that is enzymatically produced from glucoraphanin in cruciferous vegetables when the cells are disrupted, as occurs during chewing of broccoli. SFN has notable beneficial hormetic effects via activation of Nrf2. Its consumption lowers the risk of cancer and other diseases.

Symbiotic relationship: Organisms of two different species living together in a usually mutually beneficial relationship. In the context of gut health, a symbiotic relationship exists between humans and the beneficial bacteria in our gut.

Synbiont: Food ingredients or dietary supplements combining prebiotic food and probiotic bacteria for synergistic health benefits.

Telomerase: An enzyme that adds repetitive nucleotide sequences to the length of the telomere, counteracting some of the shortening that occurs during DNA replication.

Telomere: The end section of each chromosome that allows the DNA to be replicated so that each daughter cell has a copy of the DNA. A small part of the telomere is lost during each cell division, thus limiting the number of times a cell can divide. Telomere length depletion contributes to cellular aging and replicative senescence; nevertheless, lifespan is influenced by many factors.

Telomere length (TL): A measure of how long the telomeres are (usually measured in white blood cells). TL is sometimes used as one measure of biological age, but it may be more accurate to think of telomere length as a metric of chronic inflammation, causing depletion of cell cycles.

Transcription: The process by which the DNA sequence is copied into RNA.

Transcription factor: A hormone, protein, or other molecular compound that binds to a transcription factor binds to a gene's promoter (a specific DNA sequence that signals the start of a gene); it can either encourage or discourage the process of transcription, which is the first step in making a protein.

Translation: The process in which RNA is read by the ribosome to string the proper sequence of amino acids together to build a protein

TXNRD1 (Thioredoxin): A protein that reduces oxidized cysteine and is important in maintaining the response to oxidative stress of multiple organ systems. The thioredoxin system plays a critical role in redox homeostasis.

Ultrafine particulate matter: Particulate matter pollution with an aerodynamic diameter of less than 0.1 micrometers. Due to their tiny size, they can penetrate deep into the lungs and enter the bloodstream and brain. They are thus dangerous to health. They can remain airborne long distances in comparison to heavier particles, which are mostly deposited closer to the site of emissions.

Urea cycle: A metabolic pathway in the liver that helps remove waste products from the body, such as ammonia, which can then be secreted into the urine for disposal from the body. Ammonia is a toxic substance produced by the breakdown of protein.

Vascular dementia (VaD): Dementia that results from vascular injury in the brain. Typically, it is microvascular injury, and slowly progressive, but VaD can also result from microinfarcts or strokes. Alzheimer's disease commonly has a vascular component.

WBC: White Blood Cell

Werner syndrome: A genetic disease characterized by short stature and accelerated aging.

White matter lesions: Brain injury involving areas within the brain that serve to connect one area with another. These may usually be caused by vascular or ischemic injury, and more commonly seen cardiovascular risk factors include aging.

WRN DNA-repair enzyme: A DNA repair enzyme that is crucial for maintaining genome stability. WRN is a helicase involved in DNA replication and repair, which is active in telomeric regions

Xenobiotic compounds: Compounds that are not normally found in the body but rather are often manmade and frequently detrimental, such as pesticides, PFAS (per- and polyfluoroalkyl substances), and other environmental pollutants.

Virtual Index:

This book does not include an index. A digital search can be done on the book's Amazon page, going to "Read Sample" and clicking on the search icon (magnifying glass) at the top right corner. Then type in the search term.

https://www.amazon.com/dp/1938318099

Google Books provides an even better search function. The contents can be searched without any purchase. Note that the Google Play format of this book is appropriate for reading on a computer, but other than searching, would be impractical on a small-screen eReader or smartphone.

Google Play Book GGKEY:Q3JCAYRNPP7

About the Author

Dr. Lewis is board-certified in Public Health and Preventive Medicine and has over 25 years of clinical experience. He is a medical researcher and the author of several books. His goal in writing is to make complex topics accessible and to promote the understanding of science as a path to making people's lives more joyful and fulfilling. He believes that a child's work is to play and have fun, and that this should not change as we become adults.

The author would appreciate your kind comments in the Amazon or Google Books comment section for this book, as it helps more people find the book.

Amazon review:

https://www.amazon.com/dp/1938318099

Google Play Store review:

https://play.google.com/store/books/details/?id=Q3JCAYRNPP7

Link to the author's page on Amazon:

www.amazon.com/Charles-A-Lewis/e/B00OSPHQS2

If errors are noted, kindly send an explanatory message, with the page and current (1.01) edition number to:

Enteroimmunology @ gmail.com

Cover photo by J Henning

www.ingramcontent.com/pod-product-compliance
Lightning Source LLC
Chambersburg PA
CBHW061740210326
41599CB00034B/6736
9781938318092